KT-119-374

Artificial Nutrition
Support in Clinical Practice
Second Edition

Artificial Nutrition Support in Clinical Practice
Second Edition

Edited by

Jason Payne-James LLM FRCS DFM RNutr
Honorary Senior Research Fellow
Department of Gastroenterology & Nutrition
Central Middlesex Hospital,
London, UK

George K. Grimble PhD
Reader in Clinical Nutrition
School of Life Sciences
University of Surrey,
Roehampton, London, UK

David B. A. Silk MD FRCP
Consultant Physician,
Department of Gastroenterology and Nutrition,
Central Middlesex Hospital,
London, UK

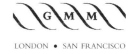

LONDON • SAN FRANCISCO

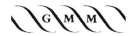

© 2001

Greenwich Medical Media Limited
137 Euston Road
London
NW1 2AA

870 Market Street, Ste 720
San Francisco, CA 94109, USA

ISBN 1 9001 51979

First published 2001

Apart from any fair dealing for the purposes of research or private study, or criticism or review, as permitted under the UK Copyright Designs and Patents Act 1988, this publication may not be reproduced, stored, or transmitted, in any form or by any means, without the prior permission in writing of the publishers, or in the case of reprographic reproduction only in accordance with the terms of the licences issued by the appropriate Reproduction Rights Organisations outside the UK. Enquiries concerning reproduction outside the terms stated here should be sent to the publishers at the London address printed above.

The rights of Jason Payne-James, George K Grimble and David BA Silk to be identified as editors of this work has been asserted by them in accordance with the Copyright Designs and Patents Act 1988.

The publisher makes no representation, express or implied, with regard to the accuracy of the information contained in this book and cannot accept any legal responsibility or liability for any errors or omissions that may be made.

A catalogue record for this book is available from the British Library.

www.greenwich-medical.co.uk

Distributed worldwide by Plymbridge Distributors Ltd and in the USA by Jamco Distribution
Typeset by Phoenix Photosetting, Chatham, Kent
Printed by MPG Books Ltd, Bodmin, Cornwall

Contents

Preface ix

Foreword xi
S P Allison

Contributors xiii

1   Metabolic response to starvation, injury and sepsis 1
    M Elia

2   Protein and amino acid metabolism in the whole body
    and in the tissues 25
    M J Rennie, D J R Cuthbertson

3   Energy metabolism 61
    J Webber, I A Macdonald

4   The liver and nutrient metabolism 81
    R A Sherwood

5   Cytokines and nutrition 93
    R F Grimble

6   Physiology of nutrient absorption and patterns of
    intestinal metabolism 107
    G K Grimble

7   The immune system and nutrition support 137
    K Bodger, R V Heatley

8   **Malnutrition in hospitalized patients** 149
    C Pennington

9   **Nutrition assessment** 165
    A Sitges-Serra, G Franch-Arcas

10 **Adult macronutrient requirements** 177
    H P Sauerwein, J A Romijn

11 **Adult micronutrient requirements** 193
    A Shenkin

12 **Paediatric nutrition requirements** 213
    P J Milla

13 **Nutrition, appetite control and disease** 225
    A Ballinger, M Clark

14 **The role of a nutrition support team** 241
    R Burnham, S Barton

15 **Hospital food as treatment** 255
    S Allison

16 **Oral diet administration and supplementation** 267
    Ib Hessov

17 **Enteral nutrition: tubes and techniques of delivery** 281
    J Payne-James

18 **Enteral diets: clinical uses and formulation** 303
    D B A Silk

19 **Complications of enteral nutrition** 333
    J Payne-James

20 **Paediatric enteral nutrition** 347
    A MacDonald, C Holden, T Johnson

21 **Home enteral tube feeding** 367
    A Micklewright, V E Todorovic

22 **Venous access for parental nutrition** 379
    D Palmer, J MacFie

23 **Parenteral nutrition substrates** 401
    P Fürst, K S Kuhn, P Stehle

24 **Parenteral nutrition formulation** 435
    M C Allwood

25 **Metabolic complications of parenteral nutrition** 445
    A Thorell, J Nordenström

26 **Paediatric parenteral nutrition** 461
    J W L Puntis

27 **Home parenteral nutrition** 485
    B J M Jones

28 **Nutrition and liver disease** 499
    C Wicks

29 **Nutrition support in trauma and sepsis** 511
    J Takala, R Suojaranta-Ylinen, O Pitkänen

30 **Nutrition support in renal disease** 523
    G Brunori

31 **Nutrition support in respiratory disease** 537
    T W Felbinger, U Suchner, K Peter, J Askanazi

32 **Nutrition and inflammatory bowel disease** 553
    M A Gassull, F Fernández-Bañares

33 **Nutrition support during the acute care of moderately or
    severely burned patients** 575
    J J Cunningham, K Prelack, R Sheridan, J P Remensnyder

34 **Nutrition support for the intensive care unit** 591
    J Wernerman

35 **Nutrition support for the surgical patient** 605
    K W E Hulsewé, M F von Meyenfeldt, P B Soeters

36   **Nutrition support in human immunodeficiency virus infection** 617
      D C Macallan, J Cotton, G E Griffin

37   **Nutrition support in patients with cancer** 639
      F Bozzetti

38   **Nutrition support in the elderly** 681
      D G Smithard, G Blandford and G K Grimble

39   **Management of patients with a short bowel** 701
      J M D Nightingale, J Lennard-Jones

40   **Nutrition support for pancreatitis** 719
      S A McClave, D A Spain

41   **The cost-effectiveness of nutrition support** 733
      C J Green

42   **The role of enteral and parenteral nutrition: enteral vs parenteral?** 759
      S M Gabe

      Index 775

Preface

The first edition of *Artificial Nutrition Support in Clinical Practice* was devised as an authoritative text for clinical practitioners who considered nutrition support to be a key part of medical therapy for hospitalized patients. Its precursor, *Nutrition Support: Theory and Practice* by the same authors ran to 25,000 copies and briefly introduced the main issues in parenteral and enteral nutrition to a wide audience. At that time, several excellent American texts had dealt with the same issues, in particular the incidence of hospital malnutrition. The editors felt that with the growth of nutrition support in Europe and Southeast Asia, there was a need for a more global approach. Practices differ from country to country and the first edition therefore covered fundamental aspects of the injury response and how nutrition support could be provided to patients in each major disease category. Not only was the need to feed patients defined but the techniques for doing so were described in detail. Thus, the reader could access authoritative accounts of, for example, the impact of disease on protein and energy metabolism as well as descriptions of techniques for intravenous and enteral tube feeding. We felt that it was also important to describe the pharmaceutical principles which underpin total parenteral nutrition (TPN) in order to put the technique into the context of nutrition support teams, where it rightly belongs.

In this new edition, authors have updated their contributions. All have been invited to provide a synthesis of underlying aspects of the disease process and how they inform clinical choices on the most appropriate methods of feeding. Furthermore, each chapter is evidence-based by referring to key clinical studies whose research technique has been able to provide answers to questions of practice.

Clinical nutrition support has advanced since the first edition and new chapters deal with the role of cytokine-driven metabolism in determining nutritional requirements (Chapter 5), the effect of disease on appetite (Chapter 13), creative application of hospital catering (Chapter 15), nutrition support in pancreatitis (Chapter 40) and whether nutrition support is cost-effective (Chapter 41). This contentious issue is vigorously debated in relation to choice of TPN or enteral nutrition where cost is perceived to be a real issue (Chapter 42). Authors have worked hard to produce authoritative and interesting contributions and have the editors' thanks for rising to the challenge.

Artificial Nutrition Support in Clinical Practice had its genesis in a small pocketbook, which comprised journal reviews originally commissioned by Professor Mike Rennie in 1989. In turn, the first edition has led to the establishment of the first European MSc in Clinical Nutrition in 1995 at University of Surrey Roehampton. The book became the curriculum for this MSc which poses two questions: -

What is the effect of disease on nutrition status?
What impact does nutrition support have on disease progression and outcome?

Research performed by students and their shared clinical expertise, together with the clinical experience of the editors has informed this new edition.

Regrettably, we have lost two dear colleagues and friends since the first edition was published. Dr Roger Rees, a gastroenterologist, had a deep and abiding interest in energy requirements and how these could best be met by enteral or parenteral feeding. Professor Mike Barnett, a pharmacist, pioneered new methods for testing the stability of existing all-in-one TPN regimens in order to devise guidelines for the safety of new formulations. This edition is dedicated to their memory.

We would also thank those who were involved in production of this edition. The team at Greenwich Medical Media have worked hard and creatively, most notably Gavin Smith, Gill Clark, Nora Naughton and Sam Gear.

JJP-J, GKG, DBAS
London
2001

Foreword

The adverse effects of malnutrition have been known since ancient times, and the importance of good nutrition in recovery from disease emphasised repeatedly over the years from the time of Hippocrates to the writings of John Hunter in the 18th and Florence Nightingale in the 19th Century. Authors such as David Cuthbertson, Moore, Wilkinson, Kinney and Hill have given us greater understanding of the metabolic changes which take place with trauma and illness and laid the foundations of modern clinical nutrition. Pioneers such as Wretland. Rhoads and Dudrick have given us the tools with which to feed patients with gastrointestinal failure, in the same sense that ventilators and dialysis machines allow us to manage respiratory and renal failure. The newer techniques of enteral feeding are now a far cry from the eel skin and pig's bladder used by Hunter in the 18th Century. This new science and technology has given fresh impetus to the subject, so that nutrition is beginning to find its rightful place in the undergraduate and postgraduate curriculum and to be recognised as an important sub-specialty.

The Editors of this book are to be congratulated on their important contribution to this process. This second edition, with its international cast of distinguished authors, will be an essential reference work for all those engaged in the nutritional care of patients. It is not just to the specialty of clinical nutrition that the book is addressed, however. It has something for all clinicians, nurses and other disciplines involved in the care of patients or the feeding of the sick. It emphasises standards of good practice in which all patients should be screened for nutritional status in the same way that vital signs and blood pressure are recorded routinely. It emphasises the responsibility which we all have to detect and treat malnutrition which, if neglected, causes so much morbidity, mortality and increased health care costs. It sets standards of practice which will form part of clinical governance and the quality of care in the future.

Simon P Allison
Professor of Clinical Nutrition, Nottingham
Chairman of ESPEN

Contributors

Simon Allison MD FRCP
Professor in Clinical Nutrition
Clinical Nutrition Unit
University Hospital
Nottingham, UK

Michael C Allwood BPharm PhD FRPharm SGB
Director
Pharmacy Academic Practice Unit
University of Derby
Derby, UK

Jeffrey Askanazi
Pain Centers Inc.
Greenville
Michigan, USA

Anne Ballinger MD MRCP
Digestive Diseases Research Centre
St Barts and the Royal London School of Medicine
and Dentistry
University of London
London, UK

Sebastian Barton MA, MD, MRCP
Consultant Physician and Gastroenterologist
Kent and Canterbury Hospital
Canterbury, UK

Gerald Blandford MBBS FRCP(C) FACP
Medical Director
The Loeb Center
Montefiore Medical Center
Professor of Medicine
Albert Einstein College of Medicine
Bronx, New York, USA

Keith Bodger MB ChB (Hons) MRCP (UK)
Clinical Lecturer in Medicine
Department of Medicine
University Clinical Departments
The Duncan Building
Liverpool, UK

Federico Bozzetti MD
Department of Surgical Oncology of the Digestive Tract
Istituto Nazionale per la Studio a la Cura dei Tumori
Milan, Italy

Giuliano Brunori MD
Consultant Nephrologist
Institute and Division of Nephrology
University and Spedali Civili of Brescia
Brescia, Italy

Rodney Burnham MA MD FRCP
Consultant Physician and Gastroenterologist
Havering Hospitals NHS Trust
Essex, UK

Michael Clark MD FRCP
Digestive Diseases Research Centre
St Bartholomew's and the Royal London School of
Medicine & Dentistry
London, UK

Barbara Clayton
Professor
Faculty of Medicine Health and Biological Sciences
University of Southampton
Biomedical Science Building
Southampton, UK

Jacqui Cotton BSc SRD PhD
Senior Dietitian
Department of Nutrition and Dietetics
St George's Hospital
London, UK

John J Cunningham PhD
Deputy Provost and Chief of Staff
University of Massachusetts Amherst
Boston, USA

Daniel J R Cuthbertson MBChB BSc MRCP
Clinical Research Fellow
Division of Molecular Physiology
School of Life Sciences
University of Dundee
Scotland, UK

Marinos Elia
Professor of Clinical Nutrition and Metabolism
Institute of Human Nutrition
University of Southhampton
Southhampton General Hospital
Southhampton, UK

Thomas W Felbinger MD
Department of Anesthesiology
Grosshadern Medical Center of the University of Munich
Munich, Germany

Fernando Fernandez-Banares
Department of Gastroenterology
Hospital Universitari Mútua de Terrassa
Senior Investigator
Hospital Universitari Germans Trias i Pujol
Badalona, Spain

Guzman Franch-Arcas MD
Staff Surgeon
General Surgery Service
Hospital de Figueres
Associate Professor of Physiology
Universitat Pompeu Fabra

Peter Fürst MD PhD
University of Hohenheim
Institute of Biological Chemistry & Nutrition
Hohenheim, Germany

Simon M Gabe MD MSc BSc MBBS MRCP
Senior Lecturer in Intestinal Failure
Consultant Gastroenterologist
St Marks Hospital
North West London Hospitals NHS Trust
London, UK

Miquel A Gassull MD PhD
Head of Department of Gastroenterology
Director of Research
Hospital Universitari Germans Triasl Pujol
Carretera Del Canyer S/M
Badalona, Spain

Ceri J Green BSc SRD PhD
Medical Information
Nutricia Health Care
Zoetermeer, The Netherlands

George E Griffin BSc PhD FRCP FRCPath FMed Sci
Professor of Infectious Diseases and Medicine
Head of Department of Infectious Diseases
St George's Hospital Medical School
London, UK

George K Grimble PhD
Reader in Clinical Nutrition
School of Life Sciences
University of Surrey Roehampton
Whitelands College
London, UK

Robert F Grimble
Professor of Nutrition
Institute of Human Nutrition
Medical and Biological Sciences Building
University of Southampton
Southampton, UK

R V Heatley MD FRCP
Consultant Physician
St. James University Hospital
Leeds, UK

Ib Hessov MD DMSc
Associate Professor of surgery and Clinical Nutrition
Department of Surgery
Aarhus University Hospital
Aarhus Amtssygehus, Denmark

Chris Holden MSc RGN RSCN
Clinical Nurse Specialist
Nutritional Care, Princess of Wales Children's Hospital,
The Birmingham Children's Hospital
Birmingham, UK

Karel W E Hulsewé MD
Department of General Surgery
University Hospital Maastricht
Maastricht, The Netherlands

Tracey Johnson BSc SRD
Senior Dietitian
Birmingham Children's Hospital
Birmingham, UK

Barry J M Jones BSc MD FRCP
Consultant Gastroenterologist
Russells Hall Hospital
Dudley
West Midlands

Katharina S Kuhn PhD
University of Hohenheim
Institute of Biological Chemistry & Nutrition
Hohenheim, Germany

John Lennard-Jones MD FRCP FRCS
Emeritus Professor of Gastroenterology
The Royal London Hospital Medical College
Emeritus Consultant Physician
St Marks Hospital
London, UK

Derek C Macallan MA PhD MRCP DTM&H
Senior Lecturer/Honorary Consultant
Department of Infectious Diseases
St George's Hospital Medical School
London, UK

Anita MacDonald PhD BSc SRD
Head of Dietetic Services
Birmingham Children's Hospital
Birmingham, UK

Ian Macdonald BSc PhD
Faculty of Medicine and Health Sciences
School of Biomedical Sciences
Medical School
Queens Medical Centre
Nottingham, UK

John MacFie MD FRCS
Department of Surgery
Scarborough NE Yorkshire Healthcare Trust
Scarborough, UK

Stephen A McClave MD
Professor of Medicine
Director of Clinical Nutrition
Division of Gastroenterology/Hepatology
School of Medicine
University of Louisville
Kentucky, USA

Bruce McElroy
Head of Aseptic Services
Royal Shrewsbury Hospital
Shrewsbury, UK

Bernard Messing MD
Service d'Hépato-Gastro-Entérologie et d'Assistance
Nutritive
Hôpital Lariboisiére-Saint-Lazare
Ambroise Paré
Paris, France

Maarten F Meyenfeldt MD, PhD
Specialist in Surgical Oncology
University Hospital Maastricht
Maastricht, The Netherlands

Anne Micklewright MSc SRD
Dietetic and Nutrition Services Manager
Queen's Medical Centre
University Hospital NHS Trust
Nottingham, UK

Peter J Milla Msc MBBS FRCP FRCPCH
Consultant Paediatric Gastroenterologist
Professor of Paediatric Gastroenterology and Nutrition
Institute of Child Health and Great Ormond Street
Hospital for Children
London, UK

Jeremy M D Nightingale MD MRCP
Consultant General Physician and Gastroenterologist
Leicester Royal Infirmary
Leicester, UK

Jörgen Nordenstrom MD PhD
Professor of Surgery
Department of Surgery
Huddinge University Hospital
Huddinge, Sweden

Diane Palmer RN BSc (Hons)
Lecturer in Nursing
University of Hull
Hull, UK

Jason Payne-James LLM FRCS DFM RNutr
Director, Forensic Healthcare Services Ltd, London, UK
Honorary Senior Research Fellow
Department of Gastroenterology & Nutrition
Central Middlesex Hospital
Middlesex, London, UK

Chris R Pennington BSc MD FRDP
Clinical Group Director
Medicine & Cardiovascular
Professor of Gastroenterology
Directorate of General Medicine
Ninewells Hospital and Medical School
Dundee, UK

Klaus Peter
Pain Centers Inc.
Greenville
Michigan, USA

Otto Pitkänen MD PHD
Critical Care Research Program
Kuopio University Hospital
Department of Anesthesiology and Intensive Care
Kuopio, Finland

Kathy Prelack, MS, RD
Research Fellow Surgery
Massachusetts General Hospital
Nutrition Support Dietitian
Shriners Hospitals For Children
Shriners Burns Hospital
Boston, USA

John W L Puntis BM (Hons) DM FRCP FRCPCH
Senior Lecturer in Paediatrics and Child Health
University of Leeds, and Consultant Paediatrician
The Children's Centre
The General Infirmary at Leeds
Leeds, UK

John P Remensnyder MD
Associate Professor in Surgery
Massachusetts General Hospital
Plastic Reconstructive Surgeon
Shriners Hospitals For Children
Shriners Burns Hospital
Boston, USA

Michael J Rennie PhD FRSE
Symmers Professor of Physiology
Division of Molecular Physiology
School of Life Science
University of Dundee
Scotland, UK

J A Romijn MD, PhD
Professor of Endocrinology
University Medical Centre
London, UK

Hans P Sauerwein
Department of Internal Medicine
Academisch Medisch Centrum
Universiteit van Amsterdam
Amsterdam, The Netherlands

Alan Shenkin BSc PhD FRCP FRCPath
Professor of Clinical Chemistry
Faculty of Medicine
Department of Clinical Chemistry
Liverpool, UK

Robert Sheridan MD
Director of Trauma and Burns
Massachusetts General Hospital
Assistant Chief of Staff
Shriners Burns Hospital
Associate Professor of Surgery
Harvard Medical School
Boston, USA

Roy Sherwood BSc MSc DPhil
Consultant Clinical Scientist
Honorary Senior Lecturer
King's College Hospital
London, UK

David Silk MD FRCP
Consultant Physician
Director
Department of Gastroenterology and Nutrition
Central Middlesex Hospital NHS Trust
London, UK

Antonio Sitges-Serra MD FRCS
Head of Department of Surgery
Hospital Universitari Del Mar
Professor of Surgery
Autonomous University of Barcelona
Barcelona, Spain

David G Smithard BSc MBBS MD FRCP
Consultant in Elderly and Stroke Medicine
William Harvey Hospital
East Kent Hospitals
Kent, UK

Peter B Soeters MD, PhD
Specialist in Gastroenterology and Clinical Nutrition
University Hospital Maastricht
Maastricht, The Netherlands

David Spain MD
Assistant Professor
Director of Surgical Critical Care
Department of Surgery
University of Louisville School of Medicine
Louisville, USA

Peter Stehle PhD
University of Bonn
Institute of Nutrition
Bonn, Germany

Ulrich Suchner
Clinic of Anesthesiology
Klinikum Großhadern off the Ludwig-Maximilians-
University of Munich
Munich, Germany

Rali Suojaranta-Ylinen MD
Department of Anaesthesiology and Intensive Care
Critical Care Research Program
Kuopio University Hospital
Kuopio, Finland

Jukka Takala MD PhD
Department of Intensive Care
Kuopio University Hospital
Institute of Child Health and Great Ormond Street
Hospital for Children
London, UK

Anders Thorell MD PhD
Karolinska Institute at Ersta Hospital
Center of Gastrointestinal Disease
Stockholm, Sweden

Vera Todorovic MBA Msc Bsc SRD
Dietetic and Nutrition Services Manager
Bassetlaw District General Hospital
Nottingham, UK

Jon Webber BMBCH MRCP
Faculty of Medicine and Health Sciences
School of Biomedical Sciences
Medical School
Queens Medical Centre
Nottingham, UK

Claire Wicks BSc SRD PhD
Formerly Chief Dietitian
Institute of Liver Studies
King's College Hospital
London, UK

Jan Wernerman MD PhD
Head of Department
Anesthesia of Intensive Care
Huddinge University Hospital
Stockholm, Sweden

Metabolic response to starvation, injury and sepsis

Marinos Elia

Starvation has often been described as producing a series of stereotyped metabolic changes, such as progressive diminution in resting and total energy expenditure, a progressive decrease in the proportion of endogenous energy derived from protein mobilisation and an increase in the proportion derived from fat and ketone bodies. However, many of the metabolic changes are neither progressive nor stereotyped. They are influenced by the age, sex and the initial body composition of the individual. Furthermore, protein oxidation and resting energy expenditure may temporarily increase before they begin to decrease,[1] and the contribution of protein oxidation to total energy expenditure in lean individuals undergoing prolonged starvation may actually increase. Similarly, the metabolic response to injury is influenced by the age, sex and nutrition status of the subject, as well as ambient temperature and interventions such as blood transfusions and use of analgaesics, sedatives and antibiotics. Whilst these are important factors, it is also necessary to understand the inter-relationships that exist between lean and fat tissues (and inter-relationship between individual organs) during starvation and injury and how these might be linked to survival.

Starvation

Short term starvation

Energy metabolism

Although prolonged starvation is associated with an absolute reduction in basal metabolic rate (BMR), which is partly due to loss of lean tissue, there is often a small absolute increase in BMR during the first 2 days of starvation (Fig. 1.1). This occurs despite a decrease in body weight and lean tissue mass (about 2%). Classic starvation studies such as that reported by Benedict[2] (included in Fig. 1.1 – square symbols) and Takahira[3] (not included in Fig. 1.1) are amongst those that reported a transient increase in BMR. The classic study of Cetti[4] is difficult to interpret because the first baseline measurement was made 1 h after breakfast, which means that dietary induced thermogenesis is likely to have influenced the results.

The temporary rise in BMR during early starvation could be due to: (a) an increase in the requirement of adenosine triphosphate (ATP) for a variety of metabolic processes, or (b) an increase in the energy equivalent of ATP as the body reduces the proportion

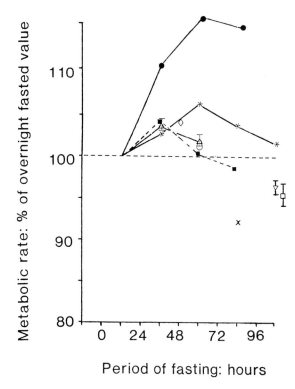

Figure 1.1 – Changes in resting energy expenditure in early starvation. The results are expressed as a percentage of overnight fasted value (100% at 12 hours). Each point represents results from a variable number of subjects ranging from one to 13. Based on Elia.[1]

of energy derived from glycogen decreases (17.52 kcal kJ/mole ATP gained) and that from fat (18.93 kcal/mole ATP gained) and ketone bodies increases.[5]

An increase in the requirement of ATP probably results from multiple metabolic processes: increased gluconeogenesis[6,7]; increased triglyceride-fatty acid cycling[8,9] which is thought to account for 1–2% of BMR in early starvation; increased protein–amino acid recycling (protein turnover) during the first 3 days of starvation;[10] and increased acetyl CoA-ketone body recycling. The last cycle occurs because ketone bodies are synthesised from acetyl CoA (AcCoA) in the liver, whilst other tissues such as muscle and brain, convert ketone bodies back to AcCoA before final oxidation. The overall cost is 1 ATP/cycle. On the basis of the rate of ketone body production and utilisation during early starvation[11] and the energy equivalent of ATP[5,12], it is estimated that this cycle alone contributes to 1–2% of BMR. After the first 1–3 days of starvation BMR decreases to values that are lower than those observed after an overnight fast.

The mechanisms are incompletely understood, but they are probably due to a combination of factors: losses of metabolically active tissues, altered proportions of tissues with different metabolic rates and changes in the metabolic rates of specific tissues.

Protein metabolism

A transient increase in nitrogen (N) excretion has frequently been observed in early starvation (Fig. 1.2).[1,2,14] Most of these studies did not take into account the change in the size of the urea pool, but the study of Elia et al.[14] reported a tendency for the blood urea concentration to rise, which would make the corrected N balance even more negative at this time. The N found in urine during early starvation does not entirely reflect increased protein oxidation, since there is a net contribution from the oxidation of free amino acids particularly glutamine (this also occurs in injury – see below). The free muscle

glutamine pool (45 g of glutamine or 15 g of N; 20–25 mmol/L intracellular water) almost halves between 12 and 72 h of starvation.[15,16] Since during this period the total urine N excretion is about 28 g (9–13 g N/day), it can be estimated that the loss of muscle glutamine corresponds to about a quarter of the urine N excretion. There is a general tendency for other amino acids to be lost from the free pool of amino acids in muscle, but some may accumulate, e.g. the branched chain amino acids. However, these other changes are relatively small compared to the loss of glutamine, which has two N atoms per molecule, in comparison with most other amino acids which have only one N atom per molecule.

Prolonged starvation

In the 19th century a number of workers, notably Chossat[17] reported that a variety of animals died from starvation after they had lost 40–50% of their body weight. The concept of lethal weight loss was developed and extended to humans. Krieger[18] suggested that the lethal level of weight loss in adults was 40% for acute starvation and 50% for semi-starvation. However, there is substantial variation in the weight loss of subjects dying of starvation (even in the subjects studied by Krieger[18]) and therefore the above figures can only be regarded as approximate. Furthermore, successful massive weight loss amounting to 65–80% of initial body weight has been described in grossly obese individuals with an initial body weight in excess of 200 kg.[1] The associated survival time during starvation can be considerably prolonged in the obese (Table 1.1) because of their excess energy stores. Autopsy studies of humans dying of starvation or semi-starvation frequently show that body fat has virtually disappeared, implying that energy reserves are linked to survival. In contrast, there is a loss of only 25–50% of most other tissues and organs, and only a small proportion of the brain and skeleton. Examples of human (typical lean subject) and non-human species dying from 'total starvation' are shown in Table 1.2. In lean humans, there is a loss of about 40% body weight before death (e.g. 41% in the subject studied by Myers[19] and 38% in the Northern Ireland fasters – Table 1.1). From this information it is possible to construct a table of the available energy reserves in lean and obese subjects (Table 1.3). It is clear that the major energy reserve is fat, for good physiological reasons. First, the energy density of endogenous fat (~9.4 kcal/g) is more than 2-fold greater than that of protein (~4.44 kcal/g) and glycogen (~4.2 kcal/g).[5] Second, the loss

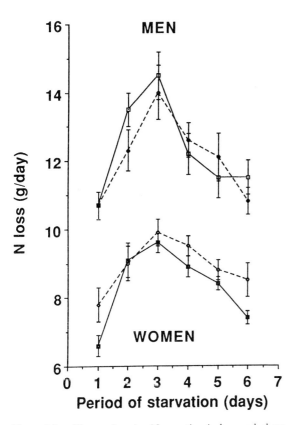

Figure 1.2 – Changes in urine N excretion in lean and obese subjects during early starvation. Solid line = lean subjects; dotted line = obese subjects; n = 12 for each point. See Elia[1] – based on Goschke et al.[13]

Table 1.1 – Effect of obesity on survival time during 'total' starvation in mice and humans.

	Survival time (days)	Author
Humans		
Lean		
($n = 9$)	57–73	Northern Ireland fasters[1]
($n = 1$) (prior gunshot wound)	43	Northern Ireland faster[1]
($n = 1$)	63	Meyers, 1917[71]
Obese (successful fasts)		
($n = 1$)	382	Stewart and Fleming, 1973[72]
($n = 1$)	315	Barnard *et al.*, 1969[73]
($n = 1$)	249	Runcie and Thomson, 1970[74]
		Thomson *et al.*, 1966[75]
		Collinson, 1967[76]
($n = 1$)	231	Barnard *et al.*, 1969[73]
($n = 1$)	210	Runcie and Thomson, 1970[74]
Several	100–200	Drenick *et al.*, 1967[77]
		Runcie and Thomson, 1970[74]
		Thomson *et al.*, 1969
		Barnard *et al.*, 1969[73]
Mice (8 weeks old)		
Lean		
Winter	4	Cuendet *et al.*, 1975[92]
Summer	8	Cuendet *et al.*, 1975[92]
Obese (ob/ob)		
Summer	> 28	Cuendet *et al.*, 1975[92]

Based on Elia.[1]

Table 1.2 – Percentage loss of organs during starvation.

	Pigeons	Cats	Rats	Dogs[a]	Man
Skeleton	3	10.4	14	5	–
Muscle	42	57.9	31	42	40.7
Brain and cord	1	2.2	3	22	6.9 (brain)
Heart	45	34.0	3	16	40.4
Spleen	71	68.5	–	57	18.4
Liver	53	59.8	54	50	28.6
Pancreas	64	55.2	–	62	48.8
Kidneys	32	50.9	–	55	49.2
Lungs	32	50.9	–	29	28.6
Fat	–	–	97	–	–

[a] Loss of fresh fat-free organs, see Elia.[1]

of 1 g of protein and glycogen is associated with the loss of up to four times more water, which is the major component of lean tissue (73% of lean tissue is water). In the examples given in Table 1.3 the energy associated with the loss of 1 g fat is 10-fold greater than the loss of 1 g fat-free tissue. Calculations based on the composition of adipose tissue which consists mainly of fat (~80% in lean subjects and up to ~90% in obese subjects) also suggests that loss of 1 g of adipose tissue is associated with the mobilisation of severalfold more metabolisable energy (7.5–8.5 kcal/g) than 1 g of other tissues. Therefore, for obvious mechanical reasons, it is advantageous to store energy as fat when food energy is readily available, and utilise fat when food energy is not available.

Table 1.3 – Hypothetical values of body composition, fuel availability and survival time in a lean 70 kg man and an obese man twice ideal body weight.

	Lean subject	Obese subject
Initial[c]		
Body weight (kg)	70.0	140.0
Fat (kg)	9.0	61.5
Protein (kg)	12.2	15.7
Glycogen (kg)	0.3	0.4
Loss during starvation		
Weight (% of initial)	38.0	69.0
Weight (kg)	26.6	96.6
Fat (kg)[a]	8.0	61.5
Protein (kg)[b]	14.0	15.7
Glycogen (kg)	0.3	0.4
Available energy during starvation		
Fat (kcal)	75,200	568,700
Protein (kcal)	17,760	33,300
Glycogen (kcal)	1,260	1,680
Total	94,220	603,680
Mean daily total energy expenditure (kcal/day)[d]	1,500	2,250
Survival time (days)	63	268

[a] Fat accounts for 30% of the loss of body weight in the lean subject and 63% of the loss in the obese subject. Fat free tissue accounts for 70% of the weight loss in the lean subject and 37% in the obese subject.
[b] Assuming 1 g N = 6.25 g protein, there is a loss of 24.0 g N.kg loss of body weight in the lean subject, and 12.4 g N/kg in the obese subject.
[c] The composition of the body in the lean subject is based on reference man (Snyder *et al.*[21]), and the excess weight in the obese individual is assumed to be 75% fat and 25% fat-free tissue, which are typical values.
[d] These are only approximate values partly because resting energy expenditure decreases to a variable extent below that predicted for normal individuals of the same weight (~25% during long-term starvation in lean individuals – Elia[1]), and partly because physical activity frequently decreases to a variable extent. Both of these changes can be regarded as adaptations.

From the information presented on the changes in body composition during starvation (Table 1.3) it is possible to make four predictions:

1. Survival is considerably longer in obese individuals than lean individuals.

2. Although lean subjects have less initial body protein than obese subjects, it is predicted that they oxidise more protein during prolonged starvation. As shown in Table 1.3 the overall protein oxidation is 2-fold greater in the lean subjects than the obese subjects (58 vs 28 g protein/day; 9.4 vs 4.5 g N/day).

3. The percentage of total energy expenditure derived from protein oxidation (p%) is greater in lean individuals. Calculations based on the figures given in Table 1.3 suggest that p% is 3-fold greater in the lean than the obese (see Table 1.4).

Table 1.4 – Per cent of total available energy derived from fat, carbohydrate and protein during starvation in lean and obese subjects[a].

	Lean subject	Obese subject
Fat	79.8	94.2
Protein	18.9	5.5
Carbohydrate	1.3	0.3

[a] Calculated from data on Table 1.2.

4. Increased physical activity during prolonged starvation will not only reduce survival time, but it will increase daily N excretion (and leave p% unaltered).

Although there is insufficient information to adequately examine the last prediction, there is sufficient data to confirm the first three predictions.

There is abundant evidence to suggest that individuals with extra energy reserves survive longer during starvation (e.g. see Table 1.1 and Keys[20]). It is also noteworthy that women, who have more per cent body fat than men, survive famines longer than men. Young children survive the shortest but this is largely related to their high resting energy expenditure which may be up to 2-fold greater (kcal/kg/day) than that of adults.

The other predictions are based on the premise that fuels are utilised in proportions that would favour prolonged survival. If obese individuals continued to oxidise protein at the same rate as in early starvation, or at the same rate as lean individuals, their lean tissues would be depleted more quickly and they would die with considerable available energy reserves (fat stores). This is obviously not the optimal physiological strategy for prolonged survival. It would therefore be advantageous for obese individuals to reduce the rate of protein oxidation (and per cent of total energy expenditure derived from protein oxidation) to a greater extent than lean individuals.

Fat-free tissue contains about 30–35 g N/kg,[21] whereas fat contains no N. If fat-free mass was preferentially catabolised the ratio of N loss to weight loss (gN/kg) would be expected to be high, and if fat was preferentially lost, the ratio will be expected to be low. Although the ratio of N loss to weight loss provides only semi-quantitative information about protein–energy inter-relationships – Figure 1.3 shows that the cumulative N loss/cumulative weight loss is lower in the obese than in the lean. There is complete separation of the two sets of results after 2 weeks, and by 1 month there is a 2-fold difference between them. More direct information about the absolute rate of protein oxidation can be obtained from the rate of urine N excretion.

Figure 1.4A shows the cumulative N excretion in lean individuals undergoing starvation, and Figure 1.4B shows that the values for groups of obese individuals fall below the dotted line, which represents the typical curve for lean individuals (derived from Fig. 1.4A). Figure 1.5A shows the changes in daily N excretion, in the obese are 2-fold lower than in the lean, and Figure 1.5B shows the corresponding values for p% are 2 to 4-fold lower than in the obese after 3 weeks of starvation[22]. This is also shown in Figure 1.6 in relation to initial body mass index (BMI) and per cent

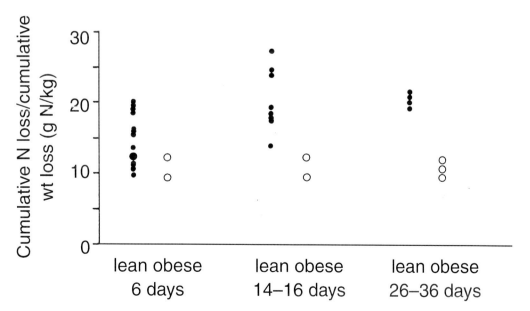

Figure 1.3 – The ratio of cumulative N loss to cumulative weight loss during starvation in lean (●) and obese (○) subjects. The small solid circles represent data from individual subjects, and the larger solid circles represent data from a group of subjects. Reproduced with permission from Elia.[1]

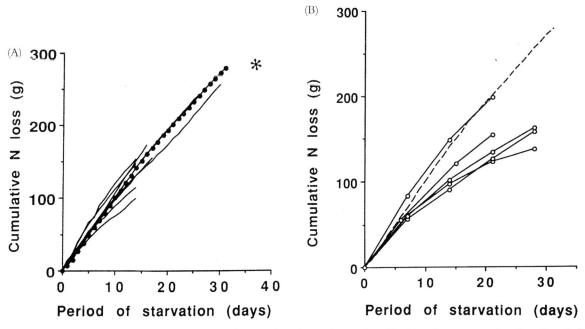

Figure 1.4 – (A) Cumulative N excretion in lean subjects undergoing total starvation. The large dots represent data from Benedict[2] and the other eight curves with small dots (some hidden behind the other curves) are derived from a variety of other starvation studies between 1905 and 1925. The asterisk represents the cumulative N loss of another subject. (B) Cumulative N loss in lean subjects (– – – – derived from A) and groups of obese subjects undergoing total starvation. Reproduced with permission from Elia.[1]

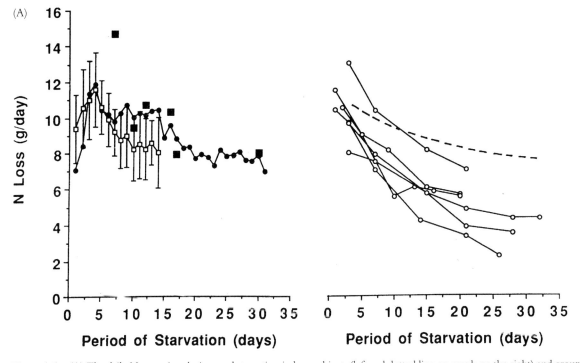

Figure 1.5 – (A) The daily N excretion during total starvation in lean subjects (left and dotted line on graph on the right) and groups of obese subjects (right).

(B)

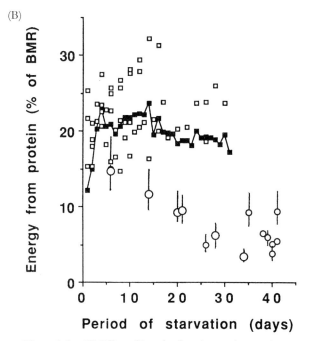

Figure 1.5 – (B) Effect of length of total starvation on the per cent contribution of protein oxidation to basal metabolic rate (BMR), in lean (solid squares – Benedict[2] and obese subjects (large circles represent results of groups of individuals and small circles represent results of individual subjects). Reproduced with permission from Elia.[1]

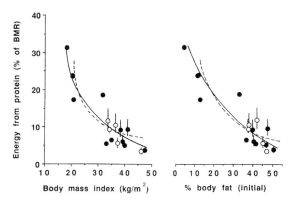

Figure 1.6 – The effect of initial BMI (left) and per cent body fat (right) on the contribution of protein oxidation to basal metabolic rate in subjects undergoing starvation (>16 days). Solid circles represent individual data (nine males, four females) and open circles group mean data. The dotted curve is a theoretical one based on calculations similar to those in Tables 1.3 and 1.4, assuming the ratio of total energy expenditure to BMR is 1.3. Reproduced with permission from Elia.[1]

body fat in individuals undergoing total starvation for more than 16 days. If the energy derived from protein oxidation is expressed in relation to total energy expenditure instead of BMR, all the values will be lower than those shown in Fig. 1.6. Furthermore, although some variability will be introduced (by effect of physical activity) this is unlikely to blur the large differences that exist between lean and obese subjects.

The above concepts developed for humans are consistent with information available from other species. For example the pig, with its copious body fat, has a value for p% that is only 7% of BMR (after 3 days of starvation) compared to 15–30% in leaner species such as dog, rabbit and man clean man).[1] Similarly, birds such as geese that have considerable body fat reserves have a particularly low value for p% during starvation compared to leaner birds.[1] A pre-mortal rise in N excretion when stores of body fat are depleted has been reported in a variety of mammals and birds.

It is also relevant to human physiology that the differences in protein economy which occur during total

starvation also occur during partial starvation.[1] Examples include the changes that occur during ingestion of low calorie or very low calorie diets for therapeutic weight reduction, and prolonged experimental semi-starvation in lean individuals. For example, in the study by Keys[20] normal subjects were semi-starved for 6 months until they lost 25% of their body weight. The leaner subjects lost a greater proportion of this weight as lean tissue[23] and had a higher value for p%. During recovery the reverse trends in body composition were obtained.

All these observations raise questions about the control mechanisms responsible for the protein–energy inter-relationships. How does excess adipose tissue produce a reduction in protein oxidation? What are the nature of the signals? How is the 'memory' retained so that those who lose a high proportion of lean to fat tissue during starvation regain a high proportion of lean to fat tissue during refeeding?[23] Why do the differences become apparent during prolonged starvation and not early starvation (first few days)? These questions remain largely unanswered and deserve further investigation.

Intermediary metabolism during starvation

The glycogen pool in the liver is lost early during starvation (Fig. 1.7), although some persists in muscle for utilisation in 'stress' or 'emergency' situations. Since the glycogen reserves are small, the tissues of the body either have to depend on alternative fuels, or

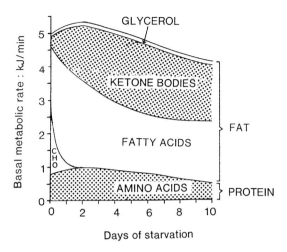

Figure 1.7 – Changes in BMR and fuel selection in a lean subject undergoing total starvation. Note the transient small increase in BMR, and the small and rapidly declining contribution of glucose (derived from glycogen) to BMR. Ketone bodies which are derived from fatty acids become a major fuel for the tissues of the body accounting for up to 40% of BMR. Reproduced with permission from Elia.[11]

they form glucose from glucogenic amino acids and the glycerol component of triglyceride (~8 g/1000 kcal during starvation). Both processes operate but the net conversion of 10 g N (62.5 g amino acids) to glucose (65% conversion) will only furnish about 40 g glucose (60 g glucose, if glycerol derived from the net oxidation of 2000 kcal triglyceride is included in the calculation)[22]. This is 4- to 5-fold less than the dietary intake of carbohydrate in a normal man in nutrient balance with an energy consumption of 2500 kcal/day, 45% of which is from carbohydrate. Lean tissues would quickly be lost if a high rate of net glucose oxidation persisted during starvation. Therefore, two important adaptations occur. First, glucose oxidation is inhibited. For example, the pyruvate dehydrogenase complex, which catalyses the first irreversible step in the oxidation of glucose carbon, is inhibited by a low insulin concentration, a rise in the AcCoA/CoA ratio (which occurs when fat oxidation predominates), and a rise in 3-hydroxybutyrate/acetoacetate ratio (which also occurs during starvation). Although it is possible for glucose to recycle through 3C fragments (glucose-lactate and glucose-alanine recycling; e.g. red blood cells, muscle, brain) this does not involve irreversible glucose oxidation. Secondly, tissues utilise energy from fatty acids, which are derived from triacylglycerol (TAG). However, the brain does not utilise fatty acids directly, partly because fatty acids do not readily penetrate the

blood–brain barrier and partly because the brain has little enzymatic potential to oxidise them. After the first few days of total starvation, ketone bodies, which are formed from fatty acids in the liver, become an important energy source for the body (Fig. 1.7) and the dominant energy source for the brain. They are water-soluble, readily cross the blood–brain barrier and undergo oxidative metabolism. However, there are differences in ketone body metabolism between lean and obese subjects[22], and these are reflected in a number of ways: their circulating concentrations (Fig. 1.8); the ratio of 3-hydroxybutyrate (β-OHB) to acetoacetate (AcAc) (Fig. 1.9), which is an index of the mitochondrial redox state; the rates of ketone body production relative to their circulating concentration (Table 1.5); and their exchange across tissues. For example, arterio-venous exchange studies undertaken by Elia *et al*[24] suggest that the contribution of ketone bodies to oxidative metabolism in the resting forearm muscle of lean individuals is about 5% after an overnight fast, 10% after 36–40 h of starvation and 20% after 60–66 h of starvation. In contrast, after 3 days of starvation ketone bodies account for up to about half of the oxygen utilised by the forearm muscle of obese individuals. However, after 3 weeks of starvation the forearms of obese individuals take up β-OHB and release some of the carbon as AcAc, with the overall result that ketone bodies account for only 18% of the O_2 utilisation,[25] or only 10% according to other studies.[26] It appears that in lean individuals the release of AcAc from forearm tissues observed at 36–40 and 60–66 h of starvation[24] occurs much earlier than in the obese.

An important factor controlling the uptake and utilisation of substrates is their circulating concentration. For example, it is believed that the major reason for ketone body utilisation by the brain is the circulating concentration of ketone bodies. However, this does not explain why the progressive rise in the circulating ketone body concentrations that occurs between 3 days and 3 weeks of starvation in the obese is associated with a decrease in ketone body uptake by the forearm (whilst non-esterified fatty acids become a more important fuel). A change in the activity of key enzymes involved in ketone body metabolism may provide a possible explanation. Another difference between lean and obese subjects during short term starvation is that glucose tolerance has been reported to deteriorate more in lean subjects than in obese subjects. Lean subjects also show a much greater increase in leucine oxidation during short term starvation, and a greater proportion of urine N in the forms of urea[22].

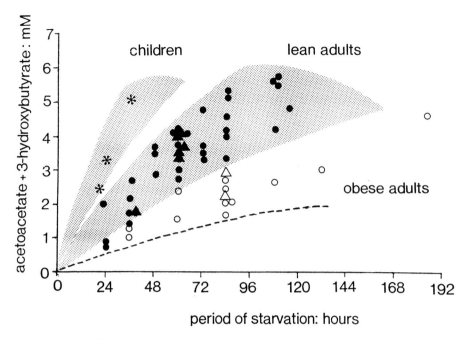

Figure 1.8 – The effect of total starvation on the circulating concentration of ketone bodies (3-hydroxybutyrate (β-OHB) plus acetoacetate (AcAc) in lean (solid symbols) and obese adults (open symbols) and children 5–7 years. Each point represents results of groups of individuals. Reproduced with permission from Elia.[11]

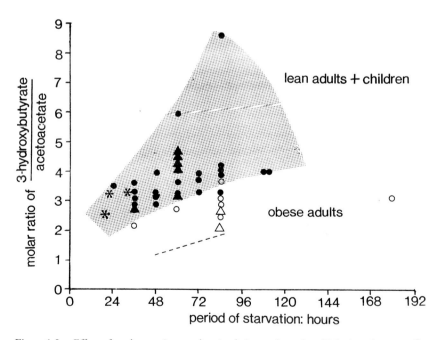

Figure 1.9 – Effect of total starvation on the circulating molar ratio of 3-hydroxybutyrate (β-OHB) to acetoacetate (AcAc) in lean (solid symbols) and obese subjects (open symbols). Reproduced with permission from Elia.[11]

Table 1.5 – Production or splanchnic release of ketone bodies 3-hydroxybutyrate (β-OHB) and acetoacetate (AcAc) in relation to their circulating concentration (and βOHB: AcAc) in lean the obese subjects undergoing short-term starvation (60–84 h).

	Period of starvation (h)	β-OHB + AcAc (mM)	β-OHB:AcAc	Splanchnic release or production (mmol/min)			Reference
				β-OHB	AcAc	β-OHB + AcAc	
Catheterisation studies							
Lean subjects (*n* = 6)	60	3.68	4.10	0.37	0.4	0.77	Bjorkman and Eriksson, 1985[78]
Lean subjects (*n* = 5)	60	4.05	4.40	0.39	0.31	0.70	Bjorkman and Eriksson, 1985[78]
Lean subjects (*n* = 16)	60–64	3.70	4.50	0.484	0.381	0.865	Eriksson et al., 1988[6]
Lean subjects (*n* = 2)[a]	80–86	3.49	2.68	0.66	0.44	1.10	Garber et al., 1974[79]
Obese subjects (*n* = 3)[a]	80–86	1.88	2.08	0.52	0.61	1.13	Garber et al., 1974[79]
Tracer studies[b]							
Lean subjects (*n* = 5)	69	4.8	2.6	–	–	1.029	Wolfe et al., 1976[80]
Obese subjects (*n* = 4)	84	2.67	2.07	0.654	0.373	1.027	Reichard et al., 1974[81]

[a] The two lean individuals (body mass index 21.3 and 22.5 kg/m²) had hypertension and cardiovascular abnormalities. The body mass index in the obese subjects ranged from 28.8 to 39.5 kg/m².

[b] Since tracer techniques are known to give higher values for rates of ketone body production than arterio-hepatic venous catheterisation (82), comparisons between lean and obese subjects should be made using the same technique.

Based on Elia.[11]

Since substrates can compete with each other, their relative circulating concentrations can affect fuel selection and utilisation by tissues. Figure 1.10 illustrates the changes in the major circulating fuels that occur during early starvation. The results are expressed in relation to the energy content of fuels because equimolar quantities of common substrates have widely different heats of combustion (glucose 669.9 kcal/mol, non-esterified fatty acids (NEFA) 2578 kcal/mol, β-OHB 479.4 kcal/mol, AcAc, 424.2 kcal/mol).[5] It can be seen that the potentially available of energy from circulating ketone bodies and NEFA increases rapidly after the start of starvation whilst that from glucose decreases (as glycogen reserves become depleted). Since circulating ketone bodies and NEFA compete with glucose for utilisation in tissues such as heart and muscle, their increased availability in blood not only has an important influence in reducing the uptake of glucose, but also in inhibiting the oxidation of glucose at the level of the pyruvate dehydrogenase complex. Lack of insulin also inhibits this complex (see above) but it activates the hormone-sensitive lipase in adipose tissue, which ensures that more NEFA are made available to the rest of the body for utilisation either directly (e.g. muscle, heart) or indirectly (e.g. brain) after they have been converted to ketone bodies by the liver.

Hyperketonaemia produces a mild metabolic acidosis and an acid urine. The body responds to this by excreting urinary ammonia (see ref.[11] for metabolic significance of this), which is to a large extent derived from glutamine. In obese individuals undergoing prolonged starvation urea may account for as little as 25% of the urine N whilst ammonia becomes the dominant nitrogenous end product. In lean individuals the urine ammonia excretion also increases but since total urine N excretion is greater in the lean than in the obese, urea continues to be the major nitrogenous end product (Fig. 1.11).

Another consequence of increased glutamine utilisation by the kidney concerns the fate of its carbon skeleton. Since the kidney can convert glutamine to glucose, this organ becomes as important a source of glucose (220 mmol/day) as the liver (250 mmol/day) during prolonged starvation in the obese.[29]

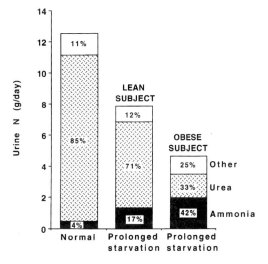

Figure 1.11 – Distribution of urine N in the fed state (normal – intake of 90 g dietary protein/day) and after 30–40 days starvation in lean and obese subjects. Data based on Elia et al.,[26] Owen et al.,[29] Benedict[2] and Cahill.[30] The data for the starving lean subject were based on Benedict[2] (day 30 of starvation). The rise in urine ammonia occurs within a few days of the start of starvation (Elia et al.,[26] Benedict,[2] Owen et al.,[29] and the absolute excretion rate at this time may be greater than in prolonged starvation.

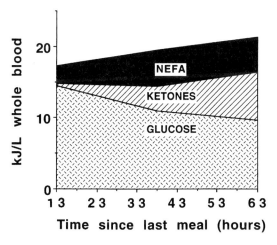

Figure 1.10 – Effect of total starvation in lean subjects on the energy content of blood glucose, ketone bodies and non-esterified fatty acids (NEFA). Reproduced with permission from Elia.[27]

Injury and sepsis

Different types and severity of injuries in individuals that differ in age, nutritional status and immune function can produce responses are variable both quantitatively and qualitatively. However, amongst the most consistent effects are an increase in BMR, a negative N balance, increased gluconeogenesis and increased synthesis of acute phase proteins.

Energy metabolism

Both the extent and duration of the increase in BMR (Figs. 1.12, 1.13) are related to the severity of injury sustained. However, this may be modified by the appearance of complications, surgical intervention, drug administration (e.g. early and appropriate use of antibiotics in sepsis), ambient temperature and specific methods of managing particular conditions. For example, the management of patients with burns has changed considerably over the last 25 years. The damaged tissue is now excised early (rather than allowed to necrose and form an eschar), sepsis associated with burn wounds is better controlled, and the ambient temperature is warmer, closer to the thermoneutral temperature. Therefore, the extent of basal hypermetabolism has decreased as new methods of treatment have become established. The changes are also affected by the age of the subjects. For example, a number of authors reported that they could not detect

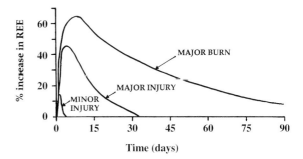

Figure 1.13 – Effect of injury severity on the magnitude and duration of basal hypermetabolism (per cent increase in resting energy expenditure (REE)).

an increase in BMR after elective surgical trauma in children especially neonates and children.[31–34] However, the first postoperative measurement in these studies was not made until 24 h after the operation. Presumably, it was felt that this would not miss an early rise in BMR, because in adults it remains elevated for a few days after elective surgical trauma. It was suggested that in infants the energy expended in healing and repair occurred at the expense of the energy expended in growth[33], so that there was little or no change in BMR. However, it now appears that there is a hypermetabolic response to elective surgical trauma in infants (accompanying other metabolic changes such as acute phase protein and cytokine responses), but the peak occurs as early as 2–4 h and lasts for less than a day (the BMR returns to normal by 12 h and is not significantly elevated above baseline at 8 h, even after major surgery) (Fig. 1.14). It also appears that the percent increase in BMR is significantly attenuated in babies less than 48 h of age compared to those greater than 48 h of age (Fig. 1.14). The reason for this difference is unknown, but it has been suggested that it may be due to secretion of endogenous opioids by the newborn infant.[38,39] The concentration of these opioids in cord blood is 5-fold higher than in the blood of resting adults.[40,41] They decrease to adult levels after 5 days.[40,41] The suggestion that opioids may modify the metabolic response to trauma has been made because exogenous opioids are known to attenuate the endocrine and metabolic response to injury and to reduce BMR.

In adults almost 60% of BMR arises from four organs (liver, kidneys, brain and heart) that account for only 5.5–6.0% of body weight.[42,43] The loss of these tissues during starvation contributes considerably to the decrease in BMR. However, animal models of injury and sepsis suggest that there is preferential preservation of the central organs,[44,45] at the expense of peripheral

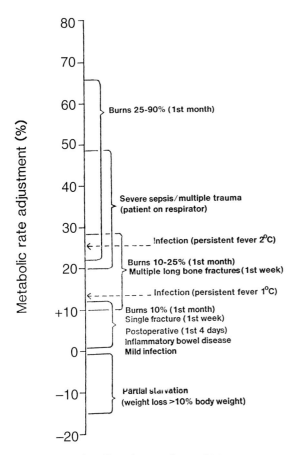

Figure 1.12 – The effect of various forms of injury on resting energy expenditure. Reproduced with permission from Elia.

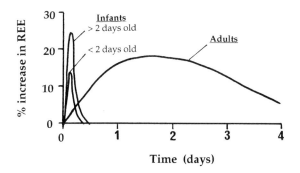

Figure 1.14 – Percent change in resting energy expenditure (REE) in infants (greater and fewer than 2 days old) and adults after elective surgery. Based on data by Pullicino and Elia M (unpublished); Carli et al.,[35] Jones et al.[36] and Jones et al.[37]

tissues such as muscle and skin[44] (a phenomenon that can be reproduced by administration of cytokines such as TNF, and hormones such as corticosteroids).[46] Indeed compared to pair fed animals, the mass and protein content of the central organs (especially the liver and lung) may show an increase of up to 50%.[45] The extent to which such changes occur in man, and the extent to which they contribute to the changes in BMR is uncertain. It is of course possible for BMR to increase rapidly after injury without a change in organ size. For example, catecholamines can produce a rise in BMR within minutes of administration, before there has been sufficient time for protein redistribution. Indeed, infusion of stress hormones (catecholamines, cortisol and glucagon) in normal subjects can reproduce the increase in BMR that occurs after injury, but they do not reproduce the large negative N balance of acute phase protein response that occurs after severe injury, nor does it reproduce a number of specific metabolic changes that occur in different tissues.[47]

Infusion of cytokines such as TNF can produce an acute phase protein response as well as a substantial increase in BMR. The metabolic processes responsible for resting energy expenditure in health and disease are poorly defined although protein synthesis, Na–K exchange across cell membranes[48] and various substrate cycles are considered to be important. The activities of some of these cycles have been assessed in health and after injury, and an estimate has been made of their contribution to BMR. Table 1.6 illustrates some of these for patients with burns, and shows that an increase in the activity of three cycles may account for almost half of the increase in BMR. A further consideration is the energy cost associated with an increase in cardiac output, which can more than double in

burned patients, and an increase in minute ventilation by up to 2- to 4-fold.

Although BMR is increased after trauma and sepsis, the energy expended in physical activity is decreased, especially after more severe disease. The overall effect is to produce little change or even a reduction in the overall energy expenditure of patients. This has important implications for nutrition support.

Nitrogen metabolism

Increased protein loss is one of the most well known effects of injury. This occurs even when a normal protein intake is maintained. Although the extent of net protein loss from the body (negative N balance) tends to be reduced when dietary protein intake is increased (at least up to 0.2–0.3 g N/kg/day), total urine N excretion is increased, implying that more energy is derived from protein oxidation. Since total energy expenditure is frequently not increased after injury (see above) the result is that the proportion derived from protein oxidation (p%) is increased. An example is given in Table 1.7 which shows that after severe head injury p% is 25–30%, which is approximately double the normal value.

The negative N balance after injury is associated with increased protein turnover, especially after more severe injury. However, neither whole body protein turnover nor N balance provide information about the tissues involved in these processes, or the subtle changes that affect individual proteins and inter-organ flux of amino acids.

Muscle is probably the main tissue that is lost after injury, and arteriovenous catheterisation studies across this tissue after severe 'injury' such as sepsis and burns, have shown an increase in the net rate of amino acid release (up to 2- to 3-fold[49]). Hormones, cytokines, metabolites and decreased muscular activity (immobilisation) are all probably involved in the net catabolism of muscle.

The increased release of amino acids by peripheral tissues is paralleled by increased uptake of amino acids by the splanchnic bed. Alanine and glutamine are the main amino acids released by muscle in health as well as injury, and the same two amino acids are the main ones extracted by splanchnic tissues. The gut extracts glutamine[50] and releases some alanine, and the liver actively utilises alanine released from both muscle and gut. Indeed, alanine is quantitatively the single most

Table 1.6 – The activity and energy cost of some substrate cycles in normal and burned subjects.

Substrate cycle	Mole ATP used/mole substrate cycled[a]	Normal subjects			Burned subjects				Reference for rates of substrate cycling
		Rate of substrate cycling mole/70 kg/day[a]	Energy cost of cycle		Rate of substrate cycling mole/70 kg/day	Energy cost of cycle		ΔEnergy cost of cycle × 100[d]	
			kcal/day[b]	%BMR[c]		kcal/day	%BMR	ΔBMR	
Protein–amino acid (protein turnover)	(4)	3.1	236	14	6.6	502	15–20	19–32	Jahoor *et al.*, 1989[83,e]
Glucose–lactate'	4	0.42	32	1.9	1.6	122	3.7–4.9	6.5–11	Wilmore and Aulick, 1978[84,f]
		0.24	18	1.1	–	–	–	–	Reichard *et al.*, 1963[85]
		0.21	16	1.0	–	–	–	–	Consoli *et al.*, 1990[86]
Triglyceride–fatty acid	8	0.12	18	0.8	0.53	81	2.9	12	Wolfe *et al.*, 1987[87,g]
		0.04	6	0.36	–	–	–	–	Elia *et al.*, 1987[87,g]
		0.13	20	1.3	–	–	–	–	Klein *et al.*, 1989[9]
Glucose–glucose 6P and Fructose 6P–	1	0.4	8	0.33	0.96	18	0.65	2	Wolfe *et al.*, 1987[87,g]
		0.29	6	0.33	–	–	–	–	Karlander *et al.*, 1986[88]
Fructose 1–6P		0.69	13	0.85	–	–	–	–	Shulman *et al.*, 1985[89]
Total									

[a] In the case of the protein–amino acid cycle, this refers to the molar rate of amino acid cycling. For the glucose–lactate cycle the molar rate refers to glucose cycling (not lactate), and for the triglyceride fatty acid cycle it refers to the triglyceride (not fatty acid).

[b] Energy cost (kcal/day) = substrate cycling rate (moles/day) × ATP used/mole substrate cycled × 19 (kcal/mole ATP).

[c] When basal metabolic rate measurements in normal adults were not available, it was assumed that they expended 1650 kcal/day (70 kg body weight).

[d] ΔEnergy cost of cycle (kcal) = energy cost of cycling in burned subjects – energy cost of cycling in normal subjects. ΔBMR = BMR of burned patients (70 kg) – BMR of normal subjects (70 kg).

[e] The burned subjects in this study (mean burn size – 65% of total surface area) were studied at 11 ± 4 days. The range in values for %BMR and for Δenergy cost cycle/ΔBMR in the burned subjects were calculated assuming metabolic rate was elevated 50–85% above normal.

[f] The range in values for %BMR and 100 × Δenergy cost cycle/ΔBMR in the burned subjects was calculated assuming metabolic rate was 50–85% above normal. The estimated rate of cycling includes cycling of lactate and other 3–carbon glycolytic products, e.g. alanine (in normal man, glucose–alanine cycling occurs at about one-half the rate of glucose–lactate cycling[87]).

[g] Both the control and burned patients in this study were a combination of adults and children. The burned subjects (74 ± 3% surface area burn) were studied 20 ± 5 days after injury when their metabolic rate was found to be 23% above normal (estimated to be ~40 kcal/kg/day compared with ~32.5 kcal/kg/day for the control subjects).
Based on Elia.[42]

Table 1.7 – Energy and protein balances and contribution of protein oxidation total energy expenditure in male subjects 3–5 days after severe head injury.

	Energy kcal/day	Protein g N/day
Intake	850 ± 849	4.6 ± 2.7
Output[b]	2247 ± 287	21.3 ± 8.8[a]
Balance	−1397 ± 648	−16.7 ± 8.1

[a] The value, which represent urine N excretion, implies that 590 kcal were derived from protein oxidation, and this accounts for 26.3% of total energy expenditure. In a normal subject in nutrient balance the value is about 15%. Total energy expenditure in normal free living young adults is greater than the values shown here, whilst protein oxidation is less.
[b] The 24-h energy expenditure was measured by continuous 24-h indirect calorimetry whilst patients were being ventilated. Based on Weekes.[91]

important amino acid extracted by the liver. In normal subjects its net fractional extraction is 45%, and this accounts for about half of the total amino acid uptake by the liver. Alanine carbon is used for hepatic gluconeogenesis whilst the N is used for urea synthesis.

The role of amino acids in the catabolic response to injury

Post-traumatic pyrexia has been incriminated in the catabolic response to injury since it stimulates a variety of metabolic processes including protein catabolism. Thus, increased protein oxidation can be regarded as part of the general hypermetabolic response to injury. However, there are other more important explanations. One of these is that there is a need to provide an increased supply of amino acids for the synthesis of acute phase proteins, leucocytes and proteins involved in healing wounds. Another is the need to provide glucose, for glucose-dependent tissues such as leucocytes and healing wounds (as well as the brain) at a time when the dietary intake of carbohydrates is reduced.

Arteriovenous catheterisation studies across burned and injured human limbs[49] have demonstrated a 5- to 10-fold increase in the uptake of glucose and release of lactate, with little change in O_2 consumption (injured legs). The wound is glycolytic,[51] and therefore derives 2 ATP per mole glucose utilised (compared to almost 20-fold more ATP when glucose is fully oxidised).[5] In a man with a 50% burn it is estimated that the wound alone utilises 200–225 g glucose/day, which is as much as the production and utilisation in a normal overnight fasted man (about 120 g for the brain and 100 g for other tissues). After an overnight fast, the proportion of glucose oxidised in the whole body is reduced in burned subjects compared to normal subjects (33% vs 65%) and about 250 g are recycled compared to about 75 g in normal subjects.

The brain will inevitably oxidise much of the glucose especially since injury is frequently associated with hyperglycaemia, whilst ketone bodies do not rise as much as expected from starvation alone[52,53] (especially after severe injury). Since the anorexia of injury results in a decreased intake of carbohydrate, glucose has to be formed endogenously, mainly from amino acids released during the catabolic process. Some of the amino acids released from peripheral tissues (muscle and skin) during the catabolic process may be used to spare and possibly increase the size of central tissues such as the liver, as has been clearly shown in animal studies.[45,54] This increase in the size of the liver is presumably related to the increased need for hepatic gluconeogenesis, synthesis of acute phase proteins and increased reticuloendothelial activity.

The three carbon glycolytic fragments (mainly lactate and alanine) which are released by the wound and other tissues such as muscle, act as gluconeogenic substrates in the liver, whilst the transfer of N from the periphery to liver is converted to urea as part of the catabolic process.

Since increased gluconeogenesis after injury is one of the most important changes that is linked to increased catabolism, the factors that control it and particularly the factors that control gluconeogenesis from alanine (the main amino acid involved in this process) are of considerable importance. In the perfused liver, uptake of gluconeogenic substrates such as lactate, glycerol and alanine[55] is concentration-dependent. In man too, the uptake of alanine and glycerol by splanchnic tissues depends on their circulating concentration, which is in turn influenced by their release from peripheral tissues. However, after 'injury' additional factors modify the gluconeogenic process. First, under normal circumstances, gluconeogenesis is suppressed by administration of glucose and by hyperglycaemia, but in injury this suppression is much less complete. Secondly, the fractional extraction of amino acids, including alanine, may be greatly increased after injury in humans (e.g. burns),[56] despite an increase in splanchnic blood flow. Thirdly, there is an increase in activity of some key gluconeogenic enzymes (animal studies). Fourthly, the circulating alanine concentration may be unchanged or even decreased, even though the release of this amino acid is increased. Finally, the rate of removal of an alanine load is increased after injury.[57] Therefore, it would appear that the catabolic effects of injury are associated and mediated by altered set points for net muscle proteolysis and for gluconeogenesis.[27]

The other major amino acid released by peripheral tissues is glutamine which carries two N per molecule compared to alanine which carries one. The two amino acids are released in approximately equimolar quantities. Together they account for about half the amino N release from muscle but they account for only ~10% of muscle protein implying that they are synthesised in muscle (the pathways are well known). Glutamine is an important fuel for the gut accounting for ~40% of its energy in the rat, but probably a smaller proportion in the human.[50] It is also an important fuel for lymphocytes and macrophages, which become activated after injury and sepsis. The mass of lymphocytes in reference man is estimated to be 1.5 kg (and 1.2 kg in women),[21] and therefore their metabolism could be quantitatively important. Glutamine is also essential for the synthesis of nucleic acids, which is important for rapidly dividing cells and newly formed tissues, which are established after trauma. The free glutamine pool in muscle rapidly becomes depleted after injury (more than half can be lost 2–3 days after severe injury, but the extent of depletion is greater in non-survivors than survivors).[58] Although both the release of glutamine by muscle, and its inter-organ flux are increased after injury, it has been suggested that the rate of production is insufficiently high for optimal tissue structure and function, and therefore this amino acid should be regarded as a conditionally essential nutrient. However, evidence for this needs to be established in a variety of situations by randomised controlled clinical trials.

Positive and negative acute phase proteins

Some of the most well known changes that occur after injury involve the acute phase proteins, which show large increments (often several-fold) in concentration in the first few days after injury. C-reactive protein (CRP), is one of the best known human acute phase proteins, since it may increase more than 50-fold after severe injury. This and several other acute phase proteins peak at about 2–4 days after elective surgical injury (Fig. 1.15). However, it takes about 6–8 h before the circulating acute phase protein concentrations begin to rise, in contrast to a variety of other metabolites and hormones, which change very quickly after the injury. Why is there such a delay, and what are the processes or signals that control production of acute phase proteins? If there is a signal for acute phase protein synthesis, one would expect

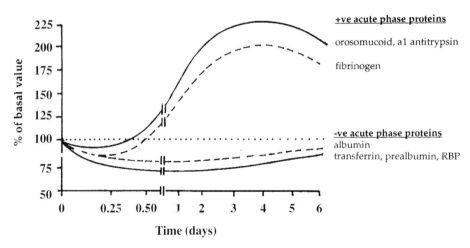

Figure 1.15 – Effect of injury (moderate elective surgical trauma or accidental long bone fractures) on the circulating concentrations of positive (orosomucoid, α1-antitrypsin and fibrinogen) and negative acute phase proteins (albumin, transferrin, pre-albumin and retinol binding protein (RBP)). Based on Myers et al.,[19] Fleck et al.,[59] Ballentyne and Fleck,[60] Colley et al.[61] and Elia et al. (unpublished). See also Shenkin et al.[62] for effect of more severe injury.

this to operate before the rise of the acute phase proteins. One of the cytokines (IL-6), which is considered to be important in mediating this response, does indeed rise and peak before the acute phase protein changes.[63]

To understand a possible biological reason for the delayed peak in the circulating acute phase protein concentration it is necessary to briefly consider the functions of some of the acute phase proteins. Fibrinogen is involved in the clotting process, and haptoglobin binds free haemoglobin (this may be released from red blood cells after crush injuries) which would otherwise block renal tubules and impair renal function. Several other acute phase proteins are protease inhibitors (e.g. α_1-antitrypsin, α_1-antichymotrypsin). Injured tissue is infiltrated with inflammatory cells, including those that scavenge and destroy damaged tissue and organisms. If the activity of proteolytic enzymes that are released locally is not checked by protease inhibitors, the damage might spread in an uncontrolled manner to surrounding tissues. Histochemical techniques have shown that some of the acute phase proteins that act as protease inhibitors are deposited close to repairing tissues. Other acute phase proteins such as CRP opsonise DNA and cell membrane debris for subsequent scavenging, whilst α-1 glycoprotein promotes fibroblast growth. Caeruloplasmin, which binds copper, also acts as an antioxidant. Therefore, the acute phase proteins are considered to be useful, encouraging and enhancing the scavenging process and helping repair. Several of these processes do not occur maximally, immediately after injury (repair is often delayed), and in this respect it is relevant that the peak concentration of acute phase proteins is delayed (see Fig. 1.15 for elective surgical injury) and prolonged after more severe injury.[62]

When the availability of amino acids is limited because of protein or protein–energy malnutrition, a number of the injury responses are attenuated, including the catabolic response (loss of N) and the acute phase protein response. Experimental data in animals demonstrate this most clearly[45,64–67] (Fig.1.16) and are supported by observations in humans.

The negative acute phase proteins

Whilst the circulating concentration of acute phase proteins increase after injury (positive acute phase response), there are also other circulating proteins such as albumin, which decrease in concentration (negative acute phase response). As the severity of

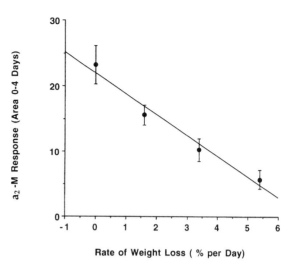

Figure 1.16 – The effect of nutritional status on the rate of weight loss prior to turpentine injection (to produce an abscess) on the acute phase response (circulating a_2-macroglobulin, which is a major acute phase protein in the rat). Reproduced with permission from Jennings and Elia.[45]

injury increases (see Fig. 1.12) the degree of hypoalbuminaemia increases. The albumin concentration may decrease by as much as 50% in the most severe cases. An understanding of the processes involved with the negative acute phase response is of some clinical importance because the response has been used to assess nutrition status.

Albumin has been widely used as a nutritional indicator, but its use for this purpose may be inappropriate, partly because it is a negative acute phase reactant, and partly because total or partial starvation uncomplicated by disease is associated with little or no change in the circulating albumin concentration. For example, there is little or no change in the circulating albumin concentration after 3 weeks of total starvation, or after 6 months of semi-starvation, in which the intake of normal subjects was restricted by 25% until they lost about 25% of their body weight.[20] Furthermore, in anorexia nervosa, the circulating concentration of albumin and other proteins such as retinol binding protein, pre-albumin and transferrin, which have also been used as nutritional indicators, are well maintained.[68,69]

Several factors could be responsible for the post-traumatic hypoalbuminaemia, including changes in protein synthesis and degradation. However, under normal circumstances the turnover of albumin is slow (normal half-life is about 3 weeks), so that the daily turnover of albumin is only 4% (15 g) of the total albumin mass (~300 g). A little less than half of the total albumin mass is located in the vascular space, and the remainder is in the extravascular space. Of considerable importance is the continuous flux of albumin from the vascular to the extravascular space, and its return into the circulation via the lymphatic system. Muscle contraction facilitates the return of lymph into the circulation. The normal transfer of albumin from the vascular to extravascular space (~5% of vascular albumin mass/h) occurs at a rate that is 10-fold greater than the rate of albumin synthesis and degradation. Therefore, factors that effect the trans-capillary escape could potentially have much greater effects on the plasma albumin concentration than changes in protein synthesis and degradation, at least in the short-term. In injury, the vascular epithelium becomes more permeable to plasma proteins and the transcapillary escape rate increases. This provides one of the most important explanations for the acute reductions in plasma albumin concentrations after injury. The more severe the injury the greater the change in vascular permeability and the greater the degree of hypoalbuminaemia. In burns, there is additional loss of albumin through the damaged skin. In contrast, studies in under-developed countries suggest that, in chronic protein–energy malnutrition with little or no associated disease, the ratio of intra- to extravascular albumin increases, although a recent study in anorexia nervosa suggests that there is little change.[70] Short-term total starvation is associated with little or no change in circulating acute phase proteins or albumin (which may actually increase as a result of mild haemoconcentration) and a decrease in the circulating concentration of proteins with a short half-life, e.g. retinol binding protein and prealbumin (Fig. 1.17). The overall pattern of changes contrasts with those which occur after injury.

Variability in response

The metabolic and clinical outcome measures of the injury response can be modified, not only by clinical management, but also by the age, sex and nutrition status of the patients. For example, there is a tendency for many aspects of the injury response (e.g. fever, N loss) to be attenuated in the elderly. The catabolic response to injury is more marked in muscular, well-nourished young men than leaner or less well-nourished individuals. (See also Fig. 1.14 for differences between neonates and adults in the hypermetabolic response to injury.) Obesity does not appear to attenuate the acute catabolic response (N loss) to injury.[71]

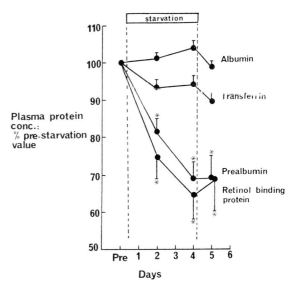

Figure 1.17 – Effect of short-term total starvation in lean subjects on the circulating concentration of selected proteins. Reproduced with permission from Elia *et al.*[28]

Hyperglycaemia (diabetes of injury) is a common feature of the injury response but imbalances between glucose production and utilisation in sepsis may occasionally lead to hypoglycaemia, especially in infants and elderly individuals suffering from severe or protracted sepsis.[53] Even experimental models of injury may produce different qualitative and quantitative tissue responses. For example, using animals trauma (including surgery) several authors have reported increased intestinal (splanchnic) utilisation of glutamine whereas endotoxaemia has been reported to reduce glutamine utilisation.[50]

Given the variability in the type and severity of injuries sustained by subjects, and the complications that may arise (renal failure, multi-organ failure, disturbances in acid base status and fluid and electrolyte status) it is not surprising that the metabolic responses are also variable. Further variability may be introduced by nutrition support, changes in ambient temperature and the treatment of the underlying condition (e.g. blood loss, sepsis).

Some clinical implications

Although many starvation studies have been carried out in the obese, this review suggests that it is not appropriate to extrapolate the findings to the lean. Survival time is much shorter in lean subjects and when injury or infection is superimposed, wasting proceeds much more rapidly and survival time is reduced even further. The very small energy reserves in premature infants born at 26–28 weeks of gestation means that survival is possible for only a few days. Therefore nutrition support becomes an urgent requirement in this situation.

In clinical practice malnutrition is usually related to disease, and therefore interactions between nutrients and disease become important considerations for repletion. Malnourished individuals have a much greater anabolic potential than normally nourished individuals and this can help establish appropriate therapies for nutrition support. Studies of total (not basal) energy expenditure following injury have also helped establish appropriate recommendations for energy intake. Furthermore, although the post-traumatic retention of fluid and salt (mediated by an increased ADH and mineralocorticoid activity) may be adaptive, especially in the 'natural' environment where water is not readily available, the injured individual may be unable to excrete a water load as easily as a normal subject. These responses should be taken into consideration during nutrition support so that fluid overload can be prevented.

Finally, although this review has largely focused on protein and energy metabolism, both injury and starvation produce important changes in vitamin mineral and trace element metabolism. For example, some of the Northern Ireland fasters developed Wernicke's encephalophathy. Deficiencies may also develop during nutritional repletion of injured and uninjured subjects if the appropriate combination of nutrients are not included in the nutritional rehabilitation regimens.

References

1. Elia M. Effect of starvation and very low calorie diets on protein-energy interrelationships in lean and obese subjects. In: Scrimshaw NS, Schurch B (eds) Protein-energy interactions. IDECG, Lausanne, 1992; pp. 249–285.

2. Benedict FG. A study of prolonged fasting. Carnegie Institute of Washington Publication, Washington DC 1915; **203**.

3. Takahira H. Metabolism during fasting and subsequent re-feeding. Imperial Government Institute for Nutrition 1925; **1**: 63–82.

4. Lehmann CF, Mueller I, Munk H, Senator H, Zuntz N. Untersuchungen an zwei hungernden Menschen. *Arch Pathol Anat Phys Klin Med* 1893; **131 (suppl)**: 1–228.

5. Elia M, Livesey G. Energy expenditure and fuel selection in biological systems: the theory and practice of calculations based on indirect calorimetry and tracer methods. *Int Rev Nutr Diet* 1992; **70**: 68–131.

6. Eriksson LS, Olsson M, Bjorkman O. Splanchnic metabolism of amino acids in healthy subjects: effect of 60 hours of starvation. *Metabolism* 1988; **37**: 1159–1162.

7. Feli P, Wen OE, Wahren J, Chaill GF. Amino acid metabolism during prolonged starvation. *J Clin Invest* 1969; **48**: 584–594.

8. Elia M, Zed C, Livesey G. The energy cost of triglyceride-fatty acid recycling in non-obese subjects after an overnight fast and four days of starvation. *Metabolism* 1987; **36**: 251–255.

9. Klein S, Peters EJ, Holland OB, Wolfe RR. Effect of short- and long-term β-adrenergic blockage on lipolysis during fasting in humans. *Am J Physiol* 1989; **257**: E65–E73.

10. Nair KS, Woolf PD, Welle SL, Matthews DE. Leucine, glucose and energy metabolism after 3 days of fasting in healthy human subjects. *Am J Clin Nutr* 1987; **46**: 557–562.

11. Elia M. The inter-organ flux of substrates in fed and fasted man, as indicated by arterio-venous balance studies. *Nutr Res Rev* 1991; **4**: 3–31.

12. Livesey G, Elia M. Estimation of energy expenditure, net carbohydrate oxidation and net fat oxidation and synthesis by indirect calorimetry. Evaluation of some errors with special reference to the detailed composition of fuels. *Am J Clin Nutr* 1989; **47**: 608–623.

13. Goschke H, Stahl M, Tholen H. Nitrogen loss in normal and obese subjects during total fast. *Klin Wochenschr* 1975; **53**: 605–610.

14. Elia M, Crozier C, Neale G. Mineral metabolism during short-term starvation in man. *Clin Chim Acta* 1984: 37–45.

15. Magnusson K, Alvestrand L, Ekman L, Wahren J. Protein and amino acid metabolism of human skeletal muscle during starvation. *Clin Nutr* 1987; **6 (suppl)**: 62.

16. Elwyn DH, Furst P, Askanazi J, Kinney JM. Effect of fasting on muscle concentrations of branched-chaim amino acids. In: Walzer M, Williamson JR (eds) Metabolism and clinical implications of branched-chain amino and keto-acids. Elsevier, Holland, 1981; pp. 547–552.

17. Chossat C. Recherches experimentales sur l'inanition. *Acad Sci Paris* 1843; 8.

18. Krieger M. Ueber die Atrophie der menschlichen Organe bei Inanition. *Z Angew Anat Konstitutionsl* 1921; **7**: 87–134.

19. Myers MA, Fleck A, Sampson B, Colley CM, Bent J, Hall G. Early plasma protein and mineral changes after surgery: a two stage process. *J Clin Pathol* 1984; **37**: 862–866.

20. Keys A, Brozek J, Henschel A, Mickelsen O, Taylor HL. The biology of human starvation. University of Minnesota Press, Minneapolis, 1950; pp. 81–535.

21. Synder WS, Cook MJ, Nasset ES, Karhausen LR, Howells GP, Tipton IH. Report of the task group on reference man. In: International commission on radiological protection. Pergamon Press, Oxford, 1975; pp. 23.

22. Elia M, Stubbs RJ, Henry CJK. Difference in gut, carbohydrate and protein metabolism between lean and obese subjects undergoing total starvation. *Obesity Research* 1999; **7**: 597–604.

23. Dulloo AG, Jacquet J, Girardier L. Autoregulation of body composition during weight recovery in humans: The Minnesota Experiment revisited. *Int J Obes* 1996; **20**: 393–405.

24. Elia M, Wood S, Khan K, Pullicino E. Ketone body metabolism in lean male adults during short-term starvation, with particular reference to forearm muscle metabolism. *Clin Sci* 1990; **78**: 579–584.

25. Owen OE, Reichard GA. Human forearm metabolism during progressive starvation. *J Clin Invest* 1971; **50**: 1536–1545.

26. Hagenfeldt L, Wahren J. Human forearm muscle metabolism during exercise VI. Substrate utilization in prolonged fasting. *Scand J Clin Lab Invest* 1971; **27**: 299–306.

27. Elia M. General integration of metabolism at the organ level. *Proc Nutr Soc* 1995; **54**: 213–232.

28. Elia M, Martin S, Price M, Hallworth J, Neale G. Effect of starvation and surgery on hand dynamometry and the circulating concentration of various proteins. *Clin Nutr* 1984; **2**: 173–179.

29. Owen OE, Felig P, Morgan AP, Wahren J, Cahill GF. Liver and kidney metabolism during prolonged starvation. *J Clin Invest* 1969; **48**: 668–675.

30. Cahill GF. Starvation in man. *N Engl J Med* 1970; **282**: 668–675.

31. Shanbhogue RLK, Jackson M, Lloyd DA. Operation does not increase resting energy expenditure in the neonate. *J Pediatr Surg* 1991; **26**: 578–580.

32. Shanbhogue RLK, Lloyd DA. Absence of hypermetabolism after operation in the newborn infant. *J Parenter Enteral Nutr* 1992; **16**: 333–336.

33. Groner JI, Brown MF, Stallings VA *et al.* Resting energy expenditure in children following major operative procedures. *J Pediatr Surg* 1989; **24**: 546–549.

34. Winthrop AL, Jones PJH, Scholler DA *et al.* Changes in the body composition of the surgical infant in the early post-operative period. *J Pediatr Surg* 1987; **22**: 546–549.

35. Carli F, Aber VR. Thermogenesis after major elective surgical procedures. *Br J Surg* 1987; **74**: 1041–1045.

36. Jones MO, Perro A, Hammond P, Lloyd DA. The metabolic response to operative stress in infants. *J Pediatr Surg* 1993; **28**: 1258–1263.

37. Jones MO, Pierro A, Hashim IA, Shenkin A, Lloyd DA. Post-operative changes in resting energy expenditure and interleukin 6 level in infants. *Br J Surg* 1994; **81**: 536–538.

38. Csontos K, Rust M, Holt V. Elevated plasma β-endorphin levels in pregnant women and their neonates. *Life Sci* 1979; **25**: 835–844.

39. Facchinetti F, Bagnoli F, Bracci R. Plasma opioids in the first hours of life. *Pediatr Res* 1982; **16**: 95–98.

40. Wardlaw SL, Stark RI, Baxi L *et al.* Plasma β-endorphin and β-lipotropin, in the human fetus at delivery: correlation with arterial pH and pO₂. *J Clin Endocrinol Metab* 1979; **49**: 888–891.

41. Panerai AE, Martini A, DiGiulio AM. Plasma β-endorphin, β-lipotropin, and metenkephalin concentrations during pregnancy in normal and drug-addicted women and their newborn. *J Clin Endocrinol Metab* 1983; **57**: 537–543.

42. Elia M. Organ and tissue contribution to metabolic rate. In: Kinney JM, Tucker HN (eds) Energy metabolism: tissue determinants and cellular corollaries. Raven Press, London, 1992; pp. 61–79.

43. Elia M. Tissue distribution and energetics in weight loss and undernutrition. In: Kinney JM, Tucker HN (eds) Physiology, stress and malnutrition: functional correlates and nutritional intervention. Lippincott-Raven, London, 1997; pp. 382–412.

44. Wusteman M, Elia M. Protein metabolism after 'injury' with turpentine: a rat model of clinical trauma. *Am J Phys* 1990; **259**: E763–E769.

45. Jennings G, Elia M. Changes in protein distribution in normal and protein deficient rats during an acute phase 'injury' response. *Br J Nutr* 1996; **76**: 123–132.

46. Lunn PG, Whitehead RG, Baker BA, Austin S. The effect of corticosterone acetate on the course of development of experimental protein energy malnutrition in rats. *Br J Nutr* 1976; **36**: 537–550.

47. McNurlan MA, Sandgren A, Hunter K, Essen P, Garlick PJ, Wernerman J. Protein synthesis rates of skeletal muscle, lymphocytes and albumin with stress hormone infusion in healthy man. *Metabolism* 1966; **45**: 1388–1394.

48. Kelly JM, McBride BW. The sodium pump and other mechanisms of thermogenesis in selected tissues. *Proc Nutr Soc* 1990; **49**: 185–202.

49. Aulick MLH, Wilmore DW. Increased peripheral amino acid release following burn injury. *Surgery* 1979; **85**: 560–565.

50. Elia M. Metabolism and nutrition of the gastro-intestinal tract. In: Bindels JG, Goedhart AC, Visser H-KA (eds) Recent developments in infant nutrition. Kluwer Academic Publishers, Boston, 1996; pp. 318–348.

51. Im MJ, Hoopes JE. Energy metabolism in healing skin wounds. *J Surg Res* 1970; **10**: 459–464.

52. Birkham RH, Lang CL, Fitkin DL, Busnardo MD. A comparison of the effects of skeletal trauma and surgery on the ketosis of starvation in man. *J Trauma* 1981; **21**: 513–519.

53. Beisel Wr, Wannemacher RW. Gluconeogenesis, ureagenesis and ketogenesis during sepsis. *J Parent Enteral Nutr* 1980; **4**: 277–285.

54. Wusteman M, Hayes A, Stirling D, Elia M. Changes in protein distribution in the rat during prolonged systemic injury. *J Surg Res* 1994; **56**: 331–337.

55. Mallette LE, Exton JH, Park CR. Control of gluconeogenesis from amino acids in the perfused liver. *J Biol Chem* 1969; **244**: 5713–5723.

56. Wilmore DW, Goodwin CG, Aulick LH, Pawanda MC, Mason A, Pruit BA. Effect of injury and infection on visceral metabolism and circulation. *Ann Surg* 1980; **192**: 491–504.

57. Elia M, Ilic V, Bacon S, Williamson DH, Smith R. Relationship between the blood alanline concentration and removal of an alanine load in various situations in man. *Clin Sci* 1980; **58**: 301–309.

58. Roth E, Fuvonics J, Muhlbacher F, Schemper M, Mauritz W, Sporn P, Fritsch A. Metabolic disorders in severe abdominal sepsis: glutamine deficiency in skeletal muscle. *Clin Nutr* 1982; **1**: 25–41.

59. Fleck A, Colley CM, Myers MA. Liver export proteins and trauma. *Br Med Bull* 1985; **4**: 265–273.

60. Ballentyne FC, Fleck A. The effect of environmental temperature (20° and 30°) after injury on the concentration of serum protein in man. *Clin Chim Acta* 1973; **44**: 341–347.

61. Colley CM, Fleck A, Goode AW, Muller BR, Myers MA. Early time course of the acute phase protein response in man. *J Clin Pathol* 1983; **36**: 203–207.

62. Shenkin A, Neuhauser M, Bergstrom J *et al.* Biochemical changes associated with severe trauma. *Am J Clin Nutr* 1980; **33**: 2119–2127.

63. Cruickshank AM, Jennings G, Fearon KH, Elia M, Shenkin A. Serum interleukin 6 (IL-6) effect of surgery and undernutrition. *Clin Nutr* 1991; **10 (suppl)**: 65–69.

64. Jennings G, Bourgeois C, Elia M. The magnitude of the acute phase protein response is attenuated by protein deficiency in rats. *J Nutr* 1992; **122**: 1325–1333.

65. Jennings G, Elia M. The acute-phase response to turpentine-induced abscesses in malnourished rats at different environmental temperatures. *Metab Clin Exp* 1992; **41**: 141–147.

66. Jennings G, Cruickshank AM, Shenkin A, Wight DG, Elia M. Effect of aseptic abscesses in protein deficient rats on the relationship between interleukin-6 and the acute phase protein α_2-macroglobulin. *Clin Sci* 1992; **83**: 731–735.

67. Jennings G, Elia M. Effect of dietary restriction on the response of α_2-macroglobulin during an acute phase response. *J Parenter Enteral Nutr* 1994; **18**: 510–515.

68. Dowd PS, Kelleher J, Walker BE, Guillou PJ. Nutritional and immunological assessment of patients with anorexia nervosa. *Clin Nutr* 1983; **2**: 79–83.

69. Martin S, Neale G, Elia M. Factors affecting maximal momentary grip strength. *Hum Nutr Clin Nutr* 1985; **39C**: 137–147.

70. Smith G, Robinson PH, Fleck A. Serum albumin distribution in early treated anorexia. *Nutrition* 1996; **10**: 677–684.

71. Jeevanandam M, Young DH, Schiller WR. Obesity and the metabolic response to severe multiple trauma in man. *J Clin Invest* 1991; **87**: 262–269.

72. Meyers AW. Some morphological effects of prolonged inanition. *J Med Res* 1917; **36**: 51 77.

73. Stewart WK, Fleming LW. Features of a successful therapeutic fast of 38 days duration. *Postgrad Med J* 1973; **49**: 203–209.

74. Barnard DL, Ford J, Garnett ES, Mardell RJ, Whyman AE. Changes in body composition produced by prolonged starvation and refeeding. *Metabolism* 1969; **18**: 546–569.

75. Runcie J, Thomson TJ. Prolonged starvation – a dangerous procedure. *Br Med J* 1970; **3**: 432–435.

76. Thomson TJ, Runcie J, Miller V. Treatment of obesity by total fasting for up to 249 days. *Lancet* 1966; **2**: 992–996.

77. Collinson DR. Total fasting for up to 249 days. *Lancet* 1967; **1**: 112.

78. Drenick EJ, Swendseid ME, Bhahd WH, Tuttle SG. Prolonged starvation as a treatment of obesity. *JAMA* 1964; **187**: 100–105.

79. Bjorkman O, Eriksson LS. Influence of a 60-h fast on insulin mediated splanchnic and peripheral glucose metabolism in humans. *J Clin Invest* 1985; **76**: 87–92.

80. Garber AJ, Menzel PH, Boden G, Owen OE. Hepatic ketogenesis and gluconeogenesis in humans. *J Clin Invest* 1974; **54**: 981–989.

81. Wolfe BM, Havel JR, Marliss EB, Kane JP, Seymour J, Ahuja SP. Effect of a 3-day fast and of ethanol on splanchinic metabolism of free fatty acids, amino acids, and carbohydrates in healthy young men. *J Clin Invest* 1976; **57**: 329–340.

82. Reichard GA, Owen OE, Haff AC, Paul P, Bortz WM. Ketone body production and oxidation in fasting obese humans. *J Clin Invest* 1974; **53**: 508–513.

83. Williamson DH, Whitelaw E. Physiological aspect of the regulation of ketogenesis. *Biochem Soc Symp* 1978; **43**: 136–161.

84. Jahoor F, Shangraw RE, Miyoshi H, Wallfish H, Herndon DN, Wolfe RR. Role of insulin and glucose oxidation in mediating the protein catabolism of burns and sepsis. *Am J Physiol* 1989; **257**: E323–E331.

85. Wilmore DW, Aulick LH. Metabolic changes in burned patients. *Surg Clin N Am* 1978; **58**: 1173–1187.

86. Reichard GA, Moury NF, Hochella NJ, Patterson AL, Weinhouse S. Quantitative estimation of the Cori cycle in humans. *J Biol Chem* 1963; **238**: 495–501.

87. Consoli A, Nurjan N, Reilly J, Bier DM, Gerich JE. Contribution of liver and skeletal muscle to alanine and lactate metabolism in humans. *Am J Physiol* 1990; **259**: E677–E684.

88. Wolfe RR, Herndon DN, Jahoor F, Miyoshi H, Wolfe M. Effect of severe burn injury on substrate by glucose and fatty acids. *N Engl J Med* 1987; **317**: 403–508.

89. Karlander S, Roovete A, Varnic M, Efendic S. Glucose and fructose-6-phosphate cycle in humans. *Am J Physiol* 1986; **251**: E530–E536.

90. Shulman GI, Ladenson PW, Wolfe MA, Ridgeway EC, Wolfe RR. Substrate cycling between gluconeogenesis and glycolysis in euthyroid, hypothyroid and hyperthyroid man. *J Clin Invest* 1985; **76**: 757–764.

91. Weekes E, Elia M. Observations on the patterns of 24 h energy expenditure and changes in body composition and gastric emptying in head injured patients. *J Parenter Enteral Nutr* 1996; **20**: 31–37.

92. Cuendet GS, Loten EG, Cameron DP, Renold AE, Marliss EB. Hormone-substrate responses to total fasting in lean and obese mice. *Am J of Physiology* 1975; **228**: 276–283.

2

Protein and amino acid metabolism in the whole body and in the tissues

Daniel J R Cuthbertson and Michael J Rennie

Introduction

Why is it important for clinicians with responsibility for nutrition support to know something about protein metabolism? The answer is that the fabric and machinery of the body are mostly made of protein, and that when people become sick and cannot eat, the protein mass of the body wastes, with potentially catastrophic consequences. Even if patients survive, wound healing and repair and rehabilitation can all be delayed if protein metabolism is not optimal.

Protein and amino acid metabolism encompasses not only protein turnover (i.e. the synthesis and breakdown of protein) but also the oxidation of amino acids to produce CO_2, ammonia and urea, the *de novo* synthesis of dispensable amino acids (e.g. alanine and glutamine by muscle), some elements of nucleic acid and ammonia metabolism, and others of carbohydrate and fat metabolism which overlap with amino acid metabolism. Protein synthesis and breakdown occur in all tissues of the body but the capacity for other metabolic functions of amino acid metabolism is distributed among several tissues, giving rise to the need for a coordinated inter-organ traffic of the amino acids. This is, to some extent, tidal in nature, depending upon the timing of meals for its size and direction between the centre and the periphery. The aim of this chapter is to provide an overview of the subject in sufficient detail to enable an understanding of what are perceived as the current questions of interest and how they might be answered. It is not meant to be an inclusive account of the biochemistry of nitrogen metabolism in mammals, and readers looking for such detail should look for it in specialised textbooks and review series.

The idea that there is something special about protein, for example that it is not a fuel like fat and carbohydrate, is a remnant of 19th century vitalist philosophy. Oddly, one of the greatest adherents to this idea, Liebig, in fact thought that protein was often a *preferred* fuel, for example during exercise, when, he believed (incorrectly!), the muscles spurned the use of fat and carbohydrate in favour of protein.[1] The well-documented craving for protein when it is lacking in our diet indicates that it is a necessary nutrient, but it is one that is also expensive and difficult to obtain in rural economies. Such facts have also contributed to the idea of the special nature of protein and its metabolism. It is of course special in many ways: protein, much more than carbohydrate or fat, is involved in the structure and function of cells, tissues

and organs. Furthermore, protein metabolism is complicated, due to the fact that there are 20 (or, including selenomethionine, 21) amino acids involved. Before reliable methods for measuring the concentrations of individual amino acids in biological material became available, protein metabolism was inevitably simplified chemically, with the result that its physiological complexity was somewhat obscured. Much of our present-day knowledge concerning amino acids has really only developed since the introduction of the automated amino acid analyser in the 1950s.

The dynamic nature of protein metabolism (Fig. 2.1) has been recognised for many years[2,3] but the methodological difficulties of determining rates of interchange of amino acids were such that many early workers concentrated on nitrogen balance – the net difference between protein intake (indicated as nitrogen content) and the nitrogenous content of body wastes. This technique was applied experimentally to the analysis of nutritional influences on the growth patterns of the young rat. However, the utility of the nitrogen balance method is limited in free-living human beings, especially children, and although it can be more easily applied in hospital patients, the most reliable results require special metabolic facilities for preparing food and collecting and analysing wastes. If used less than obsessively, the method can give incorrect results, usually overestimating positivity of nitrogen balance.[4-7]

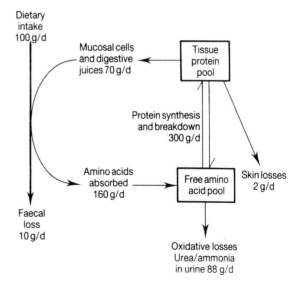

Figure 2.1 – The dynamic nature of protein metabolism and estimates of the sizes of its components. These estimates are mostly guesswork and may be in error by up to 25%.

Despite the problems, the concept is easily understood and its practical application will be difficult to replace until there is much greater access to newer methods such as those involving stable-isotope technology.[8-11]

One historical trend that has helped to inform our current views of human protein metabolism in the clinical context is the development of artificial nutrition. Only within the last 30 years has it been possible to prescribe solutions of crystalline amino acids that are sufficiently pure and of an appropriate composition to satisfy the needs of the body for maintenance of lean tissue and production of new proteins for wound healing and rehabilitation. The develop-

ment of amino acid solutions of suitable composition was only possible because of the technical developments leading to the widespread availability of the automatic amino acid analyser, which was used to monitor the effects of various candidate solutions upon blood amino acid composition[12] (Table 2.1).

Determination of body composition

Quantitative knowledge of the amounts of protein and amino acids in the body or in an organ at a given

Table 2.1 – Concentrations of amino acids in plasma, red blood cells, the muscle free amino acid pool and muscle protein, and the effects of feeding

	Plasma free amino acids (μmol/l plasma water) (n=26)		RBC free amino acids (μmol/l intracellular water) (n=24)		Muscle free amino acids (μmol/l intracellular water) (n=25)		Human muscle protein (g AA/100 g)
		SE		SE		SE	
Essential							
Histidine	87	3	120	18	592	54	2.7
Isoleucine	63	3	71	3	68	4	5.5
Leucine	120	5	137	6	133	6	7.8
Lysine	195	9	177	5	994	77	8.0
Methionine	25	1	20	3			4.7
Phenylalanine	53	2	62	2	62	3	5.4
Threonine	128	5	157	6	571	31	(ND)
Tyrosine	60	4	82	5	82	5	6.4
Valine	220	8	248	9	253	11	5.1
Tryptophan	43	2	13	1			(ND)
Non-essential							
Alanine	316	17	419	16	2250	95	5.9
Arginine	86	3	258	23	633	46	3.7
Asparagine	47	2	156	4	266	11	8.8 (incl Asp)
Citrulline	34	1	48	2	170	13	–
Glutamate	–	–	446	85	–	–	} 15.4 (incl Gln)
Glutamine	655	17	758	15	20050	514	
Glycine	248	13	544	21	1304	75	3.1
Ornithine	66	4	271	18	493	50	–
Serine	114	4	211	6	584	24	4.7
Taurine	49	3	157	28	19200	676	–
3-Methyl histidine	6	0					–
Carnitine					6130	370	–
EAA	888	26	981	23	2619	109	45.6
NEAA	1573	43	2428	43	25167	559	41.6
Total AA	2461	62	3409	56	27786	620	100
BCAA	402	15	456	17	443	19	18.4

Source: P. Fürst personal communication.
EAA, Essential amino acids; NEAA, Non-essential amino acids; BCAA, Branched-chain amino acids.

time is vital for precise studies of maintenance, growth and wasting of the lean body mass, but this information is extraordinarily difficult to obtain. Few measurements of tissue composition have been carried out on cadavers, and inevitably most of the methods for measuring the protein concentration and composition of the tissues in patients are indirect and based upon assumptions that are uncheckable.[13] There seems to be an inverse correlation between the precision and accuracy of methods for assessing body composition and their expense and availability. This is exemplified at the two extremes by neutron activation analysis (for which a nuclear reactor is required but which is the method of choice for total body N and thus body cell mass) and body impedance analysis (which, although cheap, provides derived values of lean body mass that are particularly model dependent.[13])

Methods based upon tissue biopsy are of course valuable but, with the possible exception of skin and muscle biopsies[14] (which can truly be regarded as little more invasive than blood sampling), sampling of other tissues (for example liver[15], gastrointestinal tissue,[15, 16] breast[17] and bone[18] – all of which are possible without general anaesthesia) requires specialised equipment in a hospital setting. Methods for liver export proteins,[19,20] sampled in the blood, are conceptually similar to those for fixed tissue proteins. A similar kind of approach can be used for any protein it is possible to sample, such as those secreted into the gut, and our group has done this for pepsinogen.[21]

Most of the methods currently available to us are insufficiently sensitive or precise to pick up the kind of small changes that are of great interest to scientists and clinicians, such as the alteration and the total amount of protein in the body after an overnight fast or surgical operation or a short period of sepsis. Furthermore, it is difficult to attribute any changes to particular classes of protein and to differentiate between hypothetical labile and non-labile protein pools, except in the broadest terms (e.g. possibly muscle myofibrillar vs. bone collagen protein, respectively).

For workers interested in expressing rates of protein metabolism on a lean body mass basis, it is my opinion that the best practical technique available for lean body mass is deuterium dilution (to obtain total body water[22]) with a correction for extracellular water using bromide space.[13, 23] Despite improvements in design of body impedance analysers, especially the use of different probing frequencies, the variability associated with the results is sufficiently large that they are useful only in population studies, rather than in individual patients. This is because any variation in the concentrations of electrolytes and the sizes and shapes of spaces they occupy confounds the assumptions upon which the algorithms for calculation of lean body mass are based.

Analysis of amino acids and proteins

Individual amino acids may be analysed by a variety of enzymatic methods[24] which, although usually specific and reasonably sensitive, become cumbersome for a wide range of amino acids. For some amino acids, it appears that if care is not taken to prevent non-enzymatic degradation then faulty answers may be obtained. This is particularly important for glutamine and cysteine, the concentrations of which fall, and glutamate and cystine, the concentrations of which rise, unless plasma, blood and tissue extracts are not kept frozen.

Methods using radioactive and stable-isotope tracers

Isotope dilution and dynamic isotope dilution enabling quantitation of small amounts of substances or the quantitation of their turnover have become increasingly popular over the past 10–15 years, especially since the development of user-friendly mass spectrometers in various configurations. The first use of isotope tracers for metabolic studies was by Schoenheimer and colleagues[2] using stable isotopes, analysed by cumbersome techniques. It was probably the difficulty of their analysis that hindered the more widespread use of the stable-isotope tracers, but there are other advantages.

Radioactive tracers of amino acids have been used successfully in tracing plasma amino acid turnover, but the accuracy and precision with which metabolism can be traced using radioactive amino acids is usually less than with stable-isotope amino acids. This is because measuring the extent of labelling with radioactive amino acids involves two separate processes (i.e. measurement of the rate of disintegration of the radioactive isotope and the chemical concentrations of tracer plus tracee). With stable-isotope measurement methods, the quantity analogous to the specific radioactivity is the isotope ratio and this can be obtained in a single measurement by a mass spectrometer. Liquid scintillation counters are relatively inefficient ways of measuring radioactivity (e.g. with tritium the counting efficiency is rarely above 30%) and this means that relatively high doses of amino acids would need to be used for measurement of incorporation of label into protein[9,25] unless more sophisticated methods of measurement of radioactivity become widely available. Even then, it should be recognised that in many European countries, use of radioactive tracers in normal, healthy subjects is severely limited by law. In those countries where the restrictions are less severe, ethics committees and regulatory authorities rightly demand a very good case to be made for the use of radioactive tracers[26] in adults of reproductive age; at present it is effectively impossible to study children using radioactive amino acids, but the use of stable-isotope tracers in paediatric metabolism has become almost routine.[27,28]

Tracer methods for the study of amino acid and protein metabolism have been recently reviewed.[10,11] Methods exist not only for the measurement of

turnover of amino acids in the free pool but also for their transfer between organs and incorporation of amino acids into proteins of various types. The various techniques for introducing tracers and the means of analysing them will be reviewed later.

Snapshots of protein and amino acid metabolism

The concentration of amino acids in the intracellular pool can give information that may help to interpret the overall metabolic economy under some circumstances. Realising this, many workers have measured concentrations of intracellular (chiefly intramuscular) amino acids (Tables 2.1, 2.2, Fig. 2.2). Certainly changes in, for example, glutamine, aromatic and the branched-chain amino acids can provide a valuable insight into the state of amino acid and protein metabolism.[29,30] Nevertheless it is difficult to obtain dynamic information in this way unless biopsies are taken at frequent intervals, which imposes a major limitation.

Table 2.2 – Intracellular amino acids postoperatively and in injury and disease. (From Smith & Rennie. In: Harris JB, Turnbull DM (Eds) *Muscle metabolism, Baillière's Clinical Endocrinology & Metabolism*. Baillière Tindall, London, 1990; pp 461–499)

| | Normal | Postoperative | Accidental injury | Sepsis | Uraemia | Hepatic failure | Acute pancreatitis |
			Units = μmol/L				
Ile	110	300	267	460	94	220	150
Leu	225	487	429	754	253	330	260
Val	320	682	578	940	204	500	290
Met	60	148	134	221	65	1000	60
Phe	85	201	213	387	88	460	120
Thr	770	1210	1000	1270	702	1990	670
Lys	1110	920	860	735	943	2870	950
Tyr	122	203	192	332	137	740	190
His	420	247	338	387	395	940	290
Arg	680	530	490	426	662	580	400
Ala	2860	2340	3630	4390	3480	6230	3370
Asp	1650	1640	1690	2370	2280	2090	1060
Asn	420	–	–	–	656	2170	–
Glu	3960	4530	2760	2370	4180	1470	2980
Gln	19970	9500	9140	9530	17590	30380	9760
Gly	1660	1940	1690	1910	2170	4780	1970
Orn	350	170	228	530	557	620	170
Pro	945	680	669	706	930	–	–
Ser	900	1000	1300	2520	1240	2010	930
Tau	17680	22300	19700	20100	16820	28530	25100

Reproduced with permission from reference 229.

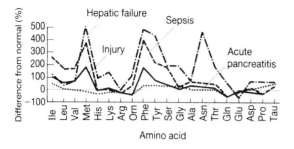

Figure 2.2 – Amino acid intramuscular concentration profiles from patients in various clinical conditions. Reproduced from Smith & Rennie. In: Harris JB, Turnbull DM (Eds) *Muscle metabolism, Baillière's Clinical Endocrinology & Metabolism.* Baillière Tindall, London, 1990; pp 461–499.

The same kind of criticism applies to other static, indirect measures of protein metabolism such as the total RNA concentration (which, being mainly due to ribosomal RNA, provides a measure of the capacity for protein synthesis), and the fraction of ribosomes that are in the polyribosome form[31,32] (i.e. engaged actively in protein synthesis), the total amount of mRNA for a particular protein, the amounts of the proteins themselves, or the capacities (V_{max}) of enzymes of protein and amino acid catabolism.[33] Nevertheless, all of these can contribute useful parts to the overall picture. It is likely that once we have identified which enzymes are important in the catabolism of protein under physiological and patho-physiological circumstances (and recent studies have made important progress in this regard[33–37]) then measurements of the amounts of the proteolytic enzymes (e.g. by western blots), their catalytic activities, and the amounts of mRNA encoding them will provide substantial insight into the control of catabolism. At the moment this remains an attractive possibility but, given the history of disappointment associated with matching the activities and amounts of lysosomal enzymes to changes in protein mass and rates of protein breakdown,[38] we should be cautious before expecting too much.

Measurement of protein turnover in human beings

The classic text by Waterlow, Garlick & Millward[3] contains a detailed account of the underlying theory. The topic has been reviewed recently by Bier[39] and Halliday,[40] who discuss the difficulties identified as a result of modern work. An investigator who is new to the field and wishes to choose a method appropriate to a particular problem must take into account a number of factors. Firstly, are the subjects to be studied in hospital or some other well-regulated environment, or are they free living? Are there any ethical considerations such as taking repeated amounts of blood from small children? Is the problem to be addressed one involving large differences between two sets of circumstances so that the variability of measurement will hardly affect the ability to detect a difference? Conversely, are the likely differences sufficiently small that great precision would be required? All of these questions should be addressed by investigators before they embark on their studies because the kind of data sought should influence the choice of method and the study design and vice versa.

There are in fact only a limited number of theoretical and practical approaches.[10,11] Compartmental analysis involves application of the tracer either as a bolus or by a constant infusion with frequent samples being required from the beginning of the tracer application until such time as a steady state is reached; such rapid sampling may in some circumstances be a limitation. Compartmental analysis will enable notional compartments (which may or may not have a physical or physiological reality) to be identified, their sizes measured, and the rates of interchange between different compartments quantified. The major limitation to compartmental analysis is, of course, that it is difficult to define a compartment into which it is impossible to introduce tracer directly or to sample its dilution except via some other compartment. The stochastic approach avoids such difficulties – by ignoring them. This approach assumes that there exists a single homogeneous well-mixed pool of amino acids into which it is possible to introduce tracer in such a way as to achieve steady labelling after a convenient time. The aim is to achieve a steady state that can be defined by as few as three samples from the free pool, taken over a period of 1–2 hours. The major disadvantage of this method is that there is no clear way of knowing, for a given study, if the assumptions have been violated and to what extent. The major advantage is that so long as a primed, constant infusion is used and the target pool is in good communication with the infused pool, then a steady state of the tracer/tracee can be achieved within a short period of time and few samples need to be obtained. A good example of the problems is the difficulty in tracing whole body glutamine metabolism because of the size of the muscle glutamine pool.[41]

Having decided upon a compartmental approach or a stochastic approach, the next major question is whether, in order to obtain an index of the turnover of the free pool, to measure the labelling of a precursor (e.g. an amino acid in the plasma) or an end-product (such as CO_2 or ammonia or urea); under certain circumstances both are required, which is more often the case with compartmental approaches (Fig. 2.3). If the plasma pool is taken as representative of the whole free amino acid pool then access to plasma needs to be easily available; this may occasionally be difficult, for example in premature infants. If an end-product such as expired CO_2 or urinary urea or ammonia is chosen then sampling, and usually analysis, becomes less difficult, but interpretation may be harder.

A variety of tracer amino acids and whole proteins have been used.[3,42–45] The constant infusion stochastic method based upon the measurement of [^{13}C]leucine in plasma and of $^{13}CO_2$ in breath is the most popular for use in normal subjects and hospital patients as the method is neither too tedious nor cumbersome to apply under a wide variety of circumstances.[44] The phenylalanine–tyrosine method[43] (which theoretically has advantages over the leucine method because oxidation does not require to be measured by collection of expired labelled CO_2) has nevertheless turned out to be somewhat unreliable under some circumstances.[46] The unreliability stems partly from the use of [D_5]phenylalanine which shows a pronounced tracer effect due to the hydrophobicity of the aromatic ring substituted with deuterons and partly also from nutritional variation in precursor–product relationships in the liver,[47] which is the major site of aromatic amino acid catabolism.

The [^{15}N]glycine ammonia end-product method has substantial practical advantages in as much as in its original form tracer was taken as a single oral dose and measurements could be made on a pooled urine sample collected over 9 hours;[48] the method has been modified (and complicated) to include a primed constant infusion of glycine[49] with measurement of isotope ratio of both urea and ammonia as end-products.[42] Unfortunately, the rates of turnover obtained with the ammonia end product method using [^{15}N]glycine as tracer are often different from those obtained with the leucine-primed constant infusion method,[50] although changes are usually (but not necessarily) in the same directions!

Dynamic methods for the measurement of regional amino acid metabolism and protein turnover

Methods based upon arteriovenous (A-V) differences

The development of the amino acid analyser made it possible for workers in the late 1960s and early 1970s to apply the methods developed by Andres, Zierler and colleagues for the study of forearm fat and carbohydrate metabolism[51] to the study of amino acid and protein metabolism. A large amount of work on the exchange of amino acids between limbs and the splanchnic bed and the blood (and later dealing with the brain, heart, lung, etc.) has provided us with much information about the net fluxes of amino acids across these tissues and organs.[52–57]

The method crucially depends upon the accurate measurement of blood flow if reliable absolute values of delivery, net exchange and production are to be obtained.[51,58] Even when blood flow measurement is possible (e.g. by plethysmography, xenon clearance or dye dilution), the errors in these measures are much greater than the analytical measures and may vitiate the calculation of accurate A-V differences of amino acids.

The A-V method provides information about delivery and net exchange but says nothing about unidirectional uptake or efflux, nor is it possible to obtain much direct information about metabolic events inside the tissue, unless products of labelled amino acids are measured. Nevertheless, it has helped to unravel the net changes that occur in a variety of circumstances including feeding and fasting, exercise, starvation and in a variety of clinical conditions, such as diabetes, uraemia, etc.[52,59–61] (Table 2.3). The use of tissue dialysis[62] to extend the range of information obtainable about amino acid metabolism is a promising technique, but one which has not yet been exploited for these purposes.

Use of indicator amino acids to obtain semi-quantitative information about protein turnover

Some amino acids, such as 3-methylhistidine or hydroxyproline, are produced as a result of post-translational modification of the proteins, i.e. histidine and proline are modified by chemical reaction after

Table 2.3 – Plasma amino acid fluxes across muscle: effects of feeding, starvation, infusion of nutrients, and exercise. (From Smith & Rennie. In: Harris JB, Turnbull DM (Eds) *Muscle metabolism, Baillière's Clinical Endocrinology & Metabolism.* Baillière Tindall, London, 1990; pp 461–499)

	Post-absorptive	Fed	Starvation (day 10)	Refeeding (AA/dextrose/lipid) nmol/min/100 g	Lipid only	+AA	+AA/insulin
Ile	−16	84	−12	68	6	21	102
Leu	−20	130	−25	98	14	25	143
Val	−18	94	7	84	19	28	146
Met	−9	–	−13	14	−1	–	–
Phe	−15	11	−14	6	−2	−1	33
Thr	−33	–	−22	3	−20	–	–
Lys	−35	74	−31	22	−10	–	–
Tyr	−13	−4	−13	6	3	−7	12
His	−21	11	−12	12	9	–	–
Arg	−20	42	−14	27	−7	–	–
Ala	−195	−14	−119	−131	−57	−45	−22
Asp	−1	−35	1	5	4	–	–
Asn	−25	–	−17	−4	−5	–	–
Glu	79	102	42	212	94	101	146
Gln	−203	172	−153	−245	−46	−221	−343
Gly	−52	−11	−75	−2	12	–	–
Orn	0	14	3	28	3	–	–
Pro	−104	–	−5	111	−26	–	–
Ser	9	–	−6	56	22	–	–
Tau	−17	−7	4	−12	–	–	–
Balance	**−709**	**330**	**−474**	**267**	**12**	**−99**	**217**

Reproduced with permission from reference 229.

the primary structure of a protein, such as actin or collagen, has been produced. Since these amino acids are not re-utilised for protein synthesis, breakdown of the protein containing them results in their release, the rate of which should be a quantitative index of the catabolism of particular proteins.[63] The measurement of 3-methylhistidine in urine is probably not as useful as was at first envisioned because of the interference with non-skeletal muscle sources of the amino acid.[64] The original concept has been successfully applied, however, to measure myofibrillar protein breakdown by monitoring limb A-V differences of the amino acid in patients with malnutrition, postoperative surgical patients and patients suffering from infection.[65–67] If longitudinal studies are carried out, enabling changes in 3-methylhistidine production to be monitored, or comparisons are made with normal subjects then it is possible to make a reasonably accurate interpretation of the likely differences in myofibrillar protein break-down between the two circumstances. The method, when originally applied,[65] was expected to provide a semi-quantitative index of changes in protein synthesis by comparing the changes in 3-methylhistidine efflux with changes in the net efflux of amino acids such as lysine, tyrosine or phenylalanine which are not metabolised in muscle, except to take part in protein turnover. However, it is now realised that myofibrillar and sarcoplasmic protein are regulated separately[33] so semi-quantitative estimates of mixed muscle protein synthesis are probably less reliable than we originally thought. This does not reduce the usefulness of the method for measurements of myofibrillar protein breakdown, and the use of labelled 3-methylhistidine for measurement of breakdown by isotope dilution[68] (see below) should make the method much more reliable.

Exchange of tracer amino acids as an index of protein turnover

A logical extension to the technique of net exchange of amino acids is to use tracers of non-metabolised amino acids in order to obtain information about protein turnover using the tracer dilution technique. This has been successfully applied to muscle and heart using phenylalanine and tyrosine[57,69] and could theoretically be applied to any tissue in which there was known to be no intermediary metabolism of the amino acid, e.g. lysine in muscle or leucine in the brain. The use of 3-methylhistidine in this way could bring a major increase in our understanding. Where the amino acid is metabolised by tissues (as are the branched-chain amino acids in muscle, or phenyl-alanine in liver) then great care has to be exercised in measuring not only the amounts of the amino acid and of its tracer but also the concentrations of the metabolites of the amino acid, i.e. in the case of leucine, CO_2 and α-ketoisocaproate (α-KIC).[70] This is obviously more difficult; calculations of amino acid metabolism based upon multiple measurements of metabolites are practically difficult and theoretically limited because of the dangers of the concatenation of errors. Nevertheless, it is possible to compare the dilution of suitable tracer amino acids with the net balance and CO_2 production to obtain values for protein synthesis, leucine oxidation, leucine trans-amination, etc., under different nutritional and hormonal conditions.[71–73] In theory the same techniques could be applied to liver, kidney, gut, etc., given the availability of an appropriate (i.e. non-metabolised) tracer amino acid and suitable methods of measurement of blood flow, and access to vessels draining the tissue bed.

Methods based upon incorporation of tracer amino acids into protein

The fractional rate of protein synthesis must be measured in terms of incorporation into protein compared to the labelling of an identifiable precursor pool, ideally the aminoacyl-tRNA for the tracer amino acid concerned. Ethical considerations limit the dose of radioactivity that can be safely applied, and it is almost impossible to use radioactive tracers to make measurements of tissue protein synthesis in people. The first measurement of tissue protein synthesis in human beings was carried out using di[15N]lysine by Halliday & McKeran who measured myofibrillar and sarcoplasmic protein turnover using a primed constant infusion protocol.[74] The methodology was later adapted to the use of [13C,15N]leucine as a tracer and this enabled whole body protein turnover to be measured simultaneously.[75] The same or similar techniques have now been applied to a wide range of measurements of protein turnover including heart, skin, gastrointestinal tract, liver, bone – indeed any tissue that can conveniently be sampled (Fig. 2.3).

The method of calculation of the fractional synthetic rate simply requires that the rate of incorporation of the tracer be linear with time; this should be checked, although sometimes it is difficult. If indeed it is linear, then, if stable-isotope tracers are used, only a single sample of the tissue protein needs to be taken at the end of the period of primed constant infusion so long as a pre-infusion sample of some other bodily protein (e.g. plasma proteins or haemoglobin) is obtained in order to set a baseline against which the enrichment of the protein of interest is measured; this works because the background value can be assumed to be similar for all proteins. Of course, if tracer has been infused at some previous time then a zero time sample is an absolute requirement.

A method developed by Zhang and colleagues,[76] and validated using arteriovenous tracer exchange methods,

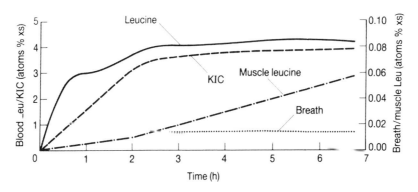

Figure 2.3 – Changes in leucine in plasma, expired CO_2 and muscle protein with time.

allows the measurement of fractional rates of protein breakdown by following the rate of dilution of tracer in the free intercellular pool by tracee amino acids released by protein breakdown after cessation of tracer infusion. If two separate tracers are used, synthesis and breakdown can be measured simultaneously.[77] The protocol involves a biopsy taken at the time of cessation of supply of one tracer plus two more taken to define the fall in the labelling of the pool and the increase in enrichment in protein from the second tracer.

The choice of tracer for incorporation studies is largely immaterial so long as it is sufficiently abundant in protein to be easily measured; it is also immaterial whether it is an essential[74, 75] or a non-essential amino acid[78] so long as the appropriate precursor pool can be identified and the precursor labelling measured. Leucine has been used as a tracer in many studies simply because it is rather abundant in protein (at about 8%) and because, being an essential amino acid, it is useful for whole body studies, especially if ^{13}C is used as then leucine oxidation is easily quantified.[75] However, for studies of proteins containing substantial amounts of other amino acids, such as albumin or collagen which contain large amounts of alanine and glycine, these amino acids should theoretically be just as good. If a ^{15}N label is to be used rather than ^{13}C then it would make sense to use amino acids such as di[^{15}N]lysine[74] or guanidino di[^{15}N]arginine for which distinctive di-labelled ions can be easily monitored. Deuterium labelling offers the possibility of making tracers with multiple hydrogen substitutions, and deuterium-labelled amino acids have found wide use. Until recently, however, with the use of high-sensitivity GC–MS methods (or by pyrolysis, see below) the determination of incorporation of free tracer into protein was impossible with deuterated tracers and still remains problematical, although it has been used by a variety of workers.[10,79] Assessment of labelling of the plasma and various precursor pools is usually carried out using gas chromatography–mass spectrometry (GC–MS) which is an appropriate method for measurement of enrichment of tracer amino acids at about 0.2–10 atoms % excess and for which the sample size is adequate (mmol–Mmol).

Where small amounts of protein are to be analysed a variety of different techniques can be applied. With any tracer amino acid labelled in the 1 carbon position or any α-amino nitrogen (with ^{13}C and ^{15}N respectively), the ninhydrin reaction can be used to recover quantitatively CO_2 or ammonia (and, by use of sodium borohydride, nitrogen) from any chemically pure tracer amino acid isolated by an appropriate method, e.g. by conventional liquid chromatography or preparative gas chromatography.[80] Very much smaller enrichments can be measured for nitrogen than for carbon because of the lower nitrogen background enrichment, but the large amount of nitrogen in the atmosphere can make this problematic if special precautions are not taken.

If continuous flow combustion methods are used,[81–83] carbon-labelled amino acids suffer the disadvantage of dilution from unlabelled carbon in the rest of the molecule (even with pure amino acids) and the burning of whole proteins is probably a non-productive approach with carbon labels. However, with ^{15}N-labelled amino acids this should be less of a problem: use of specific amino acids such as ^{15}N proline should enable quantitation of collagen turnover simply by burning collagen to produce nitric oxides and then reducing these in a continuous flow system.

Continuous flow analysis of materials isolated by chromatography and then combusted or pyrolysed to a suitable gas should be possible using carbon, oxygen, nitrogen and deuterium tracers given suitable configurations of continuous flow isotope ratio mass spectrometers.

The precursor problem

In all methods involving amino acid tracers to measure protein turnover, assumptions have to be made about the relationship between the precursor pool and the pool in which the measurements are made. These are often either uncheckable in practice or involve substantial errors that simply have to be accepted blindly. This is particularly so for the phenylalanine–tyrosine method and for the [^{15}N]glycine–ammonia or urea end-product methods. The situation appears to be much better for the primed constant infusion leucine method since there is reasonable confidence that the labelling of α-ketoisocaproate, the transamination product of leucine, is rather close to the labelling of the free amino acid pool in many tissues. According to measurements of leucyl-tRNA in muscle[84–86] and of protein exported from liver[19,47,87] we know that the assumptions cannot be too much in error (20%) for these tissues and that muscle intracellular α-KIC provides a good index of leucyl-tRNA labelling.[86] However, in skin the prolyl-tRNA labelling seems to be markedly less than the intracellular labelling, possibly because of *de novo* synthesis of proline.[88]

The whole question of precursors and their measurement is vexed, and one which is unlikely to be solved simply by improving sampling protocols or widening the range of analytes. However, the use of a novel theoretical approach to the analysis of tracer appearance in polymeric molecules (such as proteins) may in future render the need to measure precursor labelling redundant. This approach, so-called 'mass isotopomer analysis', has been successfully applied to cholesterol[89] and chances of its application for protein turnover look good.[90]

There can be no argument that the ideal precursor pool in which to measure labelling by the tracer is the aminoacyl-tRNA pool but this is difficult to sample for some tissues (e.g. for collagen-synthesising cells within bone it would be almost impossible to obtain enough aminoacyl-tRNA). Even for muscle, which is relatively accessible, substantial amounts of tissue (1–5 g) are required to make the measurement of aminoacyl-tRNA labelling.[84] When it has been done, the labelling appears to be close to that of α-KIC or that of the free intracellular pool.[84] The important thing about this information is that it *proves* that any errors in the measurement of the absolute rate of protein synthesis cannot be greater than about 20%. This is important because, as we shall see, attempts to overcome the uncertainty in the measurement of the true precursor by the use of the flooding dose produce

values[91-93] for the absolute rate of protein synthesis in various tissues that vary substantially from those obtained with the primed constant infusion protocol[94,95] and are much higher than expected given the narrow range (±10% of the plasma KIC) of possible precursor labelling (Fig. 2.4).

Theoretically, by using a large dose of labelled amino acids sufficient to bring all of the free amino acid pools to a common value of labelling, measurement of the tracer/tracee relationship in any of the free pools over time should adequately define the labelling of the precursor.[3,96] This has been done for muscle using large doses of labelled leucine and phenylalanine; the results obtained are roughly twice those obtained with the primed constant infusion method. Attempts to reconcile the difference between the two sets of values (by simultaneously making measurements of incorporation into protein of continuously infused tracer before and after giving a flooding dose of amino acids) have raised serious worries about the extent to which the flooding dose introduced artefacts in the rate of measurement of tissue protein synthesis.[94,97] It appears that, for muscle, flooding with leucine or valine causes increases in the rate of incorporation of tracer valine or phenylalanine, and the extent of the increase is sufficient to explain respectively the difference between the values obtained during the primed constant infusion method alone and the flooding dose

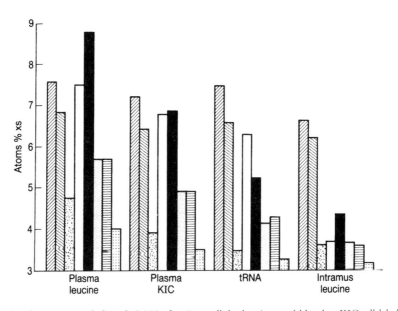

Figure 2.4 – Relationship between muscle leucyl-tRNA, free intracellular leucine, and blood α-KIC, all labelled with ^{13}C during constant infusion.

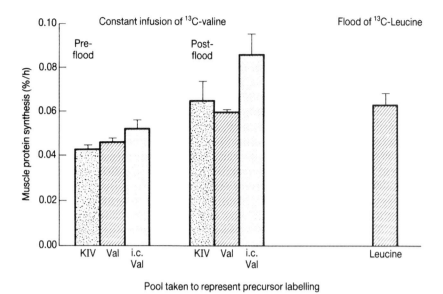

Figure 2.5 – Constant infusion of tracer valine with a flooding dose of [¹³C]leucine and the rates of muscle protein synthesis calculated from the two protocols.

method alone. This is particularly worrying because it means that the flooding dose method may artefactually cause an elevation in the rate of muscle protein synthesis measured and it may be difficult, therefore, to observe physiological elevations of protein synthesis. There are, of course, different interpretations of the results: those who use the flooding dose method have suggested that the reason the flooding dose method gives an apparent increase in the incorporation of tracer is perturbation of the tracer aminoacyl-tRNA pool. Unfortunately, no direct evidence for this belief has been obtained to date. Indeed it seems difficult to believe that the perturbation would be sufficient to account for the change since measurements of intra-muscular tracer labelling[97] do not change sufficiently or in the right direction to cause observed changes in muscle protein. Furthermore, apparent increases in the rate of incorporation of tracer as a result of the application of a flooding dose can be found for albumin[98] and for non-albumin protein (unpublished results of K Smith) in blood.

It may be, however, that the artefacts caused by the application of the flooding dose are only seen when essential amino acids are used, in muscle at least.[97] In studies in bone, the flooding dose protocol has been used with proline to obtain sensible results.[99]

The resolution of this problem must await further work but it is certainly the view of those who use the constant infusion method that (for reasons that are presently not clear) the flooding dose protocol is severely flawed, except for studies in which it is likely that there will be changes in the rate of synthesis during the time course of an infusion (e.g. in starvation[92]) or when the free pools are already equilibrated, as in TPN administration. Otherwise the values obtained are in our view unreliable.

Composition of the free and protein-bound pools of amino acid

Most (over 90%) of the amino acids in the body are present chemically combined into protein. Proteins that have major mechanical and structural roles such as actin and myosin (which comprise two-thirds of skeletal and heart muscle) and various types of collagen and keratin are present in large amounts. Muscle in adults constitutes such a large proportion (40%) of body weight that actin and myosin together make up about a quarter of all body protein, and 20% of total body protein is likely to be collagen. The protein composition of tissues naturally varies and so does the protein concentration as a percentage of total wet weight. Unfortunately there is a paucity of data concerning human body composition and the exact contribution of individual proteins to human whole body protein composition. This is one reason why it is difficult to use the factorial approach to work out protein turnover in the whole body by summing individual rates obtained in particular tissues.

The free amino acid pool and membrane transport of amino acids

The free amino acid pool contributes only a few per cent to the total of amino acids in the body.[100] The composition of the free amino acid pool in the plasma and within the intracellular compartment is the result of a variety of processes, depending upon the amino acids concerned, of *de novo* synthesis, catabolism, transamination, protein synthesis, protein breakdown and amino acid transport; no quantitative description yet exists of how these operate together to produce amino acid pools of the composition observed.

The intracellular amino acid pool is probably of the same size as the intracellular water compartment except for amino acids like taurine, for which there is evidence of complexing, possibly by binding to protein: this is the most likely explanation for the very

high concentration of taurine in the intracellular compartment in heart and skeletal muscle and in brain. Other amino acids have a distribution ratio (the concentration inside divided by that outside) across the plasma membrane which can, to some extent, be explained by whether or not they are substrates for concentrative Na-dependent transport systems (Table 2.4), which tend to accumulate amino acids intracellularly as a result of energising the transport process by the Na^+-electrochemical gradient.[101]

In the past few years many amino acid transporting proteins have been identified and isolated by molecular biological techniques.[102] The ability to discover in tissues which transporters are being expressed by Northern and western blotting and their quantification of them will make the understanding of amino acid metabolism much simpler.

A good example of an amino acid that has a high intracellular concentration is glutamine. In muscle at least, glutamine appears to be concentrated almost entirely by the Na^+-dependent system N^m, for which it is the best substrate.[101] However, histidine and asparagine which are also substrates for system N^m have much smaller distribution ratios across the membrane. This

Table 2.4 – Characteristics of amino acid transport systems present in mammalian tissues

Substrate	V_{max} (nmol/min/g muscle)	K_m (mM)	Na^+- dependence	E_m dependence	Major system	Comments
Gln	1200±200	9±1	Yes	Yes	N^m	Insulin-sensitive and pH-sensitive
Asn	1000±300	8±2	Yes	Yes	N^m	
His	230±20	1.3±0,4	Yes	Yes	N^m	Li tolerant
Ala	330±50	4±1.0	Hardly	Yes	ASC (also A and L)	Insulin- and pH-insensitive; very little A
Ser	400±60	3.4±0.5	Yes	Yes	ASC	Li-intolerant
Leu	2800±400	20±2	No	No	L	Insulin- and pH-sensitive
Val	2600±50	20±1	No	No	L	Insulin- and pH-insensitive
Ile	2600±50	18±2	No	No	L	Insulin- and pH-insensitive
Phe	3000±460	19±2	No	No	L	Insulin- and pH-insensitive
Lys	140±50	2.1±1.3	Yes	Yes	Y^+(?)	Insulin- and pH-insensitive
Pro	190±50	4.1±0.6	Yes	Yes	Pro, A	(Not done)
Glu	86±6	1.05±0.05	No		X^-_{AG}	Insulin-insensitive and pH-sensitive
Tau	0.9±0.35	7.0±2.8	Yes		β	Insulin-sensitive
3-MeHis	Most likely saturable				N^m (and/or L)	pH insensitive

The K_m values are likely to be operationally similar in human muscle. They are derived from perfusion studies and refer to transfer from blood to muscle.

can be explained partly by the fact that these amino acids are substrates for other systems, possibly including system L and system y$^+$ respectively, which are Na$^+$-independent and by whose action the concentrative effect of system N^m is lost. Where there exists the possibility of Na$^+$-independent outward flow of amino acid concentrated by a Na$^+$-dependent (secondary-active) system, there is the possibility for so-called 'tertiary amino acid transport'; the outward flow of the amino acid drives the inward flow on the same transporter of some amino acid.[101] This is probably the explanation for the fact that branched-chain amino acids and phenylalanine and tyrosine (which might be expected not to show any concentration gradient since they are mainly transported by the Na$^+$-independent systems L and T) do, in fact, exhibit a distribution ratio of greater than unity, i.e. about 1.2.

The regulation of the size of the free amino acid pool must occur as a result of the relative rates of removal of amino acids (chiefly by protein synthesis and also by catabolism of the amino acids in gluconeogenesis and ureagenesis) and addition of amino acids via protein breakdown and dietary input. In addition, for specific amino acids linked to intermediary metabolism (such as glutamate, alanine and glutamine) (Fig. 2.6) the size of the pool may be influenced by such processes as glycogenolysis and the activity of the Krebs cycle.[52,103]

It is becoming increasingly well recognised that amino acid transport may thus have an important regulatory role in altering the availability of amino acids in the free pool and thus influencing not only their own intracellular metabolism but also the metabolism of other substances and macromolecules. The case is particularly strong for the catabolism of the aromatic amino acids in liver[104] and the control of ureagenesis in liver via the availability of amino acids,[105,106] including the amplifying effect of glutamine and ammonia derived from glutaminolysis.[107] There is good evidence that anabolic effects of amino acids in glycogen and fat metabolism in liver[108] are probably mediated by osmotic mechanisms[109] and there is also some evidence that the pool size of glutamine in muscle somehow helps to promote anabolism by inhibiting protein breakdown and stimulating protein synthesis.[110,111]

The complexity of amino acid metabolism and the fact that there are 20 amino acids sharing at least six amino acid transport systems makes it difficult to partition the contributions to overall control of the free pool size between transport, intermediary metabolism and protein turnover. Nevertheless a major influence must

be the instantaneous protein balance in the whole body, since by far the biggest changes in the free amino acid pool occur as a result of factors that stimulate protein synthesis or inhibit protein breakdown. The changes occurring with starvation are a good example:[3,38] inhibition of protein synthesis and acceleration of protein breakdown markedly expand the free amino acid pool, and those amino acids showing the largest increase are normally the amino acids with the smallest contribution to the free pool and thus the biggest protein-bound:free ratio, which are the branched-chain amino acids, the aromatic amino acids and methionine. Other factors altering protein balance have predictable effects: for example feeding, which promotes anabolism, shrinks the pool, whereas diabetes, which is catabolic, expands it.

The turnover of amino acids within the free amino acid pool (or at least in the plasma pool) very much reflects the relative contribution of each amino acid to total protein, and there is a very good relationship between the plasma turnover of most individual amino acids and their composition in protein.[39] The exceptions to this are: (a) amino acids whose turnover in the plasma is much greater than expected from their composition in protein because of inter-organ trafficking (e.g. alanine and glutamine which fulfil a role as carriers of carbon and nitrogen between the musculature and the viscera); and (b) those amino acids that have a plasma turnover somewhat less than expected because much of their metabolism occurs in the intracellular pool only (e.g. glutamate).

Transport of amino acids through the blood

It is worth noting that for some amino acids, such as glutamate, the erythrocyte intracellular concentration is very much higher than that of the plasma. There is some evidence that the red blood cell participates in the cell-to-cell transfer of amino acids as blood passes through tissues,[52] particularly the kidney and the liver,[112] and this possibility should be considered for other amino acids with a high distribution ratio across the erythrocyte membrane.

Intermediary amino acid metabolism and its relationship to protein turnover

The metabolism of the 20 physiologically important amino acids is complex, and the metabolism of each is different. Therefore only a few general points that have a direct relevance to our understanding of

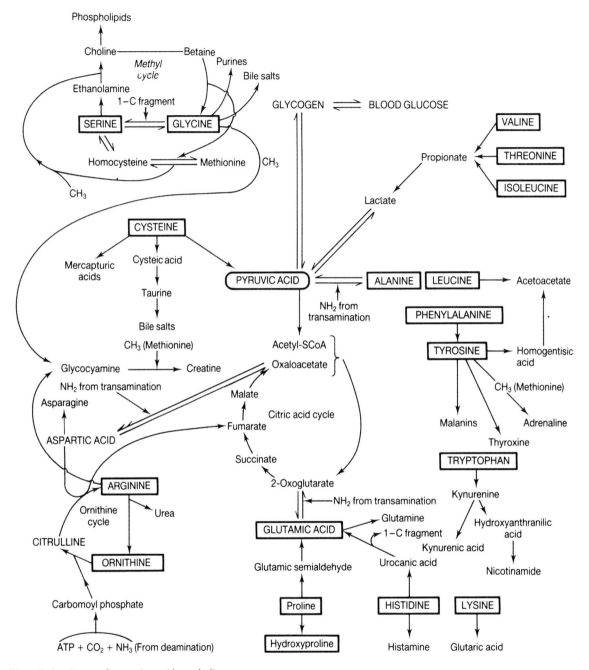

Figure 2.6a – Intermediary amino acid metabolism.

protein balance in the whole body will be emphasised. The first point concerns a division between essential and non-essential amino acids or, as they are termed in modern parlance, dispensable and non-dispensable amino acids. The classification of amino acids as essential or otherwise derives from work carried out to determine whether rats could grow on diets deficient in individual amino acids. Surprisingly little work has actually been carried out in people, and nowadays the whole concept of essentiality has become much less

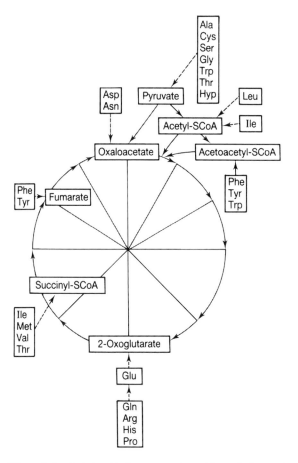

Figure 2.6b – Relationship between amino acid metabolism and the activity of the Krebs cycle.

capacity to do so. Good examples of these are glutamine, under conditions of disease and injury,[113–115] and glycine in children recovering from malnutrition.[116]

Readers are referred to textbooks of biochemistry for detailed discussion of the pathways of intermediary acid metabolism. For our purposes it is sufficient to say that most amino acids take part in reactions in which the α-amino group is lost from the carbon chain – either by oxidative deamination to form the oxo-acid or by transfer of the amino group to an oxo-acid (often 2-oxoglutarate, also called α-ketoglutarate) – to form glutamate which can then be subject to oxidative deamination. The result of this is that amino acids are converted to their oxo-acids plus ammonium ions, which are disposed of in the urea cycle. The net results of the actions of the aminotransferase enzymes and glutamate dehydrogenase tend to buffer (though not completely) the free pool concentration of many of the non-essential amino acids throughout the diurnal cycle, especially for those amino acids that have 2-oxoglutarate as a common intermediate (i.e. arginine, histidine, proline, glutamine and glutamate itself). A number of other amino acids share common intermediates, e.g.: pyruvate for alanine, glycine, serine, cysteine and tryptophan; fumarate for phenylalanine and tyrosine; succinate for valine, isoleucine and methionine, threonine; oxaloacetate for asparagine and aspartate; and acetylcoenzyme A for leucine, phenylalanine, tyrosine, lysine, tryptophan and isoleucine.

These common intermediates can be oxidised as fuel, either directly after giving rise to acetylcoenzyme A or indirectly after being converted to pyruvate; this process is important in partial or full starvation. Alternatively, when fuel supply is not limiting, they may be converted to fat (all amino acids) or to glucose (part of the carbon chain of all amino acids except leucine and lysine). All of the non-essential amino acids may be produced after transamination of their oxo-acids derived from synthesis of carbohydrate precursors such as glucose, glycogen, pyruvate, lactate, etc.

Muscle protein synthesis

Over 20 years ago McKeran and Halliday measured myofibrillar and sarcoplasmic protein turnover. Most work since then has focused on the rate of synthesis of mixed muscle protein. Rates for individual proteins may be valuable in establishing different regulatory patterns. As expected from work in animals,[117] the rate of mitochondrial protein synthesis is 95% higher than

rigid. Originally, the strict biochemical criterion was that essential amino acids were those that could not be synthesised sufficiently quickly within the body to supply adequately protein and possibly nucleic acid synthesis. Since most of the amino acids can be transaminated, what this usually comes down to is the ability or inability to synthesise a carbon chain of the amino acids. Strictly speaking, the essential amino acids are isoleucine, leucine, lysine, methionine, phenylalanine, threonine, tryptophan and valine, but it is quite likely that we should add histidine to this list, certainly in infants. In addition, if phenylalanine and methionine are present in only small amounts, then tyrosine and cysteine become essential. The concept of the 'conditional essentiality' of certain amino acids has been developed to take account of the fact that, despite the ability of the body to synthesise them, they are often required in amounts greater than the body's the rate of mixed muscle protein synthesis, whereas the synthetic rate of myosin heavy chain is 20% lower and that of actin is 61% higher respectively than the rate of mixed muscle protein.[118] No work, to date, has been reported for human subjects although this is currently the subject of investigation.

To date, there have been no applications of this technique to identify a differential response with the exception of the effects in ageing.[117]

Recommended protein and amino acid intakes

The criteria of sufficiency are not clear, because of difficulties associated with both N-balance and kinetic approaches to assessment of adequacy. Thus, recommendations as to dietary intake under different circumstances tend to err on the side of caution.[119] The subject is currently controversial.[116,120,121] There is no doubt that growing children, pregnant women and patients who are suffering from infection and cancer are likely to benefit from increased protein intakes on a per kilogram basis but it is currently impossible to give more than the broadest outlines about how much this should be. The requirements for lean tissue maintenance are likely to fall between 120 mg of protein-N/kg/day at 1 year and 96 mg of N/kg/day in adults; a 50% increment for growth, and supplements of about 6 g of protein/day for pregnancy and 11 g/day for lactation are also recommended.[119]

Tissue-specific amino acid metabolism

One of the odd features of amino acid metabolism is its tissue-specific nature. For example, although the liver has the largest mass of amino acid catabolising enzymes and contains the enzymes of the urea cycle, other tissues such as the intestine, muscle, adipose tissue and kidney also participate substantially, but specifically, in the intermediary amino acid metabolism of the whole body and therefore in the overall nitrogen economy. After a protein meal, for example, the mucosal tissue of the small intestine specifically removes the dicarboxylic acids, glutamate and aspartate, transaminating pyruvate to produce alanine. The carbon backbones of glutamate and aspartate are converted via the respective oxo-acids to pyruvate also. The rapidly dividing cells of the intestine have a requirement for glutamine as a fuel:[122,123] of the total amino acid removed from the

arterial blood by the intestine, about 50% is glutamine. This is converted to precursors of nucleic acid synthesis, or used as a fuel.

Thus the blood leaving the intestine *en route* for the liver contains more alanine and less of the dicarboxylates than might be expected. In the liver, arginine, histidine, lysine, methionine, phenylalanine, threonine and tryptophan are all catabolised reasonably effectively, but isoleucine, leucine and valine are mainly catabolised in skeletal muscle and heart. Liver and muscle both have the capacity to metabolise aspartate, glutamate, glutamine, glycine, proline and alanine. The effect of the amino acid catabolising capacity of the intestine and the liver together is to alter markedly the amount and pattern of amino acids leaving the hepatic vein compared to the hepatic artery. In a well-nourished person, accustomed to eating a diet adequate in protein, it is likely that of all the amino acids absorbed from a meal, at least half are immediately catabolised to urea, one-sixth are trapped as hepatic fixed protein or export proteins (such as albumin), and only the remainder are available to the systemic circulation.

Muscle has a particularly high capacity to synthesise alanine and glutamine from their precursors (via transamination of pyruvate and glutamine synthetase) and thus about 60–70% of the total amino acid flux leaving muscle is composed of alanine and glutamine, even though they themselves comprise only 10% of muscle protein.[52] Peripheral adipose tissue may function in a rather similar manner to muscle, being able to generate alanine and glutamine from appropriate precursors.[124]

The major role of the kidney in amino acid metabolism is the generation of ammonia from glutamine, which arises chiefly in muscle, liver and adipose tissue. The appropriate reactions are accelerated during acidosis when the diversion of amino acid-derived carbon to bicarbonate and the excretion of the amino groups as ammonia has a net benefit in counteracting acidosis.[56,125–127] The carbon chains of glucogenic amino acids, especially glutamine, can be utilised for glucogenesis in the kidney.

The rapidly dividing cells of the intestine are not the only rapidly dividing cells that require a substantial amount of glutamine; it now appears that the cells of the immune system, especially lymphocytes, also have a high requirement for glutamine as a fuel and purine and pyrimidine precursor.[128]

The patterns of amino acid metabolising enzymes in different tissues are difficult to comprehend and their biological utility puzzling. The biological advantages of the system are that when amino acids are supplied in excess of requirements they can be rapidly catabolised and the carbon chain turned into glucose or fat for fuel use or storage with the conversion of potentially toxic ammonia to urea. When the protein intake falls below maintenance requirements then amino acids released from net protein breakdown can be utilised as fuel and again the ammonia removed as urea. The enzymes involved in the catabolism of the aromatic amino acids and the branched-chain amino acids appear to be particularly active and have Km values sufficiently high that catabolism is inevitable as soon as the concentration of the amino acids in the free pool rises.[129] This is probably a protective mechanism since high concentrations of these amino acids are likely to be toxic, as can be seen in various clinical conditions (e.g. phenylketonuria) in which their catabolism is deficient.[130]

The pattern of blood amino acids

The metabolism of protein and amino acids is finely balanced and any excess or deficiency of amino acids in the diet results in the disruption of the normal pattern of amino acids in the blood. This phenomenon is not well understood despite a huge amount of work by Harper and co-workers,[131,132] but this work has provided both theoretical insights and practical tools. The recognition that deficiencies of essential amino acids lead to particular patterns is useful in using the normal pattern as the standard by which to judge the efficacy of particular diets and intravenous amino acid solutions.

Cellular biochemistry of protein synthesis and breakdown

The last 40 years have seen an explosive increase in our understanding of the cellular mechanisms of gene transcription and the expression of proteins and the various processes available for the degradation of protein. It is not the purpose of this review to attempt to reproduce what is available elsewhere; most readers will find it sufficient to read an appropriate textbook and to scan a couple of up-to-date reviews. It is probably not necessary to have a detailed understanding of the mechanisms and control of protein synthesis and breakdown although it is worth keeping in mind that fundamental advances in knowledge are often translated into practical techniques – clinically and certainly for research – in a relatively short time. Good examples of this are the use of 3-methylhistidine[133] as an indicator of myofibrillar protein breakdown[63,134,135] and the use of the polyribosome fraction[136] as an index of muscle protein synthetic rate.[31,32]

Work in cell cultures and animal studies have helped to unravel the signalling pathways that couple the extracellular growth signals (for example, amino acids or insulin) to the stimulation of protein synthesis. Most of the regulation of protein synthesis observed in pathophysiological circumstances occurs at the stage of translation initiation and is mediated by a family of proteins referred to as eukaryotic initiation factors (eIFs). Activation or inhibition of multiple initiation factors effects changes in the rate of protein synthesis. Several key regulatory proteins are of particular importance in regulating skeletal muscle growth: these are p70 S6 kinase and eIF4E. Activation of both of these proteins is involved in the stimulation of growth-related protein synthesis: p70 S6 kinase is a serine/threonine protein kinase which phosphorylates the ribosomal S6 protein, whereas EIF4E activation is modulated by the phosphorylation of its binding protein, eIF4E-BP1. Another key regulatory protein involved in the stimulation of general protein synthesis is eIF2B. Cell culture studies[137] and work in rats[138] have demonstrated activation of p70 S6 kinase and eIF4E-BP1 phosphorylation in response to amino acids. The effect of the amino acids may be independent of insulin.[138,139] eIF2 activation, again studied in rats, did not occur in response to feeding with a protein–carbohydrate mixture[140] but did occur in response to resistance exercise.[141] No work, to date, has been reported for human subjects although this is currently the subject of investigation.

Physiological control of protein turnover in the whole body

Protein turnover as a concept is a relatively modern construct.[2,142] Soon after the general acceptance of the idea of the dynamic state of metabolism, sufficient information became available not only to discern the overall pattern of protein turnover, but to put values to most of its components, at least tentatively.[3]

The use of the nitrogen balance technique[4,6,131] has provided us with many insights into the effects of nutrients and hormones on the amount of protein in the body. The most obvious influences on nitrogen balance are the total amount of dietary energy and the proportion of this that is protein. It appears that the body places a higher priority on the provision of energy to metabolic processes than to the maintenance of the protein mass; any circumstance in which total energy provision is less than requirements therefore results in negative nitrogen balance as protein is cannibalised for fuel. Under these circumstances there is a loss of protein from the lean tissues by a variety of mechanisms (see below) that liberate amino acids for utilisation as fuel directly or indirectly after conversion to glucose or ketone bodies. Consumption of a diet containing less amino acids than the minimum requirements for maintenance (i.e. replacement of obligate losses from the skin and gastrointestinal tract and the minimum oxidative amino acid losses) will result in a negative nitrogen balance that cannot be ameliorated by the provision of sufficient energy. If sufficient energy is available, provision of protein in amounts above the minimum requirements does not result in storage of protein; the excess is either used as a fuel or oxidised according to the state of energy balance and the excess nitrogen excreted as urea and ammonia. Changes in the protein composition of the diet have an effect over and above those to be expected simply on the basis of protein and energy requirements, probably because of induction and repression of amino acid oxidising enzymes, which may take a couple of days to reach a new steady state. Thus, in going from a high-protein to a low-protein diet, urinary nitrogen output falls more slowly than might be expected; in going from a low-protein to a high-protein diet, it rises more slowly. This is probably because it takes at least a few days (and possibly up to 2 weeks) for the oxidative enzymes to adapt to the availability of amino acids. It is unlikely that there is any truly labile body protein store, which was the explanation previously accepted for the lag in the pattern of nitrogen excretion observed after a change in diet. Nevertheless, it is reasonable to regard protein in the musculature as behaving rather like a protein store in as much as about 30% of muscle protein can be lost without irreparable damage.

The fall in nitrogen excretion observed during starvation[143,144] includes some measure of adaptation, probably hormonally mediated and mainly involving a decrease in thyroid hormone production which has the twin effects of decreasing energy requirements and probably also protein turnover.[37] In addition to a fall in the total amount of nitrogen excreted in the urine, its composition also changes, a smaller proportion being as urea, to allow excretion of acid as ammonium.[134,145]

Great caution should be exercised in interpreting the results of short-term nitrogen balances, particularly those carried out on free-living subjects and especially those in which no corrections are made for skin and faecal losses. The literature is full of examples of over-interpretation of nitrogen balance data leading to some very strange claims of extreme positive and negative nitrogen balances in different circumstances.

Responses of whole body protein turnover to nutrient supply

The components of whole body protein turnover, as traced by an essential amino acid such as leucine, are dietary intake and protein breakdown, which add to the free leucine pool, and protein synthesis and leucine oxidation, which remove amino acids from the free pool. The processes adding and removing amino acids from the free pool should, in the steady state, equal one another, and it is an assumption of the constant infusion stochastic method that they indeed do so. What this means is that knowledge of the dietary input and of leucine oxidation allows calculation of the rates of protein synthesis and protein breakdown.

Interpretation of the available information is difficult because of the problem that different amino acids may trace particular processes more than others; there is no perfect tracer for whole body protein turnover in people. The problem has been discussed in detail elsewhere.[146,147]

Nevertheless, there is a growing canon of information derived from apparently reliable techniques utilising the methodology based upon the use of [^{13}C]leucine as a tracer of whole body amino acid metabolism, with plasma ^{13}C α-ketoisocaproate labelling to indicate the leucine labelling at inaccessible intracellular sites. In normal healthy adult subjects these techniques give values of whole body protein turnover of about 120 mmol of leucine/kg/h in the fed state and about 90 mmol/kg/h in the overnight fasted state. These figures correspond to values of about 330 g protein/kg/day. To the extent that the labelling of plasma ^{13}C α-ketoisocaproate overestimates the true labelling of leucine at intracellular sites in which it is at equilibrium with leucine which is a substrate for protein synthesis and leucine oxidation, or produced by protein breakdown, this value will be an underestimate. Unfortunately we have no exact idea of the extent of the underestimation.

Application of this leucine model to studies carried out in the post-absorptive or fasted state and in the continually fed state suggests that the response to food depends upon the previous dietary history, especially the amount of protein in the diet.[8] Basically, food stimulates protein synthesis and decreases whole body protein breakdown in the fed state; in the fasted state protein synthesis falls and protein breakdown rises. The extent of the swing between the fed state gains and the fasted state losses depends upon the previous dietary history, the swings being greatest when protein content of the diet is highest. The mechanisms involved are unknown except that they include modulation of oxidation of essential amino acids, especially the branched-chain and aromatic amino acids, the enzymes of which are induced (in the liver of experimental animals) by a high-protein diet. Fasting for a period longer than a few hours depresses protein synthesis and breakdown and thus abolishes the food-related cycling (Fig. 2.7). Consumption of a low-protein diet for a long period diminishes the rate of cycling, and the fasted-state losses exceed the fed-state gains so that the body comes into negative

nitrogen balance. The point at which negative nitrogen balance is achieved is, of course, the point at which the body requirements exceed the nutrient intake and there is a substantial amount of controversy concerning the exact value at which dietary intake is sufficient.

Millward and co-workers[120,146,148] believe, as a result of their demonstration of the importance of the previous dietary history, that the requirement is substantially lower than the currently recommended safe intake. Bier and Young in particular, however, believe that the present recommended daily amount is unlikely to be too high, and may possibly be too low.[121]

Nutrient effects in various tissues

There is very little work available on the effect of feeding different tissues of the human body. It is possible to gain some insight by comparing the changes in the whole body with those in limb or muscle tissue investigated by the use of the tracer exchange method or by tracer incorporation into needle biopsy samples. Most of what we know, even about muscle which is most accessible in people, comes from studies carried out in experimental animals and it is not certain to what extent these are good models for adult human beings.

In skeletal muscle, the pattern of change in response to the availability and withdrawal of food is similar in direction but probably greater in extent than that

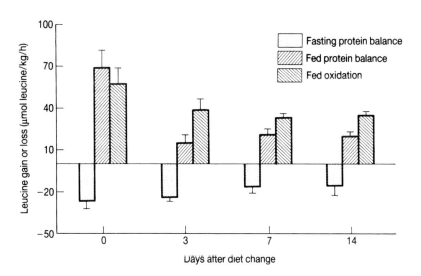

Figure 2.7 – The effects of protein intake on fed-state gains and fasted-state losses and the rates of amino acid oxidation in the two conditions.

observed in the whole body, i.e. an increase in protein synthesis during feeding with a fall in protein breakdown.[149–151] This is indicated by changes in net loss of amino acids, 3-methylhistidine and tyrosine efflux,[55,152] and also tracer exchange methods.[70,71]

It seems likely that heart behaves very much like skeletal muscle[57,153,154] but the gastrointestinal tract and the liver show changes that are probably substantially different in their pattern and mechanisms. There is some very limited information concerning rates of protein synthesis in gastrointestinal tissue during total parenteral nutrition but the data are sparse.[155] Fasting decreases protein synthesis in the gastrointestinal tissue in young growing rats and markedly stimulates protein breakdown.[156] In the liver, feeding can almost totally shut off proteolysis[157,158] and therefore it appears that a low protein synthesis does increase and decrease according to nutrient intake. The changes in protein breakdown are far more important for the regulation of the lean mass of the liver.[159,160]

Garlick and co-workers believe that the changes in protein synthesis as a result of nutrient intake decrease with the approach of adulthood so that the capacity to respond to food becomes very much less in muscle and may even be abolished.[161–166] However, since variation in whole body protein synthesis appears to be a firmly based observation in whole man it seems likely that the visceral tissue does not become as unresponsive as skeletal muscle as maturity progresses.

Nutrient and hormonal modification of protein turnover

Although energy supply has an effect on nitrogen balance, its effects on protein synthesis and breakdown are minor and appear simply to be related to the capacity for the sparing of the use of protein as a fuel.[167] Nevertheless, amino acids can increase protein synthesis in skeletal muscle[72,168] and probably decrease protein breakdown in visceral tissue.[169] The branched-chain amino acids do not appear to have lived up to their promise[170–173] as anabolic agents. It has been reported that the branched-chain amino acids may decrease protein breakdown in the human forearm[174] but this result is controversial; certainly, under other circumstances in which total amino acid availability in blood has been varied, there appears to be no effect on

skeletal muscle protein breakdown.[72,175] Branched-chain amino acids may increase the sensitivity of protein turnover to insulin[176,177] and there is the suggestion that very large doses of leucine do have some unexplained stimulatory effect on tracer amino acid incorporation into muscle and liver protein in man.[94]

Conditionally essential amino acids

In model animal preparations glutamine promotes protein synthesis and inhibits protein breakdown under some circumstances.[110,111] The concentration of glutamine is unlikely to be a factor of overriding importance, however, since in some circumstances, such as feeding a low-protein diet, glutamine concentration hardly changes under circumstances in which protein balance changes substantially.[8] Glutamine administration appears to stimulate muscle protein synthesis in normal healthy patients and in sick patients, but only by about 25%.[151] There is no doubt that glutamine administration may ameliorate the loss of nitrogen from the whole body and there are suggestions that glutamine administration may improve gut and immune function in patients undergoing elective surgical operation.[178]

Although arginine has been suggested to have major effects on wound healing, diminution of negative nitrogen balance, etc.,[179–181] no definitive effects have yet been observed concerning whole body protein synthesis, although it is claimed that arginine increases tumour protein synthesis,[17,155] probably as a result of stimulation of cell turnover. This may be beneficial if arginine can stimulate resumption of the cell cycle, rendering cells susceptible to chemotherapeutic agents (see also Ch 23).

Insulin

The effects of insulin in stimulating protein synthesis and decreasing protein breakdown are easily seen in the whole body of young animals and animals with experimental diabetes.[33] However, the exact nature of its effects on muscle is harder to describe because of the difficulty in avoiding the effect of insulin upon amino acid concentrations, which may be an independent regulator as insulin decreases muscle protein breakdown (and thus reduces availability of amino acids for protein synthesis). The inhibitory effect on muscle protein breakdown[57,182] can be easily reproduced in experiments carried out by a variety of workers[72,183,184] but there is some controversy concerning whether or not insulin increases muscle protein synthesis, some workers claiming that it does[185] and others that it does not.[57,183,186] The author's own feeling is that it does if the conditions are right and the correct experiment is carried out to observe it, and it probably does *in vivo*.[73]

The mechanisms of insulin action in stimulating protein synthesis and decreasing protein breakdown are not very well understood. Unlike the effects of insulin on glucose metabolism there is (somewhat surprisingly, considering what the textbooks say) no stimulatory effect of insulin on net amino acid transport across membranes[101] and any effects must be post-membranous in nature. The effects almost certainly include increases in aggregation of ribosomes and initiation of protein synthesis and possibly increases in translational activity.[154,187,188]

The effects on proteolysis are less well understood than the effects on protein synthesis.[33] It appears that insulin may inhibit lysosomal pathways of protein synthesis (i.e. those associated with the activities of the lysosomal proteases such as the cathepsins). It appears not to be important for regulation of non-lysosomal proteolysis such as that involved in control of the regulation of the myofibrillar apparatus in muscle, which comprises two-thirds of all muscle protein.

It seems, therefore, that the action of insulin in inhibiting proteolysis in muscle has its effect on a relatively small, rapidly turning over pool of protein,[37,189] which may be more nutritionally labile than previously thought.

Effects of other hormones on protein turnover

Thyroid and corticosteroids

In animals and man, thyroid hormone generally stimulates protein turnover:[33,190,191] in the fed state thyroid hormone stimulates protein synthesis and protein breakdown; in the fasted state the secretion of thyroid hormone *in vivo* decreases and this may be part of the adaptive response to lack of nutrient intake.[33,37]

Corticosteroids stimulate protein breakdown and inhibit protein synthesis. The effects of corticosteroids can be seen both in animals and in man in appropriate studies.[192-196] The effects of corticosteroids are, to some extent, tissue-specific since corticosteroids may stimu-

late insulin secretion which can cause hyperphagia and a decrease of splanchnic proteolysis, resulting in growth of the liver and the gastrointestinal tract at the same time that the musculature is wasting. The effects of corticosteroids on skeletal muscle are principally due to the decrease in protein synthesis[197] and an increase in the myofibrillar component of protein breakdown.[198] The effects of corticosteroids can be inhibited by the corticosteroid receptor blocking agent RU 2387.[198]

Glucagon

Glucagon is principally a hormone of fuel mobilisation and gluconeogenesis. Its effects on protein metabolism can be thought of in this context. It has no effect on skeletal muscle or heart but increases inward amino acid transport, ureagenesis and proteolysis[125,199] in the liver and thus lowers plasma amino acids. It may thus predispose to peripheral protein catabolism,[200] and the wasting of muscle seen in various conditions associated with hyperglucagonaemia may be mediated in this manner.[201,202] These are likely to contribute to the wasting of lean tissue seen in trauma, when glucagon is elevated.

Growth hormone and IGF-1

The effects of growth hormone on protein metabolism in adults are not as straightforward as might be imagined; there are some anabolic effects but they seem to be exhibited either through the insulin-like properties of the hormone (probably through its effects in stimulating the local and hepatic production of IGF-1), or only appear when the normal pattern and extent of growth hormone secretion are deranged, as in the elderly and the critically ill.[203-205] Growth hormone appears to have an acute effect in stimulating muscle protein synthesis when examined using the forearm technique,[206] but such effects must be short-lived since longer-term administration of growth hormone in healthy young adults results in no net accretion of the muscle mass or lean tissue mass.[207] Furthermore, growth hormone appears to have an anti-insulin-like effect in diminishing the potency of insulin in inhibiting protein breakdown.[208]

In critically ill patients, in whom there is a defect in growth hormone secretion, therapeutic growth hormone administration was, rather shockingly, found to be associated with greater mortality,[209] for reasons that have not been worked out. Furthermore, injury and inflammatory disease are often associated with the development of resistance to the anabolic effect of growth hormone,[210] presumably due to a down-regulation of the conversion of growth hormone to insulin-like growth factor and production of the associated binding proteins that chaperone IGF-1 in blood.

Nevertheless, administration of growth hormone to non-critically ill patients taking a hypocaloric diet results in amelioration of nitrogen losses,[211,212] probably because growth hormone has a lipolytic effect sufficiently powerful to provide enough free fatty acids to account for the energy needs of the body, thus sparing a substantial part of the use of muscle protein and allowing any exogenous amino acids to be diverted towards lean tissue synthesis and repair. Also, growth hormone can antagonise the catabolic effects of glucocorticoids.[213] It is pertinent to the discussion of the possible beneficial effects of growth hormone[214,215] that the normal pattern of growth hormone release is disturbed in acute illness, particularly in the elderly.[216–218]

Replacement growth hormone appears to increase muscle protein synthesis in the elderly.[219]

The effect of IGF-1 on protein metabolism has not been extensively studied in man. In incubated isolated muscles it stimulates protein synthesis and inhibits protein breakdown but its administration to diabetic animals or animals recovering from stunting due to malnutrition suggests that it is not a powerful anabolic agent.[220,221] However its therapeutic possibilities[216] in man may depend upon it being used in conjunction with its binding protein. The combination of IGF-1 and IGF binding protein 3 given together increases the biological half-life of IGF-1 in the mammalian body, thereby increasing its efficacy in stimulating muscle anabolism by stimulating protein synthesis.[222] Whether or not this preparation will be sufficiently cost-effective for general clinical use is, as yet, unknown.

Catecholamines

Catecholamines have a generally anabolic effect which appears to be mediated through β-receptors of an unusual kind.[223–226] The anabolic effects of catecholamines are not well understood and there is a substantial amount of confusion in the literature concerning the exact mechanisms of these effects. Furthermore, the florid protein-wasting response seen early after injury or burns,[193,227–229] which appears to require adrenaline as well as cortisol and growth hormone, is obviously a catabolic response and it is

difficult to come to a satisfactory integrated view of the role of the catecholamines in the regulation of the lean body mass.

Testosterone and other anabolic steroids

It is still reasonably common to read in the literature that there is no objective evidence that testosterone increases lean body mass, despite the easily observable differences between men and women and between young boys and young men in terms of muscle mass. In fact, there seems little doubt that massive doses of testosterone and its analogues have anabolic effects on muscle protein synthesis,[230,231] and cause large increases in muscle. The effect is even greater for some synthetic anabolic steroids that have very little prostatic activity.[232] The mechanism appears to involve, as with all steroid hormones, stimulation of the nucleus to increase the production of mRNAs and thus the stimulation of muscle protein synthesis over a period of days. There is no acute stimulation of amino acid transport or translation of pre-existing mRNAs.[233]

When anabolic steroids were administered to patients with muscle disease, it was found that, apart from patients who were hypogonadal,[234] there was little net benefit, especially in young patients with Duchenne dystrophy in whom both synthesis and breakdown seemed to be switched on.[235,236]

Role of cytokines

The role of the cytokines TNF-γ, IL-1 and IL-6 and the lymphokine interferon IFN-γ in mediating skeletal muscle proteolysis has been extensively investigated, mainly in rat skeletal muscle.

Administration to rats of the cytokines IL-1 and TNF modulates ubiquitin gene expression suggesting modulation of the protein breakdown pathway,[237–239] but no simultaneous *in vivo* measurements of proteolysis have been made. In catabolic states such as sepsis and after severe burns there are increased concentrations of the cytokines TNF-γ, IL-1 and IL-6 but blockade of their action does not normalise rates of breakdown,[240] suggesting a more complex control mechanism.

Effects of ageing on whole body and muscle protein turnover

This topic has been expanding rapidly over the past 10 years. There is no doubt that there is good evidence for a slowing of turnover of protein and that both protein synthesis and breakdown are slowed.[241] Obviously maintenance and repair processes will be slowed. In respect of both the response to food and the ability to respond to intense exercise,[242] the protein synthetic machinery seems inadequate in the elderly. There seems in addition to be accelerated oxidation of proteins, which may be a particular problem if destruction of damaged proteins is suboptimal.

Effects of disease and injury on muscle protein turnover

Two distinct patterns can be described (Fig. 2.8). In mild to moderate injury, malnutrition, immobilisation, and a variety of endocrine and other diseases that result in lean tissue wasting over a long period of time, it appears that muscle protein turnover is depressed.[243] This depression includes a fall in muscle protein synthesis and also a fall in muscle protein breakdown. Whole body protein turnover is, therefore, also depressed although in some circumstances it may be that visceral protein turnover is elevated, e.g. possibly in liver and kidney disease. Under the circumstances it makes sense that any attempts to replenish depleted cell mass should be aimed at increasing muscle protein synthesis rather than decreasing muscle protein breakdown. Certainly, in malnourished patients it is possible to achieve markedly positive protein balances by appropriate feeding of high-energy, high-protein diets, either by nasogastric tube or parenterally.[167,244]

In circumstances in which there is florid muscle wasting associated with increased whole body energy expenditure – such as in severe injury, after burns of more than about 10% of body surface area,[245,246] in florid inflammatory diseases such as polymyositis,[243] during infection,[247,248] and with some kinds of cancer[243,249] – whole body nitrogen balance is markedly negative, probably because of changes that include an increase of protein breakdown in a variety of tissues, including muscle. The evidence for this is now really quite firm but we still do not know whether muscle protein synthesis falls, as might be expected, or rises, possibly as an adaptive response to the rise in protein breakdown. Nevertheless, it appears that the major change under these circumstances of florid nitrogen loss is acceleration of lean tissue proteolysis,[250] probably including muscle proteolysis, and therefore the most likely beneficial effect will be of agents that decrease muscle protein breakdown or inhibit the proximal factors that cause it. Unfortunately, no such agent, with the possible exception of the corticosteroid blocker RU38486,[251] currently exists, so that nutritional treatment appears to be confined simply to provision of sufficient energy and of amounts of nitrogen sufficient to maintain the activities of the immune system, for wound healing and possibly the synthesis of acute-phase proteins. It is likely that aggressive treatment of the proximal cause of the muscle wasting (e.g. by anticytokine therapy) is more likely to succeed than palliative treatment to inhibit lean tissue proteolysis since the latter is probably part of an adaptive endogenous life-saving response.

Acknowledgements

Original work described in this chapter was carried out with support from UK Medical Research Council, University of Dundee and The Wellcome Trust.

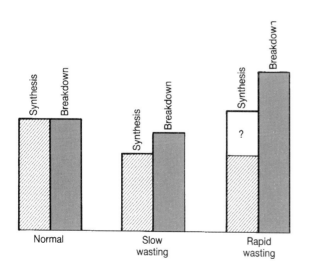

Figure 2.8 – Responses of muscle tissue to disease and injury.

References

1. Cathcart EP. The influence of muscle work on protein metabolism. *Physiol Rev* 1925; **5:** 225–243.

2. Schoenheimer R. *The dynamic state of body constituents.* Harvard University Press, Cambridge, MA, 1942.

3. Waterlow JC, Garlick PJ, Millward DJ. *Protein turnover in mammalian tissues and in the whole body.* Elsevier–North Holland, Amsterdam, 1978.

4. Hegsted DM. Balance studies. *J Nutr* 1976; **106:** 307–311.

5. Tarnopolsky MA, MacDougall JD, Atkinson SA. Influence of protein intake and training status on nitrogen balance and lean body mass. *J Appl Physiol* 1988; **64:** 187–193.

6. Hegsted DM. Assessment of nitrogen requirements. *Am J Clin Nutr* 1978; **31:** 1669–1677.

7. Mertz W. Use and misuse of balance studies. *J Nutr* 1987; **117:** 1811–1813.

8. Millward DJ, Price GM, Pacy PJH, Quevedo RM, Halliday D. The nutritional sensitivity of the diurnal cycling of body protein enables protein deposition to be measured in subjects at nitrogen equilibrium. *Clin Nutr* 1991; **10:** 239–244.

9. Halliday D, Rennie MJ. The use of stable isotopes for diagnosis and clinical research. *Clin Sci* 1982; **63:** 485–496.

10. Wolfe RR. *Radioactive and stable isotope tracers in biomedicine.* Wiley–Liss, New York, 1992.

11. Rennie MJ. An introduction to the use of tracers in nutrition and metabolism. *Proc Nutr Soc* 1999; **58:** 935–944.

12. Wretlind A. Recollections of pioneers in nutrition: landmarks in the development of parenteral nutrition. *J Am Coll Nutr* 1992; **11:** 366–373.

13. Forbes GB. *Human body composition: Growth, aging, nutrition and activity.* Springer-Verlag, New York, 1987.

14. Dietrichson P, Coakley J, Smith PEM, Griffiths RD, Helliwell TR, Edwards RHT. Conchotome and needle percutaneous biopsy of skeletal muscle. *J Neurol Neurosurg Psychiatry* 1987; **50:** 1461–1467.

15. Heys SD, Park KGM, McNurlan MA, Keenan RA, Miller JDB, Eremin O, Garlick PJ. Protein-synthesis rates in colon and liver – stimulation by gastrointestinal pathologies. *Gut* 1992; **33:** 976–981.

16. Nakshabendi IM, Obeidat W, Russell RI, Downie S, Rennie MJ. Measurement of duodenal mucosal protein synthesis after delivery of [^{13}C]leucine and [^{13}C]valine by IV and IG routes. *Clin Nutr* 1992; **11 (Suppl):** O.1.

17. Park KGM, Heys SD, Blessing K, Kelly P, McNurlan MA, Eremin O, Garlick PJ. Stimulation of human breast cancers by dietary L-arginine. *Clin Sci* 1992; **82:** 413–417.

18. Scrimgeour CM, Gibson JNA, Downie S, Rennie MJ. Collagen synthesis in human bone using stable-isotope labelled alanine and proline. *Proc Nutr Soc* 1993; **52:** 258A.

19. Olufemi OS, Humes P, Whittaker PG, Read M, Lind T, Halliday D. Albumin synthetic rates: a comparison of arginine and alpha-ketoisocaproate precursor methods stable isotope techniques. *Eur J Clin Nutr* 1990; **44:** 351–361.

20. Halliday D, Venkatesan S, Pacy P. Apolipoprotein metabolism: a stable-isotope approach. *Am J Clin Nutr* 1993; **57:** 726S–730S.

21. Corbett ME, Boyd EJS, Penston JG, Wormsley KG, Watt PW, Rennie MJ. Pentagastrin increases pepsin secretion without increasing its fractional synthetic rate. *Am J Physiol* 1995; **269:** E118–F425.

22. Schoeller DA, van Santen E, Petersen DW, Dietz W, Jaspan J, Klein PD. Total body water measurements in humans with 18O and 2H labeled water. *Am J Clin Nutr* 1980; **33:** 2686–2693.

23. Miller ME, Cappon CJ. Anion-exchange chromatographic determination of bromide in serum. *Clin Chem* 1984; **30:** 781–783.

24. Bergmeyer HU, Karlfried G. *Principles of enzymatic analysis.* Verlag Chemie, Weinheim, 1978.

25. Rennie MJ, Halliday D. The use of stable isotope tracers as metabolic probes of whole-body and limb metabolism. *Proc Nutr Soc* 1984; **43:** 189–196.

26. Keller U, Rennie MJ. Stable isotopes in clinical research. *Eur J Clin Invest* 1986; **16:** 97–100.

27. Powis MR, Smith K, Rennie M, Halliday D, Pierro A. Characteristics of protein and energy metabolism in neonates with necrotizing enterocolitis – a pilot study. *J Pediatr Surg* 1999; **34:** 5–10.

28. Chien PFW, Smith K, Watt PW, Scrimgeour CM, Taylor DJ, Rennie MJ. Protein turnover in the human fetus *in vivo* at term. *Am J Physiol* 1993; **265:** E31–E35.

29. Bergström J, Fürst P, Norée L-O, Vinnars E. Intracellular free amino acid concentration in human muscle tissue. *J Appl Physiol* 1974; **36:** 693–697.

30. Vinnars E, Bergström J, Fürst P. Influence of the postoperative state on the intracellular free amino acids in human muscle tissue. *Ann Surg* 1975; **182:** 665–671.

31. Wernerman J, von der Decken A, Vinnars E. Size distribution of ribosomes in biopsy specimens of human skeletal muscle during starvation. *Metabolism* 1985; **34:** 665–669.

32. Wernerman J, von der Decken A, Vinnars E. Polyribosome concentration in human skeletal muscle after starvation and parenteral or enteral refeeding. *Metabolism* 1986; **35:** 447–451.

33. Kettelhut IC, Wing SS, Goldberg AL. Endocrine regulation of protein breakdown in skeletal muscle. *Diabetes Metab Rev* 1988; **4:** 751–772.

34. Tischler ME, Rosenberg S, Satarug S, Henriksen EJ, Kirby CR, Tome M, Chase P. Different mechanisms of increased proteolysis in atrophy induced by denervation or unweighting of rat soleus muscle. *Metabolism* 1990; **39:** 756–763.

35. Tawa NE Jr, Kettelhut IC, Goldberg AL. Dietary protein deficiency reduces lysosomal and non-lysosomal ATP-dependent proteolysis in muscle. *Am J Physiol* 1992; **263**: E326–E334.

36. Attaix D, Aurousseau E, Combaret L *et al.* Ubiquitin–proteasome-dependent proteolysis in skeletal muscle. *Reprod Nutr Dev* 1998; **38**: 153–165.

37. Kayali AG, Goodman MN, Lin J, Young VR. Insulin and thyroid hormone-independent adaptation of myofibrillar proteolysis to glucocorticoids. *Am J Physiol* 1990; **259**: E699–E705.

38. Millward DJ, Waterlow JC. Effect of nutrition on protein turnover in skeletal muscle. *Fed Proc* 1978; **37**: 2283–2290.

39. Bier DM. Intrinsically difficult problems, the kinetics of body proteins and amino acid in man. *Diabetes Metab Rev* 1989; **5**: 111–132.

40. Pacy PJ, Cheng KN, Thompson GN, Halliday D. Stable isotopes as tracers in clinical research. *Ann Nutr Metab* 1989; **33**: 65–78.

41. Van Acker BA, Hulsewe KW, Wagenmakers AJ *et al.* Absence of glutamine isotopic steady state: implications for the assessment of whole-body glutamine production rate. *Clin Sci (Colch)* 1998; **95**: 339–346.

42. Fern EB, Garlick PJ, Waterlow JC. Apparent compartmentation of body nitrogen in one human subject: its consequences in measuring the rate of whole-body protein synthesis with ^{15}N. *Clin Sci* 1985; **68**: 271–282.

43. Clarke JTR, Bier DM. The conversion of phenylalanine to tyrosine in man. Direct measurement by continuous intravenous tracer infusions of L-[*ring*-^{2}H$_5$]phenylalanine and L-[1-^{13}C]tyrosine in the postabsorptive state. *Metabolism* 1982; **31**: 999–1005.

44. Matthews DE, Motil KJ, Rohrbaugh DK, Burke JF, Young VR, Bier DM. Measurement of leucine metabolism in man from a primed, continuous infusion of L-[1-^{13}C]leucine. *Am J Physiol* 1980; **238**: E473–E479.

45. Boirie Y, Gachon P, Corny S, Fauquant J, Maubois JL, Beaufrere B. Acute postprandial changes in leucine metabolism as assessed with an intrinsically labelled milk protein. *Am J Physiol* 1996; **271**: E1083–E1091.

46. Millward DJ, Price GM, Pacy PJH, Halliday D. Whole-body protein and amino acid turnover in man: what can we measure with confidence? *Proc Nutr Soc* 1991; **50**: 197–216.

47. Reeds PJ, Hachey DL, Patterson BW, Motil KJ, Klein PD. VLDL apoloprotein B-100, a potential indicator of the isotopic labelling of the hepatic protein synthetic precursor pool in humans: studies with multiple stable isotopically labeled amino acids. *J Nutr* 1992; **122**: 457–466.

48. Picou D, Taylor-Roberts T. The measurement of total protein synthesis and catabolism and nitrogen turnover in infants in different nutritional states and receiving different amounts of dietary protein. *Clin Sci* 1969; **36**: 283–296.

49. Jeevanandam M, Brennan MF, Horowitz GD, Rose D, Mihranian MH, Daly J, Lowry SF. Tracer priming in human protein turnover studies with [^{15}N]glycine. *Biochem Med* 1985; **34**: 214–225.

50. Golden MHN, Waterlow JC. Total protein synthesis in elderly people: a comparison of results with [^{15}N]glycine and [^{14}C]leucine. *Clin Sci* 1977; **53**: 277–288.

51. Zierler K. Theory of the use of arteriovenous concentration difference for measuring metabolism in steady and non-steady states. *J Clin Invest* 1961; **40**: 2111–2125.

52. Felig P. Amino acid metabolism in man. *Ann Rev Biochem* 1979; **44**: 993–955.

53. Elia M, Livesey G. Effects of ingested steak and infused leucine on forelimb metabolism in man and the fate of the carbon skeletons and amino groups of branched-chain amino acids. *Clin Sci* 1983; **64**: 517–526.

54. Hagenfeldt L, Eriksson S, Wahren J. Influence of leucine on arterial concentrations and regional exchange of amino acids in healthy subjects. *Clin Sci* 1980; **59**: 173–181 (Abstract).

55. Marliss EB, Aoki TT, Pozefsky T, Most AS, Cahill GF. Muscle and splanchnic glutamine and glutamate metabolism in forearm of post-absorptive and starved man. *J Clin Invest* 1971; **50**: 814–817.

56. Owen EE, Robinson RR. Amino acid extraction and ammonia metabolism by human kidney during the prolonged administration of ammonium chloride. *J Clin Invest* 1963; **42**: 273–275.

57. Barrett EJ, Gelfand RA. The in vivo study of cardiac and skeletal muscle protein turnover. *Diabetes Metab Rev* 1989; **5**: 133–148.

58. Macdonald IA. Arterio-venous differences to study macronutrient metabolism: introduction and overview. *Proc Nutr Soc* 1999; **58**: 871–875.

59. Alvestrand A, DeFronzo RA, Smith D, Wahren J. Influence of hyperinsulinaemia on intracellular amino acid levels and amino acid exchange across splanchnic and leg tissues in uraemia. *Clin Sci* 1988; **74**: 155–163.

60. Felig P, Wahren J. Amino acid metabolism in exercising man. *J Clin Invest* 1971; **50**: 2703–2709.

61. Katz A, Broberg S, Sahlin K, Wahren J. Muscle ammonia and amino acid metabolism during dynamic exercise in man. *Clin Physiol* 1986; **6**: 365–379.

62. MacLean DA, Bangsbo J, Saltin B. Muscle interstitial glucose and lactate levels during dynamic exercise in humans determined by microdialysis. *J Appl Physiol* 1999; **87:** 1483–1490.

63. Young VR, Munro HN. N'-Methylhistidine (3-methylhistidine) and muscle protein turnover: an overview. *Fed Proc* 1978; **37:** 2291–2300.

64. Rennie MJ, Millward DJ. 3-Methylhistidine excretion and the urinary 3-methylhistidine/creatinine ratio are poor indicators of skeletal muscle protein breakdown. *Clin Sci* 1983; **65:** 217–225.

65. Rennie MJ, Bennegård C, Edén E, Emery PW, Lundholm K. Urinary excretion and efflux from the leg of 3-methylhistidine before and after major surgical operation. *Metabolism* 1984; **33:** 250–256.

66. Sjölin J, Stjernström H, Henneberg S, Andersson E, Martensson J, Griman G, Larsson J. Splanchnic and peripheral release of 3-methylhistidine in relation to its urinary excretion in human infection. *Metabolism* 1989; **38:** 23–29.

67. Sjölin J, Stjernström H, Friman G, Larsson J, Wahren J. Total and net muscle protein breakdown in infection determined by amino acid effluxes. *Am J Physiol* 1990; **258:** E856–E863.

68. Rathmacher JA, Link GA, Flakoll PJ, Nissen SL. Gas chromatographic/mass spectrometric analysis of stable isotopes of 3-methylhistidine in biological fluids: application to plasma kinetics in vivo. *Biol Mass Spectrom* 1992; **21:** 560–566.

69. Jefferson LS, Li JB, Rannels SR. Regulation by insulin of amino acid release and protein turnover in the perfused rat hemicorpus. *J Biol Chem* 1977; **252:** 1476–1483.

70. Cheng KN, Dworzak F, Ford GC, Rennie MJ, Halliday D. Direct determination of leucine metabolism and protein breakdown in humans using L-[1-^{13}C,^{15}N]-leucine and the forearm model. *Eur J Clin Invest* 1985; **15:** 349–354.

71. Cheng KN, Pacy PJ, Dworzak F, Ford GC, Halliday D. Influence of fasting on leucine and muscle protein metabolism across the human forearm determined using L-[1-^{13}C,^{15}N]leucine as the tracer. *Clin Sci* 1987; **73:** 241–246.

72. Bennet WM, Connacher AA, Scrimgeour CM, Rennie MJ. The effect of amino acid infusion on leg protein turnover assessed by L-[^{15}N]phenylalanine and L-[^{13}C]leucine exchange *Eur J Clin Invest* 1990; **20:** 37–46.

73. Bennet WM, Connacher AA, Scrimgeour CM, Jung RT, Rennie MJ. Euglycemic hyperinsulinemia augments amino acid uptake by human leg tissues during hyperaminoacidemia. *Am J Physiol* 1990; **259:** E185–E194.

74. Halliday D, McKeran RO. Measurement of muscle protein synthetic rate from serial muscle biopsies and total body protein turnover in man by continuous intravenous infusion of L-[α-^{15}N]lysine. *Clin Sci* 1975; **49:** 581–590.

75. Rennie MJ, Edwards RHT, Halliday D, Matthews DE, Wolman SL, Millward DJ. Muscle protein synthesis measured by stable isotope techniques in man: the effects of feeding and fasting. *Clin Sci* 1982; **63:** 519–523.

76. Zhang XJ, Chinkes DL, Sakurai Y, Wolfe RR. An isotopic method for measurement of muscle protein fractional breakdown rate in vivo. *Am J Physiol* 1996; **270:** E759–E767.

77. Phillips S, Tipton T, Fernando AA, Wolfe RR. Resistance training reduces the acute exercise-induced increase in muscle protein turnover. *Am J Physiol* 1999; **39:** E118–E124.

78. Stein TP, Leskiw MJ, Buzby GP, Giandomenico AL, Wallace HW, Mullen JL. Measurement of protein synthesis rates with [^{15}N]glycine. *Am J Physiol* 1980; **239:** E294–E300.

79. Calder AG, Anderson SE, Grant I, McNurlan MA, Garlick PJ. The determination of low D_5-phenyl-alanine enrichment (0.002-0.09 Atom percent excess) after conversion to phenylethylamine in relation to protein turnover studies by gas-chromatography electron-ionisation mass-spectrometry. *Rapid Commun Mass Spectrom* 1993; **6:** 421–424.

80. Smith K, Scrimgeour CM, Bennet WM, Rennie MJ. Isolation of amino acids by preparative gas chromatography for quantification of carboxyl carbon ^{13}C enrichment by isotope ratio mass spectrometry. *Biomed Environ Mass Spectrom* 1988; **17:** 267–273.

81. Yarasheski KE, Smith K, Rennie MJ, Bier DM. Measurement of muscle protein fractional synthetic rate by capillary gas chromatography/combustion isotope ratio mass spectrometry. *Biol Mass Spectrom* 1992; **21:** 486–490.

82. Carraro F, Stuart CA, Hartl WH, Rosenblatt J, Wolfe RR. Effect of exercise and recovery on muscle protein synthesis in human subjects. *Am J Physiol* 1990; **259:** E470–E476.

83. Meier-Augenstein W. Use of gas chromatography-combustion-isotope ratio mass spectrometry in nutrition and metabolic research. *Curr Opin Clin Nutr Metab Care* 1999; **2:** 465–470.

84. Watt PW, Lindsay Y, Scrimgeour CM, Chien PAF, Gibson JNA, Taylor DJ, Rennie MJ. Isolation of aminoacyl tRNA and its labelling with stable isotope tracers: use in studies of human tissue protein synthesis. *Proc Natl Acad Sci USA* 1991; **88:** 5892–5896.

85. Baumann PQ, Stirewalt WS, O'Rourke BD, Howard D, Nair KS. Precursor pools of protein synthesis: a stable isotope study in a swine model. *Am J Physiol* 1994; **267:** E203–E209.

86. Ljungqvist OH, Persson M, Ford GC, Nair KS. Functional heterogeneity of leucine pools in human skeletal muscle. *Am J Physiol* 1997; **273:** E564–E570.

87. Olufemi OS, Whittaker PG, Halliday D, Lind T. Albumin metabolism in fasted subjects during late pregnancy. *Clin Sci* 1991; **81:** 161–168.

88. el-Harake WA, Furman MA, Cook B, Nair KS, Kukowski J, Brodsky IG. Measurement of dermal collagen synthesis rate in vivo in humans. *Am J Physiol* 1998; **274:** E586–E591.

89. Hellerstein MK, Neese RA. Mass isotopomer distribution analysis: a technique for measuring biosynthesis and turnover of polymers. *Am J Physiol* 1992; **263:** E988–E1001.

90. Papageorgopoulos C, Caldwell K, Shackleton C, Schweingrubber H, Hellerstein MK. Measuring protein synthesis by mass isotopomer distribution analysis (MIDA). *Anal Biochem* 1999; **267:** 1–16.

91. Smith K, Essen P, McNurlan MA, Rennie MJ, Garlick PJ, Wernerman J. A multi-tracer investigation of the effect of a flooding dose administered during the constant infusion of tracer amino acid on the rate of tracer incorporation into human muscle protein. *Proc Nutr Soc* 1992; **51:** 109P (Abstract).

92. Essen P, McNurlan MA, Wernerman J, Milne E, Vinnars E. Short-term starvation decreases skeletal muscle protein synthesis rate in man. *Clin Physiol* 1992; **12:** 287–299.

93. McNurlan MA, Essen P, Milne E *et al*. Similarity of protein synthesis rate measured with [1-¹³C]leucine and [1-¹³C]phenylalanine. *Clin Nutr* 1989; **8 (suppl):** 132, 123.

94. Smith K, Barua JM, Scrimgeour CM, Rennie MJ. Flooding with L-[1-¹³C]leucine stimulates human muscle protein incorporation of continuously infused L-[1-¹³C]valine. *Am J Physiol* 1992; **262:** E372–E376.

95. Smith K, Barua JM, Watt PW, Scrimgeour CM, Rickhuss PK, Rennie MJ. Preliminary evidence of artefactually high values of muscle protein synthesis obtained by the flooding dose technique compared to the constant infusion method. *Clin Nutr* 1991; **10 (Suppl):** O.21, 7.

96. Garlick PJ, Wernerman J, McNurlan MA, Essen P, Lobley GE, Calder GA, Vinnars E. Measurement of the rate of protein synthesis in muscle of postabsorptive young men by injection of a "flooding dose" of [1-¹³C]leucine. *Clin Sci* 1989; **77:** 329–336.

97. Smith K, Reynolds N, Downie S, Patel A, Rennie MJ. Effects of flooding amino acids on the incorporation of labelled amino acids into human skeletal muscle protein. *Am J Physiol* 1998; **275:** E73–E78.

98. Smith K, Downie SB, Watt PW, Rickhuss PK, Barua JM, Scrimgeour CM, Rennie MJ. Increased incorporation of [¹³C]valine into plasma albumin as a result of a flooding dose of leucine in man. *Clin Nutr* 1992; **11:** 77 (Abstract).

99. Rennie MJ, Meier-Augenstein W, Watt PW, Patel A, Begley IS, Scrimgeour CM. Use of continuous-flow combustion MS in studies of human metabolism. *Biochem Soc Trans* 1996; **24:** 927–932.

100. Waterlow JC, Fern EB. Free amino acid pools and their regulation. In: *Nitrogen metabolism in man*. Applied Science Publishers, England, 1981; pp 1–16.

101. Mackenzie B, Ahmed A, Rennie MJ. Muscle amino acid metabolism and transport. In: Kilberg MS, Häussinger D (Eds) *Mammalian amino acid transport: mechanism and control*. Plenum Publishing, New York, 1993; pp 195–232.

102. Taylor PM, Rennie MJ, Low SY. Biomembrane transport and inter-organ nutrient flows: the amino acids. In: Van Winkle L (Ed.) *Biomembrane transport*. Academic Press, New York, 1999; pp 295–325.

103. Wagenmakers AJM, Beckers EJ, Brouns F, Kuipers H, Soeters PB, van der Vusse GJ, Saris WHM. Carbohydrate supplementation, glycogen depletion and amino acid metabolism during exercise. *Am J Physiol* 1991; **260:** E883–E890.

104. Pogson CI, Low SY, Knowles RG, Salter M, Rennie MJ. Application of metabolic control theory to amino acid metabolism in liver In: Grunnet N, Quistorff B (Eds) *Regulation of hepatic function: Alfred Benzon Symposium 30*. Munksgaard, Copenhagen, 1990, pp 262–272.

105. Salter M, Knowles RG, Pogson CI. Quantification of the importance of individual steps in the control of aromatic amino acid metabolism. *Biochem J* 1986; **234:** 635–647.

106. Low SY, Salter M, Knowles RG, Rennie MJ, Pogson CI. Effect of L-glutamate-Â-hydrazide on the transport and metabolism of L-glutamine in rat liver cells and isolated mitochondria. *Biochem Soc Trans* 1991; **18:** 1239–1240.

107. Häussinger D. Regulation of hepatic ammonia metabolism: the intercellular glutamine cycle. *Adv Enzyme Regul* 1986; **261:** 6216–6221.

108. Lavoinne A, Baquet A, Hue L. Stimulation of glycogen synthesis and lipogenesis by glutamine in isolated rat hepatocytes. *Biochem J* 1987; **248:** 429–437.

109. Häussinger D, Lang F, Gerok W. Regulation of cell function by the cellular hydration state. *Am J Physiol* 1994; **267**: E343–E355.

110. MacLennan PA, Brown RA, Rennie MJ. A positive relationship between protein synthetic rate and intra-cellular glutamine concentration in perfused rat skeletal muscle. *FEBS Lett* 1987; **215**: 187–191.

111. MacLennan PA, Smith K, Weryk B, Watt PW, Rennie MJ. Inhibition of protein breakdown by glutamine in perfused rat skeletal muscle. *FEBS Lett* 1988; **237**: 133–136.

112. Ahlborg G, Felig P, Hagenfeldt L, Hendler R, Wahren J. Substrate turnover during prolonged exercise in man. *J Clin Invest* 1974; **53**: 1080–1090.

113. Bergström J, Fürst P, Holmström B *et al*. Influence of injury and nutrition on muscle water and electrolytes. *Ann Surg* 1981; **193**: 810–816.

114. Stehle P, Zander J, Mertes N, Albers S, Puchstein C, Lawin P, Fürst P. Effects of parenteral glutamine peptide supplements on muscle glutamine loss and nitrogen balance after major surgery. *Lancet* 1989; **i**: 270–272.

115. Vinnars E, Hammarqvist F, von der Decken A, Wernerman J. Role of glutamine and its analogs in posttraumatic muscle protein and amino acid metabolism. *J Parenteral Enteral Nutr* 1990; **14**: 1255–1295.

116. Jackson AA. Optimising amino acid and protein supply and utilisation in the newborn. *Proc Nutr Soc* 1989; **48**: 293–301.

117. Rooyackers OE, Adey DB, Ades PA, Nair KS. Effect of age on in vivo rates of mitochondrial protein synthesis in human skeletal muscle. *Proc Natl Acad Sci USA* 1996; **93**: 15364–15369.

118. Hasten DL, Morris GS, Ramanadham S, Yarasheskii KE. Isolation of human skeletal muscle myosin heavy chain and actin for measurement of fractional synthesis rates. *Am J Physiol* 1998; **275**: E1092–1099.

119. Department of Health. Dietary reference values for food energy and nutrients for the United Kingdom (Report on health and social subjects:41). HMSO, London, 1991.

120. Millward DJ, Rivers JPW. The nutritional role of indispensable amino acids and the metabolic basis of their requirements. *Eur J Clin Nutr* 1988; **42**: 367–393.

121. Young VR, Bier DM, Pellet PLA. A theoretical basis for increasing current estimates of the amino acid requirements in adult man with experimental support. *Am J Clin Nutr* 1989; **50**: 80–92.

122. Windmueller HG, Spaeth AE. Identification of ketone bodies and glutamine as the major respiratory fuels in vivo for post–absorptive rat small intestine. *J Biol Chem* 1978; **253**: 69–76.

123. Fox AD, Kripke SA, De Paula J, Berman JF, Settle RG, Rombeau JL. Effect of glutamine-supplemented enteral diet on methotrexate-induced enterocolitis. *J Parenteral Enteral Nutr* 1988; **12**: 325–331.

124. Frayn KN, Khan K, Coppack SW, Elia M. Amino acid metabolism in human subcutaneous adipose tissue in vivo. *Clin Sci* 1991; **80**: 471–474.

125. Meijer AJ, Lof C, Ramos IC, Verhoeven AJ. Control of ureagenesis. *Eur J Biochem* 1985; **148**: 189–196.

126. Kien GL, Camitta BM. Increased whole-body protein turnover in sick children with newly diagnosed leukemia or lymphoma. *Cancer Res* 1983; **43**: 5586–5592.

127. Goldstein L, Perlman DF, McLaughlin PM, King PA, Cha C-J. Muscle glutamine production in diabetic ketoacidotic rats. *Biochem J* 1983; **214**: 757–767.

128. Newsholme EA, Newsholme P, Curi R, Crabtree B, Ardawi MSM. Glutamine metabolism in different tissues. Its physiological and pathological importance. In: Kinney JM, Borum PM (Eds) *Perspectives in clinical nutrition*. Urban & Schwarzenberg, Baltimore, 1989; pp 71–98.

129. Krebs HA. Regulation of fuel supply in animals. *Adv Enzyme Regul* 1972; **10**: 406–413.

130. Seegmiller JE. Biochemical and genetic studies of an x-linked neurological disease. *Harvey Lect* 1971; **65**: 175.

131. Harper AE. Diet and plasma amino acids. *Am J Clin Nutr* 1968; **21**: 358.

132. Harper AE. Some recent developments in the study of amino acid metabolism. *Proc Nutr Soc* 1983; **42**: 437–449.

133. Asatoor AM, Armstrong MD. 3-Methylhistidine, a component of actin. *Biochem Biophys Res Commun* 1967; **26**: 168–174.

134. Young VR, Haverberg LN, Bilmazes C, Munro HN. Potential use of 3-methylhistidine excretion as an index of progressive reduction in muscle protein catabolism during starvation. *Metabolism* 1973; **22**: 1429–1436.

135. Elia M, Carter A, Bacon S, Winearls CG, Smith R. Clinical usefulness of urinary 3-methylhistidine excretion in indicating muscle protein breakdown. *Br Med J* 1981; **282**: 351–354.

136. Henshaw EC, Hirsch CA, Morton BE, Hiatt HH. Control of protein synthesis in mammalian tissues through changes in ribosome activity. *J Biol Chem* 1971; **240**: 436–441.

137. Iiboshi Y, Papst PJ, Kawasome H, Hosori H, Abraham RT, Houghton PJ, Terada N. Amino acid dependent control of p70 S6 kinase. *J Biol Chem* 1999; **274**: 1092–1099.

138. Long W, Saffer L, Wei L, Barrett EJ. Amino acids regulate skeletal muscle PHAS-I and p70 S6 kinase. *Am J Physiol* 2000; **279:** E301–E306.

139. Yoshizawa F, Kimball SR, Vary TC, Jefferson LS. Effect of dietary protein on translation initiation in rat skeletal muscle and liver. *Am J Physiol* 1998; **275:** E814–E820.

140. Yoshizawa F, Kimball SR, Jefferson LS. Modulation of translation initiation in rat skeletal muscle and liver in response to food intake. *Biochem Biophys Res Commun* 1997; **240:** 825–831.

141. Farrell PA, Fedele MJ, Hernandez J, Fluckey JD, Miller JL. Hypertrophy of skeletal muscle in diabetic rats in response to chronic resistance exercise. *J Appl Physiol* 1999; **87:** 1075–1082.

142. Munro HN. Biochemical aspects of protein metabolism. In: Munro HN, Allison JB (Eds) *Mammalian protein metabolism*. Academic, New York, 1964; p 318.

143. Cahill GF. Starvation in man. *N Engl J Med* 1970; **282:** 668–675.

144. Keys A, Brozek J, Henschel A, Mickelsen O, Taylor HL. *The biology of human starvation*. University of Minnesota Press, Minneapolis, 1950.

145. Wahren J. Extra-hepatic hepatic ammonia metabolism. In: Soeters PB, Wilson JHP, Meijer AJ, Holm E (Eds) *Advances in ammonia metabolism and hepatic encephalopathy*. Elsevier Science, Amsterdam, 1988; pp 121–129.

146. Millward DJ, Price GM, Pacy PJH, Halliday D. Maintenance protein requirements: the need for conceptual revaluation. *Proc Nutr Soc* 1990; **49:** 473–487.

147. Nair KS, Halliday D. Energy and protein metabolism in diabetes and obesity. In: Garrow J, Halliday D (Eds) *Substrate and energy metabolism*. John Libbey, London, 1985; pp 195–202.

148. Millward DJ, Rivers JPW. The need for indispensable amino acids: the concept of the anabolic drive. *Diabetes Metab Rev* 1989; **5:** 191–212.

149. Rennie MJ. Metabolic insights from the use of stable isotopes in nutritional studies. *Clin Nutr* 1986; **5:** 1–7.

150. Watt PW, Corbett ME, Rennie MJ. Stimulation of protein synthesis in pig skeletal muscle by infusion of amino acids during constant insulin availability. *Am J Physiol* 1992; **263:** E453–E460.

151. Barua JM, Wilson E, Downie S, Weryk B, Cuschieri A, Rennie MJ. The effect of alanyl glutamine peptide supplementation on muscle protein synthesis in post-surgical patients receiving glutamine-free amino acids intravenously. *Proc Nutr Soc* 1992; **51:** 115P (Abstract).

152. Albert JD, Legaspi A, Horowitz GD, Tracey KJ, Brennan MF, Lowry SF. Extremity amino acid metabolism during starvation and intravenous refeeding in humans. *Am J Physiol* 1986; **251:** E604–E610.

153. Young LH, McNulty PH, Morgan C, Deckelbaum I, Zaret BL, Barrett EJ. Myocardial protein turnover in patients with coronary artery disease. *J Clin Invest* 1991; **87:** 554–560.

154. Sugden PH, Fuller SJ. Regulation of protein turnover in skeletal and cardiac muscle. *Biochem J* 1991; **273:** 21–37.

155. Heys SD, Park KGM, Garlick PJ, Eremin O. Nutrition and malignant disease implications for surgical practice. *Br J Surg* 1992; **79:** 614–623.

156. Emery PW, Cotellessa L, Holness M, Egan C, Rennie MJ. Different patterns of protein turnover in skeletal and gastrointestinal smooth muscle and the production of N^t-methylhistidine during fasting in the rat. *Biosci Rep* 1986; **6:** 143–153.

157. Woodside KH, Mortimore GE. Suppression of protein turnover by amino acids in the perfused rat liver. *J Biol Chem* 1972; **247:** 6474–6481.

158. Pösö AR, Wert JJ Jr, Mortimore GE. Multifunctional control by amino acids of deprivation-induced proteolysis in liver. *J Biol Chem* 1982; **257:** 12114–12120.

159. McNurlan MA, Garlick PJ. Protein synthesis in liver and small intestine in protein deprivation and diabetes. *Am J Physiol* 1981; **241:** E238–E245.

160. McNurlan MA, Garlick PJ. Contribution of rat liver and gastrointestinal tract to whole-body protein synthesis in the rat. *Biochem J* 1980; **186:** 381–383.

161. Garlick PJ, McNurlan MA, McHardy KC. Factors controlling the disposition of primary nutrients. *Proc Nutr Soc* 1988; **47:** 169–176.

162. Garlick PJ, Burns HJG, Palmer RM. Regulation of muscle protein turnover: possible implications for modifying the responses to trauma and nutrient intake. *Baillière's Clin Gastroenterol* 1988; **2:** 915–940.

163. Melville S, McNurlan MA, McHardy KC, Broom J, Milne E, Calder AG, Garlick PJ. The role of degradation in the acute control of protein balance in adult man: Failure of feeding to stimulate protein synthesis as assessed by L-[1-13C]leucine infusion. *Metabolism* 1989; **38:** 248–255.

164. Volpi E, Mittendorfer B, Wolf SE, Wolfe RR. Oral amino acids stimulate muscle protein anabolism in the elderly despite higher first pass splanchnic extraction. *Am J Physiol* 1999; **277:** E513–E520.

165. Tipton KD, Ferrando AA, Philips SM, Doyle D, Wolfe R. Post-exercise net protein synthesis in human muscle from orally administered amino acids. *Am J Physiol* 1999; **276:** E628–E634.

166. Rasmussen BB, Tipton KD, Miller SL, Wolf SE, Wolfe RL. An oral essential amino acid-carbohydrate supplement enhances muscle protein anabolism after resistance exercise. *J Appl Physiol* 2000; **88:** 386–392.

167. Shaw SN, Elwyn DH, Askanazi J, Iles M, Schwarz Y, Kinney JM. Effects of increasing nitrogen intake on nitrogen balance and energy expenditure in nutritionally depleted adult patients receiving parenteral nutrition. *Am J Clin Nutr* 1983; **37:** 930–940.

168. Bennet WM, Connacher AA, Scrimgeour CM, Smith K, Rennie MJ. Increase in anterior tibialis muscle protein synthesis in healthy man during mixed amino acid infusion: studies of incorporation of 1-[13C]leucine. *Clin Sci* 1989; **76:** 447-454.

169. Gelfand RA, Glickman MG, Castellino P, Louard RJ, DeFronzo RA. Measurement of L-[1-^{14}C]leucine kinetics in splanchnic and leg tissues in humans. Effect of amino acid infusion. *Diabetes* 1988; **37:** 1365–1372.

170. Tischler ME, Desautels M, Goldberg AL. Does leucine, leucyl-tRNA, or some metabolite of leucine regulate protein synthesis and degradation in skeletal and cardiac muscle? *J Biol Chem* 1982; **257:** 1613–1621.

171. Pedersen P, Li S, Hasselgren P-O, LaFrance R, Fischer JE. Administration of balanced or BCAA-enriched amino acid solution in septic rats: Effects on protein synthesis in the liver. *Ann Surg* 1988; **208:** 714–720.

172. Hasselgren P-O, LaFrance R, Pedersen P, James JH, Fischer JE. Infusion of a branched-chain amino acid-enriched solution and α-ketoisocaproic acid in septic rats: Effects on nitrogen balance and skeletal muscle protein turnover. *J Parenteral Enteral Nutr* 1988; **12:** 244–249.

173. Buse MG, Reid SS. Leucine: a possible regulator of protein turnover in muscle. *J Clin Invest* 1975; **56:** 1250–1261.

174. Louard RJ, Barrett EJ, Gelfand RA. Effect of infused branched-chain amino acids on muscle and whole-body amino acid metabolism in man. *Clin Sci* 1990; **79:** 457–466.

175. Morrison WL, Gibson JNA, Rennie MJ. Skeletal muscle and whole body protein turnover in cardiac cachexia: influence of branched chain amino acid administration. *Eur J Clin Invest* 1988; **18:** 648–654.

176. Garlick PJ, Grant I. Amino acid infusion increases the sensitivity of muscle protein synthesis *in vivo* to insulin. *Biochem J* 1988; **254:** 579–584.

177. Flakoll PJ, Kulaylat M, Frexes-Steed M, Hourani H, Brown LL, Hill JO, Abumrad NN. Amino acids augment insulin's suppression of whole body proteolysis. *Am J Physiol* 1989; **257:** E839–E847.

178. Souba WW, Smith RJ, Wilmore DW. Glutamine metabolism by the intestinal tract. *J Parental Enteral Nutr* 1985; **9:** 608–617.

179. Barbul A. Arginine: biochemistry, physiology and therapeutic implications. *J Parental Enteral Nutr* 1986; **10:** 227-237.

180. Saito H, Trocki O, Wang SL, Gonce SJ, Jaffe SN, Alexander JW. Metabolic and immune effects of dietary arginine supplementation after burn. *Arch Surg* 1987; **122:** 784–789.

181. Visek WJ. Arginine needs, physiological state and usual diets. A re-evaluation. *J Nutr* 1986; **116:** 36–46.

182. Gelfand RA, Barrett EJ. Effect of physiological hyperinsulinemia on skeletal muscle protein synthesis and breakdown in man. *J Clin Invest* 1986; **80:** 1–6.

183. Pacy PJ, Nair KS, Ford C, Halliday D. Failure of insulin infusion to stimulate fractional muscle protein synthesis in Type I diabetic patients: anabolic effect of insulin and decreased proteolysis. *Diabetes* 1989; **38:** 618–624.

184. Bennet WM, Connacher AA, Scrimgeour CM, Jung RT, Rennie MJ. Insulin reduces skeletal muscle protein breakdown in uncontrolled Type 1 diabetes. *Clin Physiol* 1988; **6:** 347–356.

185. Bennet WM, Connacher AA, Scrimgeour CS, Jung RT, Rennie MJ. L-[^{15}N]Phenylalanine and L-[1-^{13}C]leucine leg exchange and plasma kinetics during amino acid infusion and euglycaemic hyperinsulinaemia; evidence for stimulation of muscle and whole body protein synthesis in man by insulin. *Proc Nutr Soc* 1990; **49:** 179A.

186. Arfvidsson B, Zachrisson H, Möller-Loswick A-C, Hyltander A, Sandström R, Lundholm K. The effect of insulin on skeletal muscle protein synthesis and breakdown in man. *Clin Nutr* 1989; **8(suppl):** O.72(abs), 46.

187. Kimball SR, Jefferson LS. Cellular mechanisms involved in the action of insulin on protein-synthesis. *Diabetes Metab Rev* 1988; **4:** 773–787.

188. Panniers R, Henshaw EC. A GDP/GTP exchange factor essential for eukaryotic initiation factor 2 cycling in Ehrlich ascites tumour cells and its regulation by eukaryotic initiation factor 2 phosphorylation. *J Biol Chem* 1983; **258:** 7928–7935.

189. Hasselgren P-O, James JH, Benson DW *et al*. Total and myofibrillar protein breakdown in different types of rat skeletal muscle: effects of sepsis and regulation by insulin. *Metabolism* 1989; **38:** 634–640.

190. Morrison WL, Gibson JNA, Jung RT, Rennie MJ. Skeletal muscle and whole body protein turnover in thyroid disease. *Eur J Clin Invest* 1988; **18:** 62–68.

191. Millward DJ, Bates PC, Brown JG *et al*. Physiological mechanisms for the regulation of protein balance in skeletal muscle. In: Kidman AD, Tomkins JK, Morris CA, Cooper NA (Eds) *Molecular pathology of nerve and muscle: Noxious agents and genetic lesions*. Humana Press, New Jersey, 1983; pp 315–342.

192. Southorn BG, Palmer RM, Garlick PJ. Acute effects of corticosterone on tissue protein synthesis and insulin-sensitivity in rats *in vivo*. *Biochem J* 1990; **272:** 187–191.

193. Gelfand RA, Matthews DE, Bier DM, Sherwin RS. Role of counter-regulatory hormones in the catabolic response to stress. *J Clin Invest* 1984; **74:** 2238–2248.

194. Legaspi A, Albert JD, Calvano SE, Brennan MF, Lowry SF. Proteolysis of skeletal muscle in response to acute elevation of plasma cortisol in man. *Surg Forum* 1985; **36:** 16–18.

195. Odedra BR, Millward DJ. Effect of corticosterone treatment on muscle protein turnover in adrenal-ectomized rats and diabetic rats maintained on insulin. *Biochem J* 1982; **204:** 663–672.

196. Odedra BR, Bates PC, Millward DJ. Time course of the effect of catabolic doses of corticosterose on protein turnover in rat skeletal muscle and liver. *Biochem J* 1983; **214:** 617–627.

197. Millward DJ, Odedra B, Bates PC. The role of insulin, corticosterone and other factors in the acute recovery of muscle protein synthesis on refeeding food-deprived rats. *Biochem J* 1983; **216:** 583–587.

198. Zamir O, Hasselgren P-O, Von Allmen D, Fischer JE. The effects of interleukin-1α and the glucocorticoid receptor blocker RU 38486 on total and myofibrillar protein breakdown in skeletal muscle. *J Surg Res* 1991; **50:** 579–583.

199. Almdal TP, Vilstrup H. Exogenous hyperglucagon-aemia in insulin controlled diabetic rats increases urea excretion and nitrogen loss from organs. *Diabetologia* 1988; **31:** 836–841.

200. Nair KS, Halliday D, Matthews DE, Welle SL. Hyper-glucagonemia during insulin deficiency accelerates protein catabolism. *Am J Physiol* 1987; **253:** E208–E213.

201. Wang C, Brennan WA Jr. Rat skeletal muscle, liver and brain have different fetal and adult forms of the glucose transporter. *Biochim Biophys Acta* 1988; **946:** 11–18.

202 Heindorff H, Vilstrup H, Bucher D, Billesboelle P, Thygesen V. Increased hepatic amino nitrogen con-version after elective cholecystectomy in man. *Clin Sci* 1988; **74:** 539–545.

203. Cameron CM, Kostyo JL, Adamafio NA *et al*. The acute effects of growth hormone on amino acid transport and protein synthesis are due to its insulin-like action. *Endocrinology* 1988; **122:** 471–474.

204. Ross RJM, Buchanan CR. Growth hormone secretion: its regulation and the influence of nutritional factors. *Nutr Res Rev* 1990; **3:** 143–162.

205. Pell JM, Bates PC. The nutritional regulation of growth hormone action. *Nutr Res Rev* 1990; **3:** 163–192.

206. Fryburg DA, Gelfand RA, Barrett EJ. Growth hormone acutely stimulates forearm muscle protein synthesis in normal humans. *Am J Physiol* 1991; **260:** E499–E504.

207. Yarasheski KE, Campbell JA, Smith K, Rennie MJ, Holloszy JO, Bier DM. Effect of growth hormone and resistance exercise on muscle growth in young men. *Am J Physiol* 1992; **262:** E261–E267.

208. Fryburg DA, Louard RJ, Gerow KE, Gelfand RA, Barrett EJ. Growth hormone stimulates skeletal muscle protein synthesis and antagonizes insulin's antiproteo-lytic action in humans. *Diabetes* 1992; **41:** 424–429.

209. Takala J, Ruokonen E, Webster NR, Nielsen MS, Zandstra DF, Vundelinckx G, Hinds CJ. Increased mortality associated with growth hormone treatment in critically ill adults. *N Engl J Med* 1999; **341:** 785–792.

210. Bentham J, Rodriguez-Arnao J, Ross RJ. Acquired growth hormone resistance in patients with hyper-catabolism. *Horm Res* 1993; **40:** 87–91.

211. Wilmore DW. Are the metabolic alterations associated with critical illness related to the hormonal environ-ment? *Clin Nutr* 1986; **5:** 9–19.

212. Lundeberg S, Belfrage M, Wernerman J, von der Decken A, Thunell S, Vinnars E. Growth hormone improves muscle protein metabolism and whole body nitrogen economy in man during a hyponitrogenous diet. *Metabolism* 1991; **40:** 315–322.

213. Horber FF, Haymond MW. Human growth hormone prevents the protein catabolic side effects of prednisone in humans. *J Clin Invest* 1990; **86:** 265–272.

214. Wolf RF, Heslin MJ, Newman E, Pearlstone DB, Gonenne A, Brennan MF. Growth hormone and insulin combine to improve whole-body and skeletal muscle protein kinetics. *Surgery* 1992; **112:** 284–291.

215. Hammarqvist F, Stromberg C, von der Decken A, Vinnars E, Wernerman J. Biosynthetic human growth hormone preserves both muscle protein synthesis and the decrease in muscle-free glutamine, and improves whole-body nitrogen economy after operation. *Ann Surg* 1992; **216:** 184–191.

216. Ross RJ, Miell JP, Buchanan CR. Avoiding auto-cannibalism. Consider growth hormone and insulin-like growth factor 1. *Br Med J* 1991; **303:** 1147–1148.

217. Rosen CJ. Growth hormone, IGF-I, and the elderly. Clues to potential therapeutic interventions. *Endocrine* 1997; **7:** 39–40.

218. Gibson EA, Hinds CJ. Growth hormone and insulin-like growth factors in critical illness. *Intensive Care Med* 1997; **23:** 369–378.

219. Butterfield GE, Thompson J, Rennie MJ, Marcus R, Hintz RL, Hoffman AR. Effect of rhGH and rhIGF-I treatment on protein utilization in elderly women. *Am J Physiol* 1997; **272:** E94–E99.

220. Scheiwiller E, Guler H-P, Merryweather J, Scandella C, Maerki W, Zapf J, Froesch ER. Growth restoration of insulin-deficient diabetic rats by recombinant human insulin-like growth factor 1. *Nature* 1986; **323:** 169–171.

221. Tomas FM, Knowles SE, Owens PC, Read LC, Chandler CS, Gargosky SE, Ballard FJ. Increased weight gain, nitrogen retention and muscle protein synthesis following treatment of diabetic rats with insulin-like growth factor (IGF)-I and des(1-3) IGF-I. *Biochem J* 1991; **276:** 547–554.

222. Ferrando AA Anabolic hormones in critically ill patients. *Curr Opin Clin Nutr Metab Care* 1999; **2:** 171–175.

223. Ji SQ, Orcutt MW. Effects of the beta-adrenergic agonist isoproterenol on protein accretion, synthesis, and degradation in primary chicken muscle cell cultures. *J Animal Sci* 1991; **69:** 2855–2864.

224. Martinez JA, Portillo MP, Larralde J. Anabolic actions of a mixed beta-adrenergic agonist on nitrogen retention and protein turnover. *Hormon Metab Res* 1991; **23:** 590–593.

225. Benson DW, Foley-Nelson T, Chance WT, Zhang F-S, James JH, Fischer JE. Decreased myofibrillar protein breakdown following treatment with Clenbuterol. *J Surg Res* 1991; **50:** 1–5.

226. Mantle D, Delday MI, Maltin CA. Effect of clenbuterol on protease activities and protein levels in rat muscle. *Muscle Nerve* 1992; **15:** 471–478.

227. Miles JM, Nissen SL, Gerich JE, Haymond MW. Effects of epinephrine infusion on leucine and alanine kinetics in humans. *Am J Physiol* 1984; **247:** E166–E172.

228. Wernerman J, Botta D, Hammarqvist F, Thunell S, von der Decken A, Vinnars E. Stress hormones given to healthy volunteers alter the concentration and configuration of ribosomes in skeletal muscle, reflecting changes in protein synthesis. *Clin Sci* 1989; **77:** 611–616.

229. Wernerman J, Vinnars E. The effect of trauma and surgery on interorgan fluxes of amino acids in man. *Clin Sci* 1987; **73:** 129–133.

230. Griggs RC, Kingston W, Jozefowicz RF, Herr BE, Forbes G, Halliday D. Effect of testosterone on muscle mass and muscle protein synthesis. *J Appl Physiol* 1989; **66:** E498–E503.

231. Forbes GB, Porta CR, Herr BE, Griggs RC. Sequence of changes in body composition induced by testosterone and reversal of changes after drug is stopped. *JAMA* 1992; **267:** 397–399.

232. Sheffield-Moore M, Urban RJ, Wolf SE *et al.* Short-term oxandrolone administration stimulates net muscle protein synthesis in young men. *J Clin Endocrinol Metab* 1999; **84:** 2705–2711.

233. Ferrando AA, Tipton KD, Doyle D, Phillips SM, Cortiella R, Wolfe RR. Testosterone injection stimulates net protein synthesis but not tissue amino acid transport. *Am J Physiol* 1998; **275:** E864–E871.

234. Griggs RC, Halliday C, Kingston W, Moxley RT. Effect of testosterone on muscle protein synthesis in myotonic dystrophy. *Ann Neurol* 1986; **20:** 590–596.

235. Rennie MJ, Ford C, Halliday D, Dworzak F, Gerber P, Griggs RC, Edwards RHT. Effects of anabolic steroids on muscle protein turnover in muscular dystrophy. *Cardiomiologica* 1989; **1:** 12–23.

236. Griggs RC, Rennie MJ. Muscle wasting in muscular dystrophy: decreased protein synthesis or increased degradation? *Ann Neurol* 1983; **13:** 125–132.

237. Llovera M, Carbo N, Lopez-Soriano J *et al.* Different cytokines modulate ubiquitin gene expression in rat skeletal muscle. *Cancer Lett* 1998; **133 (1):** 83–87.

238. Garcia-Martinez C, Llovera M, Agell N, Lopez-Soriano FJ, Argilles JM. Ubiquitin gene expression in skeletal muscle is increased by tumour necrosis factor alpha. *Biochem Biophys Res Commun* 1994; **201 (2):** 682–686.

239. Mansoor O, Beaufrere B, Boirie Y *et al.* Increased mRNA levels for components of the lysosomal, calcium-activated, and ATP-ubiquitin-dependent proteolytic pathways in skeletal muscle from head trauma patients. *Proc Natl Acad Sci USA* 1996; **93 (7):** 2714–2718.

240. Chang HR, Bistrian B. The role of cytokines in the catabolic consequences of infection and injury. *J Parenter Enteral Nutr* 1998; **22:** 156–166.

241. Short KR, Nair KS. The effect of age on protein metabolism. *Curr Opin Clin Nutr Metab Care* 2000; **3:** 39–44.

242. Welle S, Thornton CA. High-protein meals do not enhance myofibrillar synthesis after resistance exercise in 62- to 75-yr-old men and women. *Am J Physiol* 1998; **274:** E677–E683.

243. Rennie MJ. Muscle protein turnover and the wasting due to injury and disease. *Br Med Bull* 1985; **41:** 257–264.

244. Elwyn DH, Gump FE, Munro HN, Iles M, Kinney JM. Changes in nitrogen balance of depleted patients with increasing infusions of glucose. *Am J Clin Nutr* 1979; **32:** 1597.

245. Jahoor F, Shangraw RE, Miyoshi H, Wallfish H, Herndon DN, Wolfe RR. Roles of insulin and glucose oxidation in mediating the protein catabolism of burns and sepsis. *Am J Physiol* 1989; **257:** E1–E9.

246. Donati L, Signorini M. Nutritional effects of ornithine alpha ketoglutarate in burn patients. *Clin Nutr* 1992; **11:** 25–26 (Abstract).

247. Clowes GHA, George BC, Vilee CA, Saravis CA. Muscle proteolysis induced by a circulating peptide in patients with trauma and sepsis. *N Engl J Med* 1983; **308:** 545–552.

248. Tomkins AM, Garlick PJ, Schofield WN, Waterlow JC. The combined effects of infection and malnutrition on protein metabolism in children. *Clin Sci* 1983; **65:** 313–324.

249. Mitchell LA, Norton LW. Effect of cancer plasma on skeletal muscle metabolism. *J Surg Res* 1989; **47:** 423–426.

250. Arnold J, Campbell IT, Samuels TA *et al.* Increased whole body protein breakdown predominates over increased whole body protein synthesis in multiple organ failure. *Clin Sci* 1993; **84:** 655–661.

251. Hall-Angeras M, Angeras U, Zamir O, Hasselgren P-O, Fischer JE. Effect of the glucocorticoid receptor antagonist RU 38486 on muscle protein breakdown in sepsis. *Surgery* 1991; **109:** 468–473.

3

Energy metabolism

J Webber and IA Macdonald

Introduction

This chapter deals with the basic aspects of energy metabolism, relating to the whole body and to specific tissues, before considering the disturbances which occur in a variety of acute and chronic pathophysiological states. One common cause of confusion in this area relates to terminology, as the utilisation of fuel for energy metabolism is described as energy expenditure, metabolic rate and heat production. These terms do not have identical meanings, but the differences are not of major importance in considerations of energy metabolism in a clinical setting. For convenience, we will mainly use the term metabolic rate (MR) to describe the rate at which energy is being expended in the various metabolic processes. We feel the term thermogenesis should be used to describe the stimulation of MR above basal levels such as occurs in catecholamine stimulated thermogenesis, dietary thermogenesis. The term Basal Metabolic Rate (BMR) is frequently used to describe an individual's preprandial, resting MR. Such use is frequently incorrect, as the BMR should be determined under strictly controlled conditions and was originally used in the diagnosis of thyroid disease. It is far more useful to use the term resting metabolic rate (RMR) and precede it with terms such as fasting, postprandial etc.

Measurement of MR

Energy metabolism can only be sustained by the continuous provision of ATP and other high energy phosphate compounds. The synthesis of these compounds is linked predominantly to the complete oxidation of fatty acids, carbohydrate (mainly glucose) and amino acids (after deamination) to carbon dioxide and water with the release of some heat. As the ATP is utilised, there is additional heat release. Thus, in most situations an individual's MR can be measured from either oxygen consumption and carbon dioxide production, or from the amount of heat produced. These two approaches give rise to Indirect Calorimetry (determining MR indirectly, usually from oxygen uptake and carbon dioxide production) or Direct Calorimetry (estimating heat production by measuring heat loss and body temperature). For clinical purposes, the most appropriate methods of estimating MR are based on indirect calorimetry, and only these will be discussed here.

Respiratory gas exchange

Until recently, the commonest way of measuring gas exchange was to get the subject to wear a valved mouthpiece and noseclip, or a face mask, so that their expired air could be collected in a Douglas Bag or Spirometer. After collecting such air for 4–5 min, the oxygen and carbon dioxide contents are measured and the total volume determined so that gas exchange can be calculated from standard equations. While this technique is still widely used, especially in exercise, it is not ideal for the resting state as the mouthpiece or face mask can change the pattern of breathing[1] and may even increase MR significantly in patients with respiratory disease.[2] With such valved systems, inexperienced subjects tend to hyperventilate, so not only is the MR affected, but also the respiratory exchange ratio (carbon dioxide production/oxygen consumption) is raised, leading to potential errors in estimates of fat and carbohydrate utilisation rates.

A more satisfactory technique for assessing gas exchange in spontaneously breathing subjects is to use the ventilated canopy method originally described by Kinney.[3] This involves placing a perspex hood (or canopy) over the subject's head and drawing room air through at approximately 40 l/min. The dilution of expired air by the ventilating stream of room air means that much greater accuracy is needed in the analysis of oxygen and carbon dioxide concentrations. In addition, the analysers need to be stable over reasonable periods of time (3–4 hours) to allow continuous measurements to be made without frequent recalibration. The system also needs to be able to produce a constant, known flow rate, or have a continuous reliable measurement of flow rate. The latter is best achieved with some form of thermodilution mass flowmeter. The ventilatory stream, canopy and mixing chambers produce a delay of several seconds (usually 10–40 seconds) so it is not necessary to have rapidly responding gas analysers. As the basis of this technique is measuring the difference in gas composition between the ventilatory stream and room air, it is important to have regular measurement of the latter (at intervals of no more than 30 min) or to use differential analysers which simultaneously measure room air and the ventilating stream. The latter type of analyser is very expensive and impractical for clinical purposes. Thus, it is essential to ensure that the equipment being used regularly assesses the gas composition of the room air being inspired by the subject.

The basis of calculating gas exchange and MR from ventilated canopy and Douglas Bag methods is the same, and with both techniques MR can be derived in a variety of ways. One of the simplest methods for deriving MR from such measurements was derived for Douglas Bags by Weir[4] and subsequently used for ventilated canopy measurements.[5] This method has since been revised slightly[6] in the light of more recent estimates of the energy yield from protein oxidation. If one wishes to obtain estimates of substrate oxidation rates it is necessary to determine urinary nitrogen excretion rates at the same time as respiratory gas exchange is measured. Anyone interested in using ventilated canopy techniques to determine MR and substrate oxidation rates should ensure they are satisfied with the basis on which the measurements are made and the calculations performed. Such information is not readily obtainable with some of the commercially available systems, which is not an ideal situation.

In principle MR can be determined in ventilated patients from measurements of gas exchange. The main physiological problem in such patients is the need for a steady state to exist so that any measurements of expired air are a reliable indicator of the metabolic processes. There are also technical problems in measuring changes in oxygen content at high inspired oxygen concentrations, accurately measuring flow rates and correcting for water vapour contents and in ensuring mixed expired gas concentrations are measured.

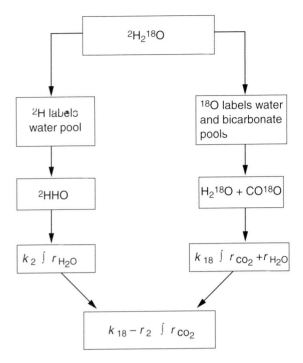

Figure 3.1 – Principle of the doubly-labelled water method. r represents production rates, k represents rate constants measured from the slope of the isotope disappearance curves. Reproduced from Murgatroyd *et al*[8] with permission of The International Journal of Obesity.

Doubly-labelled water method

This involves administering water labelled with deuterium and ^{18}O, and measuring the urinary excretion kinetics of the two tracers over time (usually 10–14 days).[7] The higher a subject's MR, the greater the CO_2 production. As some of the [18]O will end up as CO_2 due to condensation reactions, a greater MR will cause a bigger difference in the urinary excretion of deuterium compared to [18]O (Figs. 3.1, 3.2). In laboratory comparisons with continuous gas-exchange measurements, this method appears valid and reliable[9] and it may be appropriate for assessing MR in some clinical situations, provided a stable state exists over several days.

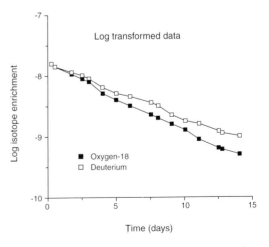

Figure 3.2 – Examples of isotope disappearance curves from a typical adult subject.

Bicarbonate–urea method

With this method labelled CO_2 (given as bicarbonate) is administered to the subject at a constant rate and is diluted by CO_2 produced endogenously by the body. The extent of isotope dilution can be used to measure the rate of CO_2 production (Fig. 3.3).[10] Initial use of labelled bicarbonate to assess energy expenditure relied upon frequent collections of breath samples and subsequent measurement of specific activity ($^{14}CO_2$) or enrichment ($^{13}CO_2$). However, CO_2 production can be more accurately calculated from the specific activity of urinary urea, into which CO_2 is incorporated in the liver. Corrections must be made for the percentage recovery of the label (approximately 95%) and for additional isotopic dilution due to splanchnic CO_2 production and formation of urea from unlabelled arginine (estimated as a correction factor of 0.85). The excretion of urea is more constant than that of bicarbonate and 24-hour collections of urine are easily made. Combining this with continuous subcutaneous infusion of $[^{14}C]$ bicarbonate using a portable infusion pump allows free-living measurements of energy expenditure to be made. The specific activity of urea is used to predict that of expired CO_2, which in turn allows calculation of net CO_2 production. This method appears to give reliable estimates of energy expenditure in free-living healthy subjects when compared with indirect calorimetry over a 24-hour period.[11] This contrasts with the doubly-labelled water method which can only provide accurate estimates over several days. Further studies using this technique in the clinical situation are awaited.

Standardisations of MR measurements and values

When making measurements of MR it is important to standardise the conditions of measurement, and to make some allowance for differences in body size between individuals. Attention should be focused on making measurements under thermoneutral (naked subjects in 29–31°C) or thermally comfortable (lightly clad to 23–25°C) conditions with subjects having fasted for 12 hours and resting supine during measurements. This will provide satisfactory baseline data to then assess responses to food ingestion, drug administration or other test situations. As far as possible, ventilated canopy methods should be used rather than valved mouthpieces and face masks. Care should be taken to ensure that measurements are made in steady state, as short periods of anaerobic metabolism, or alterations in body oxygen or carbon dioxide stores could invalidate the use of respiratory gas exchange to estimate MR.

Standardising the values obtained for an individual's body size and composition, and comparing the values with reference norms is a far more difficult problem. Instinctively, one would argue that values of MR should be standardised to a subject's fat free mass (FFM) as this represents the body's metabolically active tissue. However, differences in the amount of skeletal muscle relative to the vital organs will produce variation in the resting metabolic activity per unit FFM: those with less skeletal muscle would have a higher MR per kg FFM and vice versa. The other problem with standardising MR is that there are errors involved in the estimation of FFM such that if only a single method (e.g. bioelectrical impedance analysis (BIM), skinfold thickness, isotope dilution for body water) is used, substantial variation could arise. Where possible a combination of methods should be used to estimate FFM.

Since the late 1800s, there has been a generalised acceptance of the proposal that resting MR is predominantly determined by an organism's body surface area. This arose initially from studies of dogs performed by Rubner.[12] It is now clear that the 'law'

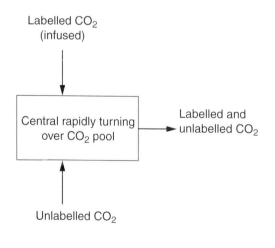

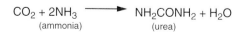

Figure 3.3 – The bicarbonate–urea method.

which developed from this work is seriously limited in its applicability as no account was taken of age or gender, and both affect the relationship between surface area and MR.[13] Nevertheless, it is still common for MR to be related to surface area. When one considers the imprecision of the available estimates of surface area[13] the use of such a method of standardisation is even more surprising.

One of the most important aspects of energy metabolism in relation to clinical practice, is to know whether a patient's MR is normal or not. In order to draw this conclusion, one needs to be able to predict the normal values for the individual. These normal values are usually related to age, gender, height, weight and surface area, or some combination of them. Elia[13] recently undertook a detailed critical analysis of some of the more common predictive equations and showed that the disagreement between the predictions could be in excess of 40% (Table 3.1). Furthermore, with any physiological variable, the variation between individuals is usually so great that the 'normal range' is substantial. The 95% confidence intervals on the normal values for MR can easily be ±15% of the mean. Thus, an individual patient (whose 'normal' state was at one extreme of the normal range) could have a change in MR of 25% and still appear to be normal. Obviously, care needs to be exercised when attempting to evaluate the normality, or otherwise, of a patient's MR. It would be better to make sequential measurements during the disease/recovery process to assess any changes in MR, and to use the values obtained to ensure that the patient received an adequate energy intake. If actual measurements of MR are not readily available, those responsible for meeting a patient's nutritional requirements should pay close attention to the problems inherent in the predictive equations for estimating energy requirements.

Metabolic rate of tissues and organs

The rate of tissue and organ metabolism of a substrate can be calculated from the product of arteriovenous difference in substrate concentration and blood flow. The same is true for tissue and organ MR, except that the 'substrate' is O_2 (or CO_2). Such measurements are only valid when a steady state exists and when blood flow can be measured accurately.

As one would expect, white adipose tissue has a low MR (Table 3.2) when measured *in vivo*[18] and *in vitro*.[19] The majority of measurements have been made on subcutaneous adipose tissue, but there is little reason to believe the other depots are substantially different. Human brown adipose tissue has been studied less frequently (mainly because it is only present in substantial quantities in neonates). The *in vitro* studies on adult human brown adipose tissue have revealed a wide range of MR values, which may be due to varying degrees of mitochondrial uncoupling occurring during the isolation procedure. However, even the lowest rate observed by Cunningham *et al.*[20] is over 30 times higher than the values observed for white adipose tissue. Nevertheless, in most situations there is only a small mass of brown adipose tissue present in the adult, so the contribution to whole body MR is of minor importance in adults. Skeletal muscle has a fairly low MR at rest[21] and potential errors in some of the techniques for assessing muscle blood flow mean that the actual resting MR may be a little lower than the values usually cited.[22] However the large mass of skeletal muscle means that it is likely to account for 20–25% of whole body MR in the resting individual.

The vital organs have the highest values of MR/kg tissue, with the heart not surprisingly the highest and the brain, kidneys and splanchnic bed being rather

Table 3.1 – Comparison of predictive equations for estimating resting MR (MJ/day) of young women of the same height (1.75 m) but different Body Mass Index (BMI) (kg/m²) (Adapted from Elia[13])

BMI	Boothby et al.[14]	Harris & Benedict[15]	Schofield[16]	Owen et al.[17]
15	5.59	5.44	5.10	4.71
30	7.50	7.28	7.72	6.09
45	8.91	9.12	10.34	7.46

Table 3.2 – Estimated tissue metabolic rates (MR) (Values are kJ/kg organ or tissue/day)

Tissue	Reference	MR
White adipose tissue	18, 19	18
Brown adipose tissue	20	600–6000
Skeletal muscle	21	50
Brain	23	1100
Heart	24	2500
Kidney	25	1700
Splanchnic bed	26	1500

similar to each other (Table 3.2). However, these average values should be viewed with caution as there is a substantial range of rates of tissue metabolism in all cases. When the size of each organ is taken into account, the proportional contributions to whole body MR for brain, splanchnic bed and skeletal muscle are each between 16 and 25% in the healthy adult.

Given the high rates of metabolism of the vital organs compared to skeletal muscle, it is readily apparent that whole body MR per unit FFM will be very dependent on the composition of the FFM. Subjects with proportionately more muscle will have a lower MR per kg FFM than those who have a larger mass of the vital organs.

Hormonal control of energy metabolism

The importance of thyroid hormones in energy metabolism has been known for many years; measure-

ments of Basal MR were routinely used in the diagnosis of hyper and hypothyroidism. There is no doubt that gross alterations in thyroid function alter the resting MR, and experimental thyrotoxicosis not only raises resting MR but also enhances the thermogenic response to infused adrenaline.[27] Interestingly, whilst mild hypothyroidism reduces resting MR by 10–15% it does not alter the thermogenic response to adrenaline.[28]

The stimulation of thermogenesis by doses of adrenaline which produce plasma levels within the physiological range, was first demonstrated by Cori & Buchwald.[29] This effect is predominantly, if not exclusively, mediated through β-adrenoceptor stimulation and is enhanced in 48-h starvation[30] and unaffected by 7 days underfeeding[31] (Fig. 3.4). The effect of adrenaline can be mimicked by other catecholamines and sympathomimetics and involves increases in MR in skeletal muscle and the splanchnic bed. The MR of skeletal muscle studied in vitro is reduced by previous β-blockade of the patient and also reduced in women with anorexia nervosa. Furthermore, skeletal

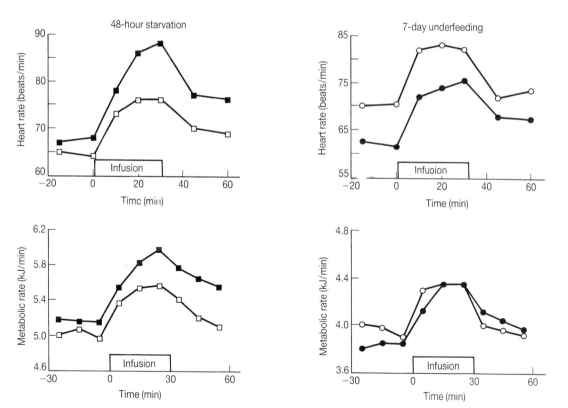

Figure 3.4 – Increases in heart rate and metabolic rate during adrenaline infusions in healthy humans in the overnight fasted state and after 48 hours of starvation. Reproduced from Mansell[30,31] with permission of The American Physiological Society.

muscle MR *in vitro* is positively correlated to thyroid status in haemodialysis patients,[32] indicating an important role for skeletal muscle in resting energy metabolism. The other catabolic stress hormones (e.g. cortisol, glucagon) will also stimulate thermogenesis, and together with a rise in adrenaline may be responsible for some of the hypermetabolism seen after injury/trauma. Recently, the effector system on which these hormones may act to alter energy expenditure has been identified as uncoupling protein-2.[33] This protein is widely expressed in human tissues and serves to uncouple mitochondrial respiration from ATP synthesis, so allowing heat generation to be the only byproduct of this process.

There is also an important effect of insulin on MR. Poorly controlled insulin dependent diabetic patients have an elevated resting MR which is normalised by improving the diabetic control.[34] It is likely this effect is more to do with elevated catabolic hormone levels, rather than the reduced insulin levels, in poorly controlled patients, with a contribution from the elevated plasma levels of the metabolic substrates (glucose, ketones, fatty acids). However, when insulin levels are raised from normal fasting levels by intravenous infusion, but glucose is infused to prevent hypoglycaemia, there is a stimulation of resting MR. Some of this thermogenic response may be blocked by propranolol, indicating a catecholamine-mediated component,[35] but some is undoubtedly due to a direct effect of insulin mediated glucose utilisation.

As with other areas of metabolism, the hormonal control of MR is complex with substantial interaction. Thus, the putative regulators should not be considered in isolation, especially in situations such as injury, trauma and undernutrition where marked changes in several hormones are likely.

Major metabolic processes and MR

Oxidation

It is obvious that as aerobic metabolism is of far greater significance than anaerobic mechanisms in the production of ATP, the oxidation of fat, carbohydrate and deaminated amino acids is of crucial importance for energy metabolism. The energy yield, oxygen consumption and CO_2 production during the oxidation of fat, carbohydrate and protein are listed in

Table 3.3. These figures illustrate the well known phenomenon of fat yielding more than twice as much energy per gram than can be derived from carbohydrate or amino acids. However, another less well recognised phenomenon is also important in that for a given MR, if the energy is derived from fat oxidation there will need to be greater ventilatory oxygen uptake and delivery of oxygen to the tissues than if carbohydrate is the fuel. Any effect of this on respiratory drive may be balanced to some extent by the raised CO_2 production from carbohydrate oxidation, but some thought should be given to such possible effects in patients with respiratory disease or a compromised peripheral circulation.

Table 3.3 – Energy yields, oxygen consumption and respiratory quotient (RQ) for the major nutrients (Values taken from Livesey & Elia[36])

	Energy yield (kJ/g)★★	Oxygen consumption (litres O_2/g)	RQ
Fat	39.50	2.015	0.710
Protein★	19.68	1.010	0.835
Carbohydrate			
Starch	17.48	0.828	1.0
Glucose	15.56	0.747	1.0
Ethanol	29.67	1.459	0.67

(★ Values are metabolisable energy, not gross energy).
★★ kcal = 4.2 × kJ.

The other points worth mentioning are that the values presented in Table 3.3 are rather generalised approximations for 'normal' dietary fat, carbohydrate and protein; there may be some minor numerical changes in some cases for enteral or parenteral feeding preparations. In addition, the values in Table 3.3 are for complete oxidation to carbon dioxide and water (after deamination in the case of amino acids). Any incomplete metabolism, such as ketogenesis from non-esterified fatty acids, gluconeogenesis from amino acids or lactate production from glucose will of course alter the relationship between energy yield, oxygen uptake and CO_2 production until the intermediate product is itself oxidised. If the product is lost from the body (e.g. in ketonuria) or the body stores of the product are not constant during a period of measurement of gas exchange, errors will arise in using indirect calorimetry data to estimate rates of fat, protein and carbohydrate oxidation. The theoretical basis of these errors is beyond the scope of this chapter; readers are directed towards the work of Livesey & Elia[36] and Ferranini[37] for a detailed consideration. However, those primarily concerned with the estimation of MR rather than substrate oxidation rates from indirect calorimetry should be reassured that the errors in the former are substantially less than the latter.

Synthesis

The energy cost of synthesising and storing fat, carbohydrate and protein depends upon the precursors used, especially for fat and carbohydrate. Thus, the cost of storing dietary fat is a small proportion of its energy content (2%) whereas the obligatory energy cost of synthesising fatty acids from glucose, and then storing the fatty acids as triacylglycerol is high (25%). Furthermore, the synthesis of fatty acids from glucose only occurs when carbohydrate intake exceeds daily energy requirements,[38] otherwise the dietary carbohydrate is used as a fuel for energy metabolism, and any fat storage is derived from dietary fat. Similarly, the storage of glycogen depends on whether the precursor is glucose or amino acids, and in the case of glucose whether the direct or indirect pathways are utilised. Recent estimates have suggested that up to 50% of postprandial glycogen storage is from glucose via the indirect pathway[39] (i.e. glucose to lactate then to glucose phosphate then glycogen) which increases the obligatory energy cost of glycogen synthesis from oral carbohydrate from an expenditure of approximately 7% (direct) to 9% (indirect) of the energy stored. If the glycogen is produced through gluconeogenesis from protein, the energy cost would be very high. However, under normal circumstances such net glycogen synthesis from protein is highly improbable.

Indirect calorimetry and respiratory gas exchange can be used to assess net rates of lipogenesis or ketogenesis. Collection of urinary nitrogen excretion to estimate rates of protein oxidation allows the non-protein respiratory quotient to be calculated. Values above 1.0 indicate lipogenesis and below 0.7 ketogenesis. The validity of indirect calorimetry under conditions of lipogenesis has been dealt with by Elia & Livesey[40] who have provided useful tables relating the actual respiratory quotient and oxygen consumption to rates of fat synthesis.

The energy cost of protein synthesis has been estimated at a minimum of 3 kJ for the formation of the peptide bonds for each gram of protein synthesised.[41] As there is substantial daily protein turnover in man (4–5 g/kg body weight/day) the energy cost of this synthesis amounts to approximately 14% of resting MR. Thus, situations in which protein synthesis is reduced (e.g. starvation) or enhanced (e.g. refeeding after weight loss) offer a potential for substantial alteration in MR. The other major synthetic processes (including cell growth and division) also involve the expenditure of substantial amounts of energy. However, these specific situations include the synthesis of fat, carbohydrate and protein and so are very difficult to separate from the energy costs of those individual processes.

Clinical aspects of energy metabolism

Having outlined the basic aspects of energy metabolism and its measurement, the following sections will consider the alterations which commonly occur clinically. In the majority of clinical situations affecting energy metabolism, the net outcome is due to a combination of the clinical event, an inadequate energy intake and enforced immobility. Thus, the metabolic events of starvation are therefore not only of relevance to itself, but also to the injured state, and must be taken into account when interpreting the changes which occur in response to injury and surgery.

Fasting/Starvation

The alterations in energy metabolism which accompany the fasting state were first demonstrated early this century.[42] The body becomes dependent on its own energy reserves and it is the composition of these which plays a major role in determining the subsequent events of starvation. In the average healthy person these reserves comprise 15 kg fat (stored as triglycerides in adipose tissue), 6 kg protein (mainly in muscle) and 0.25 kg carbohydrate (stored as glycogen in the liver and in muscle).[43] Thus, the majority of the body's energy stores are in the form of fat which confers two benefits. Firstly, triglycerides are highly chemically reduced, so the oxidative yield is twice that of carbohydrate and protein. Secondly, carbohydrates and proteins, being relatively polar compounds, are stored in association with water so further reducing their energy content per gram of tissue stored. Using the above values one can calculate that in the average 70 kg man there are 585 000 kJ of fuel in the form of fat, 100 000 kJ as protein and only about 4180 kJ as carbohydrate.

Resting metabolic rate (RMR) is around 100–125 kJ/kg body weight/day. Hence a 70 kg person will expend a minimum of 7000–8750 kJ in a day. In the normally fed state, carbohydrate will provide about half these energy requirements. However, since carbohydrate reserves only amount to 4180 kJ it is obvious that the body must change its energy substrate, for the carbohydrate will last only the first 24 hours of starvation. Rapid changes in substrate utilisation can be seen in the first few days of starvation, the respiratory exchange ratio (RER) falling from above 0.8 to around 0.7, reflecting the increasing use of fat over this time.[44]

Short-term starvation causes a transient small increase in RMR[30,45] (Fig. 3.5) which may be due to the energy costs of gluconeogenesis and ketogenesis, pathways which play an important role in adaptation to this state (see below). However, within a few days metabolic rate falls as a result of three processes: the reduced mass of metabolically active tissue, reduced physical activity, and decreased metabolic activity of the remaining body tissue. These processes reduce the rate at which energy stores are utilised (Fig. 3.6). Whilst there is uncertainty as to how the effects are mediated (changes in the sympathetic nervous system and in thyroid hormones are likely to be important), overall resting MR can fall by 30%.[42] The situation may be different in chronic energy deficiency where energy expenditure per kilogram lean body mass may not be abnormal and indeed may be elevated.[46] However, the proportions of visceral and muscle lean body mass are altered so comparisons are difficult.

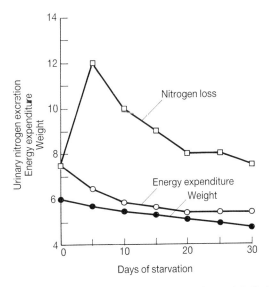

Figure 3.6 – The changes in energy expenditure (MJ/day), urinary nitrogen excretion (g/day) and weight (kg × 10⁻¹) which occur with prolonged starvation. Adapted[57].

The metabolic events of starvation are determined by the body's fuel stores and the tissue specific needs for certain preferred substrates. The brain has an obligatory requirement for glucose as a fuel, at least initially, and uses between 100 and 150 g per day.[47] The brain cannot utilise fatty acids and depends on an increased rate of gluconeogenesis to supply most of its needs once hepatic glycogen stores have been depleted. The balance of cerebral fuel requirements are met by the oxidation of ketones. Other tissues, in particular red blood cells, the lens of the eye and the renal medulla, also have an absolute need for glucose, as they receive their energy needs via the glycolytic pathway. The end products of this, lactate and pyruvate, are reconstituted into glucose in the liver by the Cori cycle with no net loss or gain of glucose, but a substantial energy expenditure through fatty acid oxidation. Gluconeogenesis, mainly from muscle protein, appears to be proceeding at a high rate even within the first day of starvation.[48,49] The liver was felt to be the main contributor to this process, but recent studies have indicated that the kidneys may contribute as much as 50% of whole body gluconeogenesis.[50]

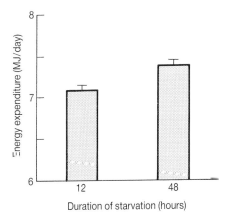

Figure 3.5 – The increase in energy expenditure seen in acute starvation. Adapted from Mansell & Macdonald.[45]

During fasting the most important regulatory signal to the body is the decline in blood glucose which leads to a reduction in insulin levels and an elevation in glucagon. These changes reduce the peripheral utilisation of glucose (preserving it for brain metabolism) and cause increased proteolysis from muscle, leading to an enhanced delivery rate of gluconeogenic precursors to the liver and kidneys.[51,52] In addition, the synthesis of alternative energy substrates (i.e. fatty acids and ketone bodies) for other tissues needs to increase. The decline in glucose and insulin levels leads to enhanced rates of lipolysis from adipose tissue[53,54] and also causes the preferential use of fat over carbohydrate for energy metabolism in muscle, kidney and the liver.[55] Lipolysis, apart from providing fatty acids for oxidation, also supplies a small amount of glycerol for hepatic gluconeogenesis.

The most dramatic change in substrate availability is the increase in plasma levels of ketone bodies, namely acetoacetate and β-hydroxybutyrate. These rise from 0.01 mmol/l to 5 mmol/l by ten days of fasting and plateau at 7 mmol/l after three weeks (Fig. 3.7), at which time their increased production rate is matched by their utilisation.[56] Ketogenesis involves the partial oxidation of fatty acids in the liver with the energy cost of this ketogenesis (and of gluconeogenesis) being provided mainly by the β-oxidation of fatty acids. The utilisation of ketones during the early stages of starvation is mainly dependent on the prevailing plasma concentrations, and occurs in the brain, and skeletal and heart muscle. By 3–4 weeks of starvation in the obese, ketones supply around 50% of the brain's energy needs and this may increase further with longer periods of starvation.[47] By contrast, in skeletal muscle,

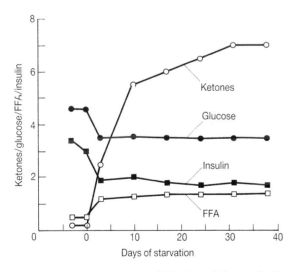

Figure 3.7 – Concentrations of blood total ketone bodies (mmol/l) and glucose (mmol/l), serum insulin (mU/l × 10⁻¹) and plasma free fatty acids (FFA)(mmol/l) in 37 obese subjects during prolonged starvation. From Owen & Reichard[56] with permission of the Israel Journal of Medical Sciences.

although ketones initially account for a considerable proportion of the substrate oxidised, by the second or third week fatty acids become the preferred fuel. These changes provide an alternative energy substrate (ketones) for the brain hence sparing protein by alleviating the need for gluconeogenesis. Any such protein sparing may be rather trivial, as the decrease in protein catabolism matches the reduction in lean body mass and concurrent decline in metabolic rate. Thus, protein catabolism, as measured by the fall in urinary nitrogen excretion during starvation, is seen to parallel the overall fall in energy expenditure.[57]

The fasting person is therefore adapted to burning fatty acids and their ketone derivatives for energy needs. Only the brain continues to oxidise glucose, albeit at a reduced rate. When exogenous glucose is supplied to such individuals endogenous glucose production is suppressed quite rapidly,[58] although the use of fat as the major energy source persists for some time.[59] In addition, in fasted and malnourished patients the provision of carbohydrate in excess of energy requirements leads to extensive lipogenesis.[60]

Modifying effects of disease states

Sepsis / Trauma / Burns

Many of the changes in energy metabolism which occur as a result of either trauma, sepsis, or burn injury are similar, differing mainly in their time course and in their relationship to the severity of the insult. These changes were originally described by Cuthbertson in patients and experimental animals with leg fractures. He proposed the concept of 'ebb' and 'flow' periods following the injury.[61] During the ebb phase immediately after the injury, energy metabolism is depressed (in direct contrast to the initial elevation in metabolic rate which occurs with fasting), and this is followed by a flow phase which is characterised by a hypermetabolic state accompanied by marked negative nitrogen balance. This catabolic state later progresses into an anabolic one as healing occurs. Should recovery not occur, the ebb phase merges into a necrobiotic one[62] and metabolism is further depressed followed by death.

The initial fall in energy metabolism takes place at a time when the so-called stress hormones, in particular adrenaline and glucagon, are rising to the high levels normally associated with increases in metabolic rate.[63] Changes in these hormones lead to the mobilisation of glucose from glycogen and of fatty acids from triglycerides. It has been difficult to demonstrate the existence of an ebb phase in man[64] and if indeed it is a clear entity it may be more related to altered thermoregulation than energy metabolism *per se*.

The flow phase has been more reliably demonstrated and studied in man. Metabolic rate is increased by about 10% above basal postoperatively, by 10–30% following long bone fractures, and by 60–100% in severe burns,[65] although the extent of the elevation may now be less marked than previously, because of modern nursing practices and analgesic strategies. Some of the increase may be accounted for by the rise in body core temperature which accompanies injury. The elevated metabolic rate does not appear to have a thermoregulatory function, because even when patients are cared for in a thermoneutral environment which reduces dry heat losses, these changes remain. This is despite the fact that the immobility and reduced nutritional intake of such patients would otherwise lead to a depressed metabolic state.[66]

The increase in energy metabolism is associated with an array of hormonal responses which occur as a result of the injury.[67] Thus, much of the short-term response can be mimicked by the infusion of catecholamines, cortisol and glucagon.[68] However, the time course of the increased energy expenditure is prolonged far beyond the measured hormonal changes even where these are relatively persistent, as in chronic sepsis. Other humoral factors such as cytokines (e.g. tumour necrosis factor (TNF), interleukin (IL) IL-1 and IL-6) are likely to play a major role in these longer term events. For example, the infusion of TNF raises metabolic rate in healthy subjects,[69] although this effect may be indirect through increased catecholamine secretion.

Increases in energy expenditure have also been well documented as a response to head injury,[70] although in these patients the use of high dose steroids and sedating drugs may modify this increase. The changes found are equivalent to those seen in patients with burns of 20%–40% of their body surface area. Head injury not unexpectedly affects the sympathetic nervous system and correlations are seen between the extent of hypermetabolism and urinary catecholamine excretion.[71] β-blockade has a significant effect in these patients to reduce the elevated metabolic rate. As in other types of trauma much of the metabolic response may be mediated by cytokines.[72]

Considerable changes in substrate turnover occur in association with the alterations in energy metabolism. Rates of glucose, fat and protein turnover are markedly increased, although their utilisation as energy substrates does not directly reflect their plasma levels.[73,74] Marked hyperglycaemia occurs in severe injury, and even in minor trauma blood glucose levels are inappropriately high for the prevailing insulin concentrations. This hyperglycaemia is mainly a result of increased glucose production, the main source of the glucose being amino acids from skeletal muscle catabolism.[75] Despite the potential increase in availability of glucose as an energy substrate, its oxidation (as shown by indirect calorimetry) does not appear much changed. Rather, the role of the elevated glucose appears to be as a substrate for glycolysis, which is the source of energy for many of the cells concerned with inflammation, immunity and healing. Glycolysis occurs at a high rate in the injured patient where the wound uses glucose preferentially for its energy requirements. Studies looking at arteriovenous differences across burned limbs show high glucose uptake with subsequent anaerobic metabolism resulting in net release of lactate. The lactate is then reconverted to glucose in the liver with no net change in glucose, but greatly enhanced turnover.[76]

Fat stores are mobilised with activation of lipolysis from adipose tissue at a rate which greatly exceeds the rate of utilisation of fat in energy metabolism.[77,78] Fat is the major energy source for injured patients, as demonstrated by fasting respiratory quotients less than 0.8,[79] but many of the fatty acids released are re-esterified to triglycerides in the liver in the critically ill.[80] The enhanced rate of substrate cycling of both glucose and fat which accompanies trauma and sepsis may be a major contributor to the hypermetabolism seen in these states,[81] and may be mediated by adrenergic processes since β-blockade reduces triglyceride–fatty acid cycling. However, the net energy costs of substrate cycling (as currently assessed by tracer methodology) account for less than 1% of total energy expenditure in healthy subjects.[82]

In the fasting state, in non-injured individuals, initial raised protein catabolic rates soon abate because of a combination of reduced energy metabolism and the presence of ketones as an alternative energy substrate for the brain. In contrast, following injury, protein breakdown continues at a high rate for the duration of the flow phase. It is tempting to speculate that this continues to provide high rates of glucose production from protein, and also the precursors required for elaboration of cells of the immune system (e.g. glutamine and nucleotides). Hyperglycaemia and hyperinsulinaemia combine to prevent an increase in ketone production, so that any protein sparing effect of ketones is lost.[83,84]

Chronic diseases

In many chronic diseases body composition undergoes significant changes and it is therefore difficult to evaluate the normality or otherwise of the energy expenditure, because there are no adequate control groups for comparison. The role of the disease state *per se* in producing measured changes in energy metabolism is often unclear. In addition to the disease, there will be effects on activity level, energy intake and the presence of coexistent conditions such as acute infections which will further modify the final measured outcome.

The difficulties in interpreting the disparate experimental data are exemplified by studies in patients with liver disease. Several studies have suggested that whereas in acute hepatitis basal energy expenditure is unchanged compared with normal controls, in chronic liver disease a hypermetabolic state may coexist.[85–88] There is however much controversy on this point, both because of the varied nature and severity of the underlying liver disease and because if metabolic rate is expressed per unit body surface area instead of per unit urinary nitrogen excretion no such difference is seen between patients with liver disease and healthy controls. Some of these conflicting results may occur because weight loss in acute disease is mainly due to decreased appetite, whereas in cirrhosis hypermetabolism and changes in body water may also play a part in weight changes.

In acute renal failure, marked hypermetabolism is often seen, but this is probably due to the underlying process (e.g. sepsis, trauma) causing the renal failure rather than being a direct consequence of the renal dysfunction.[89] There is a high incidence of wasting and weight loss in chronic renal disease. The underlying pathology may again contribute to the observed metabolic state, but it would seem that energy expenditure is unchanged from normal.[90,91] The weight loss seen is probably more due to a fall in energy intake rather than an increase in energy expenditure. It may be that on such a reduced intake, energy metabolism is depressed and this may mask an underlying hypermetabolic state.

Changes in substrate usage as well as in energy expenditure occur in many chronic diseases. In patients with cirrhosis, hepatic glycogen stores are depleted and there is a greater reliance on fat as an energy source.[92,93] After an overnight fast in these patients, tracer and indirect calorimetry studies show a pattern of substrate utilisation which is similar to that seen in normal controls after a 36–72 hour fast. In patients with chronic renal failure, as in patients with cirrhosis, resting respiratory quotients are lower than in normal controls. However, the reasons for increased use of fat as a fuel source may differ from those in cirrhosis, with uraemia having inhibitory effects on glucose utilisation.[94]

Malnutrition is marked in many patients with chronic obstructive pulmonary disease (COPD) and leads to worsening of respiratory function because of respiratory muscle weakness. Hypermetabolism has been demonstrated in several groups of patients with emphysema and weight loss,[95,96] although in those with the chronic bronchitic form of COPD this has not been shown. More recently the possible explanation behind these contradictory findings has been described. Patients with COPD had elevated RMR compared with age and height matched controls, but daily energy expenditure was unchanged.[97] Decreases in spontaneous physical activity appeared to account for this finding. Interestingly, 24–hour energy expenditure was also positively related to β_2-agonist use. Whether this increased energy expenditure reflects more severe disease and concomitant sympathetic nervous system activation,[98] or just the effects of the β_2-agonists *per se* is not clear. An increased thermic effect of food may also account for the weight loss in some patients.[98]

Much recent work in the field of energy metabolism has centred on human immunodeficiency virus (HIV) related disease. A number of studies have found an increased level of resting energy expenditure during early HIV infection, and a further elevation with the development of acquired immunodeficiency syndrome (AIDS) and accompanying active secondary infection.[99–102] However, despite these increases in resting energy expenditure, short-term weight loss is not common in early asymptomatic HIV infection[103] and indeed total energy expenditure appears to be normal in these patients.[104] There may therefore be a reduction in the other components of energy expenditure, particularly physical activity. Once secondary infections develop there is often marked weight loss due both to a further elevation in energy expenditure and a decreased energy intake.[103,105]

Utilisation of exogenous nutrients

The provision of exogenous nutrients to sick and malnourished subjects should help improve their clinical outcomes. However, it is not without its attendant risks and the nutrients may not be utilised in the sick patient as they would be in the healthy state. For many years the energy needs of acutely ill patients with burns, sepsis and multiple trauma were overestimated. Raised measured RMR was inappropriately extrapolated to reflect a raised total energy expenditure, despite low activity levels in such patients. Measurements were also performed whilst patients were being fed, thus adding the thermic effects of feeding into RMR. Overfeeding (hyperalimentation) is associated with hepatic steatosis and excess carbohydrate calories can precipitate respiratory failure in those with pre-existing respiratory disease, because of raised CO_2 production.[106] Such patients are normally utilising predominantly fat as an energy source. Substitution of this with glucose will immediately increase CO_2 production, and supplying an excess of glucose will lead to lipogenesis which generates a large amount of CO_2 (the RQ for lipogenesis is approximately 8.0). Energy needs in these patients should be supplied using up to 50% of the energy as fat,[107] but as pointed out earlier, this will require a greater oxygen uptake for the same energy expenditure.

The use of 24-hour indirect calorimetry[108] and more recently doubly-labelled water techniques[109] have demonstrated that total energy expenditure, even in acutely ill patients, is not much changed from that in healthy subjects, basal hypermetabolism being offset by reduced physical activity. RMR can therefore be a good index of total energy expenditure without other factors needing to be added in.[110]

Whilst in the starving subject the provision of glucose leads to its usage as an energy source and decreases endogenous glucose production from protein,[75] after injury there is resistance to these effects of glucose despite an exaggerated insulin response[107] (Fig. 3.8). Even when glucose is provided in excess of energy requirements there is still considerable use of endogenous fat as an energy source as reflected in non-protein respiratory quotients less than 1.[111,112] This is illustrated in Figure 3.8 where a marked difference in fat and glucose utilisation between healthy and septic patients can be seen. Since glucose oxidation is reduced whilst that of fat is enhanced, much of the

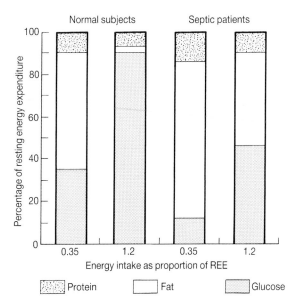

Figure 3.8 – Glucose, fat and protein oxidation in 6 normal subjects and 3 septic patients at low (0.35 × resting energy expenditure) and high (1.2 × resting energy expenditure) glucose intakes given intravenously for 3 days. Adapted.[60]

glucose provided in this situation is converted into glycogen.[113] In addition net lipogenesis may occur, with RQ values above 1 commonly found in patients receiving high rates of glucose infusion.[114] In these patients there is little benefit, and there may be harm, in providing carbohydrate at a rate which exceeds the ability to oxidise it. They should therefore receive up to 55% of their energy intake as fat.[115] In addition, exogenous glucose even in large amounts does not suppress gluconeogenesis in sepsis, but does so in fasting and malnourished subjects.[116,117] When a nitrogen source is provided as part of the nutritional support, protein catabolism still continues, although enhanced protein synthesis reduces the overall negative nitrogen balance.[118]

A number of other strategies have been proposed in order to modify energy expenditure and substrate utilisation in critically ill patients. Growth hormone has been shown to improve nitrogen balance, but does not appear to have any significant effect on fuel utilisation.[119] Medium-chain triglycerides may be more efficiently cleared and oxidised than the long-chain triglycerides found in traditional lipid emulsions.[120] However, neither of these newer nutrition support techniques, nor any others, have yet shown a marked effect on clinical outcome. It remains more important to concentrate on delivering an amount of energy and a fuel mix which meet the patient's ongoing requirements.

References

1. Askanazi J, Silverberg PA, Foster RJ, Hyman AI, Milic-Emili J, Kinney JM. Effect of respiratory apparatus on breathing pattern. *J Appl Physiol* 1980; **48:** 577–580.

2. Sridhar MK, Carter R, Reilly JJ, Banham SW, Lean MEJ. Resting energy expenditure with the ventilated hood and mouthpiece systems in patients with chronic lung disease. *Proc Nutr Soc* 1993; **52:** 6A.

3. Kinney JM, Morgan AP, Domingues FJ, Gildner KJ. A method for simultaneous measurement of gas exchange and expired radioactivity in acutely ill patients. *Metabolism* 1964; **13:** 205–211.

4. Weir JB, de V. New methods for calculating metabolic rate with special reference to protein metabolism. *J Physiol (Lond)* 1949; **109:** 1–9.

5. Fellows IW, Macdonald IA. An automated method for the measurement of oxygen consumption and carbon dioxide excretion in man. *Clin Physiol* 1985; **4:** 349–355.

6. Mansell PI, Macdonald IA. Reappraisal of the Weir equation for calculation of metabolic rate. *Am J Physiol* 1990; **258:** R1347–R1354.

7. Coward WA. The doubly-labelled ($^2H_2^{18}O$) method: principles and practice. *Proc Nutr Soc* 1988; **47:** 209–218.

8. Murgatroyd PR, Shetty PS, Prentice AM. Techniques for the measurement of human energy expenditure: a practical guide. *Int J Obesity* 1993; **17:** 549–568.

9. Ravussin E, Harper I, Rising R, Bogardus C. Energy expenditure by doubly-labelled water: validation in lean and obese subjects. *Am J Physiol* 1991; **261:** E402–E409.

10. Elia M, Fuller NJ, Murgatroyd PR. Measurement of bicarbonate turnover in humans: applicability to estimation of energy expenditure. *Am J Physiol* 1992; **263:** E676–E687.

11. Elia M, Jones MG, Jennings G, Poppitt SD, Fuller NJ, Murgatroyd PR, Jebb SA. Estimating energy expenditure from specific activity of urine urea during lengthy subcutaneous $NaH^{14}CO_3$ infusion. *Am J Physiol* 1995; **269:** E172–E182.

12. Rubner M. Uber den Einfluss der Korpergrosse auf Stoff und Kraft-wechsel. *Z Biol* 1883; **19:** 535–562.

13. Elia, M. Energy expenditure in the whole body. In: Kinney JM, Tucker HN (Eds) *Energy Metabolism: Tissue determinants and cellular corollaries*. Raven Press, NY, 1992, pp 19–59.

14. Boothby WM, Berkson J, Dunn HL. Studies of the energy metabolism of normal individuals: a standard for basal metabolism, with a nomogram for clinical applications. *Am J Physiol* 1936; **116:** 468–484.

15. Harris JA, Benedict FG. A biometric study of basal metabolism in man. Carnegie Institute of Washington, Publication No 279, Washington D.C., 1914.

16. Schofield WN. Predicting basal metabolic rate, new standards and review of previous work. *Hum Nutr Clin Nutr* 1985; **39C:** 5–41.

17. Owen OE, Kavle E, Owen RS *et al.* A reappraisal of the caloric requirements of healthy women. *Am J Clin Nutr* 1986; **44:** 1–19.

18. Coppack SW, Fisher RM, Gibbons GF, Humphreys SM, McDonough MJ, Potts SL, Frayn KN. Post-prandial substrate deposition in the human forearm and adipose tissue *in vivo*. *Clin Sci* 1990; **79:** 339–348.

19. Hallgren P, Sjostrom L, Hedlund H, Lundell L, Olbe L. Influence of age, fat cell weight and obesity on oxygen consumption of human adipose tissue. *Am J Physiol* 1989; **256:** E467–E474.

20. Cunningham S, Leslie P, Hopwood D *et al.* The characterisation and energetic potential of brown adipose tissue in man. *Clin Sci* 1985; **69:** 343–348.

21. Hlavova A, Linhart J, Prerovsky I, Ganz V, Fronek A. Leg oxygen consumption at rest and during exercise in normal subjects and in patients with femoral artery occlusion. *Clin Sci* 1966; **30:** 377–387.

22. Elia M. Organ and tissue contribution to metabolic rate. In: Kinney JM, Tucker HN (Eds) *Energy Metabolism: Tissue determinants and cellular corollaries*. Raven Press, NY, 1992, pp 61–77.

23. Kety SS, Schmidt CF. Nitrous oxide method for quantitative determination of cerebral blood flow in man: theory, procedure and normal values. *J Clin Invest* 1948; **27:** 476–483.

24. Rowe GG, Castillo C, Maxwell GM, Compton CW. Comparison of systemic and coronary hemodynamics in the normal human male and female. *Circ Res* 1959; **7:** 728–732.

25. Crosley AP, Castillo C, Rowe GG. The relationship of renal oxygen consumption to renal functions and weight in individuals with normal and diseased kidneys. *J Clin Invest* 1961; **40:** 836–842.

26. Brauer RW. Liver circulation and function. *Physiol Rev* 1963; **43:** 115–213.

27. Gelfand RA, Hutchinson-Williams KA, Bonde AA, Castellino P, Sherwin RS. Catabolic effect of thyroid hormone excess: the contribution of adrenergic activity to hypermetabolism and protein breakdown. *Metabolism* 1987; **36:** 562–569.

28. Johnson AB, Webber J, Mansell P, Gallen I, Allison SP, Macdonald IA. Cardiovascular and metabolic responses to adrenaline infusion in patients with short-term hypothyroidism. *Clin Endocrin* 1995; **43:** 747–751.

29. Cori, CF, Buchwald KW. Effect of continuous intravenous injection of epinephrine on the carbohydrate metabolism, basal metabolism and vascular system of normal men. *Am J Physiol* 1930; **95:** 71–77.

30. Mansell PI, Fellows IW, Macdonald IA. Enhanced thermogenic response to epinephrine after 48-h starvation in humans. *Am J Physiol* 1990; **258:** R87–R93.

31. Mansell PI, Macdonald IA. Underfeeding and the physiological responses to infused epinephrine in lean women. *Am J Physiol* 1989; **256:** R583–R589.

32. Fagher B. Microcalorimetric studies of resting skeletal muscle thermogenesis in human subjects. MD Thesis, University of Lund, 1988.

33. Fleury C, Neverova M, Collins S *et al.* Uncoupling protein-2: a novel gene linked to obesity and hyper-insulinaemia. *Nature Genetics* 1997; **15:** 269–272.

34. Nair KS, Halliday D, Garrow JS. Increased energy expenditure in poorly controlled Type 1 (insulin-dependent) diabetic patients. *Diabetologia* 1984; **27:** 13–16.

35. Acheson K, Jequier E, Wahren J. Influence of beta blockade on glucose induced thermogenesis in man. *J Clin Invest* 1983; **72:** 981–986.

36. Livesey G, Elia M. Estimation of energy expenditure, net carbohydrate utilisation, and net fat oxidation and synthesis by indirect calorimetry: evaluation of errors with special reference to the detailed composition of fuels. *Am J Clin Nutr* 1988; **47:** 608–628.

37. Ferranini E. The theoretical basis of indirect calorimetry: A review. *Metabolism* 1988; **37:** 287–301.

38. Acheson KJ, Schutz Y, Bessard T, Anantharaman K, Flatt JP, Jequier E. Glycogen storage capacity and de novo lipogenesis during massive carbohydrate overfeeding in man. *Am J Clin Nutr* 1988; **48:** 240–247.

39. Magnusson I, Rothman DL, Taylor R, Price TB, Katz LD, Shulman GI. Rates and pathways of liver glycogen synthesis after ingestion of a mixed meal in humans. *Diabetes* 1992; **41(suppl 1):** 187A.

40. Elia M, Livesey G. Theory and validity of indirect calorimetry during net lipid synthesis. *Am J Clin Nutr* 1988; **47:** 591–607.

41. Waterlow JC, Millward DJ. Energy cost of turnover of protein and other cellular constituents. In: Weiser W, Gnaiger E (Eds) *Energy Transformations in cells and organisms*. Georg Thieme Verlag, Stuttgart, 1990, pp. 277–282.

42. Benedict FG. A study of prolonged fasting. Carnegie Institute Publ. No. **203**, Washington DC, 1915.

43. Cahill GF Jr. Starvation in man. *New Engl J Med* 1970; **282:** 668–675.

44. Cahill GF Jr, Herrera MG, Morgan AP *et al.* Hormone-Fuel interrelationships during fasting. *J Clin Invest* 1966; **45:** 1751–1768.

45. Mansell PI, Macdonald IA. The effect of starvation on insulin induced glucose disposal and thermogenesis in humans. *Metabolism* 1990; **39:** 502–510.

46. Kurpad AV, Kulkarni RN, Sheela ML, Shetty PS. Thermogenic responses to graded doses of noradrenaline in undernourished Indian male subjects. *Br J Nutr* 1989; **61:** 201–208.

47. Owen OE, Morgan AP, Kemp HG, Sullivan JM, Herrera MG, Cahill GF Jr. Brain metabolism during fasting. *J Clin Invest* 1967; **46:** 1589–1595.

48. Rothman DL, Magnusson I, Katz LD, Shulman RG, Shulman GI. Quantitation of hepatic glycogenolysis and gluconeogenesis in fasting humans with ^{13}C NMR. *Science* 1991; **254:** 573–576.

49. Landau BR, Wahren J, Chandramouli V, Schumann WC, Ekberg K. Contributions of gluconeogenesis to glucose production in the fasted state. *J Clin Invest* 1996; **98:** 378–385.

50. Stumvoll M, Welle S, Chintalapudi U, Gutierrez O, Gerich J. Uptake and release of glucose by the human kidney: postabsorptive rates and responses to epinephrine. *J Clin Invest* 1995; **96:** 2528–2533.

51. Felig P, Owen OE, Wahren J, Cahill GF Jr. Amino acid metabolism during prolonged starvation. *J Clin Invest* 1969; **48:** 584–594.

52. Owen OE, Felig P, Morgan AP, Wahren J, Cahill GF Jr. Liver and kidney metabolism during prolonged starvation. *J Clin Invest* 1969; **48:** 574–583.

53. Jensen MD, Haymond MW, Gerich JE, Cryer PE, Miles JM. Lipolysis during fasting; decreased suppression by insulin and increased stimulation by epinephrine. *J Clin Invest* 1987; **79:** 207–213.

54. Klein S, Holland B, Wolfe RR. Importance of blood glucose concentration in regulating lipolysis during fasting in humans. *Am J Physiol* 1990; **258 (Endocrinol. Metab. 21):** E32–E39.

55. Randle PJ, Garland PB, Hales CN, Newsholme EA. The glucose and fatty acid cycle: Its role in insulin sensitivity and the metabolic disturbances of diabetes mellitus. *Lancet* 1963; **i:** 785–789.

56. Owen OE, Reichard GA Jr. Ketone body metabolism in normal, obese and diabetic subjects. *Israel J Med Sci* 1975; **11:** 560–570.

57. Henry CJK, Rivers JPW, Payne PR. Protein and energy metabolism in starvation reconsidered. *Eur J Clin Nutr* 1988; **42:** 543–549.

58. Long CL, Spencer JL, Kinney JM, Geiger JW. Carbohydrate metabolism in normal man and effect of glucose infusion. *J Appl Physiol* 1971; **31:** 102–109.

59. Elwyn DH, Kinney JM, Gump FE, Jeevanandam M, Chikenji T, Askanazi J. Metabolic and endocrine effects of fasting followed by infusion of five-percent glucose. *Surgery* 1981; **90:** 810–816.

60. Elwyn DH. The unique role of glucose in artificial nutrition: Impact of injury and malnutrition. *Clin Nutr* 1988; **7:** 195–202.

61. Cuthbertson DP. Post-shock metabolic response. *Lancet* 1942; **i:** 433–437.

62. Stoner HB. Energy metabolism after injury. In: Sevitt S, Stoner HB (Eds) *The pathology of trauma*. Royal College of Pathologists, London, 1970, pp. 47–55.

63. Frayn KN, Little RA, Maycock PF, Stoner HB. The relationship between plasma catecholamines to acute metabolic and hormonal responses to injury in man. *Circ Shock* 1985, **16:** 229–240.

64. Little RA, Stoner HB, Frayn KN. Substrate oxidation shortly after accidental injury in man. *Clin Sci* 1981; **61:** 789–791.

65. Kinney JM, Duke JH Jr., Long CL, Gump FE. Tissue fuel and weight loss after injury. *J Clin Path* 1970; **23 (Suppl. 4):** 65–72.

66. Bursztein S, Elwyn DH, Askanazi J, Kinney JM. Energy metabolism, indirect calorimetry, and nutrition. Williams & Wilkins, Baltimore, 1989.

67. Wilmore DW, Long JM, Mason AD, Skreen RW, Pruitt BA Jr. Catecholamines: Mediator of the hypermetabolic response to thermal injury. *Ann Surg* 1974; **180:** 653–669.

68. Bessey PQ, Watters JM, Aoki TT, Wilmore DW. Combined hormonal infusion simulates the metabolic response to injury. *Ann Surg* 1984; **200:** 264–281.

69. Van Der Poll T, Romijn JA, Endert E, Borm JJJ, Buller HR, Sauerwein HP. Tumor necrosis factor mimics the metabolic response to acute infection in healthy humans. *Am J Physiol* 1991; **261 (Endocrinol. Metab. 24):** E457–E465.

70. Clifton GL, Robertson CS, Grossman RG, Hodge S, Foltz R, Garza C. The metabolic response to severe head injury. *J Neurosurg* 1984; **60:** 687–696.

71. Chiolero RL, Breitenstein E, Thorin D *et al.* Effects of propranolol on resting metabolic rate after severe head injury. *Crit Care Med* 1989; **17:** 328–334.

72. McClain C, Cohen D, Phillips R, Ott L, Young B. Increased plasma and ventricular fluid interleukin-6 levels in patients with head injury. *J Lab Clin Med* 1991; **118:** 225–231.

73. Wolfe RR, Durkot MJ, Allsop JR, Burke JF. Glucose metabolism in severely burned patients. *Metabolism* 1979; **28:** 1031–1039.

74. Galster AD, Bier DM, Cryer PE, Monafo WW. Plasma palmitate turnover in subjects with thermal injury. *J Trauma* 1984; **24:** 938–945.

75. Long CL, Spencer JL, Kinney JM, Geiger JW. Carbohydrate metabolism in man: effect of elective operations and major injury. *J Appl Physiol* 1971; **31:** 110–116.

76. Wilmore DW, Aulick LH, Mason AD Jr., Pruitt BA Jr. Influence of the burn wound on local and systemic responses to injury. *Ann Surg* 1977; **186:** 444–458.

77. Carpentier YA, Askanazi J, Elwyn DH *et al.* Effects of hypercaloric glucose infusion on lipid metabolism in injury and sepsis. *J Trauma* 1979; **19:** 649–654.

78. Shaw JHF, Wolfe RR. Response to glucose and lipid infusions in sepsis: A kinetic analysis. *Metabolism* 1985; **34:** 442–449.

79. Stoner HB, Little RA, Frayn KN, Elebute AE, Tresadern J, Gross E. The effect of sepsis on the oxidation of carbohydrate and fat. *Br J Surg* 1983; **70:** 32–35.

80. Klein S, Peters EJ, Shangraw RE, Wolfe RR. Lipolytic response to stress in critically ill patients. *Crit Care Med* 1991; **19:** 776–779.

81. Wolfe RR, Herndon DN, Jahoor F, Miyoshi H, Wolfe M. Effect of severe burn injury on substate cycling by glucose and fatty acids. *N Eng J Med* 1987; **317:** 403–408.

82. Wolfe RR. Assessment of substrate cycling in humans using tracer methodology. In: Kinney JM, Tucker HN (eds) *Energy metabolism: Tissue determinants and cellular corollaries*. Raven Press, New York, 1992, pp. 507–517.

83. Birkhahn RH, Long CL, Fitkin DL, Busnardo AC, Geiger JW, Blakemore WS. A comparison of the effects of skeletal trauma and surgery on the ketosis of starvation in man. *J Trauma* 1981; **21:** 513–519.

84. Hartl WH, Jauch KW, Kimmig R, Wicklmayr M, Gunther B, Heberer G. Minor role of ketone bodies in energy metabolism by skeletal muscle tissue during the post-operative course. *Ann Surg* 1988, **207:** 95–101.

85. Shanbhogue RLK, Bistrian BR, Jenkins RL, Jones C, Benotti P, Blackburn GL. Resting energy expenditure in patients with end-stage liver disease and in normal population. *J Parenter Enteral Nutr* 1987; **11:** 305–308.

86. Schneeweiss B, Graninger W, Ferenci P *et al.* Energy metabolism in patients with acute and chronic liver disease. *Hepatology* 1990; **11:** 387–393.

87. Green JH, Bramley PN, Losowsky MS. Are patients with primary biliary cirrhosis hypermetabolic? A comparison between patients before and after liver transplantation and controls. *Hepatology* 1991; **14**: 464–472.

88. Muller MJ, Fenk A, Lautz HU *et al.* Energy expenditure and substrate metabolism in ethanol-induced liver cirrhosis. *Am J Physiol* 1991; **260 (Endocrinol. Metab. 23)**: E338–E344.

89. Hirschberg RR, Kopple JD. Energy requirements in patients with renal failure. In: Albertazzi A, Cappelli P, Di Paulo B, Evangelista M & Palmieri PF (eds) *Nutritional and pharmacological strategies in chronic renal failure*. Contrib. Nephrol. Karger, Basel, 1990; **81**: 124–135.

90. Monteon FJ, Laidlaw SA, Shaib JK, Kopple JD. Energy expenditure in patients with chronic renal failure. *Kidney Int* 1986; **30**: 741–747.

91. Schneeweiss B, Graninger W, Stockenhuber F *et al.* Energy metabolism in acute and chronic renal failure. *Am J Clin Nutr* 1990; **52**: 596–601.

92. Owen OE, Reichle FA, Mozzoli MA *et al.* Hepatic, gut, and renal substrate flux rates in patients with hepatic cirrhosis. *J Clin Invest* 1981; **68**: 240–252.

93. Owen OE, Trapp VE, Reichard GA Jr, *et al.* Nature and quantity of fuels consumed in patients with alcoholic cirrhosis. *J Clin Invest* 1983; **72**: 1821–1832.

94. Kalhan SC, Ricanati ES, Tserng KY, Savin SM. Glucose turnover in chronic uraemia: increased recycling with dimished oxidation of glucose. *Metabolism* 1983; **32**: 1155–1162.

95. Goldstein SA, Thomashow BM, Kvetan V, Ashkanazi J, Kinney JM, Elwyn DH. Nitrogen and energy relationships in malnourished patients with emphysema. *Am Rev Respir Dis* 1988; **138**: 636–644.

96. Green JH, Muers MF. The thermic effect of food in underweight patients with emphysematous chronic obstructive pulmonary disease. *Eur Respir J* 1991; **4**: 813–819.

97. Hugli O, Schutz Y, Fitting J-W. The daily energy expenditure in stable chronic obstructive pulmonary disease. *Am J Respir Crit Care Med* 1996; **153**: 294–300.

98. Hofford JM, Milakosky L, Vogel WH, Sacher RS, Savage GJ, Pell S. The nutritional status in advanced emphysema associated with chronic bronchitis. *Am Rev Respir Dis* 1990; **141**: 902–908.

99. Hommes MJT, Romijn JA, Godfried MH, Schattenkerk JKME, Buurman WA, Endert E, Sauerwein HP. Increased resting energy expenditure in human immunodeficiency virus-infected men. *Metabolism* 1990; **39**: 1186–1190.

100. Melchior J-C, Salmon D, Rigaud D *et al.* Resting energy expenditure is increased in stable, malnourished HIV-infected patients. *Am J Clin Nutr* 1991; **53**: 437–441.

101. Hommes MJT, Romijn JA, Endert E, Sauerwein HP. Resting energy expenditure and substrate oxidation in human immunodeficiency virus (HIV)-infected asymtomatic men: HIV affects host metabolism in the early asymptomatic stage. *Am J Clin Nutr* 1991; **54**: 311–315.

102. Melchior J-C, Raguin G, Boulier A *et al.* Resting energy expenditure in human immunodeficiency virus-infected patients: comparison between patients with and without secondary infections. *Am J Clin Nutr* 1993; **57**: 614–619.

103. Grunfeld C, Pang M, Shimizu L, Shigenaga JK, Jensen P, Feingold KR. Resting energy expenditure, caloric intake, and short-term weight change in human immunodeficiency virus infection and the acquired immunodeficiency syndrome. *Am J Clin Nutr* 1992; **55**: 455–460.

104. Paton NIJ, Elia M, Jebb SA, Jennings G, Macallan DC, Griffin GE. Total energy expenditure and physical activity measured with the bicarbonate-urea method in patients with human immunodeficiency virus infection. *Clin Sci* 1996; **91**: 241–245.

105. Grunfeld C, Feingold KR. Metabolic disturbances and wasting in the acquired immunodeficiency syndrome. *N Engl J Med* 1992; **327**: 329–337.

106. Askanazi J, Nordenstrom J, Rosenbaum SH, Elwyn DH, Hyman AI, Carpentier YA, Kinney JM. Nutrition for the patient with respiratory failure: Glucose vs. fat. *Anesthesiology* 1981; **54**: 373–377.

107. Wolfe RR, O'Donnell TF Jr., Stone MD, Richmand DA, Burke JF. Investigation of factors determining the optimal glucose infusion rate in total parenteral nutrition. *Metabolism* 1980; **29**: 892–900.

108. Carlsson M, Nordenstrom S, Hedenstierna G. Clinical implications of continuous measurement of energy expenditure in mechanically ventilated patients. *Clin Nutr* 1984; **3**: 103–110.

109. Pullicino E, Coward WA, Elia M. Total energy expenditure in intravenously fed patients measured by the doubly-labelled water technique. *Metabolism* 1992; **42**: 58–64.

110. Frankenfield DC, Wiles CE, Bagley S, Siegel JH. Relationships between resting and total energy expenditure in injured and septic patients. *Crit Care Med* 1994; **22**: 1796–1804.

111 Askanazi J, Carpentier YA, Elwyn DH *et al.* Influence of total parenteral nutrition on fuel utilization in injury and sepsis. *Ann Surg* 1980; **191**: 40–46.

112. Jeevanandam M, Young GH, Schiller WR. Influence of parenteral nutrition on rates of net substrate

oxidation in severe trauma patients. *Crit Care Med* 1990; **18:** 467–473.

113. Elwyn DH, Kinney JM, Jeevanandam M, Gump FE, Broell JR. Influence of increasing carbohydrate intake on glucose kinetics in injured patients. *Ann Surg* 1979; **190:** 117–127.

114. Guenst JM, Nelson LD. Predictors of total parenteral nutrition-induced lipogenesis. *Chest* 1994; **105:** 553–559.

115. Schneeweiss B, Graninger W, Ferenci P *et al.* Short-term energy balance in patients with infections: Carbohydrate-based versus fat-based diets. *Metabolism* 1992; **41:** 125–130.

116. Long CL, Kinney JM, Geiger JW. Nonsuppressability of gluconeogenesis by glucose in septic patients. *Metabolism* 1976; **25:** 193–201.

117. Long CL, Schiller WR, Geiger JW, Blakemore WS. Gluconeogenic response during glucose infusions in patients following skeletal trauma or during sepsis. *J Parent Enteral Nutr* 1978; **2:** 619–626.

118. Shaw JHF, Wolfe RR. An integrated analysis of glucose, fat, and protein metabolism in severely traumatized patients. *Ann Surg* 1989; **209:** 63–72.

119. Voerman BJ, Strack van Schijndel RJM, de Boer H, Groeneveld ABJ, Nauta JP, van der Veen EA, Thijs LG. Effects of human growth hormone on fuel utilization and mineral balance in critically ill patients on full intravenous nutritional support. *Metabolism* 1994; **9:** 143–150.

120. Jeevanandam M, Holaday NJ, Voss T, Buier R, Petersen SR. Efficacy of a mixture of medium-chain triglyceride (75%) and long-chain triglyceride (25%) fat emulsions in the nutritional management of multiple trauma patients. *Nutrition* 1995; **11:** 275–284.

4

The liver and nutrient metabolism

Roy A Sherwood

Introduction

The liver has a central role in the regulation of the metabolism of nutrients. Via bile formation, it contributes to the process of digestion and absorption. Nutrients absorbed from the gastrointestinal tract reach the liver via the portal circulation where they can be processed or stored. Most of the amino acids, carbohydrates and lipids absorbed undergo biochemical transformation in the liver before distribution to other tissues. Variations in dietary intake and the body's metabolic demands govern whether the liver processes nutrients for immediate use by other tissues or metabolises them to storage products. It serves as a store for carbohydrates in the form of glycogen and also for the fat-soluble vitamins A, D, E and K and vitamin B_{12}.

The liver is responsible for the synthesis of the majority of the circulating plasma proteins, including essential components of the coagulation system and the proteolytic enzyme inhibitor family of proteins. To achieve these varied functions the liver utilises a proportion of the nutrients to provide energy for its own macromolecular synthesis, cellular transport mechanisms and chemical transformations. Inevitably, considering the liver's prominent role in regulating the overall metabolism of the body, damage to hepatocytes through disease or by toxins causes major perturbations in many metabolic systems. Malnutrition is relatively common in patients with alcohol-induced liver disease and was originally thought to be related to poor diets associated with alcohol misuse.[1-3] It is now recognised that malnutrition is encountered in non-alcohol induced chronic liver disease and is multifactorial in its aetiology.[4,5]

Two specific areas in which nutrition plays a vital role in liver disease are the interaction between protein intake and hepatic encephalopathy[6] and the optimal nutrient intake for promotion of hepatic regeneration following hepatocellular necrosis or partial hepatectomy.[7] This chapter reviews the basic functions and mechanisms of the liver in the process of nutrient metabolism and the alterations encountered in liver disease.

Basic aspects of nutrient metabolism in the liver

Liver and energy metabolism

In order to maintain the viability of cells, a ready supply of oxidisable substrates is required for the formation of high-energy bonds. Energy supplies for the liver itself derive from fatty acids and glycerol from adipose tissue, lactate and pyruvate from skeletal muscles and alanine and certain β-keto acids from skeletal muscle produced by transamination. The liver exports two principal substrates which are oxidisable in peripheral tissues: glucose and acetoacetate (or its reduced derivative β-hydroxybutyrate). The rate of production of these substrates in the liver and their release into the circulation are dependent on a number of factors, including the endocrine system, the amount and nature of available dietary substrates and the overall energy requirements of the body.

Carbohydrate metabolism in the liver

The complex carbohydrates in the diet are mostly broken down by pancreatic and duodenal brush border enzymes to yield monosaccharides. Glucose, galactose and fructose absorbed from the gastrointestinal tract are avidly taken up by the liver via the portal circulation. The liver plays a vital role in carbohydrate metabolism as it is capable of utilising monosaccharides for immediate energy release by their incorporation into the citric acid cycle or can store them in the form of glycogen. During fasting, glucose can be released from hepatic glycogen stores by glycogenolysis, unlike muscle glycogen which does not release glucose into the circulation. In prolonged fasting the liver utilises non-carbohydrate substrates to produce glucose by gluconeogenesis, i.e. lactate, pyruvate, glycerol, propionate, alanine and other amino acids. The amino acids required for gluconeogenesis are derived from catabolism of muscle proteins, thus highlighting the interaction between the liver's roles in both carbohydrate and protein metabolism. In the fed state, the liver replenishes the muscle stores by directing alanine and the branched-chain amino acids (BCAA) to peripheral tissues for incorporation into muscle protein. These reciprocal pathways form a glucose–alanine shuttle which is modulated by dietary glucose intake and hormonal influences.

The balance in the liver of storage or production of glucose controls the blood glucose concentration within a narrow range. The key hormones regulating carbohydrate homeostasis act mainly on the liver. These include insulin, glucagon, growth hormone, glucocorticoids, catecholamines and thyroxine, all of which, except catecholamines, are also catabolised by the liver. Of these, insulin and glucagon are the most important and in the fasting state the liver contributes

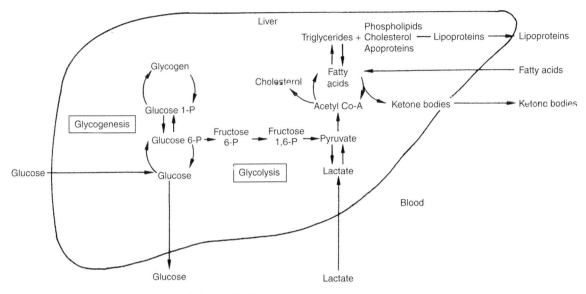

Figure 4.1 – Carbohydrate and lipid metabolism in the liver.

glucose by glycogenolysis and gluconeogenesis in response to hypoinsulinaemia and hyperglucagon-aemia.

Lipid metabolism in the liver

The liver has a major role in the synthesis, catabolism and biliary excretion of lipids, lipoproteins, phospholipids and enzymes involved in their metabolism. Neutral fats absorbed from the gastrointestinal tract are oxidised within the liver to form glycerol and free fatty acids. There is a continual exchange mechanism for free fatty acids between the liver and adipose tissue. Fatty acids in the liver may be further oxidised to acetyl coenzyme A (CoA) which can then enter the Krebs' tricarboxylic acid cycle. Alternatively, free fatty acids can be esterified to form triglycerides or other esters. In the fasting state, fatty acid synthesis is inhibited and oxidation of fatty acids occurs in preference to esterification, whilst in the fed state the reverse is true.

Cholesterol can be derived from acetate via its conversion to β-hydroxy-methylglutaryl CoA (HMG-CoA) if hepatic uptake of cholesterol from dietary sources in chylomicron remnants is sufficient to meet the body's requirements. Cholesterol and phospholipids are constituents of cell membranes and in combination with triglycerides form the circulating lipoproteins. Cholesterol is required for bile acid synthesis. Factors that regulate hepatic cholesterol synthesis include dietary cholesterol absorption, bile

acid homeostasis and the recycling of cholesterol from lipoprotein catabolism.

Protein and amino acid metabolism in the liver

Amino acid metabolism in the body is primarily controlled by the liver with contributions from peripheral tissues, particularly muscle. Following a protein meal, the amino acids absorbed from the intestine are rapidly taken up by the liver. These may be utilised in protein synthesis, gluconeogenesis or ketogenesis following deamination or transamination. Urea is the final end-product of amino acid metabolism, either formed directly from the breakdown of amino acids or via the ammonia formed during the deamination process. A classic study in dogs indicated the relative proportions of an absorbed amino acid load which were utilised for the above-mentioned purposes.[8] Although peripheral tissues require amino acids to replenish stores consumed during the fasting state, only 25% of the absorbed amino acids enter the circulation. A small proportion (6%) are utilised for the formation of plasma proteins and about 14% of the amino acid load is incorporated into proteins remaining within the liver itself. The bulk of the absorbed amino acids, however, end up as urea (57%).

The liver is the main site of catabolism for seven of the essential amino acids; the remaining three (the branched-chain amino acids, BCAA) are catabolised mainly in the peripheral muscles and the kidneys. Hepatic catabolism of amino acids is directly related to concentration. This has been clearly demonstrated for valine, leucine, lysine and threonine where the rate of hepatic catabolism rises sharply at the point where dietary supply exceeds the body's requirements, which coincides with the point where further dietary intake will raise the peripheral plasma concentration of these amino acids.[9] Regulation of amino acid homeostasis in the liver is influenced not only by dietary supply and tissue requirements but also by various hormones. Amino acids themselves stimulate insulin and adrenal corticosteroids and are, therefore, anabolic in nature.[10]

The liver produces the majority of the circulating plasma proteins, with the exception of the immunoglobulins (Table 4.1). Quantitatively, albumin is the most important of these but many other types of circulating proteins are synthesised in the liver including carrier proteins, proteolytic enzyme inhibitors and acute-phase proteins.[11] Other important proteins are those involved in the coagulation system. Fibrinogen, prothrombin and factors V, VII, IX, X, and to some extent factor VIII, are made in the liver. Conversely, inhibitors of the coagulation system, such as antithrombin III, are also synthesised in the liver. Protein synthesis occurs on polyribosomes bound to the rough endoplasmic reticulum (RER) within the hepatocytes, which comprise approximately 60% of the total cell population of the liver. Some of the albumin destined for release into the circulation is synthesised as preproalbumin containing 24 additional amino acids at the N-terminal end. The hydrophobic 'pre' portion is removed within the RER during the process of translocation. The 'pro' segment of six amino acids is removed post translocation.

Mechanisms for the regulation of hepatic plasma protein synthesis exist at various stages of the synthetic process.[12] Falls in the plasma concentration of specific proteins may reflect a decrease in synthesis or consumption of the protein at a rate greater than the maximal rate of hepatic production, e.g. haptoglobin following intravascular haemolysis. The liver is also involved in the clearance of many plasma proteins from the circulation.

Vitamin metabolism and the liver

The liver plays a vital role in the uptake, storage, metabolism and transport of both water-soluble and fat-soluble vitamins. Hepatocytes and Ito cells are involved in vitamin A metabolism and the liver acts as the storage reservoir for this vitamin. Many of the B vitamins, including thiamine, riboflavin, niacin, B_{12}, B_6, folic acid and pantothenic acid, are metabolised in the liver and are themselves essential components in various aspects of hepatic metabolism. Vitamin K is an essential requirement for the synthesis of the clotting factors and protein C and S. Absorption of the fat-soluble vitamins is dependent on normal bile production and secretion. Vitamin D is metabolised in the liver to 25-hydrocholecalciferol which is the prominent circulating form of this vitamin.

Table 4.1 – Plasma proteins secreted by the liver

Protein	Molecular weight	Principal function	Plasma concentration (g/l)
Albumin	66 000	Binding and carrier protein, osmotic regulator	35–50
α_1-antiprotease inhibitor	54 000	Elastase and trypsin inhibitor	1.0–2.0
α_2-macroglobulin	720 000	General protease inhibitor	1.5–4.0
Antithrombin III	65 000	Protease inhibitor of intrinsic coagulation system	0.15–0.3
Caeruloplasmin	134 000	Copper transport	0.15–0.6
C-reactive protein	105 000	Acute-phase reactant	<0.1
Fibrinogen	340 000	Fibrin precursor	2.0–4.5
Haptoglobin	100 000	Removal of free haemoglobin	0.8–1.8
Transferrin	80 000	Iron transport	2.0–4.0
Vitamin D binding protein	51 000	Vitamin D binding	0.3–0.35

Metabolic disturbances arising from disorders of the liver

Liver disease may cause disturbances in the metabolism of all nutrients or groups of nutrients or may itself be a consequence of altered metabolism of a specific compound or group of compounds due to an inborn error of metabolism. Detailed discussion of the latter case is beyond the scope of this chapter but specific examples will be given where appropriate.

Malnutrition

Malnutrition is a relatively common finding in patients with advanced liver disease. The majority of the early studies on the prevalence of malnutrition in liver disease were based on patients with alcohol-related liver damage and evidence of malnutrition was present in 40–60% of subjects.[3,13] The available data on the prevalence of malnutrition in non-alcohol related liver disease have now expanded and it is clear that it is a feature of liver disease generally. Fat-soluble vitamin deficiencies were observed in 40% of patients with cryptogenic cirrhosis[4] and 40% of patients with primary biliary cirrhosis and 12% of hepatitis patients were observed to be malnourished.[14] As orthotopic liver transplantation has become an accepted treatment for advanced liver disease the pre-transplant patient assessment has revealed significant loss of muscle mass in the majority of patients being assessed for transplantation for end-stage liver failure.[15] Pre-existing malnutrition at the time of transplantation is a poor prognostic factor for survival.[16] Alterations in specific metabolites may be more significant than overall nutritional state.

Carbohydrate metabolism

Abnormalities of glucose homeostasis are common in chronic liver disease, with both hypo- and hyper-glycaemia occurring regularly.[17] In the adult patient hyperglycaemia and glucose intolerance are frequently observed, associated with normal or increased circulating insulin concentrations in both the fasting state and following oral glucose loads, suggesting that insulin resistance rather than deficiency is the mechanism.[18]

Circulating C-peptide concentrations are increased following oral glucose administration, suggesting that the β-cell response of the pancreas is enhanced in

cirrhosis.[19] Impaired hepatic degradation of insulin may be the mechanism for the prolonged hyper-insulinaemia seen in patients with cirrhosis, but intra-hepatic or portosystemic shunts may also contribute.[20] The insulin resistance largely results from a defect in insulin mediated utilisation of glucose by peripheral muscles.[21] Although there are many contradictory results relating to the mechanism of this defect, it appears that the number and affinity of insulin receptors are little changed in cirrhotics but a post-receptor defect leading to reduced glycogen production may exist.[21] Glycogenolysis in the liver is appropriately suppressed by the high circulating insulin concentrations.[22] Other factors that may contribute to the apparent insulin resistance in chronic liver disease include hyperglucagonaemia[23] and increased plasma growth hormone concentrations.[24]

Hypoglycaemia is common and often persistent in acute fulminant hepatitis, but may also be seen in end-stage cirrhosis.[25] Hepatic glycogen stores are limited and can be depleted within 1–2 days of fasting. The extensive parenchymal destruction in fulminant hepatitis reduces the capacity of the liver to produce glucose via gluconeogenesis or to replenish glycogen stores. Inappropriate hyperinsulinaemia, in this case occurring acutely due to failure of hepatic insulin degradation, may contribute to the hypoglycaemia. In chronic liver disease hypoglycaemia is most often due to reduced dietary intake associated with alcohol misuse. Apart from the depletion of glycogen stores, alcohol has an inhibitory effect on hepatic gluco-neogenesis by increasing the $NADH:NAD^+$ ratio and lowering pyruvate/oxaloacetate concentrations.[26] Hypoglycaemia is a feature of several inherited metabolic disorders causing liver disease in children.

Lipid metabolism

The appearance of fat vacuoles in the liver is almost invariably due to excess accumulation of triglycerides and typically associated with alcohol misuse. There is concomitantly an increase in circulating cholesterol, free fatty acids and triglycerides. In both alcoholic and acute viral hepatitis the activities of hepatic lecithin-cholesterol acyltransferase (LCAT) and triglyceride lipases are decreased.[27,28] The reduction in LCAT activity leads to a decrease in cholesterol esterification. Plasma HDL concentrations are often decreased and VLDL may be increased. Alcohol ingestion contributes to increased plasma triglycerides by stimulating fatty acid synthesis and lowering fatty acid oxidation via the increased $NADH:NAD^+$ ratio mentioned earlier. Inhibition of lipoprotein lipases by alcohol also lowers the removal of lipoproteins from the circulation.

Eventually in chronic liver disease, decreased hepatic formation and release of lipoproteins, due to the reduced functional hepatocyte mass, causes further hepatic fat accumulation and plasma cholesterol and triglycerides begin to fall. In patients with cholestasis, either intrahepatic or due to extrahepatic biliary obstruction, increased unesterified cholesterol and phospholipid concentrations are found in plasma owing to the presence of an abnormal LDL termed lipoprotein X. This appears to originate from the reflux of bile lipoprotein into plasma where it binds with albumin to form lipoprotein X.[29]

Vitamins and liver disease

Vitamin deficiencies are commonly encountered in patients with chronic liver disease. A low dietary intake with or without malabsorption are the principal causes of the vitamin deficiencies. As the liver is the major site of storage and conversion of many vitamins to their active forms, disruption to both processes can result in deficiencies.

Water-soluble vitamins

Leevy et al. demonstrated reduced circulating concentrations of the water-soluble vitamins in 32–49% of alcoholics, the prevalence of deficiencies increasing with the severity of liver disease.[30] Folic acid was the vitamin most often found to be deficient but low serum levels of thiamine, riboflavin, nicotinic acid, B_{12} and pyridoxine were also observed in up to 25% of patients. Subsequent reports in non-alcohol related chronic liver diseases such as cryptogenic cirrhosis or hepatitis have found lower incidences of deficiencies of water-soluble vitamins than fat-soluble vitamins, with the possible exception of vitamin C.[4] Peripheral neuropathy, sometimes accompanied by Wernicke's encephalopathy, can be seen in patients with alcoholic cirrhosis due to thiamine deficiency. Administration of thiamine, whilst restoring circulating levels of thiamine, does not correct the neuropathy, suggesting that the symptoms may be related to impaired hepatic phosphorylation of thiamine.

Megaloblastic anaemia associated with folate deficiency is not uncommon in alcohol misusers with some liver impairment. Folate is stored in the liver as reduced polyglutamate forms and is converted as required to the active 5-methyl tetrahydrofolic acid, principally in hepatocytes. Studies have suggested that alcohol promotes hepatic storage of folate and reduces the enterohepatic circulation necessary for conversion to the active form.[31] The active form of vitamin B_6 compounds is the coenzyme pyridoxal-5′-phosphate (PLP) which is formed in the liver. Decreased serum PLP concentrations have been observed in chronic liver disease but rarely in acute hepatitis.[32,33] Increased PLP degradation appears to be the mechanism rather than malabsorption. Deficiencies in the other water-soluble vitamins seem to be dependent on failure of absorption or poor dietary intake.

Fat-soluble vitamins

Deficiencies of the fat-soluble vitamins A, D, E and K are seen in a high proportion of chronic liver disease patients and in acute hepatitis.[4,15] Vitamin A in plasma exists in the form of a retinol-binding protein–prealbumin complex. Deficiency of vitamin A leads to impaired dark adaptation. Reduced synthesis of both transport proteins by the liver appears to be the mechanism of the lowered circulating vitamin A concentrations in chronic liver disease, rather than poor absorption.[34] Whilst low circulating vitamin E concentrations are relatively common in patients with liver disease, there are no clear clinical sequelae attached to these deficiencies.

There has been considerable debate about the importance of vitamin D deficiency in the development of metabolic bone disease in patients with chronic liver disease, particularly PBC.[35] In both PBC and alcohol-induced liver disease, osteoporosis, and to a lesser extent osteomalacia, is a frequent finding. Plasma 25-hydroxy vitamin D concentrations are normal in early PBC, falling with progressive disease.[35] Absorption of vitamin D is impaired possibly related to the use of cholestyramine therapy, which may also disrupt the enterohepatic circulation of the hydroxylated vitamin. Oral supplementation with vitamin D has been demonstrated to restore the plasma concentration of 25-hydroxy vitamin D to normal and improves the osteomalacia but seems to have little effect on the osteoporosis, promoting the concept that the osteoporosis in PBC is due to increased bone turnover.[36] The prolongation of blood clotting times and the presence of haematomata as frank haemorrhage in liver patients may be associated with vitamin K deficiency. However, as the liver is the site for synthesis of other clotting factors, vitamin K deficiency can only be diagnosed reliably by improve-

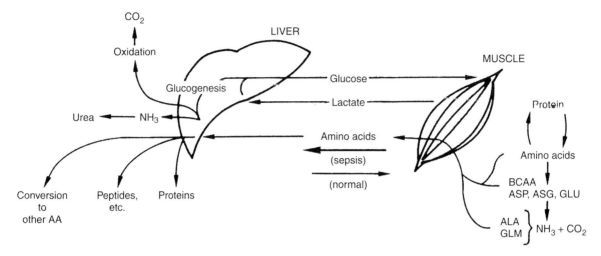

Figure 4.2 – Amino acid and carbohydrate exchange between the liver and skeletal muscle.

ment in the prothrombin time or INR (International Normalised Ratio) following administration of vitamin K.

Amino acid and protein metabolism

Changes in the plasma concentrations of amino acids and increased urinary excretion of some amino acids are found in acute and chronic liver disease, although the changes differ significantly between the two. In chronic liver disease reduced hepatic uptake of the amino acids catabolised by the liver, including tyrosine, glutamic acid and methionine, leads to increased plasma concentrations. Concurrently there is a fall in the plasma concentrations of the amino acids predominantly taken up by extrahepatic tissues, particularly the BCAAs valine, leucine and isoleucine. The altered distribution of amino acids may be related to the muscle wasting seen in patients with cirrhosis.[37] Patients with acute hepatic necrosis, however, have near normal plasma BCAA concentrations but marked elevations in all other amino acids. The degree of elevation of amino acids such as tyrosine correlates with the rise in AST, suggesting the cause is release of the amino acids from the damaged hepatocytes.

Administration of standard protein or amino acid formulae can maintain a neutral nitrogen balance in well-compensated, non-encephalopathic cirrhotics.[38] In some patients, however, protein administration can promote encephalopathy and dietary protein restriction may be necessary which can lead to a negative nitrogen balance and a reduction in lean body mass. BCAA-enriched solutions have been used, in both patients with established hepatic encephalopathy and those without, with varying degrees of success.[39] This will be discussed in more detail later in this chapter. The normal liver disposes of nitrogen from amino acids by transamination with release of ammonia, which enters the urea cycle, leading to the formation of urea. In the damaged liver, urea synthesis is reduced and ammonia can accumulate. This reduction in urea synthesis occurs earlier in cirrhotics than hyperammonaemia, hyperaminoacidaemia and hepatic encephalopathy.

Proteins synthesised by the liver (Table 4.1) are frequently decreased in patients with liver disease. A characteristic pattern of plasma proteins following electrophoretic separation can be seen in cirrhotics with reduced albumin, α_1- and α_2-globulins and increased γ-globulins (due to increased immuno-globulins). The most significant clinical manifestations are due to reduction in circulating albumin concentrations and lowered synthesis of clotting factors. Hypoalbuminaemia can promote fluid redistribution and formation of ascites. The lowered circulating albumin concentration is probably the result of a combination of reduced dietary protein intake and increased gastrointestinal losses.

The clotting factors most likely to be decreased in liver disease are factors II, VII, IX and X. Additionally, in fulminant liver failure fibrinogen and factor V may also be reduced. Prolonged clotting times and frank haemorrhage are common in severe liver disease.

Vitamin K deficiency, due to decreased intake or absorption, results in reduced synthesis of the clotting factors and can be readily corrected by the parenteral administration of vitamin K. Continued prolongation of clotting times after vitamin K repletion may indicate increased utilisation owing to disseminated intravascular coagulation and excessive fibrinolysis.

The role of nutrition in hepatic encephalopathy

The exact pathogenesis of hepatic encephalopathy remains unclear but nutritional factors may be involved in its development (Table 4.2). It is generally believed that metabolic products normally metabolised by the liver can accumulate in the brain.[6] Increased ingestion of protein, either from dietary sources or gastrointestinal bleeding, is known to precipitate encephalopathy in some patients with chronic liver disease. The toxicity of protein has been largely attributed to the production of ammonia which is not converted to urea. Although hyperammonaemia is undoubtedly associated with encephalopathy, poor correlation between arterial ammonia concentrations and the development of encephalopathy indicates that ammonia is not the sole cause.[6]

Table 4.2 – Precipitating factors for the development of hepatic encephalopathy

Excessive protein intake
Gastrointestinal bleeding
Constipation
Sepsis
Poor compliance with lactulose/fibre dietary therapy
Uraemia
Alkalosis
Some central nervous system-active drugs

It has long been known that different sources of dietary protein vary in their ability to provoke encephalopathy, meat diets causing a greater degree of encephalopathy than milk-based diets with fish being intermediate.[40] This may be related to differences in the amino acid composition of the protein sources, particularly with respect to the content of the aromatic amino acids (phenylalanine, tyrosine and tryptophan).

Tryptophan in particular has been implicated in the pathogenesis of encephalopathy, possibly through modulation of brain serotonin metabolism. The rationale of the use of BCAA-enriched formulation for the treatment of hepatic encephalopathy is partly based on competition between the BCAAs and tryptophan for passage across the blood–brain barrier. Although some studies have been unable to clearly demonstrate a benefit for BCAA-enriched preparations in encephalopathic patients, a meta-analysis of the available data showed a benefit from BCAA administration in patients with high-grade encephalopathy.[41]

The administration of a poorly absorbed disaccharide in the diet, such as lactulose, appears to be beneficial in hepatic encephalopathy. Lactulose consists of galactose and fructose and is neither degraded nor absorbed in the small intestine. It is metabolised in the colon to form organic acids by the bacterial flora. The presence of lactulose in the colon appears to increase incorporation of nitrogen into bacteria and may inhibit ammonia generation by the faecal bacteria. Similar increases in bacterial nitrogen incorporation may be seen with the use of vegetable protein diets with a high fibre content or following administration of purified protein.

Nutrition and liver regeneration

The hepatocyte is a highly differentiated cell that, unlike most other cells, retains its ability to proliferate when circumstances require. Following partial (up to 70%) hepatectomy most hepatocytes can replicate at least once. Eventually it is possible for the liver to regain most of its pre-hepatectomy mass. Although studied for many years, the mechanism involved in the initiation and progression of the hyperplasia is still poorly understood.[42] Various trophic factors activate hepatocytes from the G_0 state into an activated, pre-replicative G_1 state.[7] During this phase the hepatocyte assembles the substrates and enzymes required for DNA synthesis and cellular replication. The remaining hepatocytes, remarkably, continue to carry out liver-specific functions at virtually the same level following hepatectomy.[42] Data on the specific molecular mechanisms for the regulation of liver regeneration have been accumulated predominantly via the use of animal models, with very little information in humans.[7]

Hepatic growth factors and growth-promoting hormones (such as insulin, glucagon and gluco-corticoids) increase after liver injury and may regulate the cell growth. Most of these hormones and growth factors activate hepatic ornithine decarboxylase (ODC), the rate-limiting enzyme for polyamine synthesis, a process required for hepatocellular pro-liferation.[43] The extrahepatic effects of these factors influence the delivery of macronutrients (amino acids, lipids and carbohydrates) and micronutrients (calcium and zinc) to the hepatocyte. Adequate nutrition intake is, therefore, essential for hepatic regeneration. Starvation or protein-deficient diets depress the rate of hepatic DNA synthesis and delay the onset of synthesis for up to 16 hours in protein-deprived rats compared to control animals.[44] The amino acid composition of the diet may be important in providing the optimal substrates for regeneration. As for hepatic encephal-opathy, BCAA-enriched amino acid solutions have a better effect on cell growth than balanced amino acid formulae. Formulations high in carbohydrates and fats may also be advantageous in promoting hepatic regrowth. However, existing data do not provide definitive conclusions regarding the absolute benefit of nutritional supplementation for liver regeneration and more work is required in this area.

Summary

Chronic liver disease, particularly cirrhosis, produces significant alterations to the metabolism of carbo-hydrates, lipids and amino acids. These changes vary as the disease progresses in severity. Hypo- or hyper-glycaemia can occur together with hyperaminoacid-aemia. In the end stages of chronic liver disease or in acute hepatocellular necrosis, the changes in nutrient metabolism differ in that hypoglycaemia is more common together with reductions in lipid concen-trations. Excessive protein ingestion from either the diet or due to gastrointestinal bleeding can provoke hepatic encephalopathy by formation of ammonia. Dietary manipulation and/or the use of non-absorbed disaccharides or soluble fibre can improve existing encephalopathy. The optimal nutritional requirements for promoting hepatic regeneration have yet to be determined.

References

1. Bunout D, Gatlas V, Iturriaga H et al. Nutritional status of alcoholic patients: its possible relationship to alcoholic liver damage. Am J Clin Nutr 1983; **38**: 469–73.

2. Mendenhall CL, Anderson S, Weesner RE et al. Protein-calorie malnutrition associated with alcoholic hepatitis. Am J Med 1984; **76**: 211–22.

3. Achord JL. Malnutrition and the role of nutritional support in alcoholic liver disease. Am J Gastroenterol 1987; **82**: 1–7.

4. Morgan AG, Kelleher J, Walker BE et al. Nutrition in cryptogenic cirrhosis and chronic aggressive hepatitis. Gut 1976; **17**: 113–18.

5. McCullough AJ, Tavill AS. Disordered energy and protein metabolism in liver disease. Sem Liver Dis 1995; **11**: 265–76.

6. Mullen KD, Weber FL. Role of nutrition in hepatic encephalopathy. Sem Liver Dis 1991; **11**: 292–304.

7. Diehl AM. Nutrition, hormones, metabolism and liver regeneration. Sem Liver Dis 1991; **11**: 315–20.

8. Elwyn DH. The role of the liver in regulation of amino acid and protein metabolism. In: Munro HN (ed) Mammalian protein metabolism, vol 4. Academic Press, New York, 1970, p 523.

9. Young VR, Pellet PL. How to evaluate dietary protein. In: Barth CA, Schlimme E (eds) Milk proteins in human nutrition. Steinkopff, Darmstadt, 1989, pp 7–36.

10. Millward DJ, Jackson AA, Price G, Rivers JPW. Human amino acid and protein requirements: current dilemmas and uncertainties. Nutr Res Rev 1989; **2**: 109–32.

11. Bowman BH. Hepatic plasma proteins. Mechanisms of function and regulation. Academic Press, San Diego, 1992.

12. Mortimore GE, Poso AP. Intracellular protein catabolism and its control during nutrient deprivation and supply. Ann Rev Nutr 1987; **7**: 539–64.

13. Mills PR, Shenkin A, Anthony RS et al. Assessment of nutritional status and in vivo immune responses in alcoholic liver disease. Am J Clin Nutr 1983; **38**: 849–59.

14. Morgan MY. Enteral nutrition in chronic liver disease. Acta Clin Scand 1981; **507** (suppl): 81–90.

15. DiCecco JR, Wieners EJ, Weisner RH et al. Assessment of nutritional status in patients with end-stage liver disease undergoing liver transplantation. Mayo Clin Proc 1989; **65**: 95–102.

16. Shaw BW, Wood P, Stratta RJ et al. Stratifying the causes of death in liver transplant recipients. Arch Surg 1989; **24**: 895–900.

17. Nolte W, Hartmann H, Ramadori G. Glucose metabolism and liver cirrhosis. Exp Clin Endocrinol 1995; **103**: 63–74.

18. Petrides AS, Groop LC, Riely CA, DeFronzo RA. Effect of physiological hyperinsulinaemia on glucose and lipid metabolism in cirrhosis. *J Clin Invest* 1991; **100:** 245–51.

19. Kruszynska YT, Home PD, McIntyre N. Relationship between insulin sensitivity, insulin secretion and glucose tolerance in cirrhosis. *Hepatology* 1991; **14:** 103–11.

20. Selberg O, Burchett W, Van der Hoff J *et al*. Insulin resistance in liver cirrhosis. Positron-emission tomography scan analysis of skeletal muscle glucose metabolism. *J Clin Invest* 1993; **91:** 1897–902.

21. Barzilai G, Marchesini G, Zoli M *et al*. In vivo insulin action in hepatocellular and cholestatic liver cirrhosis. *Hepatology* 1991; **20:** 119–25.

22. Cavallo-Pelvin P, Cassader M, Bozzo C *et al*. Mechanism of insulin resistance in human liver cirrhosis. *J Clin Invest* 1985; **75:** 1659–65.

23. Smith-Laing G, Orskov H, Gore MBR, Sherlock S. Hyperglucagonaemia in cirrhosis. Relationship to hepatocellular damage. *Diabetologia* 1980; **19:** 103–8.

24. Shankar TP, Solomon SS, Duckworth WC *et al*. Growth hormone and carbohydrate intolerance in cirrhosis. *Horm Metabol Res* 1988; **20:** 579–83.

25. Felig P, Brown WV, Levine RA *et al*. Glucose homeostasis in viral hepatitis. *N Engl J Med* 1970; **283:** 1436–40.

26. Forsander OA. Influence of the metabolism of ethanol on the lactate/pyruvate ratio of rat-liver slices. *Biochem J* 1966; **98:** 244–7.

27. Blomhoff JP, Skrede S, Ritland S. Lecithin, cholesterol acyltransferase and plasma proteins in liver disease. *Clin Chem Acta* 1974; **53:** 197–207.

28. Bertram PD, Ragland JB, Sabesin SM. Accumulation of abnormal plasma lipoproteins in alcoholic hepatitis (AH) results from deficiency of enzymes of hepatic origin. *Clin Res* 1977; **25:** 307A.

29. Marzato E, Fellin R, Baggio G *et al*. Formation of lipoprotein X. Its relationship to bile compounds. *J Clin Invest* 1976; **57:** 1248–60.

30. Leevy CM, Baker H, ten Hove W *et al*. B-complex vitamins in liver disease of the alcoholic. *Am J Clin Nutr* 1965; **16:** 339–46.

31. Hillman RS, McGuffin R, Campbell C. Alcohol interference with folate enterohepatic cycle. *Clin Res* 1977; **25:** 518A.

32. Labadarios D, Roesouw JE, McConnell JB *et al*. Vitamin B$_6$ deficiency in chronic liver disease – evidence for increased degradation of pyridoxal 5′-phosphate. *Gut* 1977; **18:** 23–7.

33. Mitchell D, Wagner C, Stone WJ *et al*. Abnormal regulation of plasma pyridoxal 5′-phosphate in patients with liver disease. *Gastroenterology* 1976; **71:** 1043–9.

34. Smith FR, Goodman DS. The effects of diseases of the liver, thyroid and kidneys on the transport of Vitamin A in human plasma. *J Clin Invest* 1971; **50:** 2426–36.

35. Schaffner F, Bach N. Gastrointestinal syndromes in primary biliary cirrhosis. *Sem Liver Dis* 1988; **8:** 263–71.

36. Arnaud SB. 25-hydroxyvitamin D$_3$ treatments of bone disease in primary biliary cirrhosis. *Gastroenterology* 1982; **83:** 137–40.

37. Morrison WL, Bouchier IAD, Gibson JNA *et al*. Skeletal muscle and whole body protein turnover in cirrhosis. *Clin Sci* 1990; **78:** 613–19.

38. Munoz SJ. Nutritional therapies in liver disease. *Sem Liver Dis* 1991; **11:** 278–91.

39. Fan ST. Nutritional support for patients with cirrhosis. *J Gastroenterol Hepatol* 1997; **12:** 282–6.

40. Condon RE. Effect of dietary protein on symptoms and survival in dogs with an Eck fistula. *Am J Surg* 1971; **121:** 107–14.

41. Fischer JE. Branched chain amino acid solution in patients with liver failure. An early example of nutritional pharmacology. *J Parent Enteral Nutr* 1990; **14** (suppl 5): 5249–56.

42. Michaelopoulos GK. Liver regeneration molecular mechanisms of growth control. *FASEB J* 1991; **4:** 176–87.

43. Luk GD. Essential role of polyamine metabolism in hepatic regeneration: inhibition of tissue regeneration by difluoromethylornithine in the rat. *Gastroenterology* 1986; **90:** 1261–7.

44. McGowan J, Atryzek V, Fausto N. Effects of protein deprivation on the regeneration of rat liver after partial hepatectomy. *Biochem J* 1979; **180:** 25–35.

5

Cytokines and nutrition

Robert F Grimble

Introduction

In the last 20 years there has been increasing recognition of the importance of the pro-inflammatory cytokines, interleukin-1 and -6 (IL-1 and -6) and tumour necrosis factor-α (TNF) in health and disease. Although the molecules are part of the non-specific response to infection they modulate and facilitate many aspects of immune function. They exert a three-fold effect on the body. Firstly, they are important activators of the immune cells. They stimulate production of immunomodulatory cytokines controlling a wide range of processes designed to focus the activity of the immune system on pathogen destruction and bring about healing. These processes include: chemotaxis (IL-8), lymphocyte proliferation (IL-2) antibody isotype modulation (IL-4), red blood cell formation (IL-3) and wound healing (TGF-β). Secondly, the pro-inflammatory cytokines facilitate pathogen destruction by stimulating the production of a range of oxidant molecules and by raising body temperature to increase the rate of the biological processes which bring about elimination of invading organisms. Thirdly IL-1, IL-6 and TNF are unique among the cytokines in producing a wide range of metabolic effects. These include: muscle protein loss, fat loss, increased glucose synthesis, micronutrient redistribution and enhancement of antioxidant defences (Fig. 5.1).

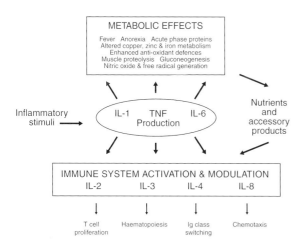

Figure 5.1 – The coordinated actions of pro-inflammatory cytokines upon the immune system and on metabolism during a normal response to infection and injury.

Beneficial effects of cytokines upon the host

Many of the effects, outlined in the previous section, are essential for the immune response. For example, bacteria are capable of multiplying at least 50 times faster than cells within the immune system. It is thus important that the immune system should not be constrained by a lack of the necessary substrates, to nourish the system, and for the synthesis of immune cells and secretory products. Glucose, glutamine and zinc are key nutrients for the system. Amino acids are necessary to synthesise additional lymphocytes and immunoglobulin during the immune response. The loss of appetite which results from IL-1 and TNF production, although appearing paradoxical, may facilitate nutrient provision to the immune system by creating a hormonal profile whereby nutrients can be released from body pools (muscle, adipose tissue and micronutrient stores) in amounts which match the requirements of the immune response (see Fig. 5.1). Once the infection has been repulsed, body stores can be repleted. An unrestrained appetite would create a hormonal response where deposition of nutrients within these pools would occur, thereby jeopardising the supply of nutrients to the immune system.

The essential nature of cytokines in recovery from inflammatory situations is indicated by the poor prognosis of malnourished patients who have a reduced ability for cytokine production.[1,2] These patients also exhibited poor wound healing as TNF-α is an important inducer of TGF-β that plays a crucial part in the process.

The pathological influence of cytokines

From the mid-1980s, evidence started to accumulate that excessive production of the pro-inflammatory cytokines underlay morbidity and mortality in a wide range of conditions involving infective organisms. The conditions included sepsis, meningitis and cerebral malaria[3,4] (Fig. 5.2). Thus cytokines are able to produce detrimental as well as beneficial effects upon patients. This concept led to the development of a number of anti-cytokine therapies, such as the administration of antibodies to

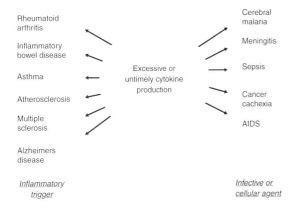

Figure 5.2 – Diseases and conditions in which pro-inflammatory cytokines produce pathological effects.

TNF and bacterial endotoxin, in treatment of seriously ill patients.

The stimuli which lead to cytokine production are not confined to invading pathogens. Evidence has also accumulated that ill defined triggers lead to the production of cytokines in a wide range of diseases including: rheumatoid arthritis, inflammatory bowel disease, psoriasis, asthma, Alzheimer's disease, multiple sclerosis and atherosclerosis (see Fig. 5.2).[5-8]

The increase in oxidant production which occurs in the presence of cytokines carries the risk that healthy tissues within the body may be damaged as well as invading organisms. Furthermore oxidants enhance production of a number of cytokines by activation of nuclear transcription factors, such as nuclear factor kappa-beta (NFκB) and NFIL-6. However, cytokines raise the level of antioxidant defences and offer a measure of protection to the hosts tissues (see Fig. 5.1). Nonetheless there is evidence of oxidant damage in a wide range of diseases and conditions in which cytokines are produced. These include: coronary artery disease, cancer, human immuno-deficiency virus (HIV) infection and alcoholic liver disease and following bone marrow transplantation, haemodialysis and open heart surgery.[9]

Further damage to the host may arise from the interaction of viruses with the mechanisms controlling cytokine production. Although IL-1 and TNF are generally antiviral in their actions, replication of HIV is enhanced by NFκB activation. Thus inflammatory stimuli which enhance IL-1 and TNF pro-

duction will indirectly increase replication of the virus.[10]

Evidence is emerging of genetic influences on cytokine production and bioactivity, which exert a pathological influence. The deleterious effects that a propensity for cytokine production has upon the host are evident in a study on children in the Gambia. Individuals who were homozygous for a variant of the TNF-α promoter region, that enhances TNF-α production, had seven times the mortality rates from cerebral malaria than children who were heterozygous.[11] In autoimmune hepatitis and pulmonary tuberculosis, similar associations have been noted between a genetic predisposition to produce IL-1 and TNF-α and pathology.[12,13] It has been hypothesised that the retention of genetic characteristics for enhanced production of cytokines within the populations gene pool may be because they bestow benefits on heterozygotes by enhancing immune function. Homozygotes exhibit the downside of this situation with increased morbidity and mortality. It is unclear, at present, whether genetic characteristics which lead to overproduction of cytokines occur in all populations and whether gene dosage effects result in a spectrum of effects ranging from improved immune function to increased risk of inflammatory disease. However a recent study on the molecular biology of the gene for the anti-inflammatory protein, interleukin 1 receptor antagonist IL-1ra (see Fig. 5.3) in inflammatory bowel disease found that less active mutant versions were more common in the colon of patients than in healthy subjects.[14]

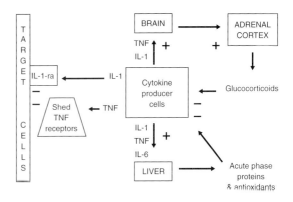

Figure 5.3 – Innate systems for controlling the production and actions of pro-inflammatory cytokines. Stimulatory actions are indicated by plus signs and inhibitory actions by minus signs. Abbreviation: IL-1ra = interleukin-1 receptor antagonist.

Biological processes underlying the effects of cytokines upon metabolism

The mechanisms underlying the metabolic changes associated with the wasting process are complex. They involve interaction between cytokines and the hypothalamus and the direct effects of IL-1 and TNF-α on peripheral tissues and liver.

Increased production of glucocorticoids and catecholamines occur due to a rise in the activity of the sympathetic nervous system and stimulation of corticotrophin-releasing factor production by the actions of cytokines on the central nervous system.[15–17] Catecholamines, glucocorticoids and cytokines enhance glycogenolysis and gluconeogenesis.[18] Studies in patients and experimental animals have shown that IL-1, TNF-α, and agents which induce production of these cytokines, stimulate skeletal muscle protein catabolism, increase glutamine synthesis and enhance efflux of glutamine and other amino acids from the tissue.[19–23] An increased supply of substrate for gluconeogenesis is thus provided from skeletal muscle. The extent to which skin and bone provide amino acids is unclear. However *in vitro* studies have shown that TNF-α and IL-1 cause bone resorption and inhibition of proteoglycan synthesis in cartilage.[24,25] *In vivo* bacterial endotoxin produces a marked reduction of protein synthesis in skin and bone of rats.[26] In studies on patients with rheumatoid arthritis, peripheral blood mononuclear cells produced greater amounts TNF and IL-1 than cells from normal subjects when stimulated with endotoxin. In addition the rheumatoid patients exhibited a reduction in lean body mass and an increase in resting energy expenditure which correlated with an increased potential for enhanced cytokine production.[27]

A rapid increase in plasma concentrations of free fatty acids and triglycerides, attached to very low density and low density lipoproteins, follows *in vivo* administration of IL-1 and TNF-α in experimental animals. The response is due to a combination of events which include enhanced lipolysis in adipose tissue and increased hepatic lipogenesis.[28]

IL-1, TNF-α and glucocorticoids are responsible for the alterations in tissue zinc concentrations that have been observed during inflammation. The cytokines cause decreased concentrations in plasma, muscle, skin and bone and an increase in liver, kidney, bone marrow and thymus.[29,30] IL-1, TNF-α and glucocorticoids exert a stimulatory effect upon the synthesis of metallothionein and may be partly responsible for the increases in tissue zinc.[31] The changes in metallothionein thus facilitate a shift in body zinc from tissues which act as a reservoir (muscle, skin, bone) to tissues where enhanced cellular activity is occurring during inflammation (thymus, bone marrow and liver).

Thus IL-1 and TNF-α directly and indirectly change metabolism to provide substrate for the immune system from endogenous sources. Such a change of nutrient supply is important, since anorexia and lethargy are among the predominant features of infected and traumatised subjects.[4]

Endogenous modulators of pro-inflammatory cytokine production and actions

When an inflammatory stimulus is encountered, a number of metabolic and cellular events occur which can lead to suppression and localisation of the production of cytokines and their subsequent actions (Fig. 5.3).

The observation that substances in the urine of febrile patients inhibited cytokine actions indicated that natural inhibitors of cytokine actions are generated during inflammation. Subsequently, a sophisticated array of control systems which modulate cytokine production and limit their impact was identified.[3] Liver, brain, adrenal cortex and immune system play major roles in the control systems. Natural inhibitors to IL-1 and TNF-α are produced in response to IL-1 and TNF-α. The inhibitor for IL-1, IL1-ra, is produced by lymphocytes and phagocytes; it exhibits a high degree of amino acid homology with IL-1 and will bind to receptors for the cytokine without leading to cellular activation. It thus competes with IL-1 in binding to receptors and decreases the sensitivity of cells to IL-1. The inhibitor for TNF-α is the extracellular domain of TNF receptors. These domains are shed into the circulation as soluble TNF receptors (sTNF-R), following binding of TNF-α to a small proportion of the receptors on the surface of target tissues. The soluble receptors compete with membrane associated TNF-α receptors, thereby reducing cellular sensitivity to the cytokine. IL1-ra and sTNF-R are present in plasma in concentrations which are well in excess, in molar terms, to concentrations of IL-1 and TNF-α and may thus exert major inhibitory influences on the biological activity of the two cytokines. Soluble forms of IL-1 receptors have been found in plasma indicating a further way in which tissue sensitivity to IL-1 may be reduced.[32] In addition to specific inhibitors for IL-1 and TNF, other cytokines downregulate IL-1 and TNF-α production. Pre-eminent among the inhibitory cytokines are IL-4 and IL-10. In addition to their direct effects on IL-1 and TNF, the inhibitory cytokines exert an indirect influence by enhancing sTNF-R and IL1-ra production.[32]

Control mechanisms arise from the actions of IL-1 and TNF upon the hypothalamo–pituitary adrenal axis. Consequently, glucocorticoids are released and suppress cytokine production by enhancing lipocortin production.[33,34] Glucocorticoids also participate indirectly in the control of cytokine production. As indicated earlier, they facilitate the release of amino acids from peripheral tissues and, in conjunction with IL-1 and IL-6, stimulate acute phase protein production by hepatocytes.[35] Some of these proteins, such as orosomucoid, alpha-2-macroglobulin, C-reactive protein and alpha-1-antichymotrypsin inhibit neutrophil activation and production of superoxide radicals and TNF-α.[36-38] Increased production of orosomucoid, caeruloplasmin and of glutathione, enhance antioxidant defences and limit the stimulatory effects of oxidant molecules on cytokine production.

Modulation of cytokine biology by nutrients

The metabolic aspects of inflammation, described earlier, are mediated by a range of secondary messengers and cell signalling mechanisms which offers broad scope for nutritional modulation.

Cytokines may have beneficial or detrimental effects, depending upon the context and amounts in which they are produced. During infection they are mostly beneficial; in cancer, chronic inflammatory disease, or in individuals infected with HIV, they may be

detrimental. Thus beneficial dietary manipulation of cytokine production and actions may be designed to facilitate, enhance or suppress events, depending upon the biological or clinical context in which they are operating.[3]

Modulation of cytokine production and biological effects of fats

Fats may exert modulatory effects by influencing the ability of cells to produce cytokines and the ability of tissues to respond to cytokines.[39,40]

Dietary fats can be divided into three broad groupings, according to the predominant types of fatty acids in their structure. Fats of animal origin from meat, eggs, cheese, milk, butter and coconut oil are classified as saturated fats. Fats from seeds and nuts such as olive, sunflower, rapeseed, corn, borage and palm oils and fats from oily fish are rich in unsaturated fatty acids. Further subdivision is possible within this group into: fats such as palm and olive oils and butter which are rich in monounsaturated fatty acids; fats, such as corn, sunflower and borage oils which are rich in polyunsaturated fatty acids of the n-6 variety (n-6 PUFAs); and fats which are rich in PUFAs of the n-3 variety which are found in abundance in oily fish and in low concentrations in green leafy vegetables.

Extensive studies have been carried out, mostly in animal models, using a number of these fats. The studies observed the effects of dietary fat on burn injury, cytokine and endotoxin-induced anorexia and fever, cytokine and endotoxin-induced changes in visceral protein metabolism and cytokine production from macrophages. In summary, fats rich in n-3 PUFAs, or n-9 monounsaturated fatty acids, or poor in n-6 PUFAs reduce responsiveness to cytokines.[40,41] Fats rich in n-6 PUFAs exert the opposite effect (Fig. 5.4). The ability of peritoneal macrophages from rats to produce IL-1 and IL-6 in response to TNF-α is greatly influenced by the dietary intake of n-6 PUFAs and total unsaturated fatty acid intake respectively. IL-1 production increased to plateau concentrations within a range of n-6 PUFA intake representing 1–4% of dietary energy, whereas IL-6 production was positively related to unsaturated fatty acid intake over a wider range of intakes.[42]

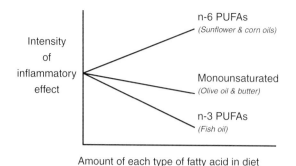

Figure 5.4 – Summary of the influence of unsaturated fatty acids on the intensity of cytokine mediated responses during infection, trauma and inflammatory disease.

The question arises as to the relevance of these observations on the effect of dietary fat in animals to clinical practice. There is a limited amount of evidence that n-6 PUFA intake may influence pro-inflammatory cytokine production in healthy subjects. The data have mostly been obtained from experiments in which discrete changes in the type of dietary fat consumed have been achieved over relatively short periods of time, and indices of immune function measured. For example, blood monocytes taken from subjects consuming a cholesterol-lowering diet, which involved a reduction in saturated fatty acid intake from 14.1 to 4% of dietary energy, and an increase from 6.1 to 8.8% in n-6 PUFAs, over a 24-week period, exhibited enhanced IL-1 and TNF-α production in response to endotoxin.[43] Smoking causes an inflammatory response by stimulating the release of pro-inflammatory cytokines from macrophages in the lung.[8] It was noted that smokers consuming n-6 PUFA intakes of greater than 7% of dietary energy had twice the concentrations of the acute phase protein, C-reactive protein than smokers with a lower intake of n-6 PUFAs.[44]

The mechanisms underlying the apparent pro-inflammatory influence of n-6 PUFAs are unknown. It is interesting to note however that, when healthy volunteers were given an n-6 PUFA rich borage oil supplement over a three month period, production of the anti-inflammatory cytokines IL-10 and IL-4 by blood mononuclear cells was halved.[45] The balance between pro- and anti-inflammatory cytokines may thus be changed by increases in n-6 PUFA intake.

An increasing body of evidence suggests that aberrant cytokine production is involved in atherosclerosis.[5]

The association of dietary fat intake with athero-sclerosis has been the subject of extensive studies. A substantial body of evidence suggests that the intake of saturated fat is positively associated with athero-sclerosis and coronary heart disease.[46]

The fat in such diets might be expected to be anti-inflammatory in nature. However, a large proportion of the saturated fat in the diet is derived from animal sources and contains cholesterol. Cholesterol may enhance cytokine production. Studies on rabbits show that IL-1 and TNF synthesis in the aorta wall, in response to an inflammatory stimulus, is enhanced by inclusion of cholesterol in diets containing saturated fat.[47] Indeed, in rats, diets containing butter were shown to have both anti-inflammatory and pro-inflammatory effects, depending upon the relative amounts of monounsaturated fatty acids and cholesterol respectively.[41,48]

As indicated earlier, malfunctioning of the immune system underlies inflammatory disease and increases mortality during the response to invasion by pathogenic organisms. The question therefore arises whether the more subtle, long-term changes which have been observed in the diet of populations, exert effects on the immune system which would alter the incidence of inflammatory disease.[49] Individuals with a genetic predisposition to inflammation might be more likely to show evidence of this effect. A key feature in the changes in dietary fat intake in the UK in the last 25 years has been a large rise in n-6 PUFA intake. A similar phenomenon has been described in the United States, Canada, Sweden, Finland, Australia, New Zealand and Japan.[50]

It has been suggested that the increase in the incidence of asthma, eczema and allergic rhinitis and regional differences within countries may relate to dietary n-6 PUFA intake.[50] For example rates of asthma are lower in Scotland and the north of England than in the south. Intakes of n-6 PUFAs were highest in the south of England. Likewise rates of asthma were lower in the former East Germany where lower intakes on n-6 PUFAs occurred, than in West Germany, where larger quantities of this nutrient were consumed. In southern Finland rates of asthma in rural children were over three times higher than in similar children from the east of the country. The levels of n-6 PUFAs in cholesterol esters were significantly greater in the former than the latter region, confirming a higher intake of n-6 PUFAs. In Japan a study conducted between 1966 and 1985 showed an increase in fat intake from 16 to 24% of dietary energy. One of the key features of this dietary change was an increase in the ratio of n-6 to n-3 PUFAs in the diet. The incidence of Crohn's disease increased dramatically during this period. Statistical analysis showed a strong positive correlation between the ratio of n-6 to n-3 PUFAs in the diet and the annual increase in numbers of newly diagnosed cases of the inflammatory disease in the population.[49]

Thus these few epidemiological studies are generally in concordance with the experimental studies in man and other species which indicate that n-6 PUFAs may exert a pro-inflammatory influence. Clearly more definitive studies are necessary before a firm conclusion can be made. However with further changes in the amounts and nature of dietary fats being likely to occur into the present millennium, in the drive to improve public health, attention should be paid to the effects of such changes on the immune system.

While the Mediterranean diet, characterised by a high monounsaturated and n-3 polyunsaturated fatty acid content, is reputed to be anti-inflammatory, little is known of the role of monounsaturated fatty acids in ameliorating symptoms in inflammatory disease. Inflammatory symptoms however are improved by fish oil, or n-3 PUFAs, in diseases such as rheumatoid arthritis, psoriasis, asthma, multiple sclerosis, Crohn's disease and ulcerative colitis.[3] Supplementation of the diet of patients with pancreatic cancer cachexia arrested weight loss.[51] The observation that fish oil reduces the ability of leucocytes from healthy subjects and rheumatoid patients to produce IL-1, IL-6 and TNF-α, may partly explain the anti-inflammatory effects.[52]

Modulation of cytokine biology by oxidants and antioxidant status

Complex antioxidant defences exist within the host. They are distributed in body fluids and within various compartments of the cell. Plasma contains a wide range of substances with antioxidant properties. These include molecules derived directly from the diet, such as vitamin E and other tocopherols, vitamin C, β-carotene and catechins, and proteins and peptides, such as glutathione, caeruloplasmin, albumin and metallothionein, which are synthesised endogenously.

Many of these substances act as antioxidants within aqueous compartments of the cell, although vitamin E and other tocopherols are the predominant antioxidants within cell membranes. Superoxide dismutase, catalase and glutathione peroxidase and reductase facilitate the processing of oxidant molecules to harmless byproducts. Clearly nutrients can contribute directly and indirectly to the robustness of antioxidant defences. In this manner they have the potential to limit the capacity of oxidants released during the inflammatory response to damage tissues of the host and to activate nuclear transcription factors. In this way, nutrients therefore limit pathological aspects of the cytokine-mediated response to infection and injury (Fig. 5.5).

A number of studies on experimental animals and human subjects illustrate this point. Oxidation of polyunsaturated fatty acids, as a result of free radical attack, leads to enhanced ethane and pentane production in respired gases. Swords et al[53] showed that although endotoxin injections produced no increase in ethane production in well-fed rats, production rates doubled in animals fed a diet that was deficient in selenium and vitamin E. Other cytokine-mediated responses to inflammatory agents are also modulated by vitamin E intake. In a study in which rats were given diets containing no vitamin E, a normal amount, or four times the normal amount, for three weeks prior to injection with endotoxin, deficient animals showed the largest anorectic response to endotoxin, the largest increase in orosomucoid and increased plasma IL-6 concentration.[54,55] Histological examination of the lungs indicated that although infiltration of the lungs by immune cells was equally intense in all dietary groups receiving endotoxin, differences existed in the saline injected controls. The deficient controls had 18 and 32% more polymorphonuclear cells in the lungs than the controls receiving diets containing normal or supernormal amounts of vitamin E respectively.[54] The data suggest that vitamin E deficiency sensitises the animals to the mild inflammatory stimuli encountered during daily activities. Thus cytokine production in response to mild chronic and acute severe exposure to inflammatory agents may be modulated when antioxidant defences are compromised by lack of vitamin E.

A similar phenomenon may occur in human subjects. Cigarette smoking provides a chronic inflammatory stimulus to the macrophage population in the lung. Indeed raised plasma acute phase protein and IL-6 concentrations have been observed in smokers,

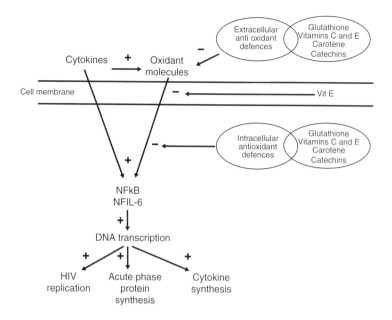

Figure 5.5 – The mechanisms for modulation of the inflammatory response and HIV replication by cytokines, oxidants and antioxidant defences. Stimulatory actions are indicated by plus signs and inhibitory actions by minus signs.

together with an enhanced capacity of whole blood samples to produce TNF-α, when stimulated with endotoxin.[56] In smokers acute phase protein concentrations correlated negatively with vitamin E intake.[44]

Influence of protein and amino acid intake on cytokine biology

The biochemical changes which occur during inflammation exert a large metabolic demand. Cytokines bring about major changes in protein and amino acid metabolism whereby amino acids are released from peripheral tissues for nutrition of cells of the immune system and the synthesis of acute phase proteins and glutathione by liver. It has been estimated that, during major infections in man, the amount of protein required to produce and maintain an increase in circulating white blood cells and acute phase proteins is approximately 45g/d.[57]

However, the supply from the peripheral tissues may not always match demands. There may be an enhanced requirement for sulphur and related amino acids following infection and trauma.[58] Severe trauma

and infection cause large decreases in plasma glycine, serine, and taurine concentrations. These changes may be due to enhanced utilisation of glycine, serine and the sulphur amino acids, methionine and cysteine, which are metabolically interrelated. Many substances produced in enhanced amounts in response to cytokines are rich in these amino acids. These include: glutathione, which consists of glycine, glutamic acid and cysteine; metallothionein, which contains glycine, serine, cysteine and methionine to a composite percentage of 56%; and a range of acute phase proteins which contain up to 25% of these amino acids in their structure. Following surgery on uninfected patients, a decrease in the ratio of urinary sulphate to nitrogen occurs, indicating preferential retention of sulphur amino acids into tissue components.[59] TNF-α may play a role in the extensive weight loss observed in patients with cancer and AIDS. In asymptomatic HIV-infected individuals, substantial reductions in GSH concentrations in plasma and lung epithelial fluid occur, which may indicate a requirement for sulphur amino acids that is not satisfied by diet or endogenous sources.[60]

The ability to increase α-2-macroglobulin in response to endogenous pyrogen in rabbits, and in response to TNF-α and turpentine abscess in rats, is impaired by low protein diets.[61 63] In rats given a turpentine abscess, the concentration of α-2-macroglobulin increased over a wide range of protein intakes of various degrees of adequacy.[63] The ability of rats fed low protein diets to increase serum orosomucoid and hepatic GSH concentrations in response to TNF-α is enhanced by dietary supplementation with glycine and cysteine respectively.[62]

In studies in rats given TNF-α, the partitioning of cysteine into hepatic protein and glutathione may depend upon the dietary sulphur amino acid intake. At low levels of intake, incorporation of cysteine into protein is favoured over incorporation into GSH to a greater extent than at high levels of intake.[3,64,65] Thus, at low intakes of sulphur amino acids, antioxidant defences may become compromised. An insufficient intake of sulphur amino acids will thereby exert a pro-inflammatory influence. In protein depleted rats given TNF-α, increases in lung GSH concentrations were only possible if cysteine and methionine was added to the diet. Infiltration of inflammatory cells into the lung, in response to the cytokine, was noted in the absence of these amino acids from the low protein diet and was prevented by their addition to the diet.[64]

The ability to maintain and enhance tissue GSH may be of particular importance in controlling cytokine production in response to inflammatory stimuli, since the stimulatory influence of oxidant molecules and TNF-α on NFκB activity is decreased by glutathione and other sulphur containing compounds.[66] Furthermore, in rats a non-lethal dose of TNF-α becomes lethal if the ability of the animal to increase and maintain GSH synthesis is prevented by administration of diethylmaleate.[67]

Glutathione, in addition to its important role as a component of antioxidant defence, can influence aspects of immune function that are related to T-lymphocytes. Normal intracellular concentrations of glutathione are required for several immune responses, including T-lymphocyte activation and proliferation and TNF and IL-2 production by macrophages. T-cell functions can be potentiated by glutathione administration in vivo.[68] However the relationship between cellular glutathione concentrations and cell numbers is complex. In healthy subjects numbers of CD4+ (suppressor) and CD8+ (helper) T lymphocytes increased in parallel with intracellular concentrations up to 30 nmol glutathione mg protein. A 75% increase in CD4+ and a 50% increase in CD8+ cells occurred over the concentration range. However numbers of both cell types declined at concentrations between 30

and 50 nmol glutathione mg protein.[69] The subjects of the study engaged in a programme of intensive physical exercise daily for four weeks. The programme resulted in a fall in glutathione concentrations in liver, muscle and blood. Individuals with glutathione concentrations in the optimal range before exercise, who experienced a fall in concentration after exercise, showed a 30% fall in CD4+ T-lymphocyte numbers. The decline in T-cells was prevented by administration of N-acetyl cysteine which did not arrest the decline in glutathione concentration. The studies therefore suggest that immune cell function may be sensitive to a range of intracellular sulphydryl compounds including glutathione and cysteine.[70]

Modulatory influence of the amount and route of nutrient delivery on cytokine biology

Anorexia is a key feature of the response to pro-inflammatory cytokines. The question therefore arises about the extent to which correction of appetite loss, by nasogastric or parenteral feeding, carries risks or benefits during an ongoing inflammatory response. Anorexia may be an unfortunate phenomenon associated with the metabolic changes induced by cytokines, or it may be an attempt to selectively avoid nutrients which might disadvantage the response of the host to pathogens. Experimental and observational data suggest that either possibility could be the case. Rats given IL-1 and a choice of casein, lard or a mixture of sucrose and cornstarch reduced intakes of the protein and fat by 57 and 68% respectively, whereas carbohydrate appetite was unaffected.[71]

Beneficial effects on immune function, morbidity and mortality were observed in burned children when additional protein in the form of whey protein was fed. The unsupplemented and supplemented diets contained 16.5 and 23% of energy as protein respectively. Improvements in neutrophil opsonic index, plasma acute phase proteins, survival and number of days with bacteraemia were noted in children fed whey protein supplements.[72]

In malnourished elderly patients showing an impaired ability to produce cytokines, dietary protein supplementation restored and enhanced production.[1] Such an enhancement carries benefits and dangers for the host if it is not part of a carefully coordinated metabolic response that disadvantages the pathogen but protects the host. Indeed enhanced mortalities have been noted in malnourished infected populations once nutrition supplementation was commenced.[73] In addition, asymptomatic infected malnourished children often become febrile during nutritional rehabilitation. The appearance of fever may indicate an enhancement of cytokine production, previously held in check by the malnourished state.[74] Similar phenomena have been observed in studies in animals. Mortality from malaria and bacterial infection is modified by alterations in specific amino acid and protein intake. Mortality in rats from *Plasmodium berghei* malaria was reduced by low protein diets but enhanced by dietary supplementation with a mixture of threonine, valine, leucine and isoleucine.[75] Likewise mortality in guinea pigs, from *Escherichia coli* and *Staphylococcus aureus* infection, was increased from 15 to 54%, over a range of protein intakes from an inadequate 5% of total dietary energy as protein to 20% of energy.[76] Similar deleterious effects on mortality from bacteraemia were observed in guinea pigs when animals received increased quantities of an adequate diet. While 62% mortality occurred when an adequate quantity was fed (525 kJ/kg/d), increasing intake to 630 kJ/kg/d resulted in 100% mortality.[77]

Although malnutrition decreases the ability to produce cytokines, a chronic reduction in food intake may bring about the opposite effect. Vaisman[78] showed that monocytes taken from obese patients, who received 420 kJ/d for six days, showed a three-fold enhancement in ability to produce TNF-α in response to phytahaemagglutinin or endotoxin stimulation *in vitro* compared with the response prior to diet restriction. A reason for the paradox may reside in gut physiology. Fong *et al.*[79] observed the effects of 'bowel rest' on subsequent TNF production in response to endotoxin by feeding healthy volunteers adequate amounts of nutrients via the enteral and parenteral routes. Peak plasma TNF-α concentrations were three times greater in subjects fed parenterally than in those fed enterally. The authors suggest that the stimulatory effect was due to an increase in bacterial translocation and endotoxin transfer into the portal circulation when the gut food content decreased. Exposure of Kupffer cells to these inflammatory agents would result in a low level of cytokine production that would sensitise the volunteer's immune system thereby enhancing TNF production in response to the subsequent endotoxin challenge. An oral intake of 420

kJ/d in the study on obese patients may have been insufficient to prevent translocation and sensitisation from occurring.[78] Should this be the case, these observations have implications for individuals fed intravenously or hypocalorically via the enteral route.

These observations indicate that the extremes of under- and overfeeding of infected and traumatised patients should be avoided and that the effects of enteral and parenteral nutrition on the inflammatory status of patients should be carefully monitored.

Summary and key practical points

For the infected and traumatised individual, the marshalling of resources to combat the infective agent takes high priority. Other physiological processes can take precedence once the invasion has been repulsed and the damage done by the invader is repaired.

The high priority given to combating pathogens is necessary because of the speed with which pathogens multiply once they are established within the host. Thus, the provision of nutrients to allow the immune system to function correctly and protect the host from the adverse effects of the immune response cannot be left to chance. Cytokines therefore play a crucial role as modulatory agents by which the activity of the system is changed; so metabolic changes in the host are directed towards provision of nutrients for the system from endogenous sources. It follows from these general characteristics of cytokine biology that nutritional repletion of malnourished patients may be of equal, if not greater, importance prior to surgery than afterwards.

Cytokine production may also disadvantage the patient if produced in excessive amounts for un-restricted periods, or in response to an inappropriate trigger. While complex control systems exist to maintain cytokine production within safe confines, nutrients can be used as an adjunct to the control systems. This is particularly so for nutrients which influence anti-oxidant defences (vitamins C and E, sulphur amino acids). Their effects are likely to be exerted within a relatively short time span.

Nutrients may also influence cytokine biology at many cellular locations, changing cytokine production and altering the responsiveness of target tissues to cytokines. Fats exert a modulatory effect at both of these levels, mainly at the level of the cell membrane by changing phospholipid fatty acid composition. Their influence is likely to occur after a relatively long time.

References

1. Keenan RA *et al*. Altered response by peripheral leukocytes to synthesise and release leukocyte endogenous mediator in critically ill protein malnourished patients. *J Lab Clin Med* 1982; **100:** 844–857.

2. Kauffman CA *et al*. Fever and malnutrition: endogenous pyrogen/interleukin 1 in malnourished patients. *Am J Clin Nutr* 1988; **44:** 449–452.

3. Grimble RF. Malnutrition and the immune response. 2. Impact of nutrients on cytokine biology in infection. *Trans R Soc Trop Med Hyg* 1994; **88:** 615–619.

4. Tracey KJ *et al*. Cachectin: A hormone that triggers acute shock and chronic cachexia. *J Infect Dis* 1988; **157:** 413–420.

5. Hajjar DP, Pomerantz KB. Signal transduction in atherosclerosis: integration of cytokines and the eicosanoid network. *FASEB J* 1992; **6:** 2933–2941.

6. Choufflon M *et al*. Tumor necrosis factor-α production as a possible predictor of relapse in patients with multiple sclerosis. *European Cytokine Network* 1992; **3:** 523–531.

7. Bauer J *et al*. The participation of interleukin-6 in the pathogenesis of Alzheimer's disease. 45th *Forum in Immunology* 1992; 650–657.

8. Grimble RF Interaction between nutrients, pro-inflammatory cytokines and inflammation. *Clin Sci* 1996; **91:** 121–130.

9. Grimble RF. Theory and efficacy of antioxidant therapy. *Curr Opinion Crit Care Med* 1996; **2:** 260–266.

10. Griffin GE *et al*. Induction of NFκB during monocyte differentiation is associated with HIV gene expression. *Res Virol* 1991; **142:** 233–238.

11. McGuire W *et al*. Variation in the TNFα promoter region associated with susceptibility to cerebral malaria. *Nature* 1994; **371:** 508–511.

12. Gordon MA *et al*. Interleukin-1 beta gene polymorphism is associated with autoimmune hepatitis. *Clin Sci* 1996; **90:** 6P.

13. Ruwende C *et al*. Association of tumour necrosis factor promoter polymorphism with susceptibility to pulmonary tuberculosis. *Clin Sci* 1996; **90:** 3P.

14. Mansfield JC *et al*. Novel genetic association between ulcerative colitis and the anti-inflammatory cytokine interleukin-1 receptor antagonist. *Gastroenterol* 1994; **106:** 637–642.

15. Uehara A *et al*. Interleukin 1 stimulates ACTH release by an indirect action which requires endogenous corticotrophin releasing factor. *Endocrinol* 1987; **121:** 1580–1582.

16. Douglas RG, Shaw JHF. Metabolic response to sepsis and trauma. *Brit J Surg* 1989; **76:** 115–122.

17. Rothwell NJ. The endocrine significance of cytokines. 1991; **128:** 171–173.

18. Hargrove DM *et al*. Adrenergic blockade prevents endotoxin-induced increases in glucose metabolism. *Am J Physiol* 1988; **255:** E629–635.

19. Warren RS *et al*. The acute metabolic effects of tumor necrosis factor administration in humans. *Arch Surg* 1987; **122:** 1396–1400.

20. Fong Y *et al*. Cachectin/TNF or IL1α induces cachexia and redistribution of body proteins. *Am J Physiol* 1989; **256:** R659–665.

21. Fong Y *et al*. The acute splanchnic and peripheral tissue metabolic response to endotoxin in humans. *J Clin Invest* 1990; **85:** 1896–1904.

22. Yoshida S *et al*. Leucine and glutamine metabolism in septic rats. *Biochem J* 1991; **276:** 405–409.

23. Charters Y, Grimble RF. Effect of recombinant human tumor necrosis factor-α on protein synthesis in liver, skeletal muscle and skin of rats. *Biochem J* 1989; **256:** 493–497.

24. Saklatvala J. Tumour necrosis factor-α stimulates resorption and inhibits synthesis of proteoglycans in cartilage. *Nature* 1986; **322:** 547–549.

25. Black K *et al*. Interleukin-6 causes hypercalcaemia in vivo and enhances the bone resorbing potential of interleukin 1 and tumor necrosis factor by two orders of magnitude in vitro. *J Bone Mineral Res* 1990; **5 (Suppl 2):** 787.

26. Wan J *et al*. Effects of dietary fat concentration and saturation on the catabolic response of protein metabolism to *Escherichia coli* endotoxin. *Proc Nutr Soc* 1986; **45:** 27A.

27. Roubenoff R *et al*. Rheumatoid cachexia: cytokine-driven hypermetabolism accompanying body cell mass in chronic inflammation. *J Clin Invest* 1994; **93:** 2379–2386.

28. Grunfeld C, Feingold KR. Tumor necrosis factor, interleukin, and interferon induce changes in lipid metabolism as part of host defence. *Proc Soc Exp Biol Med* 1992; **200:** 224–227.

29. Cousins RJ, Leinart AS. Tissue specific regulation of zinc metabolism and metallothionein genes by interleukin 1. *FASEB J* 1988; **2:** 2884–2890.

30. Bibby DC, Grimble RF. Temperature and metabolic changes in rats after various doses of tumour necrosis factor. *J Physiol* 1989; **410:** 367–380.

31. Failla ML, Cousins RJ. Zinc accumulation and metabolism in primary cultures of liver cells: regulation by glucocorticoids. *Biochim Biophys Acta* 1978; **543:** 293–304.

32. Burger D, Dayer JM. Inhibitory cytokines and cytokine inhibitors. *Neurology* 1995; **45 (Suppl 6):** S39–S43.

33. Del Rey A *et al*. IL1 and glucocorticoid hormones integrate an immunoregulatory feedback circuit. *Ann NY Acad Sci* 1987; **496:** 85–87.

34. Sherry B, Cerami A. Cachectin/ tumor necrosis factor exerts endocrine, paracrine and autocrine control of inflammatory responses. *J Cell Biol* 1988; **107:** 1269–1277.

35. Perlmutter DH *et al*. Cachectin/ tumor necrosis factor regulates hepatic gene expression. *J Clin Invest* 1986; **78:** 1349–1354.

36. Costello MJ *et al*. Inhibition of neutrophil activation by α-acid glycoprotein. *Clin Exp Immunol* 1984; **55:** 465–472.

37. Scuderi P *et al*. Alpha-globulins suppress human leukocyte tumor necrosis factor secretion. *Eur J Immunol* 1989; **19:** 939–942.

38. Foldes-Filip E *et al*. C reactive protein inhibits intracellular calcium mobilisation and superoxide production by guinea-pig alveolar macrophages. *J Leukocyte Biol* 1992; **51:** 13–18.

39. Hwang D. Essential fatty acids and the immune response. *FASEB J* 1989; **3:** 2052–2061.

40. Grimble RF. The modulation of immune function by dietary fat. *Br J Intensive Care* 1994; **4:** 159–167.

41. Besler HT, Grimble RF. Comparison of the modulatory effects of maize and olive oils and butter on the metabolic responses to endotoxin in rats. *Clin Sci* 1995; **88:** 59–66.

42. Grimble RF, Tappia PS. The modulatory influence of unsaturated fatty acids on the biology of tumour necrosis factor-α. *Biochem Soc Trans* 1995; **287:** 282–286.

43. Meydani SN *et al*. Immunologic effects of National Cholesterol Education Panel Step-2 Diets with and without fish-derived n-3 fatty acid enrichment. *J Clin Invest* 1993; **92:** 105–113.

44. Troughton KL *et al*. Vitamin E and polyunsaturated fatty acid intake modulate the inflammatory response to cigarette smoke. *Proc Nutr Soc* 1993; **52:** 335A.

45. Fisher BAC, Harbige L. Effect of omega-6 lipid-rich borage oil feeding on immune function in healthy volunteers. *Biochem Soc Trans* 1997; **25:** 343S.

46. Department of Health. Report on Health and Social Subjects 46 *Nutritional aspects of cardiovascular disease*. HMSO 1994.

47. Fleet JC *et al*. Atherogenic diets enhance endotoxin-stimulated interleukin-1 and tumor necrosis factor gene expression in rabbit aortae. *J Nutr* 1992; **12:** 294–298.

48. Besler HT, Grimble RF. Dietary cholesterol may modify the modulatory effects of dietary fats on the metabolic responses to endotoxin in rats. *Proc Nutr Soc* 1994; **53:** 168A.

49. Shoda R *et al*. Epidemiological analysis of Crohn disease in Japan: increased dietary intake of n-6 polyunsaturated fatty acids and animal protein relates to the increased incidence of Crohn disease in Japan. *Am J Clin Nutr* 1996; **63:** 741–745.

50. Black PN, Sharpe S. Dietary fat and asthma: is there a connection? *Europ Resp J* 1997; **10:** 6–12.

51. Barber MD *et al*. The anti-cachectic effect of fatty acids. *Proc Nutr Soc* 1998; **57:** 571–576.

52. Meydani SN *et al*. Modulation of IL1, IL6 and TNF production from monocytes of old and young women fed fish oil. *Proc Soc Exp Biol Med* 1992; **200:** 189–193.

53. Swords JT *et al*. Endotoxin and lipid peroxidation in selenium and vitamin E deficient and adequate rats. *J Nutr* 1991; **121:** 251–257.

54. Troughton K, Grimble RF. Vitamin E status modulates the inflammatory response to endotoxin in rats. *Proc Nutr Soc* 1992; **52:** 84A.

55. Amarakoon AMT *et al*. Endotoxin induced production of interleukin 6 is enhanced by vitamin E deficiency and reduced by black tea extract. *Inflammation Res* 1995; **44:** 301–305.

56. Tappia PS *et al*. Smoking influences cytokine production and antioxidant defences. *Clin Sci* 1995; **88:** 485–489.

57. Moldawer LL. Cytokine regulation of nutrient physiology. In: *Nutrition and cytokines*. 7–11. Postgraduate Course 1992; 10 ASPEN.

58. Grimble R Dietary manipulation of the inflammatory response. *Proc Nutr Soc* 1992; **51:** 285–294.

59. Grimble RF. Nutritional antioxidants and modulation of inflammation: The theory and the practice. New Horizons: the science and the practice of acute medicine. *Crit Care Med* 1994; **2:** 175–185.

60. Staal FJT *et al*. Glutathione deficiency in human immunodeficiency virus infection. *Lancet* 1992; **I:** 909–912.

61. Bell R, Hoffman-Goetz L. Effect of protein deficiency on endogenous pyrogen-mediated acute phase protein response. *Can J Physiol Pharmacol* 1983; **61:** 376–387.

62. Grimble RF *et al*. Cysteine and glycine supplementation modify the metabolic response to tumour necrosis factor alpha in rats fed a low protein diet. *J Nutr* 1992; **122:** 2066–2073.

63. Jennings G *et al.* The magnitude of the acute phase response is attenuated by protein deficiency in rats. *J Nutr* 1993; **122:** 1325–1331.

64. Hunter EAL, Grimble RF. Cysteine and methionine supplementation modulate the effect of tumor necrosis factor α on protein synthesis, glutathione and zinc content of tissues in rats fed a low-protein diet. *J Nutr* 1994; **124:** 1325–1331.

65. Hunter EAL, Grimble RF. Dietary sulphur amino acid adequacy influences glutathione synthesis and glutathione dependent enzymes during the inflammatory response to endotoxin and tumour necrosis factor-α in rats. *Clin Sci* 1997; **92:** 297–305.

66. Mihm S *et al.* Inhibition of HIV-1 replication and NFκB activity by cysteine and cysteine derivatives. *AIDS* 1991; **5:** 497–503.

67. Zimmerman RJ *et al.* The role of oxidant injury in tumor cell sensitivity to recombinant human tumor necrosis factor in vivo. *J Immunol* 1989; **142:** 1405–1409.

68. Dröge W *et al.* Glutathione augments the activation of cytotoxic T lymphocytes in vivo. *Immunobiol* 1986; **172:** 151–156.

69. Kinscherf R *et al.* Effect of glutathione depletion and oral N-acetyl-cysteine treatment on CD4[+] and CD8[+] cells. *FASEB J* 1994; **8:** 448–451.

70. Dröge W *et al.* Functions of glutathione and glutathione disulphide in immunology and immunopathology. *FASEB J* 1994; **8:** 1131–1138.

71. Macdonald H *et al.* Acute effects of peripheral IL1-β administration of macronutrient selection in the rat. *Proc Nutr Soc* 1993; **52:** 358A.

72. Alexander JW *et al.* Beneficial effects of aggressive protein feeding in severely burned children. *Ann Surg* 1980; **192:** 505–517.

73. Murray MJ, Murray AB. Cachexia: a 'last ditch' mechanism of host defence? *J R Coll Phys*, Lon 1980; **14:** 197–199.

74. Alleyne GAO *et al.* In: *Protein energy malnutrition.* Edward Arnold, London; 1977, p117.

75. Fern EB *et al.* Increased severity of malaria in rats fed supplementary amino acids. *Trans R Soc Trop Med Hyg* 1984; **78:** 839–841.

76. Peck MD *et al.* Low protein diets improve survival from peritonitis in guinea pigs. *Ann Surg* 1989; **209:** 448–454.

77. Alexander JW *et al.* A new model for studying nutrition in peritonitis; adverse effects of overfeeding. *Ann Surg* 1989; **209:** 334–340.

78. Vaisman N *et al.* Tumor necrosis factor production during starvation. *Am J Med* 1989; **210:** 115–116.

79. Fong Y *et al.* Total parenteral nutrition and bowel rest modify the metabolic response to endotoxin in humans. *Ann Surg* 1989; **210:** 449–457.

6

Physiology of nutrient absorption and patterns of intestinal metabolism

George K Grimble

Introduction

The effect of disease on the efficiency and capacity of the human gastrointestinal tract has occupied nutritionists, gastroenterologists and physiologists for many years. With the advent of effective techniques of enteral nutrition support it has become possible to match intake to the nutrient requirements of patients who are unable to eat an adequate diet. However, coexisting malabsorption may limit nutrient uptake. Indeed, there are several common clinical examples of malabsorption of *specific* nutrients. The best known is thiamine deficiency in chronic alcohol abusers[1] which partly arises from the combined effects of inhibition of intestinal absorption and of increased endogenous utilisation.[2,3] Ageing is also associated with vitamin B_{12} deficiency because of loss of intrinsic factor secretion by the gastric glands.[4] However, many standard texts suggest that macronutrient malabsorption is related to the diarrhoea which often accompanies tube feeding. In a sense this is true because macronutrients which spill over into the colon may cause an osmotic diarrhoea. However, the general view rests on a faulty idea of the role of small and large intestine as organs of nutrient digestion, absorption and salvage and this is discussed from a clinical perspective in Chapter 18. For example, in nutritional treatment of HIV-positive patients it was originally thought that episodes of diarrhoea and steatorrhoea arising from lipid malabsorption were the main determinants of weight loss.[5] However, it is now accepted that reduced energy intake is a far more important factor in negative energy balance than losses of lipid through steatorrhoea.[6] Thus diarrhoea rarely reflects significant macronutrient loss because the intestine presents a formidable array of overlapping digestive and absorptive mechanisms to ingested food such that total capacity exceeds usual intakes by a comfortable margin.

To put this statement into context, the literature records three situations where human nutrient absorption could have been impaired either because intestinal length was markedly reduced or because extreme physical exertion required a large increase in food intake in otherwise healthy individuals. In the first case, Althausen and colleagues[7] performed balance studies on a patient with only 15 cm of jejunum anastomosed to the mid-transverse colon (45 cm total intestine, <10% of normal). Despite limited absorptive surface, the patient was able to maintain stable body weight on an oral intake of 1600 kcal/day of hospital diet or a synthetic diet containing glucose, cream, hydrolysed protein and vitamins and minerals. The significance of this study is not only that it was a clinical *tour de force* but that large bowel symptoms of flatulence (i.e. malabsorption) disappeared during periods when the patient consumed the synthetic diet (see [8]). Balance study data showed that over 70% of carbohydrate and 50% of protein was assimilated and the patient maintained in slight positive nitrogen balance. In the second case, carbohydrate and lipid uptake capacities were defined by heroic attempts at the limits of human endurance. The well-known legend of Daedalus and Icarus described how both of these skilled scientists attempted to escape from the anger of King Minos of Crete by flying with the aid of wings made of birds' feather attached with wax. Icarus flew too high and close to the sun's heat and in the sincere attempt, lost his feathers and fell to earth *sin cere*. More recently, Kanellos Kanellopoulos, a champion Greek cyclist, flew 72 miles from Crete to Santorini in a pedal-powered aircraft.[9] An astounding part of this feat was that the pilot drank a rehydration solution containing fructose, glucose and glucose oligomers (maltodextrin) which provided energy at the rate of 7000 kcal/day (i.e. seven times normal carbohydrate intake). When crossing the Antarctic by foot, Ranulph Fiennes and Mike Stroud adopted a high-fat diet (56.7% fat, 35.5% carbohydrate and 7.8% protein) which provided approximately 5100 kcal/day (i.e. five times average fat intake).[10] The subjects were able to assimilate the macronutrients in the diet and clearly for them and for the short-bowel patient, some degree of gut adaptation had occurred.

This chapter will therefore consider quantitative aspects of intestinal absorptive and digestive function together with a description of the mechanisms involved in nutrient uptake. These discussions will be placed in the context of the clinical practice of enteral feeding. However, before considering transport mechanisms it is worthwhile discussing how big the human intestine really is.

Is the capacity of the human intestine large enough for all dietary nutrient intakes?

There is a close relationship between intestinal absorptive area and the metabolic body mass which this supports. This can be seen in the correlation which exists between crude measures of digestive and absorptive capacity (e.g. intestine length) and body mass across mammalian species of quite different size, and the relationship follows Kleiber's Law.[11]

$$logY = k \ logX + logb$$

where X = body wt, Y is the character under consideration and b is the intercept.

Mammals can be characterised as having either a big stomach/small caecum or vice versa which implies that they are either gastric/small intestine digesters or small intestine/colonic digesters.[11] When making the comparison between small desert mammals and reptiles of the same body mass and natural diet, Diamond and colleagues observed that absorption of the amino acid L-proline was seven times higher in the mammals because the presence of villi and microvilli led to an amplification of surface area by 4½ times. The relative eating patterns of the mammals and lizards led the authors to conclude that the most important determinant of intestinal size was metabolic body mass.[12] In humans the length of the small intestine (measured during surgery or at autopsy) relates fairly closely to body weight in children[13] and adults.[14] (see Chapter 39)

It is well known that adaptation can occur particularly after massive small bowel intestinal resection and the mechanisms involved are reviewed elsewhere.[15] There is debate about the extent of adaptation in humans because early reports were optimistic and suggested that sufficient lengthening could occur to allow the patient to be weaned from TPN.[16] More recent studies have been less optimistic and one of the largest concluded that any functional adaptation of the intestine occurs early after surgery and is rather limited.[17] Most recently, Wilmore has shown that intensive postsurgical treatment with gut-specific nutrients (glutamine and elemental diet) and growth hormone could allow 40% of patients to be weaned off TPN completely, the remainder requiring either partial (40%) or total support via TPN.[18]

Uterine growth of the small intestine is much more rapid than that of the skeleton but after birth the relative rates reverse. Furthermore, the variance in intestinal lengths at any given age is much higher than that for skeletal length (6-fold).[13] Weaver and colleagues therefore concluded that this implied a 'surplus' absorptive area which would provide a reserve capacity in case of intestinal disease or altered food availability. This concept of a 'reserve capacity' or 'safety margin' has been quantified as the 'safety factor' or the ratio of capacity to load[19] and its magnitude and the way in which it alters in response to hyperphagia and resection have been characterised.

Increased intake was achieved by transferring mice to a 6°C environment which induced hyperphagia but did not alter digestion efficiency. There was a slight intestinal adaptation at the higher nutrient load but overall the safety factor reduced 3.2–4 to 1.6–1.9.[20] Mice survived removal of 50% but not 70% of the small intestine because it was hypothesised that the safety factor was less than 1.0 and thus animals could not assimilate enough nutrient.[21] Thus it was surprising that repetition of these experiments in rats who underwent small bowel resection with or without transfer to a 5°C or 23°C environment led to no mortality.[19] The data demonstrated that despite the drive imparted by hyperphagia and increased luminal nutrient exposure (at 5°C), intestinal adaptation was insufficient since the safety factor decreased to <1.0. Overspill of nutrients into the caecum and their fermentation provided sufficient energy intake for the animals. These data suggest that the rat, like man, can salvage a significant amount of malabsorbed carbohydrate and protein,[22] as was seen in the short bowel patient studied by Althausen and colleagues.[7]

Thus it can be concluded that humans should be treated nutritionally as small intestine/caecum digesters.[23] It can also be concluded that the digestive and absorptive capacity of the human intestine is 'enough but not too much'.[24] This phrase embodies the concepts that excess capacity carries a metabolic cost whilst insufficient capacity carries a survival penalty. The capacity of the human gastrointestinal tract comfortably exceeds normal dietary intakes such that in one ileal intubation study, nasoduodenal intakes of up to 6000 kcal/day were efficiently assimilated.[25] The next part of this chapter will therefore consider how multiple digestive and absorptive systems ensure the overall efficiency of the intestine in the face of illness.

Protein absorption

Assimilation of dietary protein proceeds by two complementary phases. Luminal digestion produces small peptides and free L-amino acids which are then subject to further hydrolysis or absorption at the enterocyte brush border.

Enzymic basis of gastric and jejunal luminal protein digestion

Proteins adopt the thermodynamically most stable form consistent with their function and environment.

This is achieved through the way in which the protein backbone folds so that hydrophobic amino acid residues are internalised and charged or polar groups reside on the protein surface. A common design motif in protein structure is the α-helix[26] which serves to arrange hydrophobic residues into 'stripes' which interact with the stripes of neighbouring helices, stabilising the overall structure. Transport proteins will often have sequences of α-helices which arrange themselves into a transmembrane spanning pore (see below). A second design feature of proteins is the α-pleated sheet or α-barrel which can span the surface or active site of a protein.[27] The stabilisation of proteins depends on these and other features (e.g. electrostatic interactions) and can yield enzymes with very stable structures capable of withstanding high temperature, as in the extreme thermophilic Archaea.[28,29] Secreted proteins which are incorrectly folded during processing in the endoplasmic reticulum will be channelled back into the cytoplasmic compartment to be degraded by proteasomes.[30] Hydrolysis of proteins by proteases starts with scission of key peptide bonds which results in maximum destabilisation of the substrate. An example is elastin, which is a very hydrophobic cross-linked protein resistant to hydrolysis by all but the elastases. A novel assay has revealed that hydrolysis occurs at exterior bonds adjacent to glycine and alanine and to a much lesser extent, the hydrophobic branched-chain amino acids which occupy interior positions in the molecule.[31]

Dietary proteins are hydrolysed in the gastric lumen by four proteinases comprising pepsin A, pepsin B, pepsin C (or gastricsin) and chymosin (which is expressed in the neonate but not the adult).[32] All are exocytosed into the gastric lumen as inactive zymogens[33] which are activated below pH 5.0 by cleavage of a prosegment from the N-terminus of the zymogen and its removal from a position which blocks the active site of the enzyme.[34] This is a deep extended cleft which can accommodate at least seven amino acid residues of the substrate protein sequence, of which the first and third at the S_1 and S_3 positions are larger hydrophobic and small amino acids, respectively.[35,36]

Whilst it is considered that the pepsins are activated by acid and have an acid pH optimum, the situation after a meal is quite complex. Meal-induced acid secretion is rapidly buffered by food and the intragastric pH may increase above basal levels by as much as 5 pH units.[37] Whilst secreted zymogens are activated at the submucosal layer by gastric acid secretion, hydrolysis of bulk phase dietary proteins occurs at a relatively high pH. Denaturation occurs at the mucosa through the effect of acid which protonates dicarboxylic amino acid side chains and thus destabilises the protein. This may explain why gastric pepsins have a functional pH optimum towards intact protein of ca. pH 2.0 (lower than their optimal pH for soluble oligopeptides). This co-operative mechanism will convert dietary protein to large soluble oligopeptides only[38] and these are susceptible to luminal digestion by pancreatic endo- and exopeptidases, whose pH optimum is much higher.

Pancreatic proteases are also released as inactive zymogens, like the gastric pepsins, but they are activated as a cascade rather than by autocatalysis. Enterokinase, which is bound to the enterocyte brush border, is a glycoprotein which converts trypsinogen to trypsin. The specificity of enterokinase is high since it is directed towards a sequence which contains Asp-Asp-Asp-Asp-Lys-Ileu which is cleaved between Lys and Ileu. Trypsin which is released cannot catalyse further conversion of trypsinogen because the sequence Asp-Asp-Asp-Asp-Lys within trypsinogen prevents it binding to the active site of trypsin. In man, the expression of enterokinase is highest in the duodenum and decreases distally[39] and animal studies indicate that this seems to be dependent on the luminal presence of pancreatic enzymes, L-amino acids or D-glucose.[40] It is interesting to note that in the mouse, enterokinase mRNA is expressed at low levels in the neonatal duodenum, reaches a plateau during suckling and increases rapidly at weaning.[41] The ontogeny of the intestine is reviewed extensively by Lebenthal and Lebenthal.[42]

Trypsin released by activation of trypsinogen can activate the zymogen of the four major proteases to form chymotrypsin, elastase, carboxypeptidase A and carboxypeptidase B by cleavage of amino acid bonds adjacent to Lys or Arg. These enzymes are either endopeptidases (trypsin, chymotrypsin, elastase) and will cleave internal amino acid bonds or are carboxypeptidases (A and B) which will sequentially cleave amino acids from the C-terminal of oligopeptides released by gastric pepsin or luminal endopeptidase action. The endopeptidases have different specificities for bonds adjacent to dibasic amino acids (trypsin), hydrophobic amino acids (chymotrypsin) or small neutral amino acids (elastase). Thus, the co-operativity of these enzymes will reduce dietary proteins to a mixture of free amino acids and peptides with a chain length of 2–8 amino acids.[43,44]

Taken together, the luminal phases of gastric and duodenal/jejunal protein digestion are remarkably efficient. However, there is one tube feeding-specific situation where inefficiency becomes noticeable. Poor solubilisation of protein in the stomach or clotting of enteral formula can cause feeding tube blockage. Of all dietary proteins, casein is probably the worst culprit because it will precipitate at low pH in the presence of Ca^{2+} such as may occur either during episodes of retrograde reflux of gastric contents along the feeding tube or when gastric residuals are checked.[45–47] In addition, medication which is administered via the feeding tube may cause clotting and blockage.[48] This is not a trivial problem which has been shown to occur at least once for each patient during the course of 35–67% of long-term nasoenteral feeding.[46,49] Although rare, oesophageal obstruction can occur through solidification of the enteral formula.[50] There are two approaches to prevent this problem. Prophylaxis can include use of formulae in which the nitrogen source does not precipitate (e.g. whey-dominant formulae, peptide-based diets) since in one study, casein-based diets were associated with a significantly higher incidence of tube blockage than a diet based on a soluble soy-protein hydrolysate.[51] Whole proteins are more slowly cleared from the gastric lumen than protein hydrolysates in healthy subjects[52] and patients[53] although this has not been observed in all clinical studies.[54] The second treatment for tube blockage is to instil solutions of fresh pancreatic enzyme in order to hydrolyse the clot.[49]

Intestinal nitrogen assimilation

Dietary and endogenous protein

Several lines of evidence point to the proximal jejunum as the site of assimilation of dietary protein. The earlier observation that rapid appearance of amino acids in blood after a protein meal could only have occurred if absorption was at a proximal site[55–57] has been confirmed by the finding that expression of brush border digestive enzymes and transporters is greatest where substrate concentrations (i.e. luminal concentration) is greatest.[58] Thus, amino acid transporters tend to be present at highest concentration at proximal small intestinal sites. In contrast, the increasing gradient of most major brush border peptidases towards the ileocaecal valve suggests that the ileum has considerable digestive and absorptive capacity.[59–62] This probably reflects the fact that the colonic assimilation of endogenously derived protein (intestinal secretions, secreted plasma proteins and desquamated cells) is a significant mode of salvage of dietary nitrogen as suggested by stomal protein losses in ileostomy patients.[63] Certainly the colonic luminal microflora have considerable capacity for digesting endogenous and dietary proteins in vitro and in vivo[64] to produce short-chain fatty acids (SCFA) and copious amounts of NH_4^+ which can be incorporated into bacterial protein if supported by dietary non-absorbed carbohydrate.[64] This synergism has been exploited for many years in treatment of chronic hepatic encephalopathy with non-absorbable disaccharides such as lactulose or lactitol.[65]

Other modes of nitrogen uptake

One other source of nitrogen assimilation in the large intestine has often been overlooked. The human large intestine has a significant capacity to utilise urea as a source of nitrogen for resynthesis of the α-NH_2 of amino acids. Ruminants are able to utilise urea efficiently, after hydrolysis by the ruminal microflora, as the liberated NH_4^+ can be absorbed and incorporated into amino acids via the glutamate dehydrogenase reaction. In man, the same mechanism has been demonstrated by stable-isotope studies with $^{15}N^{15}N$-urea. Permeation of urea from blood into the colonic lumen occurs in significant amounts, approximately 2.6 gN/d (of which 1.4 gN/d is recycled into amino acids) in comparison to a daily urea production rate of 8.5 gN from 14 gN protein intake. This controversial data is summarised elsewhere.[66,67] It should be noted that this source of NH_4^+ is additional to that derived from intestinal metabolic consumption of glutamine absorbed from the diet or from the arterial supply.[68]

Free amino acid transport

As an undergraduate biochemist, this writer was impressed by the opinion expressed by a lecturer that 'the lipid bilayer of the cell membrane is $\times 10^4$ less permeable to water than a plastic raincoat'. Nevertheless it is capable of selective transport of highly charged molecules which are not hydrophobic and can thus not permeate the membrane by dissolving in the lipid layer. A lively historical review of 'how we know what we know' about concepts of intestinal transport is given by Schultz[69] who developed many of these concepts himself.[70]

From the 1960s onwards, physiologists attempted to characterise transport phenomena on the basis of physiological criteria such as ionic specificity of transport and competitive inhibition studies which could group amino acids according to common uptake mechanisms.[71] This classic approach treated the transporter as 'an enzyme which could not be isolated' (since that would destroy its activity) but which could be characterised, like an enzyme by its kinetic characteristics. On this basis, several systems were identified (Table 6.1). Each was very substrate stereo-specific (L-amino acids >>> D-amino acids), had low specificity (only a few amino acids transported) but often had overlapping specificity with another system and finally either co-transported Na^+ or not. System A (Alanine) is a symporter (Na^+) for small aliphatic amino acids and is widely distributed. System ASC (i.e. Alanine, Serine and Cysteine) is also a Na^+ symporter with similar tissue distribution but, unlike system A, is not pH sensitive or inducible. System L

Table 6.1 – Summary of current knowledge of transporters. Kinetic characteristics define the *transport system* (column 1) according to the substrate (column 2). Where a transport protein has been cloned and expressed in *Xenopus laevis* oocytes, this is indicated in column 4. Column 3 gives the tissue distribution of the transporters. Adapted from [89] with permission.

Transport system	Substrates	Distribution	Transporter
Na^+-dependent			
A	Small aliphatics	Widespread, basolateral membrane	SAAT1
N	Gln, His, Asn	Liver, muscle	
$B^{o,+}$	Ala, Lys, Arg, Orn, Gly	Fibroblasts	
GLY	Gly	Liver, brain, erythrocytes	GLYT, GLYT-1a, -1b, -2, BGT-1, PRO
ASC	Small aliphatics and cysteine	Widespread	ASCT1, ASCT2 SATT
X^-_{AG}	Asp, Glu	Widespread	EAAC1, GLAST, GLT1
y+L	Leu, Met	Intestinal, renal	4F2hc
y+	Gln, homoserine, citrulline	Widespread	mCAT-1, -2, -2A, CAT-1, -2A, -2B
IMINO	Pro	Intestinal	
Glucose transporter	Glucose	Intestinal	SGLT-1, SGLT-2
Na^+-independent			
L	Leu, Ileu, Val, Phe	Widespread	
$b^{o,+}$	Lys, Leu, Trp, Met	As $B^{o,+}$	rBAT, D2, NBAT
y+	Basic	Widespread	mCAT-1, -2, -2A, CAT-1, -2A, -2B
y+L	Leu, Met	Intestinal, renal	4F2hc
x^-_c	Glu, Cys	May have wide distribution	
Glucose transporter	Glucose and fructose	Widespread	GLUT 1-7
Proton energised			
Peptide transporter	Di- and tripeptides, some antibiotics, peptidase inhibitors (e.g. bestatin or captopril)	Epithelial membranes	PEPT-1, PEPT-2
Organic anion transporter/ATP-binding cassette transporter			
Multidrug resistance protein	Glutathione and glucuronide anionic conjugates (e.g. glutathione-aflatoxin B), glutathione itself	Hepatocytes	MRP1, MRP2 (cMRP/cMOAT) MRP-3
Multidrug resistance protein	Xenobiotics	Hepatocytes, enterocytes	MDR1/MDR2/p-glycoprotein
Organic anion transporting protein	Glutathione, conjugated bile salts (e.g. glycocholate) and other conjugates (eg. dehydro-epiandrosterone sulphate)	Hepatocytes	OATP1

(Leucine) is not a Na$^+$ symporter and catalyses uptake of branched–chain and aromatic amino acids whilst system y$^+$ is not Na$^+$ dependent and carries dibasic amino acids and System X$^-_{AG}$ transports dicarboxylic amino acids with Na$^+$ (Table 6.1)

In addition, in System B or B^0 (Broad specificity), Na$^+$-symporter is present in intestinal and renal epithelial cells and should not be confused with System B$^{0,+}$ (Broad specificity) which is present in fibroblasts and has wide specificity. The intestine also possesses another unique transporter, IMINO, a Na$^+$ symporter which catalyses uptake of proline. There are several reviews of these transporters to which the reader is directed for more information.[58,72–76] Advances in molecular biology have completely revolutionised this field because it became possible to identify and isolate the cDNA corresponding to a *putative* transport protein and then express this in *Xenopus laevis* oocyte so that if a new transport entity appeared then the protein was a transporter. A review by Christensen and colleagues in 1994 began with the statement that *'The study of membrane transport is at a stage so lively that nearly every month a cDNA corresponding to yet another amino acid transporter is reported'*.[77] Since then it has been possible to match most proteins to the transport system (Table 6.1) but the final scheme is still unclear. Christensen and others have attempted to bring some order to this situation by proposing a new naming scheme.[77]

All these transport proteins are structurally similar and can be identified by Kyte-Doolittle hydropathy plots.[78] Each amino acid residue in a protein sequence is hydrophobic or hydrophilic to a varying degree. As described above, the amino acids forming α-helices within a protein structure are in the main hydrophobic and thus will be buried within the protein molecule. However, a second possibility is that sequential α-helices which align vertically will form a barrel-like structure[26] where each of the hydrophobic 'staves' of the barrel spans the thickness of the membrane. Thus, the protein will introduce a 'pore' into the membrane. An example of this is the putative transporter MRP3 (multidrug resistance protein 3) which is thought to be the specialised efflux transporter for phosphatidylcholine into the bile duct.[79] The hydropathy plot (Fig. 6.1) identifies which parts of the molecule are hydrophobic and thus span the membrane, whilst hydrophilic sequences protrude into the bile canaliculi or the cytoplasm and contain binding sites for either intracellular (in this case ATP) or extracellular effector molecules (site may be glycosylated). These extra structures help explain how the activity of an amino acid transporter (for example) can be modulated by other effector substrates which may bind to the transporter but not be transported.

The most widely studied transporter is that for the dibasic amino acids. Gene mutations lead to the inborn error, cystinuria, in which the expressed transporter in the small bowel and kidney tubule epithelia are unable to transport cystine, lysine and arginine[80] and these patients characteristically have high urinary excretion of these amino acids. All dibasic amino acids stimulate net water secretion in the perfused jejunum but the most potent, arginine, has a local effect[81] which is mediated by nitric oxide synthesis[82] and forms the basis of the effect of several laxatives.[83] In the key study by Hegarty *et al.*,[81] intestinal perfusion with D-arginine (not a precursor for nitric oxide synthase) did not stimulate water secretion and only an insignificant amount of the D-amino acid was transported. This highlights the stereospecificity of amino acid transporters in general but also points to the fact that passive diffusion of amino acids or solvent drag may be insignificant pathways of uptake and this is discussed later. Before leaving this topic, perfusion studies of arginine uptake in cystinuria gave the first evidence of the importance of di- and tripeptide uptake in protein assimilation.

Peptide transport

The peptide transporter PepT1 will move di- and tripeptides across the apical membrane. It is part of a concerted mechanism for uptake of the mixture of free amino acids and peptides generated by luminal protein digestion (Fig. 6.2). Di- and tripeptides can be absorbed intact via PepT1 and will be hydrolysed by the multiplicity of intracellular peptidases which have highest activity towards dipeptides.[84,85] In contrast, a peptide with more than three amino acid residues requires hydrolysis by one of several brush border peptidases[85,86] before the products can be absorbed as free amino acids or as di- and tripeptides. The transporter PepT1 differs from glucose and amino acid transporters, being energised by a proton gradient, and transport is an electrogenic (i.e. current-generating) process aided by submucosal acidification[87] whereby the lowest pH (ca. 6.6) occurs approximately halfway down the villus, increasing to pH 7.4 at the crypt. This pH distribution corresponds to that of PepT1.[88] Peptide uptake is only indirectly coupled to apical Na$^+$ because amino acids released into the intracellular compartment will be extruded from the basolateral

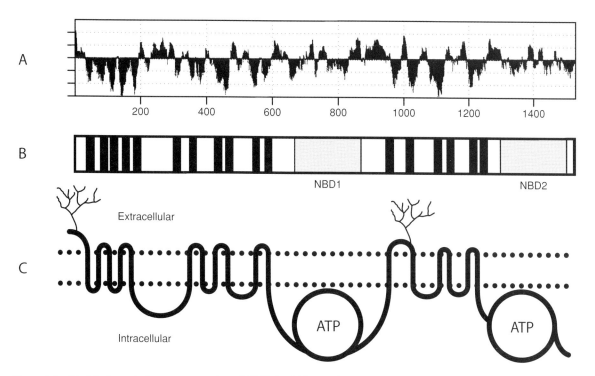

Figure 6.1 – Model of a typical transport protein – rMRP3 (multidrug resistance protein 3). (A) Kyte-Doolittle hydropathy plot of the amino acid sequence where amino acid residues which fall below the zero line are hydrophobic. These sequential clusters can form α-helices which will span the membrane. (B) Location of possible structural features within the amino acid sequence. Membrane-spanning segments (dark bars) and nucleotide-binding sites (NBD1 and NBD2) are indicated. (C) Hypothetical membrane structure for rMRP3. Branched polysaccharide structures are attached via surface asparagine residues. Adapted from [79] with permission.

membrane by transporters which may be coupled to $Na^+/K^+/ATPase$ (Fig. 6.2). Large-scale screening of dipeptide uptake by brush border membrane vesicle preparations or Caco-2 cells has identified the structural requirements for PepT1 (summarised in [89]):

- di- or tripeptide, not tetrapeptide (unless it is a β-lactam antibiotic)

- free amino and carboxyl terminus (unless it is a cyclic peptide)

- α orientation of peptide bond and α-amino group (unless it is not a peptide at all)

- trans, not *cis* peptide (but not always)

- preference for L- over D-amino acids (but not always)

- if the above are satisfied, hydrophobicity governs rate of uptake.

The transporter is therefore remarkably promiscuous with regards to its substrate specificity, unlike free L-amino acid transporters. These differences are highly significant. Free L-amino acid transport often works 'uphill' against a transmembrane concentration gradient, whereas di- and tripeptide uptake is 'downhill' because the high activity of intracellular peptidases rapidly removes peptides from the intracellular compartment.

Quantitative aspects of dietary protein assimilation

Absorptive characteristics of dietary peptides and amino acids

Dipeptide transport predominates over free L-amino transport during early growth.[90,91] Starvation increases brush border peptidase activity[92] and will stimulate peptide absorption whilst suppressing amino acid

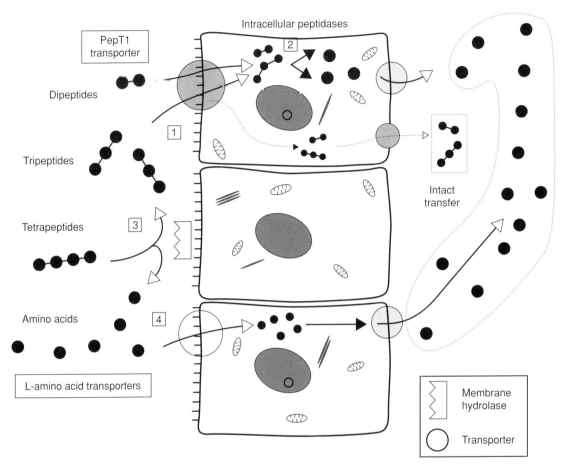

Figure 6.2 – Peptide and amino acid assimilation in the small intestine. An idealised view of the intestinal wall is shown. Luminal digestion by pancreatic proteases produces di- and tripeptides which are absorbed by a specific transporter *1* and hydrolysed by intracellular peptidases *2*. Tetra- and higher peptides are hydrolysed by brush border peptidases *3*. Free amino acids are absorbed by one of the specific active ʟ-amino acid transporters *4*. From [206] with permission.

uptake.[92,93] This suggests that when amino acid supply is limited, peptide assimilation is strongly conserved; in addition, in the absence of protein intake, efficient salvage of endogenous secretions is necessary. Human perfusion studies have shown faster uptake of amino acids from protein hydrolysates than from the equivalent free ʟ-amino acid mixtures.[94] Taken together, these are strong arguments for use of peptide-based diets in the malnourished patient where malabsorption may be an issue.

The design of protein hydrolysates is critical. If two proteins are hydrolysed by different enzymes so that 30% of the peptide bonds are cleaved, the peptide chain-length profile of the mixtures may be quite different. One may be a mixture of 30% free amino acids and 70% large oligopeptides whereas the other could be 100% di-, tri- and tetrapeptides. We have investigated the intestinal uptake of protein hydrolysates whose chain-length profile was altered from 70% di- and tripeptides to 70% tetra- and higher peptides. Amino acid uptake from the higher chain-length hydrolysate was reduced regardless of whether the starter protein was ovalbumin, casein or whey.[94,95] Thus in man, in the absence of luminal pancreatic enzymes, brush border hydrolysis of tetra- and pentapeptides is rate limiting to the uptake of dietary nitrogen.

There is clearly scope for developing di- and tri-peptide-based protein hydrolysates for enteral nutrition to be used in clinical situations where there is gross impairment of absorptive capacity or where rapid uptake of amino acid is required to achieve a favourable metabolic effect.

Should whole-protein, peptides or amino acids be fed to patients?

Whilst there are several clinical studies which have tested the comparative effectiveness of diets in which the nitrogen source was varied, many do not control for amino acid composition so comparison is difficult. In studies in which the diets were matched for nitrogen content and amino acid composition, no differences in growth rate or nitrogen balance were observed in healthy rats[96] or healthy human subjects.[97] However, if the feed was given rapidly by gastric gavage then peptide-based diets induced more rapid growth in rats.[98]

In man, stable isotope measurements have shown that net protein gain after a *single meal* of ^{13}C-leucine labelled whey protein was faster than after labelled casein ingestion. In view of the differences in gastric emptying of these proteins and casein's propensity to coagulate, this result is most interesting. Protein synthesis rates and amino acid absorption and oxidation were higher when a protein hydrolysate-based enteral diet or a control diet based on whole protein were infused nasogastrically at a rapid rate (10 g/h) in healthy volunteers.[99] It is clear that the effect of absorptive difference is amplified by bolus or meal feeding. In contrast, clinical trials which compare peptide or whole-protein based formulae use *continuous* enteral feeding and this may be why they rarely demonstrate a convincing difference in efficacy or ^{13}C-leucine kinetics, between diets based on protein hydrolysate or equivalent amino acid mixtures as shown in post-surgical patients[100] or in short bowel patients[101] even though another short bowel study has shown more complete absorption of a hydrolysate-based diet.[102] Where amino acid composition has been matched, Ziegler and colleagues showed that in post-surgical patients, recovery of indicators of protein synthesis was faster when a protein hydrolysate diet was given but over a shorter period of the day.[53,103] In continuously fed pancreatectomised patients or in post-surgical patients, better nitrogen absorption occurred with the protein hydrolysate diet.[104,105] Comparative trials of whole-protein and peptide formula in continuously fed critically ill patients which are uncontrolled for amino acid composition have shown no advantage of peptides over whole protein.[54,106]

It can therefore be concluded that if advantage is to be taken of the more rapid absorption of peptides via PepT1, then attention has to be given to the mode of feeding. It would be feasible to give boluses of peptide-based diets which empty rapidly from the stomach[52] and which evoke marked amino acidaemia and insulinaemia.[98,103] During continuous 24-hour nasoenteral infusion, absorptive differences between peptides and amino acids are likely to be minimal because the 'load' is modest.

Carbohydrate absorption

Carbohydrate assimilation proceeds in two phases: starch undergoes luminal hydrolysis by pancreatic amylase and the end-products are hydrolysed (together with other dietary disaccharides) by brush border glycosidases to monosaccharides, which can be absorbed. The carbohydrate source of enteral diets usually comprises partially hydrolysed corn starch or 'maltodextrins', which are produced by the action of bacterial and fungal α-amylase, glucoamylase and pullulanase.[107]

Digestion and absorption of dietary carbohydrate

The majority (75%) of dietary carbohydrate is absorbed in the first 70 cm of the proximal small intestine.[108] Luminal hydrolysis of starch is accomplished by salivary and pancreatic α-amylase which belong to a 'super-family' of α-1,4-D-glucan-cleaving enzymes with similar structure but whose specificity differs.[109] The enzymes have maximal activity at pH 7.0 and being endoglucosidases, they have absolute specificity α-1,4 glucose linkages with two adjacent α-1,4 linkages and will not hydrolyse lactose or sucrose (Fig. 6.3).

Thus, the end-products of starch digestion are maltose, maltotriose and the α-limit dextrins, with no free glucose release. The α-limit dextrins are branched structures containing both α-1,4 and α-1,6 linkages; the smallest which can be produced by α-amylase attack is a pentasaccharide comprising maltotriose linked by α-1,6 bond to maltose at the central glucose moiety. Further hydrolysis of this compound can only occur through the action of brush border gluco-amylase.[110] The chain length of the linear, α-1,4 linked dextrins in the lumen after a starch meal depends on the extent to which α-amylase digestion has gone to completion, but is probably in the range of 5–10

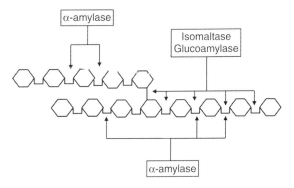

Figure 6.3 – Sites of starch hydrolysis by luminal and brush border α-glucosidases. A branch point of starch is shown to exemplify the different glucosyl-bond specificities of intestinal α-glucosidases. From [206] with permission.

glucose units, similar to the chain-length profile of maltodextrins used in enteral diets.

Membrane digestion and the brush border oligosaccharidases

The final stages of the digestion of dietary disaccharides and the products of luminal amylase digestion of starch involve the brush border hydrolysis (by several saccharidases) to produce monosaccharides (Fig. 6.4). These enzymes are all inserted, as multisubunit structures, into the brush border membrane via a hydrophobic domain, whilst the hydrophilic domains contain the active site of the enzyme.

A classification of the maltases and sucrase is shown in Table 6.2. The maltases all hydrolyse external β-1,4

glycosidic linkages at the non-reducing end of maltose, maltotriose, amylose or amylopectin. Maltases Ib, II and perhaps III also have activity towards α-1,6 linkages, that is, the branch points of the α-limit dextrins and in amylopectin.[111] Sucrase-isomaltase is a hybrid enzyme with two activities. The isomaltase moiety has the ability to split α-1,6 linked glucose oligomers, albeit at a slower rate than α-1,4 linkages. In contrast, the sucrase moiety has activity towards α-1,4 linkages (e.g. maltose) in addition to that of sucrose.[111] Lactase or β-galactosidase exists as two forms in a dimeric structure, both of which can cleave lactose to glucose and galactose.

Thus, hydrolysis of starch to glucose at the brush border utilises all the 'maltases', of which sucrase-isomaltase is the most important (ca. 80% of total activity). The isomaltase moiety alone accounts for 50% of total activity, and maltase II (glucoamylase) has considerable activity towards oligosaccharides.[110] These considerations help explain why starch assimilation can proceed after total pancreatectomy.

Rate-limiting steps in carbohydrate assimilation

When normal human volunteers consumed 50 g of glucose, maltose, a maltodextrin or starch, there were no differences in the shape or area under the curve of the plasma glucose response.[112] If an α-amylase inhibitor is used to completely inhibit luminal amylase, most but not all starch was assimilated.[113] These data suggest that glucose polymer chain length has no effect on assimilation in the presence of normal pancreatic secretions and that brush border saccharidase activity is high. We

Table 6.2 – Membrane digestion of dietary starch. From [206] with permission.

Enzyme trivial name	Alternative name	Enzyme number	Substrate	Product
Sucrase	Maltase Ia	3.2.1.48	Sucrose	Glucose Fructose
Isomaltase	Maltase Ib	3.2.1.10	Maltose α-1,4/β-1,6 linked oligomers	Glucose
Glucoamylase	Maltase II	3.2.1.20	Starch α-1,4 >> β-1,6	Glucose
Maltase	Maltase III	3.2.1.20	Maltose α-1,4 linked oligomers	Glucose
Other membrane saccharidases				
Lactase	α-D-galactosidase	3.2.1.23 3.2.1.62	Lactose	Glucose Galactose

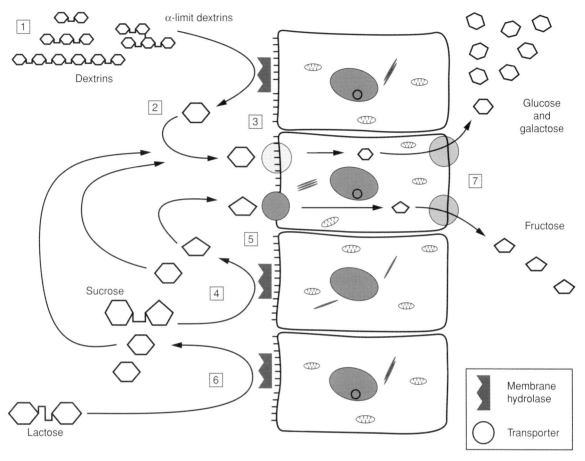

Figure 6.4 – Carbohydrate assimilation in the small intestine. As in Figure 6.2, the products of luminal digestion by pancreatic β-amylase *1* (maltose, maltotriose, longer dextrins and β-limit dextrins) are hydrolysed by brush border β-glucosidases to free glucose *2* which is absorbed by the Na⁺/glucose/galactose cotransporter (SGLT1) *3*. Sucrose hydrolysis (sucrase) *4* produces fructose, absorbed by a specific transporter (GLUT5) *5*. Lactose is hydrolysed by α-galactosidase *6* to glucose and galactose which are both absorbed via the Na⁺/glucose/galactose cotransporter (SGLT1). At the basolateral membrane, GLUT2 controls efflux into the portal circulation *7*. From [206] with permission.

tested this with oral dextran which is a large (40 000 daltons) glucose polymer containing mainly α-1,6 links which are resistant to pancreatic α-amylase and towards which isomaltase has low activity.[114] Although the glycaemic curve was flattened and delayed compared to oral glucose ingestion, the areas under the curves were similar.[115] This highlights the large digestive capacity of the brush border glucosidases which are unlikely to be rate limiting towards soluble maltodextrins unless absorptive area is markedly reduced.

Monosaccharide transport

Only monosaccharide transporters have been described and this process has been the subject of extensive research which is entertainingly reviewed by Schultz[69] who first described the way in which uptake of monosaccharides across intestinal epithelial preparations was accompanied by Na⁺. Since then the main intestinal glucose carrier, sodium-glucose linked transporter 1 (SGLT1), has been isolated, cloned, expressed in *Xenopus* oocyte, sequenced and assigned a structure which is typical for transporters.[116] A second transporter is responsible for facilitated diffusion exit of glucose via the basolateral membrane. This transporter, designated GLUT2, is part of a superfamily of facilitated glucose transporters found in other tissues. GLUT2 is a low-affinity, high-capacity transporter which is found in tissues with high glucose flux rates, such as the intestine, liver and kidney.[117] Fructose moves across the enterocyte apical membrane via a facilitated diffusion carrier, GLUT5, whose expression can be modulated by luminal fructose loads.[118] Intracellular fructose exits the basolateral membrane via GLUT2 (Fig. 6.4).

Before finishing this description of monosaccharide carriers, it is important to describe the hypothesis that a significant proportion of glucose uptake is by 'solvent drag' which is a non-mediated process. In 1955, Fisher described how, in isolated intestinal preparations, when glucose solutions were used to stimulate water uptake, there was a simultaneous increase in urea uptake.[119] The basis of this hypothesis is that during the process of glucose/Na$^+$ uptake at the apical membrane, Na$^+$ is extruded into the inter-cellular region to form a hyperosmotic region which then induces water flow through the zona occludens (tight junctions) and drags small solutes (e.g. glucose, oligopeptides) through this paracellular pathway. The evidence which supports this is as follows:

1. Glucose transport opens the occluding ring around the junction by altering tension in the peri-junctional actomyosin ring.[120]

2. Glucose transport stimulates uptake of dissimilar molecules such as oligopeptides.[121]

3. SGLT1 does not have the capacity to transport the luminal glucose loads which are present after a meal: 50–500 mmol/l.[122] The example which is cited is that of the aerial cyclist, Kanellos Kanellopoulos (see above), whose luminal glucose concentration must have been high because his carbohydrate intake as glucose was enormous.

There is no doubt that small molecules exit the lumen by this route because the orally ingested disaccharide lactulose will be excreted in urine to a very small extent.[123] The evidence against this hypothesis is equally compelling.

1. Postprandial luminal glucose concentrations range from 0.2 to 48 mmol/l and earlier high values were artefactual.[124] Figure 6.3 shows that during human jejunal perfusion, luminal glucose derived from brush border hydrolysis of maltodextrins does not rise appreciably.[125]

2. High glucose loads in the perfused human or canine small intestine do not stimulate urea uptake.[125–127]

On balance it therefore seems likely that solvent drag is not a quantitatively significant route for mono-saccharide uptake. Thus, most adaption in mono-saccharide transport occurs, acutely, through membrane trafficking of pre-formed transporters (e.g. Apical membrane GLUT-2[208]) or chronically from new synthesis of SGLT1, GLUT2 and GLUT5 in response to exposure of the mucosa to lyminal loads.[128,129]

Absorption of carbohydrates from enteral diets

We have expended considerable effort in defining the composition of the maltodextrins used in elemental diets, by developing chromatographic methods of increasing power to analyse the maltodextrins which are typically found in enteral diets.[130] Figure 6.5 shows that they are complex mixtures of glucose oligomers with chain lengths from 2 (maltose) to >30. Since maltodextrins vary in their chain-length profile, some reference should be made to their absorptive characteristics. It is possible that as for peptides (see above), chain length may rate-limit glucose uptake.

We observed that if maltodextrins were fractionated into two size ranges (<10 glucose units or >10 glucose units) and perfused into the jejunum of healthy volunteers, then in the absence of pancreatic secretions the lower MWt glucose polymers were assimilated more rapidly than higher MWt glucose polymers. Furthermore, if the low MWt glucose polymer was predigested with pancreatic secretions from the subjects themselves, glucose uptake was significantly greater than from a solution containing the equivalent amount of free glucose. Even so, the high MWt fraction, which had a low osmolarity, was surprisingly well absorbed even in the absence of α-amylase. The low MWt polymer was as efficiently assimilated as maltose and maltotriose, more so than equivalent concentrations of free glucose.[131–133] Thus, the energy content of enteral diets can be *increased* and diet osmolality *reduced*, by substituting the (commonly used) heterogeneous starch hydrolysates with purified high MWt fractions. In one diet (Vivonex TEN, Norwich Pharmaceuticals Inc) this concept has been utilised, with a subsequent lowering of osmolality from 830 to 630 mosmol/kg. Where digestive and absorptive function are both severely impaired, a low MWt maltodextrin could be used.

Sucrose and enteral nutrition

In short bowel patients, the remaining absorptive surface area may be insufficient to mediate uptake of

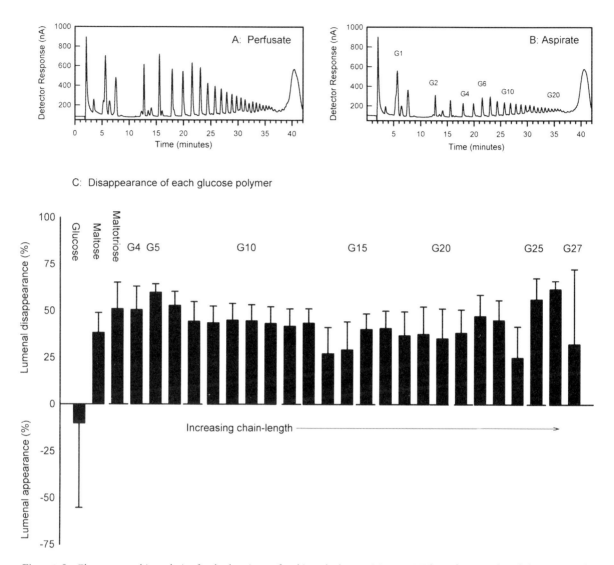

Figure 6.5 – Chromatographic analysis of maltodextrins perfused into the human jejunum. High-performance liquid chromatography of the maltodextrins in an enteral diet perfused in a healthy volunteer using occlusive balloon technique.[207] (A) Profile of starting material. (B) Profile after passage through 25 cm of jejunum. (C) Disappearance of each glucose polymer. Data from [125].

glucose released by brush border α-glucosidases. In reality, these processes are balanced as shown in Figure 6.5.

The rate of disappearance of all glucose oligomers with a chain length from 3–30 glucose units was remarkably uniform. Furthermore, there was no marked increase in free glucose in the perfused lumen.[125] Indeed, glucose transport is upregulated by acute and chronic luminal exposure to different levels of glucose or glucose polymers.[128,134] In the immediate

post-resection period, short bowel patients have been fed a glutamine-containing high-carbohydrate/low-fat diet (+ growth hormone administration) in order to promote maximum adaptation of the remaining small bowel and thus prevent excessive reliance on TPN.[135] Jejunal studies have shown that if glucose transport from glucose polymers is saturated, sugar absorption can be enhanced if the disaccharide sucrose is added.[136] This is because fructose released from sucrose by brush border hydrolysis can be absorbed via GLUT5. The linkage between brush border hydrolysis of sucrose and absorption of the mono-saccharides fructose and glucose absorption appears to confer a kinetic advantage on fructose uptake, since in one study 8/10 subjects malabsorbed 50 g of fructose while none malabsorbed 100 g of sucrose.[137] Thus the addition of sucrose to enteral diets can further enhance carbohydrate uptake.

Fat absorption

Dietary fat assimilation by the intestine is a complex process which involves several steps which (i) partially digest fat, (ii) emulsify it, (iii) mix it with detergent, cholesterol and phospholipid, (iv) react the micellar mixture with a lipase, (v) release fatty acids, (vi) translocate these across the enterocyte membrane, (vii) resynthesise triglycerides and (viii) translocate these into the lymphatic system. The major dietary fats are triglycerides, cholesterol and the fat-soluble vitamins. Triglycerides (TG) are fatty acid triesters of glycerol, which may contain long chain fatty acids (C16–C18 – long chain triglycerides, LCT) or medium chain fatty acids (C6–C12 – medium chain triglycerides, MCT) and enteral diets may be designed with increased amounts of MCT, for reasons which will be explained.

The important thing about this complex process is that it is still not completely understood. This is because the substrate for the process (a fatty acid) is hydrophobic and exists in free solution only at very low concentrations. Thus, lipids and fatty acids are mostly bound to or within macromolecular structures (e.g. micelles, transport proteins) during transport from one body compartment to another and the significance of all these structures is not yet known. In contrast, glucose, being water soluble, may freely permeate cellular compartments and cross membranes via one of the GLUT series transporters.[138] Several of the steps increase the rate of a reaction which may be rather slow when carried out on oil-in-water droplets. Thus, exogenous (e.g. bile acids) or endogenous (fatty acids, monoglycerides released *in situ*) chemical emulsificants produce an emulsion with high surface area/volume for efficient enzyme hydrolysis and which can permeate the unstirred water layer adjacent to the brush border membrane of the enterocyte.

The first phase in emulsification occurs in the stomach by mechanical action and lingual lipase partially hydrolyses some TG to free fatty acid and diglyceride

(DG).[139] Transfer of gastric contents, rich in fat, to the duodenum has two consequences.

1. H^+-stimulated secretin stimulates pancreatic water and HCO_3^- secretion into the duodenum, raising the pH to 6–7.

2. Luminal free fatty acids in the duodenum stimulate cholecystokinin-pancreozymin (CCK-PZ) release by duodenal epithelial cells. This signals contraction of the gall bladder and release of bile acids into the intestinal lumen.

The higher pH of the duodenal contents aids in further emulsification and facilitates the action of pancreatic lipase. At pH 6–7, bile salts are soluble in water but above a certain concentration (critical micellar concentration) will form pure bile salt micelles. Fatty acids, monoglycerides and phospholipids interdigitate with this structure, forming mixed micelles with a hydrophobic core and hydrophilic outer surface.[140,141] Pancreatic lipase would not be able to hydrolyse triglycerides within the micelles were it not for colipase which binds tightly to micellar surfaces, acting as an electrostatic anchor for lipase which has considerable specificity for the 1,3 positions of TG.[142] Osmotic pressures generated within the micelle by extensive TG hydrolysis cause budding of smaller micelles from the surface of these structures. The resulting smaller micelles are then available for uptake of MG and fatty acids at the microvilli surface. Diffusion of lipid-rich micelles across the unstirred water layer is important because at physiological pH, free long chain fatty acids do not exist free in solution except at very low concentration but will form insoluble aggregates.[143] It is postulated that heparin can act as a bridge to bind pancreatic lipase to the brush border of the enterocyte, thus ensuring that fatty acids released in this way are in closest proximity to the apical membrane.[144] Finally, two distinct mucosal acid- and alkaline-active intestinal lipases have been demonstrated in the lysosomal and cytosolic compartments of villus tip enterocytes, that is, those most actively engaged in absorption and transport of dietary lipid.[145,146] The exact mode of transport of fatty acids across the membrane is still unclear[143] and there are two possible mechanisms.

1. The acidic microenvironment adjacent to the brush border membrane is important in promoting lipid absorption since protonation of fatty acids allows their diffusion through the membrane. Within the enterocyte, the higher intracellular pH results in their ionisation, thus reducing the likelihood of back-diffusion.[147]

2. Fatty acids bind to fatty-acid binding protein (iFABP) which is a transmembrane protein[148] which translocates the fatty acid into the cytoplasmic compartment. Most recently, it has been shown that site-directed mutations which prevent fatty acid binding to iFABP do not lead to fat malabsorption in mice.[149]

Within the enterocyte, fatty acids are transferred by their specific cytoplasmic carrier proteins to the smooth endoplasmic reticulum for re-esterification to TG. These TG are transferred, along with cholesterol, phospholipids and fat-soluble vitamins, to the Golgi apparatus where they combine with apolipoproteins to form chylomicrons and very low density lipoproteins. The Golgi apparatus is transferred to the enterocyte lateral membrane and fuses with it. Subsequent rupture of the fused vesicle by exocytosis results in the release of lipid into the lymphatic system. The rate-limiting step in this process is transfer of lipid from endoplasmic reticulum to Golgi apparatus.[150]

Although probably not of any clinical significance, not all the neutral lipid absorbed from the lumen of the intestine is destined for packaging and transport via the lymphatic in chylomicrons.[151] Experimental animal studies indicate that nearly half of neutral lipids may be transported out of the enterocytes via the portal vein. These are postulated to require prior hydrolysis by a specific, non-pancreatic, alkaline-active lipase.

Medium chain triglycerides appear to 'short-circuit' some of these processes because they are more water soluble than LCT and may either be absorbed intact or undergo considerably more rapid lipase hydrolysis than LCT, with subsequent direct uptake of MG and fatty acid.[152] There is no absolute requirement for mixed micelle formation with bile acids and, within the enterocyte, short and medium chain fatty acids are generally not re-esterified to TG and incorporated into chylomicrons but may be released directly into the portal circulation where they bind to albumin.

Absorption of water and electrolyte

Table 6.3 lists the approximate values of water and electrolytes handled by the normal gut in a 24 h period. As can be seen, the combined totals of fluid from the diet and secretions from the salivary glands, stomach, pancreas, biliary tree and intestinal mucosa account for about 9 litres which enter the small intestine. Of this, about 1–5 litres pass the ileocaecal valve, less than 200 ml escaping into the stool.[153] There are no specific active transport processes for the absorption of water. The intestinal mucosa acts as a semipermeable membrane through which water flows in either direction in response to differences in osmotic pressure. Thus, luminal nutrient digestion renders the bulk phase hypertonic and water moves from the intestinal fluid into the gut lumen;[154] nutrient absorption, however, renders it more hypotonic such that water is absorbed along with these solutes. In this way, the luminal contents are adjusted to near isotonicity throughout the small bowel.

Mucosal permeability varies along the length of the intestine, being highest in the jejunum, intermediate

Table 6.3 – Approximate quantities of water and electrolytes handled by the intestine each day in healthy subjects.

	Water (ml)	Sodium (mmoles)	Chloride (mmoles)	Potassium (mmoles)
Input				
Diet	1500	150	150	80
Gut secretions	7500	1000	750	40
Total	9000	1150	900	120
Absorption				
Small intestine	7500	950	800	110
Colon	1350	195	97	−3
Output	150	5	3	13

in the ileum and lowest in the colon. Therefore, the jejunum effects the rapid equilibration of osmotic pressure gradients created by the digestion and absorption of nutrients. The lower permeability of the colonic mucosa prevents water from leaking back into the lumen when the mainly ionic solutes are actively absorbed. Water has difficulty passing across the lipid membrane of the epithelial cells and it is now clear that most of it passes between cells rather than through them.[155]

Therefore, the differences in permeability throughout the intestine depend on the different permeabilities of the 'tight' junctions between cells. It has been calculated that the pores through which water passes in the jejunum are about twice the diameter of those in the ileum.[154] Thus, water absorption in the upper intestine is determined largely by absorption of nutrients; however, in the ileum, and particularly in the colon, the absorption of salt is the main driving force for water absorption and resulting dehydration of colonic contents.

Electrolytes

The gut has extremely efficient mechanisms for conservation of Na^+ intake because, of the 1000 mmol of sodium chloride entering the upper intestine each day, only 5 mmol is excreted in normal stool. In the duodenum and upper jejunum, simple diffusion of sodium and chloride occurs down concentration gradients producing luminal concentrations similar to those in plasma. When a sodium chloride solution that is isotonic with plasma is perfused in the normal human jejunum, no net uptake of sodium or chloride ions occurs.[156] Sodium uptake is, however, stimulated in the presence of glucose, amino acids, di- and tripeptides as well as bicarbonate ions through the action of Na^+-nutrient cotransporters (see above). Bicarbonate is removed as CO_2 by reaction with actively secreted hydrogen ions. Hydrogen ion is secreted by exchange with absorbed sodium on a specific cation exchange carrier. In addition to nutrient and bicarbonate-stimulated absorption in the jejunum, sodium and chloride ions are also thought to move in response to solvent drag (see above). A lower luminal nutrient concentration in the ileum results in the greater significance of active absorption processes, such as ion exchange of H^+ and Cl^- for HCO_3^-.[155] The ileal mucosa is less permeable to ions than in the jejunum so, once absorbed, only limited back-diffusion occurs into the lumen.

In the colon 1.5–2.6 litres of water are absorbed daily, compared to a reserve capacity of three to four times this amount. It is only when this absorptive capacity is overwhelmed, acutely, that diarrhoea results.[157] The absorption of water is determined largely by absorption of sodium and chloride ions and SCFA.[158,159] The presence of active Na^+ transport can be shown by the presence of a transmembrane potential difference (30–40 mV) across the mucosa. An electrically neutral exchange of chloride absorption for bicarbonate secretion has been demonstrated also in the human colon. SCFA, mainly acetate, propionate and butyrate, are generated within the lumen as a consequence of the bacterial fermentation of unabsorbed dietary carbohydrate and fibre. SCFA are avidly absorbed and one component of their absorption stimulates sodium uptake, the other is by passive permeation of protonated species.[158]

Water malabsorption and diarrhoea

The characteristics of diarrhoea associated with tube feeding in patients have been quite carefully defined within the last 20 years. Several causative factors (apart from diarrhoeal infections) have been identified. There is a close association between diarrhoea and concurrent antibiotic therapy[160] and not the lactose content of enteral feeds or the rate of infusion.[161] Diarrhoea may also be potentiated by the stimulatory effect of continuous nasogastric feeding on colonic water and electrolyte secretion (discussed in Chapter 18). Net water uptake in the small intestine can be maximised if sufficient Na^+ (>90 mmol/l) is included in the enteral diet.[136] Malabsorbed carbohydrate and protein will generate osmotically active monosaccharide and amino acids which may undergo fermentation to SCFA. Whilst unfermented monosaccharides present in the colon can potentiate diarrhoea,[162] their fermentation products (SCFA) stimulate water and Na^+ uptake. Oral antibiotics which inhibit colonic bacteria may thus contribute to the diarrhoea encountered in enterally fed patients by reducing SCFA production.[163] One interesting report has demonstrated the link between carbohydrate malabsorption and impaired salvage in enterally fed patients, because a rise in breath-H_2 concentrations preceded the onset of diarrhoea by several hours.[164] These factors are summarised in Table 6.4.

Table 6.4 – Causes of non-infectious diarrhoea in enterally-fed patients.

Causative agents		Mechanism	Suggested solution
Inappropriate feeding techniques	Too rapid diet infusion (e.g. bolus feeding)	Will result in high 'load' which overwhelms the digestive or absorptive capacity of the small intestine	Use lower infusion rate
	Too slow diet infusion	Fails to elicit postprandial motility response (i.e. slowing of transit)	Use higher infusion rate (e.g. cyclical feeding)
Impaired digestive or absorptive function		Malabsorption of nutrients	Use predigested diets or enzyme supplements
Low sodium content in enteral diet		Poor water and Na$^+$ uptake in small intestine	Increase Na$^+$ to > 90 mmol/l
Antibiotics		Inhibition of colonic fermentation of malabsorbed carbohydrate or protein	

Substrate utilisation by the intestine

Arginine

Arginine metabolism by the intestine is most interesting because during the weaning period, a feature of the intestine (i.e. to markedly alter the pattern of amino acids which are absorbed) becomes switched on.[165] Arginine has unique properties. It is an essential nutrient for several species, and its absence from the diet will lead either to depressed growth rates in young rats and dogs[166,167] or to death from hyperammonaemic coma in the cat.[168] This is because reduced intramitochondrial arginine supply may limit the rate at which NH_4^+ is converted to urea. This was discovered during early development of intravenous amino acid solutions because infusion of mixtures deficient in arginine led to hyperammonaemia, which was reversed on addition of arginine.[169] Arginine in a mixture of amino acids infused into the duodenum gut is converted almost quantitatively into ornithine and citrulline[170] and this is converted back to arginine in the kidney.[171] Some citrulline can be formed from glutamine in the rat[172] and in subjects fed enterally with a glutamine-enriched diet, there was increased renal arginine synthesis. This explains why arginine is not an essential amino acid in orally fed humans.

However, several studies have shown that arginine has interesting properties. First, it potently stimulates both insulin and growth hormone secretion.[173,174] Second, daily supplements given to healthy volunteers stimulate lymphocyte responsiveness to mitogens.[175] In the clinical setting, arginine supplements have been tested. Healing of a standardised wound was more rapid[176] whilst in healthy elderly subjects supplementation led to improved protein balance and plasma insulin-like growth factor.[177] Some of these effects are mediated through nitric oxide, which is produced from arginine since blockade of this pathway reverses the beneficial effects of arginine on mortality in burned/septic mice.[178] In a thorough review, Brittenden and colleagues present the evidence for use of arginine as adjunct therapy in cancer patients, because of its immunostimulatory effects.[179]

Nucleotides

These exist in a normal diet but are absent from most enteral formulae apart from those for infants.[180] For such a minor dietary component they have surprisingly far-reaching effects. Thus, removal of nucleotides from the diet of rats leads to considerable loss of the machinery of protein synthesis (i.e. ribosomes) from the liver and a smaller loss of DNA from the gut mucosa.[181,182] They can be synthesised *de novo* from amino acids such as glutamine and from other small molecules, such as formate. Alternatively, nucleotides released by intracellular turnover of RNA or DNA can be salvaged by removal of the ribose moiety and its replacement with 5-phosphoribosyl-1-phosphate (PRPP) to form a new nucleotide monophosphate. Dietary sources of nucleotides enter the nucleotide pool via this route.

Nucleotide supplementation has been shown to have beneficial effects on the intestine in models of TPN-induced atrophy or lactose-induced chronic diarrhoea.[183–185] More rapid growth was observed in small-for-gestational-age infants receiving formula milk supplemented with nucleotides[186] whilst episodes of diarrhoea in children were also reduced.[187] This might be taken to show that nucleotides are conditionally essential nutrients but this is unlikely because the amount required to show an effect is so small in itself and in relation to whole-body flux of nucleotides. In addition, the intestine and liver form a barrier to dietary nucleotides because adenosine and uridine are almost completely degraded. It is more likely that dietary nucleotides exert their effect through purinergic signalling[188] and suppression of tumour necrosis factor release by lymphocytes in gut-associated lymphatic tissue.[189]

Glutamine

Windmueller[190] observed that the intestine is capable of high rates of oxidation of glutamine, glucose and α-hydroxybutyrate from arterial or luminal sources. Consumption of glutamine and β-hydroxybutyrate were proportional to infused load[191] and this led to the idea that glutamine is a 'preferred fuel' for the gastrointestinal tract. From a metabolic point of view, this property seems to be shared by all cell types with a rapid rate of turnover[192] and high rates of glucose and glutamine metabolism may be required not only for energy generation but also to provide precursor for ribose and purines involved in nucleic acid synthesis.[193] Stable isotope studies in pigs have shown that glutamate absorbed from a protein meal was not only the single biggest contributor to gut energy production but was also precursor to glutathione, arginine and proline in the intestine. In contrast, arterial glutamine provided only 15% of CO_2.[194]

It is outside the scope of this chapter to deal with clinical studies of glutamine supplementation which are described in Chapter 23.

Perspectives

Protein assimilation

A significant proportion of dietary N is absorbed in the form of di- and tripeptides. The transporter PepT1 has been cloned and its distribution along the gut and along the villus axis has been investigated. There are also several specific transporters for L-amino acids, which, together with PepT1, provide an efficient, duplicated system for capture of dietary amino acids. Since pancreatic and other secretions overspill past the main site of luminal protein hydrolysis (i.e. duodenum and jejunum) and are, by their nature, resistant to pancreatic proteolytic attack, the coupling of peptide uptake to brush border peptidases with different specificity provides an efficient means of salvage. It is therefore interesting that starvation, which suppresses amino acid transport, upregulates PepT1[93] as do chemotherapeutic agents like 5-fluorouracil which suppresses the other macronutrient transporters.[88] Since dietary protein assimilation is a jejunal event whereas endogenous protein secretions are assimilated more distally, any adaptation which will occur in the remaining intestine after resection has more limited scope for maintenance of protein assimilation.[195,196]

A second reason for duplication is that peptide transport serves to relieve competition for transport between free amino acids which share the same carrier. This may be especially true in cases where poor protein quality and malabsorption coexist with a high requirement for essential amino acid residues (e.g. rapid growth in infants).

Carbohydrate assimilation

The molecular biology of monosaccharide transporters is now well understood and more traditional physiological methods have defined the reserve capacity of the small intestine towards carbohydrates. Current knowledge suggests that it is 2–3 times the maximum nutrient intake which is likely to be used in enteral feeding and would comfortably exceed the necessary intake of a hypermetabolic, severely burned patient. Where absorptive function has been severely reduced by distal small bowel resection, remaining reserve capacity is often sufficient to allow complete assimilation of carbohydrate[7,197] as opposed to protein.[63] The reason for this difference is that carbohydrate assimilation is primarily duodenal and jejunal, as shown by the negative longitudinal distribution gradient for the brush border disaccharidases and the Na^+-glucose cotransporter.[198,199]

Fat assimilation

Normal lipid digestion and absorption depend on several mechanisms, the most important of which appear to be adequate luminal levels of pancreatic lipase and bile salts, as well as sufficient absorptive area. In some patients, one or several of these factors may be limiting and diets containing excessive amounts of LCT should be avoided to prevent essential fatty acid and vitamin deficiency caused by competition for uptake by other long chain fatty acids.[200] Such patients include those with severe exocrine pancreatic insufficiency (chronic pancreatitis and cystic fibrosis[201]), severe abnormalities of intestinal mucosa (untreated coeliac disease) or extensive small bowel resection. Although MCT has been proposed as an efficiently absorbed fat source in these cases[202,203] it does not contain linoleic acid and exclusive use of MCT may provoke essential fatty acid deficiency.[204] It may therefore be better to use combination therapy of diets containing mixtures of MCT and LCT, as well as oral, enteric-coated pancreatic enzyme supplements which

enhance utilisation of LCT and MCT and reduce steatorrhoea.[201,205]

Intestinal metabolism

The interrelationship between the intestine and other organs is much clearer, especially with respect to amino acid nitrogen organ flows in health and disease. The current view is that the small intestine is a net consumer of glutamine, derived mainly from the liver and skeletal muscle. During long-term starvation, muscle is the main provider of glutamine. Several schemes have been proposed to account for this. It is thought that the high requirement for *de novo* synthesis of purines and pyrimidines is one reason for this flow. In addition, the intestine is dependent on liver *de novo* synthesis of adenine for RNA and DNA synthesis.

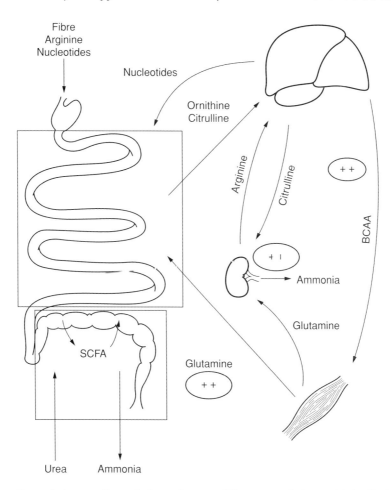

Figure 6.6 – Interorgan flows of substrates. Flows of substrate between different organs is shown. ++ signifies increased flow in septic, traumatised or acidotic patients. BCAA – branched-chain amino acids. From [206] with permission.

The intestine is also a net producer of ornithine and citrulline which is resynthesised into arginine by the kidney. Considerable amounts of circulating urea-nitrogen can be diffused into the large intestine to be hydrolysed by luminal bacteria. This appears to serve two purposes. The first is that liberated NH_4^+ can be reabsorbed and reincorporated into the α-NH_2 nitrogen pool and may provide a means of recycling the α-NH_2 groups of the deamidating amino acids (e.g. glycine). Second, luminal NH_4^+ provides a nitrogen source for luminal bacteria and will be excreted in stool. SCFAs generated during luminal fibre fermentation are an energy source for the colon (especially butyrate) and their absence will result in impaired function (see above). Finally, dietary nucleotides have specific effects on the intestine which are not related to substrate loading but may arise from purinergic signalling. This is summarised in Figure 6.6. These considerations have led to a renaissance of research into the intestine which is no longer viewed as an inert absorptive tube but rather an organ whose metabolism is central to metabolic homeostasis.

References

1. Majumdar SK, Shaw GK, O'Gorman P, Aps EJ, Offerman EL, Thomson AD. Blood vitamin status (B1, B2, B6, folic acid and B12) in patients with alcoholic liver disease. *Int J Vitamin Nutr Res* 1982; **52**(3): 266–71.

2. Thomson AD, Baker H, Leevy CM. Patterns of ^{35}S-thiamine hydrochloride absorption in the mal-nourished alcoholic patient. *J Lab Clin Med* 1970; **76**(1): 34–45.

3. Cook CC, Hallwood PM, Thomson AD. B Vitamin deficiency and neuropsychiatric syndromes in alcohol misuse. *Alcohol Alcohol* 1998; **33**(4): 317–36.

4. Carmel R. Cobalamin, the stomach, and aging. *Am J Clin Nutr* 1997; **66**(4): 750–9.

5. Kapembwa MS, Fleming SC, Griffin GE, Caun K, Pinching AJ, Harris JR. Fat absorption and exocrine pancreatic function in human immunodeficiency virus infection. *Q J Med* 1990; **74**(273): 49–56.

6. Carbonnel F, Beaugerie L, Abou Rached A *et al.* Macronutrient intake and malabsorption in HIV infection: a comparison with other malabsorptive states. *Gut* 1997; **41**(6): 805–10.

7. Althausen TL, Uyeyama K, Simpson RG. Digestion and absorption after massive resection of the small intestine. I. utilization of food from a 'natural' versus a 'synthetic' diet and a comparison of intestinal absorption tests with nutritional balance studies in a patient with only 45 cm of small intestine. *Gastroenterology* 1949; **12**: 795–807.

8. Hammer HF, Fine KD, Santa Ana CA, Porter JL, Schiller LR, Fordtran JS. Carbohydrate malabsorption. Its measurement and its contribution to diarrhea. *J Clin Invest* 1990; **86**: 1936–44.

9. Nadel ER. The limits of human performance: project Daedalus. *Res Q Exerc Sport* 1996; **67**(3 suppl): S71–S72.

10. Stroud MA, Jackson AA, Waterlow JC. Protein turnover rates of two human subjects during an un-assisted crossing of Antarctica. *Br J Nutr* 1996; **76**(2): 165–74.

11. Martin RD, Chivers DJ, MacLarnon AM, Hladnik CM. Gastrointestinal allometry in primates and other mammals. In: Jungers WL (ed) Size and scaling in primate biology. Plenum Press, New York, 1985; pp. 61–89.

12. Karasov WH, Solberg DH, Diamond JM. What transport adaptations enable mammals to absorb sugars and amino acids faster than reptiles? *Am J Physiol* 1985; **249**: G271–G283.

13. Weaver LT, Austin S, Cole TJ. Small intestinal length: a factor essential for gut adaptation. *Gut* 1991; **32**(11): 1321–3.

14. Lennard-Jones JE. Nutrition support in short-bowel syndrome. In: Payne-James JJ, Grimble GK, Silk DBA (eds) Artificial nutrition support in clinical practice. Edward Arnold, London, 1995.

15. Robinson MK, Ziegler TR, Wilmore DW. Overview of intestinal adaptation and its stimulation. *Eur J Pediatr Surg* 1999; **9**(4): 200–6.

16. Scheflan M, Galli SJ, Perrotto J, Fischer JE. Intestinal adaptation after extensive resection of the small intestine and prolonged administration of parenteral nutrition. *Surg Gynecol Obstet* 1976; **143**(5): 757–62.

17. Cosnes J, Carbonnel F, Beaugerie L *et al.* Functional adaptation after extensive small bowel resection in humans. *Eur J Gastroenterol Hepatol* 1994; **6**: 197–202.

18. Wilmore DW. Growth factors and nutrients in the short bowel syndrome. *J Parent Ent Nutr* 1999; **23**(5 suppl): S117–S120.

19. O'Connor TP, Lam MM, Diamond J. Magnitude of functional adaptation after intestinal resection. *Am J Physiol* 1999; **276**(5 Pt 2): R1265–R1275.

20. Toloza EM, Lam M, Diamond J. Nutrient extraction by cold-exposed mice: a test of digestive safety margins. *Am J Physiol* 1991; **261**: G608–G620.

21. Hammond KA, Lam M, Lloyd KC, Diamond J. Simultaneous manipulation of intestinal capacities and nutrient loads in mice. *Am J Physiol* 1996; **271**(6 Pt 1): G969–G979.

22. Nyman M, Asp NG, Cummings J, Wiggins H. Fermentation of dietary fibre in the intestinal tract: comparison between man and rat. *Br J Nutr* 1986; **55**: 487–96.

23. Stevens CE, Hume ID. Contributions of microbes in vertebrate gastrointestinal tract to production and conservation of nutrients. *Physiol Rev* 1998; **78**(2): 393–427.

24. O'Connor TP, Diamond J. Ontogeny of intestinal safety factors: lactase capacities and lactose loads. *Am J Physiol* 1999; **276**(3 Pt 2): R753–R765.

25. Bowling TE, Raimundo AH, Grimble GK, Silk DBA. Colonic secretory effect in response to enteral feeding in humans. *Gut* 1994; **35**(12): 1734–41.

26. Efimov AV. Complementary packing of alpha-helices in proteins. *FEBS Lett* 1999; **463**(1–2): 3–6.

27. Perona JJ, Craik CS. Evolutionary divergence of substrate specificity within the chymotrypsin-like serine protease fold. *J Biol Chem* 1997; **272**(48): 29987–90.

28. Cowan DA. Thermophilic proteins: stability and function in aqueous and organic solvents. *Comp Biochem Physiol A Physiol* 1997; **118**(3): 429–38.

29. Cowan DA. Protein stability at high temperatures. *Essays Biochem* 1995; **29**: 193–207.

30. Cresswell P, Hughes EA. Protein degradation: the ins and outs of the matter. *Curr Biol* 1997; **7**(9): R552–5.

31. Mecham RP, Broekelmann TJ, Fliszar CJ, Shapiro SD, Welgus HG, Senior RM. Elastin degradation by matrix metalloproteinases. Cleavage site specificity and mechanisms of elastolysis. *J Biol Chem* 1997; **272**(29): 18071–6.

32. Hersey SJ. Cellular basis of pepsinogen secretion. In: Forte JG, Schultz SG (eds) Handbook of physiology, section 6, volume III (salivary, gastric, pancreatic, and hepatobiliary secretion). American Physiological Society, Washington, 1989.

33. Tao C, Yamamoto M, Mieno H, Inoue M, Masujima T, Kajiyama G. Pepsinogen secretion: coupling of exocytosis visualized by video microscopy and [Ca^{2+}]i in single cells. *Am J Physiol Gastrointest Liver Physiol* 1998; **274**(6): G1166–G1177.

34. Richter C, Tanaka T, Yada RY. Mechanism of activation of the gastric aspartic proteinases: pepsinogen, progastricsin and prochymosin. *Biochem J* 1998; **335** (Pt 3): 481–90.

35. Fujinaga M, Chernaia MM, Tarasova NI, Mosimann SC, James MN. Crystal structure of human pepsin and its complex with pepstatin. *Protein Sci* 1995; **4**(5): 960–72.

36. Shintani T, Nomura K, Ichishima E. Engineering of porcine pepsin. Alteration of S1 substrate specificity of pepsin to those of fungal aspartic proteinases by site-directed mutagenesis. *J Biol Chem* 1997; **272**(30): 18855–61.

37. Stein HJ, Kauer WKH. Methods in disease: investigating the gastrointestinal tract. Greenwich Medical Media, London, 1998.

38. Foltmann B. Pepsin, chymosin and their zymogens. In: Desnuelle P, Sjöström H, Norén O (eds) Molecular and cellular basis of digestion. Elsevier, Amsterdam, 1986; pp. 491–505.

39. Antonowicz I, Lebenthal E. Developmental pattern of small intestinal enterokinase and disaccharidase activities in the human fetus. *Gastroenterology* 1977; **72**(6): 1299–303.

40. Bett NJ, Grant DAW, Magee AI, Hermon-Taylor J. Induction and maintenance of mucosal enterokinase activity in proximal small intestine by a genetically determined response to mediated sodium transport. *Gut* 1981; **22**: 804–11.

41. Yuan X, Zheng X, Lu D, Rubin DC, Pung CY, Sadler JE. Structure of murine enterokinase (enteropeptidase) and expression in small intestine during development. *Am J Physiol* 1998; **274**(2 Pt 1): G342–G349.

42. Lebenthal A, Lebenthal E. The ontogeny of the small intestinal epithelium. *J Parent Ent Nutr* 1999; **23**(5 suppl): S3–S6.

43. Desnuelle P. Chemistry and enzymology of pancreatic endopeptidases. In: Desnuelle P, Sjöström H, Norén O (eds) Molecular and cellular basis of digestion. Elsevier, Amsterdam, 1986; pp. 195–211.

44. Puigserver A, Chapus C, Kerfelec B. Pancreatic exopeptidases. In: Desnuelle P, Sjöström H, Norén O (eds) Molecular and cellular basis of digestion. Elsevier, Amsterdam, 1986; pp. 235–247.

45. Hofstetter J, Allen LV Jr. Causes of non-medication-induced nasogastric tube occlusion. *Am J Hosp Pharm* 1992; **49**(3): 603–7.

46. Powell K, Marcuard SP, Farrior ES, Gallagher ML. Aspirating gastric residuals causes occlusion of small-bore feeding tubes. *J Parent Ent Nutr* 1993; **17**: 243–6.

47. Yeoh D, Zhao XT, Sanders SL, Elashoff JD, Bonorris G, Lin HC. Bile salt inhibits acid-promoting feeding tube occlusion. *Nutr Clin Pract* 1996; **11**(3): 105–7.

48. Scanlan M, Frisch S. Nasoduodenal feeding tubes: prevention of occlusion. *J Neurosci Nurs* 1992; **24**(5): 256–9.

49. Marcuard SP, Stegall KS. Unclogging feeding tubes with pancreatic enzyme. *J Parent Ent Nutr* 1990; **14**(2): 198–200.

50. Turner JS, Fyfe AR, Kaplan DK, Wardlaw AJ. Oesophageal obstruction during nasogastric feeding. *Intensive Care Med* 1991; **17**(5): 302–3.

51. Viall C, Porcelli K, Teran JC, Varma RN, Steffee WP. A double-blind clinical trial comparing the gastro-intestinal side effects of two enteral feeding formulas. *J Parent Ent Nutr* 1990; **14**: 265–9.

52. Calbet JA, MacLean DA. Role of caloric content on gastric emptying in humans. *J Physiol* (Lond) 1997; **498**(Pt 2): 553–9.

53. Ziegler F, Ollivier JM, Cynober L *et al*. Efficiency of enteral nitrogen support in surgical patients: small peptides v non-degraded proteins. *Gut* 1990; **31**: 1277–83.

54. Mowatt-Larssen CA, Brown RO, Wojtysiak SL, Kudsk KA. Comparison of tolerance and nutritional outcome between a peptide and a standard enteral formula in critically ill, hypoalbuminemic patients. *J Parent Ent Nutr* 1992; **16**: 20–4.

55. Craft IL, Geddes D, Hyde CW, Wise IJ, Matthews DM. Absorption and malabsorption of glycine and glycine peptides in man. *Gut* 1968; **9**(4): 425–37.

56. Chung YC, Kim YS, Shadchehr A, Garrido A, MacGregor IL, Sleisenger MH. Protein digestion and absorption in human small intestine. *Gastroenterology* 1979; **76**: 1415–21.

57. Silk DBA, Chung YC, Berger KL *et al*. Comparison of oral feeding of peptide and amino acid meals to normal human subjects. *Gut* 1979; **20**: 291–9.

58. Stevens BR. Amino acid transport in intestine. In: Kilberg MS, Häussinger D (eds) Mammalian amino acid transport. Plenum Press, New York, 1992; pp. 149–163.

59. Skovbjerg H. Immunoelectrophoretic studies on human small-intestinal brush-border proteins. *Biochem J* 1981; **193**: 887–90.

60. Triadou N, Bataille J, Schmitz J. Longitudinal study of the human intestinal brush border membrane proteins: distribution of the main disaccharidases and peptidases. *Gastroenterology* 1983; **85**: 1326–32.

61. Bai JPF. Influences of regional differences in activities of brush-border membrane peptidases within the rat intestine on site-dependent stability of peptide drugs. *Life Sci* 1993; **53**(15): 1193–201.

62. Bai JPF. Distribution of brush-border membrane peptidases along the rabbit intestine: implication for oral delivery of peptide drugs. *Life Sci* 1993; **52**(11): 941–7.

63. Chacko A, Cummings JH. Nitrogen losses from the human small bowel: obligatory losses and the effect of physical form of food. *Gut* 1988; **29**(6): 809–15.

64. Mortensen PB, Holtug K, Bonnen H, Clausen MR. The degradation of amino acids, proteins, and blood to short-chain fatty acids in colon is prevented by lactulose. *Gastroenterology* 1990; **98**: 353–60.

65. Morgan MY. The treatment of chronic hepatic encephalopathy. *Hepatogastroenterology* 1991; **38**: 377–87.

66. Jackson AA. Nitrogen trafficking and recycling through the human bowel. In: Fürst P, Young VR (eds) Proteins, peptides and amino-acids in enteral nutrition. Karger, Basel, 2000; pp. 89–108.

67. Jackson AA. Salvage of urea-nitrogen and protein requirements. *Proc Nutr Soc* 1995; **54**(2): 535–47.

68. Häussinger D. Hepatic glutamine transport and metabolism. *Adv Enzymol Relat Areas Mol Biol* 1998; **72**: 43–86.

69. Schultz SG. A century of (epithelial) transport physiology: from vitalism to molecular cloning. *Am J Physiol Cell Physiol* 1998; **274**(1): C13–C23.

70. Schultz SG, Curran PF. Coupled transport of sodium and organic solutes. *Physiol Rev* 1970; **50**: 637–72.

71. Christensen HN. Methods for distinguishing amino acid transport systems of a given cell or tissue. *Fed Proc* 1966; **25**(3): 850–3.

72. Argiles JM, López-Soriano FJ. Intestinal amino acid transport: an overview. *Int J Biochem* 1990; **22**(9): 931–7.

73. Devés R, Boyd CAR. Transporters for cationic amino acids in animal cells: discovery, structure, and function. *Physiol Rev* 1998; **78**(2): 487–545.

74. McGivan JD, Pastor-Anglada M. Regulatory and molecular aspects of mammalian amino acid transport. *Biochem J* 1994; **299**(Pt 2): 321–34.

75. Munck LK, Munck BG. Amino acid transport in the small intestine. *Physiol Res* 1995; **44**(2): 335–46.

76. Palacín M, Estévez R, Bertran J, Zorzano A. Molecular biology of mammalian plasma membrane amino acid transporters. *Physiol Rev* 1998; **78**(4): 969–1054.

77. Christensen HN, Albritton LM, Kakuda DK, MacLeod CL. Gene-product designations for amino acid transporters. *J Exptl Biol* 1994; **196**: 51–7.

78. Kyte J, Doolittle RF. A simple method for displaying the hydropathic character of a protein. *J Mol Biol* 1982; **157**(1): 105–32.

79. Ortiz DF, Li S, Iyer R, Zhang X, Novikoff P, Arias IM. MRP3, a new ATP-binding cassette protein localized to the canalicular domain of the hepatocyte. *Am J Physiol* 1999; **276**(6 Pt 1): G1493–G1500.

80. Milliner DS. Cystinuria. *Endocrinol Metab Clin North Am* 1990; **19**: 889–907.

81. Hegarty JE, Fairclough PD, Clark ML, Dawson AM. Jejunal water and electrolyte secretion induced by L-arginine in man. *Gut* 1981; **22**: 108–13.

82. Mourad FH, Andre EA, O'Donnell LJD, Clark ML, Farthing MJG. L-arginine, nitric oxide, and intestinal secretion: studies in rat jejunum in vivo. *Gut* 1996; **34**: 539–44.

83. Gaginella TS, Mascolo N, Izzo AA, Autore G, Capasso F. Nitric oxide as a mediator of bisacodyl and phenolphthalein laxative action: induction of nitric oxide synthase. *J Pharmacol Exptl Ther* 1994; **270**(3): 1239–45.

84. Sterchi EE, Woodley JF. Peptide hydrolases of the human small intestinal mucosa: distribution of activities between brush border membranes and cytosol. *Clin Chim Acta* 1980; **102**(1): 49–56.

85. Nicholson JA, Peters TJ. Subcellular distribution of hydrolase activities for glycine and leucine homo-peptides in human jejunum. *Clin Sci Mol Med* 1978; **54**: 205–7.

86. Tobey N, Heizer W, Yeh R, Huang TI, Hoffner C. Human intestinal brush-border peptidases. *Gastroenterology* 1985; **88**: 913–26.

87. Daniel H, Herget M. Cellular and molecular mech-anisms of renal peptide transport. *Am J Physiol* 1997; **273**(1 Pt 2): F1–8.

88. Tanaka H, Miyamoto KI, Morita K et al. Regulation of the PepT1 peptide transporter in the rat small intestine in response to 5-fluorouracil-induced injury. *Gastroenterology* 1998; **114**(4): 714–23.

89. Grimble GK. Mechanisms and regulation of peptide and amino acid transport. In: Fürst P, Young VR (eds) Proteins, peptides and amino-acids in enteral nutrition. Karger, Basel, 2000; pp. 63–88.

90. Guandalini S, Rubino A. Development of dipeptide transport in the intestinal mucosa of rabbits. *Pediatr Res* 1982; **16**: 99–103.

91. Miller PM, Burston D, Brueton MJ, Matthews DM. Kinetics of uptake of L-leucine and glycylsarcosine into normal and protein malnourished young rat jejunum. *Pediatr Res* 1984; **18**(6): 504–8.

92. Vazquez JA, Morse EL, Adibi SA. Effect of starvation on amino acid and peptide transport and peptide hydrolysis in humans. *Am J Physiol* 1985; **249**: G563–G566.

93. Ogihara H, Suzuki T, Nagamachi Y, Inui K, Takata K. Peptide transporter in the rat small intestine: ultra-structural localization and the effect of starvation and administration of amino acids. *Histochem J* 1999; **31**(3): 169–74.

94. Grimble GK. The significance of peptides in clinical nutrition. In: Olson RE, Bier DM, McCormick DB (eds) Annual review of nutrition, volume 14. Annual Reviews Inc, Palo Alto, 1994; pp. 419–447.

95. Grimble GK. Protein hydrolysates as vehicles for the application of di- and tripeptides in clinical nutrition. In: Grimble GK, Backwell FRC (eds) Peptides in mammalian protein metabolism: tissue utilisation and clinical targeting. Portland Press, London, 1997; pp. 119–139.

96. Itoh H, Kishi T, Chibata I. Comparative effects of casein and amino acid mixture simulating casein on growth and food intake in rats. *J Nutr* 1973; **103**: 1709–15.

97. Moriarty KJ, Hegarty JE, Fairclough PD, Kelly MJ, Clark ML, Dawson AM. Relative nutritional value of whole protein, hydrolysed protein and free amino acids in man. *Gut* 1985; **26**: 694–9.

98. Monchi M, Rérat AA. Comparison of net protein utilization of milk protein mild enzymatic hydrolysates and free amino acid mixtures with a close pattern in the rat. *J Parent Ent Nutr* 1993; **17**: 355–63.

99. Beaufrère B, Vidal C, Cayol M et al. Protein metabolism during enteral nutrition with a high protein or peptide diet in healthy subjects. *Clin Nutr* 1993; **12** (suppl 2): 6.

100. Velasco N, Long CL, Nelson KM, Blakemore WS. Whole-body protein kinetics in elective surgical patients receiving peptide or amino acid solutions. *Nutrition* 1991; **7**: 28–32.

101. Rees RG, Grimble G, Halliday D, Ford C, Silk DBA. Influence of orally administered amino acids and peptides on protein turnover kinetics in the short-bowel syndrome. *Gut* **28**: A1397.

102. Cosnes J, Evard D, Beaugerie L, Gendre JP, Le Quintrec Y. Improvement in protein absorption with a small-peptide-based diet in patients with high jejunos-tomy. *Nutrition* 1992; **8**(6): 406–11.

103. Ziegler F, Nitenberg G, Coudray-Lucas C, Lasser P, Giboudeau J, Cynober L. Pharmacokinetic assessment of an oligopeptide-based enteral formula in abdominal surgery patients. *Am J Clin Nutr* 1998; **67**(1): 124–8.

104. Steinhardt HJ, Wolf A, Jakober B et al. Nitrogen absorption in pancreatectomised patients: protein versus protein hydrolysate as substrate. *J Lab Clin Med* 1989; **113**: 162–7.

105. Donald P, Miller E, Schirmer B. Repletion of nutritional parameters in surgical patients receiving peptide versus amino acid elemental feedings. *Nutr Res* 1994; **14**: 3–12.

106. Heimburger DC, Geels VJ, Bilbrey J, Redden DT, Keeney C. Effects of small-peptide and whole-protein enteral feedings on serum proteins and diarrhea in critically ill patients: a randomized trial. *J Parent Ent Nutr* 1997; **21**(3): 162–7.

107. Pedersen S, Norman BE. Enzymatic modification of food carbohydrates. In: Andrews AT (ed) Chemical aspects of food enzymes. Royal Society of Chemistry, London, 1987; pp. 156–187.

108. Johansson C. Studies of gastrointestinal interactions: VII. Characteristics of the absorption pattern of sugar, fat and protein from composite meals in man: a quantitative study. Scand J Gastroenterol 1975; **10**: 33–42.

109. MacGregor EA, Svensson B. A super-secondary structure predicted to be common to several α-1,4-D-glucan-cleaving enzymes. Biochem J 1989; **259**: 145–52.

110. Gray GM. Starch digestion and absorption in non-ruminants. J Nutr 1992; **122**(1): 172–7.

111. Norén O, Sjöström H, Danielsen EM, Cowell GM, Skovbjerg H. The enzymes of the enterocyte plasma membrane. In: Desnuelle P, Sjöström H, Norén O (eds) Molecular and cellular basis of digestion. Elsevier, Amsterdam, 1986; pp. 35–365.

112. Wahlqvist ML, Wilmshurst EG, Murton CR, Richardson EN. The effect of chain length on glucose absorption and the related metabolic response. Am J Clin Nutr 1978; **31**: 1998–2001.

113. Layer P, Rizza RA, Zinsmeister AR, Carlson GL, DiMagno EP. Effect of a purified amylase inhibitor on carbohydrate tolerance in normal subjects and patients with diabetes mellitus. Mayo Clin Proc 1986; **61**: 442–7.

114. Dahlqvist A. Rat-intestinal dextranase: localization and relation to the other carbohydrases of the digestive tract. Biochem J 1963; **86**: 72–6.

115. Grimble GK, Denholm EE, Gabe SM, Debnam ES. Differences in the glycaemic response to dextran and maltodextrin ingestion in man. Proc Nutr Soc 1997; **56**(2): 225A.

116. Wright EM, Loo DD, Panayotova-Heiermann M et al. 'Active' sugar transport in eukaryotes. J Exptl Biol 1994; **196**: 197–212.

117. Thorens B. Glucose transporters in the regulation of intestinal, renal, and liver glucose fluxes. Am J Physiol 1996; **270**(4 Pt 1): G541–G553.

118. Corpe CP, Basaleh MM, Affleck J, Gould G, Jess TJ, Kellett GL. The regulation of GLUT5 and GLUT2 activity in the adaptation of intestinal brush-border fructose transport in diabetes. Pflügers Arch 1996; **432**(2): 192–201.

119. Fisher RB. The absorption of water and of some small solute molecules from the isolated small intestine of the rat. J Physiol (Lond) 1955; **130**: 655–64.

120. Pappenheimer JR. Physiological regulation of epithelial junctions in intestinal epithelia. Acta Physiol Scand 1988; **571**(suppl): 43–51.

121. Atisook K, Madara JL. An oligopeptide permeates intestinal tight junctions at glucose-elicited dilatations. Implications for oligopeptide absorption. Gastroenterology 1991; **100**: 719–24.

122. Pappenheimer JR. On the coupling of membrane digestion with intestinal absorption of sugars and amino acids. Am J Physiol 1993, **265**(3 Pt 1): G409–17.

123. Travis S, Menzies I. Intestinal permeability: functional assessment and significance. Clin Sci 1992; **82**: 471–88.

124. Ferraris RP, Yasharpour S, LLoyd KCK, Mirzayan R, Diamond JM. Luminal glucose concentrations in the gut under normal conditions. Am J Physiol 1990; **259**: G822–G837.

125. Grimble GK, Guilera Sarda M, Sesay HF et al. The influence of whey hydrolysate peptide chain length on nitrogen and carbohydrate absorption in the perfused human jejunum. Clin Nutr 1994; **13** (suppl): 46.

126. Lane JS, Whang EE, Rigberg DA et al. Paracellular glucose transport plays a minor role in the unanesthetized dog. Am J Physiol 1999; **276**(3 Pt 1): G789–G794.

127. Fine KD, Santa Ana CA, Porter JL, Fordtran JS. Effect of D-glucose on intestinal permeability and its passive absorption in human small intestine in vivo. Gastroenterology 1993; **105**: 1117–25.

128. Debnam ES, Denholm EE, Grimble GK. Acute and chronic exposure of rat intestinal mucosa to dextran promotes SGLT1-mediated glucose transport. Eur J Clin Invest 1998; **28**(8): 651–8.

129. Shu R, David ES, Ferraris RP. Luminal fructose modulates fructose transport and GLUT-5 expression in small intestine of weaning rats. Am J Physiol 1998; **274**(2 Pt 1): G232–G239.

130. Grimble GK. Ion chromatography in clinical research: a neglected technique? Analyt Proc 1992; **29**: 468–70.

131. Jones BJM, Brown BE, Spiller RC, Silk DBA. Energy dense enteral feeds – the use of high molecular weight glucose polymers. J Parent Ent Nutr 1981; **5**: 567.

132. Jones BJM, Brown BE, Loran JS et al. Glucose absorption from starch hydrolysates in the human jejunum. Gut 1983; **24**: 1152–60.

133. Jones BJM, Higgins BE, Silk DBA. Glucose absorption from maltotriose and glucose oligomers in the human jejunum. Clin Sci 1987; **72**(4): 409–14.

134. Dyer J, Hosie KB, Shirazi-Beechey SP. Nutrient regulation of human intestinal sugar transporter (SGLT1) expression. Gut 1997; **41**(1): 56–9.

135. Byrne TA, Persinger RL, Young LS, Ziegler TR, Wilmore DW. A new treatment for patients with short-bowel syndrome. Growth hormone, glutamine, and a modified diet. Ann Surg 1995; **222**(3): 243–54.

136. Spiller RC, Jones BJM, Silk DBA. Jejunal water and electrolyte absorption from two proprietary enteral feeds in man: importance of sodium content. *Gut* 1987; **28**(6): 681–7.

137. Rumessen JJ, Gudmand-Høyer E. Absorption capacity of fructose in healthy adults. Comparison with sucrose and its constituent monosaccharides. *Gut* 1986; **27**: 1161–8.

138. Zierler K. Whole body glucose metabolism. *Am J Physiol Endocrinol Metab* 1999; **276**(3): E409–E426.

139. Hamosh M, Klaeveman HL, Wolf RD, Scow RD. Pharyngeal lipase and digestion of dietary triglyceride in man. *J Clin Invest* 1975; **55**: 908–13.

140. Roda A, Gioacchini AM, Manetta AC, Cerre C, Montagnani M, Fini A. Bile acids: physico-chemical properties, function and activity. *Ital J Gastroenterol* 1995; **27**(6): 327–31.

141. Hauton JC, Domingo N, Martigne M *et al.* A quantitative dynamic concept of the interphase partition of lipids: application to bile salt-lecithin-cholesterol mixed micelles. *Biochimie* 1986; **68**(2): 275–85.

142. Ayvazian L, Crenon I, Hermoso J, Pignol D, Chapus C, Kerfelec B. Ion pairing between lipase and colipase plays a critical role in catalysis. *J Biol Chem* 1998; **273**(50): 33604–9.

143. Hamilton JA. Fatty acid transport: difficult or easy? *J Lipid Res* 1998; **39**(3): 467–81.

144. Bosner MS, Gulick T, Riley DJ, Spilburg CA, Lange LG. Heparin-modulated binding of pancreatic lipase and uptake of hydrolyzed triglycerides in the intestine. *J Biol Chem* 1989; **264**(34): 20261–4.

145. Rao RH, Mansbach CM. Acid lipase in rat intestinal mucosa: physiological parameters. *Biochim Biophys Acta* 1990; **1043**(3): 273–80.

146. Rao RH, Mansbach CM. Alkaline lipase in rat intestinal mucosa: physiological parameters. *Arch Biochem Biophys* 1993; **304**(2): 483–9.

147. Shiau Y. Mechanism of intestinal fatty acid uptake in the rat: the role of an acidic environment. *J Physiol (Lond)* 1990; **421**: 463–74.

148. Sacchettini JC, Gordon JI. Rat intestinal fatty acid binding protein. A model system for analyzing the forces that can bind fatty acids to proteins. *J Biol Chem* 1993; **268**(25): 18399–402.

149. Vassileva G, Huwyler L, Poirier K, Agellon LB, Toth MJ. The intestinal fatty acid binding protein is not essential for dietary fat absorption in mice. *FASEB J* 2000; **14**(13): 2040–6.

150. Mansbach CM, Nevin P. Intracellular movement of triacylglycerols in the intestine. *J Lipid Res* 1998; **39**(5): 963–8.

151. Mansbach CM, II, Dowell RF, Pritchett D. Portal transport of absorbed lipids in rats. *Am J Physiol* 1991; **261**(3 Pt 1): G530–G538.

152. Chow BP, Shaffer EA, Parsons HG. Absorption of triglycerides in the absence of lipase. *Can J Physiol Pharmacol* 1990; **68**(4): 519–23.

153. Phillips SF, Giller J. The contribution of the colon to electrolyte and water conservation in man. *J Lab Clin Med* 1973; **81**: 733–46.

154. Fordtran JS, Rector FC, Jr., Ewton MF, Soter N, Kinney J. Permeability characteristics of the human small intestine. *J Clin Invest* 1965; **44**: 1935–44.

155. Turnberg L. Cellular basis of diarrhoea. The Croonian lecture 1989. *J R Coll Physicians Lond* 1991; **25**: 53–62.

156. Silk DBA, Fairclough PD, Park NJ *et al.* A study of relations between the absorption of amino acids, dipeptides, water and electrolytes in the normal human jejunum. *Clin Sci Mol Med* 1975; **49**: 401–8.

157. Debongnie JC, Phillips SF. Capacity of the human colon to absorb fluid. *Gastroenterology* 1978; **74**: 698–703.

158. Ruppin H, Bar-Meir S, Soergel KH, Wood CM, Schmitt MG. Absorption of short chain fatty acids by the colon. *Gastroenterology* 1980; **78**: 1500–7.

159. Devroede GF, Phillips SF, Code CF, Lind JF. Regional differences in rates of insorption of sodium and water from the human large intestine. *Can J Physiol Pharmacol* 1971; **49**: 1023–9.

160. Keohane PP, Attrill H, Love M, Frost P, Silk DB. Relation between osmolality of diet and gastrointestinal side effects in enteral nutrition. *Br Med J* 1984; **288**(6418): 678–80.

161. Rees RGP, Keohane PP, Grimble GK, Frost PG, Attrill H, Silk DBA. Tolerance of elemental diet administered without starter regimen. *Br Med J* 1985; **290**: 1869–70.

162. Hammer HF, Santa Ana CA, Schiller LR, Fordtran JS. Studies of osmotic diarrhea induced in normal subjects by ingestion of polyethylene glycol and lactulose. *J Clin Invest* 1989; **84**: 1056–62.

163. Rao SS, Edwards CA, Austen CJ, Bruce C, Read NW. Impaired colonic fermentation of carbohydrate after ampicillin. *Gastroenterology* 1988; **94**: 928–32.

164. Homann H-H, Kemen M, Mumme A, Bauer KH, Zumtobel V. The role of carbohydrate malabsorption in the pathogenesis of diarrhea during postoperative enteral nutrition. *J Clin Nutr Gastroenterol* 1992; **7**: 54–9.

165. Reeds PJ, Burrin DG, Stoll B, Van Goudoever JB. Role of the gut in the amino acid economy of the host. In: Fürst P, Young VR (eds) Proteins, peptides and amino-acids in enteral nutrition. Karger, Basel, 2000.

166. Milner JA. Metabolic aberrations associated with arginine deficiency. *J Nutr* 1985; **115:** 516–23.

167. Barbul A. Arginine, biochemistry, physiology and therapeutic implications. *J Parent Ent Nutr* 1986; **10:** 227–38.

168. Morris JG, Rogers QR. Ammonia intoxication in the near-adult cat as a result of a dietary arginine deficiency. *Science* 1978; **199:** 431–2.

169. Fahey JL. Toxicity and blood ammonia rise resulting from intravenous amino acid administration in man: the protective effect of L-arginine. *J Clin Invest* 1957; **36:** 1647–55.

170. Rérat A, Simoes-Nuñes C, Mendy F, Roger L. Amino acid absorption and production of pancreatic hormones in non-anaesthetised pigs after duodenal infusions of a milk enzymic hydrolysate or of free amino acids. *Br J Nutr* 1988; **60:** 121–36.

171. Brosnan JT. The 1986 Borden award lecture. The role of the kidney in amino acid metabolism and nutrition. *Can J Physiol Pharmacol* 1987; **65:** 2355–62.

172. Lund P. Glutamine metabolism in the rat. *FEBS Lett* 1980; **117** (suppl): K86–K92.

173. Merimee TJ, Lillicrap DA, Rabinowitz D. Effect of arginine on serum levels of human growth hormone. *Lancet* 1965; **ii:** 668–70.

174. Floyd JC, Fajans SS, Conn JW, Knopf RF, Rull J. Stimulation of insulin secretion by amino acids. *J Clin Invest* 1966; **45:** 1487–502.

175. Barbul A, Sisto DA, Wasserkrug HL, Efron G. Arginine stimulates lymphocyte immune response in healthy human beings. *Surgery* 1981; **90:** 244–51.

176. Barbul A, Lazarou SA, Efron DT, Wasserkrug HL, Efron G. Arginine enhances wound healing and lymphocyte immune responses in humans. *Surgery* 1990; **108:** 331–7.

177. Hurson M, Regan MC, Kirk SJ, Wasserkrug HL, Barbul A. Metabolic effects of arginine in a healthy elderly population. *J Parent Ent Nutr* 1995; **19**(3): 227–30.

178. Gianotti L, Alexander JW, Pyles T, Fukushima R. Arginine-supplemented diets improve survival in gut-derived sepsis and peritonitis by modulating bacterial clearance: the role of nitric oxide. *Ann Surg* 1993; **217:** 644–54.

179. Brittenden J, Heys SD, Ross J, Eremin O. Nutritional pharmacology: effects of L-arginine on host defences, response to trauma and tumour growth. *Clin Sci* 1994; **86:** 123–32.

180. Cosgrove M. Perinatal and infant nutrition. Nucleotides. *Nutrition* 1998; **14**(10): 748–51.

181. López-Navarro AT, Ortega MA, Peragon J, Bueno JD, Gil A, Sánchez-Pozo A. Deprivation of dietary nucleotides decreases protein synthesis in the liver and small intestine in rats. *Gastroenterology* 1996; **110**(6): 1760–9.

182. López-Navarro AT, Bueno JD, Gil A, Sánchez-Pozo A. Morphological changes in hepatocytes of rats deprived of dietary nucleotides. *Br J Nutr* 1996; **76**(4): 579–89.

183. Kishibuchi M, Tsujinaka T, Yano M et al. Effects of nucleosides and a nucleotide mixture on gut mucosal barrier function on parenteral nutrition in rats. *J Parent Ent Nutr* 1997; **21**(2): 104–11.

184. Bueno J, Torres M, Almendros A et al. Effect of dietary nucleotides on small intestinal repair after diarrhoea. Histological and ultrastructural changes. *Gut* 1994; **35**(7): 926–33.

185. Iijima S, Tsujinaka T, Kido Y et al. Intravenous administration of nucleosides and a nucleotide mixture diminishes intestinal mucosal atrophy induced by total parenteral nutrition. *J Parent Ent Nutr* 1993; **17:** 265–70.

186. Cosgrove M, Davies DP, Jenkins HR. Nucleotide supplementation and the growth of term small for gestational age infants. *Arch Dis Child* 1996; **74:** F122–F125.

187. Brunser O, Espinoza J, Araya M, Cruchet S, Gil A. Effect of dietary nucleotide supplementation on diarrhoeal disease in infants. *Acta Paediatr* 1994; **83:** 188–91.

188. Roman RM, Fitz JG. Emerging roles of purinergic signaling in gastrointestinal epithelial secretion and hepatobiliary function. *Gastroenterology* 1999; **116**(4): 964–79.

189. Grimble GK, Westwood OM. Nucleotides as immunomodulators in clinical nutrition. *Curr Opin Clin Nutr Metab Care* 2001; **4:** 57–64.

190. Windmueller HG. Enterohepatic aspects of glutamine metabolism. In: Mora J, Palacios R (eds) Glutamine: metabolism, enzymology and regulation. Academic Press, New York, 1980; pp. 235–257.

191. Souba WW, Smith RJ, Wilmore DW. Glutamine metabolism by the intestinal tract. *J Parent Ent Nutr* 1985; **9:** 608–17.

192. McKeehan WL. Glycolysis, glutaminolysis and cell proliferation. *Cell Biol Int Rep* 1982; **6:** 635–49.

193. Newsholme EA, Newsholme P, Curi R. The role of the citric acid cycle in cells of the immune system and its importance in sepsis, trauma and burns. In: Kay J, Weitzman PDJ (eds) Krebs' citric acid cycle: half a century and still turning. Biochemical Society Symposium 54. The Biochemical Society, London, 1987; pp. 145–161.

194. Reeds PJ, Burrin DG, Stoll B, Jahoor F. Intestinal glutamate metabolism. *J Nutr* 2000; **130**(4S suppl): 978S–982S.

195. Curtis KJ, Sleisenger MH, Kim YS. Protein digestion and absorption after massive small bowel resection. *Dig Dis Sci* 1984; **29**: 834–40.

196. Bristol JB, Williamson RCN. Nutrition, operations, and intestinal adaptation. *J Parent Ent Nutr* 1988; **12**: 299–309.

197. McIntyre PB, Fitchew M, Lennard-Jones JE. Patients with a high ileostomy do not need a special diet. *Gastroenterology* 1986; **91**: 25–33.

198. Haase W, Heitmann K, Friese W, Ollig D, Koepsell H. Characterization and histochemical localization of the rat intestinal Na(+)-D-glucose cotransporter by monoclonal antibodies. *Eur J Cell Biol* 1990; **52**: 297–309.

199. Skovbjerg H. Immunoelectrophoretic studies on human small intestinal brush border proteins – the longitudinal distribution of peptidases and disaccharidases. *Clin Chim Acta* 1981; **112**: 205–12.

200. Dodge JA, Yassa JG. Essential fatty acid deficiency after prolonged treatment with elemental diet. *Lancet* 1980; **ii**: 1256–7.

201. Bronstein MN, Sokol RJ, Abman SH *et al.* Pancreatic insufficiency, growth, and nutrition in infants identified by newborn screening as having cystic fibrosis. *J Pediatr* 1992; **120**: 533–40.

202. Dodge JA. Nutrition in cystic fibrosis: a historical overview. *Proc Nutr Soc* 1992; **51**: 225–35.

203. Durie PR, Pencharz PB. Cystic fibrosis: nutrition. *Br Med Bull* 1992; **48**: 823–46.

204. Pettei MJ, Daftary S, Levine JJ. Essential fatty acid deficiency associated with the use of a medium-chain-triglyceride infant formula in pediatric hepatobiliary disease. *Am J Clin Nutr* 1991; **53**: 1217–21.

205. Hamosh M, Mehta NR, Fink CS, Coleman J, Hamosh P. Fat absorption in premature infants: medium-chain triglycerides and long-chain triglycerides are absorbed from formula at similar rates. *J Pediatr Gastroenterol Nutr* 1991; **13**: 143–9.

206. Grimble GK. Physiology of nutrient absorption and patterns of intestinal metabolism. In: Payne-James JJ, Grimble GK, Silk DBA (eds) Artificial nutrition support in clinical practice. Edward Arnold, London, 1995; pp. 73–97.

207. Grimble GK, Duncan HD. Intestinal perfusion techniques. In: Preedy VR, Watson RR (eds) Methods in disease: investigating the gastrointestinal tract. Greenwich Medical Media, London, 1998; pp. 27–40.

208. Kellett GL. The facilitated component of intestinal glucose absorption. *J Physiol* 2001; **531**: 585–95.

Introduction

A broad spectrum of nutritional deficiencies is encountered in clinical practice, ranging from life-threatening protein-energy malnutrition (PEM) to subclinical deficiencies of individual micronutrients. The relationship between nutrition, immune function and disease is complex, though there is little doubt that nutritional depletion *per se* can profoundly effect immunocompetence. In fact, malnutrition is probably the commonest cause of secondary immunodeficiency world wide, and is not restricted to developing countries.[1]

Effects of nutrition status on immune function

Protein-energy malnutrition (Table 7.1)

Protein-energy malnutrition provides a vivid illustration of the deleterious effects of inadequate nutrition on the host immune system. Studies of malnourished children in the developing world have been a major source of data, providing sad testimony to the harmful effects of malnutrition on the body's resistance to disease.[3-6] In the severely malnourished there is gross macroscopic evidence of adverse effects on lymphoid tissues, with involution of the thymus and a reduction in the weight of tonsils, lymph nodes and spleen.[7] Reduced peripheral T-cell counts (CD3+, CD4+ and CD8+) have been observed[1] and poor primary recall and delayed cutaneous hypersensitivity responses reported.[8,9] Anergy to tuberculin in BCG vaccination has been observed in malnourished children.[10] Lymphocyte responses may be attenuated in PEM, with evidence of reduced *in vitro* lymphocyte transformation in response to T-cell mitogens,[11,12] reduced production of T-cell cytokines such as IL-2 and IFN-γ,[13] and (in animal studies) impaired responsiveness of lymphocytes to cytokine stimulation.[14] Circulating B-cell counts and immunoglobulin levels may be normal in PEM,[15] and antibody response to measles vaccination was not found to be depressed in malnourished Mali children.[16] Although absolute natural killer (NK) cell numbers may be elevated,[15] NK activity may be reduced in children with kwashiorkor/marasmus.[11] Alterations in monocyte phagocytic activity are reported,[15] polymorphonuclear function may be reduced,[17] and pro-inflammatory cytokine release is depressed in PEM.[18] Reduced complement activity may also occur.[19,20] Many of the immunological abnormalities observed in PEM can be partly or completely restored by nutritional repletion.[8,11]

Individual nutritional components

Amino acids

Whilst a severely restricted dietary protein intake (as seen in cases of PEM) undoubtedly leads to profound effects on immunological function, less is known about the role of individual amino acids in maintaining immunocompetence. The reduced cellular immunity resulting from lymphoid atrophy observed in animals deprived specifically of branched-chain or sulphur-containing amino acids[21] are very similar to the changes observed in paediatric PEM. *In vitro* studies have demonstrated that the amino acid, arginine, has immunostimulatory and thymotrophic properties, enhancing the production of T-helper cells and stimulating the production and release of interleukin-2.[22] Glutamine is a very important metabolic fuel for lymphocytes and monocytes, and has been shown *in vitro* to be vital for lymphocyte and macrophage proliferation, differentiation of B- and T-cells, antibody production and macrophage phagocytic activity.[23]

Nucleotides

Normal immune functioning may require dietary intake of ribonucleic acid (RNA), with dietary nucleotides being involved in the regulation of a range of cellular immune responses.[24] In a murine model, a diet free of nucleotides resulted in reduced interleukin-2 production, decreased cell-mediated immunity, increased allograft rejection and reduced resistance to infection whereas administration of RNA significantly improved host immune responsiveness and host survival to a septic challenge.[25]

Table 7.1 – Effects of protein-energy malnutrition on immune function[2]

Lymphoid tissues	↓
Lymphocyte numbers	↓
Humoral immunity	Variable
Cellular immunity	↓
Lymphocyte proliferation	↓ or normal
Phagocyte function	↓ or normal

Lipids

Dietary lipids may influence immune function by changing the fluidity of cell membranes, as suggested over 80 years ago.[26] Animals injected with cholesterol supplements show suppressed phagocytic function, whilst methylation of cellular phospholipids, which facilitates lymphocyte mitogenesis, chemotaxis in neutrophils and the release of histamine from mast cells and basophils is increased.[27] Artificial lipid micelles (as in the lipid emulsions used in intravenous feeding) may also alter lymphocyte function.[28,29]

Ω-6 polyunsaturated fatty acids (PUFAs) are essential dietary components which are found in animal fat, acting as precursors of eicosanoid metabolites such as prostaglandins, lipoxins, thromboxanes and leukotrienes. Fatty acids found in fish oils belong to the Ω-3 class, and promote different cytoproliferative effects, often anti-inflammatory in nature. Prostaglandin E_2 has been suggested as an important factor in immunosuppression following major injury. Enteral feeds rich in Ω-3 PUFAs result in a suppression of prostaglandin E_2 synthesis, and have been shown in some animal studies to improve immune parameters and/or survival after injury or endotoxin challenge.[30–32] In burns patients Ω-3 PUFAs diminished immunosuppression secondary to blood transfusion, reduced infectious complications and improved survival.[33] However, excess polyunsaturates can suppress cell-mediated immunity,[34] and diets high in Ω-3 fatty acids may lead to the generation of lipid peroxides and consumption of the free-radical scavenger, vitamin E, potentially aggravating oxidative stress in critical illness.[23]

Iron

Iron deficiency is one of the commonest forms of single micronutrient deficiency to occur in the absence of other accompanying forms of malnutrition. In experimental animals, iron deficiency has been shown to lead to increased susceptibility to infections[35] but human studies have been less consistent.[36] Many studies, however, indicate that iron deficiency adversely affects cellular immune function and phagocytic activity.[37–39] There is little agreement on the effects of iron deficiency on total lymphocyte numbers or on mitogen responses, suggesting that iron deficiency may have a differential effect on lymphoid subpopulations.[40] No significant abnormalities have been reported in association with iron deficiency in serum immunoglobulin concentrations, salivary IgA levels, or consistently in other parameters of humoral immune function.[37]

Zinc

The trace metal zinc is a constituent of a number of cellular enzymes which participate in a wide variety of metabolic processes including carbohydrate, lipid, protein and nucleic acid synthesis or degradation. Zinc undoubtedly plays a pivotal role in cell-mediated immunity. Even short periods of zinc deprivation in humans and animals can cause thymic hypoplasia or atrophy and premature involution of the spleen and lymph nodes,[41–43] with lymphopaenia and increased proportions of circulating immature T-cells. Animal studies have demonstrated that zinc deficiency results in decreased $CD4^+$ cell activity, decreased mitogen responsiveness, cutaneous anergy, a reduction in the long-term memory of T-cells, decreased NK cell activity and reduced monocyte cytotoxicity.[44–49] Complete reversal of some of these changes has also been shown on repletion of zinc.[45–48]

In man, zinc deficiency may occur in a variety of circumstances. Acrodermatitis enteropathica is an hereditary zinc-deficiency disease in which there is defective proximal intestinal absorption of zinc and hypozincaemia. In this condition, T-cell numbers are reduced and mitogen-induced proliferation and delayed cutaneous hypersensitivity responses are all depressed.[50] These abnormalities are corrected by zinc supplementation. A similar picture of impaired cellular immunity, reversible on repletion, is seen in patients who receive prolonged total parenteral nutrition without adequate zinc supplementation.[51,52] In patients with Down's syndrome, low serum zinc levels accompanied by impaired delayed cutaneous hypersensitivity responses, lymphocyte transformation and phagocyte function have been improved by zinc supplements.[53] Zinc excess, however, can also reduce immune function.[54]

Other minerals and trace elements

Although deficits in magnesium have not been reported to cause immunological abnormalities in human subjects, rodents fed diets moderately deficient in magnesium for extended periods of time exhibit marked changes, including leucocytosis, mast cell degranulation, and even leukaemia and lymphoma.[55–60] Selenium, calcium and copper deficiency are all associated with abnormal immune responses, although the significance of such observations is unclear.[61–66] Excess lead, cadmium, chromium, mercury, nickel, gold, vanadium and iodine can all suppress various immune responses but their clinical significance is limited.[67,68]

Vitamins *(Table 7.2)*

Water-soluble vitamins

Off all essential micronutrients, vitamin C has undoubtedly generated the greatest interest concerning its interaction with host defence mechanisms and the immune system. The high ascorbic acid concentration of leukocytes and lymphocytes, and its rapid expenditure during infection and phagocytosis, suggest that this vitamin has a vital role in supporting immune function.[70] Exogenous administration of vitamin C has been shown to improve neutrophil function and the motility of monocytes.[71,72] The relationship between vitamin C and lymphocyte function is not clearly defined. Studies in animal models suggest that severe vitamin C deficiency is associated with depressed T-lymphocyte mitogenic responses which can be reversed by ascorbate supplementation.[73–75] In man, withdrawal of dietary vitamin C, or supplementation, does not appear to affect absolute lymphocyte numbers nor subsets, but supplementation may enhance mitogen–induced lymphocyte transformation.[76,77] No consistent pattern has been found for the effect of vitamin C on humoral immunity, although supplementation has been shown to increase serum immunoglobulins.[78]

Deficiencies of folic acid lead to a reduction of host resistance and to impaired lymphocyte functions in both man and experimental animals.[2,79] In animal models, pyridoxine deprivation causes atrophy of lymphoid tissues, lymphopaenia, inhibition of cell mediated immunity, and humoral responsiveness to a variety of test antigens. In fact, isolated pyridoxine deficiency causes more profound effects on immune system function than deficiencies of any other B group vitamin.[80]

Fat-soluble vitamins

Two of the fat-soluble vitamins, vitamins A and E, have recognised effects on immune system function. An association between vitamin A status and immune function has been suggested by various studies.[81] Deficiency of vitamin A appears to predispose to an increased susceptibility to infection and to increased rates of morbidity and mortality.[81,82] In animal models, vitamin A deficiency affects both humoral and cellular immunity.[83–85] Recent evidence shows that T-cell subpopulations, cytokines and antibody subclasses are all affected by vitamin A. The immune defects caused by vitamin A deficiency may be due to alterations in the glycoproteins of the lymphocyte membrane, an adverse effect on helper T-cell function or related to the important role of vitamin A in maintaining the functional integrity of epithelial surfaces.[86]

Vitamin E is believed to play an important role as an antioxidant, a scavenger of free radicals and a stabiliser of cellular membranes. In animal studies, vitamin E administration appears to protect against bacterial infection and improves measures of cellular and humoral immune function.[87,88] In man, defects in cellular immunity have been observed.[89]

Table 7.2 – Effects of specific vitamin deficiencies on parameters of immune function[2,69]

Parameter	Vit C	Folate	Vit B₁	Vit B₆	Vit A	Vit E
Lymphoid tissue		↓	↓	↓	↓	↓
Antibody response			↓	↓	↓	↓
Peripheral blood lymphocytes			↓	↓	↓	
Delayed hypersensitivity response	↓		↓	↓		
Neutrophil phagocytosis	↓	↓				
Monocyte function	↓				↓	↓
Lymphocyte proliferation		↓		↓	↓	↓

Nutrition and immune dysfunction in clinical practice

In an individual patient, there are potentially many factors influencing the integrity of the immune system. Immunological abnormalities may be a primary feature of a specific disease state, a result of associated single or multiple nutritional deficiencies, or may be secondary to a range of additional factors including drugs, infection, neoplasia, tissue trauma, burns, septic shock and anaesthetic/surgical procedures.[90-93]

Immunosenescence

Nutrition has been suggested as a critical determinant of immunocompetence and risk of illness in old age. Ageing is accompanied by changes in T-cell subgroups (characteristically a reduction in CD4$^+$-cells), decreased lymphocyte proliferative responses to mitogens, reduced natural killer cell activity, and reduced polymorph chemotactic responses.[94] Simultaneous assessment of nutritional status and immune responses with subsequent analysis of correlation in elderly subjects has suggested a role for nutritional deficiencies in immunosenescence.[95,96] Nutrition advice and supplementation in elderly subjects has been shown to result in improvements in mitogen-induced lymphocyte stimulation response, natural killer cell activity, enhanced cutaneous hypersensitivity and increased interleukin-2 production.[94]

Medical and surgical in-patients

Under-nutrition has been reported to affect 30–50% of all patients with medical conditions in hospital.[97] Patients most affected are those with longstanding chronic diseases, especially those affecting the liver, kidneys or gut. Whilst numerous studies have demonstrated immune dysfunction in malnourished hospitalised patients, a positive correlation between nutritional deprivation and depressed immunocompetence has yet to be well documented, except in some patients with liver disease and in the elderly.[98] What is clear is that even relatively short periods of under-nutrition can result in depressed immunity, especially cellular. Studies of adult PEM in hospitalised patients with acute and chronic illnesses have shown depressed skin reactivity,[99-101] impaired B-lymphocyte function,[99] and either depressed[99] or normal[100] mitogen transformation to phytohaemagglutinin (PHA), pokeweed mitogen and concanavalin A. Reduced interleukin-1 production has been reported in chronically malnourished patients[102,103] which may account for the common observation of attenuated febrile responses to infection in such patients. Upregulation of MHC class II molecule expression by monocytes in response to IFN-γ *in vitro* is impaired in malnourished surgical patients and improved by nutrition repletion with TPN.[104]

There is no doubt that under-nourishment in surgical patients impairs resistance to infection.[105] In one of the earliest surgical studies of its kind,[106] postoperative survival was shown to be directly related to nutritional status in patients receiving surgical treatment for peptic ulcer disease. Whilst a third of patients who had lost weight prior to surgery died (frequently from infective complications), mortality in better nourished patients was only one-tenth of this figure. The commonest complication of surgery in the malnourished patient appears to be sepsis.[107-109] Cachexia commonly arises during any critical illness, and results from a combination of factors including malnutrition, immobility and hypercatabolism.[23] The degree of weight loss occurring during acute illness is correlated with mortality.[110]

Recent interest has focused on the use of nutritional supplements specifically formulated to 'boost' immune function during critical illness, such as after major surgery. To date, data are limited on the efficacy of this so-called 'immunonutrition' on infectious morbidity or mortality in man. The use of enteral feeds supplemented with arginine, Ω-3 PUFAs and RNA has been studied in postoperative patients. In one study,[111] lymphocyte responsiveness was restored, and infectious and wound complications reduced in patients given the supplemented formulation compared with those receiving standard diet after surgery for upper gastrointestinal cancer. In another study[112] comparing the supplemented enteral feed against an isonitrogenous control diet, T-cell numbers, B-lymphocyte indices, immunoglobulin M and G levels and interferon-gamma production after PHA stimulation were higher in the supplemented patients.

Cancer patients

Patients with cancer appear to be especially at risk of infection, and may or may not suffer from nutritional depletion. Diminished immunocompetence very frequently occurs irrespective of the nutritional status. Fatal infections are a common cause of death in cancer patients, affecting about 50% of those dying from solid tumours.[113] Indices of nutritional status have a predictive role in relation to immunological reactivity in cancer patients, and both factors have prognostic significance. Skin test reactivity to a variety of antigens and *in vitro* tests of cell-mediated immunity are commonly reduced in patients with cancer, and often related to nutrition deficiencies. Those patients who have reduced immune parameters, notably indices of cell-mediated immunity and reduced circulating lymphocyte numbers, and who also suffer nutritional depletion, tend to have greater postoperative morbidity and mortality.[114-116] In patients with cancer, correction of nutritional deficiencies has been reported in some investigations to improve parameters of immune competence, improve tumour response to chemotherapy, and reduce postoperative complications.[117-119]

Inflammatory bowel disease

Many nutritional disturbances can occur in patients with inflammatory bowel disease, particularly those with Crohn's disease, which may have profound effects on morbidity and even mortality.[120,121] A number of clinical features seen in Crohn's disease, such as poor wound healing, fistula formation, muscle wasting, hypoalbuminaemia, weight loss and impaired immunocompetence are shared with other conditions in which nutritional depletion is a prominent feature. It is reasonable to conclude that malnutrition is a leading cause of such clinical features in Crohn's disease.[120] Malnutrition occurring in patients with inflammatory bowel disease is usually a result of reduced dietary intake rather than malabsorption *per se*, except where there has been extensive small bowel disease or resection.[122] Anorexia is common in all chronic inflammatory conditions and may result from increased production of cytokines, which exert diverse effects on body metabolism.[123] Serum TNF-α levels, for example, are elevated in inflammatory bowel disease,[124] and clinical responses with TNF-α antibodies may be mediated by similar mechanisms.[125]

It has been suggested that certain antigenic food items may trigger an inflammatory response provoking relapse in patients with Crohn's disease.[122] Non-antigenic elemental diets can produce a response in acute Crohn's disease[126] and complete 'bowel rest' through the use of intravenous feeding (TPN) may benefit some patients with steroid-resistant disease.[122]

Both treatments appear to exert similar immunosuppressive effects in patients with Crohn's disease.[127]

Total parenteral nutrition

There is little doubt that parenteral nutrition is beneficial to many severely malnourished patients who cannot tolerate enteral feeding. However, the use of TPN is not without its complications, particularly infection, which may reflect immunological changes. TPN has been reported to alter both specific and non-specific immune functions, often exerting immunosuppressive effects.[128-130] Individual components of the feed may be responsible for some of the observed immunological changes, such as the specific immunosuppressive effect of certain lipid emulsions.[131] The cessation of enteral feeding is also a possible contributing factor in TPN-associated immune dysfunction and infective complications, resulting from the development of mucosal atrophy, bacterial overgrowth, and (possible) gut translocation of bacteria or endotoxin in patients subjected to prolonged fasting.[23]

Conclusions

There can be little doubt that control of nutritional balance is of crucial importance in maintaining the integrity of the normal immune response. In a wide range of animal experiments, pan-nutritional depletion or specific isolated nutritional defects show a clear association with abnormal immune parameters. The evidences of links between the two phenomena have been strengthened when immune responsiveness has been corrected by individual nutritional replenishment.

In the clinical setting these close associations have been difficult to prove, since pure nutrient deficiencies seldom exist in isolation from disease states which may themselves directly influence immune functioning. Nevertheless, there is compelling evidence that malnutrition *per se* diminishes immune competence and increases the risks of sepsis. Evidence that nutritional repletion in man can rectify these defects is less well proven than in animal models, but even so is reasonably convincing. Clarification of the immunological effects of nutritional repletion in the clinical setting will require carefully controlled trials in specific and well defined disease states. The insights provided by such studies into the links between nutrition and immunocompetence have the potential to benefit the management of a wide and varied range of clinical conditions.

References

1. Puri S and Chandra RK. Nutritional regulation of host resistence and predictive value of immunological tests in assessment of outcome. *Pediatr Clin North Am* 1985; **32**: 499–516.

2. Dowd PS, Heatley RV. The influence of undernutrition on immunity. *Clin Sci* 1984; **66**: 241–248.

3. Chandra RK and Newberne PM. Nutrition, Immunity & Infection: *Mechanisms of Interactions*. Plenum, New York: 1977.

4. Lindtjorn B, Alemu T, Bjorvatn B. Nutritional status and risk of infection among Ethiopian children. *J Trop Pediatr* 1993 Apr; **39(2)**: 76–82.

5. Isaack H, Mbise RL, Hirji KF. Nosocomial bacterial infections among children with severe protein energy malnutrition. *East Afr Med J* 1992 Aug; **69(8)**: 433–436.

6. Alwar AJ. The effect of protein energy malnutrition on morbidity and mortality due to measles at Kenyatta National Hospital, Nairobi (Kenya). *East Afr Med J* 1992 Aug; **69(8)**: 415–418.

7. Christou, N. Perioperative nutritional support: Immunological defects. *J Parenter Enter Nutr* 1990; **14**: 186S-196S.

8. Neumann CG, Lawlor GJ, Stiehm ER, *et al.* Immunological responses in malnourished children. *Am J Clin Nutr* 1975; **28**: 89–104.

9. McMurray DN, Loomis SA, Casazza LJ, Rey H, and Miranda R. Development of impaired cell-mediated immunity in mild and moderate malnutrition. *Am J Clin Nutr* 1981; **34**: 68–77.

10. Udani PM. BCG vaccination in India and tuberculosis in children: newer facets. [Review] *Indian J Pediatr* 1994 Sep–Oct; **61(5)**: 451–462.

11. Salimonu LS, Ojo-Amaize E, Johnson AOK, Laditan AAO, Akinwolere AOA and Wigzell H. Depressed natural killer cell activity in children with protein-calorie malnutrition. *Cell Immunol* 1983; **82**: 210–215.

12. Chandra RK. Lymphocyte subpopulations in human nutrition: cytotoxic and suppressor cells. *Paediatr* 1977; **59**: 423–427.

13. Bradley J, Xu X. Diet, age and the immune system. *Nutr Rev* 1996; **54**: S43–S50.

14. Hoffman-Goetz L, Keir R, Young C. Modulation of cellular immunity in malnutrition: effect of interleukin 1 on suppressor T cell activity. *Clin Exp Immunol* 1986 Aug; **65(2)**: 381–386.

15. Kahan BD. Nutrition and host defence mechanisms. *Surg Clin North Am* 1981; **61**: 557–570.

16. Dao H, Delisle H, Fournier P. Anthropometric status, serum prealbumin level and immune response to measles vaccination in Mali children. *J Trop Pediatr* 1992 Aug; **38(4)**: 179–184.

17. Chandra RK, Chandra S and Ghai OP. Chemotaxis, random motility and mobilization of polymorphonuclear leukocytes in malnutrition. *J Clin Pathol* 1976; **29**: 224–227.

18. Grimble RF. Malnutrition and the immune response 2. Impact of nutrients on cytokine biology in infection. [Review] *Trans R Soc Trop Med Hyg* 1994 Nov–Dec; **88(6)**: 615–619.

19. Haller L, Zubler RH, Lambert PH. Plasma levels of complement components and complement haemolytic activity in protein energy malnutrition. *Clin Exp Immunol* 1978; **34**: 248–252.

20. Ozkan H, Olgun N, Sasmaz E, Abacioglu H, Okuyan M, Cevik N. Nutrition, immunity and infections: T lymphocyte subpopulations in protein–energy malnutrition. *J Trop Pediatr* 1993 Aug; **39(4)**: 257–260.

21. Gross RL and Newberne PM. Role of nutrition in immunologic function. *Physiol Rev* 1980; 188–302.

22. Barbul, A. Arginine: Biochemistry, physiology and therapeutics. *J Parenter Enter Nutr* 1986; 227–238.

23. O'Leary MJ and Coakley JH. Nutrition and immunonutrition. *Br J Anaesth* 1996; **77**: 118–127.

24. Carver JD, Cox WI, Barness LA. Dietary nucleotide effects upon murine natural killer cell activity and macrophage activation. *J Parenter Enter Nutr* 1990; **14**: 18–22.

25. Fanslow WC, Kulkharni A, Van Buren CT, Rudolph F. Effect of nucleotide restriction and supplementation on resistance to experimental murine candidiasis. *J Parenter Enter Nutr* 1988; **12**: 49–52.

26. Dewey K, Nuzum F. The effect of cholesterol on phagocytosis. *J Infect Dis* 1914; **15**: 472–482.

27. Hirata F, Axelrod J. Phospholipid methylation and biological signal transmission. *Science* 1980; **209**: 1082–1090.

28. Sedman PC, Ramsden CW, Brennan TG, Guillou PJ. Pharmacological concentrations of lipid emulsions inhibit interleukin-2-dependant lymphocyte responses in vitro. *J Parenter Enter Nutr* 1990; **14**: 12–17.

29. Sedman PC, Somers SS, Ramsden CW, Brennan TG, Guillou PJ. Effects of different lipid emulsions on lyphocyte function during total parenteral nutrition. *Br J Surg* 1991; **78**: 1396–1399.

30. Alexander JW, Saito H, Trocki O, Ogle CK. The importance of lipid type in the diet after burn injury. *Ann Surg* 1986; **204**: 1–8.

31. Mascioli EA, Iwasa Y, Trimbo S, Leader L, Bistrian BR, Blackburn GL. Endotoxin challenge after menhaden oil diet: effect on survival in guinea pigs. *Am J Clin Nutr* 1989; **49**: 277–282.

32. Barton RG, Wells CL, Carlson A, Singh R, Sullivan JJ, Cerra FB. Dietary omega-3 fatty acids decrease mortality and Kupffer cell prostaglandin E_2 production in a rat model of chronic sepsis. *J Trauma* 1991; **31:** 768–773.

33. Gottschlich MM, Jenkins M, Warden GD, Baumer T, Havens P, Snook JT, Alexander JW. Differential effects of three enteral dietary regimens on selected outcome variables in burns patients. *J Parenter Enter Nutr* 1990; **14:** 225–236.

34. Uldall *et al.* Linoleic acid and transplantation. *Lancet* 1975; **2(7925):** 128–129.

35. Baggs RB, Miler SA. Defect in resistence to *Salmonella typhimurium* in iron-deficient rats. *J Infect Dis* 1974; **130:** 409–411

36. Strauss RG. Iron deficiency, infections and immune function: a reassessment. *Am J Clin Nutr* 1978; **31:** 660–666.

37. Nalder BN, Mahoney AW, Ramakrishnan R, Hendricks DG. Sensitivity of the immunological response to the nutritional status of rats. *J Nutr* 1972; **102:** 535–542.

38. Bhashkaram C, Reddy V. Cell mediated immunity in iron and vitamin deficient children. *Br Med J* 1975; **iii:** 522.

39. Rothenbacher H, Sherman AR. Target organ pathology in iron deficient suckling rats. *J Nutr* 1980; **110:** 1648–1654.

40. Soyano A, Candellet D, Layrisse M. Effect of iron deficiency on the mitogen-induced proliferative response of rat lymphocytes. *Int Arch Aller Appl Immun* 1982; **69:** 353–357.

41. Fraker PJ, Despasquale-Jardieu P, Zwickl CM, Luecke RW. Regeneration of T-cell helper function in zinc deficient adult mice. *Proc Nat Acad Sci USA* 1978; **75:** 5660–5664.

42. Gross RL, Osdin N, Fong L, Newberne PM. Depressed immunological function in zinc-deprived rats as measured by mitogen response of spleen, thymus and peripheral blood. *Am J Clin Nutr* 1979; **32:** 1260–1265.

43. Chandra RK, Au B. Single nutrient deficiency and cell mediated immune responses. 1: Zinc. *Am J Clin Nutr* 1980; **33:** 736–738.

44. Fraker PJ, Haas SM and Luecke RW. Effect of zinc deficiency on the immune response of the young adult A/J mouse. *J Nutr* 1977; **107:** 1889–1895.

45. Fernandes G, Nair M, Onoe K, Tanaka T, Floyd R, Good RA. Impairment of cell mediated immunity functions by dietary zinc deficiency in mice. *Proc Nat Acad Sci USA* 1979; **76:** 457–461.

46. Frost P, Rabbani P, Smith J, Prasad A. Cell-mediated cytotoxicity and tumour growth in zinc deficient mice. *Proc Soc Exp Biol Med* 1981; **167:** 333–337.

47. Berger NA and Skinner AM. Characterisation of lymphocyte transformation induced by zinc ions. *J Cell Biol* 1974; **6:** 45–55.

48. Beach RS, Gershwin ME, Hurley LS. Gestational zinc deprivation in mice: persistence of immunodeficiency for three generations. *Science* 1982; **218:** 469–471.

49. Zanzonico P, Fernandes G and Good RA. The differential sensitivity of T-cell and B-cell mitogenesis to in vitro zinc deficiency. *Cell Immunol* 1981; **60:** 203–211.

50. Endre L, Katona Z, Gyurkkovits K. Zinc deficiency in cellular immune deficiency in acrodermatitis enteropathica. *Lancet* 1975; **i:** 1196.

51. Pekarek RS, Sandstead HH, Jacob RA, Barcome DF. Abnormal cellular immune responses during acquired zinc deficiency. *Am J Clin Nutr* 1979; **32:** 1466–1471.

52. Allen JI, Key NE, McClain CJ. Severe zinc deficiency in humans: association with a reversible T-lymphocyte dysfunction. *Ann Int Med* 1981; 95:154–157.

53. Bjorksten B, Back O, Gustavson KH, Hallmans G, Hagglof B, Tarnvik A. Zinc and immune function in Down's Syndrome. *Acta Paediatr Scand* 1980; **69:** 183–187.

54. Chandra RK. Excessive intake of zinc impairs immune responsiveness. *J Am Med Assoc* 1984; **252:** 1443–1446.

55. Kashiwa HK, Hungerford GF. Blood leukocyte response in rats fed a magnesium deficient diet. *Proc Soc Exper Biol Med* 1958; **99:** 441–443.

56. Hungerford GF, Karson EF. The eosinophilia of magnesium deficiency. *Blood* 1960; **16:** 1642–1650.

57. McCreary PA, Battifora HA, Laing GH, Hass GM. Protective effect of magnesium deficiency on experimental allergic encephalomyelitis in the rat. *Proc Soc Exper Biol Med* 1966; **121:** 1130–1133.

58. McCreary PA, Battifora HA, Hahneman BM, *et al.* Leukocytosis, bone marrow hyperplasia and leukaemia in chronic magnesium deficiency in the rat. *Blood* 1967; **29:** 683–690.

59. Battifora HA, McCreary PA, Hahneman BM, *et al.* Chronic magnesium deficiency in the rat: studies of chronic myelogenous leukamia. *Arch Path* 1968; **86:** 610–620.

60. Bois P. Effect of magnesium deficiency on mast cells and urinary histamine in rats. *Br J Exper Path* 1963; **44:** 151–155.

61. Mulhern SA, Morris VC, Vessey AR, Levander OA. Influence of selenium and chow diets on immune function in first and second generation mice. *Fed Proc* 1981; **40:** 935.

62. Spallholz JE, Martin JL, Gerlach ML, Heinzerling RH. Immunologic responses of mice fed diets supplemented with selenite selenium. *Proc Soc Exp Biol Med* 1973a; **143:** 685–689.

63. Spallholz JE, Martin JL, Gerlach ML, Heinzerling RH. Enhanced immunoglobulin M and immunoglobulin G antibody titres in mice fed selenium. *Infect Immunol* 1973b; **8:** 841–842.

64. Hui DY, Berebitsky GL, Harmony JAK. Mitogen-stimulated calcium ion accumulation by lymphocytes: influence of plasma lipoproteins. *J Biol Chem* 1979; **254:** 4666–4673.

65. Korchak HM, Smolen JE. The role of calcium movements in human neutrophil (PMN) activation. *Fed Proc* 1981; **40:** 753.

66. Omole TA, Onawunmi AO. Effect of copper on growth and serum constituents of immunized and non-immunized rabbits infected with *Trypanosoma Brucei*. *Ann Parasitol* (Paris) 1979; **54:** 495–506.

67. Koller LD. Immunosuppression produced by lead, cadmium and mercury. *Am J Veter Res* 1973; **34:** 1457–1458.

68. Waters MD, Gardner DE, Aranyi C, Coffin DL. Metal toxicity for rabbit alveolar macrophages in vitro. *Environ Res* 1975; **9:** 32–47.

69. Beisel WR. Single nutrients and immunity. *Am J Clin Nutr* 1982; **35 (Suppl):** 417–468.

70. Thomas WR, Holt PG. Vitamin C and immunity: an assessment of the evidence. *Clin Exp Immunol* 1978; **32:** 370–379.

71. Smith WB, Shohet SB, Zagajeski E, Lubin BH. Alteration in human granulocyte function after in vitro incubation with L-ascorbic acid. *Ann NY Acad Sci* 1975; **25:** 329–338.

72. Stankova L, Gerhardt NB, Nagel L, Bigley RH. Ascorbate and phagocyte function. *Infect Immunol* 1975; **12:** 252–256.

73. Zweiman B, Schoenwetter WF, Hildreth EA. The effect of the scorbutic state on tuberculin hyper-sensitivity in the guinea pig. I: Passive transfer of tuberculin hyper-sensitivity. *J Immunol* 1966; **96:** 296–300.

74. Kalden JR, Guthy EA. Prolonged skin allograft survival in vitamin C–deficient guinea pigs. *Eur Surg Res* 1972; **4:** 114–119.

75. Fraser RC, Pavlovic S, Kurahara CG, *et al*. The effect of variations in vitamin C intake on the cellular immune response of guinea pigs. *Am J Clin Nutr* 1978; **33:** 839–847.

76. Anderson R, Oosthuizen R, Maritz R, *et al*. The effects of increasing weekly doses of ascorbate on certain cellular and humoral immune functions in normal volunteers. *Am J Clin Nutr* 1980; **33:** 71–76.

77. Vilter RW, Woolford RM, Spies TD. Severe scurvy: a clinical and hematologic study. *J Lab Clin Med* 1946; **31:** 609–630.

78. Siegel BV, Morton JI. Vitamin C and the immune response. *Experientia* 1977; **33:** 393–397.

79. Gross RL, Reid JVO, Newberne PM, Burgess B, Marston R, Hift W. Depressed cell-mediated immunity in megaloblastic anaemia due to folic acid deficiency. *Am J Clin Nutr* 1975; **28:** 225–232.

80. Axelrod AE, Trakatellis AC. Relationship of pyridoxine to immunological phenomena. *Vitam Horm* 1964; **22:** 591–607.

81. Rumore MM. Vitamin A as an immunomodulating agent. *Clin Pharm* 1993 Jul; **12(7):** 506–514

82. Darip *et al*. Effect of vitamin A deficiency on susceptibility of rats to *Angiostrongylus cantonensis*. *Proc Soc Exp Biol Med* 1979; **161(4):** 600–604.

83. Krishnan S, Bhuyan UN, Talwar GP, Ramalingaswami V. Effect of vitamin A and protein calorie undernutrition on immune responses. *Immunology* 1974; **27:** 383–392.

84. Nauss KM, Mark DA, Suskind RM. The effect of vitamin A deficiency on the in vitro cellular immune response of rats. *J Nutr* 1979; **109:** 1815–1823.

85. Brown KH, Rajan MM, Chakraborty J, Aziz KMA. Failure of a large dose of vitamin A to enhance the antibody response to tetanus toxoid in children. *Am J Clin Nutr* 1980; **33:** 212–217.

86. Harbige LS. Nutrition and immunity with emphasis on infection and autoimmune disease. *Nutr Health* 1996; **10(4):** 285–312.

87. Nockels CF. Protective effects of supplemental vitamin E against infection. *Pediatr Proc* 1979; **38:** 2134–2138.

88. Oski FA. Vitamin E: a radical defense. *N Engl J Med* 1980; **303:** 454–455.

89. Kelleher J. Vitamin E and the immune response. *Proc Nutr Soc* 1991; **50:** 245–249.

90. Tarnawski A, Batko B. Antibiotics and processes. *Lancet* 1973; **i:** 674–675.

91. Mullin TJ, Kirkpatrick JR. The effects of nutritional support on immune competence in patients suffering from trauma, sepsis, or malignant disease. *Surgery* 1981; **90:** 610–614.

92. Munster AM, Winchurch RA, Birmingham WJ, Keeling P. Longitudinal assay of lymphocyte responsiveness in patients with major burns. *Ann Surg* 1980; **192:** 772–775.

93. Howard RJ, Simmons RL. Acquired immunologic deficiencies after trauma and surgical procedures. *Surg Gynecol Obstet* 1974; **139:** 771–782.

94. Chandra RK. Nutrition and immunity in the elderly. *Nutr Rese Rev* 1991; **4:** 83–95.

95. Chavrance M, Brubacher G, Herberth B, Vernes G, Mitstacki T, Dete F, *et al*. Immunological and nutritional status among the elderly. In: *Nutrition, Immunity and Illness in the elderly*. Chandra RK (Ed). Pergamon, New York: 1985.

96. Sakamoto M, Ooyamma T, Tango T, Nishioka K. Association of nutritional indices and immunological parameters in elderly patients, including those with cancer. In: Chandra RK (Ed). *Nutrition, Immunity and Illness in the Elderly*. Pergamon, New York: 1985.

97. Bistrian BR, Blackburn GL, Vitale J, Cochran D, Naylor J. Prevalence of malnutrition in general medical patients. *J Am Med Ass* 1976; **235:** 1567–1570.

98. Chandra RK. Immunology of nutritional disorders. In: *Current Topics in Immunology*, vol 12. Edward Arnold, London; 1980: 76–87.

99. Law DK, Dudrick SJ, Abdou NI. Immunocompetence of patients with protein-calorie malnutrition: the effects of nutritional repletion. *Ann Int Med* 1973; **79:** 545–550.

100. Bistrian BR. Cellular immunity in adult marasmus. *Archiv Int Med* 1977; **137:** 1408–11.

101. Chandra RK, Baker M, Kumar V. Body composition, albumin levels and delayed cutaneous cell-mediated immunity. *Nutr Res* 1985; **5:** 679–684.

102. Keenan RA, Moidawer LL, Yang RD, Kawamura I, Blackburn GL, Bistrian BR. An altered response by peripheral leukocytes to synthesis or release of leuco-cyte endogenous mediator in critically ill, protein-malnourished patients. *J Lab Clin Med* 1982; **100:** 844–857.

103. Kauffman CA, Jones PG, Kluger MJ. Fever and mal-nutrition: endogenous pyrogen/interleukin-1 in mal-nourished patients. *Am J Clin Nutr* 1982; **36:** 127–130.

104. Welsh FK, Farmery SM, Ramsden C, Guillou PJ, Reynolds JV. Reversible impairment in monocyte major histocompatibility complex class II expression in malnourished surgical patients. *JPEN J Parenter Enter Nutr* 1996 Sep; **20(5):** 344–348.

105. Law DK, Dudrick SJ, Abdou NI. The effects of protein-calorie malnutrition on immuno-competence of the surgical patient. *Surg Gynecol Obstet* 1974; **139:** 257–266.

106. Studley HO. Percentage of weight loss: a basic indi-cator of surgical risk in patients with chronic peptic ulcer. *J Am Med Assoc* 1936; **106:** 458.

107. Rhoads JE, Alexander LE. Nutritional problems of surgical patients. *Ann NY Acad Sci* 1955; **63:** 268.

108. Cannon PR. Protein metabolism and resistance to infection. *J Michigan Med Soc* 1944; **43:** 323.

109. Mullen JL, Gertner MH, Buzby GP, Goodhart GL, Rosato EF. Implication of malnutrition in the surgical patient. *Arch Surg* 1979; **114:** 121–125.

110. Detsky AS. Parenteral nutrition—is it helpful ? *N Engl J Med* 1991; **325:** 573–575.

111. Daly M, Liekerman MD, Goldfine J, Shou J, Weintraub F, Rosato EF, Lavin P. Enteral nutrition with supplemental arginine, RNA and omega-3 fatty acids in patients after operation: immunologic, metabolic and clinical outcomes. *Surgery* 1992; **112:** 56–57.

112. Kemen M, Senkal M, Horman H-H, Mumme A, Dauphin A-K, Baier J, *et al*. Early post-operative enteral nutrition with arginine, omega-3 fatty acids and ribonucleic acid-supplemented diet versus placebo in cancer patients: an immunologic evaluation of impact. *Crit Care Med* 1995; **23:** 652–659.

113. Inagaki J, Rodriquez V, Bodey GP. Causes of death in cancer patients. *Cancer* 1974; **33:** 568–573.

114. Daly JM, Dudrick SJ, Copeland EM. Evaluation of nutritional indices as prognostic indicators in the cancer patient. *Cancer* 1979; **43:** 925–931.

114. Dionigi P, Dionigi R, Nazari S, Bonoldi AP, Griziotti A, Pavesi F, *et al*. Nutritional and immunological evaluations in cancer patients: relationship to surgical infections. *J Parenter Enter Nutr* 1980; **4:** 351–356.

115. Brookes GB, Clifford P. Nutritional status and general immune competence in patients with head and neck cancer. *J R Soc Med* 1981; **1:** 132–139.

117. Copeland EM, Daly JM, Guinn E, Dudrick SJ. Effects of protein nutrition on cell-mediated immunity. *Surg Forum* 1976; **27:** 340–342.

118. Haffejee AA, Angorn IB, Brian PP, Duursma J, Baker LW. Diminished cellular immunity due to impaired nutrition in oesophageal carcinoma. *Br J Surg* 1978; **65:** 480–482.

119. Bozzetti F, Cozzaglio L, Villa ML, Ferrario E, Trabattoni D. Restorative effect of total parenteral nutrition on natural killer cell activity in malnourished cancer patients. *Eur J Cancer* 1995; **31A(12):** 2023–2027.

120. Heatley RV. Nutritional implications of inflammatory bowel disease. *Scand J Gastroenterol* 1984 Nov; **19(8):** 995–998.

121. Heatley RV. Assessing nutritional state in inflam-matory bowel disease. *Gut* 1986 Nov; **27 Suppl 1:** 61–66.

122. O'Keefe SJD. Nutrition and gastrointestinal disease. *Scand J Gastroenterol* 1996; **31 suppl 220:** 52–59.

123. Grimble RF. Nutrition and cytokine action. *Nutr Res Rev* 1996; **3:** 193–210.

124. Murch SH, Lamkin VA, Savage MO, Walker-Smith JA, MAcDonald TT. Serum concentrations of tumour necrosis factor alpha in childhood chronic inflammatory bowel disease. *Gut* 1991; **32:** 913–917.

125. Heatley RV. Nutritional replenishment as an alternative to TNF-alpha in Crohn's disease. [Letter] *Lancet* 1997; 349 [In press].

126. O'Morain C, Segal A, Levy AJ. Elemental diet as a primary treatment of acute Crohn's disease: a controlled trial. *Br Med J* 1984; **288:** 1859.

127. O'Keefe SJD, Ogden J, Rund J, Potter P. Steroids and bowel rest versus elemental diet in the treatment of patients with Crohn's disease: the effects on protein metabolism and immune function. *J Parenter Enter Nutr* 1989; **13(5):** 455–460.

128. Alverdy JC, Burke D. Total parenteral nutrition: iatrogenic immunosuppression. *Nutrition* 1992 Sep; **8(5):** 359–365.

129. Pomposelli JJ, Bistrian BR. Is total parenteral nutrition immunosuppressive? *New Horiz* 1994 May; **2(2):** 224–229.

130. Gogos CA, Kalfarentzos F. Total parenteral nutrition and immune system activity: a review. *Nutrition* 1995 Jul; **11(4):** 339–344.

131. Guillou PJ. The effects of lipids on some aspects of the cellular immune response. *Proc Nutr Soc* 1993 Feb; **52(1):** 91–100.

8

Malnutrition in hospitalised patients

Chris Pennington

Introduction

The development of disease may be accompanied by a loss of appetite or inability to eat, and in some cases intestinal malfunction associated with the impaired absorption of nutrients. The consequent starvation leads to impaired organ function and tissue wasting. Tissue wasting, which is accelerated through the metabolic effects of the inflammatory mediators, is the feature which identifies clinical malnutrition. However, detrimental effects of starvation precede such measurable changes in body structure (Fig. 8.1).

Malnutrition is common in hospital patients, but clinicians fail to recognise it. Consequently many patients do not receive appropriate treatment. This is one reason why nutrition status declines in the majority of patients who are admitted to hospital, with detrimental effect on clinical outcome. Nutrition status can be improved by nutrition support in the majority of patients when there is more rapid recovery from disease and surgery. Unfortunately nutrition support is often poorly managed, which results in significant complications and increased morbidity.

This chapter addresses the problems of disease associated malnutrition with particular reference to prevalence and clinical significance. The recognition and management of malnutrition are briefly reviewed, but these topics are covered in more detail elsewhere in the book.

The recognition of malnutrition in the clinical setting

There is evidence that malnutrition escapes recognition in many affected patients. In an early study of 105 surgical patients only 22 had a comment on their nutrition state in their case record, and only 17 had been weighed at any time during their hospital stay.[1] A study of 500 consecutive hospital admissions revealed that 104 of 200 malnourished patients had no nutrition information recorded in their cases notes.[2] This suggests that the recognition of nutritional impairment is regarded as unimportant, a view supported by a study in which 450 nurses and 319 junior doctors in 70 hospitals were surveyed. Only 34% of the doctors knew if the patients had been weighed and 60% of the remainder considered weight to be unimportant.[3] Similar information was obtained in a recent Danish Study.[3a] The failure to recognise that patients are malnourished is the reason why affected patients are not referred for nutrition support. Only 10 of 55 malnourished patients who had been in hospital for more than one week were referred for nutrition assessment and treatment.[2] In recent studies 8 of 18[2a] and 41 of 161[2b] malnourished patients were referred for nutritional management. The failure to identify patients who are at risk of nutrition depletion may be one reason why the nutrition status of the majority of patients declines during their hospital stay.

Unfortunately we lack adequate tools for the measurement of this condition. Body mass index (BMI), the weight in kg divided by the height in (metres)^2 is the gold standard for defining nutrition category. A BMI of 19 or below signifies undernutrition, and 25 or above excessive weight.[4] The measurement of height will determine growth velocity in the child, a sensitive marker of nutrition and disease[5] (Fig. 8.2). Measurement of mid-arm muscle circumference and triceps

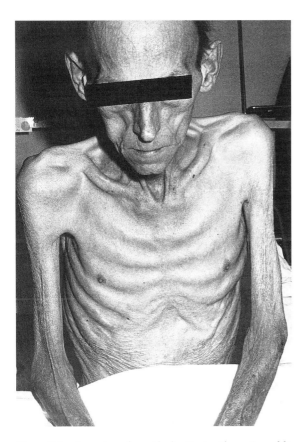

Figure 8.1 – Severely malnourished patient with wasting of fat and muscle.

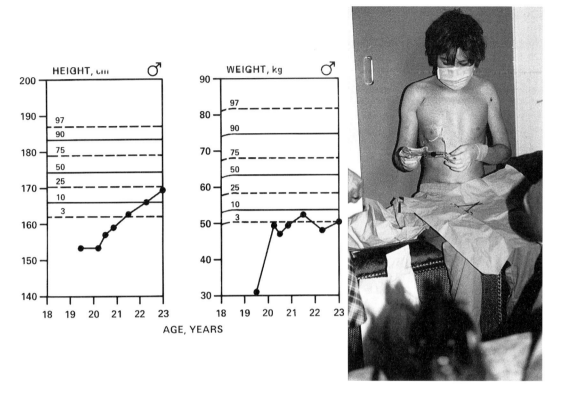

Figure 8.2 – A twenty-year-old patient with short bowel due to Crohn's disease. Malnutrition has resulted in growth retardation. At presentation he was the height of an average 11-year-old. With home parenteral nutrition he grew to reach normal height.

skinfold thickness will help to identify tissue wasting of muscle and fat.[6] Serial measurements of weight and anthropometry can be used to chart nutritional progress under some circumstances over prolonged periods. However, reliance on weight and structural change is frequently inadequate and may be misleading. Impairment of organ function develops with starvation before significant structural change can be measured, and nutritional deprivation is especially likely to be overlooked in the obese patient during hospital illness. Thus such measurements need to be interpreted in relation to the diet over the previous few weeks. Furthermore parameters such as weight and arm circumference are influenced by hydration status, which varies considerably during the course of significant illness, and the techniques of anthropometry are prone to inter-observer error. Bioelectrical impedance analysis can provide more accurate information about body composition in the normal subject,[7] however disturbance of water and electrolyte metabolism in the ill patients and patients with organ failure limit the usefulness of this technique.

Older studies employed albumin and other serum protein measurements.[8] The concentration of these synthetic proteins is influenced by the acute phase response, and changes in hydration and vascular permeability. Whereas hypoalbuminaemia is a marker of surgical risk,[9] it is not a true indicator of nutrition status, and normal serum concentrations are maintained in starving patients who are not stressed, for example in anorexia nervosa, until the terminal phases of illness.[9] Clearly there is no single laboratory marker of nutrition status. However the laboratory has an important role in the identification of single nutrient deficiencies, such as iron, folate, and some vitamins and trace elements. This is especially important during the monitoring of nutrition support in the patient with chronic intestinal failure.

There is a need for functional measurements of nutrition status. Hand grip dynamometry and pulmonary function tests are employed by some as measurements of muscle function;[10] both have obvious limitations. These include patient cooperation and the presence of underlying pulmonary disease.

Thus many authorities advocate simple nutrition screening which will identify patients who are either at risk, or who have established nutrition depletion, and who merit nutrition assessment. Screening might include questions about reduction in food consumption, normal weight and weight loss, accompanied by the measurement of weight and height.[3] Nutrition screening can be undertaken as part of the admission process by the nursing staff.[11] Patients who are identified as being at risk can then undergo more detailed assessment.

The prevalence of malnutrition in hospital patients

Many studies of the prevalence of malnutrition in hospital patients, defined by anthropometric criteria,

have been published during the last 20 years. Some of the more important studies are summarised in Table 8.1.

Bistrian and colleagues surveyed all 131 surgical patients in an urban municipal hospital. There was evidence of malnutrition in 48%.[12] A second study was undertaken in general medical patients in which 250 patients were examined in three surveys. The prevalence of malnutrition was 44%. Greater reduction in arm circumference was demonstrated in the surgical patients, whereas the medical patients had lower values for skinfold thickness.[13] In 1977 Hill and colleagues[1] used weight, arm muscle circumference and serum albumin, to determine nutrition status in 105 surgical patients, and also reported malnutrition in 50% of these patients. These surveys all demonstrated that almost half of the patients within surgical and medical wards were affected by some degree of nutrition depletion.

Other studies have assessed nutrition status on admission to hospital (Table 8.2). The incidence of mal-

Table 8.1 − Prevalence of malnutrition in hospital patients.

Study	Year	Number of patients	Type of patients	% malnourished
Bistrian et al.[12]	1974	131	general surgical	50.0
Bistrian et al.[13]	1976	251	general medical	44.0
Hill et al.[1]	1977	105	general surgical	50.0

Table 8.2 − Incidence of malnutrition on admission to hospital.

Study	Year	Number of patients	Type of patients	% malnourished
Willard et al.[14]	1980	200	general medical general surgical	31.5
Bastow et al.[15]	1983	744	orthopaedic surgical	52.8
Zador and Truswell[16]	1989	84	general surgical	14.0
Larsson et al.[21]	1990	501	care of elderly	28.5
Cederholm et al.[17]	1993	200	general medical	20.0
McWhirter and Pennington[2]	1994	500	general medical general surgical, orthopaedic, surgical, respiratory medicine, care of elderly	40.0
Giner et al.[19]	1996	129	intensive care	43
Kelly et al.[23]	2000	219★	general medical general surgical	13★
Edington et al.[26]	2000	850	all medical all surgical	20†

★ 219 of 337 patients examined.
† 850 of 1611 patients.
In both cases more severely ill patients who were at greater risk of malnutrition were not assessed.

nutrition was 31% in 200 consecutive non-obstetric admissions to a community hospital.[14] A large study of 744 elderly women with fracture neck of femur reported 255 as thin and 138 as very thin on the basis of anthropometric measurements which were respectively 1−2, and more than 2 standard deviations below the mean for that population.[15] One report suggested a lower incidence of malnutrition, 14%, in patients on admission to a general or vascular surgical unit.[16] However, emergency admissions were excluded and many patients were unavailable for examination. In a Swedish study of 205 acute medical admissions without cancer 20% of patients were classified as malnourished.[17] The nutrition status was assessed in 100 patients who were admitted to hospital with an acute stroke; 16% were malnourished.[18] A study of 500 admissions (100 consecutive admissions to general surgery, general medicine, respiratory medicine, orthopaedic surgery, and care of the elderly) found that 40% of patients were malnourished and 27% had evidence of moderate or severe malnutrition.[2] In the most recent studies, malnutrition was evident in 13% and 20% of patients admitted to general hospitals.[2a,2b] However, in both studies the more severely ill patients were not examined, thus underestimating the size of the problem.

Thus malnutrition is common at the time of admission; data have also been obtained on the change of nutrition status during hospital stay. Significant reduction in nutrition parameters was reported in 401 malnourished patients who did not receive nutrition support during their hospital stay of at least three weeks.[20] The proportion of patients with malnutrition who were in hospital with an acute stroke increased from 16% on admission to 23% on discharge.[20] In a study of 501 patients admitted to a geriatric ward, those patients who did not receive nutrition supplements exhibited a decline in nutrition status with increased morbidity.[21] Of 500 hospital admissions to five major acute specialities who were nutritionally assessed, 112 were in hospital for more than 1 week and were examined on discharge. Weight loss occurred in 72 (64%) of these patients. Furthermore, in comparison with the normally nourished, more of the patients who were malnourished on admission lost weight, and their weight loss was proportionately greater.[2] A similar proportion of patients lost weight during their hospital stay in a study of 568 patients who were admitted to hospital in Dublin.[21a] In another study comparing the efficacy of oral supplements with supplemental nasogastric feeding in malnourished patients, the malnourished control group who

received normal hospital treatment continued to deteriorate nutritionally.[22] Nutrition assessment of patients who were admitted to an intensive care unit suggested that inadequate management led to nutritional depletion during their hospital stay prior to admission to the unit.[19] Forty-three of 129 patients were depleted on admission.

Thus many patients are malnourished on admission; there is a tendency for hospital patients to lose weight during their hospital stay, and this particularly applies to those patients who are malnourished on admission. The observation that weight loss continued for 8 weeks after discharge in patients who had undergone curative surgical procedures[23] emphasises the importance of appropriate nutrition assessment of all hospital patients. In this study mean weight loss increased from 3.6% of admission weight at discharge to 9.8% by week 8. A community study of patients with chronic disease and cancer revealed a prevalence of malnutrition of 10%.[24] These studies emphasise the need to consider the nutrition parameters during the entire patient journey from symptom onset through the convalescence to cure. The period in hospital is a decreasing component of this journey.

The pathogenesis of malnutrition in hospital patients

The syndrome of malnutrition develops because of relative starvation, which often occurs in association with the metabolic response to stress. Relative starvation may arise through lack of nutrients compounded by increased nutrition requirements. Factors associated with inadequate nutrient provision include: anorexia, the failure to provide the patient with food, an inability to eat and impaired digestive and absorptive function. Several of these factors may be present at the same time.

Depression and chronic illness lead to anorexia. Anorexia may arise through the effects of cytokines on the central nervous system, chronic pain and drug therapy. For example opiates delay gastric emptying and may cause nausea. The feeding of patients in hospital has been reviewed.[25] The selection of 'healthy' high fibre and low energy foods from menu cards by patients in whom illness promotes a desire to adopt what is perceived as a healthy lifestyle may not be appropriate for the patient's needs. Guidance is needed in food selection. Food is only available for limited periods during the day in many hospital wards. Thus, when meals are missed because of investigative or therapeutic procedures, there is no opportunity to provide additional meals.[26] One study found that approximately 20% of hospital meals were missed in various hospital wards for these reasons.[27] Not all patients have access to food brought in from outside the hospital.

Assistance with feeding may be needed, particularly in patients with eating difficulties and other disabilities such as severe rheumatoid arthritis and cerebrovascular disease. Some patients who were observed for 7 consecutive days were consistently unable to reach their food because it was placed beyond their reach. Visits by medical staff or phlebotomists at mealtimes can significantly reduce the consumption of food.[28] In a geriatric unit where the meals that arrived on the ward were theoretically adequate for the patients needs, 40% of the food provided was wasted.[29] Unless arrangements are in place for the monitoring of food consumption this cause of malnutrition may be overlooked.

In critical illness energy requirements may change. However, in most patients energy requirements are not increased; previous studies overestimated energy needs, and increased demands through illness are often matched by reduced mobility in the patient.[30] Nevertheless accelerated tissue wasting is a feature of severe illness. The humoral response does not account for the observed metabolic changes,[1,31] which may be attributable to the actions of cytokines. These small proteins, interleukins, tumour necrosis factor, and interferons, are released from immune cells and cancer cells. Cytokines share multiple activities.[32] These include anorexia, pyrexia, release of amino acids from muscle tissue, increased glucose transport, the stimulation of hepatic lipid secretion, reduced albumin synthesis, increased vascular permeability, immune cell availability and the promotion of acute phase protein synthesis. Immobility is another important factor in the development of muscle wasting in critically ill patients. Malnutrition is also a consequence of intestinal failure. Patients with multiorgan failure and critical illness suffer from impaired intestinal digestive and absorptive capacity, and the cytokine response may be driven through increased intestinal permeability to toxins, in addition to microbial translocation. There are claims of improved intestinal barrier function with some form of jejunal feeding in these critically ill patients with gastric stasis. Chronic intestinal failure can accompany a range of disorders, notably short bowel syndrome, inflam-

matory bowel disease, radiation enteritis and motility disorders. Some patients cannot maintain fluid and electrolyte balance, others require parenteral nutrition to ensure adequate feeding.

Specific nutrient deficiencies accompany some forms of gastrointestinal disease. Thus vitamin B_{12} deficiency is associated with atrophic gastritis and disease of the terminal ileum, while iron and folate depletion are particularly common in patients with gluten enteropathy. Patients with small intestinal disease may become deficient in magnesium, and those with high output jejunostomies lose large amounts of zinc.

Clinical consequences of malnutrition

Starvation will ultimately lead to the death of the patient. The negative effects of nutrition depletion augment the adverse influences of disease and may contribute to a patient's demise before death from starvation. During the Irish hunger strike 10 of 30 subjects died by 70 days, when there was an average weight loss of 38%. The time taken to reach the critical weight when death ensues is prolonged during semi-starvation, but significantly reduced in the stressed patient.[33] Furthermore many hospital patients are already nutritionally depleted on admission.

Malnutrition adversely affects organ function.[34] Malnourished patients may be apathetic and appear uncooperative. Muscle strength is reduced and muscles fatigue more readily. Such impairment can be demonstrated during fasting in obese subjects for merely two weeks, before there are any changes in the conventional parameters of nutrition assessment.[35,36] Such changes may delay patient mobilisation following surgery, but they can have other important consequences. Respiratory muscle strength and maximum voluntary ventilation were significantly reduced in a study of 16 malnourished patients without respiratory disease.[37] Clearly the need for artificial ventilation, and the ability to wean from ventilation may well be influenced by respiratory muscle impairment in the malnourished subject. Impairment of cardiac function through malnutrition has also been documented.[38]

The ageing process, underlying disease and malnutrition influence the immune system. Protein energy malnutrition in children is associated with thymic atrophy. Similar changes also occur in other lymphoid tissues. There may also be impaired anti-body production and phagocyte function.[39,40] Malnutrition adversely affects thermoregulation.[39,41] This may be an important factor in the genesis of hypothermia in the elderly population.

Specific nutrient deficiencies lead to well recognised syndromes. Examples include thiamine and Wernicke's encephalopathy, folate and megaloblastic anaemia, ascorbic acid and scurvy. Vitamin B_{12} deficiency will also lead to a macrocytic megaloblastic anaemia; it can also cause neurological deficits, which classically present as subacute combined degeneration of the cord. Deficiency syndromes have occurred during prolonged artificial nutrition support when early nutrient solutions were deficient in certain micronutrients such as selenium.[42,43] Selenium depletion has been associated with myopathy and cardiomyopathy.

Many studies attest to the fact that morbidity is increased in the malnourished patient, especially in surgical practice. Studley reported deaths following surgery for peptic ulcer disease in 1 out of 28 patients who had lost less than 20% of their body weight (mean 12.6% weight loss) compared to 6 out of 18 patients who had lost more than 20% body weight (mean 26.1% weight loss).[44] In a study of 80 patients who were undergoing surgery, protein depletion, determined by neutron activation analysis, was documented in 39. The depleted patients, who were similar in other respects, had impaired respiratory function, increased propensity to pneumonia and prolonged hospital stay.[45] In another study 365 patients underwent abdominal surgery for malignant disease; complications and death respectively occurred in 72% and 23% of those who were malnourished, and 29% and 4% in patients who were not malnourished. The difference was not related to the type and extent of tumour, or the nature of the procedure. Malnutrition was identified in 55 of 129 patients who were admitted to an intensive care unit. The incidence of complications and the number of patients who were not discharged from hospital were both greater in patients who were malnourished on admission. Significantly, the impact of malnutrition was greater in the patients who were less ill.[19] Another study of patients in intensive care reported reduced survival in those in whom the body mass index was below the 15th centile when stratified according to illness severity.[46] Malnourished elderly patients had a longer hospital stay than those who received nutrition support.[47,48] The death rate in 501 elderly patients at 6 months was 18.6%, but reduced to 8.6% in those who received nutrition supplements. In a study of 100 patients with acute stroke, the length of stay was related to the nutrition status.[18]

Benefits of nutrition support

Studies demonstrate that nutrition management can improve nutrition status. There is also data to show that this translates into improved outcome.

Nutrition status

Nutrition status was improved in elderly patients by increasing the energy density of hospital food.[49] This may well be the most cost-effective approach for the majority of patients. A prospective study of patients who were malnourished on admission to hospital demonstrated nutritional improvement in those patients randomised to the nutrition support groups (63% with oral supplements and 68% with supplemental nasogastric feeding), and deterioration in 73% of the control patients who received conventional nutrition management. Food consumption was the same in all three groups.[22] However, nutrition recovery with oral supplements may be slow and incomplete, especially in the elderly with an acute phase response.[50] The intestinal tract may be impaired in the surgical patient. In a study of patients who had lost weight on account of malignant disease, post-operative parenteral nutrition prevented a further decline in muscle protein in association with the surgery.[51] A study of mildly malnourished post-operative surgical patients demonstrated improved nutrition outcomes when oral supplements were administered, in particular the progressive decline for 2 months after discharge was avoided.[23,52]

Clinical outcome

The most important end-point in relation to the value of the prevention or correction of nutrition depletion is the recovery from disease. There have been many studies which established the role of nutrition support in different patient populations. There is no benefit from the routine use of nutrition support in patients who are not malnourished or at risk of malnutrition.[53,54]

Preoperative parenteral nutrition in patients with gastrointestinal carcinoma was associated with a significant reduction in major complications and mortality. This was attributed to the prevention of nutritional decline during the preoperative hospital stay.[55] The value of preoperative nutrition support was further assessed by giving depleted patients 10 days of enteral or parenteral feeding. There were depleted and non-depleted control groups. The depleted controls had more septic complications than the non-depleted controls. Artificial nutrition support, by enteral nutrition or parenteral nutrition, led to a significant reduction in major complications in patients who had lost more than 10% of their body weight.[54] Similarly the severely depleted patients in the Veterans Affairs study of preoperative parenteral nutrition demonstrated a reduction of non-infective complications and this was in spite of methodological questions about potentially excessive nutrient provision and the route of nutrient administration (many of these patients were able to eat and could have received enteral nutrition). In a recent study of appropriate postoperative parenteral nutrition in patients who were undergoing surgery for cancer, nutritional support reduced mortality as well as morbidity.[55a]

The use of immediate postoperative parenteral nutrition, as opposed to introducing parenteral nutrition after one week if oral intake had not been established, was assessed in a study of 35 patients who were undergoing radical cystectomy. Early parenteral nutrition was associated with a reduction of hospital stay of 7 days.[56] (Table 8.3). In another study of 300 patients, mortality and morbidity were reduced by the use of parenteral nutrition in patients who were unable to eat for 14 days.[56a]

The use of prophylactic parenteral nutrition in patients who received bone marrow transplantation reduced nutrition depletion and was associated with improved survival and time to relapse in the treated group.[57]

Early feeding with oral supplements in unselected postoperative patients reduced the incidence of complications following major gastrointestinal surgery during the hospital phase, no benefit from supplements was observed in these patients after discharge from hospital.[52] However another study in which patients with mild malnutrition were studied demonstrated improved nutrition status, hand grip dynamometry and quality of life in the patients randomised to receive oral supplements. The intervention group required fewer antibiotic prescriptions.[23] Supplemental nasogastric feeding reduced hospital mortality and length of stay in malnourished orthopaedic patients with fracture neck of femur.[47] In another study of patients with fracture neck of femur oral supplements (254 kcal per day) reduced the

Table 8.3 – Randomised controlled studies which examined the influence of nutrition support on the length of hospital stay (LOS). Adapted from Booth and Morgan 1995.

Study	Patient group	Nutrition management	Reduction of LOS Days
Bastow et al. 1983[47]	122 elderly women, fracture neck of femur	Nocturnal nesogastric supplementary EN	9 (in very thin group)
Askanazi et al. 1986[56]	35 radical cystectomy	Postoperative PN	7
Delmi et al. 1990[48]	59 elderly with fracture neck of femur	Oral supplements postoperatively	16
Rana et al. 1992[76]	40 patients undergoing moderate or major abdominal surgery	Oral supplements postoperatively	3.3
Eisenberg et al. 1993[50]	459, 86% general surgical, 14% general medical	Preoperative PN	0
MacBurney et al. 1994[78]	43 bone marrow transplant patients	Glutamine supplemented PN	7
Bower et al. 1995[68]	368 intensive care patients	Early EN with formula supplemented with arginine, nucleosides, and fish oil	8 (in patients who tolerated at least 821 ml per day.
Keele et al. 1997[52]	100 patients following moderate or major abdominal surgery	Postoperative supplements	0

complication rate, including bed sores and cardiac failure, and the mortality, an effect which was sustained 6 months after the fracture.[48] A large study of 501 elderly patients demonstrated that the use of a 400 kc calorie oral supplement greatly reduced mortality at 6 months from 18.6 to 8.6% compared to the control group.[21] Patients with chronic illness who attended a nutrition support clinic demonstrated that restitution of body weight and lean body mass is associated with significant improvement of quality of life indices.[58]

Thus artificial nutrition support in prevention and management of nutrition depletion benefits nutrition status and recovery from disease.

The provision of nutrition support

Artificial nutrition support is available in the form of oral supplements, enteral tube feeding and parenteral nutrition. It is used to prevent or treat malnutrition. In future specific nutrients may also be employed to modify the inflammatory response. Increasing attention is now paid to the route of administration and the nature of the nutrients administered.

Nutrition support in the malnourished and critically ill patient

Enteral feeding stimulates the gut-associated immune function. Furthermore the intestinal mucosa is dependent on luminal nutrition and glutamine is an important fuel.[59] Enteral feeding has physiological and clinical advantages, is less expensive and avoids the complications associated with parenteral nutrition. Studies comparing enteral and parenteral nutrition in surgical patients indicate fewer complications and a reduced number of infective complications in the patients who received enteral nutrition.[60,61]

Nutrition support in the starving and malnourished patient will lead to an anabolic response through increased protein synthesis. In the severely malnourished patient a switch of energy source from endogenous lipid to exogenous carbohydrate may be one explanation for the dramatic reduction in the serum concentrations of phosphate, magnesium and potassium, which move into the cell under the influence of insulin. Under such circumstances increased provision of these nutrients will be required.

This is described as the refeeding syndrome.[62] Hypocaloric feeding in the initial phase may reduce the incidence of metabolic problems in such patients.

In the stressed patient, who is septic or traumatised, nutrition support may increase protein synthesis but protein degradation remains high and anabolism cannot be achieved with conventional solutions.[63] Maintaining body structure pending resolution of the underlying disease process is the goal. Increasing nitrogen and energy intakes above normal requirements in an attempt to induce an anabolic response is ineffective, hazardous and wasteful.[55] Energy requirements have been estimated at 30–35 kcal (126–146 Kj)/kg per day, any increase in metabolic demand is balanced by reduced physical activity in these ill patients.[30] In an attempt to prevent or reverse tissue wasting in critically ill patients three approaches are under evaluation: the use of anabolic agents, novel substrates and antioxidants.

Anabolic agents reverse the defect in amino acid transport in these patients. Growth hormone, which increases protein synthesis, and IGF-1, which reduces protein degradation, have a complimentary effect. Their opposing influences on blood glucose concentrations circumvent hyperglycaemia and hypoglycaemia which respectively occur when each agent is used alone.[64] However, benefit from the use of these compounds has not been demonstrated.

Lipid solutions provide a useful energy source, which reduces the glucose load and associated respiratory and hepatic complications, and correct essential fatty acid deficiency. Concern has been expressed about the potential immunosuppressive properties of conventional lipid solutions.[39] However, there has been no convincing evidence of increased susceptibility to infection in patients who are receiving lipid containing parenteral nutrition. Another concern about conventional long chain lipid solutions is the effect on pulmonary haemodynamics and gas exchange in the septic patient. This has been attributed to the increased formation of prostanoids. There is no evidence that when conventional solutions are used in the recommended doses, and infused as part of a mixed solution, that this effect is observed. Nevertheless mixed lipid solutions containing medium chain triglycerides have been introduced and structured lipids are being developed. The substitution of MCT for some LCT has been shown to reduce the production of some proinflammatory cytokines.[65] An increase in the ratio of omega 3 to omega 6 fatty acids leads to the synthesis of eiconasoids with less inflammatory potency.[66,67] This may also be useful in the management of the cancer patient. Some studies have suggested that the use of enteral feeds enriched with arginine, fish oil and nucleosides reduce the length of stay in intensive care and in hospital when used in patients who are critically ill.[68] The role of these formulations awaits further evaluation, especially because in some studies unfavourable outcome was observed.

The suggestion that intestinal permeability with translocation contributes to the cytokine response in critically ill subjects has led to the appraisal of glutamine in parenteral nutrition solutions.[69] Many animal experiments suggest that the provision of glutamine may preserve intestinal integrity and protect against intestinal translocation of microorganisms, in addition to an effect on immune function. Because of considerations of stability this is difficult to achieve, although peptide solutions are undergoing evaluation.[70,71] In spite of these theoretical considerations there are relatively few studies at present which support the role of parenterally administered glutamine in the clinical situation. Nevertheless in a study of critically ill patients the administration of glutamine dipeptide in the parenteral nutrition solution appeared to improve absorptive capacity compared to the control group.[71] The use of glutamine was associated with improved outcome with reduced infection and fluid retention in bone marrow transplant recipients,[72] and in another study there was a reduction in long-term mortality in patients discharged from the intensive care unit.[73] However the role of IgA in preventing bacterial adherence and cytokine generation may also be important. The production of secretory IgA has been linked to cholecystokinin which is released in response to enteral stimulation by whole protein and long chain triglycerides LCT, not by elemental diets and parenteral nutrition. This may be one reason why early enteral feeding, compared to parenteral feeding, is associated with fewer postoperative septic complications. Ornithine alpha keto glutarate, which may facilitate the release of growth hormone and insulin and the synthesis of glutamine and arginine, is being evaluated as a nutrition substrate.

Free radicals are generated by the inflammatory response. They may have a role in the killing of microorganisms, cell signalling and the reduction of cell volume by the opening of potassium channels, which may be the signal for the catabolic response.

Nevertheless, free radicals also cause tissue damage, which is minimised by antioxidants. The requirement for antioxidants, selenium and vitamins A, E and C is increased in catabolic patients although amounts that should be supplied are uncertain.[74] A study in burn patients suggested that the provision of additional antioxidants is associated with a reduced incidence of infection.[75]

Oral supplements

Swedish studies have demonstrated that nutrition goals can be achieved in some patients by the adequate provision of conventional food.[49] Within the UK there has been concern about inadequate hospital food, and the fact that it is not readily available.[26] Oral supplements are convenient, complete nutrient solutions with various flavours. They are used between meals to increase oral nutrient intake. The perception that they suppress the appetite and are taken in preference to the hospital diet is false; a significant increase in nutrient consumption with improved nutrition status can be achieved in many patients.[22] The use of these products in the postoperative period led to improved outcome.[23] The role of oral supplements has recently been reviewed.[76]

Enteral tube feeding

Tube feeding may be necessary with profound anorexia, and nocturnal tube feeding is a useful method of fully exploiting residual bowel function in patients with intestinal failure and cystic fibrosis. It is an essential method of nutrient delivery with disorders of eating or swallowing. Many of these patients suffer from chronic neurological disease, such as cerebrovascular disease and motor neurone disease; others have chronic oropharyngeal disease. The recognition that following abdominal surgery small intestinal function returns rapidly led to the use of naso-enteral feeding with simultaneous gastric aspiration. Not only does this technique avoid the expense and complications of parenteral nutrition in these ill patients, it may protect the intestinal integrity and reduce enteric associated sepsis.[77] This led to the concept of minimal enteral feeding, emphasising the potential value of some nutrient delivery to the intestine even though intestinal function was inadequate and required supplemental parenteral nutrition. Similarly there is evidence to suggest that patients with burns have a better outcome with early enteral feeding rather than total parenteral nutrition.[78]

When enteral tube feeding is required for more than 2–4 weeks the use of a percutaneous gastrostomy should be considered.[79,80] These devices are commonly inserted endoscopically, but for patients in whom endoscopy is not possible or advisable, e.g. with carcinoma of the upper alimentary tract, or severe respiratory impairment in patients with neuro-muscular disorders, radiological placement under screening should be considered. PEG represents a useful development and leads to improved nutrition care by ensuring the more effective delivery of nutrient solutions when compared to nasogastric tubes.[81] A significant improvement in the nutrition status of a group of mentally handicapped patients was observed following the adoption of PEG feeding: all had previously received nasogastric feeding for at least 3 months.[82] Although the procedure is occasionally associated with complications such as stomal infection and peritonitis, complications of nutrient delivery are reduced and nutrition management simplified.

Parenteral nutrition

Parenteral nutrition is required when the intestine is unavailable or intestinal function is inadequate. The realisation that nutrient needs are less than previously estimated, and the development of the all-in-one lipid containing nutrient solution has facilitated the administration of parenteral nutrition by the peripheral vein. Many studies have demonstrated that adequate nutrition support can be provided for up to 2 weeks at least by peripheral parenteral nutrition.[83,84] This avoids potentially serious complications associated with the insertion and use of central feeding catheters. The addition of low dose heparin and hydrocortisone in the nutrient bag, and nitrate patches over the vein, may delay the onset of thrombophlebitis.[85–87] However not all authorities accept the need for these measures.

Management of nutrition support

There is convincing evidence that artificial nutrition support is suboptimal in many of our hospitals. Many studies attest to the high complication rate of nutrient delivery. There is evidence that some of these complications, such as catheter related sepsis, can be avoided when nutrition management is undertaken by nutrition support teams.[88] The majority of hospitals in the UK still do not have access to such multi-disciplinary teams.[80] Whereas it is possible to minimise complications of treatment by the application of standard protocols, data suggest that even with established nutrition advisory groups standards of treat-ment are unsatisfactory. A 6-month study of artificial nutrition support in a teaching hospital in which an advisory group had introduced nutrition management protocols illustrates this point. The estimated nutrient requirements were received by only 50% of enterally and parentally fed patients. The deficit arose because of inappropriate prescription and failure to deliver the prescribed nutrients. Complications occurred in 47% of patients who were fed enterally, and 36% of patients who received parenteral feeding. The latter included catheter related infection in 5 of 49 patients who were receiving central parenteral nutrition.[89]

Summary and key practical points

Malnutrition is common in hospital patients; many patients are malnourished on admission and nutritional depletion affects the majority of patients during their stay in hospital. Malnutrition frequently escapes recognition because nutrition status is not routinely assessed.

Malnourished patients are at risk of increased morbidity, mortality and delayed recovery from illness because of the effect of nutrition depletion on organ and immune function.

Screening patients on admission to hospital will identify those who are at risk and who require formal nutrition assessment. The use of artificial nutrition support, which should be given by the enteral route wherever possible, can prevent the development of nutrition depletion, or improve nutrition status in the majority of patients. Nutrition support should be offered before significant depletion has occurred not only because the restoration of nutrition status takes a long time, but also because such restoration may not be possible in the stressed patient in whom the reduction in the rate of tissue wasting is the only achievable outcome with conventional nutrition management.

The optimum use of nutrition is most likely to occur with a nutrition support team to ensure the efficient use of this therapeutic modality with the minimum morbidity due to treatment complications.

References

1. Hill GL, Blackett RL, Pickford I *et al.* Malnutrition in surgical patients – an unrecognised problem. *Lancet* 1977; **(i):** 689–692.

2. McWhirter JP, Pennington CR. The incidence and recognition of malnutrition in hospital. *Brit Med J* 1994; **308**: 945–948.

2a. Kelly IE, Tessier S, Cahil A *et al*. Still hungry in hospital: identifying malnutrition in acute hospital admissions. *Quarterly Journal of Medicine* 2000; **93**: 93–98.

2b. Edington J, Boorman J, Durrant ER *et al*. Prevalence of malnutrition on admission to four hospitals in England. *Clin Nutr* 2000; **19**(3): 191–195.

3. Lennard-Jones JE, Arrowsmith H, Davison C, Denham AF, Micklewright A. Screening by nurses and junior doctors to detect malnutrition when patients are first assessed in hospital. *Clin Nutr* 1995; **14**: 336–340.

3a. Rasmussen HH, Kondrup J, Ladefoged K *et al*. Clinical Nutrition in Danish Hospitals: a questionnaire-based investigation among doctors and nurses. *Clin Nutr* 1999; **18**: 153–158.

4. Gregory J, Foster K, Turner H & Wiseman M. *Dietary and Nutritional Survey of British Adults*. London: H.M. Stationery Office, 1990.

5. Widdowson EN. Intra-uterine growth retardation in a pig – organ size and cellular development at birth and after growth to maturity. *Biol Neonate* 1971; **19**: 329–340.

6. Heymsfield SB, McManus MCC, Smith J, Stevens V, Nixon DW. Anthropometric measurements of muscle mass: revised equations for calculating bone free arm muscle area. *Am J Clin Nutr* 1982; **36**: 680–690.

7. Lukaski HC, Johnson PE, Bolonchuk WW, Lykken GI. Assessment of fat free mass using Behr electrical impedance measurement of the human body. *Am J Clin Nutr* 1985; **41**: 810–817.

8. Fleck A, Colley CM, Myres MA. Liver export proteins in trauma. *Brit Med Bull* 1985; **41**: 265–273.

9. Anderson CF, Wochers DN. The utility of serum albumin values in the nutritional assessment of hospitalised patients. *Mayo Clin Proc* 1982; **57**: 181.

10. Webb AE, Newman LA, Taylor M, Keogh JB. Hand grip dynamometry as a predictor of post-operative complications. Reappraisal using age standardised grip strengths. *J Parent Enter Nutr* 1989; **13**: 30–33.

11. Reilly EN, Martineau JK, Moran A, Kennedy H. Nutritional screening-evaluation and implementation of a simple nutritional risk score. *Clin Nutr* 1995; **14**: 269–274.

12. Bistrian BR, Blackburn GL, Hallowell E, Heddle R. Protein status of general surgical patients. *J Am Med Assoc* 1974; **235**: 858–860.

13. Bistrian BR, Blackburn GL, Vitale J, Cochran D, Naylor J. Prevalence of malnutrition in general medical patients. *J Am Med Assoc* 1976; **235**: 1567–1570.

14. Willard MD, Gilsdorf RB, Price RA. Protein-calorie malnutrition in a comminuty hospital. *J Am Med Assoc* 1980; **243**: 1720–1722.

15. Bastow MD, Rawlings J, Allison SB. Under-nutrition, hypothermia and injury in elderly women with fracture neck of femur: An injury response to altered metabolism? *Lancet* 1983; **(i)**: 143–145.

16. Zador DA, Truswell AS. Nutritional status on admission to a general surgical ward in a Sydney hospital. *Aust New Z J Med* 1987; **17**: 234–240.

17. Cederholm T, Jagren C, Hellstrom K. Nutritional status and performance capacity in internal medical patients. *Clin Nutr* 1993; **12**: 8–14.

18. Axelsson K, Asplund K, Norburg A, Alafuzoff I. Nutritional status in patients with acute stroke. *Acta Medica Scand* 1988; **224**: 217–224.

19. Giner M, Laviano A, Meguid MM, Gleason JR. In 1995 a correlation between malnutrition and poor outcome in critically ill patients still exists. *Nutrition* 1996; **12**: 23–29.

20. Pinchcofsky GD, Kaminski NV. Increasing malnutrition during hospitalisation: Documentation by nutritional screening programme. *J Am Col Nutr* 1985; **4**: 471–479.

21. Larsson J, Unosson N, Ek AC, Nilsson L, Thorslund S, Bjurulf P. Effect of dietary supplement on nutritional status and clinical outcome in 501 geriatric patients – a randomised study. *Clin Nutr* 1990; **9**: 179–184.

21a. Corish C, Flood P, Mulligan S, Kennedy NP. Undernutrition seems less frequent among patients in Dublin. *Clin Nutr* 1998; **17** (suppl 1): 31–32.

22. McWhirter JP, Pennington CR. A comparison between oral and nasogastric supplements in malnourished patients. *Nutrition* 1996; **12**: 502–506.

23. Beattie AH, Prach A, Baxter JP, Pennington CR. An evaluation of the use of enteral nutritional supplements post operatively in malnourished surgical patients. 2000. *Gut* **46**: 813–818.

24. Edington J, Kon P, Martyn CN. Prevalence of malnutrition in patients in general practice. *Clin Nutr* 1996; **15**: 60–63.

25. McGlone PC, Dickison JWT, Davis GJ. The feeding of patients in hospital: A review. *J R Soc Health* 1995; 282–288.

26. Garrow J. Starvation in hospitals. *Brit Med J* 1994; **308**: 934.

27. Eastwood M. Hospital food. *New Engl J Med* 1997; **336**: 1261.

28. Dickerson JWT. Hospital induced malnutrition: a cause for concern. *Professional Nurse* 1986; 293–296.

29. Stephen AD, Beigg CL, Elliot ET, MacDonald IA, Allison SP. Food provision wastage and intake in elderly hospital patients. *Proc Nut Soc* 1997; **56:** 220A.

30. Elia M Changing concepts of nutrient requirements in disease: Implications for artificial nutritional support. *Lancet* **(i):** 1995; 1279–1284.

31. Frayn KN. Hormonal control of metabolism in trauma and sepsis. *Clin Endocrinol* 1986; **24:** 577–599.

32. Tracy KJ. TNF and other cytokines in the metabolism of septic shock and cachexia. *Clin Nutr* 1992; **11:** 1–11.

33. Allison S. Malnutrition in hospitalised patients, assessment of nutritional support. In: Payne-James J, Grimble G, Silk D (Eds) *Artificial Nutritional Support in Clinical Practice.* Edward Arnold, London, 1995, pp. 115–126.

34. Keys A, Brozek J, Henschel A. The biology of human starvation. Minneapolis University of Minnesota Press, 1950.

35. Lopez J, Russell DM, Whitwell J, Jeejeebhoy K. Skeletal muscle function in malnutrition. *Am J Clin Nutr* 1982; **36:** 602–610.

36. Jeejeebhoy KN. Bulk or bounce – the object of nutritional support. *J Parent Enter Nutr* 1988; **12:** 539–545.

37. Arora NS, Rochester DF. Respiratory muscle strength in maximal voluntary ventilation in undernourished patients. *Am Rev Resp Dis* 1982; 1265–1268.

38. Heymsfield SB, Bethell RA, Ansley JD, Gibbs DM, Felner JM, Nutter ON. Cardiac abnormalities in cachectic patients before and during nutritional repletion. *Am Heart J* 1978; **95:** 584–593.

39. Hill GL. Disorders of nutritional metabolism in clinical surgery: understanding management. Churchill Livingstone, London, 1992.

40. Animashaun A, Hill GL. Body composition research: Implications for the practice of clinical nutrition. *J Parent Ent Nutr* 1992; **16:** 197–218.

41. Mansell PI, Fellows IW, MacDonald IA, Allison SP. Restoration of normal thermal regulation following weight gain in undernourished patients. *Q J Med* 1990; **76:** 817–829.

42. Cohen HJ, Brown MR, Hamilton D. Glutathiane peroxidase and selenium deficiency in patients receiving home parenteral nutrition. Time course for development of deficiency and repletion of enzyme activity in plasma and blood cells. *Am J Clin Nutr* 1989; **49:** 132–141.

43. Yagi M, Tani T, Hashimoto T, Shimisu K, Nagakawa T, Miwa K, Miyazaki I Four cases of selenium deficiency in four cases of post-operative long-term enteral nutrition. *Nutrition* 1996; **12:** 40–43.

44. Studley HO. Percentage of weight loss – a basic indicator of surgical risk in patients with chronic peptic ulcer. *J Am Med Assoc* 1936; **106:** 458–460.

45. Windsor JA, Hill GL. Risk factors for post operative pneumonia. The importance of protein depletion. *Ann Surg* 1988; **17:** 181–185.

46. Galanos A, Pieper CF, Kussin PS, Winchell MT *et al.* Relationship of body mass index to subsequent mortality among seriously ill hospitalised patients. *Critl Care Med* 1997; **25:** 1962–1968.

47. Bastow MD, Rawlings J, Allison SP. Benefits of supplementary tube feeding after fractured neck of femur: A randomised control trial. *Brit Med J* 1983; **287:** 1589–1592.

48. Delmi M, Rapin CH, Bengoa JM, Delmas PD, Vasey H, Bonjour JP. Dietary supplementation in elderly patients with fractured neck of femur. *Lancet* 1990; **335:** 1013–1016.

49. Olin AO, Osterberg B, Hadell K, Armyr I, Jerstrom S, Ljungqvist O. Energy enriched hospital food to improve energy intake in elderly patients. *J Parent Enter Nutr* 1996; **20:** 93–97.

50. Cederholm TE, Hellstrom KH. Reversibility of protein-energy malnutrition in a group of chronically ill elderly out-patients. *Clin Nutr* 1995; **14:** 81–87.

51. Petersson B, Hultzman E, Andersson K, Wernerman J. Human skeletal muscle protein: Effect of malnutrition, elective surgery and total parenteral nutrition. *Clin Sci* 1995; **88:** 479–484.

52. Keele AM, Bray M, Emery P, Duncan H, Silk D. Two phased randomised controlled clinical trial of post-operative dietary supplements in surgical patients. *Gut* 1997; **40:** 393–399.

53. Veterans Affairs Total Parenteral Nutrition Cooperative Study Group. Pre-operative total parenteral nutrition in surgical patients. *N Engl J Med* 1991; **325:** 525–532.

54. Von Meyenfeld MF, Meijerink WJHJ, Rouflard MJ, Buil-Maassen NTHJ, Soeters PB. Perioperative nutritional support – a randomised clinical trial. *Clin Nutr* 1992; **11:** 180–186.

55. Muller JM, Brenner U, Dienst C, Pichlmaier H. Pre-operative parenteral feeding in patients with gastro-intestinal carcinoma. *Lancet* 1982; **1:** 68–71.

55a. Bozzetti F, Gavazzi C, Miceli R *et al.* Perioperative total parenteral nutrition in malnourished gastrointestinal cancer patients: a randomised clinical trial. *J Parenter Enter Nutr* 2000; **24:** 7–14.

56. Askanazi J, Starker PN, Olsson C et al. Effect of immediate post-operative nutritional support on the length of hospitalisation. *Ann Surg* 1986; **203:** 236–239.

56a. Sandstrom R, Drott C, Hyltander A et al. The effect of post operative intravenous feeding (TPN) on outcome following major surgery evaluated in a randomised study. *Ann Surg* 1993; **217:** 185–195.

57. Weisdorf SA, Lysne J, Wynd D et al. Positive effect of prophylactic total parenteral nutrition on longterm outcome of bone marrow transplantation. *Transplantation* 1987; **43:** 833–838.

58. Jamieson CP, Norton B, Day T, Lakeman M, Powell-Tuck J. The quantitative effect of nutritional support on quality of life in out-patients. *Clin Nutr* 1996; **16:** 25–28.

59. Bengmark S. Econutrition and health maintenance – a new concept to prevent GI inflammation, ulceration and sepsis. *Clin Nutr* 1996; **15:** 1–10.

60. Kudsk KA, Groce MA, Fabian TC et al. Enteral versus parenteral feeding. *Ann Surg* 1992; **215:** 503–513.

61. Moore FA, Feliciano DV, Andrassy RJ et al. Early enteral feeding compared with parenteral reduces post operative septic complications. *Ann Surg* 1992; **216:** 172–183.

62. Solomon SN, Kirby DS. The refeeding syndrome: A review. *J Parent Enter Nutr* 1990; **14:** 90–95.

63. Askanazi J, Carpentier YA, Elwyn DH et al. Influence of total parenteral nutrition on fuel utilisation in injury and sepsis. *Ann Surg* 1980; **191:** 40–46.

64. Kupfer SR, Underwood LE, Baxter RC, Clemmons DR. Enhancement of the anabolic effects of growth hormone and insulin like growth factor 1 by use of both agents simultaneously. *Am Soc Clin Invest* 1993; **91:** 391–396.

65. Gogos CA, Zoumbos N, Makri M, Kalfarentzos F. Medium and long chain triglycerides have different effects of the synthesis of tumour necrosis factor by human mononuclear cells in patients under total parenteral nutrition. *J Am Coll Nutr* 1994; **13:** 40–44.

66. Wernerman J, Tucker HN. Future nutritional goal in the intensive care unit. In: Kinney JM, Tucker HN (Eds) *Organ Metabolism and Nutrition*: Ideas for future critical care. Raven Press, New York, 1994; **40:** 481–495.

67. Meydani SN. Effect of (n-3) polyunsaturated fatty acids on cytokine production and their biological function. *Nutrition* 1996; **12:** S8–S14.

68. Atkinson S, Sieffert E, Bihari D et al. A prospective randomised double-blind clinical trial of enteral immunonutrition in the critically ill. *Crit Care Med* 1998; **26:** 1164–1172.

69. Van der Hurst RRWJ, Van Kreel BK, Van Meyenfeldt MF et al. Glutamine and the preservation of gut integrity. *Lancet* 1991; **341:** 1363–1365.

70. Furst P, Albers S, Stehle P. Glutamine containing dipeptides in parenteral nutrition. *J Parent Enter Nutr* 1990; **14 (4Suppl):** S124–S188.

71. Tremel G, Kienle B, Weilemann LS, Stehle P, Furst P. Glutamine dipeptide – Supplemented parenteral nutrition maintains intestinal function in the critically ill. *Gastroenterol* 1994; **107:** 1595–1601.

72. Zeigler TR, Young LS, Benfell K. Clinical and metabolic efficacy of glutamine supplemented parenteral nutrition after bone marrow transplantation. A randomised double blind control study. *Ann Int Med* 1992; **116:** 821–828.

73. Griffiths RD, Jones C, Palmer TEA. Six month outcome of critically ill patients given glutamine supplemented parenteral nutrition. *Nutrition* 1997; **13:** 295–302.

74. Grimble G. Nutritional antioxidants and the modulation of inflammation: Theory and practice. *New Horizons* 1994; **2:** 175–185.

75. Berger MM, Spertini F, Shenkin A et al. Clinical, immune, and metabolic effects of trace element supplements in burns: a double blind placebo controlled trial. *Clin Nutr* 1996; **15:** 94–96.

76. Stratton RJ, Elia M. A critical, systematic analysis of the use of oral nutritional supplements in the community. *Clin Nutr* 1999; **18:** Suppl 2: 29–84.

77. Gardiner KR, Kirk SJ, Rowlands BJ. Novel substrates to maintain gut integrity. *Nutr Res Rev* 1995; **8:** 43–66.

78. MacBurney M et al. A cost evaluation of glutamine supplemented parenteral nutrition in adult bone marrow transplant patients. *JADA* 1994; **94:** 1263–1266.

78a. Kudsk KA. Gut mucosal nutritional support – Enteral nutrition as primary therapy after multiple system trauma. *Gut* **(Suppl 1)** 1994; S52–S54.

79. Gauderer NWL, Ponsky JL, Izand RJ. Gastrostomy without laparotomy: The percutaneous endoscopic technique. *J Paediatr Surg* 1980; **15:** 872–875.

80. Payne-James J. Enteral nutrition: Tubes and techniques of delivery. In: Payne-James J, Grimble G, Silk D (Eds) *Artificial Nutritional Support in Clinical Practice*. Edward Arnold, London, 1995, pp. 197–214.

81. Park RHR, Allison MC, Lang J, Russell R. Randomised comparison of percutaneous endoscopic gastrostomy and nasogastric tube feeding in patients with persisting neurological dysphagia. *Brit Med J* 1992; **304:** 1406–1409.

82. Wicks C, Gimson A, Lavianos V *et al.* Assessment of percutaneous endoscopic gastrostomy feeding tube as part of an integrated approach to enteral feeding. *Gut* 1992; **33:** 613–616.

83. Madden N, Alexander DJ, McMahon MJ. Influence of catheter type on the occurrence of thrombophlebitis. *Lancet* 1992; **339:** 101–103.

84. Payne-James J, Khawaja HT. First choice for total parenteral nutrition: The peripheral route. *J Parent Enter Nutr* 1993; **17:** 468–471.

85. Khawaja HT, Campbell MJ, Weaver PC. Effect of transdermal glyceryl trinitrate on the survival of peripheral intravenous infusions: a double blind clinical study. *Brit J Surg* 1988; **75:** 1212–1215.

86. Madden N, Alexander DJ, Mellor E, McMahon M. A randomised study of the effects of osmolality and heparin with hydrocortisone on thrombophlebitis in peripheral intravenous nutrition. *Clin Nutr* 1991; **10:** 309–314.

87. Tighe MJ, Wong C, Martin IG, McMahon MJ Do heparin, hydrocortisone, and glyceryl trinitrate influence thrombophlebitis during full intravenous nutrition via a peripheral vein. *J Parent Enter Nutr* 1995; **19:** 507–509.

88. Burnham WR. The role of the nutrition support team. In: Payne-James J, Grimble G, Silk D (Eds) *Artificial Nutritional Support in Clinical Practice.* Edward Arnold, London; 1995; pp. 175–186.

89. McWhirter JP, Hill K, Richards J, Pennington CR. The use, efficacy and monitoring of artificial nutritional support in a teaching hospital. *Scot Med J* 1995; **40:** 179–183.

9

Nutrition assessment

Antonio Sitges-Serra and Guzmán Franch-Arcas

For clinical practitioners, malnutrition in hospitalised patients can be defined as an abnormal body composition with functional impairment of different organs, due to chronic or acute reduction of calorie and protein intake, which worsens the clinical outcome. The fact that malnutrition is a disorder of the quantity and distribution of the body components gives the rationale for discussing nutrition assessment; that is, the qualification and quantification of the nutritional status of a given patient.

When dealing with nutrition assessment strategies, it must be emphasised that we are looking at methods and techniques which can better predict morbidity and mortality related to nutritional depletion. Thus, we will focus on those nutrition assessment methods that have been shown to have a significant prognostic value. Finally, the reader must be aware that nutrition assessment cannot be used as the only predictor of outcome as, in many instances, factors other than the nutrition status (surgical skill, organ dysfunction, iatrogenic complications, etc.) may be more relevant in determining the outcome of patients.[1]

History

The predictive value of weight loss and low plasma proteins in surgical patients was identified over 50 years ago by Studley[2] and subsequently by Rhoads & Alexander.[3] Increasing awareness among surgeons and physicians of the relationship between malnutrition and clinical outcome has encouraged the development of the new field of nutrition assessment. The introduction of 'nutritional parameters or markers' to assess the nutrition status of hospitalised patients was pioneered by American authors during the 1970s.[4–6] Methods imported from nutrition studies carried out in the Third World were applied to hospitalised patients with different and often controversial results. Investigators were looking at specific parameters or combination of parameters that would have prognostic value in order to guide the indications of artificial nutrition and improve the clinical outcome of patients. These 'objective' assessments based on quantitative criteria have been and are being widely used, although consensus on which are the best nutrition markers or risk formulae is lacking.

Objective nutrition assessment has been criticised by Jeejeebhoy's group[7] on the following grounds:

- It does not distinguish between nutrition-related and disease-related abnormal parameters.

- Plasma proteins commonly measured in nutrition studies (albumin and transferrin) have long half-lives and do not accurately reflect changes in food intake.

- Reference values vary considerably among healthy individuals.

These authors claim that an experienced clinician can accurately qualify the nutritional status of his patients by taking the appropriate medical history and performing an appropriate physical examination. This common-sense approach has served to counterbalance the abuse and commercialisation of 'objective assessment' and has correctly emphasised the value of a medical history and physical examination of the patient. However, in our opinion, some form of simple parametrical nutrition assessment is required for the following reasons:

- Although biochemical markers are influenced by the underlying pathology, they still have prognostic relevance.

- It assists in identifying the indications for artificial nutrition and in monitoring its efficacy.

- It allows the comparison and grouping of patients for scientific analysis.

- It makes it possible to qualify malnutrition in specific disease states.

- Subjective assessment cannot accurately predict hypoalbuminaemia.

- It allows the relationship between the severity of malnutrition and its complications to be established.

Aims of nutrition assessment

Malnutrition influences negatively the outcome of many diseases and treatments (i.e. surgery, intensive chemotherapy). Prolonged starvation should not be allowed in the hospital setting. Therefore, clinicians dealing with severely ill patients, patients requiring aggressive surgical or medical therapy or patients at high risk for developing malnutrition (e.g. gastrointestinal malignancies, complicated pancreatitis) must implement a simple nutrition assessment protocol to evaluate the degree and type of malnutrition and help to determine whether nutrition support is indicated. Such a protocol must be explained to all the medical and nursing staff so that they can promptly identify patients who are at risk of malnutrition. Thus, the principal aim of an objective nutrition assessment must be to provide the health care worker with simple guidelines to allow a decision to be made about the implementation of artificial nutrition.

A second aim of nutrition assessment is to quantify and qualify malnutrition. A weight loss of 10% has different influences on clinical outcome dependent on whether hypoalbuminaemia is present or absent.[8] Death rates increase in proportion to the amount by which albumin concentration falls.[4]

A third aim of nutrition assessment is to enable the health care worker to better determine nutrition requirements: body weight is required to calculate the energy requirements in the Harris–Benedict formulae. The presence of oedema is a contraindication to the administration of sodium. Patients with signs of dehydration and increased blood urea nitrogen require extra water. Some patients may show overt signs of vitamin deficiency.

The fourth aim of nutrition assessment is to provide the means for the clinician to monitor the efficacy of nutrition support.

Finally, nutrition assessment makes it possible to evaluate scientifically metabolic abnormalities present with common diseases, to compare outcome of patients among different institutions and to analyse the metabolic effects of artificial nutrition. In essence, it may act as a form of audit.

Methods for nutrition assessment

Nutrition assessment allows determination of the alterations in body composition parameters and the resulting associated organ function impairment that may adversely influence clinical outcome. Several markers of the quantitative status of different body compartments are useful for nutrition assessment because, if certain parameters are exceeded, complications may occur and/or the response of the organism to a given complication (particularly of the infectious type) is impaired. The ideal method for assessing human body composition should be relatively inexpensive, minimally invasive and should yield highly reproducible and accurate results.

Most traditional methods of body composition analysis are based upon the two compartments model in which the body is divided into fat and fat-free mass. This model assumes that the water, protein and mineral proportions in the fat-free mass are constant as well as the hydration coefficient.[9] However, for nutritional purposes the body should be regarded as divided into four compartments: water, protein and minerals (the three constituents of the fat-free mass), and body fat (Fig. 9.1). The use of this model necessitates independent assessment of at least three of the compartments: fat, protein and water, all of which are directly influenced by nutrition intake.

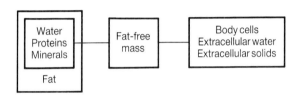

Figure 9.1 – Constituents of the body which form the biological basis of nutrition assessment.[9]

Whole-body assessment

The past medical and dietary history, a physical examination and accurate investigation of the primary illness are fundamental to nutrition assessment. Vomiting, dysphagia and/or anorexia, may cause drastic reductions in calorie and protein intakes leading to weight loss, the severity of which will depend on the time period elapsed between the onset of symptoms and the start of treatment. A history of chronic diarrhoea may signal malabsorption and/or inflammatory bowel disease, both of which are commonly associated with weight loss and hypo-albuminaemia. In the absence of renal, heart or liver disease, the presence of oedema or ascites is a marker of pronounced hypoalbuminaemia. Absolute sodium excess imposes a modified nutrition regimen with no sodium and water restriction. Weakness and apathy are often seen in patients with advanced weight loss.[7] Overt signs of specific vitamin or trace mineral deficiencies are uncommon but should be looked for particularly in alcoholic and geriatric patients in whom deficit of the B vitamin complex, folate and iron are often observed.

By far the most important parameter measuring whole-body status is actual weight and the percentage of weight loss over usual pre-illness weight. As suggested by Studley's pioneering work,[2] for weight loss alone to be relevant as a prognostic factor, it should be at least 15–20%. In our own work with gastric cancer patients submitted for major gastric surgery without preoperative nutrition,[11] those having lost 20% or more of their usual weight had a threefold higher postoperative mortality compared to those who did not lose as much weight (23 vs. 7%). However the oft-quoted division line of 10% did not identify populations with different mortality rates. Windsor & Hill[8] have found that a weight loss of 10% has no prognostic relevance unless associated with hypoalbuminaemia (<32 gl), impaired mental status or organ dysfunction. If those factors were present the patients suffered more septic complications, a higher prevalence of pneumonia and a longer hospital stay. Most of the patients in this high risk group had malignant disease of the gastrointestinal tract.

Body fat

Fat stores are significantly diminished in chronic malnutrition. Unfortunately, direct measurement of total body fat is still not possible. Prompt neutron activation analysis of carbon requires long irradiation periods and this limits application of the technique to research work.[2] The simplest way to assess the body fat compartment is by measuring the triceps skinfold thickness (TSF) which correlates reasonably well with total body fat.[13] When the dermis is felt between the finger and the thumb on pinching the triceps and biceps skinfolds – the so called positive finger-thumb test – fat losses of up to 60–70% have occurred.[14] Body impedance also gives a good estimate of total body fat in healthy individuals but its value in severely depleted patients has not been convincingly proven. Of all the anthropometric values, the TSF is the one having shown some influence on outcome. However, the variation of TSF between sexes and in the general healthy population is such that, as an isolated parameter, it is of little value. Furthermore, although it is a component of the prognostic nutrition index (PNI) it contributes to less than 10% of its final value[15] and therefore its routine use is controversial. On the other hand, it may be very useful in serial nutrition assessment of a given patient over a period of months (i.e., home parenteral nutrition, rehabilitation from severe malnutrition).

Albumin and visceral proteins

The body cell mass is the most relevant body compartment from the metabolic point of view. It contains the cellular proteins which carry out the synthetic, electrochemical and transport work and it contains the heat producing tissues. From the functional point of view, the body cell mass can be divided into two compartments: visceral and muscle protein.

The visceral protein compartment is the body component which more definitely influences clinical outcome. This compartment is assessed in daily clinical practice using the serum albumin and transferrin concentration and the total lymphocyte count. These non-specific markers can be considered to reflect the general functional status of the main parenchymatous organs and the immune system. Visceral protein markers have been used either in isolation or in combination to predict morbidity and mortality with notable success. Specifically, serum albumin concentrations has been shown by many to be an accurate predictor of complications and death.[1,8,11,16–18] Albumin concentration contributes to almost 60% of the final value of the Prognostic Nutritional Index.[15] A serum albumin concentration below 35 g/l reflects a non-specific impairment of the body's ability to cope with major illness, surgical intervention or a septic complication. Anergic patients have lower serum albumin concentrations than immunocompetent individuals.[11,16,17]

While the prognostic ability of serum albumin concentration is largely undisputed, controversy still remains concerning the pathogenesis of hypo-albuminaemia and whether it is in any way related to malnutrition.[18] Bentdal et al.[19] found that patients with anorexia nervosa had normal levels of serum albumin despite a mean weight loss of 30% of the premorbid weight. However, these authors did not measure the total albumin mass. Redistribution of albumin with a reduction of the rather large extravascular mass of albumin may occur in chronic starvation although hard data to support this assertion are lacking. Normal serum albumin concentrations in marasmic patients are thought to be due to channelling of muscle derived amino acids to the liver to support albumin synthesis.[20]

Gastric cancer patients are at risk of presenting with low serum albumin concentrations. Hypoalbuminaemia is most often seen with patients with large tumours and in those over 70 years of age. This suggests that losses through the gastrointestinal tract, and metabolic adaptation to these losses, are important in the pathogenesis of hypoalbuminaemia. In pancreatic cancer, an acute phase response (defined as the presence of high levels of C-reactive protein) is associated with hypoalbuminaemia; this suggests that a persistent neoplastic/inflammatory focus may secrete mediators which act on the liver to reduce the hepatic synthesis of albumin.[21] Finally, both in chronic malnutrition and in acute stress, hypoalbuminaemia is closely related to extracellular fluid expansion, a condition which itself may have a deleterious effect on wound healing, gas transport and the function of different organs.[22,23]

Thus, hypoalbuminaemia is a complex multifactorial phenomenon and the mechanisms by which it influences outcome are also complex. Subjective nutrition assessment cannot accurately predict whether a given non-stressed patient with chronic malnutrition has hypoalbuminaemia, and this gives further support to the inclusion of this important biochemical marker in nutrition assessment.

Transferrin is used as a visceral protein marker. Nutrition formulae or prognostic indices often incorporate transferrin (or the total iron binding capacity of plasma). Transferrin values are particularly reliable in the absence of iron-deficiency anaemia. In patients with gastrointestinal malignancies and iron-deficiency anaemia due to chronic blood loss, transferrin values may be spuriously high and do not properly reflect the advanced degree of malnutrition often observed in these patients. Prealbumin and retinol-binding protein (RBP) are plasma proteins with shorter half-lives and thus, theoretically, may better reflect chronic food deprivation or the effects of refeeding. However, their use has been limited because they have not proved to perform better than albumin in outcome prediction and they are not measured routinely in many hospitals.

Muscle protein

Skeletal muscle is an important reserve of amino acids available for mobilisation in times of stress and starvation. Static parameters reflecting the muscle protein mass or the lean body mass (LBM) are not good predictors of outcome. Total urine creatine, creatinine-height index (CHI) and arm muscle circumference (AMC) have not found a definite place in nutrition assessment protocols or in formulae of nutritional risk. However, parameters of muscular function have been shown in some studies to predict complications and death.

Total body protein (TBP) can be measured by prompt neutron activation of body nitrogen[24] although we agree

with Garrow et al.[25] in that 'it is probably the nature, distribution and concentration of protein rather than its absolute amount, which determines clinical outcome'. Only a few institutions, mostly research centres, have the facilities required for this type of analysis.

Since malnutrition is characterised by a loss of body skeletal protein, the assessment of muscular strength has been proposed as a suitable marker to assess quantitatively the degree of protein depletion. Klidjian et al.[26] standardised hand grip strength from measurements obtained in 284 healthy patients admitted for minor operations or as day cases at their unit. In 225 patients admitted for elective major abdominal operations they proved that hand grip strength was a more sensitive predictor of postoperative complications than indices of body protein stores such as weight loss, weight related to height, skinfold thickness, arm muscle circumference and serum albumin. About half of their patients (20 out of 44) with a hand grip strength below 85% of standard values developed complications, while out of 58 patients with a hand grip strength above 85% only three did. Furthermore, in that series, well established markers of surgical risk, considered alone (e.g. serum albumin below 35 g/l) were not better predictors of postoperative complications than hand grip strength. To make hand grip strength measurements more reliable, Webb et al.[10] proposed a derived sex and age-related standard grip strengths from 247 healthy volunteers to predict postoperative complications. They found, in agreement with Klidjian and coworkers,[26] that a hand grip strength below 85% of normal was the best predictor (in terms of sensitivity and specificity, Fig. 9.2).

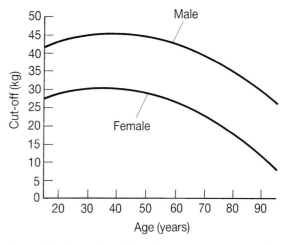

Figure 9.2 – Lower limit for hand grip strength in preoperative patients according to age and sex.[10]

In another study conducted among surgical patients, Windsor et al.[27] showed that measurement of voluntary hand grip strength of the non-dominant hand correlated with TBP as measured by prompt gamma in vivo neutron activation analysis. However, their 'protein index' (measured TBP divided by predicted TBP) correlated weakly with hand grip strength (r = 0.56). Although a decrease in hand grip strength can be a disease related phenomenon due to pain, circulatory changes, drug administration and/or decreased motivation to perform the test,[28] these factors do not necessarily detract from the potential usefulness of hand grip strength measurements. Despite that, however, other studies have yielded disappointing results, either because of the fluctuations of grip strength[29] or the inability to reproduce the initially favourable results.[30] Hand grip strength remains a simple and reliable method for detecting preoperative protein depletion and predicting postoperative complications and studies on its value should be pursued.

Other authors have investigated the contraction and relaxation patterns of the adductor pollicis muscle in response to an electrical stimulus of the ulnar nerve at the wrist, in an attempt to develop a more sensitive and specific test of muscle function less dependent on patient cooperation. Initial reports[31] with this technique in two models of starvation and refeeding in humans (anorectic patients and the starving obese), suggest that refeeding improves muscle function assessed in this way. Zeiderman & McMahon[32] have investigated the usefulness of this test in predicting postoperative complications and suggested that it may be a better predictor of postoperative complications than other parameters of muscular function such as arm muscle circumference and hand grip strength. However, as with many anthropometric parameters, the scatter of normal values for the normal population is too wide and in Zeiderman's paper there is too much overlap between the control and the patient population. Thus, the prognostic ability of adductor pollicis electromyographic patterns remains controversial.

Body water compartments

Starvation, stress and refeeding induce important alterations in body water compartments. In a study with volunteers submitted to partial starvation, Keys[33] found that extracellular water volume (ECW), assessed by the distribution space of thiocyanate, remained constant after a mean weight loss of 24%. Extracellular fluid relatively increased from 23 to 34% of the body weight, without any significant increase in absolute values. Other studies have confirmed the presence of a relative ECW expansion in chronic malnutrition.[34–36] Conversely, acutely ill patients with sepsis or trauma show an absolute increase in ECW. Elwyn et al.[34] found a mean excess of 3.7 litres of ECW in a series of postoperative and depleted patients. Shizgal[37] made a similar observation in malnourished cancer patients who showed an increased ratio of total exchangeable sodium to total exchangeable potassium, revealing an absolute increase of the ECW.

The expansion of the ECW has several undesirable consequences. Interstitial oedema may be detrimental for organ function particularly for the lung.[38] Hypervolaemia may precipitate heart failure in susceptible individuals. Oedema may also impair wound healing. Pharmacokinetics of many drugs (antibiotics, dopamine, antiarrhythmics) may be altered due to the considerable increase of their distribution space.[39] Finally, hypoalbuminaemia increases surgical risk. Tellado et al.[40] have clearly shown that expansion of the extracellular fluid in relation to exchangeable potassium (Na_e/K_e) positively and closely correlates to mortality in ill surgical patients. The risk of extracellular fluid over-expansion is higher in those patients with a physiologically small ECW; namely, thin adults (40–45 kg), very obese short and aged frail individuals. In these cases, the volume of the extracellular compartment can be as low as 10 litres,[41] so a rapid infusion of just 2.5 litres of saline represents a 25% increase in the size of this compartment.

Several mechanisms have been proposed to explain the ECW expansion in malnutrition and stress:[23]

- Activation of water- and sodium-retaining mechanisms by hypovolaemia and pain

- Increased capillary permeability and 'albumin leak' to the interstitium

- Aggressive fluid therapy during resuscitation

- Excessive administration of water and sodium (including TPN solutions) during the post-traumatic flow phase

- Hypoalbuminaemia due to haemodilution

- Administration of high-glucose/low-protein diets.

Methods to assess the volume of the body water compartments

Non-invasive, cheap and clinically applicable methods to assess body water compartments are awaited. Fluid therapy is still largely based on haemodynamic measurements and fluid balance sheets. These are not accurate enough to predict total body water and its compartmental distribution. Errors in balance methods tend to be cumulative and ill patients submitted to prolonged intensive treatment often develop complications due to water and sodium excess. Artificial nutrition can also induce changes in body water distribution, and those caring for patients receiving nutritional support should be familiar with water and electrolyte disturbances.

Clinical examination

Physical examination may offer direct signs revealing alterations in water compartments. Presence of oedema demonstrates an expansion of the ECW with absolute sodium excess. It is worth noting that for oedema to develop the ECW has to expand up to 10% of the body weight (i.e., in a 60 kg man, the ECW must expand at least 6 litres for oedema to be clinically detectable); thus, overt oedema often implies a 50–100% expansion of the ECW.[35] Daily weighing during refeeding will also detect inappropriate water retention, a common finding in severely depleted patients receiving total parenteral nutrition (TPN).[23,42–44] In an experimental model of malnutrition and intravenous refeeding, we have demonstrated that weight changes during the initial week of therapy are largely dependent on water and sodium balance.[45] In the clinical setting, increasing weight and decreasing serum albumin concentrations develop in about half the patients treated with standard TPN regimens because of severe preoperative depletion. This seems to predispose to major postoperative complications.[42,44] Thus, proper monitoring of weight and fluid balance is essential in oedematous and depleted patients to monitor the efficacy of artificial nutrition.

Dilution techniques

The simultaneous intravenous injection of different isotope tracers represents the most established approach to body water compartment analysis. Bauer et al.[46] described a dual beta-tracer technique using ^{35}S-sulphate with a dual gamma-tracer technique using [125]radioiodinated labelled human serum albumin and ^{51}Cr tagged red blood cells for determining plasma volume and red blood cells mass. Shizgal[47] described a similar methodology but substituted ^{35}S-sulphate with [22]SNa. However, the use of these radioactive tracers is contraindicated in children and women of reproductive age or in repeated determinations in a short

period of time. Currently, the use of stable isotopes (deuterium, bromide) or non-isotopic tracers (i.e., sodium bromide) is being expanded as newer techniques for their assay in aqueous solutions are available. In our experience[36] the reliability of ECW volume assessment by determining the bromide dilution space with an spectrophotometric technique is comparable to that obtained using ^{35}S-sulphate. Furthermore, bromide has a very satisfactory flat equilibrium slope in comparison with the very steep one of thiosulphate. In Moore's experience,[48] the bromide dilution volume proved to be the most reproducible. However, as also pointed out by Moore, since these dilutional methods have an overall random error of ±2–4%, their use over short periods of time (less than 30 days) is limited by the magnitude of the expected changes in the compartments under investigation.

Body impedance analysis

The basis for the use of body impedance analysis (BIA) was established by Thomasset[49] who first observed changes in the bio-electric tissue characteristics as a function of fluctuations of the extracellular electrolyte concentrations. Hoffer et al.[50] state:

'Impedance of simple geometric systems is a function of conductor length and configuration, conductor cross-sectional area and signal frequency; using a fixed signal and a relatively constant conductor configuration, the impedance becomes a function of conductor length and cross section or conductor volume.'

Conductive pathway is directly related to the percentage of water. Accordingly, conductivity is higher across hydrated tissue. Fat-free mass is hydrated but fat is mostly anhydrous. This is why the resistance that tissues offer to electrical current (i.e. their impedance), is essentially an index of total body water. In fact, equations to calculate fat-free mass and extracellular water used in current impedance systems are derived from densitometry or isotope dilution technique studies in normal subjects. Thus, these equations are not necessarily representative of starved or hospitalised populations and clinical application of impedance measurements is still controversial. BIA is not an accurate technique for measuring changes in total body water[51] over short periods of time and this seems to have discouraged researchers looking for an accurate bedside method for body composition analysis.[52]

Albumin as a marker of the ECW changes

Although serum albumin has been traditionally considered a parameter of malnutrition, chronic food deprivation does not result in hypoalbuminaemia until the very advanced terminal phase. In many cases hypoalbuminaemia reflects ECW expansion rather than an absolute decrease of the albumin mass. Studies by Mullins & Bell[53] have demonstrated a redistribution of albumin following ECW expansion with crystalloids. This phenomenon is likely to represent an increase of the interstitial space available for albumin rather than a primary endothelial injury. These authors have shown that an expanded interstitial volume is associated with excessive hydration of the interstitial gel matrix and an increased mass of extravascular albumin. Thus, increased ECW would result in hypoalbuminaemia by increasing the albumin distribution space.

That this may be indeed the case in clinical practice is further supported by Symreng's studies[54] which showed that patients with gastric carcinoma and hypoalbuminaemia had an increased ECW. On the other hand, patients with normal serum albumin concentration did not exhibit ECW expansion. Furthermore, these authors could demonstrate an inverse correlation between serum albumin and total muscle water. Starker et al.[42] observed that half of their surgical patients receiving TPN increased their weight, due to positive water and sodium balances, and had a concomitant decrease of their serum albumin levels. We have made similar observations in non-stressed patients with gastrointestinal malignancies receiving preoperative TPN in whom there was a close positive correlation between weight changes and sodium balances and an inverse correlation between weight gain and serum albumin concentrations.[44] Thus, albumin concentration indirectly reflects the volume of extracellular water and should be interpreted in the light of ECW changes both before or during artificial nutrition.

Prognostic nutrition indices

The grouping of nutrition parameters in formulae derived from stepwise regression analysis was pioneered by Buzby et al[5] in an attempt to improve the sensitivity of nutrition assessment in predicting postoperative complications and death. These authors described a Prognostic Nutritional Index based on four nutritional markers which were shown to be independent predictors of outcome. Thus:

PNI (% risk) = 158 − 16.6 (albumin, g/l) − 0.78 (TSF, mm)
− 0.2 (transferrin, mg/dl) − 5.8 (delayed hypersensitivity tests, 0–2)

PNI values above 50 are associated with increased morbidity and mortality in some surgical populations with high nutritional risk. For example in gastric cancer patients, mortality in the high risk PNI group was almost tenfold that of patients with low PNI.[11] However, the predictive value of PNI was much less in oesophageal carcinoma where factors other than nutrition may be more relevant concerning the final outcome.[55]

The Sheffield team[56] aimed to eliminate the skin tests from the PNI formula because they did not add significantly to the final PNI value, were cumbersome to perform and their relation to nutrition per se was controversial. Furthermore, they substituted the transferrin values for those of total iron binding capacity, a technique most commonly performed routinely in many hospitals. Thus:

PI (Sheffield) = 150 − 1.66 (alb, g/l) − 0.78 (TSF, mm) − 0.53 (TIBC, mg/dl)

Finally, Rainey-Macdonald et al.[15] were able to eliminate TSF from the formula since it contributed to less than 10% of the final value of the PNI. Thus these authors proposed a two variable formula:

PI (R−M) = 1.20 (alb, g/dl) + 0.013 (transferrin, mg/dl) − 6.43
(Negative or positive values indicate mortality or survival respectively)

Seltzer et al.[57] were, in fact, the first to propose the use of a two variable 'Instant Nutritional Assessment'. Combining the presence or absence of hypoalbuminaemia (albumin below 35 g/l) and/or lymphopaenia (lymphocytes below 1500 mm³) these authors could predict the increase likelihood of complications and death. Thus:

Alb <35 g/l = complications × 4; death × 6
Lymphocytes < 1500 = complications × 1.8 (NS); death × 4
Alb < 35 g/l and lymphocytes < 1500 = complications × 4; death × 20.

From the history and mathematical analysis of these formulae, it appears that their main strength lies in the assessment of the so-called 'visceral protein' and, particularly, of albumin.

Conclusion: a proposal for nutrition assessment

Nutrition assessment must combine clinical evaluation with objective measurements of those body compartments the integrity of which is particularly relevant to clinical outcome. Sophisticated research techniques for body composition analysis are not available in the majority of institutions and a renewed effort should be made by researchers to improve our means to accurately quantify the different body compartments at the bedside. There is also a definite need for new functional parameters related to organs whose function is altered by food deprivation. Meanwhile, most nutrition assessment protocols will continue to implement simple measurements which, if correctly interpreted, may be very useful in guiding the indications and monitoring the efficacy of nutrition support. Based on current evidence we propose the parameters in Table 9.1 should be looked for and recorded in all patients when considering the necessity of artificial nutrition support.

This assessment technique can be used by any nutrition team. It should be an integral part of the overall clinical care of all hospitalised patients, and should be used and recorded in the notes at the time of admission or initiation of treatment. Those patients at risk of malnutrition and those already malnourished can by these means be managed with appropriate nutrition support.

References

1. Pettigrew RA, Burns HJG, Carter DC. Evaluating surgical risk: the importance of technical factors determining outcome. *Br J Surg* 1987; **74:** 791–794.

2. Studley HO. Percentage of weight loss: a basic indicator of surgical risk in patients with chronic peptic ulcer. *J Am Med Assoc* 1936; **106:** 458–460.

3. Rhoads JE, Alexander CE. Nutritional problems of surgical patients. *Ann NY Acad Sci* 1955; **63:** 268–275.

4. Blackburn GL, Bistrian BR, Maini BS, Schlamm HT, Smith MF. Nutritional assessment of the hospitalized patient. *JPEN* 1977; **1:** 11–22.

5. Buzby GP, Mullen JL, Matthews DC, Hobbs CL, Rosato EF. Prognostic nutritional index in gastrointestinal surgery. *Am J Surg* 1980; **139:** 160–167.

6. Grant J, Custer PB, Thurlow J. Current techniques of nutritional assessment. *Surg Clin N Am* 1981; **61:** 437–463.

7. Baker JP, Detsky AS, Wesson DE, Wolman SL, Stewart S, Whitewell J, Langer B, Jeejeebhoy KN. Nutritional assessment. A comparison of clinical judgement and objective measurements. *N Engl J Med* 1982; **306:** 969–972.

8. Windsor JA, Hill L. Weight loss with physiologic impairment: A basic indicator of surgical risk. *Ann Surg* 1988; **207:** 290–296.

9. Mackie A, Hannan WJ, Tothill P. An introduction to body composition models used in nutritional studies. *Clin Phys Physiolog Meas* 1989; **10:** 297–310.

Table 9.1 – Nutrition assessment

Type of assessment	Parameters to be recorded
Clinical history and examination	In particular, dietary history, concurrent disease, evidence of loss of fat, loss of muscle, dehydration, oedema
Whole body	Actual weight, % loss from normal weight (risk if above 15%), weight changes during refeeding (risk if weight gain is too rapid and/or excessive)
Fat	TSF
Muscle protein	Hand grip strength (risk if below 85%, age and sex matched)
Visceral protein	Albumin (risk if <35 g/l) Lymphocytes (risk <1200 mm^3) Albumin concentration changes during refeeding (risk if it decreases) Transferrin or total iron binding capacity optional
Extracellular water compartment	Albumin, physical examination (risk: oedema)

10. Webb AR, Newman LA, Taylor M, Keogh JB. Hand grip dynamometry as a predictor of postoperative complications: reappraisal using age standardized grip strengths. *JPEN* 1989; **13**: 30–33.

11. Sitges-Serra A, Gl MJ, Rafecas A, Franch G, Jaurrieta E. Nutritional issues in gastric cancer patients. *Nutrition* 1990; **6**: 171–173.

12. Kyere K, Oldroyd B, Oxby CB, Burkinshaw L, Ellis RE, Hill GL. The feasibility of measuring total body carbon by counting neutron inelastic scatter gamma rays. *Phys Med Biol* 1982; **27**: 805–817.

13. Shizgal HM. Nutritional assessment with body composition measurements. *JPEN* 1987; **11(suppl 5):** 42–44.

14. Hill GL. *Disorders of nutrition and metabolism in clinical surgery*. Churchill Livingstone, Edinburgh, 1992, p.98.

15. Rainey-Macdonald CG, Holliday RL, Wells GA, Donner AP. Validity of a two-variable nutritional index for use in selecting candidates for nutritional support. *JPEN* 1983; **7**: 15–20.

16. Harvey KB, Moldawer LL, Bistrian BR, Blackburn G. Biological measures for the formulation of a hospital prognostic index. *Am J Clin Nutr* 1981; **34**: 2013–2022.

17. Christou NV, Tellado-Rodríguez J, Chartrand L. Estimating mortality risk in preoperative patients using immunologic, nutritional and acute phase response variables. *Ann Surg* 1989; **210**: 69–77.

18. Nogués R, Sitges-Serra A, Sancho JJ, Sanz F, Monne J, Girvent M, Gubern JM. Influence of nutrition, thyroid hormones and rectal temperature on in-hospital mortality of elderly patients with acute illness. *Am J Clin Nutr* 1995; **61**: 597–602.

19. Bentdal O, Froland SS, Askevold F, Bjoro K, Larsen S. Nutritional assessment of anorexia nervosa. Analysis of anthropometric and biochemical variables to evaluate patients at risk. *Clin Nutr* 1988; **7**: 95–99.

20. Smith G, Robinson PH, Fleck A. Serum albumin distribution in early treated anorexia nervosa. *Nutrition* 1996; **12**: 677–684.

21. Falconer JS, Fearon KCH, Plester CE, Ross JA, Carter DC. Cytokines, the acute-phase response, and resting energy expenditure in cachectic patients with pancreatic cancer. *Ann Surg* 1994; **219**: 325–331.

22. Sitges-Serra A, Franch-Arcas G, Guirao X, García-Domingo M, Gil MJ. Extracellular fluid expansion during parenteral refeeding. *Clin Nutr* 1992; **11**: 63–68.

23. Guirao X, Franch G, Gil MJ, García-Domingo MI, Girvent M, Sitges-Serra A. Extracellular volume, nutritional status and refeeding changes. *Nutrition* 1994; **6**: 558–561.

24. Beddoe AH, Streat SJ, Hill GL. Evaluation of an in-vivo prompt gamma neutron activation facility for body composition studies in critically ill intensive care patients: results on 41 normals. *Metabolism* 1984; **33**: 270–280.

25. Garrow JS, Fletcher K, Halliday D. Body composition in severe infantile malnutrition. *J Clin Invest* 1965; **44**: 417–425.

26. Klidjian AM, Foster KJ, Kammerling RM, Cooper A, Karran SJ. Relation of anthropometric and dynamometric variables to serious postoperative complications. *Br Med J* 1980; **281**: 899–901.

27. Windsor JA, Hill GL. Grip strength: a measure of the proportion of protein loss in surgical patients. *Br J Surg* 1988; **75**: 880–882.

28. Martin S, Neale G, Elia M. Factors affecting maximal mommentary grip strength. *Clin Nutr* 1985; **39**: 137–147.

29. Young VL, Pin P, Kraemer BA, Gould RB, Nemergut L, Pellowski M. Fluctuations in grip and pinch strength among normal subjects. *J Hand Surg* 1989; **14A**: 125–129.

30. Griffith CDM, Whyman M, Bassey EJ, Hopkinson BR, Makin GS. Delayed recovery of hand grip strength predicts postoperative morbidity following major vascular surgery. *Br J Surg* 1989; **76**: 704–705.

31. Jeejeebhoy KN, Detsky AS, Baker JP. Assessment of nutritional status. *JPEN* 1990; **14(Suppl.):** 193–196.

32. Zeiderman M, McMahon MJ. The role of objective measurement of skeletal muscle function in the preoperative patient. *Clin Nutr* 1989; **8**: 161–166.

33. Keys A, Brozek J, Henschel A, Mickelson O, Taylor HL. *The biology of human starvation*. University of Minnesota Press, Minneapolis, 1950.

34. Elwyn DH, Bryan-Brown WB, Shoemaker WC. Nutritional aspects of body water dislocation in postoperative and depleted patients. *Ann Surg* 1975; **182**: 76–85.

35. Kinney JM, Weissman CH. Forms of malnutrition in stressed and unstressed patients. *Clin Chest Med* 1986; **7**: 19–28.

36. Franch-Arcas G, Guirao G, Gil MJ, Sitges-Serra A. Changes in corrected bromide space due to simple starvation in rabbits. A validated technique for measuring extracellular water. *Clin Nutr* 1990; **9(suppl):** 72–73.

37. Shizgal HM. Body composition of patients with malnutrition and cancer. Summary of methods of assessment. *Cancer* 1985; **55**: 250–253.

38. Harms BA, Pahl AC, Radosevich BS, Starling JR. The effects of hypoproteinemia and volume expansion on lung and soft tissue transvascular fluid filtration. *Surgery* 1989; **105**: 605–614.

39. Tormo C, Abad FJ, Rochera-Oms CL, Parra V, Jiménez V. Critically-ill patients receiving total parenteral nutrition show altered amikacin pharmacokinetics. *Clin Nutr* 1995; **14:** 254–259.

40. Tellado JM, García-Sabrido JL, Hanley JH, Shizgal HM, Christou NV. Predicting mortality based on body composition analysis. *Ann Surg* 1989; **209:** 81–87.

41. Moore FD. *The body cell mass and its supporting environment.* Saunders, Philadelphia, 1963, pp. 167–168.

42. Starker PM, Lasala PA, Askanazi J, Gump FE, Forse RA, Kinney JM. The response to TPN. A form of nutritional assessment. *Ann Surg* 1983; **198:** 720–721.

43. Sitges-Serra A, Gil MJ, Martínez-Ródenas F. The influence of TPN formulation on the metabolic response to pre-operative refeeding in depleted patients. *Br J Clin Pract* 1988; **42(Suppl. 63):** 133–137.

44. Gil MJ, Franch G, Guirao X, Oliva A, Herms R, Salas E, Girvent M, Sitges-Serra A. Response of severely malnourished patients to preoperative parenteral nutrition: a randomized clinical trial of water and sodium restriction. *Nutrition* 1997; **13:** 26–31.

45. Franch G, Gil MJ, Guirao X, Sitges-Serra A. Water and sodium metabolism during intravenous refeeding in the malnourished rabbit. *Clin Nutr* 1991; **10(Suppl.):** 58–64.

46. Bauer JH, Willis LR, Burt RW, Grim CE. Volume studies. II. Simultaneous determination of plasma volume, red cell mass, extracellular fluid, and total body water before and after volume expansion in dog and man. *J Lab Clin Med* 1975; **86:** 1009–1017.

47. Shizgal HM. Body composition and nutritional support. *Surg Clin North Am* 1981; **61:** 729–741.

48. Moore FD. Energy and the maintenance of the body cell mass. *JPEN* 1980; **4:** 228–260.

49. Thomasset A. Propriétés bio-electriques des tissues mesurés de l'impédance et clinique signification des courbes obtenues. *Lyon Medical* 1962; **21:** 107–118.

50. Hoffer EC, Meador CK, Simpson DC. Correlation of whole-body impedance with total body water volume. *J Appl Physiol* 1969; **27:** 531–534.

51. Jebb SA, Elia M. Assessment of changes in total body water in patients undergoing renal dialysis using bio-electrical impedance analysis. *Clin Nutr* 1991; **10:** 81–84.

52. Pullicino E, Coward WA, Elia M. The potential use of dual frequency bioimpedance in predicting the distribution of total body water in health and disease. *Clin Nutr* 1992; **11:** 69–74.

53. Mullins R, Bell DR. Changes in interstitial volume and masses of albumin and IgG in rabbit skin and skeletal muscle after saline volume loading. *Circ Res* 1982; **51:** 305–311.

54. Symreng T, Larsson J, Möller P. Muscle water and electrolytes in relation to nutritional status in gastric carcinoma. *Clin Nutr* 1985; **4:** 115–120.

55. Sitges-Serra A, Minguella JL, Rafecas A, Oms L, Valverde J, Jaurrieta E. Preoperative nutritional status and postoperative outcome in patients with carcinoma of the esophagus. *Nutrition* 1990; **6:** 167–168.

56. Simms JM, Smith JAR, Woods HF. A modified prognostic index based upon nutritional parameters. *Clin Nutr* 1982; **1:** 71–79.

57. Seltzer MH, Slocum BA, Cataldi-Belcher EL. Instant nutritional assessment. *JPEN* 1979; **3:** 157–159.

10

Adult macronutrient requirements

Hans P Sauerwein and JA Romijn

Introduction and definition

Macronutrients are defined as anabolic substrate (protein) and energy substrates (carbohydrates and lipids). The physiological effect of these macronutrients is dependent on both the absolute and the relative amounts given and on the subject to whom they are administered. If the amounts of macronutrients provided fall below the Recommended Daily Allowances (RDA), breakdown of tissues takes place to supply the metabolic energy needs of the body. Provision of increased amounts of macronutrients will result in stimulation of synthesis of body constituents and of oxidation of different substrates. This adaptation to increasing macronutrient supply increases to a point above which excess protein intake will be catabolised and excess glucose and fat will be stored as fat.

Nutrient intake modifies both macromolecular synthesis and substrate oxidation to a different extent. As a result nutrition goals in patients differ from those in healthy individuals. In healthy subjects the main aim of provision of macronutrients is maintenance of lean body mass (LBM). In sick subjects the aim is different, because illness has a catabolic influence on metabolism.[1] The aims of nutrition support should be not only to *prevent* loss of lean body mass, but also, if possible, to maximise healing and wound repair. The RDA for macronutrients for sick patients should be optimal, without producing adverse side-effects through excess oxidative load.

Adult energy requirements

All organisms obey the first and second law of thermodynamics, and the first is the law of conservation of energy. This states that energy can neither be created nor destroyed, but only converted from one form into another. Supplying an organism with inadequate amounts of energy results in tissue mobilisation to make up the energy deficit. In contrast, calories provided in excess of energy requirements are stored as glycogen or fat. This is undesirable unless the goal of nutrition is replenishment of lost fat stores. Fat synthesis is a costly process, consuming 23% of the original calories contained in its carbohydrate precursor, glucose.[2] Moreover, fat synthesis from dietary

energy substrates eventually results in obesity[2-4] or storage of fat in inappropriate organs such as the liver.[5] Therefore, energy *balance* is the target in healthy subjects as well as patients. It can be seen that hyperalimentation (the provision of substrates in *excess* of actual needs) serves no clinically relevant purpose and is probably harmful.

Energy balance means that intake and expenditure of energy are in equilibrium. By estimating the energy contained in carbohydrate, fat and protein, and the efficiency of digestion and absorption, energy intake can be estimated. When all factors are considered, energy values of 4, 9 and 4 kcal/g are obtained for carbohydrate, fat and protein respectively.[6] Energy expenditure is the unknown variable.

Energy expenditure comprises three major components: resting energy expenditure (REE), metabolic requirements of exercise, and the thermic effects of food (post-prandial thermogenesis) (Ch. 3). The actual value of post-prandial thermogenesis depends on the substrate: 5–10% for carbohydrate, 0–3% for fat, 20–30% after a protein meal. For mixed diets, a value of 10% is usually assumed.[2] However, recent data suggest that dietary input may not be very thermogenic if intake is modest, or when food is given to a very malnourished subject.[7] Consequently REE and the thermic effect of exercise are the main components of energy expenditure. Many attempts have been made to establish normal values for both components, and this has been reviewed.[8] Emphasis has been placed on REE because it is easier to measure and it is usually the largest component of total energy expenditure.

Predictive equations for REE are reasonably accurate in healthy male and female caucasians, the most frequently used being that of Harris and Benedict:

> Males: REE = 66 + (13.7 × body weight) + (5.0 × height) − (6.8 × age)
>
> Females: REE = 665 + (9.6 × body weight) + (1.7 × height) − (4.7 × age)

Length is expressed in centimetres, body weight in kilograms and age in years. Comparison of the results of the Harris–Benedict equations and the actual measurements of REE obtained by various authors reveals that the calculated values are approximately 5% higher than the measured values in men and 5–10% in women.[8]

However, these equations are invalid in patients

because REE is increased in many diseases.[9,10] Therefore nomograms have been constructed to predict the effect of different diseases on REE.[10–11] In these nomograms the influence of different diseases on REE is given as the mean of data obtained in groups of patients with those diseases. However, often a wide inter-individual variability is found even in an apparently homogeneous group.[12] Calculations of REE based on a nomogram can therefore easily result in either significant over-feeding or under-feeding in individual patients. It is preferable to measure energy expenditure itself, rather than relying on estimates based on nomograms.

Measurement of energy expenditure

Total daily energy expenditure in a free-living subject can be measured either by integrated heart-rate measurements or by the doubly labelled water method. With (in)direct calorimetry, total daily energy expenditure can be measured in a respiration chamber, but this hampers daily activity. REE can also be measured by calorimetry, but these values give no clue about the metabolic requirements of daily activity.

The doubly-labelled water method

Assessment of energy expenditure (and thus of energy requirements) should not be limited to the measurement of REE. The provision of energy should cover total daily energy requirements, including that for physical activity. Energy expenditure in free-living conditions has been estimated from calorimetric determination of different activities and from estimates of times spent undertaking each of these daily activities. The techniques have limited sensitivity and cannot be applied to patients.

Total daily energy expenditure can be measured by the doubly-labelled water technique.[13–18] The method is based on the relationship between water metabolism and respiration. Oxygen, expired as carbon dioxide, is in isotopic equilibrium with oxygen in body-water. After a loading dose of H_2O, the decline in the enrichment of isotopic oxygen in body-water is a reflection of both H_2O and CO_2 output, whereas the decrease in isotopic hydrogen in body-water relates only to H_2O output. The difference between the elimination rates of the two isotopes is proportional to CO_2 pro-

duction, which can be converted to O_2 consumption, using an appropriate respiratory quotient (RQ) estimate. Energy expenditure can then be computed, based on O_2 consumption in a manner similar to that used in traditional calorimetry (see below). The advantage of this technique over classic calorimetry is that the subject can be ambulant and it is only necessary to sample body-water for isotopic analysis occasionally (once a week for up to 3 weeks).[15]

Estimation of energy expenditure

The doubly-labelled water method has shown that the metabolic requirements of exercise have a major impact on total daily energy expenditure (Fig. 10.1). In free-living young adults, total daily energy expenditure exceeds REE by about 100%, whereas the figure is about 25% in sedentary people.[16,19] This concurs with the finding that measurements in a respiration chamber, with restricted physical activity, give values for energy expenditure about 20% lower than those obtained in subjects admitted to wards for study purposes, because of increased physical activity such as walking and game-playing.[20]

Although simple in concept, analysis of samples for the doubly-labelled water method requires expensive analytical mass spectrometers, available in only a few research centres. Therefore, total adult energy expenditure (and consequently energy requirements) is rarely measured clinically by this method.

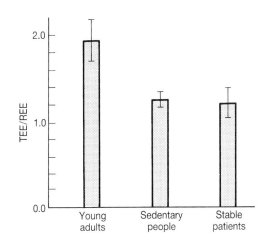

Figure 10.1 – Increase in daily total energy expenditure (TEE) over resting energy expenditure (REE).

Direct calorimetry

The body requires the production of energy for maintenance of life. Energy is produced from oxidation of substrates. Oxygen is consumed and heat, work and CO_2 are produced. Because energy cannot be destroyed, the production of work will eventually result in the production of heat. Direct measurement of heat production, or the combined measurement of oxygen consumption and CO_2 production, are therefore both possible methods for measuring energy expenditure. Direct calorimetry measures energy expenditure from heat loss. In this technically difficult method the subject is placed in a thermally isolated chamber and the dissipated heat is measured precisely. Therefore *indirect* calorimetry (which calculates energy expenditure from measured O_2 consumption and CO_2 production) is the most frequently used technique for measuring energy expenditure.

Indirect calorimetry

Indirect calorimetry measures gas exchange: O_2 uptake (VO_2) and CO_2 release (VCO_2). The amount of CO_2 exchanged by use of 1 litre of oxygen depends on the substrate (Table 10.1). Since a mix of metabolic 'fuels' is generally being oxidised, it is assumed that combustion of 1 litre of oxygen is equivalent to the production of 4.85 kcal. Energy expenditure (EE), or metabolic rate, can thus be calculated from the following equation:

$$EE = VO_2 \times 4.85$$

with EE in kcal/min and VCO_2 in 1/min. In this equation a constant value for the energy equivalent of oxygen is assumed, which is correct only when the fuel mix is constant. Because the amount of CO_2 produced from combustion of carbohydrate, fat or protein is different, a more precise value for EE can be obtained by including VCO_2 and urinary nitrogen excretion (N) in the calculation of EE. Urinary nitrogen excretion is a reflection of protein oxidation:

$$EE = 3.91 \, VO_2 + 1.10 \, VCO_2 - 1.93 \, N$$

with VO_2 and VCO_2 in 1/min and N in g/min.

Table 10.1 – Calorie equivalent of oxygen.

	kcal/l
Amino acids	4.96
Palmitate	4.66
Glucose	5.02

VO_2 and VCO_2 can be measured in a respiration chamber or by the ventilated hood system. The respiration chamber is a small air-tight room in which the subject can move around relatively freely. This is not suitable for studies in patients, as the subject must be completely isolated during measurements. Therefore the method most frequently used for indirect calorimetry is the open-circuit ventilated hood system. The subject lies in bed and a perspex box is placed over his head. The box is supplied with a constant flow of air and the inspiratory and expiratory concentrations of O_2 and CO_2 and airflow are measured by very sensitive analysers. It is obvious that with this technique only REE can be measured. For assumptions and limitations of the technique the reader is referred to excellent reviews.[21–24]

The influence of disease on resting energy expenditure

In addition to REE and the metabolic expenditure of exercise, disease itself adds further variation to EE. In the clinical setting, reduction in EE due to the loss of LBM or pre-existing starvation are balanced against increases due to fever or inflammation (see Ch. 3). For the purposes of this discussion, these influences will be ignored.

Indirect effects of disease on REE

Loss of lean body mass

The main factor determining REE is lean body mass. When individual differences in LBM are accounted for, REE is constant in healthy young adults.[25] Loss of LBM will itself result in a decrease in REE. This accounts for the decrease in metabolic rate of the elderly who have lost 'active' cellular mass (i.e. LBM).[26–28] Loss of LBM (especially muscle mass) induced by the underlying disease or by concomitant anorexia will lower REE.[29,30]

Fever and ambient temperature

The thermodynamic treatment of reaction kinetics by van'tHoff led to the empirical observation that for every 10°C rise in temperature, the reaction velocity increases 2–3-fold. In mammals an increase in body temperature of 1°C also results in 13% increase in energy expenditure, although inter-individual variation is considerable.[31] Thus, for example, a pyrexia of 40°C will cause a 40% increase in energy expenditure.

Ambient temperature also has an influence on oxygen consumption. If the environmental temperature exceeds the skin temperature, sweating is the only defence mechanism to prevent a rise in body temperature. This can be an important loss of energy since 1g of water lost by evaporation represents energy expenditure of 0.58 kcal.

Paradoxically, a low ambient temperature also has an important influence on energy expenditure. Of the mechanisms of adaptation to heat loss (vasoconstriction, inhibition of sweat secretion and shivering), shivering increases energy expenditure. Clinical studies have shown that an environmental temperature above 23–26°C reduces the metabolic response to trauma,[32,33] and insulation with blankets or bedclothing is therefore desirable when temperatures lower than this are encountered.[33]

Direct effects of disease on REE

REE in patients tends to be higher than in healthy subjects. The degree of hypermetabolism is related to the degree and intensity of illness, being most pronounced in severe diseases like haemorrhagic pancreatitis, blunt trauma, sepsis and extensive burns (Fig. 10.2). Only in the more recent studies on REE in these patient groups have appropriate controls been included. However, the results in these studies are comparable to earlier data in which measured REE was compared with values calculated with prediction equations like the Harris–Benedict formula,[10] showing that these equations give a reasonable estimate of REE in healthy subjects. Studies in patients with severe diseases used body weight instead of LBM in their calculations. This may not be a major problem as REE measurements in these patients, who were presumably previously healthy, were usually done within a few days of injury or disease onset. In more chronically ill patients (such as those with cirrhosis, or AIDS) a decrease in LBM can be expected. Therefore only studies in which LBM was measured and compared with appropriate controls are included in Fig. 10.2. The data clearly show that increases in REE can occur in these chronic diseases.

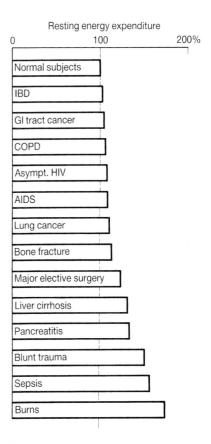

Figure 10.2 – Influence of disease on resting energy expenditure, measured in post-absorptive state (PAS) after 16 hours of fasting. Only studies with appropriate control groups are included. IBD = inflammatory bowel disease; COPD = chronic obstructive lung disease. (Adapted[33, 36–48])

It is unknown whether energy expenditure related to physical activity is influenced by the mere existence of disease, except for its obvious influence (i.e. limitation) on the amount of activity. The few studies in patients in which total daily energy expenditure was measured using the doubly-labelled water method suggest that disease itself has no great influence on the metabolic requirements of exercise, as the increase in expenditure above REE was the same as in sedentary people (± 20%).[34,36]

Summary

Many variables influence total daily energy expenditure. The data in the literature suggest that it is 20% above REE in patients unless the patient has a very active lifestyle. As disease influences REE in a rather unpredictable way, *measurement* of REE is preferable to its estimation. When measurement is impossible, calculation of REE multiplied by a disease-related percentage (Fig. 10.2) is better than making no estimation at all. However, it should be realised that there is a wide inter-individual variation in REE, and the provision of energy in excess of measured or calculated energy requirements has never been shown to be of any benefit.

Adult protein requirements

Traditionally, the requirements of protein have been related to nitrogen balance, which represents the difference between intake and loss of nitrogen (particularly in urine). However, this approach to determining protein requirements is not correct as it does not relate to the effect of protein administration on whole-body protein metabolism.

The goal of defining adult protein requirements has proved elusive because of the complexity of protein metabolism. This complexity is reviewed in detail in Chapters 2 and 3. However, for the sake of this discussion one point should be made. It is that, on average, daily dietary amino acid intake is a third of the daily rate at which amino acids in body protein turn over.

Protein requirements in healthy adults

In general, two methods have been employed to quantify the effect of protein intake on protein metabolism. Firstly, nitrogen balance represents the difference between nitrogen intake and nitrogen loss from all sources; secondly, tracer techniques enable quantification of protein synthesis and breakdown.

From nitrogen balance studies, approximate minimum requirements of dietary protein in healthy subjects have been derived. During consumption of a protein-free diet (with adequate calories), net protein catabolism decreases progressively to a plateau value after 1–2 weeks.[52] This plateau represents the obligatory loss of protein. Using this approach, and taking into consideration individual variations in protein catabolism, it has been estimated that in the region of 0.45 g/kg(BW)/day would represent the obligatory protein loss (and consequently the theoretical minimum amount of dietary protein) that is needed for maintenance of LBM.[53] In practice, however, the

average amount of high-quality protein that is needed to maintain nitrogen balance appears to be equivalent to about 130–140% (~0.6 g/kg/day) of the total obligatory nitrogen losses. When individual variability (to cover 95% of the population) is taken into account, protein requirements become about 0.75 g/kg(BW)/day.[53]

Current estimates of essential amino acid requirements provided by FAO/WHO/UNU (Table 10.2) are based on the results of nitrogen balance studies performed during feeding of mixtures of purified amino acids with variable amounts of essential amino acids.[54] However, in recent years these recommendations have been debated.[55]

Table 10.2 – Adult requirements for essential amino acids (mg/ kg/day).

Histidine	8–12
Isoleucine	10
Leucine	14
Lysine	12
Met + cystine	13
Phe + tyrosine	14
Threonine	7
Tryptophan	3.5
Valine	10
Total	94

% of average protein requirement (= 600) 16%

There are several shortcomings in the design of individual studies. These include factors such as excessive energy intake, methodological problems of nitrogen balance studies and persistent over-estimation of nitrogen balance. Several recent reports have evaluated the requirements of essential amino acids by measurement of amino acid fluxes and amino acid oxidation in response to graded levels of amino acid uptake. Amino acid requirement was *defined* as the intake of the essential amino acid that was just needed to balance the minimum irreversible loss of the amino acid via oxidation. These studies of amino acid metabolism have suggested that current recommendations of essential amino acids have underestimated actual requirements.[55] However, these tracer studies are also subject to criticism.[56] Consequently, the requirements of essential amino acids require further evaluation. Nevertheless, it should be realised that the average requirement of high-quality protein (egg) to maintain nitrogen balance in the presence of adequate amounts of energy substrates contains three times the current requirements of essential amino acids.[56] It is therefore unlikely that an adequate intake of protein will result in deficiency of amino acids.

The sources of protein and energy intake have to be considered in the evaluation of protein requirements. Traditionally, whole-egg protein has served as a standard composition of protein and has been a guideline in the formulation of amino acid mixtures for parenteral nutrition. However, protein requirements (reflected in the amount of protein required to maintain nitrogen balance) are different when other protein sources are used. For instance, the minimum amount of rice protein (or of wheat gluten) required to achieve nitrogen balance is higher than of whole egg protein, owing to differences in utilisation.[42]

Energy intake is another factor influencing protein requirement.[57] As long as the energy in the diet matches the energy expenditure, increasing intake of dietary proteins improves nitrogen balance. When energy intake becomes limiting, increasing protein intake has no further effect. The data on adult protein requirements are based on considerations on the minimal amounts of protein needed to maintain nitrogen balance. The question arises, especially in patient care, as to the optimal requirement of dietary protein. Indirect data for answering this question can be obtained from studies employing tracer techniques enabling quantification of net protein synthesis and breakdown. These studies have shown that, in healthy subjects, whole-body protein synthesis is a function of dietary protein intake. Maximum stimulation of protein synthesis occurs at a dietary protein intake of 1.5–1.7 g/kg(BW)/day (when provided with an adequate amount of energy substrates).[58] Intake above this level will not stimulate synthetic rates any further but merely results in catabolism of the excess protein and increased urea excretion. Studies using the nitrogen balance technique have also indicated that nitrogen balance improves (although minimally so) when protein intake is increased above the minimum requirements.[57] Nutrition modulation influences protein synthesis with little change in breakdown in skeletal muscle.[59] For other tissues this relationship is less clear. It may well be that the optimal amount of dietary protein is higher than the minimum amount necessary to maintain nitrogen balance, depending on the condition and the activity of the subject. However,

on combining the results of both approaches, it can be deduced that the optimal adult protein requirement is somewhere between 0.75 (the minimum requirement) and 1.5–1.7 g/kg/day.

Protein requirements in disease

The effect of disease on protein metabolism is characterised by net protein catabolism, owing to differences between protein synthesis and breakdown rates. This is seen as a negative nitrogen balance. The pathophysiological mechanism of this catabolic reaction is related to the severity of disease. During minor illnesses (e.g. after elective surgery) the negative nitrogen balance is associated mainly with a decreased protein synthesis rate, whereas protein breakdown is hardly affected.[60] In critical illness, however, net protein catabolic rate can be markedly stimulated, by relatively higher increases in protein breakdown rates than in synthesis rates, resulting in the rapid decrease of LBM.[61] In addition, ill patients do not show the adaptation to progressive starvation (with its associated nitrogen loss) seen in healthy subjects, which enhances the catabolic effect of disease.

It should be noted that this catabolic response is a net phenomenon. In some tissues (e.g. muscle) protein breakdown is clearly present, whereas in some organs (e.g. liver) mixed reactions may occur, with increases in the synthesis rate of some proteins (e.g. acute-phase proteins) and decreases in the synthesis rate of others (e.g. albumin).

What are the protein requirements of patients? The emphasis must be on optimal rather than *minimal* amounts of dietary proteins. Unfortunately a clear clinical or physiological end-point for the determination of optimal protein requirements is not available. Only studies documenting the effects of dietary protein content on nitrogen balance or on protein kinetics have been published. From these studies it is clear that in patients with severe conditions (e.g. major burns, sepsis) net protein synthesis cannot be achieved, despite the administration of large amounts of protein given together with adequate amounts of glucose and lipids (Fig. 10.3).[62] Therefore, the catabolic effects of disease on LBM cannot be manipulated merely by nutrition. The goal in these patients can only be to decrease net protein catabolic rates as much as possible rather than to try to achieve net protein synthesis. The available data suggest that net protein catabolic rates are lowest during administration of 1.5–2 g/kg/day of protein with adequate amounts of energy substrates.[62–63]

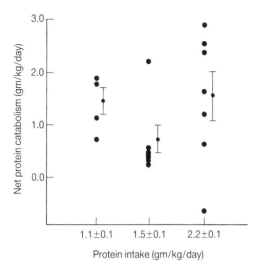

Figure 10.3 – Rates of net protein catabolism calculated from urea turnover data in septic patients receiving total parenteral nutrition (glucose ≈ 3.5 mg/kg/min) at three rates of protein intake. Individual values + mean rate of net protein catabolism with SEM. Adapted[62] with permission.

Administration of proteins exceeding this quantity result only in increased protein catabolism.

Adult glucose requirements

Glucose requirement in healthy adults

Adult requirements of glucose are not clearly defined in healthy subjects. One study showed that 10-day infusion of amino acids in an amount equivalent to 60 g of protein together with fat or glucose, at or above caloric expenditure, maintained nitrogen balance.[64] However, there are indications that maintenance of LBM may not be as efficient with a carbohydrate-free diet as there is a tendency for a slightly negative nitrogen balance when lipid is the only energy source.

An estimate of the optimal amount of dietary carbohydrate can be made as follows. Glucose, administered either orally or intravenously, is oxidised only in part. As increasing amounts of glucose are given the absolute rate of glucose oxidation increases but only to a certain level; when the rate of glucose infusion exceeds 4–5 g/kg/day, glucose oxidation is not further stimulated.[43,65–70] The excess of glucose that is

not oxidised is stored as glycogen but, because the glycogen storage capacity is about 15 g/kg, a massive intake of carbohydrate (>500 g/day) will after a few days result in substantial *de novo* lipid synthesis.[71] However, the primary goal of providing energy substrates in a balanced diet is the provision of substrates for oxidation, not for storage. Therefore, in predominantly sedentary healthy subjects a carbohydrate intake of 4–5 g/kg/day seems to be optimal, the actual amount depending on the level of physical activity.

The administration of carbohydrates, but not of lipids, will induce insulin secretion. Carbohydrates thus may have an advantage over fat, because insulin is a key anabolic hormone. Insulin inhibits glucose production, it stimulates glucose uptake in insulin-dependent tissues,[72] it inhibits lipolysis[73] and protein breakdown, and it stimulates protein synthesis by stimulating amino acid uptake in cells.[74] Insulin also stimulates glucose oxidation, with dose–response characteristics comparable to its effect on proteolysis.[65,75] Infusion of glucose at 4–5 g/kg(BW)/day results in plasma insulin levels of 20–30 μU/ml, which is in the same range as post-prandial insulin levels. Table 10.3 shows that the absolute gain in energy derived from glucose oxidation in healthy subjects is not impressive at plasma insulin levels higher than 25 mU/I, whereas the amount of glucose that will be stored is large. In addition to its influence on glucose oxidation, at insulin levels up to 30 μU/ml a significant anabolic effect on protein metabolism will be exerted.[76]

Table 10.3 – Mean rates for disposal, oxidation and storage of glucose in relation to plasma insulin concentrations in healthy subjects.

Plasma insulin (μU/ml)	Glucose disposal (g/70 kg/day)	Glucose oxidation (g/70 kg/day)	Glucose storage (g/70 kg/day)
22	315	281	34
34	580	307	273
39	624	327	297
49	671	443	228
80	890	408	482

Adapted[65,69,75]

Adult glucose requirements in healthy sedentary subjects can realistically be set at 4–5 g/kg/day, equivalent to 50% of the total energy requirement.

Glucose requirements in disease

In patients, REE may be only slightly increased – with the exception of critically ill patients (Fig. 10.2). Therefore, requirements for energy substrates are usually comparable to those in healthy sedentary subjects.

In almost all diseases (except for AIDS) glucose metabolism is characterised by insulin resistance.[77–87] Most of the studies on insulin resistance in disease have dealt with its effect on glucose production and glucose tissue uptake. When healthy and sick subjects are compared, infusion of similar amounts of glucose results in higher plasma glucose levels in patients, corresponding to their decreased glucose oxidation rate (Table 10.4) which can be overcome by exogenous infusion of insulin. Euglycaemic clamp studies reveal normal rates of glucose oxidation with plasma insulin concentrations in the range 45–90 μU/ml.[43,83,84,92] In healthy subjects, comparable glucose infusion rates without additional insulin result in similar glucose oxidation rates with insulin levels of only 2530 μU/ml. Thus it appears that when the quantity of glucose considered to be optimal in healthy subjects (4–5 g/kg/day) is given to patients and euglycaemia is maintained with additional insulin, glucose oxidation will be comparable to that in healthy subjects. The higher insulin concentration obtained in patients may have an additional advantage. Plasma insulin levels of 45–90 μU/ml induce a substantial suppression of proteolysis in healthy subjects.[43,74,80,93,94] However, it is not known whether these concentrations are also the optimal ones for patients because no dose–response curves have been published. The few publications dealing simultaneously with the effects of insulin on glucose and protein metabolism in insulin-resistant states suggest that the effect of insulin on protein metabolism is more or less maintained despite a marked resistance to insulin's effect on glucose metabolism.[81,94–96]

Table 10.4 – Glucose oxidation (expressed as percentage of tissue uptake) during infusion of glucose at 4 mg/kg/day.

Normal subjects	30–40
Elective surgery	20
Pancreatitis	20
Sepsis	20
Sepsis + cancer	10

Adapted[88–92]

In summary then, energy needs in sedentary/bed-ridden patients will hardly ever exceed 2500 kcal/day in an average 70 kg subject. The adult glucose requirement can be set at 4–5 g/kg/day, equivalent to approximately 50% of total daily energy expenditure. For optimal utilisation of glucose, exogenous insulin may be required to maintain euglycaemia.

Adult lipid requirements

Lipid requirements in healthy adults

Non-protein requirements are provided by carbohydrates and lipids, mainly triglycerides. As discussed in the section on adult glucose requirement, the optimal amount of glucose can be set at 4–5 g/kg/day. Lipid requirement can be calculated by subtracting energy derived from dietary glucose and protein from total energy expenditure and thus is about 1–1.5 g/kg/day. Unlike this indirect method, direct calculation of lipid requirement does not result in a clearly defined amount. The minimum requirement of lipid is reflected by the amount that is necessary to prevent deficiency of essential fatty acids (e.g linoleic and linolenic acid), which are necessary for the normal functioning of all tissues. An average daily provision of 3–4.5% of total calories as fat appears to be sufficient for prevention of this deficiency.[97] The maximum amount of lipids that can be administered is represented by total non-protein energy requirements. However, the utilisation of lipids, which are usually given as triglycerides, is difficult to evaluate owing to the complex nature of lipid metabolism. Lipids will be mainly presented to the peripheral tissues as triglycerides, as chylomicrons (containing absorbed triglycerides) or as very low density lipids (VLDL) (triglycerides secreted by the liver). Administration of lipids that completely cover non-protein energy requirements result in high plasma concentration of non-esterified fatty acids (NEFA), triglycerides and cholesterol.[98] Provision of lipids in amounts that largely cover total non-protein requirements results in a negative nitrogen balance even when given with adequate amounts of dietary protein.[64,99] Although this period of negative nitrogen balance lasts for about 5–8 days, it suggests that a diet consisting only of lipids and protein is less balanced than a lipid-carbohydrate-protein diet. For these reasons lipid requirements as derived from the indirect approach (1–1.5 g/kg/day), outlined in the first paragraph of this section, seem appropriate.

Lipid requirements in disease

Lipid requirements of patients can be calculated in the same way as has been described for healthy subjects, giving an equivalent requirement (1.5 g/kg/day). In disease there is an additional reason to be careful with the provision of dietary fat. One of the metabolic features of disease is stimulation of lipolysis, resulting in an increased availability of NEFA (Fig. 10.4). The administration of dietary glucose has a negative feedback on endogenous glucose production by stimulation of endogenous insulin secretion. Such a feedback system does not exist for fat metabolism because provision of lipids does not suppress lipolysis directly or indirectly. The release of NEFA into the bloodstream in healthy subjects after an overnight fast is equivalent to the dietary provision of 30–60 g of triglycerides per day.[47,89,100–103] In patients this amount is frequently much higher (Fig. 10.4). When exogenous fat is provided on top of this high endogenous lipolytic rate, extremely high levels of triglycerides and NEFAs can be expected. In a mixed diet containing glucose and protein, insulin secretion will be stimulated and lipolysis inhibited.[73] With the recommended glucose infusion rate (4–5 g/kg/day), NEFA release in healthy subjects will be suppressed to values equivalent to 10–20 g of triglyceride.[92,103,104] As stated before, one of the metabolic features of disease is insulin resistance.[77,84] No dose–response characteristics for the effect of insulin on lipolysis have been published for most diseases. Nevertheless a few studies in critically ill patients suggest that, despite stimulation of insulin secretion by provision of the recommended amount of glucose (with insulin levels up to 40–90 µU/ml), the equivalent of 40-100 g of triglycerides per day is still released as NEFA.[89,92,97,100,101]

Therefore, disease presents an invidious situation with respect to lipid metabolism and lipid requirements. The provision of an optimal diet will not result in adequate suppression of lipolysis. Dietary and endogenous lipids will compete for oxidation and re-esterification of the excess may occur. Therefore, in more critically ill patients lower amounts of exogenous lipids may be required. This inefficient metabolism of lipids will presumably persist until the disease severity decreases.

In summary, the optimal amount of fat in disease can be set at 1–1.5 g/kg(BW)/day, with lower values for the more critically ill patients (0.8–1.0 g/kg/day).

Acknowledgement

We acknowledge substantial secretarial support given by I. L. Jonker.

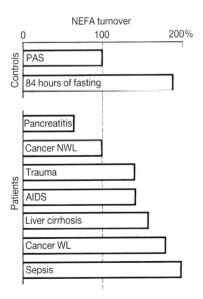

Figure 10.4 – Influence of disease on NEFA turnover. Measurements were done in the post-absorptive state (PAS) (for explanation see Fig. 10.2). Only studies with appropriate controls are included. NEFA = non-esterified fatty acid; NWL = not-weight losing; WL = weight-losing. (Adapted)[47,89,100,102]

References

1. Watters JM, Wilmore DW. The metabolic response to trauma and sepsis. In: DeGroot LJ (ed) *Endocrinology.* W.B. Saunders, Philadelphia, 1989; pp. 2367–2393.

2. Flatt JP. The biochemistry of energy expenditure. In: Bray GA (ed) *Obesity Research,* vol 2. Newman Publishing, London; 1978: 211–228.

3. Sims EA, Danforth E. Expenditure and storage of energy in man. *J Clin Invest* 1987; **79:** 1019–1025.

4. Acheson KJ, Schutz Y, Bessard T, Ravussin E, Jequier E, Flatt JP. Nutritional influences on lipogenesis and thermogenesis after a carbohydrate meal. *Am J Physiol* 1984; **246:** E62–70.

5. McGill DB, Jeejeebhoy KN. Longterm total parenteral nutrition. *Gastroenterology* 1974; **64:** 195–197.

6. Durschlag RP, Smith RJ. Principles of nutritional management. In: Becker KL (ed) *Principles and Practice of Endocrinology and Metabolism.* J.B. Lippincott, Philadelphia, 1990; pp. 1032–1038.

7. James WPT. From SDA to DIT to TEF. In: Kinney JM, Tucker HN (eds) *Energy Metabolism: Tissue Determinants and Cellular Corollaries.* Raven Press, New York, 1992; pp. 163–186.

8. Elia M. Energy expenditure in the whole body. In: Kinney JM, Tucker HN (eds) *Energy Metabolism: Tissue Determinants and Cellular Corollaries.* Raven Press, New York, 1992; pp. 19–59.

9. Duke JH, Jorgenson JB, Broell JR, Long L, Kinney JM. Contribution of protein to caloric expenditure following injury. *Surgery* 1970; **68:** 168–174.

10. Elwyn DH. Nutritional requirements of adult surgical patients. *Crit Care Med* 1980; **8:** 9–20.

11. Wilmore DW. *The Metabolic Management of the Critically Ill.* Plenum Medical, New York, 1977; pp. 36.

12. Carli F, Aber VR. Thermogenesis after major elective surgical procedures. *Br J Surg* 1987; **74:** 1041–1045.

13. Schoeller DA, Ravussin E, Schutz Y, Acheson KJ, Baertschi P, Jequier E. Energy expenditure by doubly-labelled water: validation in humans and proposed calculation. *Am J Physiol* 1986; **250:** R823–830.

14. Westerterp KR, Brouns F, Saris WHM, ten Hoor F. Comparison of doubly labelled water with respirometry at low- and high-activity levels. *J Appl Physiol* 1988; **65:** 53–56.

15. Riumallo JA, Schoeller D, Barrera G, Gattas V, Uauy R. Energy expenditure in underweight, free-living adults: impact of energy supplementation as determined by doubly labelled water and indirect calorimetry. *Am J Clin Nutr* 1989; **49:** 239–246.

16. Schulz S, Westerterp KR, Brijck K. Comparison of energy expenditure by the doubly labelled water technique with energy intake, heart rate and activity recording in man. *Am J Clin Nutr* 1989; **49:** 1146–1154.

17. Heini A, Schutz Y, Diaz E, Prentice AM, Whitehead RG, Jequier E. Free-living energy expenditure measured by two independent techniques in pregnant and non-pregnant Gambian women. *Am J Physiol* 1991; **261:** E9–17.

18. Ravussin E, Harper IT, Rising R, Bogardus C. Energy expenditure by doubly labelled water: validation in lean and obese subjects. *Am J Physiol* 1991; **261:** E402–409.

19. Roberts SB, Heyman MB, Evans WJ, Fuss P, Tsay R, Young VR. Dietary energy requirements of young adult men, determined by using doubly labelled water method. *Am J Clin Nutr* 1991; **54:** 499–505.

20. Ferraro R, Boyce VL, Swinburn B, DeGregorio M, Ravussin E. Energy cost of physical activity on a metabolic ward in relationship to obesity. *Am J Clin Nutr* 1991; **53:** 1368–1371.

21. Ravussin E, Lillioja S, Anderson TE, Christin L, Bogardus C. Determinants of 24-hour energy expenditure in man: methods and results using a respiration chamber. *J Clin Invest* 1986; **78:** 1568–1578.

21a. Reid CL, Carlson GC. Indirect calorimetry: a review of clinical applications. *Curr Opinion in Clin Nutr and Metabolic Care* 1998; **1:** 281–286.

22. Jequier E, Felber JP. Indirect calorimetry. *Clin Endocrin Metab* 1987; **4:** 911–937.

22a. McClare SA, Kleber MJ, Lowen CC. Indirect calorimetry: can this technology impact patient outcome? *Curr Opinion in Clin Nutr and Metabolic Care* 1999; **2:** 61–67.

23. Ferrannini E. The theoretical basis of indirect calorimetry: a review. *Metabolism* 1988; **37:** 287–301.

24. Simonson DC, DeFronzo RA. Indirect calorimetry: methodological and interpretative problems. *Am J Physiol* 1990; **258:** E399–412.

25. Welle S, Nair KS. Relationship of resting metabolic rate to body composition and protein turnover. *Am J Physiol* 1990; **258:** E990–998.

26. Ravussin E, Bogardus C. Relationship of genetics, age and physical fitness to daily energy expenditure and fuel utilization. *Am J Clin Nutr* 1989; **49:** 968–975.

27. Fukagawa N, Bandini LG, Young JB. Effect of age on body composition and resting metabolic rate. *Am J Physiol* 1990; **259:** E233–238.

28. Vaughan L, Zurlo F, Ravussin E. Ageing and energy expenditure. *Am J Clin Nutr* 1991; **53:** 821–825.

29. Zurlo F, Larson K, Bogardus C, Ravussin E. Skeletal muscle metabolism is a major determinant of resting energy expenditure. *Am J Clin Invest* 1990; **86:** 1423–1427.

30. Kinney JM. Indirect calorimetry in malnutrition: nutritional assessment or therapeutic reference. *J Parent Enter Nutr* 1987; **11:** 90S–94S.

31. Dubois EF. *Basal Metabolism in Health and Disease,* 2nd edn. Lea & Febiger, Philadelphia; 1924.

32. Tilstone WJ. The effects of environmental conditions on the metabolic requirements after injury. In: Lee HA (ed) *Parental Nutrition in Acute Metabolic Illness.* Academic Press, London, 1974: pp. 197–210.

33. Wilmore DW. *The Metabolic Management of the Critically Ill.* Plenum Medical, New York, 1977; pp. 57–83.

34. Goran M, Peters EJ, Herndon DN, Wolfe RR. Total energy expenditure in burned children using the doubly labelled water technique. *Am J Physiol* 1990; **259:** E576–585.

35. Pullicino EA, Coward WA, Elia M. Energy expenditure in intravenously fed patients using doubly-labelled water, 24-hour whole-body calorimetry and bedside calorimetry. *Clin Nutr* 1991; **10 (suppl 2):** 114.

36. Kusner RF, Schoeiler DA. Resting and total energy expenditure in patients with inflammatory bowel disease. *Am J Clin Nutr* 1991; **53:** 161–165.

37. Nixon DW, Kutner M, Heymsfield S *et al.* Resting energy expenditure in lung and colon cancer. *Metabolism* 1988; **37:** 1059–1064.

38. Weston PMT, King RFGJ, Goode AW, Williams NS. Diet-induced thermogenesis in patients with gastro-intestinal cancer cachexia. *Clin Sci* 1989; **77:** 133–138.

39. Fredrix EWHM. Energy metabolism in cancer patients. Thesis, University of Maastricht, 1990.

40. Schols A. Nutritional depletion and physical impairment in patients with chronic obstructive pulmonary disease. Thesis, University of Maastricht, 1991.

41. Hommes MJT, Romijn JA, Endert E, Sauerwein HP. Resting energy expenditure and substrate oxidation in asymptomatic human immunodeficiency virus (HIV) infected men. *Am J Clin Nutr* 1991; **54:** 311–316.

42. Hommes MJT, Romijn JA, Godfried MH *et al.* Increased resting energy expenditure in HIV-infected men. *Metabolism* 1990; **39:** 1186–1193.

43. Henderson AA, Frayn KN, Galasko CSB, Little RA. Dose-response relationships for the effects of insulin on glucose and fat metabolism in injured patients and control subjects. *Clin Sci* 1991; **80:** 25–32.

44. Carli F, Aber VR. Thermogenesis after major elective surgical procedures. *Br J Surg* 1987; **74:** 1041–1045.

45. Muller MJ, Fenk A, Lautz HU *et al.* Energy expenditure and substrate metabolism in ethanol-induced liver cirrhosis. *Am J Physiol* 1991; **260:** E338–344.

46. Shaw JHF, Wolfe RR. Glucose, fatty acid and urea kinetics in patients with severe pancreatitis. *Ann Surg* 1986; **204:** 665–672.

47. Shaw JHF, Wolfe RR. An integrated analysis of glucose, fat and protein metabolism in severely traumatized patients. *Ann Surg* 1989; **209:** 63–72.

48. Jeevanandam M, Young DH, Schiller WR. Glucose turnover, oxidation and indices of recycling in severely traumatized patients. *J Trauma* 1990; **30:** 582–589.

49. Christensen HN. Free amino acids and peptides in tissues. In: Munro HN, Allison JB (eds) *Mammalian Protein Metabolism,* vol 1. Academic Press, New York, 1964; pp. 105–124.

50. Waterlow JC, Garlick PJ, Millward DJ. *Protein Turnover in Mammalian Tissues and in the Whole Body.* Elsevier/North Holland, Amsterdam; 1978.

51. Munro HN, Crim MC. The proteins and amino acids. In: Shils ME, Young VR (eds) *Modern Nutrition in Health and Disease.* Lea & Febiger, Philadelphia, 1988; pp. 1–37.

52. Borst JGG. Protein catabolism in uraemia: effects of protein free diet, infection and blood transfusion. *Lancet* 1948; **i:** 824–825.

53. WHO/FAO/UNU report. *Energy and Protein Requirements.* WHO, Technical Report Series 724, Geneva; 1985.

54. Rose WC. The amino acid requirements in adult man. *Nutr Abs Rev* 1957; **27:** 631–647.

55. Young VR, Bier DM, Pellett PL. A theoretical basis for increasing current estimates of the amino acid requirements in adult man, with experimental support. *Am J Clin Nutr* 1989; **50:** 80–92.

56. Millward DJ, Rivers JPW. The nutritional role of indispensable amino acids and the metabolic basis for their requirements. *Eur J Clin Nutr* 1987; **42:** 367–393.

57. Calloway DH, Spector H. Nitrogen balance as related to caloric and protein intake in active young man. *Am J Clin Nutr* 1955; **2:** 405–412.

58. Jeevanandam M, Lowry SF, Horowitz GD, Legaspi A, Brennan MF. Influence of increasing dietary intake on whole body protein kinetics in normal man. *Clin Nutr* 1986; **5:** 41–48.

59. Rennie MJ, Edwards RHT, Halliday D, Matthews DE, Wolman SL, Millward DJ. Muscle protein synthesis measured by stable isotopes in man: the effect of feeding and fasting. *Clin Sci* 1982; **63:** 519–523.

60. Crane CW, Picou D, Smith R, Waterlow JC. Protein turnover in patients before and after elective orthopaedic operations. *Br J Surg* 1977; **64:** 129–133.

61. Birkhahn RH, Long CL, Fitkin D, Jeevanandam M, Blakemore WS. Whole body protein metabolism due to trauma in man, as estimated by L[15 N] alanine. *Am J Physiol* 1981; **241:** E64–71.

62. Shaw JHF, Wildbore M, Wolfe RR. Whole body protein kinetics in severely septic patients. *Ann Surg* 1987; **205:** 288–294.

63. Cerra F, Hirsch J, Mullen K, Blackburn G, Lutker W. The effect of stress level, amino acid formula, and nitrogen dose on nitrogen retention in traumatic and septic stress. *Ann Surg* 1987; **205:** 282–287.

64. Wolfe BM. Substrate-endocrine interactions and protein metabolism. *J Parent Enter Nutr* 1980; **4:** 188–194.

65. Henry RR, Thoburn AW, Beerdsen P, Gumbiner B. Dose-response characteristics of impaired glucose oxidation in non-insulin dependent diabetes mellitus. *Am J Physiol* 1991; **261:** E132–140.

66. DeFronzo RA, Jacot E, Jequier E, Maeder E, Wahren J, Felber JP. The effect of insulin on the disposal of intravenous glucose. *Diabetes* 1981; **30:** 1000–1007.

67. Jacot E, DeFronzo RA, Jequier E, Maeder E, Felber JP. The effect of hyperglycemia, hyperinsulinemia and route of glucose administration on glucose oxidation and glucose storage. *Metabolism* 1982; **31:** 922–930.

68. Thiebaud D, Jacot E, DeFronzo RA, Maeder E, Jequier E, Felber JP. The effect of graded doses of insulin on total glucose uptake, glucose oxidation and glucose storage in man. *Diabetes* 1982; **31:** 957–963.

69. Ferrannini E, Locatelli L, Jequier E, Felber JP. Differential effects of insulin and hyperglycemia on intracellular glucose disposition in humans. *Metabolism* 1989; **38:** 459–465.

70. McMahon MM, Marsh HM, Rizza RA. Comparison of extracellular and net glucose oxidation measured isotopically and by indirect calorimetry during high and low glucose turnover. *Am J Clin Nutr* 1991; **53:** 1138–1142.

71. Acheson KJ, Schutz Y, Bessard T, Anatharaman K, Flatt JP, Jequier E. Glycogen storage capacity and *de novo* lipogenesis during massive carbohydrate overfeeding in man. *Am J Clin Nutr* 1988; **48:** 240–247.

72. Rizza RA, Mandarino LJ, Gerich JE. Dose response characteristics for effects of insulin on production and utilization of glucose in man. *Am J Physiol* 1981; **240:** E630–639.

73. Nurjhan N, Campbell PJ, Kennedy FBP, Miles JM, Gerich JE. Insulin dose-response characteristics for suppression of glycerol release and conversion to glucose in humans. *Diabetes* 1986; **35:** 1326–1331.

74. Castellino P, Luzi L, Simonson DC, Haymond M, DeFronzo RA. Effect of insulin and plasma amino acid concentrations on leucine metabolism in man. *J Clin Invest* 1987; **SO:** 1784–1793.

75. Fukagawa NK, Minaker KI, Rowe JW *et al*. Insulin-mediated reduction of whole body protein breakdown: dose-response effects on leucine metabolism in post-absorptive men. *J Clin Invest* 1985; **76:** 2306–2311.

76. Tessari P, Pehling G, Nissen SL *et al*. Regulation of whole-body leucine metabolism with insulin during mixed-meal absorption in normal and diabetic humans. *Diabetes* 1988; **37:** 512–519.

77. Black PR, Brooks DC, Bessey PQ, Wolfe RR, Wilmore DW. Mechanisms of insulin resistance following injury. *Ann Surg* 1982; **196:** 420–435.

78. Cavallo-Perin P, Cassader M, Bozzo C *et al*. Mechanism of insulin resistance in human liver cirrhosis. *J Clin Invest* 1985; **75:** 1659–1665.

79. Copeland GP, Leinster SJ, Davis JC, Hipkin J. Insulin resistance in patients with colorectal cancer. *Br J Surg* 1987; **74:** 1031–1036.

80. Church JM, Hill GL. Impaired glucose metabolism in surgical patients improved by intravenous nutrition: assessment by the euglycemia-hyperinsulinemic clamp. *Metabolism* 1988; **37:** 505–509.

81. Alvestrand A, DeFronzo RA, Smith D, Wahren J. Influence of hyperinsulinaemia on intracellular amino acid levels and aminoacid exchange across splanchnic and leg tissues in uraemia. *Clin Sci* 1988; **74:** 155–163.

82. Shangraw RE, Jahoor F, Miyoshi H *et al*. Differentation between septic and post-burn insulin resistance. *Metabolism* 1989; **38:** 983–989.

83. Yki-Jarvinen H, Sammalkorpi K, Koivisto VA, Nikkila EA. Severity, duration and mechanisms of insulin resistance during acute infections. *J Clin Endocrin Metab* 1989; **69:** 317–323.

84. Brandl LS, Frediani M, Oleggini M *et al*. Insulin resistance after surgery: normalization by insulin treatment. *Clin Sci* 1990; **79:** 443–450.

85. Hommes MJT, Romijn JA, Endert E, Eeftinck Schattenkerk JKM, Sauerwein HP. Insulin sensitivity and insulin clearance in HIV infected men. *Metabolism* 1991; **40:** 651–656.

86. Sauerwein HP, Pesola GR, Godfried MH, Levinson MR, Jeevanandam M, Brennan MF. Insulin sensitivity in septic cancer-bearing patients. *J Parent Enter Nutr* 1991; **15:** 653–658.

87. Cersossimo E, Pisters PWT, Pesola GR *et al*. The effect of graded doses of insulin on peripheral glucose uptake and lactate release in cancer cachexia. *Surgery* 1991; **109:** 459–467.

88. Wolfe RR, O'Donnell TF, Stone MD, Richmond DA, Burke JF. Investigation of factors determining the optimal glucose infusion rate in total parenteral nutrition. *Metabolism* 1980; **29:** 892–900.

89. Shaw JHF, Wolfe RR. Glucose, fatty acid and urea kinetics in patients with severe pancreatitis. *Ann Surg* 1986; **204:** 665–672.

90. Shaw JHF, Wolfe RR. Determinations of glucose turnover and oxidation in normal volunteers and septic patients using stable and radio-isotopes: the responses to glucose infusion and total parenteral feeding. *Aust NZ J Surg* 1986; **56:** 785–791.

91. Humberstone DA, Shaw JHF. Isotopic studies during surgical convalescence. *Br J Surg* 1989; **76:** 154–158.

92. Sauerwein HP, Pesola GR, Groeger JS, Jeevanandam M, Brennan MF. Relationship between glucose oxidation and FFA oxidation in septic cancer-bearing patients. *Metabolism* 1988; **37:** 1045–1050.

93. Flakoll PJ, Kulaylat M, Frexes-Steed M *et al*. Amino acids augment insulin; suppression of whole-body proteolysis. *Am J Physiol* 1989; **257:** E839–837.

94. Fukagawa NK, Minaker KL, Rowe JW, Matthews DE, Bier DM, Young VR. Glucose and amino acid metabolism in aging man: differential effects of insulin. *Metabolism* 1988; **37:** 371–377.

95. Shangraw RE, Stuart CA, Prince MJ, Peters EJ, Wolfe RR. Insulin responsiveness of protein metabolism in *vivo* following bedrest in humans. *Am J Physiol* 1988; **255:** E548–58.

96. Brooks DC, Bessey PQ, Black PR, Aoki TT, Wilmore DW. Insulin stimulates branched chain amino acid uptake and diminishes nitrogen flux from skeletal muscle of injured patients. *J Surg Res* 1986; **40:** 395–405.

97. Burr LH, Dunn GD, Brennan MF. Essential fatty acid deficiency during parenteral nutrition. *Ann Surg* 1981; **193:** 304–311.

98. Wolfe BM, Ney DM. Lipid metabolism in parenteral nutrition. In: Rombeau JL, Caldwell MD (eds) *Parenteral Nutrition*. W.B. Saunders, Philadelphia, 1986; pp. 72–100.

99. Wolfe BM, Culebras JM, Sim AJW, Ball MR, Moore FD. Substrate interaction in intravenous feeding. *Ann Surg* 1977; **186:** 518–540.

100. Shaw JHF, Wolfe RR. Fatty acid and glycerol kinetics in septic patients and in patients with gastrointestinal cancer. *Ann Surg* 1987; **205:** 368–376.

101. Hommes MJT, Romijn JA, Endert E, Eeftinck Schattenkerk JKM, Sauerwein HP. Basal fuel homeostasis in symptomatic human immundeficiency virus infection. *Clin Sci* 1991; **80:** 359–365.

102. Romijn JA, Endert E, Sauerwein HP. Glucose and fat metabolism during short-term starvation in cirrhosis. *Gastroenterology* 1991; **100:** 731–737.

103. Jensen MD, Haymond MW, Gerich JE, Cryer PE, Miles JM. Lipolysis during fasting. *J Clin Invest* 1987; **79:** 207–213.

104. Bonadonna RC, Group LC, Zych K, Shank M, DeFronzo RA. Dose-dependent effect of insulin on plasma free fatty acid turnover and oxidation in humans. *Am J Physiol* 1990; **259:** E736–750.

11

Adult micronutrient requirements

Alan Shenkin

Introduction

Micronutrients can still be regarded as a 'Cinderella subject' in clinical nutrition. Of papers presented at international congresses, only a small proportion are concerned with micronutrients, the vast majority dealing with the major energy and amino acid components of the diet.

This may be for several reasons. Micronutrients are difficult to measure and therefore there is relatively little knowledge of requirements, especially in disease. Secondly, the effects of altering micronutrient intake often appear small in comparison with the more obvious effects of altering major nutrient intake. However, there is now a growing awareness that micronutrients have wide-ranging effects, far beyond the simple prevention of deficiency states. The interaction of disease on micronutrient requirements, both in terms of the effects of disease on the requirement, and the role of micronutrients in prevention of disease states, is now being extensively re-examined.

The term 'micronutrients' includes two main classes of nutrient substances required in the diet in very small amounts: the essential inorganic micronutrients (or trace elements) and the essential organic micronutrients (or vitamins). Other dietary micronutrients, such as co-enzyme Q, lipoic acid and carnitine, which

can be synthesised in the body and which are not recognised as being essential in artificial nutritional support, will not be included in this review. The major minerals of sodium, potassium, calcium, magnesium and phosphorus will also not be included.

Effects of suboptimal micronutrient intake

Every essential micronutrient has been initially identified as a result of the development of a clinical deficiency state (subsequently confirmed by biochemical evidence of deficiency), which is uniquely reversible by addition to the diet of that individual micronutrient. Such major clinical end-points may take months or even years to develop, and it is inevitable that patients will pass through various phases of impaired micronutrient status, of increasing severity, before this end-point is reached (Fig. 11.1).[1] It is becoming increasingly apparent that such conditions, often referred to as 'subclinical deficiency', are associated with some impairment in function, particularly of the immune system[2] and of the free radical scavenging mechanisms.[3] This might leave the individual at increased risk of developing a disease process such as infection, neoplastic disease, or coronary artery disease.[4] Controlled confirmation of

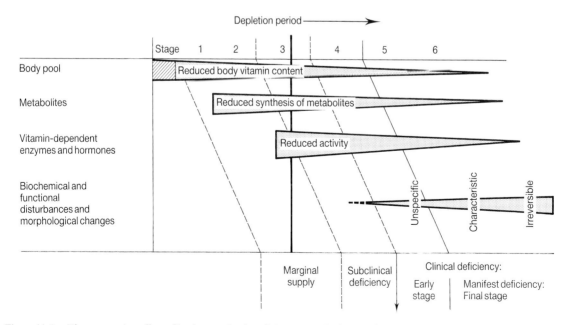

Figure 11.1 – The progressive effect of inadequate intake of vitamins (and of essential trace elements). Reproduced from Fidanza, p. 188[1] with permission.

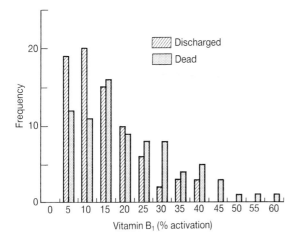

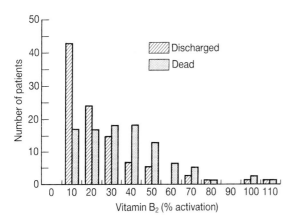

Figure 11.2 – Vitamin B_1 and B_2 status in relation to outcome in patients admitted to an intensive therapy unit. An abnormal vitamin B_1 status is defined as an activation of RBC trans-ketolase of greater than 25%, and abnormal vitamin B_2 status as activation of glutathione reductase of greater than 60%.[13,14] Reproduced with permission.

the specific effects of individual micronutrients is limited, but general observations convince us that on a population basis low intakes are associated with an increased incidence of disease.[5] Whether an *increased* intake which will normalise nutrition status will *reduce* the incidence of disease is as yet unproven.

Some recent studies have shed light on this. A trial of a multivitamin and trace element supplement in apparently healthy elderly individuals led to reduced infective illness over a one year period, and was associated with improved indices of lymphocyte

function.[6] Vitamin A supplements reduced infectious complications of measles.[7] Moreover, a trial of selenium supplements alone led to a reduction in lung, colorectal and prostate tumours but not in skin tumours.[8] Selenium (Se) is not only important in anti-oxidant defences, but also it specifically improves cytotoxic lymphocyte and natural killer cell functions.[9] An intriguing observation is that deficiency of a micronutrient (Se) may lead to the mutation of a harmless form of Coxsackie B virus to a harmful form, which might then cause cardiomyopathy.[10] This observation might explain why only a small proportion of all Se deficient patients develop symptoms.[11,12] It also has possible implications for other micronutrient deficiencies.

An example of subclinical deficiency in critically ill patients is shown in Fig. 11.2, where the vitamin B_1 and B_2 status at the time of admission to an intensive care unit is plotted in relation to outcome. Those patients who subsequently died had a greater incidence of abnormal vitamin B_1 status, and a poorer vitamin B_2 status despite being within the reference range.[13,14] None of the patients had clinical signs of deficiency. These results led to all subsequent patients receiving a bolus injection of water-soluble vitamins on admission to the intensive care unit.[13] Furthermore, in severely burned patients, a supplement of zinc, copper and selenium, designed to replace the extensive losses through the skin, has led to reduced infectious complications.[15]

Such observations therefore make it very difficult to recommend levels of intake which are optimal for the range of functions in which micronutrients are involved.

Effects of large intakes of micronutrients

A number of studies have suggested that some micronutrients (especially the water-soluble vitamins such as vitamin C and vitamin B_6) taken in doses much larger than those required to prevent depletion, may have clinical effects in prevention or treatment of disease states.[5] Recent studies have yielded contradictory results. A trial of high dose vitamin E supplements (400–800 mg) in patients with proven heart disease led to a reduced incidence of not-fatal myocardial infarction over a one-year period.[16] Moreover, in a trial of vitamin E supplements in a healthy elderly population, an intake of 200 mg/day led to an increased antibody response to hepatitis B vaccine, and increased delayed hypersensitivity skin response.[65] On the other hand, a six-year trial of low dose vitamin E (50 mg) and β-carotene had no effect on heart disease,[17] and this trial, and a further trial of β-carotene and retinyl palmitate[18] led to a higher risk of lung cancer. It seems clear therefore that when high dose micronutrients have an effect, this is more pharmacological than nutritional. However much more work is required to identify the types of high dose supplement which are associated with clinical benefit, and which types expose the individual to an increased risk of disease.

Functions of micronutrients

The micronutrients have two main functions (Fig. 11.3). Firstly, they have a key role in intermediary metabolism, as cofactors or coenzymes in enzyme catalysed reactions. Thus many of the trace elements (such as zinc or copper) either function as cofactors which activate the enzyme activity, or are an integral part of the prosthetic group of the enzyme itself. In general, the water-soluble vitamins have roles as co-enzymes, taking an active part in enzyme catalysed reactions. For both of these groups of substances, enzyme activity (and therefore the activity of a metabolic pathway) may be modulated by the availability of the micronutrient. In disease states, the metabolism of the major substrates is significantly increased, and therefore the requirements for micronutrients are also increased.

A second, and more recently identified, role for the micronutrients is as part of the free-radical scavenging system. Oxidative metabolism generates a family of reactive oxygen species (superoxide, hydroxyl, hydroperoxy) some of which contain unpaired electrons, and these have the potential to cause significant chemical damage owing to their high degree of chemical activity.[3,4] When oxidative metabolism is increased as a result of the metabolic response to disease, the production of such RUS is also increased. In the ischaemia–reperfusion syndrome which accompanies many surgical procedures, organs such as intestinal mucosa or myocardium are subjected to prolonged ischaemia and are then reperfused. The subsequent tissue damage is at least in part due to a burst of superoxide free radicals generated in endothelial cells.[19] The major oxidative damage is to the

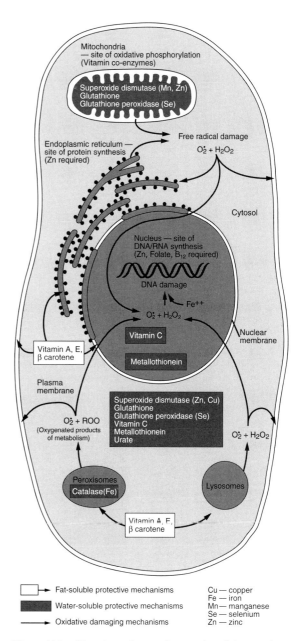

Figure 11.3 – Vitamins and trace elements in cellular metabolism. Modified from 'Clinical micronutrition, Gidden & Shenkin *Nursing Times*, 1997; **93 Suppl. 6.**

polyunsaturated fatty acid (PUFA) components of the various membrane structures, including intracellular nuclear membrane and cell membranes. Free-radical scavengers protect tissues from such oxidative damage. In addition there may be direct free-radical attack on DNA, causing strand breakage and formation of hydroxylated bases.[20]

A number of free-radical scavenging mechanisms exist. These include enzyme catalysed reactions which can remove some of the reactive oxygen species. Examples are copper and zinc in the form of cytoplasmic superoxide dismutase, and manganese in mitochondrial superoxide dismutase, these enzymes disposing of superoxide radicals.[21] Selenium in the form of the enzyme glutathione peroxidase will remove hydroperoxy compounds.[22] Vitamin C also has strong reductive activity[23] and is involved in recycling vitamin E.[4] Low vitamin C status is common in critically ill patients.[24] On the other hand, polyunsaturated substances such as vitamin E, vitamin A and beta-carotene can react directly with the free-radical species. It seems that the enzymes and vitamin C are particularly important in the cytoplasm and mitochondria, whereas the fat-soluble vitamins function within lipid components of cell membranes. Technical problems in measuring production and disposal of RUS have caused particular difficulty in quantifying and characterising this function.

The interaction of micronutrients with certain drugs may be important. Propofol, a lipid soluble anaesthetic agent which is widely used in intensive care, has antioxidant properties similar to vitamin E.[25]

Effects of disease on micronutrient requirements

Apart from the requirement for an increased intake of micronutrients to cope with the increase in metabolic rate and the increase in free-radical production, disease can affect micronutrient metabolism in two main ways. Firstly, there may be reduced absorption of any of the micronutrients in association with generalised malabsorption due to short gut, loss of integrity of intestinal mucosa (e.g. in coeliac disease or prolonged intravenous nutrition), or disorders of gastrointestinal motility. There may also be more specific malabsorption of particular micronutrients, such as fat-soluble vitamins in fat malabsorption, or vitamin B_{12} in pernicious anaemia. Rarely, there may be an inborn error of absorption (e.g. zinc in acrodermatitis enteropathica). Secondly, there may be an increased loss of water-soluble micronutrients, by such means as diarrhoea, nasogastric aspirate, fistula fluids, or renal dialysis. One extreme of the scale of this loss can be seen in burn injury where the amount of zinc, copper and selenium lost through the skin may be many times greater than that through all other routes.[26,27]

Patients requiring nutrition support therefore have an increased requirement for micronutrients. There may already be a significant whole-body deficit as a result of increased losses and inadequate replacement, and there is a continued need for an intake greater than that in health. The necessary intake for each patient cannot be predicted, and although the mixtures of micronutrients present in tube feeds and in intravenous additives may be adequate for the majority of patients, some patients may still require additional amounts of individual micronutrients (e.g. zinc, selenium or water-soluble vitamins).

Such additional intake is most likely to be required during the period of anabolism which follows a catabolic illness.[28] At this time of rapid protein synthesis and new tissue growth, micronutrient supply may become limited and an acute deficiency state may develop (e.g. a zinc deficiency rash[29] or selenium deficiency myopathy[30]).

Differences between enteral and parenteral requirement for micronutrients

Micronutrients, especially trace elements, show substantial variation in the efficiency with which they are absorbed and utilised within the body. The bioavailability is highly variable, often being low (less than 50%) and unpredictable. Factors which affect bioavailability include the nature of the diet. Examples include whether iron is present as haem or as inorganic iron, whether there are additional factors present in the diet (e.g. phytate) which may limit absorption, or whether other trace elements in the diet may compete for absorption. Iron, copper, and zinc may all compete with one another for absorption.[31] Moreover, the effectiveness of absorption and utilisation may be altered by the previous dietary supply, by the rate of net anabolism or catabolism, and by systemic and local endocrine or cytokine factors.[32]

It is therefore difficult to predict the requirements in parenteral infusions from the perceived enteral requirements. The effectiveness of intravenous supply may also be affected by inadequate or inappropriate binding to specific carrier proteins through bypassing the carrier mechanism at the gut. Additionally, bioavailability of trace elements in parenteral nutrition may vary as a result of provision of a trace element in an inappropriate inorganic state or valency (e.g. Cr^{6+} rather than Cr^{3+}), by complexes of trace elements to amino acids[33] or amino sugars which are lost in the urine,[34] or by interaction of inorganic cations with anionic species in the infusion leading to precipitation.[35]

Recommended intakes of micronutrients

The aforementioned variation in bioavailability partly explains the difficulty in establishing recommendations for intakes of micronutrients in health.[32,36] When coupled with the effects of disease the problem is magnified, and so recommendations for intakes in artificial nutrition are usually regarded as 'broad brush'. The problem is not too difficult for those micronutrients (such as most water-soluble vitamins) where there is a wide safety margin between effectiveness and toxicity. However, for the fat-soluble vitamins and for many trace elements (such as selenium) there is a relatively narrow margin of safety and caution is required to prevent overdosage. This is also true for nutrients where homeostasis is achieved by controlling absorption from the gut. Intravenous provision bypasses this normal control mechanism and intravenous supplements (e.g. of iron) must therefore be used with caution.[37] The object of supply by both enteral and parenteral routes is to achieve an intake into the circulation which will permit optimal tissue function, whilst preventing subclinical, or overt, deficiency or toxicity states (Fig. 11.4).

The Expert Panel on Dietary Reference Values in the UK has issued guidelines regarding nutrient intake.[32] For many nutrients, especially the major ones, the panel set an estimated average intake for the population, together with the mean plus two standard deviations (the reference nutrient intake RNI); 2.5% of the normal population has a requirement greater than this. They also set a lower reference nutrient intake at the mean minus two deviations, this being a value below which intake would be inadequate for 97.5% of the normal population. For most of the micronutrients it was not possible to set each of these values, and recommendations only for the upper limit,

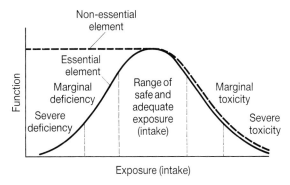

Figure 11.4 – Biological dose–response curves. All essential and non-essential elements (and fat-soluble vitamins) have toxic properties if intake is excessive. Depletion of all essential nutrients can be described by variants of the left-hand side of the curve.

that is the RNI, were made. These data are included in Tables 11.1 and 11.2 as the estimated oral requirement in health.

For some micronutrients, about which there is even less data but which nonetheless have important functions in humans, estimated safe intakes were proposed, at which there is little risk of deficiency and below the level at which there may be side-effects of toxicity. Such micronutrients include biotin, vitamins E and K, and the trace elements manganese, molybdenum and chromium.

Similar guidelines have been produced in the US, where the recommended daily allowance (RDA) is defined as the 'level of intake judged to be adequate to meet the known needs of practically all healthy persons'.[36] Because of the skewed distribution of requirements for many micronutrients, the US expert group tended to recommend a higher allowance of all micronutrients to ensure all normal individuals are included. For example, the RNI for zinc in males in the UK is 9.5 mg/day, whereas the RDA is 15 mg/day in the USA; the vitamin C recommendations are 40 mg/day in the UK and 60 mg/day in the USA.

Assessment and monitoring of micronutrient status

The problem of provision would not be so great if there were accurate and relatively simple tests which

Table 11.1 – Essential organic micronutrients (vitamins)

	Biochemical function	Effects of deficiency	Postulated subclinical deficiency	Main oral intake	Homeostasis	Risk of toxicity	Effects of toxicity
Vitamin A	Growth and development. Differentiation of tissues	Xerophthalmia. Impaired dark adaptation[56,57]	Increased risk of certain neoplasms[5] infections	Vegetables, especially carrots supply carotene. Fish oils, liver supply retinol	Poor. Extensive liver stores	Moderate	Liver disease. Skin rash
Vitamin D	Calcium absorption. Differentiation of macrophages	Osteomalacia in adults. Rickets in children	Effects on immune status[58,59]	Fish oils. Vegetable oils (Synthesis in skin)	Poor	High	Increased serum calcium. ? Role in bone disease of TPN[60,61]
Vitamin E	Antioxidant of membrane	Haemolytic anaemia in infants.[62] Central and peripheral neuropathy[63] Myopathy[64]	Increased risk of ischaemic heart disease, and cancer[4,5] Impaired immune function[65]	Vegetable oils	Poor	Low	Not known
Vitamin K	γ-carboxylation synthesis of coagulation factors, coagulation inhibitors and bone osteocalcin[66]	Bleeding disorders. ? Bone disorders[66]	Not known	Green vegetables. Beef liver. Gut flora	Poor	Low with natural Vitamin K	Few
B₁ (thiamin)	Decarboxylation in carbohydrate, fat and alcohol metabolism	Beri-beri with neurological, cardiac effects.[68] Wernicke-Korsakov syndrome[69]	Impaired immune function[70]	Germ of cereals, pulses. Yeast	Excess excreted in urine	Low	Anaphylaxis rarely. Chronic very high intake is toxic[32]
B₂ (riboflavin)	Oxidative metabolism	Lesions of lips, tongue and skin[72]	Possibly impaired immune function[70]	Liver, milk eggs, vegetables	Excess excreted in urine	Low	Not known

Effects of disease on requirements	Oral requirements per day[32]	Amount in 2000 Kcal tube feeds†	IV requirements/ recommendations per day[54,55]	Assessment of status[44,51]	Reference values[44,51]	Comments
Not known	M-300–700 µg RE F-250–600 µg RE	1000–2160 µg	1000 µg RE/day*§° as retinol, or retinol palmitate	Plasma retinol (C) Plasma retinol binding protein (C) Liver biopsy retinol (B)	1.3–3.0 µmol/l 30–60 mg/l	Fall in retinol during acute phase response due to fall in retinol binding protein
Not known	0 if <65 yr 10 µg if >65 yr	8.5–14.6 µg	5 µg*§ 200IU, 5.5 µg° ergocalciferol	Serum Ca/P/ alkaline phosphatase (A) Serum 25-hydroxy vit D (A) (Rarely, 1,25-dihydroxy vit D) (B)	5–25 µg/l, winter 10–60 µg/l, summer	
Not known	Related to PUFA M->4 mg F->3 mg	20–64 mg	10 mg*§, 11.2 mg° α tocopherol equivalents IV fat emulsions contain different amounts of α tocopherol	Plasma tocopherol/ cholesterol (A)	<2.25 µmol/ mmol	Vitamin E is transported in LDL
Increased in liver disease and fat malabsorption.[67] Problems in patients on anticoagulants	1 µg/kg	100–200 µg	150 µg*	Prothrombin time (A) Plasma phylloquinone (B) Results should be expressed per mmol triglyceride[66]	0.7–4.9 nmol/l	Time consuming assay
Increased with metabolic rate	0.4 mg/ 1000 kcal	1.4–3.4 mg	3.0 mg*§, 3.5 mg°	RBC transketolase (A) Blood thiamine (B) Urine thiamine/ creatinine (B)	High activation suggests deficiency 94–159 µmol/l 5.0–157 µmol/ mmol	Deficiency may occur and is reversed rapidly[71]
Increased with metabolic rate	M:1.3 mg F:1.1 mg	2–6 mg	3.6 mg*§, 4 mg° Sensitive to ultraviolet light	RBC glutathione reductase (A) Blood FAD (B) Urine riboflavin/ creatinine (A)	High activation suggests deficiency 210–350 nmol/l 11–45 nmol/mmol	

Table 11.1 – (continued).

	Biochemical function	Effects of deficiency	Postulated subclinical deficiency	Main oral intake	Homeostasis	Risk of toxicity	Effects of toxicity
B$_6$ (pyridoxine)	Transamination of amino acids	Anaemia in children. Lesions of lips and skin in children/adult	Premenstrual symptoms.[73] Carpal tunnel syndrome	Liver, whole grain cereals	Excess excreted in urine	Moderate	Neuropathy. Max intake 10mg/day
Niacin	NAD/NADP in oxidative metabolism	Pellagra – rash, weakness and diarrhoea	Not known	Meat, fish, cereals, yeast Tryptophan	Excess excreted in urine	Moderate	Hepatotoxicity. Cutaneous vasodilatation
Vitamin B$_{12}$	Recycling of folate coenzymes. Valine metabolism	Megaloblastic anaemia. Demyelination of neurones	Not known	Animal products, milk	Not known Extensive liver stores	Low	Not known
Folate	Single carbon transfer – purine/ pyrimidine metabolism	Megaloblastic anaemia. Growth retardation. Pancytopenia in IVN[76]	Neural tube defects in pregnancy. Elevated homocysteine[77]	Liver, green vegetables	Excess excreted in urine	Low	Reduced zinc absorption
Biotin	Carboxylase reactions – lipogenesis/ gluconeogenesis	Scaly dermatitis.[78,79] Hair loss	Not known	Most foods. Intestinal	Excretion in urine bacteria	Low	Not known
Vitamin C (ascorbic acid)	Antioxidant. Absorption of iron	Scurvy. Impaired wound healing[80]		Citrus fruits	Excretion in urine	Low	Oxalate stones Diarrhoea

would permit an assessment of the present status of each individual micronutrient, and which would allow the effectiveness and adequacy of provision of that particular micronutrient to be monitored during artificial nutrition. Such tests reflecting whole-body status are not readily available.

The most frequently used biochemical tests in assessment are the measurement of the micronutrient in plasma and serum. For some micronutrients this may provide a reasonable index of the status for that nutrient (e.g. vitamin B$_{12}$) whereas for others it may reflect the adequacy of recent intake (e.g. folate or selenium). The plasma concentration may also be helpful in reflecting excess provision of elements such as manganese and chromium.[11] For many other nutrients, interpretation of such measurements is seriously limited.

Firstly, since plasma only represents about 5% of total body water, the state of the nutrient within the intracellular compartment in most body tissues is not known. This is especially important for those nutrients which have substantial stores (e.g. vitamin A in the liver), or where there is a marked difference in content within different tissues (e.g. trace elements[38]).

Effects of Disease on requirements	Oral requirements per day[32]	Amount in 2000 Kcal tube feeds†	IV requirements/ recommendations per day[54,55]	Assessment of status[44,51]	Reference values[44,51]	Comments
Related to protein requirements	15 µg/g protein	2–13.8 mg	4.0 mg*§, 4.5 mg°	RBC transaminase (A)	High activation suggests deficiency	
				Blood pyridoxal phosphate (B)	39–98 nmol/l	Less interference by disease than for transaminase
				Urine 4 – pyridoxic acid (B)	Population specific	
Increase with metabolic rate	6.6 mg/ 1000 kcal	18–45 mg	40 mg*§, 46 mg°	Urine N-methyl nicotinamide (B)	>2.5 mg/24 h	Rarely measured
				Blood niacin (B)	>30 µmol	
Not known	1.5 µg	3–15 µg	5.0 µg*§, 6 µg°	Serum Vitamin B12 (A)	150–520 pmol/l	
				Serum homocysteine [74](B) or cystathionine[75](B)		
Not known	200 µg	340–880 µg	400 µg*§, 414 µg° May interact with copper	Serum folate (A)	>3 µg/l	
				RBC folate (A)	>150 µg/l	
				Serum homocysteine[74,75]		
Not known	10–200 µg	100–660 µg	60 µg*§, 69 µg°	Serum biotin (B)	>0.5 nmol/l	Rarely assayed
				Urine biotin (B)	120–240 nmol/ 24 h	
Increased – amount not known	40 mg	100–300 mg	100 mg*§, 125 µg° Readily oxidised in infusion mixture	Leucocyte Vit C (B)	>0.1 µmol/10⁸ cells	Plasma conc. falls in injury or infection[44]
				Plasma Vit C (C)	>11 µmol/l	

† The range of amounts in various tube feeds, including Ensure (Abbott, Maidenhead, UK), Nutrison (Nutricia Clinical, Wilts, UK), Fresubin (Fresenius, Birchwood, Warrington, UK), Clinifeed (Nestlè, Surrey, UK), Elemental 028 (Scientific Hospitals Supplies (SHS) Int. Ltd, Liverpool, UK)
* The amount present in Vitalipid N (Fresenius Kabi)
§ The amount present in MVI-12 (Astra Zeneca)
+ The amount present in Solivito N (Fresenius Kabi))
° The amount present in Cernerit (Baxter)
RE – Retinol equivalents
PUFA – Polyunsaturated fatty acids
(A) – tests which are widely available and clinically useful
(B) – good markers of status but of limited availability
(C) – tests of little value in assessing status

Secondly, the concentration in plasma can alter rapidly during redistribution between body components due to the acute phase response to trauma or infection. An example is the uptake of zinc or iron into the liver in response to the induction of synthesis of metallo-thionein[39] and ferritin[40] respectively, and release of copper from the liver in the form of caeruloplasmin. These changes in plasma concentration clearly do not reflect changes in whole-body status.[41] Thirdly, there may be changes in the binding proteins within plasma. A fall in serum albumin for whatever cause will inevitably be associated with a fall in serum zinc, and similarly a fall in retinol binding protein, which is typical either in the acute-phase response or in malnutrition, will lead to a fall in serum retinol, although there may be adequate stores of retinol within the liver.[42]

On the other hand, provided there is no acute phase response to injury, infection or other inflammatory stimulus, it may be possible to interpret changes in serum or plasma concentration of these nutrients. This may be the case in many patients receiving long-term nutrition support where the serum zinc does broadly reflect the amount of zinc intake.[11,43] Hence an assessment of the acute-phase response, by

Table 11.2 – Essential inorganic micronutrients (trace elements)

	Biochemical function	Effects of deficiency	Postulated subclinical deficiency	Main oral intake	Homeostasis	Risk of toxicity	Effects of toxicity
Zinc	Enzymes of intermediary metabolism and protein synthesis. Structural proteins controlling gene transcription	Growth retardation.[83] Diarrhoea. Skin rash.[29] Immune deficiency[84]	Loss of appetite.[85] Impaired wound healing	Red meat, unrefined flour. Usually about 30% absorbed – less in high fibre diet	Regulation by gut absorption and faecal loss	Moderate	Acute – nausea/ vomiting. Chronic – copper and iron deficiency
Copper	Cytochrome oxidase. Superoxide dismutase. Neuroactive amines (e.g enkephalins)	Hypochromic anaemia.[88] Neutropenia. Subperiosteal bleeding.[89] Cardiac arrhythmia	Not known	Green vegetables, fish, liver. About 35–70% absorbed	Mainly excreted in bile. Little in urine	Low	Chronic toxicity – similar to Wilson's Disease
Selenium	Glutathione peroxidase – protection against oxidative damage. Thyroxine deiodinase	Skeletal myopathy.[92] Cardio-myopathy.[93] Macrocytosis.[94] Pseudo-albinism[94]	Increased risk of neoplastic disease	Cereals, fish, meat. About 65% absorbed	Mainly excreted in urine	High	Nail dystrophy. Gastrointestinal intestinal upset
Manganese	Mitochondrial superoxide dismutase, arginase, co-factor for hydrolases, kinases	Lipid abnormalities.[96] Anaemia		Tea, cereals green vegetables. Low absorption	Biliary excretion	Low	Chronic inhalation toxicity. Possibly neurological damage[97,98]
Chromium	Organic complex – insulin activity – lipoprotein metabolism. Gene expression	Glucose intolerance.[101] Weight loss.[102,103] Peripheral neuropathy[104]		Yeast, meat, whole grain	Urine excretion	Low	Hexavalent form can cause renal or liver damage
Molybdenum	Xanthine oxidase in DNA metabolism. Sulphite oxidase in S metabolism	Intolerance to sulphur amino acids.[107] Tachycardia, visual upset		Meat, vegetables. Common pathway with copper absorption	Urine excretion	Low	Impaired copper absorption. Altered purine metabolism

Effects of disease on requirements	Oral requirements/ recommendations per day[32]	Amount in 2000 Kcal tube feed†	IV requirements/ recommendations per day[47,55,81,82]	Assessment of status[44,51]	Reference values[44,51]	Comments
Increased loss in fistula/ diarrhoea.[86] Increased urine loss in hypercatabolism[87]	M-5.5–9.5 mg (85–145μmol) F-4.0–7.0 mg (60–110μmol)	13–36 mg	3.2–6.5★ mg (50–100★ μmol)	Plasma zinc – alone (C) with albumin and C-reactive protein (A) Leucocyte zinc[45] (B) Alkaline phosphatase (C) Hair zinc (C)	12–18 μmol/l 35–55 g/l <10 mg/l LRV LRV LRV	Plasma Zn falls in acute phase reaction
Increased loss in biliary fistula.[90] Reduced excretion in obstructive jaundice	1.2 mg (19 μmol)	2–3.4 mg	0.3–1.3★ mg (5–20★ μmol)	Plasma copper/ caeruloplasmin with CRP (A) Liver copper (B) Cu, Zn superoxide dismutase[91] Factor VIII Cyt c oxidase	10–25 μmol/l 150–300 mg/l <10 mg/l LRV LRV	Plasma Cu increases in acute phase reaction
Not known ? increased	M-40–75 μg (500–900 nmol) F-40–60 μg (500–800 nmol)	30–130 μg	30★–60 μg (400★–800 nmol)	Plasma Se (A)[95] Rbc glutathione peroxidase (A) Urine Se (B) Whole blood Se (B) Platelet glutathione peroxidase (B)	0.8–2.0 μmol LRV LRV >0.2 μmol/l LRV	Pre-illness Se status varies depending on total Se intake. Depletion may be asymptomatic
Reduced excretion in cholestasis[99]	>1.4 mg (26 μmol)	2.4–8 mg	0.2–0.3★ mg (3–5★ μmol)	Plasma Mn (B) Mitochondrial superoxide dismutase (C)[100] Whole blood Mn (B)	7–27 nmol/l LRV 73–255 nmol/l	Deficiency state not confirmed in man
Not known	>25 μg (500 nmol)	30–200 μg	10★–20 μg (200★–400 nmol) Variably present as contaminant of albumin and amino acid solutions[105,106]	Plasma Cr (B) Glucose tolerance (C)	2–10 nmol/l	Contamination free blood sampling
Not known	50–400 μg (0.5–4 μmol)	74–240 μg	19 μg (400★nmol)	Urine xanthine[107] (B) hypoxanthine (B) sulphite (B) Plasma Mo (B)	LRV LRV LRV LRV	Rarely measured

Table 11.2 – continued).

	Biochemical function	Effects of deficiency	Postulated subclinical deficiency	Main oral intake	Homeostasis	Risk of toxicity	Effects of toxicity
Iron	Haemoglobin Myoglobin Cytochrome system	Anaemia	Possibly increased resistance to infection[37]	Meat, fish Haem iron better absorbed (about 30%). Non-haem iron absorption increased by Vit C	Regulation of gut absorption	Moderate	Acute toxicity potentially fatal. Chronic toxicity leads to haemosiderosis
Iodine	Thyroxine and triiodothyronine – cellular metabolism	Hypothyroidism in adults. Cretinism in infants. Goitre		Milk, sea food	Mainly excreted in urine	Low	Toxic nodular goitre
Fluoride	Bone mineralisation as calcium fluorapatite		Dental caries	Tea, drinking water	Urine excretion	Moderate	Acute toxicity may be fatal. Chronic toxicity leads to fluorosis of teeth and bone

measurement of a typical acute-phase reactant such as C-reactive protein, may facilitate interpretation (Fig. 11.5).

For some micronutrients, measurements on erythro-cytes or white blood cells can yield useful information which reflects whole-body status, and the processing of the cells themselves may not be too difficult. Thus measurement of the activation of red cell enzymes such as transketolase gives an index of thiamine status, red cell transaminase indicates vitamin B_6 status, and red cell glutathione peroxidase indicates selenium status.[44] Similarly, red cell folate has been widely used as a good index of whole-body folate status. On the other hand, leucocyte measurements have been demonstrated to provide a good index of body status for vitamin C[44] and for zinc,[45] although preparation of the white cells is more difficult. Urinary excretion of vitamins, or their metabolites, has been helpful in

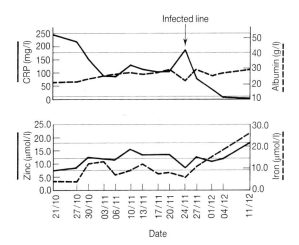

Figure 11.5 – Development and resolution of an acute-phase response leads to changes in serum CRP (reference range < 10 mg/l), with reciprocal changes in serum albumin (40–52 g/l), serum zinc (12–18 μmol/l) and serum iron (9–30 μmol/l).

Effects of disease on requirements	Oral requirements/ recommendations per day[32]	Amount in 2000 Kcal tube feed†	IV requirements/ recommendations per day[47,55,81,82]	Assessment of status[44,51]	Reference values[44,51]	Comments
Increased in blood loss	M-4.7–8.7 mg (80–160 µmol) F-8.0–14.8 mg (140–260 µmol)	18–27 mg	1.2 mg★ (20 µmol★) + blood transfusion as required[108,109]	Serum iron/ IBC (C) Serum ferritin with CRP (A) Bone marrow iron (B)	>16% saturation >12 µg/l <10 mg/l	Serum Fe concentration falls in APR– care needed not to exceed IBC
Not known	140 µg (1.1 µmol)	120–220 µg	131 µg (1 µmol★)	SerumT₄ (A) T₃ (A) TSH (A)	70–155 nmol/l 1.4–3.2 nmol/l 0.2–4.0 mu/l	
Not known	0.05 mg/kg (3 µmol/kg)	NR – 1.6 mg	0.95 mg (50 µmol★)	Urine excretion	LRV	Provision in nutritional support is controversial

† The range of amounts present in various tube feeds, including Ensure (Abbott, Maidenhead, UK), Nutrison (Nutricia Clinical, Wilts, UK), Fresubin (Fresenius, Birchwood, Warrington, UK), Clinifeed (Nestlè Clinical, Surrey, UK), Elemental 028 (Scientific Hospital Supplies (SHS) Int. Ltd., Liverpool, UK)
★ The amount present in the commonly used intravenous trace elements additive Additrace (Fresenius Kabi))
LRV – local reference values required
(A) – tests which are widely available and clinically useful
(B) – good markers of status but of limited availability
(C) – tests of little value in assessing status
NR – not reported

population studies but is rarely useful in the individual patient.

Commonly used tests for the micronutrients, together with some of their limitations, are summarised in Tables 11.1 and 11.2. Despite this extensive test list, it is likely that the only micronutrients which require regular assessment are zinc, copper, selenium, iron and folate. Other micronutrients are only assessed when there is a specific indication.

A summary of micronutrient metabolism and biochemistry

Tables 11.1 and 11.2 provide an overview of the properties and requirements of micronutrients.

Inevitably such a summary is highly selective and a limited bibliography which focuses on deficiency and supply during nutrition support is therefore provided for most of the entries.

It is interesting to note the differences between the oral and intravenous recommendations which arise from the following considerations:

- The oral recommendations are those for a healthy adult. Most adults requiring artificial enteral nutrition have a higher requirement for micro-nutrients, and indeed many tube feeds provide amounts at least twice these recommendations.

- Absorption from the oral diet is variable.

- Patients requiring intravenous nutrition are more likely to have a degree of depletion on commencing feeding, and may be more seriously ill than those receiving enteral nutrition.

These recommendations are only general guidelines, but in practice they provide a good starting point for assessing the intake of the individual. Specific patients may, however, have requirements different from these, especially when the intravenous route is used.

Ultra-trace elements

Apart from the essential trace elements summarised in Table 11.2, there are many others which have been considered to be essential in plants and some laboratory animals, but which have not been convincingly proven to be essential in man,[32,36] although they may be beneficial. Elements in this category include nickel, silicon, tin, vanadium, boron and arsenic.[46] For the purposes of nutrition support it is generally considered that if there is a need for such elements, adequate amounts will be obtained from contaminants of the other nutrients provided. Analysis of most artificial nutrients reveals a wide range of contaminating elements.[47]

Provision of micronutrients during nutrition support

Most of the preparations currently used as tube feeds in the UK now contain adequate amounts of micronutrients for the typical patient. These amounts are considerably in excess of the recommendations shown in the tables for intake in the oral diet in health. Additives of selenium, chromium and molybdenum have been made recently to many, to ensure that they are suitable for long-term use. If patients require additional supplements, either because of a pre-existing depletion or because of continued losses, care must be taken not to inhibit absorption of other elements in the diet (e.g. iron supplements may reduce zinc absorption[48]). Supplements should either be given separately from the rest of the feed, or a mixture of elements provided.

From the parenteral point of view, interactions within the nutritive mixture must be minimised. Thus infusions of trace elements and vitamins should ideally be separate to avoid oxidation of ascorbic acid under the action of copper.[49] Oxidation of ascorbic acid can also be minimised if multi-layered bags are used instead of the more oxygen permeable ethyl vinyl acetate bags.[50] Complete nutritive mixtures have been demonstrated to be as effective as separate infusions in short-term feeding.[51] The vitamins and trace elements are therefore usually added to the mixture immediately before infusion. This also minimises the possibility of absorption of fat-soluble vitamins onto the plastic bag and infusion set,[52] and the potential for photo-degradation of vitamins under the action of ultraviolet light.[53] This can be further minimised by addition of the vitamins to the fat emulsions, usually as part of an 'all-in-one' mixture, where the turbidity provides protection.

Conclusions

Micronutrients are an essential part of the diet, and preparations now exist to ensure that all patients receiving either enteral or parenteral nutrition have a broadly adequate intake. Difficulties still remain in assessing whole-body status of many of the micronutrients, especially in the critically ill patient. Thus patients may not receive an intake optimal for their own condition, and they run a variable risk of developing a subclinical deficiency syndrome. Prevention of this may be important not only in minimising complications in the short term, but also in maintaining long-term health in the growing number of patients requiring prolonged nutrition support. Continued effort is therefore required to identify the requirements of the individual patient. This will require new approaches to the study of metabolism, tissue function and outcome in relation to micronutrient status.

References

1. Fidanza F, Brubacher GB. Vitamin nutritive methodology. In: Fidanza F (Ed) *Nutritional Status Assessment*. Chapman & Hall, London, 1991; pp. 186–191.

2. Chandra RK. Nutrition and the immune system. *Proc Nut Soc* 1993; **52:** 77–84.

3. Furst P. The role of antioxidants in nutritional support. *Proc Nut Soc* 1996; **55:** 945–961.

4. Halliwell B. Free radicals, antioxidants, and human disease: curiosity, cause, or consequence? *Lancet* 1994; **344:** 721–724.

5. Gaby SK, Bendich A, Singh VN, Machlin LJ. Vitamin intake and health – A scientific review. Marcel Dekker, New York, 1991; pp. 1–217.

6. Chandra RK. Effect of vitamin and trace-element supplementation on immune responses and infection in elderly subjects. *Lancet* 1992; **340:** 1124–1127.

7. Glasziou PP, Mackerras DEM. Vitamin A supplementation in infectious diseases: a meta-analysis. *Br Med J* 1993; **306:** 366–369.

8. Clark LC, Combs GF, Turnbull BW *et al.* Effects of selenium supplementation for cancer prevention in patients with carcinoma of the skin. *J Am Med Assoc* 1996; **276:** 1957–1963.

9. Kiremidjian-Schumacher L, Roy M, Wishe HI, Cohen MW, Stotzky G. Supplementation with selenium and human immune cell functions II. Effect on cytotoxic lymphocytes and Natural Killer Cells. *Biol Trace El Res* 1994; **41:** 115–127.

10. Beck M, Shi Q, Morris VC, Levander OA. Rapid genomic evolution of a non-virulent Coxsackie virus B₃ in selenium deficient mice results in selection of identical isolates. *Nature Med* 1995; **1:** 433–436.

11. Shenkin A, Fell GS, Halls DJ, Dunbar PM, Holbrook IB, Irving MH. Essential trace element provision to patients receiving home intravenous nutrition in the United Kingdom. *Clin Nutr* 1986; **5:** 91–97.

12. Rannem TRJE, Ladefoged K, Hylander E *et al.* The effect of selenium supplementation on skeletal and cardiac muscle in selenium-depleted patients. *JPEN* 1995; **19:** 351–355.

13. Cruickshank AM, Telfer ABM, Shenkin A. Thiamine deficiency in the critically ill. *Intens Care Med* 1988; **14:** 384–387.

14. Shenkin SD, Cruickshank AM, Shenkin A. Subclinical riboflavin deficiency is associated with outcome of seriously ill patients. *Clin Nutr* 1989; **8:** 269–271.

15. Berger MM, Spertini F, Shenkin A *et al.* Trace element supplementation modulates pulmonary infection rates after major burns: a double-blind placebo-controlled trial. *Am J Clin Nutr* 1998; **68:** 365–371.

16. Stephens NG, Parsons A, Schofield PM *et al.* A randomised controlled trial of Vitamin E in patients with coronary disease: The Cambridge Heart Antioxidant Study (CHAOS). *Lancet* 1996; **347:** 781–786.

17. The Alpha-Tocopherol, Beta-Carotene Cancer Prevention Study Group. The effect of vitamin E and beta-carotene on the incidence of lung cancer and other cancers in male smokers. *New Eng J Med* 1994; **330:** 1029–1035.

18. Omenn GS, Goodman GE, Thornquist MD *et al.* Effects of combination of beta carotene and vitamin A on lung cancer and cardiovascular disease. *N Engl J Med* 1996; **334:** 1150–1155.

19. Schiller HJ, Reilly PM, Bulkley GB. Antioxidant therapy. *Crit Care Med* 1993; **21:** S92–S102.

20. Shigenaga MK, Ames BN. Assays for 8-hydroxy-2-deoxyguanosine: a biomarker of in vivo oxidative DNA damage. *Free Radic Biol Med* 1991; **10:** 211–216.

21. Dreosti IE. The physiological biochemistry and antioxidant activity of the trace elements copper, manganese, selenium and zinc. *Clin Biochem Rev* 1991; **12:** 127–129.

22. Diplock AT. Metabolic and functional defects in selenium deficiency. *Phil Trans Roy Soc Lond* 1981; **294:** 105–117.

23. Levine M. New concepts in the biology and biochemistry of ascorbic acid. *New Engl J Med* 1986; **314:** 892–902.

24. Schorah CJ, Downing C, Piripitsi A *et al.* Total vitamin C, ascorbic acid, and dehydroascorbic acid concentrations in plasma of critically ill patients. *Am J Clin Nutr* 1996; **63:** 760–765.

25. Aarts L, van der Hee R, Dekker I *et al.* The widely used anesthetic agent propofol can replace α-tocopherol as an antioxidant. *FEBS Lett* 1995; **357:** 83–85.

26. Bayer-Berger MM, Cavadini C, Mansourian R *et al.* Zinc, copper and selenium cutaneous loss and balances in burn patients. *J Trace Elem Exper Med* 1989; **2:** 208.

27. Berger MM, Cavadini C, Bart A *et al.* Selenium losses in 10 burned patients. *Clin Nutr* 1992; **11:** 75–82.

28. Tasman-Jones C, Kay RH, Lee SP. Zinc and copper deficiency with particular reference to parenteral nutrition. In: Nybus M (Ed) *Surgery Annual* 1978; Appleton, New York, pp. 23–52.

29. Kay RG, Tasman-Jones C, Pybus J, Whitney R, Black H. A syndrome of acute zinc deficiency during total parenteral alimentation in man. *Ann Surg* 1976; **183:** 331–340.

30. Van Rij AM., Thompson CD., McKenzie JM, Robinson MF. Selenium deficiency in total parenteral nutrition. *Am J Clin Nutr* 1979; **32:** 2076–2085.

31. O'Dell BL. Bioavailability of trace elements. *Nutr Rev* 1984; **42:** 301–308.

32. Panel on Dietary Reference Values, Department of Health. Dietary reference values for food energy and nutrients for the United Kingdom. HMSO, London, 1991.

33. Berthon G, Matuchansky C, May PM. Computer simulation of metal ion equilibria in biofluids. 3: Trace metal supplementation in total parenteral nutrition. *J Inorg Chem* 1980; **13:** 63–73.

34. Stegink LD, Freeman DB, Den Besten L, Filer LJ. Maillard reaction products in parenteral nutrition. *Prog Food Nutr Sci* 1981; **5:** 265–278.

35. Hall SB, Duffield JR, Williams DR, Barnett MI, Cosslett AG. Computer program for safety assessment and optimization of parenteral nutrition formulations based on chemical speciation analysis. *Nutrition* 1992; **8:** 167–176.

36. Food and Nutrition Board, National Research Council. *Recommended dietary allowances, 10th edn.* National Academy Press, Washington, 1991.

37. Weinberg ED. Iron and infection. *Microbiol Rev* 1978; **42:** 45–66.

38. Martin BJ, Lyon TDB, Fell GS. Comparison of inorganic elements from autopsy tissue of young and elderly subjects. *J Trace Elem Elect Hum Dis* 1991; **5:** 203–211.

39. Cousins RJ. Absorption, transport and hepatic metabolism of copper and zinc: special reference to metallothionein and ceruloplasmin. *Physiol Rev* 1985; **65:** 238–309.

40. Konijn AM, Carmel N, Levy R, Hershko C. Ferritin synthesis in inflammation. II: Mechanisms of increased ferritin synthesis. *Br J Haematol* 1981; **49:** 361–370.

41. Fraser WD, Taggart DP, Fell GS *et al.* Changes in iron, zinc and copper concentrations in serum and in their binding to transport proteins after cholecystectomy and cardiac surgery. *Clin Chem* 1989; **35:** 2243–2247.

42. Olson JA. New approaches to methods for the assessment of nutritional status of the individual. *Am J Clin Nutr* 1982; **36:** 1160–1168.

43. Malone M, Shenkin A, Fell GS, Irving MH. Evaluation of a trace element preparation in patients receiving home intravenous nutrition. *Clin Nutr* 1989; **8:** 307–312.

44. Sauberlich HE. Laboratory tests for the assessment of nutritional status. CRC Press. Boca Raton, 2nd ed, 1999.

45. Goode HF, Kelleher J, Walker BE. The effects of acute infection on indices of zinc status. *Clin Nutr* 1991; **10:** 55–59.

46. Neilsen FN. How should dietary guidance be given for mineral elements with beneficial actions or suspected of being essential? *J Nutr* 1996; **126:** 2377S–2385S.

47. Jacobson S, Wester PO. Balance study of twenty trace elements during total parenteral nutrition in man. *Br J Nutr* 1977; **37:** 107–126.

48. Solomons NW, Pineda O, Viteri F, Stanstead HH. Studies in the bioavailability of zinc in humans: mechanisms of the intestinal interactions of non-heme iron and zinc. *J Nutr* 1983; **113:** 337–349.

49. Allwood MC. Factors affecting the stability of ascorbic acid in total parenteral nutrition infusions. *J Clin Hosp Pharm* 1984; **6:** 75–85.

50. Allwood MC, Brown PE, Ghedini C, Hardy G. The stability of ascorbic acid in TPN mixtures stored in a multi-layered bag. *Clin Nutr* 1992; **11:** 284–288.

51. Shenkin A, Fraser WD, McLelland AJD, Fell GS, Garden OJ. Maintenance of vitamin and trace element status in intravenous nutrition using a complete nutritive mixture. *J Parent Enter Nutr* 1987; **11:** 238–242.

52. Gillis J, Jones G, Penchary P. Delivery of vitamins A, D and E in total parenteral nutrition solutions. *J Parent Enter Nutr* 1983; **7:** 11–14.

53. Allwood MC, Kearney MCJ. Compatibility and stability of additives in parenteral nutrition admixtures. *Nutrition* 1998; **14:** 697–706.

54. American Medical Association, Department of Food and Nutrition. Multivitamin preparations for parenteral use: a statement by the Nutrition Advisory Group. *J Parent Enter Nutr* 1979; **3:** 258–265.

55. Shenkin A. Clinical aspects of vitamin and trace element metabolism. Bailliere's *Clin Gastroenter* 1988; **2:** 765–798.

56. Main ANH, Mills PR, Russell RI *et al.* Vitamin A deficiency in Crohn's disease. *Gut* 1983; **24:** 1169–1175.

57. Howard L, Chu R, Freman S, Mintz H, Oversen L, Wolf B. Vitamin A deficiency from long-term parenteral nutrition. *Ann Int Med* 1980: **93:** 576–577.

58. Gray TK, Cohen MS. Vitamin D, phagocyte differentiation and immune function. *Surv Immunol Res* 1985; **4:** 200–212.

59. Manolagas SC, Hustmeyer FG, Yu XP. 1,25-dihydroxy vitamin D_3 and the immune system. *Proc Soc Exp Biol Med* 1989; **191:** 238–245.

60. Koo WWK. Parenteral nutrition related bone disease. *J Parent Ent Nutr* 1992; **16:** 386–394.

61. Verhage AH, Cheong WK, Allard JP, Jeejeebhoy KN. Increase in lumbar spine bone mineral content in patients on long-term parenteral nutrition without vitamin D supplementation. *JPEN* 1995; **6:** 431–436.

62. Ritchie JH, Fish MB, McMasters V *et al.* Edema and hemolytic anemia in premature infants: a vitamin E deficiency syndrome. *New Engl J Med* 1968; **279:** 1185–1190.

63. Howard L, Oversen L, Satya Marti S, Chu R. Reversible neurological symptoms caused by vitamin E deficiency in a patient with short bowel syndrome. *Am J Clin Nutr* 1982; **36:** 1243–1249.

64. Bieri JG, Farrell PM. Vitamin E. *Vit Horm* 1976; **34:** 31–75.

65. Meydani SN, Meydani M, Blumberg JB, Lynette LS, Siber G *et al.* Vitamin E supplementation and in vivo immune response in healthy elderly subjects – A randomised controlled trial. *J Am Med Assoc* 1997; **277:** 1380–1386.

66. Shearer MJ. Vitamin K metabolism and nutrition. *Blood Rev* 1992; **6:** 92–104.

67. Ansell JE, Kumar R, Deykin D. The spectrum of vitamin K deficiency. *J Am Med Assoc* 1977; **238:** 40–42.

68. La Selve P, Demolin P, Holzapfel L, Blanc PL, Teyssier G, Robert D. Shoshin beriberi: an unusual complication of prolonged parenteral nutrition. *J Parent Ent Nutr* 1986; **10:** 102–103.

69. Nadel AM, Burger PC. Wernicke encephalopathy following prolonged intravenous therapy. *J Am Med Assoc* 1976; **235:** 2403–2405.

70. Chandra RK. Immunology of nutritional disorders. Edward Arnold, London, 1980; pp. 1–110.

71. Anderson SH, Charles TJ, Nicol AD. Thiamine deficiency at a district general hospital: report of five cases. *Quart J Med* 1985; **216:** 15–19.

72. Duhamel JF, Ricour C, Dufier JL *et al.* Deficit en vitamin B₂ et nutrition parenteral exclusive. *Arch Fr Pediatr* 1979; **36:** 342–346.

73. Gaby SK. Vitamin B₆. In: Gaby SK, Bendich A, Singh VN, Machlin LJ (Eds) *Vitamin Intake and Health*. Marcel Dekker, New York, 1991; pp. 163–174.

74. Stabler SP, Marcell PD, Podell ER, Allen RH, Savage DG, Lindenbaum J. Elevation of total homocysteine in the serum of patients with cobalamin or folate deficiency detected by capillary gas chromatography-mass spectrometry. *J Clin Invest* 1988; **81:** 466–474.

75. Stabler SP, Lindenbaum J, Savage DG, Allen RH. Elevation of serum cystathionine levels in patients with cobalamin and folate deficiency. *Blood* 1993; **81:** 3404–3413.

76. Tennant GB, Smith RC, Leinster SJ, O'Donnell JE, Wardrop CAJ. Amino acid infusion induced depression of serum folate after cholecystectomy. *Scand J Haemat* 1981; **27:** 333–338.

77. Naurath HJ, Joosten E, Riezler R, Stabler SP, Allen RH, Lindenbaum J. Effects of vitamin B₁₂, folate and vitamin B₆ supplements in elderly people with normal serum vitamin concentrations. *Lancet* 1995; **346:** 85–89.

78. Mock DM, Lorimer AA, Liebman WM, Sweetman K, Baker H. Biotin deficiency: an unusual complication of parenteral nutrition. *New Engl J Med* 1981; **304:** 820–823.

79. Innis SM, Allardyce DB. Possible biotin deficiency in adults receiving long-term total parenteral nutrition. *Am J Clin Nutr* 1983; **37:** 185–187.

80. Gaby SK, Singh VN. Vitamin C. In: Gaby SK, Bendich A, Singh VN, Machlin LJ (Eds) *Vitamin Intake and Health*. Marcel Dekker, New York, 1991; pp. 103–161.

81. American Medical Association. Guidelines for essential trace element preparations for parenteral use. *J Am Med Assoc* 1979; **241:** 2051–2054.

82. Department of Food and Nutrition, American Medical Association. Working conference on parenteral trace elements. *Bull NY Acad Med* 1984; **60:** 115–212.

83. Aggett PJ. Severe zinc deficiency. In: Mills CF (Ed) *Zinc in Human Biology*. Springer Verlag, London, 1989; pp. 259–279.

84. Shankar AH, Prasad AS. Zinc and immune function: the biological basis of altered resistance to infection. *Am J Clin Nutr* 1998; **68:** 447S–463S.

85. Solomon NW, Ruz M, Castillo-Durgh C. Putative therapeutic roles for zinc. In: Mills CF (Ed) *Zinc in Human Biology*. Springer Verlag, London, 1989; pp. 297–321.

86. Wolman SL, Anderson GH, Marliss EB, Jeejeebhoy KN. Zinc in total parenteral nutrition: requirements and metabolic effects. *Gastroenterology* 1978; **76:** 458–467.

87. Davies JWL, Fell GS. Tissue catabolism in patients with burns. *Clin Chim Acta* 1974; **51:** 83–92.

88. Dunlap WM, James GW, Hume DM. Anaemia and neutropenia caused by copper deficiency. *Ann Int Med* 1974; **80:** 470–476.

89. Karpel JT, Peden VH. Copper deficiency in long-term parenteral nutrition. *J Pediatr* 1972; **80:** 32–36.

90. Shike M, Roulet M, Kurian R, Whitewell J, Stewart S, Jeejeebhoy KN. Copper metabolism and requirements in total parenteral nutrition. *Gastroenterology* 1981; **81:** 290–297.

91. Milne DB, Nielsen FH. Effects of a low copper diet on copper status indicators in post-menopausal women. *Am J Clin Nutr* 1996; **63:** 358–364.

92. Mansell PI, Rawlings J, Allison SP *et al.* Reversal of a skeletal myopathy with selenium supplementation in a patient on home parenteral nutrition. *Clin Nutr* 1987; **6:** 179–183.

93. Johnson RA, Baker SS, Fallon JT *et al.* An occidental case of cardiomyopathy and selenium deficiency. *New Engl J Med* 1981; **304:** 1210–1212.

94. Vinton N, Dahlstrom K, Strobel C, Ament M. Macrocytosis and pseudoalbinism: manifestations of selenium deficiency. *J Paediatr* 1988; **111:** 711–717.

excessive body fluid losses, such as occur with polyuria or diarrhoea. The minimum fluid requirements for metabolism are 40–50 ml/kg/day, and water intake may be restricted to this amount in those circumstances where a reduced fluid intake is desirable, such as in renal failure or heart failure.

Vitamin requirements

A vitamin is an organic substance occurring in minute quantities which may be supplied in the diet or synthesised from essential dietary precursors. Vitamins are essential for specific metabolic functions to proceed normally and the body has variable stores of them. There are relatively small stores of the water-soluble vitamins, especially the B complex, whereas there are large stores of the fat-soluble vitamins A, D, E and K. Some B vitamins (thiamine, riboflavin, pyridoxine and nicotinic acid) are required for energy metabolism; ascorbic acid and vitamin E for oxidative defences; vitamin K for blood coagulation, and vitamin D for adequate mineralisation of bones. Vitamin A has a large number of functions but is particularly related to control of the composition of the extracellular basement membranes of tissues.

Requirements for vitamins present a number of problems which are largely associated with their stores and their function. Often, recommended daily allowances (RDA) have been derived from the amount required to prevent a deficiency disease and then multiplied by a so-called 'safety factor'. The RDAs for the paediatric population are shown in Table 12.2.

Vitamin deficiency disorders occur particularly in the growing infant and less commonly in adolescence. With the exception of conditions related to vitamins D, E and K, diseases due to deficient intake of

vitamins almost never occur in the UK in infants born at term. Rickets and osteomalacia due to inadequate vitamin D intake still occur mainly in the Asian immigrant population.[21]

Vitamin deficiencies are usually the result of insufficient vitamin intake or malabsorptive conditions such as cystic fibrosis, protracted diarrhoea or short-gut syndrome. Rarely is one vitamin alone deficient; where a recognisable deficiency is identified, a severe lack of the vitamin can be assumed and may be in association with other subclinical vitamin deficiencies.

Treatment involves the use of a comprehensive vitamin supplement. In the Third World, vitamin deficiencies are relatively common, vitamin A deficiency being in particular a major cause of blindness and a risk factor for diarrhoeal diseases.

Vitamin toxicity is confined mainly to the fat-soluble vitamins A and D, of which there are relatively large stores in the body. Toxicity is usually the result of excessive vitamin supplementation.

In the growing infant, human milk provides adequate nutrition for the first months of life. A healthy mother who has a nutritionally adequate diet and has been exposed to sunlight will be able to provide her baby with a milk which contains adequate quantities of all known vitamins. Proprietary infant formulae which meet the recommended compositional guidelines[19] contain added vitamins. However, when mixed feeding is introduced — and particularly once the infant changes from infant milk formulae to cow's milk — there is a greater risk of vitamin D deficiency in particular, and a supplement of vitamins A, D and C is recommended. The standard 'five drops per day' dose of children's vitamin A, D and C supplementation

Table 12.2 – Recommended daily amounts of vitamins.

Age range	Thiamin (mg)	Riboflavin (mg)	Nicotinic acid (mg)	Ascorbic acid (mg)	Vitamin A (µg)	Vitamin D (µg)	Vitamin E (µg)
0–6 m	0.3	0.4	5	20	450	7.5	3
6–12 m	0.3	0.4	5	30	450	7.5	4
1–3 y	0.5	0.7	8	20	300	10	5
4–6 y	0.7	0.9	10	20	300	10	6
7–10 y	0.9	1.2	14	20	400	10	7
10–17 y	1.2	1.7	18	25	500–750	10	10

Derived from DHSS[8] – 1985 and NRC – 1980[9].

contains 200 μg of vitamin A, 20 mg of vitamin C and 7.5 μg of vitamin D. For the older child, vitamins are plentifully supplied in a mixed diet which includes cow's milk, cereals, fruits, vegetables, meat, eggs, butter and margarine.

In children who are treated with a therapeutic diet in which there is great restriction of natural foods, it has been shown that rashes and failure to thrive can result from deficiency of vitamins such as choline chloride, panthothenic acid, vitamin K, vitamin E, biotin, vitamin B_{12} and folic acid.[22] These vitamins are not commonly present in multivitamin supplements[23] and thus for therapeutic diets a comprehensive vitamin supplement is recommended.

Mineral and trace element requirements

A mineral is considered nutritionally essential when a subject who is deprived of it develops reproducible features which can be prevented or reversed by supplementation with physiological amounts of that mineral. Mineral elements are commonly divided into minerals and trace elements, but there are no specific guidelines for their classification. In general, the term 'trace element' is used to indicate a mineral for which the requirement is measured in quantities of less than 1 mg. The essential minerals for man include: calcium, phosphorus, sulphur, magnesium, sodium, potassium, chlorine, iron, zinc, copper, manganese, iodine, cobalt, molybdenum, chromium and selenium. Others such as nickel, fluorine, tin, vanadium, silicon and arsenic have been reported essential in other mammals but direct evidence of a nutrition requirement in man is awaited.[24]

The paediatric nutrition requirements for minerals and trace elements are well established and are shown in Table 12.3.

Our knowledge of the functions of many of the trace elements is incomplete. However, it would appear that they have an essential role in a large number of enzyme activities, usually as an integral part of the enzyme where these are metallo proteins. Zinc in alkaline phosphatase and copper in cytochrome oxidase are typical examples.

The dietary intake of minerals is greatly influenced by the choice of foods and by their origins. The selenium content of diet, for example, is determined by that element's existence in the soil in which crops and root vegetables are grown. It is also clear that a number of physicochemical properties of diet will influence uptake and utilisation of trace elements: for example, the phosphate content, particularly in the form of phytate, reduces the bioavailability of iron, zinc and copper.[24] The casein content of milk reduces the bioavailability of zinc. Interactions between trace elements may also have a bearing on uptake: for example, iron supplements may inhibit zinc uptake.[25] Similarly, high copper intakes may result in zinc deficiency; and conversely, oral zinc supplements may be used in the management of Wilson's disease in which copper is handled abnormally.[26]

The effects of starvation in infants and young children

Infants and children are particularly susceptible to the effects of starvation. The small pre-term infant of 1 kg body weight contains only 1% fat and 8% protein and has a non-protein caloric reserve of only 460 kJ/kg. As fat and protein content rise with increasing size, the non-protein caloric reserve increases steadily to 920

Table 12.3 – Recommended daily amounts of minerals and trace elements.

Age range	Iron (mmol)	Calcium (mmol)	Phosphorus (mmol)	Zinc (μmol)	Copper (μmol)	Selenium (μmol)	Manganese (μmol)	Molybdenum (μmol)	Chromium (μmol)
0–6 m	0.11	15	7.7	46	10	0.3	11	0.45	0.5
6–12 m	0.11	15	11.6	76	14	0.5	15	0.60	0.8
1–3 y	0.13	15	26	153	20	0.6	22	0.75	0.9
4–6 y	0.18	15	26	153	25	1.0	32	1.0	1.7
7–10 y	0.18	15	26	153	35	1.5	45	2.0	2.4
10–17 y	0.22	17.5	39	299	40	1.5	68	2.25	2.4

Derived from NRC – 1980[9] and Aggett & Davies.[24]

kJ/kg in a one-year-old child of 10.5 kg.[27] If it is assumed that all non-protein and one-third of the protein content of the body is available for caloric needs at a rate of 210 kJ/kg/day in infants and children, estimates of the duration of survival during starvation and semi-starvation may be made. Thus, a small pre-term baby has sufficient reserve to survive only 4 days of starvation, and a large pre-term baby has enough for only 12 days. Clearly infants are at a considerable disadvantage compared with adults, and early recourse to parenteral nutrition is essential when impaired gastrointestinal function precludes enteral nutrition.

Areas of controversy

Fetal and neonatal nutrition determines health in adult life

There is now a growing and emerging body of evidence that suggests that nutrition in early life has permanent consequences for long-term health and development. If this occurs at a critical period of growth, i.e. during a period of rapid cell divisions, then nutrition may exert a long lasting or permanent effect on their physiology and metabolism. Lucas has coined the term 'programming' for this form of metabolic entrainment.[28] Widdowson & McCance[1] showed that even brief periods of under-nutrition at a critical period may permanently reduce the numbers of cells in particular organs at such times. For the central and enteric nervous systems the critical period of growth is from 25–26 weeks gestation through to 18 months post term. Thus under- or malnutrition during this time may 'programme' the later performance of both the central and enteric nervous systems.

However programmable changes may not be restricted to the nervous system but also involve the cardiovasculature and other organs of the body. Barker has provided persuasive evidence that coronary heart disease and the related disorders of stroke, diabetes and hypertension have their origins in programmed changes of the human fetus and young infant.[29]

A number of studies have shown the following general features of programming in the human infant:

- In pre-term infants, the period of nutritional sensitivity extends post term and throughout infancy.

- Infants born at full term remain sensitive to nutrition programming through at least the first year of life.

- In infants born small for gestational age at term, the adverse long-term effects of poor fetal growth may be ameliorated by nutrition management in infancy.

- Specific nutrient status of long chain polyunsaturated fatty acids, Ca, Fe, PO_4 and energy may have selective long-term programming effects in infancy.

- Non-nutrient factors in human milk may also programme health and developmental outcomes.

Observational studies on both whole milks and specific nutrients have shown effects on the central nervous system. Breast feeding gives the infant advantages in cognitive and intellectual development compared to infants fed formula milk. In pre-term infants there is at least a 10-point advantage by the time they reach the age of 7.5–8 yrs.[6] A randomised controlled pilot study of a nutrient enriched formula showed both improved catch-up growth and motor development.

Two specific nutrients may have important effects on growth and development: iron and long chain polyunsaturated fatty acids (LC-PUFA).

Iron

Iron deficiency anaemia is a major problem in infants and young children with a world-wide prevalence of 43% with a higher prevalence in developing (51%) than developed regions (12%). In the UK iron deficiency is the most common nutrition disorder during early childhood. The National Diet and Nutrition Survey of 1995 found that 12% of children aged 18–30 months were anaemic, especially those from Asian ethnic groups. It is clear that this is largely due to an inadequate supply of absorbable iron from the diet. The consequences of this are growth faltering due to reduced appetite and food intake, hair and nail changes, a minor degree of malabsorption and, most seriously, impairment of mental and psychomotor development.[30] Although iron treatment reverses anaemia, impaired cognitive function has been reported 4–5 years later by same. If such developmental delay is shown to be irreversible then prevention of iron deficiency must be a high priority. It is clear that the iron availability of infant diets is marginal and in many inadequate from the age of 4–6 months on. Current information on the bioavailability of iron in infant weaning foods is insufficient to predict the effects that different feeding regimes might have, though the effects of cow's milk feeds before the age of 1 year, macrobiotic diets and tea drinking are well known to result in poor iron status. Clearly early detection of iron deficiency is required and supplementary iron is required by those affected. Recent studies have suggested that 30 mg Fe given twice weekly is as effective as a daily dose in those with iron deficiency anaemia.

Long chain polyunsaturated fatty acids

In the past, it has been assumed that the supply of linoleic and α-linolenic acid can completely fulfil the body's requirements for polyunsaturated fatty acids in every age-group, including newborn and premature infants. Recent studies have shown, however, that this assumption might not hold true for premature infants. *In utero*, longer chain polyunsaturates with 20–22 carbon atoms and 2–6 double bonds seem to be preferentially transferred from mother to fetus during the last trimester. Such long chain polyunsaturates (LCP) are required for the synthesis of different prostaglandins, thromboxanes, leukotrienes and for membrane synthesis in growing tissue, particularly in the brain and retina. There is an increasing body of evidence to show that visual function and brain development is influenced by the LCP status of infants born prematurely.[31-33]

As a result there is now a drive to introduce specialised formulae for premature infants supplemented with long chain polyunsaturates.

Practical applications

Nutrition assessment of children

Infants and children are in a precarious nutritional state compared with adults. Specific nutrition deficiencies occur earlier and are often more florid. Assessment of nutrition status therefore provides an important baseline against which to judge the effects of therapy, and may be divided into: the assessment of past and present dietary intake, clinical examination, anthropometric measurements and laboratory assessment.

Measurement of dietary intake

A number of methods are available, including dietary recall, dietary history, dietary questionnaire, estimated food record, weighed dietary record and duplicate meal analysis. Although the analysis of duplicate diets is the most accurate way of assessing intake, the method is time-consuming and requires the back-up of a specialist nutrition laboratory. Consequently, dietary recall and estimated food record or a weighed dietary record are the approaches most commonly used in clinical practice. Dietary recall is the most common.[34] In this method, the mother recalls her child's diet over a 24-hour period. The accuracy of this method is partly dependent on the skill of the interviewer and is more accurate in developing countries where there are fewer different types of food to recall.

In the estimated food record method, the subject keeps a dietary diary recording the amounts of food consumed and when they are eaten. Quantities are normally estimated in household measures and are later translated to numeric values by the investigator. The weighed dietary record is obtained by providing the subject with dietary scales and each item of food eaten is weighed prior to consumption. Waste food is similarly recorded and thus the amount of each food consumed can be calculated. If the mother is suitably motivated, this type of procedure can produce accurate results.

Clinical examination

This is the least objective of all forms of assessment and abnormal signs do not necessarily indicate current deficiency. Laboratory evidence is necessary to substantiate any clinical observations.

Anthropometry

Growth being a major characteristic of children, and dependent on an adequate supply of nutrients, anthropometric measurements are particularly important in nutrition assessment. Somatic measurements are of most value when performed sequentially. A fall-off in the rate of growth is one of the earliest indicators of malnutrition. A single value, however, gives little indication of whether the situation is improving or deteriorating, and a value within the normal range may be abnormal if it represents a large fall from a previously higher growth rate.

Measurement of weight provides an indication of present nutrition status while height indicates the previous long-term dietary history. Standards for weight and height of UK infants and children have been published by Tanner *et al.*[35] Growth charts[2] (Fig. 12.1) based on these data are extremely helpful in the recognition of children who are small for age but well proportioned, and children who have disproportionately low weight for height, i.e. they are acutely malnourished or wasted. However, an accurate chronological age is essential when using such growth charts.

Measurement of skinfold thickness provides a means of assessing subcutaneous fat stores[36] whilst upper arm circumference (when used in conjunction with TSF) gives an indication of arm muscle area and hence skeletal muscle mass.[37]

Laboratory assessment

Laboratory investigations provide an objective assessment of nutrition status and are useful in the detection of early physiological adaptation to malnutrition and the recognition of specific mineral and vitamin deficiencies. Plasma albumin concentration is useful in assessing protein energy malnutrition (PEM) in children and has the advantage of being widely available. However, albumin has a long plasma half-life, and in the marasmic form of PEM, plasma levels tend to be maintained until malnutrition is severe and clinically overt.[38] Some other proteins (such as transferrin and retinol binding protein) have a shorter half-life, but these tests are not as widely available and the levels of transferrin are raised in the presence of iron deficiency which often creates difficulty in interpretation.

Tests of cell-mediated immunity are commonly abnormal in malnutrition and intrauterine growth retardation. Cell-mediated immunity may be abnormal as a result of deficiencies of folic acid, pyridoxine, vitamin A and trace elements such as zinc and selenium. A lymphocyte count and assessment of *in vivo* delayed hypersensitivity to *Candida* are useful indications of cell-mediated immunity.[39]

Earlier tests of nutrition status based on urine collection for 24 hours or more have an inherent disadvantage in infants and children. Although theoretically easy, it is often extremely difficult in practice to obtain reliably complete and uncontaminated samples. Thus, estimation of urinary creatinine height index, urinary hydroxyproline creatinine ratio and urine 3-methyl histidine estimation have not found lasting favour. Alternative grading systems of nutrition status have been proposed[40] but have never become really popular. However, they have some merit in that they permit identification of children nutritionally at risk and indicate the degree of nutrition support likely to be required. Further consideration should be given to such systems.

Summary

In infants and children diet must provide sufficient nutrients not only for the maintenance of body tissues but also for growth and normal development. Somatic growth is bimodal, with faster growth occurring in infancy and adolescence; however, other organs may have single critical periods of growth and differentiation. The inadequate provision of nutrition at such times may have far reaching later effects with evidence that major adult health disorders such as cardiovascular disease and diabetes having their origins in fetal malnutrition. The provision of good nutrition for pregnant mothers and infants is likely to be the single most effective health measure available to us in the millennium.

References

1. Widdowson EM, McCance RA. The determinants of growth and form. *Proc Roy Soc Lond* 1974; **185:** 1–17.

2. Tanner JM, Whitehouse RH. Clinical longitudinal standards for height, weight, height velocity, weight velocity and stages of puberty. *Arch Dis Child* 1976; **51:** 170–175.

3. Prader A, Tanner JM, van Harnack GA. Catch-up growth following illness or starvation. *J Paediat* 1963; **5:** 646–651.

4. Metkoff J. Maternal nutrition and fetal growth. In: McLaren DS, Burman D (eds) Textbook of Pediatric Nutrition. Churchill Livingstone, Edinburgh, 1982; pp. 18–38.

5. Grand RJ, Watkins JB, Torti F. Development of the human gastrointestinal tract: a review. *Gastroenterology* 1976; **70:** 790–810.

6. Lucas A, Marley R, Cole TJ, Lister G, Leeson-Payne C. Breast milk and subsequent intelligence quotient in children born pre-term. *Lancet* 1992; **339:** 261–264.

7. Forbes GB. Nutritional requirements in adolescence. In: Suskind RM (ed) Textbook of Paediatric Nutrition. Raven Press, New York; 1981, 381–391.

8. DHSS. Recommended Daily Amounts of Food Energy and Nutrients for Groups of People in the United Kingdom. Report 15. HMSO, London; 1979.

9. US National Research Council. Food and Nutrition Board Recommended Dietary Allowances. 9th rev edn. National Academy of Sciences, Washington, DC; 1980.

10. World Health Organisation. Energy and protein requirements: Report of a joint FAO/WHO adhoc expert committee. WHO Technical Report 522. WHO, Geneva; 1973.

11. Ashworth A, Bell R, James WPT, Waterlow JC. Caloric requirements of children recovering from protein calorie malnutrition. *Lancet* 1968; **2:** 600–613.

12. Ashworth A. Growth rates in children recovering from protein calorie malnutrition. *Br J Nutr* 1969; **23:** 835–845.

13. Sturman JA, Gaull G, Raiha NCR. Absence of cystathionase in human fetal liver. Is cystine essential? *Science* 1970; **169:** 74–76.

14. Panteliadias C, Jurgens P, Dolif D. Amino-saurende-dorf Fruh-und-Neugeborener unter den Bedingungen der Parenteralen Ernahrung. *Infus Ther Klin Ernahrung* 1975; **2:** 65–68.

15. Jurgens P, Dolif D. Experimental results of parenteral nutrition with amino acids. In: Wilkinson AW (ed) *Parenteral Nutrition*. Churchill Livingstone, Edinburgh; 1972.

16. Evans E, Witty R. An assessment of methods used to determine protein quality. *Wld Rev Nutr Dietet* 1978; **32:** 1–26.

17. Berman D. Nutrition in early childhood. In: McLaren DS, Berman D (eds) *Texbook of Paediatric Nutrition*. 2nd edn. Churchill Livingstone, Edinburgh, 1982; pp. 39–73.

18. American Academy of Paediatrics Committee on Nutrition. Commentary on breast-feeding and infant formulas, including proposed standards for formulas. *Paediatrics* 1976; **57:** 278–285.

19. DHSS. Artificial Feeds for the Young Infant. Report 18. HMSO, London; 1980.

20. FAO-WHO. 1980. Dietary fats and oils in human nutrition. FAO of the United Nations, Rome; 21–37.

21. DHSS. Rickets and Osteomalacia. Report 19. HMSO, London; 1980.

22. Mann TP, Wilson KM, Clayton BE. A deficiency state in infants on synthetic foods. *Arch Dis Child* 1965; **40:** 364–375.

23. Tripp JH, Francis DEM, Knight JA, Harries JT. Infant feeding practices: a cause of concern. *Br Med J* 1979; **2:** 707–709.

24. Aggett PJ, Davies NT. Some nutritional aspects of trace metals. *J Inher Metab Dis* 1983; **6:** 22–30.

25. Thorn JM, Aggett PJ, Dells HT, Clayton BE. Mineral and trace metal supplement for use with synthetic diets based on comminuted chicken. *Arch Dis Child* 1978; **53:** 931–938.

26. Van Caillie-Bertrand M, Dagenhart HJ, Visser HKA, Sinaasappel M, Bouquet J. Oral zinc sulphate for Wilson's disease. *Arch Dis Child* 1985; **60:** 656–659.

27. Heird WC, Driscoll JM, Schullinger JN, Grebin B, Winters RW. Intravenous alimentation in paediatric patients. *J Paediat* 1972; **80:** 351–372.

28. Lucas A. Programming by early nutrition in man. In: Bock GR, Whelan J (ed) The Childhood Environment and Adult Disease. John Wiley, Chichester, 1991; pp. 38–55.

29. Barker DJ. The fetal and infant origins of adult disease. *British Medical Journal* 1990; **301:** 1111.

30. Loyoff B, Jimeney E, Wolf AB. Long term developmental outcome of infants with iron deficiency. *N Engl J Med* 1991; **325:** 687–694.

31. Carlson SE, Cooke RJ, Peeples JM, Werkman SH, Tolley EA. Docosahexanoate and eicosapentanoate status of pre-term infants: relationship to visual accurity in Ω-3 supplemented and unsupplemented infants. *Paediat Res* 1989; **25:** 285a.

32. Carlson SE, Werman SH, Rhodes PG, Tolley EA. Visual acuity development in healthy preterm infants: effects of marine oil supplementation. *Am J Clin Nutr* 1993; **58:** 35–42.

33. Uauy R, Birch D, Birch E, Tyson J, Hoffman D. Are omega-3 fatty acids required for normal eye and brain development in the very low birthweight infant? In: Koletzko B, Okken A, Rey J, Salle B, Van Biervliet JP (eds) Recent Advances in Infant Feeding. New York: Georg Thieme Verlag, New York, 1992; pp. 13–22.

34. Rutishauser IH, Frood JD. The effect of a traditional low-fat diet on energy and protein intake, serum albumin compensation and bodyweight in Ugandan pre-school children. *Br J Nutr* 1973; **29:** 261–268.

35. Tanner JM, Whitehouse RH, Takaishi M. Standards from birth to maturity for height, weight, height velocity and weight velocity: British children, parts 1 and 2. *Arch Dis Child* 1966; **41:** 454–71 and 613–635.

36. Tanner JM, Whitehouse RH. Revised standards for triceps and subscapular skin folds in British children. *Arch Dis Child* 1975; **50:** 142–145.

37. Gurney JM, Jelliffe DB. Arm anthropometry in nutritional assessment: nomogram for rapid calculation of muscle circumference and cross-sectional and fat areas. *Am J Clin Nutr* 1973; **26:** 912–915.

38. Coward WA, Whitehead RG, Lunn PG. Reasons why hypoalbuminaemia may or may not appear in protein energy malnutrition. *Br J Ntr* 1977; **38:** 89–94.

39. Chandra RK. Immunocompetence as a functional index of nutritional status. *Br Med Bull* 1981; **37:** 89–94.

40. Hattner JAT, Kerner JA. Nutritional assessment of the paediatric patient. In: Kerner JA (ed) Manual of Parenteral Nutrition. Wiley Medical, New York, 1983; pp. 19–60.

13

Nutrition, appetite control and disease

Anne Ballinger and Michael Clark

Introduction

Under stable conditions most adults maintain a relatively narrow range of body weight despite psychological and environmental influences. This suggests that a system exists to precisely regulate energy intake and body weight. This system comprises a complex network of integrated peripheral and central pathways which utilise chemical, endocrine and neuroregulatory pathways. The nature of appetite research dictates that much of our knowledge has been gained from animal experiments, although the peripheral pathways that have been studied appear similar in humans. The feeding of mammals is a discontinuous process in which periods of eating are interspersed with periods where no food is taken. These periods are regarded as meals and inter-meal intervals. A state of 'hunger' leads an animal to seek and ingest food. The food once ingested initiates a series of signals which induce a state of 'satiety' which inhibits hunger or feeding during the inter-meal interval. Ingestion of certain foods may only produce satiety for that particular nutrient. For instance, a food deprived rat will drink a certain volume of glucose solution which produces satiety for that solution which persists over at least the ensuing 20–30 minutes. Feeding is inhibited if the rat is offered further glucose during this period of satiety but vigorous feeding resumes if the rat is offered a different type of food such as milk. This phenomenon of so-called sensory-specific satiety may explain why many of us crave a high carbohydrate pudding after eating a main course of mixed nutrients which has created a feeling of satiety and indeed may even not have all been eaten. Most of the processes which follow eating have a negative influence on food ingestion and create a negative feedback loop which tends to inhibit further eating. This is in contrast to the generally positive feedback provided by the signals which are generated by the sight and smell of food before food ingestion.

Initiation of feeding and intake of food during a *single meal* is controlled by a series of overlapping mediating processes which originate in the periphery and are integrated in the brain. These *short-term regulators* of food intake are superimposed on a background of *long-term control* that works, at least in part, by monitoring fat mass with integration of these signals predominantly in a well defined area in the base of the brain, the hypothalamus (Fig. 13.1).

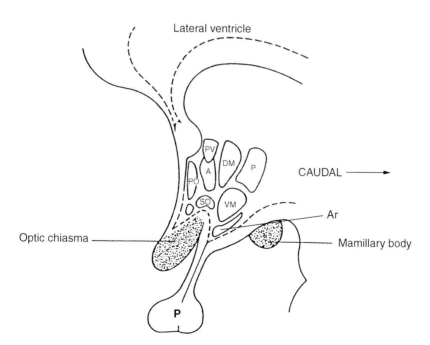

Figure 13.1 – Sagittal section through the third ventricle and hypothalamus. The hypothalamus forms the lateral walls and floor of the third ventricle and sits above the pituitary gland (**P**). The principal nuclei of the human hypothalamus are shown. PV, para-ventricular; PO, preoptic; A, anterior; DM, dorsomedial; P, posterior; SO, supreoptic; VM, ventromedial; Ar, arcuate.

Stable weight: a precise balance of energy intake and expenditure

Maintenance of a stable body weight requires a precise balance of energy intake and energy expenditure i.e. the number of kilojoules (kJ) ingested must equal the amount used to maintain physiologic functions.

Weight gain

Weight gain occurs when there is a positive energy balance which may arise as a result of an increase in energy intake, a decrease in energy expenditure, or a combination of the two. Total energy expenditure is the sum of resting energy expenditure (REE also known as the resting metabolic rate) and activity energy expenditure. In many studies of body weight, resting energy expenditure is the only parameter which has been measured but it is the total energy expenditure which is the key determinant of energy balance. Self-reported food intake in obese subjects would suggest that obesity results from a reduction in energy expenditure because they invariably report low levels of energy intake. However, carefully conducted research contradicts these predictions and has shown that total energy expenditure is actually substantially raised in obese adults and children.[1,2] It is likely that the higher energy cost to perform weight-bearing activities in obese subjects may explain, at least in part, the increased energy expenditure. Amatruda et al[3] also demonstrated that weight reduced individuals have the same resting metabolic rate as controls and this therefore could not explain their greater propensity to regain weight. In summary, therefore, weight gain is always due to an increase in energy intake. The exception to this are the few cases in which obesity results from a metabolic cause such as hypothyroidism in whom a reduced energy expenditure plays a part.

Weight loss

Wasting is a common accompaniment to many chronic inflammatory conditions, cancer and acquired immunodeficiency syndrome (AIDS). Wasting in these conditions is associated with depression, anxiety and impaired quality of life. Significant weight loss also portends a poor patient prognosis in terms of tolerance to treatment and survival.[4] Furthermore, extreme inanition may be a direct cause of mortality for some patients with advanced cancer and wasting.

Chronic inflammatory conditions

Weight loss is a feature of chronic inflammatory conditions and in our own clinical practice we see this most frequently in association with inflammatory bowel disease (IBD), namely Crohn's disease and ulcerative colitis. Weight loss achieves the greatest significance in children with IBD in whom it is associated with delayed linear growth and a failure to achieve expected height in adult life with implications for social and psychological development. Puberty may also be delayed, in some cases this may not occur until their twenties unless the inflammatory disease is controlled. The potential causes of weight loss and growth retardation in IBD include malabsorption of nutrients from the inflamed gut, steroid treatment, increased energy expenditure or a reduced energy intake secondary to a loss of appetite (anorexia). Of these reduced energy intake has been identified as the single most important factor leading to weight loss and has been documented to be only 42–82% of expected values.[5,6] Experimental studies have implicated the pro-inflammatory cytokines, tumour necrosis factor-α (TNF-α, previously called cachectin), interleukin-1β (IL-1β) and interleukin-6 (IL-6), released from inflammatory cells, in causation of anorexia in these disease states.[7,8] In an animal model for human Crohn's disease administration of an IL-1 antagonist into the brain partially reversed the anorexia and weight loss which occurs with the development of colitis.[9] This would suggest that IL-1 is responsible, at least in part, for the reduction in food intake in this model and, furthermore that it may be acting by an interaction with the central feeding pathways which are discussed in detail below.

AIDS

Early studies suggested that resting energy expenditure was increased in AIDS patients and weight loss with wasting could be attributed to this. Further studies have shown however that *total* energy expenditure is lower than expected in patients with AIDS[10] even at times of rapid weight loss. Records of food intake showed that energy intake was only a mean of 5586 kJ/day during periods of rapid weight loss compared with 11 634 kJ/day during periods of stable weight. This study, which also showed a higher resting energy expenditure in AIDS patients, showed that intake rather than total energy expenditure is the key determinant of energy balance in these patients.

Cancer

Both a reduction in energy intake and an increase in energy expenditure may contribute to weight loss in cancer patients. Data from some of the tumour models would suggest that, in contrast to HIV infection, a reduction in energy intake is not the main mechanism leading to weight loss. In the murine MAC16 model, a chemically induced, transplantable adenocarcinoma of the colon, there is progressive weight loss but without an accompanying decrease in food intake when compared with that of non-tumour bearing mice.[11] However, this model has a poor resemblance to the clinical condition in that the tumour mass reaches 20–33% of host body weight before weight loss is observed. In contrast to the results from some of these animal models a reduction in energy intake is thought to be the main mechanism leading to weight loss in patients with cancer. Loss of appetite was present in 85% of patients and was the second most frequent symptom in almost 300 consecutive cancer patients admitted to one unit.[12] The energy intake of patients with cancer and weight loss has been documented from 24-h dietary recall and shown to be markedly reduced at only about 50% of predicted values.[13] An increase in REE in cancer patients has been shown in some studies[14,15] but total energy expenditure has not been measured. Cancer patients may prove to be similar to patients with HIV infection and have increased resting energy expenditure but a low or normal total energy expenditure. Similar to inflammatory disease, it is thought that cancer-associated anorexia may also be cytokine mediated. Anti-TNF antibodies and a receptor antagonist against IL-1 ameliorate the manifestations of cancer cachexia in mice.

In summary, weight loss is a common feature in patients with chronic inflammatory and malignant conditions. An increase in REE has been demonstrated in these conditions and suggested to account for the weight loss. However, as discussed previously total energy expenditure is the key determinant of energy balance. Furthermore, a simple calculation shows that the increase in resting energy expenditure which has been measured in these studies simply could not account for the degree of weight loss. For instance, the difference in REE between healthy individuals and patients with advanced AIDS who are losing weight (> 3 kg/month) is 168 kJ/day.[10] Over a 1-month period this amounts to a total of 35 280 kJ. However weight loss of > 3 kg requires an energy expenditure of 70 988 kJ or more in excess of intake. Thus to summarise, the cause of weight loss in these chronic conditions is due entirely or in part (possibly in the cancer patients) to loss of appetite and a reduction in energy intake.

Control of appetite in health

The control of appetite is achieved in the short term by meal-to-meal variation in food intake which responds to the body's immediate metabolic needs and is heavily influenced by psychosocial factors. Short-term control is superimposed on a complex system which regulates energy balance in the long-term and relies on key hypothalamic feeding pathways to integrate these control mechanisms.

Long-term regulation of appetite and body weight

The identification of genes responsible for the distinct obesity syndromes in the rat and mice models has been a huge leap forward in the understanding of appetite control and energy balance (Table 13.1). One of

Table 13.1 – The five monogenic murine models of obesity.

Mouse model	Gene	Normal gene product	Tissue expression of protein
Obese	*ob*	*ob* protein (leptin)	Adipose tissue
Diabetes	*db*	leptin receptor	Hypothalamus, choroid plexus
Tubby	*tub*	hypothalamic protein	Hypothalamus
Obese yellow	A^y	agouti protein	Exclusively within the hair follicle in normal mice
			Widespread ectopic expression in mutants
Fat	*fat*	carboxypeptidase E	Endocrine/neuroendocrine tissues

MSH = melanocyte-stimulating hormone

these, the *ob* gene and its protein product, the *ob* protein (leptin), has generated an enormous amount of research. The results of these studies largely fulfil predictions that were made from a series of experiments which began over 40 years ago.

The lipostat theory of body weight control

Gordon Kennedy proposed the 'lipostat' theory of body weight control.[16] He suggested that an increase in fat mass somehow signals to the brain that the body is overweight and leads to a reduction in food intake and an increase in energy expenditure. A reduction in fat mass, whether by a reduction in food intake or surgical removal (lipectomy), would lead to food seeking behaviour, increased food intake when available and decreased energy expenditure. These compensatory mechanisms would therefore tend to restore fat mass and body weight to its set point.

Strong support for this 'set point' theory was obtained from cross-circulation experiments in which two mice are joined together surgically so that they share a common blood supply (parabiosis). In these experiments excessive forced feeding and an increase in fat mass by one mouse in the pair caused decreased feeding and weight loss in the other member of the pair.[17] These results suggested that in response to an increase in fat mass there was increased production of a fat derived satiety signal in the member of the pair which fed excessively. This would normally inhibit further eating and restore body weight back to its set point. However, in this experimental situation the satiety factor also gained access to the second animal, via the circulation, and led to reduced food intake and weight loss in this animal.

Destruction of a critical area of the hypothalamus in one member of the pair led to excessive weight gain in the affected animal with reduced feeding and loss of weight in the other. Hervey[17] proposed that destruction of this hypothalamic nucleus rendered the affected rat insensitive to the circulating satiety signals. However, as body fat accumulated in these animals a circulating satiety signal produced hypophagia and eventually death by starvation in the other member of the pair with an intact hypothalamus.

Further support for a fat-derived circulating satiety signal was obtained from cross-circulation experiments in animals with genetic obesity.[18] The *ob/ob* mouse eats continuously and weighs approximately three times as much as normal mice. When paired with a normal animal in parabiotic experiments the *ob/ob* mouse eats less and gains less weight. Together with the data from previous experiments these results were consistent with a circulating factor that regulates energy intake and metabolism and is deficient in the *ob/ob* mouse.

The *ob* protein and *ob* receptor in mice

The long search for this satiety signal ended in 1994 when Zhang *et al*[19] reported that they had identified and sequenced the gene responsible for obesity in the *ob/ob* mouse. The *ob* gene encodes a protein of 167 amino acids (*ob* protein or leptin) which is expressed exclusively in fat tissue. The common strain of *ob/ob* mouse has a mutation of the *ob* gene which results in the production of a short and non-functional protein. Thus, in the absence of functioning leptin the feeding control centres of these animals perceive incorrectly that the fat mass is low. This results in continuous eating and weight gain which leads to extreme obesity and premature death.

Shortly after the *ob* gene was cloned it was shown that daily injections with recombinant leptin caused a reduction in food intake and loss of weight in the *ob/ob* mouse and to a lesser degree in normal weight animals.[20,21] When both treated and untreated *ob/ob* mice were given equal amounts of a low-calorie diet, the leptin treated mice lost more weight.[21] This demonstrates that leptin-induced weight loss in free feeding animals is due to an increase in energy expenditure as well as a reduction in food intake. It is thought that neural signals which emanate from the hypothalamus and are transmitted by the sympathetic nervous system to brown adipose tissue result in activation of uncoupling protein and increased energy expenditure. The mode of action of leptin is reflected in the obese syndrome of *ob/ob* mice which is due predominantly to excessive food intake but also to inappropriately decreased energy expenditure. This is therefore in contrast to the situation seen in obese humans where, as discussed previously, energy expenditure is increased and obesity results entirely from an increase in energy intake.

Where does leptin act?

In the *ob/ob* mouse a reduction in food intake and body weight is seen when much smaller doses (compared to doses injected peripherally) of leptin are injected into the cerebral ventricles suggesting that one or more areas in the brain is the most likely target for leptin.[22] This may at first seem unlikely as leptin is a 167 amino acid protein and its size would normally exclude it from crossing the blood–brain barrier and passing into the brain. However, a form of the leptin receptor is expressed in the choroid plexus (vascular folds in the cerebral ventricles) and may be involved in transporting leptin from the blood to the brain. The intense expression of the leptin receptor in the hypothalamus would support the proposed central site of action. The proposed mode of action of leptin is summarised in Figure 13.2 and discussed in more detail in a later section of this chapter.

Mutations in the receptor for leptin

Inability to respond to leptin characterises the *db/db* mice (Table 13.1) which, like the *ob/ob* mouse, shows early onset obesity with persistently excessive food intake and reduced energy expenditure. Unlike the *ob/ob* mouse there is no response to exogenous administration of leptin because of a mutation in the leptin receptor gene which results in production of an abnormal receptor which cannot respond normally to leptin binding. Identification of the defects in this hormone-receptor pair, the *ob/ob* and *db/db* mice, has therefore helped to define a feedback loop which, at least in mice, is crucial in the long-term regulation of nutrient intake and energy balance.

The *ob* gene and leptin in humans

Leptin is also expressed and secreted by fat cells in humans. Similar to the results found in animals leptin circulates in the blood where the plasma levels are very closely and positively correlated with fat mass.[23–26] This relationship (Fig. 13.3) holds true even at the extremes of fat mass such as in anorexia nervosa and highly trained lean athletes.[27,28] The human *ob* gene has now also been cloned and shown to be 84% identical to the mouse gene and situated on chromosome 7. In contrast to the obese mouse, no mutations in the *ob* gene were found in obese subjects suggesting that any

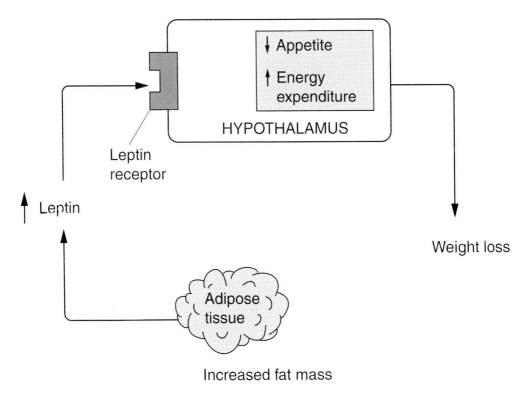

Figure 13.2 – The proposed mode of action of leptin. In response to weight gain and an increase in fat mass there is increased synthesis and release of leptin from fat cells. This leads to increased circulating concentrations of leptin which is transported from the blood into the brain; here it binds to hypothalamic receptors and alters the activity of key feeding pathways. The final result is a reduction in food intake and in some animals an increase in energy expenditure. These changes tend to restore fat mass to its 'set point'.

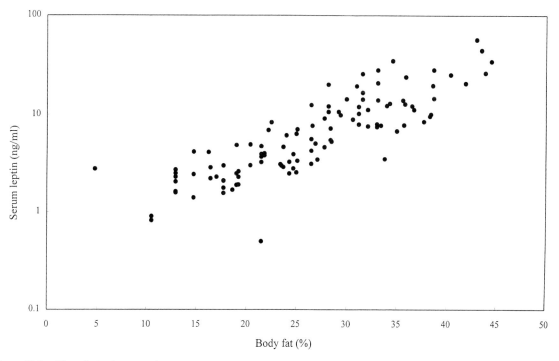

Figure 13.3 – The relation between the percentage of body fat and the serum leptin concentration in 107 subjects. There is a close and positive correlation with fat mass.

defect, if there is one in these individuals, lies elsewhere.[29] However, only a small number of patients were included in this study and it remains possible that a small but unidentified fraction of obese humans have a functionally significant mutation in the *ob* gene.

The vast majority of obese humans follow a predicted pattern and have high circulating concentrations of leptin appropriate for their fat mass. It has therefore been suggested that overeating and obesity in humans may be a result of resistance to leptin. This could arise either because leptin cannot gain sufficient access to the brain, or because access to the brain is normal but the hypothalamic receptor is unresponsive to leptin. Caro *et al*[30] have investigated the first hypothesis and found a 30% increase in the amount of leptin in the cerebrospinal fluid (CSF) of obese compared with lean subjects despite 318% higher serum leptin in the obese individuals. Expressed differently the CSF/serum leptin ratio in lean individuals was 4.3-fold higher than that in obese individuals. The authors suggest that the system which transports leptin from the periphery into the brain may be defective in obese individuals. Future studies will be needed to determine whether this finding does indeed contribute to obesity in humans.

Other factors released peripherally which control body weight

The studies in the *ob/ob* mice point to the crucial role of leptin in the control of body weight. However, several other circulating factors have been proposed to control food intake and energy homeostasis. Insulin, like leptin, circulates at levels proportionate to fat mass and can enter the brain through specific blood–brain barrier insulin receptors. Insulin injected into the hypothalamus causes reduced energy intake, increased energy expenditure and weight loss – similar effects to those seen after administration of leptin. *In vitro* insulin increases leptin synthesis and protein release from isolated fat cells.[31] The functional link between leptin and insulin, if any, in the control of food intake and energy balance is not known.

Hypothalamic control of food intake and energy balance

Feeding is predominantly controlled by integratory centres in the hypothalamus. Peptides and neurotransmitters are usually divided into those which stimulate feeding and those which inhibit feeding (Fig. 13.4). This division is largely based on the results of animal

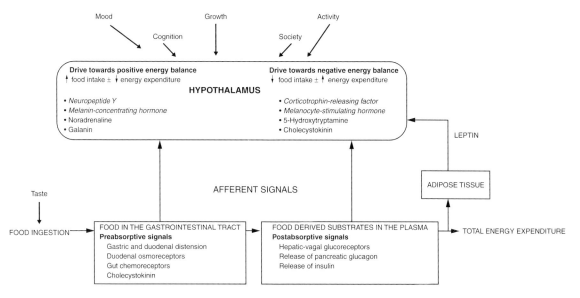

Figure 13.4 – Interaction of the central and peripheral feeding pathways implicated in the control of food intake and energy balance. Peptides in italics are those which are thought to mediate the central actions of leptin. This system is heavily influenced by a variety of external factors such as taste of food, mood and place of eating.

experiments where the peptides and neurotransmitters of interest have been injected into specific hypothalamic nuclei and the feeding response observed. Subsequently for many of these factors their physiological role in the control of appetite has been identified from experiments using specific inhibitors.

Peptides and neurotransmitters which lead to an increase in food intake

Neuropeptide Y

The exact mechanisms mediating the weight reducing effects of leptin are not completely understood. However the actions are mediated, at least in part, by inhibition of synthesis and release of neuropeptide Y (NPY), the most potent known stimulator of appetite.[32]

NPY is a 36-amino acid peptide which is found in most brain regions and at particularly high concentrations in the hypothalamus. Within the hypothalamus NPY is synthesised virtually exclusively in neurones in the arcuate nucleus which mostly terminate in the paraventricular nucleus, the major site of NPY release (see Fig. 13.1). NPY injected into the paraventricular nucleus is a potent stimulus to feeding and induces insatiable hyperphagia; chronic administration produces obesity.[33] A physiological role for NPY in control of appetite and energy balance is supported by the observation that levels of NPY and its messenger RNA (mRNA) correlate with the normal feeding cycle in rodents. Before the onset of feeding there is an increase in NPY mRNA (which usually indicates increased protein synthesis) in the arcuate nucleus, and increased tissue protein concentrations and release of NPY from the paraventricular nucleus; it would seem likely that these changes may play a part in initiating feeding. This hypothesis is supported by the observation that central injection of antibodies directed against NPY (and hence blocking its action) delays the normal onset of feeding.

Increased activity of NPY is thought to be one factor which mediates the hyperphagia in the *ob/ob* mouse. Increased levels of NPY mRNA in the arcuate nucleus and enhanced secretion of NPY from the paraventricular nucleus have been found in the obese mice compared to their lean litter mates. Furthermore, administration of leptin to *ob/ob* mice suppresses NPY expression in the arcuate nucleus and reduces feeding. Leptin has also been shown to act directly on NPY-expressing cells *in vitro* to inhibit release of NPY.[32] Taken together these results suggest that the NPY neurone is likely to be a key target for leptin.

To further define the role of NPY in leptin deficient mice Erickson et al[34] generated ob/ob mice which were also deficient for NPY. They demonstrated that, in the absence of NPY, ob/ob mice are less obese because of reduced food intake and increased energy expenditure. These results implicate NPY-containing neural pathways as mediators of the hyperphagia and hypometabolism resulting from chronic deficiency of leptin. Melanin-concentrating hormone which is also overexpressed in ob/ob mice is proposed as a further candidate to mediate the central actions of leptin.

The physiological role of NPY in normal weight animals may be to restore energy balance after a period of reduced food intake and energy deficit. The arcuate nucleus-paraventricular projection is stimulated by conditions of energy deficit and weight loss such as fasting.[35-37] These conditions increase the synthesis of NPY in the arcuate nucleus and also lead to increased release of NPY from the paraventricular nucleus. In food-deprived rats which have lost weight, the activity of the arcuate nucleus-paraventricular projection only returns to normal when overeating has restored body weight to control values.[38] NPY is therefore suggested to drive hunger and hyperphagia in these states and thus return body weight to its set point. Confirmatory evidence for the role of NPY in energy deficient states has been gained from experiments which demonstrated that destruction of NPY neurones prevented the food intake stimulation usually induced by a 12-hour fast in the rat.[39]

Galanin

Galanin is a 29-amino acid peptide which was first isolated from porcine intestine. In the brain, galanin-like immunoreactivity has been shown to be predominantly localised to the hypothalamus-hypophysial region. The physiological role of neuronal galanin in the central nervous system has not been established but its presence in brain areas concerned with regulation of ingestive behaviour suggests a potential role in feeding regulation. When injected into the paraventricular nucleus, but not other hypothalamic sites, galanin increases food intake in satiated animals.[41,41] Further experiments also showed an increase in food intake after galanin injection in fasted animals.[42] This suggests that galanin is acting by activation of feeding behaviour and not by suppression of satiety signals which are presumably not initially operative in fasted animals. A physiological role for galanin in feeding behaviour would be more convincing if galanin antagonists or anti-galanin antibodies had been shown to produce a reduction in food intake. Furthermore a relationship between galanin expression and nutrient status has not been shown. These studies should be performed before the role of galanin in feeding behaviour can be defined.

Melanin-concentrating hormone

New hypothalamic peptides which may influence feeding behaviour are still being discovered although their exact physiological role is not yet known. Qu and co-workers[43] used differential display polymerase chain reaction to identify mRNAs that are differentially expressed in the hypothalamus of ob/+ heterozygotes compared with ob/ob mice. In the obese mice they found overexpression of NPY as reported previously and also overexpression of mRNA which encodes for the neuropeptide melanin-concentrating hormone (MCH). This 19-amino acid neuropeptide is synthesised and released almost exclusively from the lateral hypothalamus. Fasting increased expression of MCH mRNA in both normal and obese animals by factors of four and three respectively. Administration of MCH into the lateral ventricle at the beginning of the feeding cycle doubled caloric consumption. The overexpression of MCH in obese mice, the change in expression with nutritional status and the increase in feeding after administration of MCH all suggest a physiological role for this peptide in feeding behaviour. It is possible that MCH may stimulate feeding by antagonism of the anorexigenic peptide, melanocyte-stimulating hormone. Further experiments will be necessary to define the interaction between leptin and MCH and also to clarify the role of MCH in feeding behaviour in normal weight animals.

Other peptides which stimulate feeding

Noradrenaline has been shown to enhance feeding when injected into the paraventricular nucleus by a mechanism that involves α_2 postsynaptic adrenergic receptors.[44] It is thought that α_2 adrenergic receptors stimulate feeding by blocking the release of a feeding inhibitor and the most likely candidate is corticotrophin-releasing factor. The observation that opioid antagonists, such as naloxone, increase feeding in a single meal suggest that the endogenous opioids modulate feeding behaviour.[45] However, they do not appear to regulate long-term feeding as chronic administration of opioid antagonists do not result in weight loss in humans.

Peptides and neurotransmitters which reduce food intake

Serotonin

The hypothalamic peptides discussed so far act principally to initiate feeding. Other peptides, when administered into the brain seem principally to inhibit feeding and these are summarised in Figure 13.4. Pharmacological, biochemical and behavioural evidence has accumulated in animals in support of the belief that brain serotonin (5-HT) has an inhibitory influence over feeding behaviour.[46,47] There are additional studies which indicate a potential role for 5-HT in control of human eating behaviour as well. Serotonin is found in various peripheral regions and is particularly concentrated in the gastrointestinal tract. While there is evidence that peripheral 5-HT systems may play some role in mediating the anorexic actions of serotonergic agonists it is believed that brain 5-HT which is dense within the hypothalamus is most critically involved in feeding regulation.

Injection of 5-HT into the ventricles or hypothalamus of mice reduces food intake in a subsequent test meal. In these studies the paraventricular nucleus has been found to be most sensitive to the administration of 5-HT and at doses that are 100- to 1000-fold lower than doses used with peripheral injection. After central 5-HT administration, animals display a significant decrease in the size and duration of meals, as well as a reduced rate of eating. However, the latency to meal onset and the frequency of meals are not affected.[48] These results suggest that endogenous 5-HT may influence primarily the termination of feeding (i.e. via induction of satiety) rather than initiation of feeding which is controlled by other neuropeptides such as NPY and MCH. Changes in the metabolism of brain 5-HT in animals experiencing different nutritional states have been found and this would support the role of 5-HT as a physiological regulator of food intake. This is also suggested by the observation that 5-HT antagonists increase feeding and lead to weight gain.[49] In addition drugs such as dexfenfluramine which mimic the effects of 5-HT, by releasing 5-HT from serotonergic nerve endings and inhibiting its neuronal reuptake in the central nervous system, inhibit feeding and induce weight loss in animals and humans.

Genetic manipulation of serotonergic function in mice have confirmed that 5-HT does indeed have a role in the control of feeding. These studies point to an important function of 5-HT in the long-term regu-

lation of energy balance and they have also indentified the receptor subtype which modulates feeding. Mutant mice lacking functional 5-HT$_{2c}$ receptors develop obesity which is entirely due to increased food consumption.[50]

Corticotrophin–releasing factor

Corticotrophin-releasing factor (CRF) is expressed at high levels in neurones of the paraventricular nucleus which project to the median eminence and autonomic centres in the brain stem. CRF neurones are closely surrounded by NPY terminals and some CRF neurones project close to the NPY cell bodies. The effects of CRF are diammetrically opposed to those of NPY. Injection into the paraventricular nucleus causes profound suppression of food intake and can inhibit feeding induced by NPY.[51] In contrast to NPY, CRF activity in the paraventricular nucleus increases with feeding and decreases with fasting.[35] The opposing actions of NPY and CRF on food intake and energy balance together with their close anatomical proximity in specific hypothalamic regions that control food intake suggest that the balance between these two systems may be an important determinant of energy homeostasis. This hypothesis is supported by the observation that CRF inhibits NPY synthesis and NPY-induced feeding is enhanced in CRF-deficient rats. Overall these observations suggest that CRF neurones normally tonically inhibit the arcuate nucleus-paraventricular NPY projection.

Melanocyte–stimulating hormone

Yellow-agouti mouse mutants are named for their bright yellow fur but they are also obese (Table 13.1). In this model there is widespread expression of the agouti protein which is normally exclusively expressed within the hair follicle and induces a switch in melanocytes from eumelanin to phaeomelanin synthesis by antagonism of the melanocyte-stimulating hormone (MSH) receptor. A series of experiments suggests that ectopic agouti peptide expression induces obesity by chronic inhibition of MSH on hypo-thalamic melanocortin-4 receptors.[52,53] A role for MSH in feeding behaviour is supported by the observation that MSH agonists inhibit food intake in normal and obese animals whereas MSH antagonists have the opposite effect. Very high circulating concentrations of leptin in the yellow-agouti mouse mutants and melanocortin-4 receptor knockout mice suggest that a functioning melanocortin-4 receptor may be necessary to respond to leptin.

Other anorectic peptides

Central administration of thyrotropin releasing hormone (TRH) and its breakdown product, cyclo-histidyl-proline-diketopiperzaine (cHis-Pro) inhibit food intake and long-term central infusions result in weight loss. However, it is possible that TRH produces its effects on weight loss by increasing sympathetic nervous system outflow and increasing metabolic rate. Calcitonin gene-related peptide decreases food intake after central administration but this may be secondary to its aversive effects rather than a specific effect on appetite.[54]

Summary

Therefore, in summary there are two groups of peptides and neurotransmitters involved in the control of feeding behaviour. One group stimulate feeding and in the long-term tend to promote weight gain. Others reduce food intake and lead to weight loss. It would seem likely that these groups do not work in isolation and body weight depends on the balance between the two systems.

Short-term regulation of appetite control

The neurotransmitters which have been discussed previously have been shown to have a central role in the regulation of energy balance over long periods. Some of these have also been shown to influence feeding behaviour in single meal experiments. There are additional mechanisms, predominantly originating in the gastrointestinal tract, which appear only to influence the short-term regulation of food intake i.e. meal-to-meal variation. However, the response of short-term signals to food ingestion is influenced by long-term regulators. For example, after a period of food deprivation these short-term signals would be less influenced by food ingestion which would lead to greater than usual food intake during each meal until body weight is restored.

Gastric distension, accomplished either by eating or balloon inflation, results in a feeling of 'fullness' and a reduction in food intake which is thought to be mediated by hormonal mechanisms. However, the pleasant feeling of satiety which is experienced after a meal requires additional signals from the gastro-intestinal tract and these are generated by the presence of food in the upper intestine.[55] Intraduodenal, but not intravenous, infusion of lipid in both animals and man will induce feelings of satiety and a reduction in food intake.[56,57] This suggests that the effects of the lipid infusion are related to nutrient receptor mechanisms in the gut rather than due purely to postabsorptive influences on eating behaviour. Cholecystokinin (CCK) has come under close scrutiny as a potential mediator of gut derived satiety signals. Luminal nutrients are potent stimulants of cholecystokinin (CCK) from I cells which are predominantly situated in the intestinal crypts of the duodenum and proximal jejunum. Experiments in both animals and humans have shown that an intravenous infusion of CCK, which reproduces postprandial plasma concentrations, will reduce food intake in a subsequent test meal.[58,59] Furthermore administration of trypsin inhibitors or amino acids before a meal will induce release of CCK and reduce subsequent calorie consumption.[60,61] These experiments provide support that CCK is a physio-logical satiety peptide in both animals and humans. It is thought that CCK initiates its action in the periphery and subsequently information is relayed to the brain by a combination of CCK- and non-CCK containing pathways including the vagus nerve, nucleus tractus solitarius, area postrema and the para-ventricular nucleus of the hypothalamus.

Intravenous infusion of another gut derived peptide, bombesin, increases satiety ratings and reduces food intake in humans.[62] However, this may have been a pharmacological rather than physiological action and further studies are needed to clarify the role of bombesin in regulation of food intake.

Postingestive signals generated by nutrients absorbed from the digestive tract are also thought to act on putative receptors in the satiety system. These signals include circulating amino acids and simple sugars such as glucose. The latter may act by releasing glycogen from the liver and increasing plasma concentrations which then somehow signals to the central feeding centres.

Mechanisms of anorexia in disease

As was discussed in the introductory paragraphs of this chapter weight loss in chronic disease results from a reduction in food intake secondary to anorexia. The continuing anorexia despite progressive weight loss suggests that there is a failure in the regulatory mech-anisms which would normally lead to consumption of extra calories after a period of semistarvation. A greater understanding of the mechanism of anorexia in these disease states may help in the development of specific and targeted treatments to reverse anorexia and promote weight gain.

We have explored the hypothesis that anorexia in chronic inflammatory disease results from plasma concentrations of leptin which are inappropriately high for the percentage body fat. This hypothesis developed from studies *in vitro* which showed that pro-inflammatory cytokines (previously discussed as potential mediators of anorexia and weight loss in chronic inflammatory disease) released leptin from isolated fat cells.[63] In our studies we found that patients with IBD and AIDS had raised plasma concentrations of TNF but serum leptin was not raised compared to healthy controls matched for body fat.[64,65] In the AIDS patients serum leptin was actually lower than expected suggesting a compensatory response to extreme weight loss. These results are thus in contrast to those predicted from the animal studies and do not support a role for leptin in mediating anorexia and weight loss associated with chronic inflammatory and infectious diseases.

In the Yoshida sarcoma rat model tumour growth is accompanied by anorexia and progressive weight loss. In tumour-bearing animals there is a decrease in NPY concentrations and an increase in CRF concentrations compared to controls.[66] These results are opposite to those expected in weight losing animals who would normally show increased NPY and reduced CRF concentrations which would stimulate feeding in an attempt to restore body weight. It is thought that pro-inflammatory cytokines may lead to impaired NPY activity and failure of CRF activity to be suppressed in response to weight loss. These changes may contribute to the anorexia and wasting which are seen in this model.

Conclusions

In the last few years there has been enormous progress in our understanding of appetite control in health. From this we have developed some insight into the potential mediators of anorexia associated with disease states. Future studies will identify other mediators and clarify exactly which of these mediators play key roles in causation of anorexia. This will hopefully allow investigators to develop targeted and specific treatments to correct anorexia which would undoubtedly improve the prognosis and quality of life for many patients.

References

1. Maffeis C, Zaffanello M, Pinelli L *et al*. Total energy expenditure and patterns of activity in 8–10-year-old obese and nonobese children. *J Paediatr Gastroenterol Nutr* 1996; **23**: 256–261.

2. Prentice AM, Black AE, Coward WA *et al*. Energy expenditure in overweight and obese adults in affluent societies: an analysis of 319 doubly-labelled water measurements. *Eur J Clin Nutr* 1996; **50**: 93–97.

3. Amatruda JM, Statt Mc, Welle SL. Total and resting energy expenditure in obese women reduced to ideal body weight. *J Clin Invest* 1993; **92**: 1236–1242.

4. DeWys WB, Begg C, Lavin PT *et al*. Prognostic effect of weight loss prior to chemotherapy in cancer patients. *Am J Med* 1980; **69**: 491–497.

5. Kelts DG, Grand RJ, Shen G *et al*. Nutritional basis of growth failure in children and adolescents with Crohn's disease. *Gastroenterology* 1979; **76**: 720–727.

6. Kirschner BS, Klich JR, Kalman SS *et al*. Reversal of growth retardation in Crohn's disease with therapy emphasizing oral nutritional restitution. *Gastroenterology* 1981; **80**: 10–15.

7. Oliff A, Defeo-Jones D, Boyer M *et al*. Tumors secreting human TNF/cachectin induce cachexia in mice. *Cell* 1987; **50**: 555–563.

8. Black K, Garrett R, Mundy R. Chinese hamster ovarian cells transfected with the murine interleukin-6 gene cause hypercalcaemia as well as cachexia, leukocytosis and thrombocytosis in tumor-bearing nude mice. *Endocrinology* 1991; **128**: 2657–2659.

9. McHugh KJ, Collins SM, Weingarten HP. Central interleukin-1 receptors contribute to suppression of feeding after acute colitis in the rat. *Am J Physiol* 1994; **266**: R1659–R1663.

10. Macallan DC, Noble C, Baldwin C *et al*. Energy expenditure and wasting in human immunodeficiency virus infection. *N Engl J Med* 1995; **333**: 83–88.

11. Bibby MC, Double JA, Sahira AA *et al*. Characterization of a transplantable adenocarcinoma of the mouse colon producing cachexia in recipient animals. *JNCI* 1987; **78**: 539–546.

12. Bruera E. Clinical management of anorexia and cachexia in patients with advanced cancer. *Oncology* 1992; **49**: 35–42.

13. Fearon KHC. The mechanisms and treatment of weight loss in cancer. *Proc Nutr Soc* 1992; **51**: 251–265.

14. Fredrix EW, Soeters PB, Wouters EF *et al*. Effect of different tumour types on resting energy expenditure. *Cancer Res* 1991; **51**: 6138–6141

15. Hyltander A, Drott C, Korner U *et al*. Elevated energy expenditure in cancer patients with solid tumours. *Eur J Cancer* 1991; **27**: 9–15.

16. Kennedy GC. The role of depot fat in the hypothalamic control of food intake in the rat. *Proc R Soc* 1953; **140**: 578–592.

17. Hervey GR. The effect of lesions in the hypothalamus in parabiotic rats. *J Physiol* 1958; **145**: 336–352.

18. Hausberger FX. Parabiosis and transplantation experiments in hereditary obese mice. *Anat Rec* 1959; **130**: 313.

19. Zhang Y, Proenca R, Maffei M *et al.* Positional cloning of the mouse obese gene and its human homologue. *Nature* 1994; **372**: 425–432.

20. Halaas JL, Gajiwala KS, Maffei *et al.* Weight-reduction effects of the plasma protein encoded by the obese gene. *Science* 1995; **269**: 543–546.

21. Pelleymounter MA, Cullen MJ, Baker MB *et al.* Effects of the obese gene product on body weight regulation in *ob/ob* mice. *Science* 1995; **269**: 540–543.

22. Campfield LA, Smith FJ, Guisez Y *et al.* Recombinant mouse ob protein: evidence for a peripheral signal linking adiposity and central neural networks. *Science* 1995; **269**: 546–549.

23. Considine RV, Sinha MK, Heiman ML *et al.* Serum immunoreactive-leptin concentrations in normal-weight and obese humans. *N Engl J Med* 1995; **334**: 292–295.

24. Frederich RC, Hamann A, Anderson S *et al.* Leptin levels reflect body lipid content in mice: evidence for diet-induced resistance to leptin action. *Nature Med* 1995; **1**: 1311–1314.

25. Hassink SG, Sheslow DV, de Lancey E. Serum leptin in children with obesity: relationship to gender and development. *Paediatrics* 1996; **98**: 201–203.

26. Maffei M, Halaas J, Ravussin E *et al.* Leptin levels in human and rodent: measurement of plasma leptin and ob mRNA in obese and weight-reduced subjects. *Nature Med* 1995; **1**: 1155–1161.

27. Grinspoon S, Gulick T, Askari H *et al.* Serum leptin levels in women with anorexia nervosa. *J Clin Endocrinol Metab* 1996; **81**: 3861–3863.

28. Hickey MS, Considine RV, Israel RG *et al.* Leptin is related to body fat content in male distance runners. *Am J Physiol* 1996; **271**: E938–940.

29. Considine RV, Considine EL, Williams CJ *et al.* Evidence against either a premature stop codon or the absence of obese gene mRNA in human obesity. *J Clin Invest* 1995; **95**: 2986–2988.

30. Caro JF, Kolaczynski JW, Nyce MR *et al.* Decreased cerebrospinal-fluid/serum leptin ratio in obesity: a possible mechanism for leptin resistance. *Lancet* 1996; **348**: 159–161.

31. Wabitsch M, Jensen PB, Blum WF *et al.* Insulin and cortisol promote leptin production in cultured human fat cells. *Diabetes* 1996; **45**: 1435–1438.

32. Stephens TW, Basinski M, Briston PK *et al.* The role of neuropeptide Y in the antiobesity action of the obese gene product. *Nature* 1995; **377**: 530–532.

33. Zarjevski N, Cusin I, Vettor R *et al.* Chronic intracerebroventricular NPY administration to normal rats mimics hormonal and metabolic changes of obesity. *Endocrinol* 1993; **133**: 1753–1758.

34. Erickson JC, Hollopeter G, Palmiter RD. Attenuation of the obesity syndrome of *ob/ob* mice by the loss of neuropeptide Y. *Science* 1996; **274**: 1704–1707.

35. Brady LS, Smith MA, Gold PW *et al.* Altered expression of hypothalamic neuropeptide mRNAs in food restricted and food deprived rats. *Neuroendocrinology* 1990; **52**: 441–447.

36. Sahu A, Kalra PS, Kalra SP. Food deprivation and ingestion induce reciprocal changes in neuropeptide Y concentration in the paraventricular nucleus. *Peptides* 1988; **9**: 83–86.

37. Williams G, Gill JS, Lee YC *et al.* Increased neuropeptide Y concentrations in specific hypothalamic regions of streptozocin-induced diabetic rats. *Diabetes* 1989; **38**: 321–327.

38. Davies L, Marks JL. Role of hypothalamic NPY gene expression in body weight regulation. *Am J Physiol* 1994; **266**: R1687–R1691.

39. Burlet A, Grouzmann E, Musse N *et al.* The immunological impairment of arcuate neuropeptide Y neurons by ricin A chain produces persistent decrease of food intake and body weight. *Neuroscience* 1995; **66**: 151–159.

40. Kyrkouli SE, Stanley BG, Hutchinson R *et al.* Peptide-amine interactions in the hypothalamic paraventricular nucleus: analysis of galanin and neuropeptide Y in relation to feeding. *Brain Res* 1990; **521**: 185–191.

41. Smith BK, York DA, Bray GA. Effects of dietary preference and galanin administration in the paraventricular or amygdaloid nucleus on diet self-selection. *Brain Res Bull* 1996; **39**: 149–154.

42. Schick RR, Soheyla S, Zimmermann JP *et al.* Effect of galanin on food intake in rats: involvement of lateral and ventromedial hypothalamic sites. *Am J Physiol* 1990; **264**: R355–R361.

43. Qu D, Ludwig DS, Gammeltoft S *et al.* A role for melanin-concentrating hormone in the central regulation of feeding behaviour. *Nature* 1996; **380**: 243–247.

44. Goldman CK, Marino L, Leibowitz SF. Post synaptic alpha-2 noradrenergic receptors mediate feeding induced by paraventricular nucleus injection of norepinephrine and clonidine. *Eur J Pharmacol* 1985; **115**: 11–19.

45. Holtzman SG. Behavioural effects of separate and combined administration of naloxone and d-amphetamine. *J Pharmacol Exp Ther* 1974; **189:** 51–60.

46. Blundell JE. Serotonin and appetite. *Neuropharmacology* 1984; **23:** 1537–1551.

47. Garratini S, Samanin R. D-Fenfluramine and salbutamol: two drugs causing anorexia through different neurochemical mechanisms. *Int J Obesity* 1984; **8 (Suppl 1):** 151–157.

48. Leibowitz SF, Shor-Posner G. Hypothalamic monoamine systems for control of food intake: analysis of meal patterns and macronutrient selection. In: *Psychopharmacology of eating disorders: theoretical and clinical advances.* Raven, New York, 1986.

49. Simpson RJ, Lawton DJ, Watt MH *et al*. Effect of zimelidine, a new antidepressant, on appetite and body weight. *Br J Clin Pharmacol* 1981; **11:** 96–98.

50. Tecott LH, Sun LM, Akana SF *et al*. Eating disorder and epilepsy in mice lacking 5-HT$_2$ serotonin receptors. *Nature* 1995; **374:** 542–546.

51. Glowa J, Barrett J, Russell J. Effects of CRF on appetitive behaviours. *Peptides* 1992; **13:** 609–621.

52. Huszar D, Lynch CA, Fairchild-Huntress V *et al*. Targeted disruption of the melanocortin-4 receptor results in obesity in mice. *Cell* 1997; **88:** 131–141.

53. Fan W, Boston BA, Kesterson RA *et al*. Role of melanocortinergic neurons in feeding and the *agouti* obesity syndrome. *Nature* 1997; **385:** 165–168.

54. Krahn DD, Gosnell BA, Levine AS. The effect of calcitonin-gene related peptide on food intake involves aversive mechanisms. *Biochem Behav* 1986; **24:** 5–7.

55. Read N, French S, Cunningham K. The role of the gut in regulating food intake in man. *Nutr Rev* 1994; **52:** 1–10.

56. Greenberg D, Gibbs J, Smith GP. Infusions of lipid into the duodenum elicit satiety in rats while similar infusions into the vena cava do not (abstract). *Appetite* 1989; **12:** 213.

57. Welch IMcL, Saunders K, Read NW. The effect of ileal and intravenous infusions of fat emulsions on feeding and satiety on human volunteers. *Gastroenterology* 1985; **89:** 1293–1297.

58. Ballinger AB, McLoughlin L, Medbak S *et al*. Cholecystokinin is a satiety hormone in humans at physiological postprandial concentrations. *Clin Sci* 1995; **89:** 375–381.

59. Calingasan N, Ritter S, Ritter R *et al*. Low-dose near-celiac arterial cholecystokinin suppresses food intake in rats. *Am J Physiol* 1992; **263:** R572–R577.

60. Ballinger AB, Clark ML. L-phenylalanine releases cholecystokinin and is associated with reduced food intake in humans: Evidence for a physiological role of CCK in control of eating. *Metabolism* 1994; **43:** 735–738.

61. Hill AJ, Peikin SR, Ryan CA *et al*. Oral administration of protease inhibitor II from potatoes reduces energy intake in man. *Physiol Behav* 1990; **48:** 241–246.

62. Lieverse RJ, Jansen JBMJ, Masclee AAM *et al*. Bombesin reduces food intake after a preload in man by a cholecystokinin-independent mechanism. *Clin Sci* 1993; **85:** 277–280.

63. Sarraf P, Frederich RC, Turner EM *et al*. Multiple cytokines and acute inflammation raise mouse leptin levels: potential role in inflammatory anorexia. *J Exp Med* 1997; **185:** 171–175.

64. Ballinger AB, Hallyburton EM, Besser R, Alstead EM, Farthing MJG. Serum leptin in inflammatory bowel disease (IBD): implications for the pathogenesis of anorexia and weight loss (abstract). *Gut* 1997; **40:** 74.

65. Kelly P, Ballinger AB, Luo N, Pobee JOM, Farthing MJG. Leptin dysregulation in Africans with 'slim disease' (abstract). *Gastroenterology* 1977; **112:** 885.

66. McCarthy HD, McKibbin PE, Perkins AV *et al*. Alterations in hypothalamic NPY and CRF in anorexic tumor-bearing rats. *Am J Physiol* 1993; **264:** E638–E643.

15

Hospital food as treatment

Simon Allison

16

Oral diet administration and supplementation

Ib Hessov

The oral route for nutrition support is little understood and the most under-utilised in hospitals when prevention or reversal of malnutrition is being considered.[1] However, if the patient is conscious and if the gastrointestinal tract is functioning the oral route is cheap, does not require sophisticated technology and has no life-threatening complications.

The best use of the oral route for nutrition support will only be achieved with adequate nutrition education of doctors and nurses who may then motivate the patient to reach appropriate nutrition targets. Paradoxically, knowledge about the nutrient value of normal food is often sparse compared to the knowledge about intravenous nutrition and enteral products.

Hospital food

In contrast to food consumed by the average person, food recommended by Health Authorities is rich in fibre, vitamins and minerals but poor in refined sugars, fat and energy (Table 16.1). In many countries the basic hospital food is very similar to the food recommended for healthy people – presumably because many patients are those with diabetes, heart attack and obesity-related diseases. For these patients and for all the well nourished individuals with good appetite such recommendations are appropriate.

But is such food also appropriate for sick undernourished patients with poor appetite? No studies in patients have compared the nutrient intake from normal solid food with different energy densities but certainly it is difficult for undernourished patients to consume voluminous portions of food. Is it possible to increase energy intake in these patients by either enriching the diet with energy or by manipulating diet

Table 16.1 – Percentage energy distribution in the average Danish diet,[2] in the Nordic recommendations,[3] and in standard hospital diet in Denmark.[4]

	Average diet %	Recommended diet %	Hospital diet %
Protein	13	10–15	13
Fat	43	30	30
Carbohydrate	44	55–60	57
Alcohol	3	–	–

composition? This topic has been extensively studied in healthy volunteers.

Effects of the physical state of food and energy density on satiety and food intake

When the same food is served in either solid or liquid form the rate of consumption of the liquid form is faster and the meal duration shorter than for the solid.[5,6] After both liquid and solid test meals the appetite is suppressed for two to three hours with a maximum satiety at between 30 minutes and two hours after the food intake.[5,7] Studies on the importance of the physical state (liquid/solid) of the food on satiety are conflicting.[5,6] If two test meals containing 60 g of available carbohydrate as apple (482 g) or apple juice (469 ml) were compared, the lowest satiety was found after the fibre-free juice.[5] This is in agreement with studies demonstrating that a fibre-rich breakfast resulted in reduced energy consumption from the following lunch, as well as from the breakfast alone when compared to a fibre-poor breakfast.[7,8] Conversely, soup has been shown to be more effective in producing satiety, as measured by food intake reduction, when compared with the same amount of energy given as solid food.[6]

The importance of energy density on energy intake

Contrary to the conflicting studies mentioned above there is agreement between studies on the effect of energy consumption from simple meals on satiety and on total consumption. Mixed meals, solid food and liquid supplements with a high energy content reduce appetite more than those with low energy content.[6,7,9,10] In most of the studies[6,7,9] the high energy food also suppressed energy consumption from a subsequent test meal. Nevertheless consumption of an energy-rich meal results in higher overall total daily energy intake. If test subjects were served a fibre-poor midday meal rich in fat and refined sugar giving approximately 2.0 MJ in excess of normal, the subjects consumed about 2.0 MJ extra that day and continued to do so for the entire 14-day study period.[11] Also, consumption of one litre of soda water with 2.3 MJ high-fructose corn syrup resulted in an increase in total energy consumption as it only decreased other voluntary food intake the same day by 0.8 MJ.[10] This is in agreement with a study demonstrating substantial weight loss on a low-energy diet compared with high-energy foods.[12]

Effects of food composition on satiety and food intake

The satiating effect of protein, carbohydrate and fat appears the same in some studies.[7,13] Others have described that protein has a greater depressor effect on appetite and hunger, and on subsequent energy intakes than fat and carbohydrates.[14,15] However, a Swedish study showed that protein enrichment of the hospital food resulted in a substantial increase in both protein consumption and in energy intake.[16] Some studies seem to indicate that high-fat diets tend to increase energy intake.[9,13,17]

Thus healthy volunteers, who received continuous intravenous (IV) nutrition consumed twice as much energy from liquid meals on days when they were given IV fat emulsions compared with days when they were given iso-energetic glucose infusions.[18] Additionally, high-fat diets gave rise to less intensive satiety than high-carbohydrate diets of equal energetic value,[19] and excess of fat surreptitiously added to meals leads to increased daily energy consumption.[11,17,20]

Conclusions from studies in healthy volunteers

The statements listed in Table 16.2 summarise the data available. The question remains whether these results are also valid for undernourished patients with poor appetite. Data are available for liquid supplements (see below), but data concerning solid food are lacking. Most health care workers would agree, however, that it is difficult for the undernourished sick patient to consume large bulky portions of food. Unfortunately, fibre-rich low-energy diets are just that. Thus a diet based on recommendations for the healthy population

Table 16.2 – Relevance of the nature of food on energy intake in healthy individual.

1. A fibre-rich low energy diet results in lower energy consumption and weight loss.
2. A high-energy solid meal suppresses appetite more than a low-energy meal but results finally in an increased daily energy intake.
3. High energy liquid supplements before meals induce satiety but nevertheless the daily energy intake increases.
4. The degree of hunger or satiety is often unrelated to the amount of food subsequently consumed.
5. IV nutrition based on glucose suppresses voluntary food intake.

is probably inappropriate for the undernourished anorectic patient.

A practical strategy for feeding undernourished patients could therefore follow these recommendations.

- For the severely undernourished patient a high-energy high-protein diet should be given in the full knowledge that this diet is rich in fat and refined sugars and poor in fibre.

- An energy-rich basic diet may be convenient for those who are severely undernourished after acute illness or for those who are undernourished because of chronic illness (e.g. cancer or chronic obstructive pulmonary disease). However, many undernourished patients can increase their nutrition intake only by oral supplements consumed between the main meals (see below).

- As IV nutrition suppresses food intake it is not rational to use IV nutrition as a supplement!

Recently it has officially been recommended[4] that Danish hospital kitchens offer two different basic hospital diets to the wards: a standard diet, and a diet for the under-nourished (Table 16.3). This means that the staff in the ward have to decide which diet is appropriate for each patient.

Table 16.3 – Percentage energy distribution in the two recommended basic hospital diets in Denmark.[4]

	Standard diet	Diet for the under-nourished
Protein	13	18
Fat	30	40
Carbohydrate	57	42

Oral supplements

Patients' knowledge about the nutrient content in food is often sparse. It is therefore worth explaining to the undernourished patient about the energy and protein contents in what may be considered nourishing food (Table 16.4) compared with the oral supplements offered him by the hospital (Table 16.5). Many patients are very surprised by the very low nutrient value of soups. A strong, tasty meat soup, or a tasty vegetable soup, is not at all rich in nutrients. Only

Table 16.4 – Comparative energy and protein contents in drinks (200 ml) soups (200 ml) and snacks.

	Energy kJ	Protein g
Lager	306	0
Stout	310	0
Red wine	588	0
Irish coffee	978	1
Beef soup (clear)	24	1
Vegetable soups (clear)	380	2
Oatmeal	400	3
Chocolate (25 g)	565	2
Peanuts (20 g)	522	5
Pommes frites (25 g)	408	1
Cookies (20 g)	252	2
Apple (large)	147	0
Carrot (10 cm)	125	1

Table 16.5 – Comparative energy and protein content in drinks and liquid supplements (200 ml) available in the ward.

	Energy kJ	Protein g
Apple juice	364	0
Orange juice	566	1
Protein juice	560	7
Light beer	234	0
Milk	538	7
Quarg drink	780	14
Cocoa quarg drink	722	9
Fortimel® Nutricia Clinical, Wilts, UK	840	20
★Addera®	720	8

★ Manufacturer is Semper

soups thickened with energy-rich and protein-rich nutrients such as milk products and egg will contain satisfactory amounts of nutrients. Again, surprisingly to many, neither are strong beer, red wine, an apple or a carrot worth taking as a supplement for the undernourished.

Every ward should have a list showing the energy and protein content in available drinks and supplements. Table 16.5 shows the energy and protein content in refreshing drinks and supplements served in my own department. It enables both staff and patient to decide what is worth drinking and what is not.

Home-made oral supplements

Some of the oral supplements in Table 16.5 are made in the kitchen from milk products, quarg and egg. From clinical experience and from controlled studies[21,,22] we know that many patients like these drinks, and if they drink a glass (200 ml) between main meals and one before bed time the protein intake may increase by 30–40 g per day. All hospitals should have some home-made supplements available and arrange to offer the patients the recipies at discharge (Tables 16.6, 16.7).

Intolerance to lactose and intolerance to the taste of milk prevent a widespread use of home-made supplements. Milk constitutes a large percentage of these supplements and those individuals with lactose intolerance need to be identified. There are patients with known lactose intolerance, but also some patients demonstrate a temporary lactose intolerance following fasting and intravenous nutrition or after gastrointestinal disease or surgery involving the gastrointestinal tract.

Table 16.6 – Recipe for cocoa quarg★ drink (722 kJ, 9 g protein).

150 ml cocoa milk
3 spoons of quarg★ 5% (30 g)
4 spoons of maltodextrin
1 spoon of cream 36%

Table 16.7 – Recipe for quarg★ drink (780 kJ, 14 g protein).

1 egg (60 g)
1 spoon of sugar (12 g)
4 1/2 spoons of quarg★ 5% (45 g)
150 cc of buttermilk
2 spoons of orange juice

★ Quarg is a low fat cream cheese (12 g protein and 280 kJ in 100 ml)

Commercial oral supplements

Two principally different industrial products are listed in Table 16.5. The first (Fortimel Nutricia Clinical, Wilts, UK) contains all vitamins and minerals in recommended amounts and are based on intact protein. The protein juice, based on enzymatically hydrolysed peptides, is only an energy-protein supplement.

The technical problem with protein in commercial liquid diets is the low solubility often resulting in an unpleasant appearance and in a rather high viscosity.[23] When a protein is hydrolysed the solubility increases and the viscosity of the solution is reduced. Unfortunately, the result is often a penetrating bitter taste. This palatability problem depends on the amino acid composition of the protein and the degree of hydrolysis.[23–25] It is predominantly the hydrophobic amino acids which are responsible for the bitter taste. These amino acids are mainly placed in the structural centre of the protein and will therefore not influence the taste when the supplements are based on un-hydrolysed intact protein.

With increasing hydrolysis the bitter taste increases. Therefore, pure amino acid solutions will always have some degree of unpalatability. In peptide solutions bitterness has also been a practical problem but today it is possible by means of sophisticated enzymatic approaches to obtain a peptide solution with a specific degree of hydrolysis.[23,25] Thus it is possible to produce aqueous protein-rich supplements without an unpleasant taste. In the near future a variety of tasty aqueous juice-like supplements with a protein content between 4 g and 10 g per 100 ml should be available for the undernourished patient.

Palatability of oral supplements

Palatability is defined as 'the hedonic response' of the individual to the flavour of the food to be ingested,[1] and flavour, broadly defined, includes smell, taste, temperature and viscosity.

Palatability studies are often performed by taste panels of healthy people, who imbibe only 10 ml of the test drink. Although a high palatability rating is necessary for the patients' choice of supplements, the result of taste studies will only give us a slight impression of the applicability in the clinical setting. Thus, high palatability ratings in undernourished patients do not necessarily imply high volume intake or good compliance.[26] One reason may be the monotony in diet repetition.[27,28] However several clinical studies have demonstrated that this is not a common explanation. When first accepted during a week, most patients will continue to take the same amount of supplements for months.[29–35]

Not unexpectedly, all amino acid solutions are rated poorly in spite of all attempts to disguise taste using flavoured additives.[1] Amino-acid based supplements are not generally to be recommended for the under-nourished patient. In contrast, flavoured commercial supplements based on intact protein or on peptides have received high palatability rating in many studies.[1,26,36]

Who needs oral supplements?

All undernourished patients capable of eating spontaneously may benefit from oral supplements. However, in many surgical departments patients are not allowed to eat normally because of the belief that postoperative intestinal decompression decreases the patients' abdominal discomfort as well as the incidence of complications. The traditional postoperative regimen has therefore consisted of decompression via a nasogastric tube until passage of flatus, followed by stepwise return to normal food. However, controlled studies have made it clear that this regimen is not necessary after the majority of abdominal operations including surgery on the intestine.[37]

Are postoperative nasogastric tubes necessary?

After an abdominal operation propulsive peristaltic waves are seen in the small intestine after a few hours.[38,39] In fasting patients non-propulsive activity can be recorded in the colon after 40–48 hours and flatus passes after 4–5 days. There are no controlled clinical studies demonstrating what happens to the postoperative colon, when stimulated by food intake. Studies on immediate postoperative enteral or oral feeding[22,37]) suggest that delayed gastric emptying is far more clinically relevant than delayed colon activity. After abdominal operations (e.g. cholecystectomies) a near normal emptying of the stomach can be demonstrated after 24 hours in most patients.[40]

The primary reason for delay in the return of gastric function is the use of systemically administered opioids.[41] It has now been shown that the recovery of gastrointestinal function depends on the choice of postoperative analgesia and that epidural analgesia with bupivacaine and low dose morphine in combination give the best postoperative pain relief and accelerate the recovery of gastrointestinal function.[41]

The frequency of nausea and vomiting is high after abdominal operations but controlled clinical studies have shown that the incidence is very little influenced by whether nasogastric decompression is used or not. Indeed, the routine use of nasogastric tubes increases the risk of lung complications. In a meta-analysis of 3964 patients, nasogastric decompression reduced the risk of abdominal distention (11–8%) and vomiting (14–10%) but increased the incidence of postoperative atelectasis (3–6%), fever (7–11%) and pneumonia (3.6–6.1%).[42]

The most important question for the surgeon is whether decompression diminishes the risk of an anastomotic bowel leak. In the biggest study on animals[43] no differences were seen in anastomotic disruption; early enteral feeding in both nutritionally depleted and well nourished animals have clearly shown an increased DNA-synthesis and improved anastomotic strength.[44–46] These data from animal experiments lend support to the assumption that early enteral feeding may be not only harmless but positively beneficial in the presence of bowel anastomosis in man.

Early oral feeding after surgery

After some operations involving the upper gastrointestinal tract, especially after oesophagus resections, total gastrectomies and pancreatic operations, oral food is not allowed during the first days because of the anastomoses performed. In these patients early enteral feeding through a jejunostomy tube is often recommended. After nearly all other gastrointestinal operations patients can be fed orally from the first day after surgery.

The first principle is 'keep it simple' (Table 16.8). Specific rules as to how much patients may drink per hour in different situations are not necessary. Often the patient is better aware than the doctor of what he or she can tolerate and what he would like to drink and eat. Therefore, the second principle is 'let the patient decide when and what and how much to drink

Table 16.8 – Four principles in postoperative oral nutrition.

1. Keep it simple
2. Let the patient decide, when and what and how much to drink and eat.
3. Teach the patient about the nutritional value of the supplements.
4. Encourage the patient to achieve his or her requirements.

and eat'. As the hospital staff know more about postoperative nutrition than the patients, it is important to inform them about what is best, and this can be done by giving a list showing the content of energy and protein in available supplements (principle 3). Thereafter encourage them to achieve their own requirements (principle 4).

Nutrition after intestinal surgery

After elective surgery on the rectum, colon and small bowel the feeding regimen summarised in Table 16.9 is recommended. These patients have no nasogastric tube since it should be removed at the end of the operation and they may drink as soon as they are awake after the operation. Protein-rich refreshing drinks are allowed immediately. If systemic opioids are avoided in favour of epidural analgesia with bupivacaine[41] the average patient will drink 2 l on the following day and the routine IV drip should be removed. A full liquid diet is given on that day and the patient may choose between all the liquid supplements available in the department. Normal solid food is given when the patient is inclined to eat, which is usually by day 2 or 3. The staff should encourage the patient to drink at least 200 ml of liquid supplements between main meals at first and thereafter increase the protein energy consumption from the supplements either by increasing the volume or by choosing more nutrient-dense products (Table 16.5).

Many patients vomit during the first days but small volume vomiting is not an indication for a tube and does not contraindicate drinking or eating.

Early oral nutrition is safe after bowel surgery[47,48] and results in substantial nutritional intakes during the first

Table 16.9 – Feeding regimen after intestinal surgery and after all major surgery not involving the upper GI tract.

Day 0	The stomach tube is removed at the end of the operation. Give free aqueous liquids including protein soft drinks.
Day 1	Full liquid diet including all liquid supplements. Stop IV supply in the morning. Drink 2 litres.
Day 2 (or when the patients want it)	Full solid diet including supplements between main meals.

four postoperative days.[22,49] In the first controlled study performed[22] patients consumed an average of 26 g protein daily during the first four postoperative days. A recent study showed that by combining the principles in Table 16,8 with an optimal epidural analgesia[41] the average patient could drink 2 l at day one and meet nutritional requirements at day 3 or 4 after colorectal surgery.[49]

However, many surgical patients are still offered a traditional postoperative regimen which includes nasogastric decompression until bowel sounds are heard, whereupon clear liquids are given before a normal diet is allowed. At this point (usually at day 3 or 4) the staff should encourage the patients to drink a glass of one of the energy-rich and protein-rich drinks 3 times a day. By doing so the majority of patients will consume about 40 g protein by day 5 after surgery. The additional oral intake will result in an improved nitrogen balance and in reduced weight losses (about 2 kg instead of 4 kg). Two controlled studies have shown that the prescription of oral dietary supplements after major gastrointestinal surgery also resulted in less reduction in muscle function and in a lower incidence of serious infections.[50,51] In both studies oral sip feeding was first allowed after removal of the stomach tube.

If the patient does not accept the protein enriched drinks (Table 16.5) because of the taste or thick consistency he or she can choose milk or more aqueous commercial products.

Nutrition after surgery not involving the gastrointestinal tract

After the majority of minor operations patients can eat normal hospital food from the first postoperative day and it is not necessary to give any supplements.

After major retroperitoneal operations and abdominal operations not involving the GI tract, the stomach tube is not necessary, and nearly all patients will drink and consume a soup the first postoperative day (see Table 16.9). This is also valid after major gynaeco-logical surgery (e.g. radical hysterectomies with pelvic and retroperitoneal lymph node dissection). This statement is at odds with the recommendations in many textbooks which claim that nasogastric suction is necessary because a compulsory postoperative intestinal paralysis develops, often lasting for many days. In this hospital we have not used a stomach tube

after radical hysterectomies since 1987. Instead we have fed the patients.

When solid food is offered to these patients, they normally will accept it from day 2. Our regimen has been evaluated under controlled conditions in patients undergoing radical hysterectomies.[52] As expected it resulted in improved energy and protein intake when compared to a regimen including nasogastric decompression.

Feeding elderly patients in the orthopaedic department

Many elderly patients need an operation for femoral neck fracture. The majority of these patients have a very low nutritional intake while they are in hospital,[53] and many are already undernourished at admission.[54] A UK study showed that it was the undernourished patients who had the longest mobilisation time and the highest mortality.[55] Furthermore it was shown[55] that when the patients' total intake of nutrients was increased by about 2.8 MJ and 20 g of protein per day, the patients gained mobility more quickly. The extra nutritional intake in this study was administered by overnight tube feeding. Subsequently two French groups have obtained similar results using oral supplements.[56,57] In the first study, the use of a single commercial supplement increased the daily intake of energy by 1.2 MJ (23%) and the protein intake from 34 to 49 g per day. An identical increase in energy and protein consumption was demonstrated in elderly Danish women with fractured neck of the femur who were offered an oral supplement based on hydrolysed soy protein.[58] The studies demonstrated that elderly and very elderly patients can improve their spon-taneous nutritional intake by very simple measures. If undernourished orthopaedic patients are offered a variety of supplements instead of a single one, their nutritional intake may improve even more.

Preoperative feeding instead of overnight fasting

Both animal and clinical studies suggest that the overnight fasting routine may add to the metabolic stress of the operation.[59] Insulin resistance develops following surgery[60] and this insulin resistance is reduced in about 50% of patients if, instead of over-night fasting before operation, they receive 300 g of glucose as an IV infusion.[61] Older studies have shown improved protein metabolism when patients are given high preoperative doses of glucose[62] or glucose plus insulin.[63]

In many countries patients are now allowed to drink clear fluids up to 3 hours before operation.[64] A carbohydrate drink results in an insulin response similar to that after a normal meal[65] and recently it was shown that 400 ml of isotonic carbohydrate drink taken 3 hours before an operation passed through the stomach in 90 minutes.[66] Thus preliminary studies suggest that preoperative isotonic carbohydrate drinks may not only add to the patient's well-being but also reduce inappropriate postoperative insulin resistance.

Oral supplementation after discharge from hospital

Surgical patients with moderate weight losses will not regain their preoperative weight for 3–4 months after elective operations.[51,67–69] In a Danish study spontaneous food intake after discharge was almost the same as in the healthy population in the same geographical area.[69] This might explain the slow regain of body mass. In two studies of patients with small to moderate weight losses, an intervention group had full access to protein-rich supplements for 4 months.[51,69] These patients increased their protein and energy intakes, regained their body mass in 2 months,[51,69] and DEXA-scanning studies revealed that nearly all the weight gain was due to regain of lean body mass and not fat mass.[69] Unfortunately muscle function, work capacity and well-being was not influenced by the dietary intervention.[51,70]

Regain of lean body mass is therefore substantially accelerated if patients are instructed to increase their protein intake from 1.0 to 1.5 g protein per kg per day by drinking protein-rich supplements, and this may be important for patients with major weight losses.

Effects of oral supplements on geriatric patients

Malnutrition and inappropriate food intake are common in elderly patients both at home and in hospital.[53,72–74] Studies have taught us that morbidity is reduced and mobilisation time shortened in patients receiving nutritional intervention.[55–57] In an extensive Swedish study[73,74] of 501 geriatric patients, half the group was randomised to receive 2 glasses (1.6 MJ) of oral supplementation per day. After 26 weeks there was a lower incidence of malnutrition, reduced

mortality rate and a significantly higher level of activity in the supplemented group. The study did not state if the total nutritional intake improved or not. However, other studies from similar populations have shown that use of a single oral commercial supplement will improve the average energy intake by 0.8-1.6 MJ.[71,75] Thus there are good reasons to believe that in long-term geriatric care, nutritional oral supplements as part of the diet may help to maintain or improve nutritional status and functional health.

Oral nutrition in chronic pulmonary disease

Severe malnutrition in chronic obstructive pulmonary disease is a common phenomenon and weight loss in these patients is a bad prognostic sign which goes hand in hand with a deterioration in lung function. These patients have increased energy requirements and in good periods they spontaneously have a high energy consumption.[29–31] Despite this, nearly all controlled studies show that it is possible to increase both the energy and protein intake by means of oral supplements. In three studies all patients were compliant with study goals, which meant drinking up to 700 ml of either whole milk protein[30] or hydrolysed soy protein.[26,28] All three studies lasted 12 weeks, no taste fatigue was observed and the average weight gains were 1.5, 1.7 and 2.4 kg respectively. Fat-free mass increased in the study, where it was measured,[29] and the serum albumin increased significantly in all the studies. In a placebo controlled study[31] no changes in function or well-being were seen, while an improvement in maximal voluntary ventilation was seen after 6 weeks in one study.[29] In the investigation with the highest weight gain patients also improved respiratory muscle and hand grip strength as well as general well-being and 6-minutes walking distance.[30]

It can be concluded that patients in a very poor physical condition because of severe lung disease may also improve nutritional intake as well as nutritional condition and perhaps well-being and function by means of oral supplements. One would expect these severely undernourished patients to drink about 600 ml supplying 2.4 MJ and 30 g of protein per day.

Oral supplements for the cancer patient

Liquid foods are frequently offered to patients with cancer who complain of poor appetite, early satiety and weight loss. In some of the few studies of long-term intake, poor compliance occurs in 30–40%. This is often evident during the first week of supplementation.[26,32] It is claimed that food aversion and taste fatigue resulting in decreasing intake is a special problem in cancer patients but the few studies of long-term intake of supplements have not found taste fatigue to be a significant problem. If cancer patients do accept a supplement they usually continue to consume the same amounts week after week.[32–35]

Although a single study has shown that a partially hydrolysed and slightly acidic product resulted in a higher nutritional intake after 2 months in weight loosing cancer patients than a product based on intact milk protein,[35] protein-based commercial products have contributed with significant increases of energy and protein in other long-term studies.[33,34] If accepted by the cancer patient 1.6–2.4 MJ and 20–40 g protein will usually be consumed daily from a single supplement offered.

Does sip feeding reduce the consumption of solid food?

As shown in Table 16.2 the consumption of high-energy drinks in healthy man increases the total daily energy intake.

Many studies in different undernourished patient populations have convincingly demonstrated that sip feeding between the main meals does not alter the overall solid food intake. No changes in solid food intake were observed in those with femoral neck fractures[56,58] in geriatric patients[75] or after radical hysterectomy[52] and an improvement in main meal intake was the surprising result following major GI surgery.[50]

It is difficult to decide from the literature whether there is an advantage or not in giving oral supplements with very high energy and/or protein density. Only one single controlled study has compared anorectic patients' nutritional intake, when a supplement, of either nutrient dense or standard concentration was given. No differences in total nutritional intake were observed between the two groups.[36]

Conclusions from studies in undernourished patients

From the literature the following conclusions may be drawn:

- Most undernourished patients, who are able to drink can improve their nutritional intake substantially by use of liquid supplements.

- Amino-acid based supplements are not tasty and are not well accepted by the sick as oral supplements.

- Supplements based on intact proteins and on peptides both rate highly in palatability studies.

- High palatability ratings do not necessarily imply good compliance or high volume intakes.

- Supplements based on both intact protein and on peptides from enzymatically hydrolysed protein have been consumed in reasonable volumes in long-term studies without signs of taste fatigue.

- One supplement can lead to an extra intake of 2.4 MJ and 20–40 g protein daily in the average patient. A higher nutritional intake may be expected from a selection of supplements.

- Poor compliance, at a rate of 30–40%, may be seen in cancer patients during the first week of supplementation.

- Oral liquid supplements do not suppress the total nutritional intake from the main meals.

How to control the food intake

A fluid balance sheet is mandatory for ill patients. Similarly, undernourished patients, patients at risk for malnutrition and those receiving nutritional therapy should have a food record sheet for calculation of their energy and protein consumption.

In hospitals and other institutions this can be put into practice as follows. The patient is given a food-intake record sheet in the morning. The patient, his relatives, and the nursing staff note all food and drinks taken during the day on the sheet; for example: 1/2 hamburger, 2 potatoes, and 1/4 half-pint of sauce; 1 slice of rye bread with cheese; 1 cup of coffee with milk; 1/2 bar of chocolate, etc. The next morning a completed record sheet is sent to the kitchen, where the energy and protein consumption is calculated from national food-composition tables either by the dietician or by catering staff.

This simple record has been compared with the time-consuming precise weighing method[76] in a very large study of 603 one-day food intake records in a surgical department.[77] When the accuracy of 3-day records was compared, the calculation based on the simple record gave a correct assessment of the energy and protein intake within 200 kcal and 10 g of protein in 85–90% of the patients. This degree of accuracy is satisfactory for clinical use.

When the use of such a simple record becomes routine in the ward, the interest in and the attention paid to the importance of the patient's proper food intake will automatically increase. The staff and the patient in collaboration can control whether dietary manipulation leads to a satisfactory nutrient intake or not. If not, patients who need tube feeding will be detected earlier and their acceptance of the tube may be increased when they are aware of how poor their oral intake is.

Recommendations for wards with undernourished patients

- A high-energy high-protein diet should be available for undernourished patients.

- Every ward should offer the undernourished a selection of liquid supplements comprising drinks or sip feeds with different viscosity, taste and nutrient density.

- All health care staff should have knowledge about energy and protein recommendations for sick people and about the nutrional value of hospital food and available supplements.

- Written instructions containing information about the energy and protein content of the supplements given in the ward are shown to the patient and discussed.

- The staff – not least the doctors – must encourage the patients to take adequate supplements.

- Weigh undernourished patients twice a week. Ask them to be responsible for weighing themselves. Then it will be done.

- A food record sheet is filled in and calculated daily for all patients thought to have an inadequate nutritional intake.

- If the patient does not improve and the food intake is still insufficient, progress to tube feeding.

- At the time of discharge from hospital, the patient must be assessed as to whether nutrition therapy is still required. If so, appropriate advice is given with recipies on the preferred supplements. Follow-up may be continued in the community.

References

1. Settle RG. Defined formula diets: Palatability and oral intake. In: Rombeau, Caldwell (eds) *Enteral and tube feeding*. WB Saunders, Philadelphia, 1984; pp. 212–227.

2. Haraldsdottir J, Holm L, Jensen JH, Møller A. *Danskernes kostvaner 1985.* Levnedsmiddelstyrelsen. København 1987.

3. Pedersen AN, Ovesen L. Recommendations for the diet in Danish institutions (in Danish). *Levnedsmiddelstyrelsen*, Copenhagen, 1995.

4. Hygiejnekomiteens ernæringsudvalg. Sygehuskost i Danmark. *Ugeskr Læg* 1981; **143:** 2760–2762.

5. Haber GB, Heaton KW, Murphy D. Depletion and disruption of dietary fibre. Effects on satiety, plasma-glucose, and serum-insulin. *Lancet* 1977; **2:** 679–682.

6. Kissileff HR. Effects of physical state (liquid-solid) of foods on food intake: procedural and substantive contributions. *Am J Clin Nutr* 1985; **42:** 956–965.

7. de Graff C, Hulshof T, Weststrate JA *et al.* Short-term effects of different amounts of protein, fats, and carbo-hydrates on satiety. *Am J Clin Nutr* 1992; **55:** 33–38.

8. Levine AS, Tallmann JAR, Grace MK *et al.* Effect of breakfast cereals on short term food intake. *Am J Clin Nutr* 1989; **50:** 1303–1307.

9. Rodin J. Comparative effects of fructose, aspartame, glucose, and water preloads in calorie and macro-nutrient intake. *Am J Clin Nutr* 1990; **51:** 428–435.

10. Tordoff MG, Alleva AM. Effect of drinking soda sweetened with aspartame or high-fructose corn syrup on food intake and body weight. *Am J Clin Nutr* 1990; **51:** 963–969.

11. Mattes RD, Pierce CB, Friedman MI. Daily caloric intake of normal-weight adults: response to changes in dietary energy density of a luncheon meal. *Am J Clin Nutr* 1988; **48:** 214–219.

12. Duncan KH, Bacon JA, Weinsier RL. The effect of high and low energy density diets on satiety, energy and eating time of obese and non-obese subjects. *Am J Clin Nutr* 1983; **37:** 763–767.

13. Barkeling B, Rössner S, Björvell H. Efficiency of a high-protein meal (meat) and a high carbohydrate meal (vegetarian) on satiety measured by automated computerized monitoring of subsequent food intake, motivation to eat and food preferences. *Int J Obes* 1990; **14:** 743–75l.

14. Hill AJ, Blundell JE. Comparison of the action of macronutrients on the expression of appetite in lean and obese human subjects. *Ann N Y Acad Sci* 1990; **580:** 529–531.

15. Rolls BJ, Hetherington M, Burley VJ. The specificity of satiety: the influence of different macronutrient contents on the development of satiety. *Physiol Behav* 1988; **43:** 145–153.

16. Isaksson B, Edlund B, Gelin LE *et al.* The value of protein-enriched diet in patients with peptic ulcer. *Acta Chir Scand* 1959/60; **118:** 418–427.

17. Blundell JE. Appetite disturbance and the problems of overweight. *Drugs* 1990; **39:** 3: 1–19.

18. Gil KM, Skei B, Kvetan V *et al.* Parenteral nutrition and oral intake: Effect of glucose and fat infusions. *JPEN* 1991; **15:** 4: 426–432.

19. Van Amelsvoort JMM, Van Stratum P, Kraal JH, Lussenburg RN, Houfsmulle VMT. Effects of varying the carbohydrate: fat ratio in a hot lunch on post-prandial variables in male volunteers. *Br J Nutr* 1989; **61:** 267–283.

20. Lissner L, Levitsky DA, Strupp BV *et al.* Dietary fat and regulation of energy intake in human subjects. *Am J Clin Nutr* 1987; **46:** 856–892.

21. Solem G, Olesen ES, Amdrup E. Protein and caloric intake before and after gastrectomy and removal of the colon. *Nord Med* 1963; **70:** 1103–1108.

22. Wara P, Hessov I. Nutritional intake after colorectal surgery: A comparison of a traditional and a new post-operative regimen. *Clin Nutr* 1985; **4:** 225–228.

23. Adler-Nissen J. Relationship of structure to taste of peptides and peptide mixtures. In: Feeney RE, Whitaker JR (eds) *Protein tailoring for food and medical uses.* Marcel Dekker, New York, 1986; pp 97–122.

24. Grimble GK, Silk DBA. The nitrogen source of elemental diets – an unresolved issue? *Nutr Clin Pract* 1990; 227–230.

25. Grimble GK, Silk DBA. Peptides in human nutrition. *Nutr Research Rev* 1989; **2:** 87–108.

26. Ovesen L. Palatability and intake of two commercial liquid diets in patients with poor appetite. *Eur J Clin Nutr* 1991; **45:** 273–275.

27. Cabanac M, Rabe EF. Influence of a monotonous food on body weight regulation in humans. *Physiol Behav* 1976; **17(4):** 675–678.

28. Garb JL, Stunkard AJ. Taste aversions in man. *Am J Psychiatry* 1974; **131:** 1204–1207.

29. Nørregård O, Tottrup A, Saack A *et al.* Effect of oral nutritional supplements to adults with chronic obstructive pulmonary disease. *Clin Resp Physiol* 1987; **23:** suppl. 12: 388.

30. Efthimiou J, Fleming J, Gomes C *et al.* The effect of supplementary oral nutrition in poorly nourished patients with chronic obstructive pulmonary disease. *Am Rev Respir Dis* 1988; **137:** 1075–1082.

31. Otte KE, Ahlburg P, D'Amore F, Stellfeld M. Nutritional repletion in malnourished patients with emphysema. *JPEN* 1989; **13:** 152–156.

32. Brown MS, Buchanan RB, Karran SJ. Clinical observations on the effects of elemental diet supplementation during irradiation. *Clin Radiol* 1980; **31:** 19–20.

33. Moloney M, Moriarty M, Daly L. Controlled studies of nutritional intake in patients with malignant disease undergoing treatment. *Hum Nutr: Appl Nutr* 1983; **37A:** 30–35.

34. Arnold C, Richter MP. The effect of oral nutritional supplements on head and neck cancer. *Int J Radiation Oncology Biol Phys* 1989; **16:** 1595–1599.

35. Ovesen L, Allingstrup L. Different quantities of two commercial liquid diets consumed by weightlosing cancer patient. *JPEN* 1992; **16:** 275–278.

36. Ovesen L. The effect of a supplement which is nutrient dense compared to standard concentration on the total nutritional intake of anorectic patients. *Clin Nutr* 1992; **11:** 154–157.

37. Hessov I. Oral feeding after uncomplicated abdominal surgery. *Br J Clin Prac* 1988; **42:** 63–75–79.

38. Wells G, Rawlinson K, Tinckler L *et al.* Postoperative gastrointestinal motility. *Lancet* 1964; **ii:** 4–10.

39. Naclas MM, Younis MT, Roda CP *et al.* Gastro-intestinal motility studies as a guide to postoperative management. *Ann Surg* 1972; **17:** 510–522.

40. Ingram DM, Sheiner HJ. Postoperative gastric empty-ing. *Br J Surg* 1981; **68:** 572–576.

4l. Kehlet H. Multinodal approach to control post-operative pathophysiology and rehabilitation. *Br J Anaesth* 1997; **78:** 606–617.

42. Cheatham ML, Chapman WC, Key SP *et al.* A meta-analysis of selective versus routine nasogastric decompression after elective laparotomy. *Ann Surg* 1995; **221:** 469–478.

43. Bauer JJ, Gelernt IM, Salley BA *et al.* Is routine postoperative nasogastric decompression really necessary? *Ann Surg* 1985; **201:** 233–236.

44. Moss G, Bifrenbaum A, Bova F *et al.* Postoperative metabolic pattern following immediate total nutritional support: hormone levels, DNA synthesis, nitrogen balance and accelerated wound healing. *J Surg* 1976; **21:** 383–393.

45. Daly JM, Vars HM, Dudrick SJ. Effects of protein depletion on strength of colonic anastomoses. *Surg Gynecol Obstet* 1972; **134:** 15–21.

46. Ward MWN, Danzi M, Lewin MR *et al*. The effects of subclinical malnutrition and refeeding on the healing of experimental colonic anastomoses. *Br J Surg* 1982; **69:** 308–310.

47. Reisman P, Teoh TA, Cohen SM *et al*. Is early oral feeding safe after elective colorectal surgery. *Ann Surg* 1995; **222:** 73–77.

48. Ortiz HM, Armendariz P, Karnoz C. Is early postoperative feeding feasible in elective colon and rectal surgery. *Int J Colorect Dis* 1996; **11:** 119–121.

49. Henriksen MG, Hansen HV, Hessov I. Early oval nutrition after elective culorectal surgery influence of balanced analgesia and enforced mobilisation. *Nutrition* 2001; submitted.

50. Rana SK, Bray J, Menzics-Gorv N *et al*. Short term benefits of postoperative oral dietary supplements in surgical patients. *Clin Nutr* 1992; **11:** 337–344.

51. Keele AM, Bray MJ, Emery PW *et al*. Two phase randomised controlled clinical trial of postoperative oral dietary supplements in surgical patients. *Gut* 1997; **40:** 393–399.

52. Hessov I, Larsen KR, Sondergaard K. Improved early alimentation after radical hysterectomies without the traditional use of a stomach tube. *Acta Obstet Gynecol Scand* 1988; **67:** 225–228.

53. Hessov I. Energy and protein intake in elderly patients in an orthopedic surgical ward. *Acta Chir Scand* 1977; **143:** 145–149.

54. Mansell PI, Rawlings J, Allison SP *et al*. Low anthropometric indices in elderly females with fractured neck of femur. *Clin Nutr* 1990; **9:** 190–194.

55. Bastow MD, Rawlings J, Allison SP. Benefits of supplementary tube feeding after fractured neck of femur: a randomised controlled trial. *Br Med J* 1993; **287:** 1589–1592.

56. Delmi M, Rapin CH, Bengoa JM *et al*. Dietary supplementation in elderly patients with fractured neck of the femur. *Lancet* 1990; **335:** 1013–1016.

57. Tkatch L, Rapin CH, Rizzoli R *et al*. Benefits of oral protein supplementation in elderly patients with fracture of the proximal femur. *J Am Coll Nutr* 1992; **11:** 519–525.

58. Møller-Madsen B, Tottrup A, Hessov I, Jensen J. Nutritional intake and nutritional status of patients with fracture of the femoral neck: Value of oral supplements. *Acta Orthop Scand* 1998; **59:** suppl. 227: 48.

59. Hessov I, Ljungqvist O. Perioperative oral nutrition. *Curr Opin Clin Nutr Metab Care* 1998; **1:** 29–33.

60. Brandi LS, Frediani M, Oleggini M *et al*. Insulin resistance after surgery: Normalization by insulin treatment. *Clin Sci* 1990; **79:** 443–450.

61. Ljungqvist O, Thorell A, Gutniak M *et al*. Glucose infusion instead of preoperative fasting reduces postoperative insulin resistance. *J Am Coll Surg* 1994; **178:** 329–336.

62. Grove PJ, Dennison A, Royle GT. The effect of preoperative glucose loading on postoperative nitrogen loading. *Br J Surg* 1984; **71:** 635–637.

63. Woolfson AMJ, Heatley RW, Allison SP. Insulin to inhibit protein catabolism after injury. *N Engl J Med* 1979; **300:** 14–17.

64. Eriksson LI, Sandin R. Fasting guidelines in different countries. *Acta Anaesth Scand* 1996; **40:** 971–974.

65. Gutniak M, Grill V, Efendic S. Effects of composition of mixed meals low- versus high-carbohydrate content, on insulin, glucagon and somatostatin release in healthy humans and in patients with NIDDM. *Diabetes Care* 1986; **9:** 244–249.

66. Nygren J, Thorell A, Jacobsen H *et al*. Preoperative gastric emptying; the effects of anxiety and carbohydrate administration. *Ann Surg* 1995; **222:** 728–734.

67. Fasth S, Hulten L, Magnusson O *et al*. The immediate and long-term effects of postoperative total parenteral nutrition on body composition. *Int J Colorectal Dis* 1987; **2:** 139–145.

68. Hill GL, Douglas RG, Schroeder D. Metabolic basis for the management of patients undergoing major surgery. *World J Surg* 1993; **17:** 146–153.

69. Jensen MB, Hessov I. Dietary supplementation at home improves the regain of lean body mass after surgery. *Nutrition* 1997; **13:** 422–430.

70. Jensen MB, Hessov I. Randomisation to nutritional intervention at home did not improve postoperative function, fatigue or well being. *Br J Surg* 1997; **84:** 113–118.

71. Elmståhl S, Steen B. Hospital nutrition in geriatric longterm care medicine: II. Effects of dietary supplements. *Age Ageing* 1987; **16:** 73–80.

72. Elmståhl S. Hospital nutrition in geriatric long-stay medicine. Dietary intake, body composition and the effects of experimental studies. *Näringsforskning* 1988; **32:** 141–152.

73. Larsson J, Unosson M, Ek AG *et al*. Effects of dietary supplement on nutritional status and clinical outcome in 501 geriatric patients – a randomised study. *Clin Nutr* 1990; **9:** 179–84.

74. Unosson M, Larsson J, Bjurulf P. Effects of dietary supplement on functional condition and clinical outcome measured with a modified Norton scale. *Clin Nutr* 1992; **11:** 134–139.

Introduction

For the purposes of this chapter, enteral nutrition will refer to the administration of nutrients by tubes or other devices direct into some part of the gastro-intestinal (GI) tract. The term has been used to include specific nutrients (e.g. sip feeds) given by the oral route but this aspect of enteral nutrition is dealt with in Chapter 16.[1] Over the years many different techniques of tube feeding have been described and the use of a rectal or intraoesophageal tube was a common means of feeding inmates of asylum hospitals in the latter half of the 19th century. Such tubes were made of rubber or gum elastic and the administration of feed was made without patient consent. The issue of consent remains – for different reasons – of great relevance today and a number of authors have addressed concerns about the value of tube feeding in specific patient groups (e.g. those with advanced dementia) and the need for all those involved in care to be aware of the perceived versus actual benefits.[2,3]

It was only in the mid 1970s that the techniques of what is now commonly understood by the term 'enteral nutrition' were clearly established. One of the first reports clearly outlining the concept of whole liquid diets administered via specifically designed tubes by continuous pump administration was published by Dobbie and Hoffmeister in 1976.[4] By the 1990s it was firmly established that parenteral and enteral nutrition were complementary and not competing therapies and their respective roles within the spectrum of nutrition support have in the last decade become much better defined.[5]

It is also true that the best way of administering additional nutrients to the majority of nutritionally compromised (or potentially compromised) patients is by oral feeding. Often patients are capable of oral consumption of adequate nutrient requirements but may require advice or help to assist swallowing or to increase palatability of prescribed diets.

For those patients (in hospital or in the community) with functioning GI tracts, other routes and techniques of enteral administration are required. There are now only a few situations when a malnourished or potentially malnourished patient with a functioning GI tract cannot have a tube appropriately placed.

For the purposes of defining the optimum feeding techniques, patients may be divided into two main groups: those with a self-limiting acute illness or pathology who may only require shorter term feeding (for a few days or weeks) and those with other chronic pathology which requires longer term or indefinite feeding.

When a decision has been made that enteral nutrition is required, a number of key points need to be addressed and assessed. These are listed in Table 17.1.

Table 17.1 – Factors to be considered for enteral nutrition

Access route
Type of tube
Complications
Enteral diet (see Chapter 18)
Delivery systems
Reservoirs
Giving sets
Mode of delivery
Continuous/intermittent/bolus
Starter regimens
Monitoring
Complications (see Chapter 19)

The paediatric patient is considered in more detail in Chapter 20.

Access routes

Once a decision has been made that enteral nutrition is indicated, the access route is mainly decided according to whether a patient is considered to require short- or long-term feeding, although other factors (see below) may influence the choice. Generally, feeding for less than four weeks may be considered short term and more than four weeks long term.[1] Figure 17.1 illustrates a decision-making path for the determination of access routes.

A wide variety of enteral access routes are now available (see Table 17.2). The different types of tubes may be variously placed by nurse, dietitian, endoscopist, radiologist or surgeon. The type of short- or long-term tube placed will often be dependent on the local expertise available.

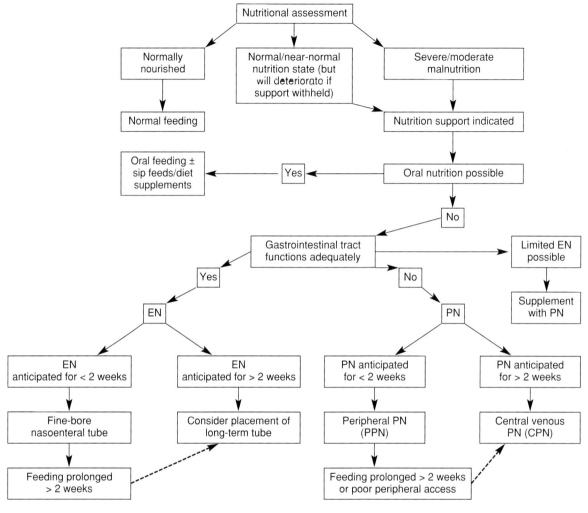

Figure 17.1 – Determination of routes of access in nutrition support (enteral route in bold).

Short-term enteral feeding

Fine-bore nasoenteral tubes

Most hospitalised patients receive interventional nutrition support for less than 4 weeks[6] – most by the enteral route. For most of these patients the best method of enteral delivery is a fine-bore nasogastric feeding tube (FBT), generally made from soft polyurethane or silicone elastomer and with a diameter under 3 mm. Polyvinyl chloride tubes are predominantly used for feeding for 14 days at maximum, because of being more prone to compli-

cations such as cracking.[7] Complications such as rhinitis, pharyngitis, oesophagitis, oesophageal strictures, gastritis and erosion-related upper gastrointestinal haemorrhage were previously associated with the use of larger bore (> 12F) Ryle's or Levin-type tubes which should not now be used in clinical practice. If for physical reasons (e.g. diameter of tube compared with diameter of nostril) the tube substantially occludes the airway, then respiratory failure may be precipitated in certain patient groups (the elderly or very young) as a result of difficulty in initiating oral breathing.[8] Wider-bore tubes have certain other disadvantages and Noviski *et al.*[9] have shown that the presence of a 12F nasogastric tube compared with an 8F tube caused significant increases in the numbers of

Table 17.2 – Access routes for enteral feeding

Short-term feeding
    Fine-bore nasoenteral tubes (FBT):
        nasogastric ★
        nasoduodenal ★
        nasojejunal
    Double-lumen nasoenteral tubes:
        gastric aspiration/jejunal feeding
Longer term feeding
    Cervical pharyngostomy:
        percutaneous cervical (PCP)
    Cervical oesophagostomy
    Gastrostomies:
        surgical (SG)
        percutaneous
            endoscopic (PEG) ★
            fluoroscopic (FPG or PFG) ★
        laparoscopic gastrostomy (LG)
    Duodenostomy:
        percutaneous endoscopic (PED)
    Jejunostomy:
        surgical jejunostomy (SJ)
        percutaneous endoscopic (PEJ)
        direct percutaneous endoscopic jejunostomy (DPEJ)
        jejunal tubes through PEG (PEGJ)
        needle catheter jejunostomy (NCJ) ★
        cuffed tube jejunostomy (CTJ)
        subcutaneous jejunostomy (SCJ)
    Buttons
    Ports

★ Indicates the most widely used techniques

gastric reflux episodes lasting more than 5 minutes and of the percentage time with an oesophageal pH less than 4.

Per-nasal insertion of FBTs with wire stylets should be done by staff trained in the technique because of the small but definite risk of pneumothorax as a result of malposition and subsequent oesophageal or pulmonary perforation causing pneumothorax.[10–14] Treatment may be straightforward if the complication is recognised early but delay may result in the development of effusion, empyema, hydrothorax or respiratory failure[15–18] which may be fatal or need surgical intervention.[19] If difficulty is experienced when siting an FBT, the wire stylet must not be removed and re-inserted because it is in these situations that stylet penetration of the FBT (either through the wall or exiting via a sideport) itself and then the oesophagus or other viscus is most likely to occur.[20] A recent report recognises that the effects may not present until some days later.[21]

FBT malposition at the time of insertion occurs in under 5% of patients but is generally into the trachea or bronchi.[6,22] If placement of the FBT within the bronchus is unrecognised then accidental intrapulmonary aspiration of feed may occur which may be fatal if unrecognised at an early stage. Patients most at risk for such a complication are those who are obtunded or have altered swallowing or a diminished gag reflex. In patients who are alert and orientated, correct positioning of the tube can be confirmed by syringe aspiration of gastric contents (pH <3) and auscultation of the epigastrium, although there are few data from controlled trials supporting the efficacy of such practices.[23] If aspiration of gastric contents or auscultation are unsuccessful, X-ray confirmation of the position of the tube is essential and must, in any case, be undertaken routinely in all patients with altered consciousness, altered cough or gag reflex or in those who are mechanically ventilated. Both chest and abdominal films may be required to confirm position.[24,25] The use of pH-sensing feeding tubes as a means of confirming position and assessing whether position has been maintained has been shown to be cost effective (about 25% of the cost of endoscopic placement) but unfortunately is of no use in the presence of drugs which alter intragastric pH, thus limiting their role.[26]

In the ventilated patient the presence of a cuffed endotracheal tube has been said to prevent potential FBT malposition into the trachea but a number of authors have shown that this is not the case.[27,28] Indeed, the presence of a cuffed endotracheal tube may actually increase the risk. It is in these situations that an FBT with a tip widened by the addition of a weight may be of use as perforation will be less likely (see Fig. 17.2). X-rays may be misinterpreted and what appears to be correct FBT siting may in fact be extraoesophageal placement into the left main bronchus. Extra information about placement may be obtained by confirming acidic pH of any aspirated gastric contents.[29] If doubt remains or aspirate cannot be obtained, then X-ray tube contrast studies may be deemed appropriate. Fatal intracranial misplacement of FBTs has been reported and patients with facial injuries are particularly at risk.[30] For patients with mechanical abnormalities of the upper airways (e.g. nasal septal deviation, obstructing neoplasms or after oropharyngeal surgery), insertion under direct vision with a flexible nasopharyngoscope has been recommended.[28] Dranoff and colleagues[30] describe an effective system of placement using a 'through the scope' placement of a tube via the transnasal route.

They consider this technique particularly useful in the critically ill, where accurate siting is particularly important; indications for using this technique included pneumonia, coagulopathy and high gastric residual volumes.

The most common complication causing interruption of the enteral feeding regimen is unplanned or non-elective extubation of FBTs, which occurs in up to 60% of patients. Fifty per cent of all FBTs are accidentally or deliberately removed by patients and about 5% by staff (e.g. when turning a patient or during physiotherapy). About 4% are vomited up and an occasional tube has to be removed because of unsalvageable blockage. Only about 20% of the total are electively removed because the patient has been able to start oral nutrition. About 10% are removed because of the patient's death.[31]

Secure fixing of the tube to the nose and face with good adhesive tape and subsequent regular (twice-daily) examination is the best way of keeping

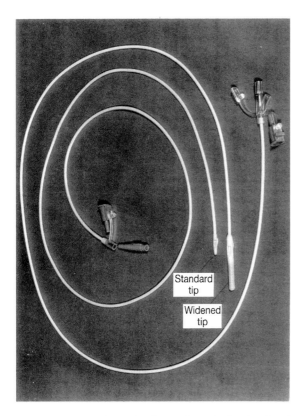

Figure 17.2 – Fine-bore tubes showingh standard and widened tip.

unplanned extubation to a minimum. A few cumbersome and bulky fixation devices have been described which generally involve 'anchoring' of the tube by means of an additional piece of tubing passing behind the posterior part of the nasal septum. For obvious reasons (cosmesis and comfort) these are not widely used.[32,33,34]

Infants (see also Chapter 20), because of their small size, are liable to develop nasal obstruction and nasal mucosal oedema with FBTs placed per nasally. For such individuals, appliances have been described which stabilise tubes placed into the stomach via the oropharyngeal route, so avoiding the complications.[35] If nasal intubation is essential in infants (to allow sucking), then the smallest possible FBT should be used and the opposite nostril must remain unobstructed.[36]

Nasoduodenal or jejunal tube placement

Some patients receiving enteral delivery of nutrients may be at increased risks of enteral diet regurgitation and/or pulmonary aspiration of feed.[22,37] Such patients and those with documented gastric atony or gastroparesis for any reason should be considered for postpyloric duodenal or jejunal feeding which may assist in reducing those risks. Examples of such patient groups are listed in Table 17.3. The incidence of pulmonary aspiration is low (2.4%)[38] and although excess morbidity and mortality are rare, steps should be taken to avoid them.[39] In addition to the higher risk groups in Table 17.3, Mullan and co-workers[40] have identified that the likelihood of a patient developing pulmonary aspiration is significantly less in an intensive care unit (ICU) than in a general ward. This is probably because of better standards (and frequency of nursing and pulmonary care).

Table 17.3 – Possible increased risk of diet regurgitation and aspiration

Diabetics with neuropathy
Hypothyroidism
Neuromotor deglutition disorders
Neurosurgical patients
Impaired gastrointestinal motility
Neuromuscular blocking agents
Postabdominal surgery
Recumbency
The elderly
Ventilated patients

Additionally it has been shown that ICU patients fed by jejunal tube receive a higher proportion of their daily caloric intake, have significantly greater increases in serum prealbumin concentrations and lower rates of pneumonia than those fed intragastrically.[41]

Successful placement of fine-bore tubes beyond the pylorus remains a problem.[42] Clearly the FBT must be long enough to reach the duodenum/jejunum (approximately 110 cm in an adult) and many such tubes are now available. In a series of 882 fluoroscopically placed FBTs, an 86.6% success rate in positioning the tip of the tube distal to the third part of the duodenum was achieved.[38] Malposition occurs in less than 2% of fluoroscopically placed tubes[22] and placement time is quick, an average fluoroscopy time of 5.3 minutes having been reported.[43] 'Peel-away' sheaths with a torque catheter[44] and guidewire duodenal/jejunal placement have also been successfully described.[45,46]

Endoscopic FBT placement can be done by:

- Using an endoscope to visualize tube positioning.

- Siting a guidewire with the endoscope and advancing the FBT over the guidewire.

- A 'pull-along' technique where a suture is attached to the distal end of an FBT and endoscopic forceps pull the tube into the small bowel.

- A 'push-technique' using specially designed forceps to grab the FBT directly and push the tube into the small bowel.[47–50]

Damore and colleagues[51] utilised a newly designed 'through-the-scope' enteral tube and found the technique simple, precise and reproducible. Techniques of utilising ultrasound, external magnetic guidance and 'through the tube' fiberoptics have also been described.[52,53] The techniques allowing accurate placement under direct vision or using appropriate placement technology appears to be the most appropriate for the critically ill and other 'at-risk' groups who require postpyloric feeding; however, it is most appropriate to use what is available locally in terms of expertise and equipment.[54]

Prokinetic drugs[55,56] can promote gastric emptying and theoretically can facilitate the passage of the end of the FBT through the pylorus, although their main benefit in achieving duodenal placement appears to be for specific patient groups such as diabetics with neuropathy. A recent study within a medical ICU compared the effect of cisapride, metoclopramide, erythromycin and placebo in promoting gastric emptying in patients intolerant of enteral nutrition. Results showed that single enteral doses of metoclopramide and cisapride were effective for promoting gastric emptying, metoclopramide having a faster onset.[57] Some of the impaired emptying in such patients may relate to the use of morphine, as a study has demonstrated impaired antroduodenal motility in mechanically ventilated patients.[58]

Prospective randomised controlled trials have consistently failed to demonstrate any advantage of adding weights (up to 8 g) to the distal end of an FBT, in terms of both ability to pass into the duodenum or jejunum or when considering how long the tube remains in place.[59,60] These studies demonstrate that less than 50% of 110 cm enteral tubes will pass spontaneously through the pylorus and this incidence is unaffected whether the patient is mobile or bedridden. Thus, there remains no evidence from controlled clinical studies that these modifications offer any advantage in practical terms in either the duration of tube usage or the incidence of spontaneous transpyloric passage.

If the decision has been made that an adult patient requires duodenal or jejunal feeding, then enteral tube positioning should be achieved at the earliest opportunity by either endoscopic or fluoroscopic positioning, depending on specialist expertise available, to prevent delay in instituting the feeding regimen.

Double-lumen (dual-function) tubes

For patients with short- to medium-term gastric stasis or gastroparesis, the use of double-lumen nasoenteral tubes, with ports for concurrent gastric aspiration and postpyloric (duodenal or jejunal) feeding, should be considered[61,62] (see Fig. 17.3). There is undoubtedly a role for these tubes in the postoperative patient (when the tube can be sited at laparotomy) or the recumbent ventilated ICU patient for short-term feeding. One study explored the use of such tubes placed at endoscopy with the assistance of fluoroscopy (with a mean placement time of 20 minutes), with clinical and radiographic evidence of adequate gastric decompression. Within 72 hours most patients were receiving 90% of their nutrition needs.[63] Another use is for the patient with proximal GI tract fistulae, perforations or anastomotic leaks. If the aspiration ports are placed (endoscopically or fluoroscopically) adjacent to the defect, adequate local drainage and concomitant

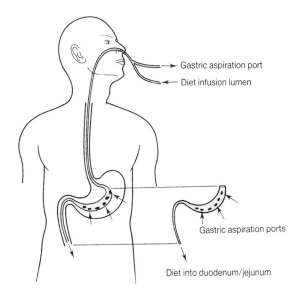

Gastric aspiration port

Diet infusion lumen

Gastric aspiration ports

Diet into duodenum/jejunum

Figure 17.3 – Double-lumen nasoenteral tube *in situ* (modified from Moss 1984[62]). Note jejunal infusion and gastric aspiration ports.

feeding are ensured.[64] When the defect has closed or gastric function returns, the double-lumen tube may be replaced by a standard fine-bore nasogastric tube if feeding is still required.

Longer term feeding

In terms of practicality, comfort and cosmesis, it is now well recognised that FBT intubation is not the ideal route for longer term (> 3–4 weeks) or indefinite feeding. Other routes of enteral administration may be more appropriate and other factors need to be taken into account. The material from which the tube is made may have particular relevance in the longer term fed patient. Recent studies examined the effect of feeds containing different amounts of MCT oil on silicone feeding tubes. The authors showed that the silicone of such tubes is significantly affected over an eight-week period and the authors advised that the type of feed should be taken into account in long-term feeding using silicone gastrostomy tubes.

Cervical pharyngostomy or oesophagostomy

These routes have been used by surgeons operating on the head and neck (including nose and larynx). For both cervical pharyngostomy and oesophagostomy the external part of the FBT exits from the neck (avoiding the mouth, nose and upper airways) and passes through the skin into the oesophagus or pharynx.[65] The cervical oesophagostomy was developed as a technique for feeding patients with oropharyngeal cancer and adapted for patients with neurological disease, trauma to the face and after oromaxillary surgery. Placement of cervical pharyngostomy percutaneously (PCP) using local anaesthetic has been described[66] and requires a certain confidence in one's knowledge of the anatomy of the anterior triangle of the neck. Such techniques have not become widespread as methods of long-term feeding in part because of the acceptance of the technique of percutaneous gastrostomy (PG).

Gastrostomy

Endoscopic gastrostomy

The placement of a tube through the abdominal wall directly into the stomach for either temporary or permanent delivery of enteral feed or drainage of gastric contents is termed a gastrostomy. Historically a gastrostomy was created surgically either during other abdominal surgery or as a separate procedure and was commonly fashioned for long-term administration of feed for patients with incurable disorders of deglutition (e.g. motor neurotic disease, multiple sclerosis). Thus a laparotomy was often needed and this may have required the administration of a general anaesthetic.

A simplified technique of gastrostomy was described in 1980 by Gauderer and colleagues[67] by which the gastrostomy tube was inserted percutaneously under endoscopic control using local anaesthesia. This technique was called percutaneous endoscopic gastrostomy (PEG) and two main (and many lesser) methods of placement have been described. The first method is the 'direct stab' technique in which the endoscope is passed and the stomach inflated with air. The endoscopist then watches a cannula entering the stomach having been inserted directly through the anterior abdominal wall. A guidewire is then passed through the cannula into the stomach. A gastrostomy tube may then be introduced into the stomach through a 'peel-away' sheath.[68]

The second PEG insertion method is the transoral 'pull or push-through' technique, whereby a guidewire or suture is brought out of the stomach by the endoscope (after transabdominal, through-cannula insertion) and is either attached to a gastrostomy tube or the tube is pushed over the guidewire. The abdominal end of the wire is then pulled (or the tube pushed), advancing the gastrostomy tube down through the mouth, pharynx, oesophagus and into the stomach. Continued traction (or pushing) advances the tube through the anterior abdominal wall until the tube buffer abuts the gastric wall (Fig. 17.4). Multiple modifications of both techniques are available, but the morbidity rates are all similar. It has been shown that a smaller bore (12F) tube performs as well as a larger (20F) PEG in a prospective randomised study, suggesting that the smaller bore is more appropriate (in terms of size and comfort).[69]

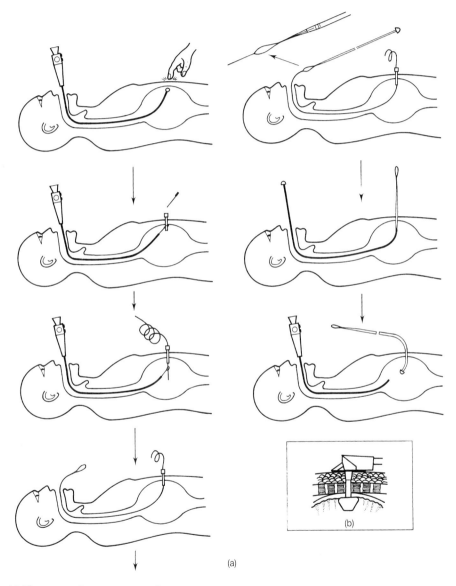

Figure 17.4 – **(a)** Placement of percutaneous endoscopic gastrostomy: (i) finger pressure on anterior abdominal wall noted by endoscopist; (ii) needle and cannula inserted into stomach through anterior abdominal wall after local anaesthesia; (iii) guidewire threaded through cannula and grasped by endoscopic forceps or snare; (iv) endoscope withdrawn with guidewire; (v) guidewire attached to gastrostomy tube; (vi) guidewire and tube are pulled back through mouth, oesophagus and stomach to exit on anterior abdominal wall; (vii) endoscope re-passed to confirm site of placement of retention device. **(b)** Retention device loosely abuts gastric mucosa – position maintained by external fixation device.

PEG has become increasingly recognised as the technique of choice for placing gastrostomies in patients who require long-term enteral nutrition and usage in the UK and elsewhere in Europe has become widespread in many patient groups, including neurological rehabilitation[70] and adjunctive enteral nutrition in cystic fibrosis.[71] PEG placement should now be considered as a concurrent procedure for any patient undergoing elective tracheostomy. Other examples include brain-damaged (traumatic and vascular) and ventilated ICU patients as PEG placement clears the oropharynx of tubes and may reduce the incidence of upper respiratory tract infections (e.g. acute sinusitis) without minimal insertion-related morbidity.[72,73,74] The safety of placement of such tubes in patients with Crohn's disease has been demonstrated, with an acceptable complication risk and in particular no development of either peristomal disease or prolonged gastrocutaneous fistulae after removal.[75]

Bad patient selection for placement of PEGs may result in early dislodgement of tubes by patients and therefore conditions such as psychosis or dementia should be considered relative contraindications to PEG insertion.[76] In some patient groups, such as those with dysphagic stroke, early placement (within 2 weeks of the stroke) with appropriate selection can be a very useful therapeutic intervention, with patients attaining a reasonable level of function in daily activities.[77]

PEG has proved to be cost effective with a satisfactorily low morbidity (less than 10%) and mortality (2%) when compared with the conventional surgical placement,[78,79] with a failure (of placement) rate of about 5%. A prospective 4-year study of a heterogeneous group of 210 patients had a 0% procedure-related mortality with 20% 'mild' complications (including pyrexia, local bleeding, local ulceration, leakage, tube occlusion and tube fracture) and 3.8% severe (gastric perforation, localised peritonitis, pulmonary aspiration during procedure, wound infection).[80] In a relatively high-risk group (cystic fibrosis patients with severe pulmonary disease), the complication rate was acceptable.[71] Two of the cohort of 54 had respiratory depression during the procedure, whilst 13% developed late complications. One patient had the tube removed because of pain when feeding (cause undetermined) and one patient had tube displacement. Ten of the cohort had lesser problems including local pain, low-grade sepsis and tube occlusion.

PEG does have procedure-specific complications. Necrotising fasciitis and intra-abdominal wall abscesses are potentially fatal complications that have been recorded.[76,78] Streptococcal bacteraemia has been reported secondary to an infected stoma site and *Candida albicans* colonisation of the PEG tube itself has been recognised.[80] The need for prophylactic antibiotics at the time of PEG insertion to reduce the incidence of insertion-related infections has been confirmed in a randomised, double-blind trial,[81] although some users only provide antibiotics for those at risk of endocarditis.[82] The same group found that paracetamol suppositories were appropriate analgesia in the majority of cases.

Pneumoperitoneum (normally benign) occurs to a greater or lesser degree in up to 38% of PEG placements. This normally resolves spontaneously but may be present for up to 5 weeks after insertion.[83]

It had been believed that the timing of endoscopy might affect the occurrence or degree of pneumoperitoneum but a study has shown that the timing has no effect.[84] The development of persistent pneumoperitoneum in the mechanically ventilated patient suggests the possibility of concurrent pathology, such as unrecognised tracheo-oesophageal fistula.[85] The first case of stomal seeding of tumour cells was reported in 1992 in a patient with a pharyngeal squamous cell carcinoma.[86] With increasing use of both enteral nutrition and PEGs in the palliation of malignant disease, it is possible that this complication will be seen more frequently in the future. Intestinal obstruction has been caused by the buffer on the distal end of the tube[87] and oesophageal obstruction has occurred after attempted removal of the distal end perorally.[88] Subcutaneous emphysema has been observed (which must be distinguished from necrotising fasciitis) and may result from inability of leaked insulation air (at endoscopy) to discharge around the PEG tube. A skin incision of adequate size must always be made to allow egress of insufflated air. If subcutaneous emphysema develops it may take 3 weeks to settle completely.[89]

Spontaneous tube extrusion or displacement has been recorded and it is now clear that complications such as these (including fasciitis and local infection) may be caused by excess local pressure of the retaining buffer on the gastric wall when the tube is first sited.[90,91,92] Occasionally early failure of the balloon or buffer occurs. If this happens before a mature stoma tract has formed (<2 weeks after insertion, although this may be longer, especially in patients on steroids)[93] then replacement may be difficult to achieve, although the use of a Seldinger guidewire and endoscopy to allow replacement of the recently inserted PEG has been successfully used.[94]

Variations of normal anatomy tend to account for the reports of gastrocolic fistula or misplacement in the colon.[95,96] Rotation of the stomach and colonic penetration at PEG insertion in the paediatric population (because of immature mesenteric attachments) may cause gastrocolic or colocutaneous fistulae which become manifest with faeculent vomiting.[97] If prolonged diarrhoea or vomiting develops after PEG placement or the PEG malfunctions, then confirmation of correct placement should be done using radio-opaque media to identify the problem.

Most of these complications may be avoided by strict attention to insertion protocols and post-insertion care plans, which should be agreed at a local level.

For those patients at risk of diet regurgitation and aspiration, conversion of PEG to jejunostomies (PECJ) by passing specially adapted FBTs through the PEG lumen may now be achieved in a number of ways,[98] in order to try to reduce the risk of gastric aspiration, although that risk cannot be completely avoided.[99] Any technique of conversion should ideally maintain the function of gastric aspiration as well as jejunal feeding. In some cases this is achieved by using tubes originally designed for other purposes but commercial kits are now available to convert PEGs to PEGJs.

Fluoroscopically guided percutaneous gastrostomy (FPG)

The percutaneous placement of gastrostomies under fluoroscopic guidance was first described in 1983 and as the morbidity and mortality compare favourably with PEG and surgical gastrostomy, has become increasingly used.[102,103]

The technique requires air insufflation of the stomach through a nasogastric tube and external puncture of the stomach. Of 158 patients who had FPGs placed, major morbidity was 6% (including peritonitis, haemorrhage, sepsis and tube migration) and minor morbidity was 12%. FPG has also been used to place gastrostomies in patients with ascites or peritoneal dialysis, both of which are relative contraindications for the endoscopic technique.[104]

Removal of percutaneous enterostomies
Removal of PEGs, PEDs, PEGJs or FPGs is depen-

dent on the individual design. Some require cutting externally as the internal buffer cannot be retrieved from within the stomach and this ultimately passes out per rectum. For most patients this is a perfectly acceptable method of removal.[105] This technique may be dangerous in individuals who have previously undergone abdominal surgery as the buffer may cause visceral perforation, particularly if the bowel is fixed by adhesions.[106] Such tubes can be withdrawn at endoscopy and various authors have described different ways of achieving this, even using balloon angioplasty catheters.[107] However, PEGs that can be removed without the need for endoscopy (e.g. by external traction) may have advantages in terms of ease of use and cost savings.[108]

Laparoscopic gastrostomy

Not surprisingly, with the upsurge in laparoscopic surgery, it was not going to be long before laparoscopic gastrostomy was performed. These techniques may be particularly useful in patients with mechanical or obstructing upper airway lesions. Placement of a standard large-bore gastrostomy tube can be undertaken ensuring the stomach is apposed to the abdominal wall[109] (Fig. 17.5) or a Depage-Janeway permanent gastrostomy may be fashioned.[110] The main disadvantages are the need for urinary catheterisation

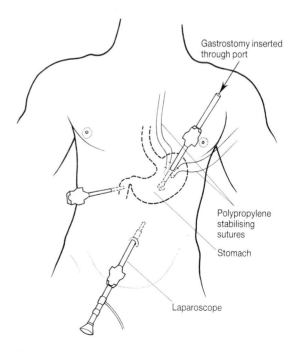

Figure 17.5 – Laparoscopic gastrostomy (after Murphy *et al.*[109]).

(to empty the bladder) and the time taken for the procedure. Additionally, general anaesthesia will be needed for more patients than when endoscopic or fluoroscopic techniques are used.

Endoscopic duodenostomy/jejunostomy

For patients who have had previous oesophagogastric surgery, access to the gut may be achieved by a direct approach into small bowel. Direct percutaneous endoscopic duodenostomies and jejunostomies (PED and PEJ) have been used but in general the results are unsatisfactory because complications such as displacement or leakage are common.[100] Shike and colleagues (100) described six direct PEJs inserted using a 160 cm endoscope allowing siting of tubes 60 cm distal to the ligament of Treiz. Despite the technical difficulties of this approach it appeared superior to the PEGJ-type conversion. Occasionally siting of PEGs or PEJs in the complex patient may be facilitated by use of imaging techniques such as scanning.[100,101]

Jejunostomy

Surgical jejunostomies (SJ) may be fashioned at laparotomy as a separate operative procedure or concurrently during surgery for other abdominal procedures. A 1992 series describes the placement of 100 SJs for enteral feeding.[111] Fifty per cent of the indications were for neurological disease and the postpyloric route was chosen to reduce the risk of gastric aspiration. There was a 21% 30-day mortality (mainly due to cardiopulmonary failure). Only one death was due to aspiration of feed. Ninety-four per cent of cases were performed under general anaesthetic. Twelve per cent of patients had tube-related complications which included wound infection, inadvertent tube removal and small bowel obstruction.

Clearly correct patient selection for SJ is paramount and, as recently suggested for PEGs, when deciding if a procedure justified, not only must the risks of the procedure and the benefits be included in assessment but also the 30-day survival of the patient due to the underlying disease.[112] Holmes and colleagues have shown that larger surgical jejunostomies (e.g. the Witzel tube jejunostomy) causes more major complications than needle catheter jejunostomies,[113] although they have been used successfully and with low morbidity for delivering immediate postoperative feeding in patients with non-traumatic intestinal perforations and peritonitis.[114] However, a number of cases of small bowel necrosis have been described in

patients with feeding jejunostomies inserted by the modified Witzel technique. In each case the necrosis was preceded by progressive abdominal pain, distension and high nasogastric output. Clearly this triad of signs should be looked for in any patient undergoing such feeding.[115]

The technique of needle catheter jejunostomy (NCJ) using a fine catheter to access the jejunum through the anterior abdominal wall, described by Delaney and Garvey in 1973,[116] is still considerably underused.[117] For NCJ a fine catheter is inserted into the jejunum and brought through the anterior abdominal wall, away from the laparotomy wound, to facilitate postoperative enteral feeding. NCJ is generally performed in association with major gastrointestinal surgery to provide access for enteral feeding if there are peroperative technical problems or if a prolonged convalescence is anticipated. The technique has a low morbidity with a major complication rate of 1%.[118] The complications appear to be primarily intraperitoneal leakage of infusions (in 1.5% of patients),[119] jejunostomy dislodgement or bowel obstruction. Other complications (which apply to any type of jejunostomy) have been reported, including small bowel perforation[120] and knotting of tubes.[121] Cyst-like intramural gas collections have been observed in the intestinal wall after NCJ insertion, and it is believed these represent a benign form of pneumatosis intestinalis.[122]

NCJ should be considered for patients who:

- Are malnourished at the time of surgery.
- Are undergoing major upper gastrointestinal surgery.
- May receive adjuvant radio- or chemotherapy after surgery.
- Are undergoing laparotomy after major trauma.[125,126]

De Gottardi and others report a large series of patients receiving NCJ feeding after major abdominal surgery. Although minor catheter-related complications (catheter luminal obstruction, local cellulitis) were common (26%), they concluded that NCJ gave safe and effective access for postoperative feeding but recommended that meticulous insertion technique and postoperative management were essential.[125]

Should problems with blockage arise, the use of a Seldinger wire, a track dilator and a 'peel-away' sheath will allow conversion of an NCJ into a standard-size jejunostomy.[126] The use of standard-size jejunostomies has recently been reported in a small series of post-operative patients and complications were few (clogging and tube dislodgement occurring most frequently). A modified cuffed-tube jejunostomy (CTJ) using a single-cuff Tenckhoff catheter sited within a Witzel-type tunnel in the jejunum has been described, with only one tube (out of 150 placed) requiring premature removal because of complications.[127] Shike described the placement of 150 direct percutaneous endoscopic jejunostomies using an endoscope; 86% were placed successfully, the remaining 14% failing because of either tight gastric outlet or proximal bowel obstruction. Of those successfully placed, 122 were used for feeding and seven for drainage. There were three major complications requiring surgery – severe gastric bleeding, abdominal wall abscess and colonic perforation – a low number considering that most patients had undergone major upper gastrointestinal surgery.[128]

Buttons

Button devices (skin-level gastrostomies or jejunostomies) have become increasingly popular as the cosmetic and practical advantages have been recognised. These devices can be placed in mature stoma or placed primarily. Primary placement is a useful technique although complications such as migration into the stoma track may occur at an early stage, particularly in the presence of infection. However, successful initial placement and retention and usage for well over 1 year are to be expected,[129] even in complex patients such as those on peritoneal dialysis.[130] Apart from the very important cosmetic benefits for the patient, they are less likely to be pulled out, clogged or dislodged.[131] Laparoscopic insertion of gastrostomy buttons has been described with 100% successful placement and with a mean placement time of 15 minutes if not concurrent with another procedure.[132]

Ports

For the patient with intra-abdominal malignancy for whom jejunostomy feeding may subsequently be necessary due to obstruction, the placement of a subcutaneous jejunostomy (SCJ) might be appropriate. This technique involves placing an access port (more commonly used for venous access) in the abdominal wall with a connecting catheter allowing delivery of nutrition (should it eventually be required) into the jejunum. The patient has no external tube visible.[133] The system has been used with different types of

patients including those with advanced oesophageal cancer who received a port at the time of oesophagectomy and lymph node resection. The main problem is the blockage of small-bore needles required to access the port but authors report use for up to 1 year without permanent obstruction.

Prevention of tube blockage

Any feeding tube may become blocked with feed and an untreated blockage will necessitate tube replacement. All tubes should be flushed through with water on a regular basis, whether a diet infusion is continuous or intermittent. Manufacturers' guidelines differ but a minimum of twice-daily flushing of the tube is essential. If build-up of solidified diet is observed, instillation into the tube of agents such as chymotrypsin or papain may salvage a partially or totally obstructed tube.[134] The use of a guidewire to 'declog' should be avoided, as the tube (and thus anatomical structures) can be perforated.

Administration techniques

It is important that all centres which use enteral nutrition should have a fixed protocol on enteral infusion. Spain and colleagues showed that having an infusion protocol improved delivery of calories, appropriateness of feed and advancement of feeding.[135] Most problems arose as a result of physician reluctance to use protocols. The detail of the protocol may vary widely from unit to unit. General guidelines for any patient receiving enteral nutrition are given below and should be adapted according to specialty, skill base and local need. In certain disease states different recommendations may be advised and the relevant chapter in this book should be consulted to establish whether guidelines specific to that disease are given.

Reservoirs, giving sets and contamination

In recent years the proportion of critically ill patients being fed by the enteral route has increased and this increase has highlighted the possibility of infectious episodes in these patients being directly related to the administration of enteral diet.[136] Often these patients are immunologically compromised and many have been prescribed H2-blockers or antacids to raise intragastric pH[137] or are receiving antibiotics which may predispose to infection by Gram-negative bacilli.[138] Other investigators have observed a high incidence of gastric and tracheal colonisation in ventilated patients receiving enteral nutrition.[139]

The risk of infectious episodes secondary to enteral nutrition-related bacterial contamination in neonatal, transplant, oncology, HIV/AIDS and other immuno-suppressed patients is thus a cause for concern. It has been shown that bacterial colonisation and infectious complications that develop in some patients can be directly related to the ingestion or administration of contaminated enteral diet.[140–143] Sources of contamination must be eliminated and it has been possible to identify a number of areas where enteral diet contamination may originate[144] (see Table 17.4). The use of commercially prepared feeds is a major factor in reducing the incidence of diet contamination, although diets requiring reconstitution or dilution have an increased risk of contamination.[145,146]

Commercial production and packaging of feed do not guarantee sterility. Most diets will support bacterial growth once contaminated and as these diets are often ideal culture media, rapid bacterial proliferation may occur.[147] It has been shown that acidification of enteral diet formulae (pH = 3.5) prevents gastric colonisation in critically ill patients.[148] Sterile gloves must be worn during preparation of enteral diet delivery systems.[149]

Table 17.4 – Potential sources of contamination of feed

Endogenous
From patient

Exogenous
From diet components
Kitchen environment
Mixing utensils
During transfer to reservoir
Suboptimal storage conditions
Handlers (nursing, dietetic, medical)
Ward environment
Air and dust

Delivery systems
Administration sets:
   reservoir
   giving set
   enteral tube

Until recently the possibility of ascending (or retro-grade) bacterial contamination originating from the patient and colonising the enteral diet container had been noted in a single report,[150] and indeed, it is often not considered an important source of diet contamination.[151] Retrograde contamination of diet containers from enteral tube via the giving set may be of considerable significance, with almost 25% of enteral diet reservoirs being colonised in this manner by 48 hours,[152] and this has now been confirmed in clinical studies.[153] The role of the guidewire withdrawal after tube placement has also now been recognised as contributing to the development of endogenous contamination.[154] The development of closed, prefilled, sterile administration systems (when diet does not require transfer from its supply container) has been shown to be successful in preventing exogenous bacterial contamination (Fig. 17.6), with substantial and significant reduction in colonisation of containers.[155] The enteral tube itself may become colonised and in turn act as a source for contamination.[78,147]

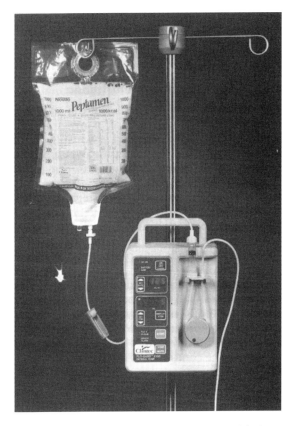

Figure 17.6 – Closed administration system for enteral feeding – reduces risk of contamination as transfer of diet not required.

The 'hang time' of enteral feeding reservoirs and giving sets has been shown to influence the degree of contamination. Periods of longer than 24 hours are not permissible,[152,156] particularly in warm climates, as an increased ambient temperature will speed bacterial multiplication. A recent study has shown that 26.9% of enteral diets administered to patients were contaminated and those patients were twice as likely to develop symptoms such as vomiting, abdominal pain and diarrhoea.[157]

Extra vigilance should be undertaken in the critically ill and the immunocompromised patient. For such patients it would seem appropriate to advocate the administration of diets by continuous infusion, from a sterile closed administration system, with a change of giving set at least every 24 hours. All handling must be undertaken using sterile gloves. Mechanical means of preventing diet regurgitation or reflux up giving sets may have a role to play and further studies may clarify the influence of regular irrigation or replacement of colonised enteral tubes. Commercially prepared sterile enteral diets are presented most commonly in 500 ml containers. Larger reservoirs are now available and will result in an increase in the ratio of administered diet to prescribed diet[158,159] because the nursing care and handling are simplified. However, the ever-increasing use of enteral nutrition in immunocompromised patients means that the same rigour is applied to control of infection in enteral nutrition as that already applied in parenteral nutrition. The use of established means of identification and hazards such as the Hazard Analysis Critical Control Point (HACCP) has been suggested as the most appropriate way forward but has yet to be widely utilised.[160]

Continuous versus intermittent versus bolus administration

Bolus feeding of enteral diets was the standard method of administration for many years. A volume of 200–400 ml of feed was instilled into the stomach via a nasogastric tube over a period of time ranging from 15 minutes to 1 hour. There is now substantial evidence to show that this is a poor method of administering enteral diet, because it has greater incidence of side-effects such as bloating and diarrhoea, in addition to which a considerable amount of nursing time is required and feeds may often be accidentally omitted.[161]

A recent randomised study has shown significant increases in diarrhoea, with apparent increases in both non-elective extubation and aspiration pneumonia in an intermittently fed group. Interestingly, tube blockage was more common in the continuous group despite similar anticlogging regimens.[162] A continuous overnight infusion followed by disconnection during the day may be the optimal technique, as nutritional parameters may be additionally improved in this way.[163] A study within an ICU demonstrated that continuous 24-hour feeding which stopped gastric pH lowering might be a factor in the earlier development of gastric bacterial colonisation and advised that the intermittent approach may allow decreases in gastric pH, delaying the onset of colonisation.[164] The intermittent approach should be the technique of choice for patients on home enteral nutrition, as it allows them a substantial part of the day free from infusion apparatus.

If a continuous 24-hour administration regimen is chosen then the access route may have relevance. A study comparing the use of PEG versus PEGJ in the administration of enteral feed to trauma patients established that nutritional goals were achieved more rapidly by using the PEGJ route, although no reduction in length of hospital stay was noted.[165] For those patients being enterally fed via jejunostomy tubes prior to surgery, Moncure and colleagues have shown that feeds need not be discontinued until surgery starts, rather than stopping feeding some hours before. Using this approach, protein and calorie intake is maximised which is of particular importance in those with malnutrition.[166]

Starter regimens

Controlled clinical trials have convincingly demonstrated that the use of starter regimens (either by diluting the feed or reducing the volume) only results in limiting the intake of diet in the first few days of feeding, thereby prolonging the length of negative nitrogen balance.[167,168] The incidence of gastrointestinal side-effects is unchanged when a full-strength, full-volume diet is used to commence enteral nutrition. Dilutional starter regimens should therefore not be used routinely.

Commencing enteral feeding

Access to the gut having been gained by the appropriate route and the appropriate diet having been chosen, enteral nutrition may then commence. For those patients who are immobile or confined to bed and those with altered consciousness, it is good practice to have the patient sitting at an angle of 30–45° to help reduce the risk of regurgitation and aspiration. In most adult patients with no other metabolic or fluid balance problems, between 2 and 2.5 litres of diet should be prescribed on a daily basis. This volume can be infused from day 1. Only in a small percentage (<10%) are lower infusion rates initially required. Subtle differences in infusion rates may be made irrelevant by large inaccuracies in enteral pump infusion rates which have shown a variation between 53% and 107% of the amount of prescribed feed.[169] It is essential to establish the degree of accuracy of a pump prior to use and to have regular review and assessment of performance.

Approximately 70% of critically ill patients in ICUs tolerate enteral feeding. The patients in whom enteral nutrition is likely to be inappropriate are those with major abdominal sepsis or very major gastrointestinal surgery. In most cases, if these patients require nutrition support, TPN is appropriate. Patients on ventilators often have absent bowel sounds; this in itself is not a contraindication to enteral nutrition, although sadly it is often regarded as such. Enteral nutrition is, however, contraindicated in the presence of gross abdominal distension.

In the first 24 hours of enteral infusion, gastric aspiration is undertaken every 2–3 hours. If the residual gastric volume is above 200 ml from a per-nasal FBT or above 100 ml from a gastrostomy, then it is possible that enteral nutrition is not being tolerated. Further observation and assessment should be undertaken before stopping feeding.[170]

Monitoring

A patient receiving enteral nutrition support should be monitored closely. Patients most likely to develop problems are those with major concurrent illnesses rather than those to whom enteral nutrition is being administered to preserve nutritional status.

A diet chart enables an accurate record of the patient's actual versus prescribed intake to be kept and the chart will allow correction of intake problems to be undertaken. These charts are also of importance during the changeover from enteral feeding to peros nutrition.

Weighing is the simplest and most valuable way to ensure that the enteral nutrition regimen prescribed for a particular patient is satisfactory. A steady increase in weight of 1–2 kg per week suggests adequate nutrition in those requiring body mass repletion. Basic

haematological and biochemical parameters should be measured daily at the commencement of enteral nutrition. Once nutrition support has been stabilised, then weekly measurements are reasonable.

Initially, close monitoring of the plasma potassium, phosphate[171] and glucose are important, particularly in the severely malnourished patient. In patients on long-term feeding, vitamin levels or trace element levels may be required if clinically indicated (see Chapter 11). The plasma proteins albumin, transferrin and thyroid-binding prealbumin can all be useful markers for indicating a response to nutrition support over a period of time. Urinary urea levels allow an estimate of nitrogen excretion to be made (to estimate nitrogen balance) although this is not as accurate as direct determination of urine nitrogen.[172] Anthropometric and dynamometric measurements are often considered as research tools but they can offer sensitive and effective measurement of the efficacy of nutrition support.

Summary

This chapter has highlighted the important points that need to be considered when the enteral route is chosen to provide nutrition support to the nutritionally compromised patient. Enteral nutrition has become a technologically advanced medical therapy in the last 20 years and as clinical nutrition continues to develop, further advances will be made. For now, with the range of access routes and delivery systems available and with the wealth of information derived from basic and clinical research, there should be no excuse for failing to provide enteral nutrition in a safe and cost-effective manner (see Table 17.5).

Table 17.5 – Optimising enteral nutrition

Adopt same standards for enteral nutrition as for TPN
Monitor (and audit) by nutrition support team
Identify most appropriate route of access
Confirm tube placement (if in doubt, X-ray)
Check placement regularly during course of feeding
Regularly cleanse and flush tubes
Use closed diet system when possible (avoids 'exogenous' contamination)
Use large-volume reservoirs to minimise handling
Undertake all handling with sterile gloves
'Hang time' never > than 24 hours
Avoid starter regimens
Use continuous infusion in preference to bolus
Adopt regular nutrition assessment

References

1. British Association of Parenteral and Enteral Nutrition. Current perspectives on enteral nutrition in adults. BAPEN, London, 1999.

2. Finucane TE, Christmas C, Travis K. Tube feeding in patients with advanced dementia. *JAMA* 1999; **282:** 1365–70.

3. Mitchell SL, Lawson FME. Decision-making for long-term tube feeding in cognitively impaired elderly people. *CMAJ* 1999; **160:** 1705–9.

4. Dobbie RP, Hoffmeister JA. Continuous pump-tube hyperalimentation. *Surg Gynecol Obstet* 1976; **143:** 273–6.

5. Suchner U. Enteral versus parenteral nutrition: effects on gastrointestinal function and metabolism: background. *Nutrition* 1998; **14:** 76–81.

6. Payne-James JJ, de Gara CJ, Grimble GK *et al*. Artificial nutrition support in hospitals in the United Kingdom, 1991: second national survey. *Clin Nutr* 1992; **11:** 187–92.

7. Dewar H. Nasogastric tube audit: standard setting and review of specification. *Journal of Human Nutrition and Dietetics* 1997; **10:** 313–15.

8. Hernandez OG, Nelson S, Haponik EF, Lopez A, Summer W. Obligate nasal breathing in an elderly woman: increased risk of nasogastric tube feeding. *J Parent Enteral Nutr* 1988; **12:** 531–2.

9. Naviski N, Yehuda Y, Serour F. Does the size of naso-gastric tube affect gastroesophageal reflux in children? *J Paediatric Gastroenterology and Nutrition* 1999; **29:** 448–51.

10. Olbrantz KR, Gelfand D, Choplin R, Wu EC. Pneumothorax complicating enteral feeding tube placements. *J Parent Enteral Nutr* 1985; **9:** 210–11.

11. Idar S, Meguid MM. Pneumothorax following attempted nasogastric intubation for nutritional support. *J Parent Enteral Nutr* 1984; **8:** 450–2.

12. Hand RW, Kempster M, Levy JH, Rogol PR, Spirn P. Inadvertent transbronchial insertion of narrow-bore feeding tubes into the pleural space. *JAMA* 1984; **251:** 2396–7.

13. James RH. An unusual complication of passing a narrow bore nasogastric tube. *Anaesthesia* 1978; **33:** 716–18.

14. Balogh GJ, Adler SJ, VanderWoude J, Glazer HS, Roper C, Weyman PJ. Pneumothorax as a complication of feeding tube placement. *Am J Roentgenol* 1983; **141:** 1275–7.

15. Torrington KG. Fatal hydrothorax and empyema complicating a malpositioned nasogastric tube. *Chest* 1981; **79:** 240–2.

16. Hendry PJ, Akyurekli Y, McIntyre R, Quarrington A, Keon WJ. Bronchopleural complications of nasogastric feeding tubes. *Crit Care Med* 1986; **14:** 892–4.

17. Katelaris PH. Pleuropulmonary complications of fine-bore nasoenteric feeding tubes. *Aus NZ J Surg* 1991; **61:** 39–42.

18. Wendell GD, Lenchner GS, Promisloff RA. Pneumothorax complicating small-bore feeding tube placement. *Arch Intern Med* 1991; **151:** 599–602.

19. Scholten DJ, Wood TL, Thompson DR. Pneumothorax from nasoenteric feeding tube insertion. *Am Surg* 1986; **52:** 381–5.

20. Saltzberg DM, Goldstein M, Levine GM. Feeding tube-induced pneumothorax. *J Parent Enteral Nutr* 1984; **8:** 714–16.

21. Simon T, Fink AS. Current management of endoscopic feeding tube dysfunction. *Surg Endosc* 1999; **13:** 403–5.

22. McWey RE, Curry NS, Schabel SI, Reines HD. Complications of nasoenteric feeding tubes. *Am J Surg* 1988; **155:** 253–7.

23. Metheny N. Measures to test placement of nasogastric and nasointestinal feeding tubes: a review. *Nurs Res* 1988; **37:** 324–9.

24. Valentine RJ, Turner WW. Pleural complications of enteric feeding tubes. *J Parent Enteral Nutr* 1985; **9:** 605–7.

25. Rolfe I. Complications associated with the insertion of narrow bore feeding tubes. *Med J Aust* 1990; **152:** 108.

26. Berry S, Orr M, Schoettker P *et al*. Intestinal placement of pH sensing nasointestinal feeding tubes. *J Parent Enteral Nutr* 1994; 67–70.

27. Muthuswamy PP, Patel K, Rajendran R. Isocal pneumonia with respiratory failure. *Chest* 1982; **81:** 390.

28. Kiwak MG. Entriflex feeding tube: need for care in using it. *Am J Roentgenol* 1984; **143:** 1341–2.

29. Widmann WD. Complications of nasoenteric tubes. *JAMA* 1985; **254:** 54.

30. Bouzarth WF. Intracranial nasogastric tube insertion. *J Trauma* 1978; **18:** 818–19.

31. Keohane PP, Attrill H, Silk DBA. Clinical effectiveness of weighted and unweighted 'finebore' nasogastric feeding tubes in enteral nutrition: a controlled clinical trial. *J Clin Nutr Gastroenterol* 1986; **1:** 189–93.

32. McDonald E, Daggett M, Swint E. A comparison of four holding devices for anchoring nasogastric tubes. *J Neurosurg Nurs* 1982; **14:** 90–3.

33. Tophill PR, Finan PJ. An improved method for securing nasogastric tubes. *Ann Roy Coll Surg Engl* 1988; **70:** 282.

34. Sax HC, Bower RH. A method for securing naso-gastric tubes in uncooperative patients. *Surg Gynecol Obstet* 1987; **164**: 471–2.

35. Erenberg A, Nowak AJ. Appliance for stabilising oro-gastric and orotracheal tubes in infants. *Crit Care Med* 1984; **12**: 669–70.

36. Stocks J. Effect of nasogastric tubes on nasal resistance during infancy. *Arch Dis Child* 1980; **55**: 17–21.

37. Kiver KF, Hayes DP, Fortin DF, Mains BS. Pre- and post-pyloric enteral feeding: analysis of safety and complications. *J Parent Enteral Nutr* 1984; **8**: 95.

38. Gutierrez GD, Balfe DM. Fluoroscopically guided nasoenteric feeding tube placement: results of a 1 year study. *Radiology* 1991; **178**: 759–62.

39. Winterbauer RH, Durning RB, Barron E. Aspirated nasogastric feeding solution detected by glucose strips. *Ann Int Med* 1981; **95**: 67–8.

40. Mullan H, Roubenoff RA, Roubenoff R. Risk of pulmonary aspiration among patients receiving enteral nutrition support. *J Parent Enteral Nutr* 1992; **16**: 160–4.

41. Montecalvo MA, Steger KA, Farber HW *et al.* Nutritional outcome and pneumonia in critical care patients randomized to gastric versus jejunal feedings. *Crit Care Med* 1992; **20**: 1377–87.

42. McLean GK, Meranze SG, Burke DR. Inadvertent tracheobronchial placement of feeding tubes. *Radiology* 1989; **163**: 278.

43. Grant JP, Curtas MS, Kelvin FM. Fluoroscopic place-ment of nasojejunal feeding tubes with immediate feeding using a non-elemental diet. *J Parent Enteral Nutr* 1983; **7**: 299–303.

44. Cardoza JD, Jeffrey RB. Nasojejunal feeding tube placement in immobile patients. *Radiology* 1988; **166**: 893.

45. McLean GK, Meranze SG, Burke DR. Enteric alimentation: a radiologic approach. *Radiology* 1986; **160**: 555–6.

46. Hatfield DR, Beck JL. An improved technique for feeding tube placement. *Radiology* 1981; **1** (141): 823.

47. Payne-James JJ, Loft DE, Silk DBA. Novel endoscopic grasping forceps for enteral tubes. *J Clin Nutr Gastroenterol* 1990; **4**: 199–201.

48. Rives DA, LeRoy JL, Hawkins ML, Bowden TA. Endoscopically assisted nasojejunal feeding tube place-ment. *Am Surg* 1989; **55**: 88–91.

49. Lewis BS, Mauer K, Bush A. The rapid placement of jejunal feeding tubes: the Seldinger technique applied to the gut. *Gastrointest Endosc* 1990; **36**: 139.

50. Stark SP, Sharpe JN, Larson GM. Endoscopically placed nasoenteral feeding tubes. *Am Surg* 1991; **57**: 203–5.

51. Damore LJ, Andrus CH, Hermann VM *et al.* Prospective evaluation of a new through-the-scope nasoduodenal enteral feeding tube. *Surg Endosc* 1997; **11**: 460–3.

52. Gabriel SA, Ackermann RJ, Castresana MR. A new technique for placement of nasoenteral feeding tubes using external magnetic guidance. *Crit Care Med* 1997; **25**: 641–5.

53. Grathwohl KW, Gibbons RV, Dillard TA *et al.* Bedside videoscopic placement of feeding tubes: development of fiberoptics through the tube. *Crit Care Med* 1997; **25**: 629–34.

54. Huerta G, Puri VK. Nasoenteric feeding tubes in critically ill patients (fluoroscopy versus blind). *Nutrition* 2000; **16**: 264–7.

55. Kittinger JW, Sandler RS, Heizer WD. Efficacy of metoclopramide as an adjunct to duodenal placement of small-bore feeding tubes: a randomised, placebo-controlled double-blind study. *J Parent Enteral Nutr* 1987; **11**: 33–7.

56. Whatley K, Turner WW, Dey M *et al.* When does metoclopramide facilitate transpyloric intubation? *J Parent Enteral Nutr* 1984; **8**: 679–81.

57. MacLaren R, Kuhl DA, Gervasio JM *et al.* Sequential single doses of cisapride, erythromycin, and meto-clopramide in critically ill patients intolerant to enteral nutrition: a randomised, placebo-controlled, crossover study. *Crit Care Med* 2000; **28**: 438–44.

58. Bosscha K, Nieuwenhuijs VB, Vos A *et al.* Gastrointestinal motility and gastric tube feeding in mechanically ventilated patients. *Crit Care Med* 1998; **26**: 1510–17.

59. Payne-James JJ, Doherty J, Rees RG, Silk DBA. 7 g weighted vs unweighted enteral tubes – spontaneous transpyloric passage and tube performance: a random-ised controlled trial. *Clin Nutr* 1990; **9**: 109–12.

60. Levenson R, Turner WW, Dyson A, Zike L, Reisch J. Do weighted nasoenteric feeding tubes facilitate duodenal intubations? *J Parent Enteral Nutr* 1988; **12**: 135–7.

61. Lee SM. The use of double-lumen tubes in upper gastrointestinal surgery. *Am Surg* 1980; **141**: 363–5.

62. Moss G. Efficient gastroduodenal decompression with simultaneous full enteral nutrition: a new gastrostomy catheter technique. *J Parent Enteral Nutr* 1984; **8**: 203–7.

63. Baskin WN, Johanson JF. An improved approach to delivery of enteral nutrition in the intensive care unit. *Gastrointest Endosc* 1995; **42**: 161–5.

64. Mathus-Vliegen EMH, Tytgat GNJ. The role of endoscopy in the correct and rapid positioning of feeding tubes. *Endoscopy* 1983; **15**: 78–84.

65. Klopp CT. Cervical oesophagostomy. *J Cardiovasc Surg* 1951; **21**: 490.

66. Gaggiotti G, Orlandoni P, Boecoli G, Caporelli SG, Patrizi SG, Masera N. A device to perform percutaneous cervical pharyngostomy (PCP) for enteral nutrition. *Clin Nutr* 1989; **8**: 273–5.

67. Gauderer MWL, Ponsky JL, Izant RJ. Gastrostomy without laparotomy: a percutaneous endoscopic technique. *J Ped Surg* 1980; **15**: 872–5.

68. Russell TR, Brotman M, Norris F. Percutaneous gastrostomy: a new simplified and cost-effective technique. *Am J Surg* 1984; **148**: 133–5.

69. Duncan HD, Bray MJ, Kapadia SA *et al.* Prospective randomised comparison of two different sized percutaneous endoscopically placed gastrostomy tubes. *Clin Nutr* 1996; **15**: 317–20.

70. Fertl E, Steinhoff N, Schofl R *et al.* Transient and long-term feeding by means of percutaneous endoscopic gastrostomy in neurological rehabilitation. *Eur Neurol* 1998; **40**: 27–30.

71. Williams SGJ, Ashworth F, McAlweenie A *et al.* Percutaneous endoscopic gastrostomy feeding in patients with cystic fibrosis. *Gut* 1999; **44**: 87–90.

72. Slezak FA, Kofol W. Combined tracheostomy and percutaneous endoscopic gastrostomy. *Am J Surg* 1987; **154**: 271–3.

73. Vaughan JR, Scott JS, Edelman DS, Unger SW. Tracheostomy: a new indication for percutaneous endoscopic gastrostomy tube placement. *Am Surg* 1991; **57**: 214–15.

74. Finucane P, Aslan SM, Duncan D. Percutaneous endoscopic gastrostomy in elderly patients. *Post-grad Med J* 1991; **67**: 371–3.

75. Mahajan L, Oliver L, Wyllie R *et al.* The safety of gastrostomy in patient's with Crohn's disease. *Am J Gastro* 1997; **92**: 985–8.

76. Ditesheim JA, Richards W, Sharp K. Fatal and disastrous complications following percutaneous endoscopic gastrostomy. *Am Surg* 1989; **55**: 92–6.

77. James A, Kapur K, Hawthorne AB. Long-term outcome of percutaneous endoscopic gastrostomy feeding in patients with dysphagic stroke. *Age & Ageing* 1998; **27**: 671–8.

78. Deitel M, Bendago R, Spratt EH *et al.* Percutaneous endoscopic gastrostomy by the pull and introducer methods. *Can J Surg* 1988; **31**: 102–4.

79. Stiegmann G, Goff JS, Silas D, Pearlman N, Sun J, Norton I. Endoscopic versus operative gastrostomy: final results of a prospective randomised trial. *Gastrointest Endosc* 1990; **36**: 1–5.

80. Loser C, Wolters S, Folsch UR. Enteral nutrition via percutaneous endoscopic gastrostomy (PEG) in 210 patients. *Dig Dis Sci* 1998; **43**: 2549–57.

81. Jain NK, Larson DE, Schroeder KW *et al.* Antibiotic prophylaxis for percutaneous endoscopic gastrostomy: a prospective double-blind clinical trial. *Ann Intern Med* 1987; **107**: 824–8.

82. Behrens R, Lang T, Muschsweck H *et al.* Percutaneous endoscopic gastrostomy in children and adolescents. *J Pediatr Gastroenterol Nutr* 1997; **25**: 487–91.

83. Payne-James JJ, Bray J, Rana SK, Silk DBA. Occult peristomal abscess associated with percutaneous endoscopic gastrostomy. *Clin Nutr* 1990; **9**: 289–90.

84. Pidala MJ, Slezak FA, Porter JA. Pneumoperitoneum following percutaneous endoscopic gastrostomy: does the timing of panendoscopy matter? *Surg Endosc* 1992; **6**: 128–9.

85. Nath GD, Goodgame R, Saeed ZA, Graham DY. Pneumoperitoneum: a preventable complication of PEG in mechanically ventilated patients. *Gastrointest Endosc* 1991; **37**: 84–5.

86. Huang DT, Thomas G, Wilson WR. Stomal seeding by percutaneous endoscopic gastrostomy in patients with head and neck cancer. *Arch Otolaryngol Head Neck Surg* 1992; **118**: 658–9.

87. Waxman I, AI-Kawas FH, Bass B, Glouderman M. PEG ileus: a new cause of small bowel obstruction. *Dig Dis Sci* 1991; **36**: 251–4.

88. Colletti RB, Hebert C. Esophageal obstruction after incomplete removal of a PEG tube. *Gastrointest Endosc* 1991; **37**: 211–12.

89. Stathopoulos G, Rildberg MA, Harig JM. Subcutaneous emphysema following PEG. *Gastrointest Endosc* 1991; **37**: 374–6.

90. Behrle KM, Dekovich AA, Ammon HV. Spontaneous tube extrusion following percutaneous endoscopic gastrostomy. *Gastrointest Endosc* 1989; **35**: 56–8.

91. Chung RS, Schertzer M. Pathogenesis of complications of percutaneous endoscopic gastrostomy. *Am J Surg* 1990; **56**: 134–7.

92. Pesarini AC, Dittler HJ. Feeding tubes perforation as a complication of percutaneous endoscopic gastrostomy. *Endoscopy* 1992; **24**: 235.

93. Eisdorfer RM, DiLorenzo JC, Miskowitz P. A complication of PEG change. *Gastrointest Endosc* 1991; **37**: 108.

94. Esker AH, Hall CH. Replacement of the damaged percutaneous endoscopic gastrostomy feeding tube in the immature tract. *Gastrointest Endosc* 1990; **36**: 389.

95. Saltzberg DM, Anand K, Juvan P, Joffe I. Colocutaneous fistula: an unusual complication of percutaneous endoscopic gastrostomy. *J Parent Enteral Nutr* 1987; **11**: 86–7.

96. Bui HD, Dang CV, Schlater T, Nghiem CH. A new complication of percutaneous endoscopic gastrostomy. *Am J Gasser* 1988; **83**: 448–51.

97. Stefan MM, Holcomb GW, Ross AJ. Cologastric fistula as a complication of percutaneous endoscopic gastrostomy. *J Parent Enteral Nutr* 1989; **13**: 554–6.

98. Shike M, Wallach C, Likier H. Direct percutaneous endoscopic jejunostomies. *Gastrointest Endosc* 1991; **37**: 62–5.

99. DiSario JA, Foutch PG, Sanowski RA. Poor results with percutaneous endoscopic jejunostomy. *Gastrointest Endosc* 1990; **36**: 257–60.

100. Sanchez RB, Van Sonnenverg E, D'Agostino HB *et al.* CT guidance for percutaneous gastrostomy and gastro-enterostomy. *Radiology* 1992; **184**: 201–5.

101. Mirich DR, Gray RG. Infracolic percutaneous gastro-jejunostomy. *Cardiovasc Intervent Radiol* 1990; **12**: 340–1.

102. Tao HH, Gillies RR. Percutaneous feeding gastros-tomy. *Am J Roentgenol* 1983; **141**: 793–A.

103. Halkier BK, Ho CS, Yee ACN. Percutaneous feeding gastrostomy with the Seldinger technique: review of 252 patients. *Radiology* 1989; **171**: 359–62.

104. Hicks ME, Surratt RS, Picus D, Marx MV, Lang EV. Fluoroscopically guided percutaneous gastrostomy and gastroenterostomy: analysis of 158 cases. *Am J Roentgenol* 1990; **154**: 725–8.

105. Pearce CB, Goggin PM, Collett J *et al.* The cut and push method of percutaneous endoscopic gastrostomy tube removal. *Clin Nutr* 2000; **19**: 133–5.

106. Campbell TA, Drabek GA, Tatum H, Lytlen GH. Removal of gastrostomy tubes. *JAMA* 1992; **268**: 1270.

107. Glass-Royal M, Teitelbaum GP, Joseph GJ, Matsumoto AH, Barth KH. Non-endoscopic tech-niques for manipulating Sacks-Vine gastrostomy tubes. *Cardiovasc Intervent Radiol* 1990; **12**: 346–9.

108. Payne-James JJ, Kapadia S, Loft DE, Silk DBA. Early experience with the Bower PEG tube. *J Roy Coll Surg Edin* 1992; **37**: 34–7.

109. Murphy C, Rosemurgy AS, Albrink MH, Carey LC. A simple technique for laparoscopic gastrostomy. *Surg Gynecol Obstet* 1992; **174**: 424–5.

110. Cossa JP, Marmuse JP, Lecomte P *et al.* Gastrostomie tubulee sous coelioscopie. *Presse Med* 1992; **21**: 1519–21.

111. Weltz CR, Morris JB, Mullen JL. Surgical gastrostomy in aspiration risk patients. *Ann Surg* 1992; **215**: 140–5.

112. Kirby DF. To PEG or not to PEG – that is the costly question. *Mayo Clin Proc* 1992; **67**: 1115–17.

113. Holmes JH, Brundage SI, Yuen P-C *et al.* Complications of surgical feeding jejunostomy in trauma patients. *J Trauma* 1999; **47**: 1009–12.

114. Singh G, Ram P, Khanna SK. Early postoperative feeding in patients with non-traumatic intestinal perforation and peritonitis. *J Am Coll Surg* 1998; **187**: 142–6.

115. Lawlor DK, Inculet RI, Malthaner RA. Small-bowel necrosis associated with jejunal tube feeding. *Can J Surg* 1998; **41**: 459–62.

116. Delaney HM, Carnevale NJ, Garvey JW. Jejunostomy by a needle catheter technique. *Surgery* 1973; **73**: 786–90.

117. Hoover HC. Needle catheter jejunostomy: friend or foe? *Mayo Clin Proc* 1988; **636**: 28–9.

118. Page CP. Needle catheter jejunostomy. *Contemp Surg* 1981; **19**: 29–47.

119. Blebea J, King TA. Intraperitoneal infusion as a complication of needle catheter feeding jejunostomy. *J Parent Enteral Nutr* 1985; **9**: 758–9.

120. Sorensen VJ, Rafidi F, Obeid FN. Perforation of the small bowel after insertion of feeding jejunostomy: a case report. *J Parent Enteral Nutr* 1987; **11**: 202–4.

121. Butsch JL. A knotty problem with a feeding jejunos-tomy tube. *Arch Surg* 1986; **121**: 736.

122. Thomas L, Cohen AJ, Omiya B, McKenzie R, Tominga G. Pneumatosis intestinalis associated with needle catheter jejunostomy tubes: CT findings and implications. *J Comput Assist Tomogr* 1992; **16**: 418–19.

123. Heberer M, Bodoky A, Iwatschenko P, Harder F. Indications for needle catheter jejunostomy in elective abdominal surgery. *Am Surg* 1987; **153**: 545–52.

124. Sarr MG, Mayo S. Needle catheter jejunostomy: an unappreciated and misunderstood advance in the care of patients after major abdominal operations. *Mayo Clin Proc* 1988; **63**: 565–72.

125. De Gottardi A, Krahenbuhk L, Farhadi J *et al.* Clinical experience of feeding through a needle catheter jejunostomy after major abdominal operations. *Eur J Surg* 1999; **165**: 1055–60.

126. Antinori CH, Andrew C, Villanueva DT *et al.* A tech-nique for converting a needle-catheter jejunostomy into a standard jejunostomy. *Am J Surg* 1992; **164**: 68–9.

127. McGonigal MD, Lucas CE, Ledgerwood AM. Feeding jejunostomy in patients who are critically ill. *Surg Gynecol Obstet* 1989; **168:** 275–7.

128. Shike M, Latkany L, Gerdes H *et al.* Direct percutaneous endoscopic jejunostomies for enteral feeding. *Gastrointest Endosc* 1996; **44:** 536–40.

129. Treem WR, Etienne NL, Hyams JS. Percutaneous endoscopic placement of the 'button' gastrostomy tube as the initial procedure in infants and children. *J Pediatr Gastroenterol Nutr* 1993; **17:** 382–6.

130. Coleman JE, Watson AR, Rance CH *et al.* Gastrostomy buttons for nutritional support on chronic dialysis. *Nephrol Dial Transplant* 1998; **13:** 2041–6.

131. Shike M, Wallach C, Gerdes H, Hermann Zaidins M. Skin-level gastrostomies and jejunostomies for long-term enteral feeding. *J Parent Enteral Nutr* 1989; **13:** 648–50.

132. Rothenberg S, Bealer JF, Chang JHT. Primary laparoscopic placement of gastrostomy buttons for feeding tubes. *Surg Endosc* 1999; **13:** 995–7.

133. Maruyama M, Ebuchi M, Sugano N *et al.* Subcutaneously implanted enteral nutrition port. *J Parent Enteral Nutr* 1997; **21:** 238–40.

134. Nicholson LJ. Declogging small-bore feeding tubes. *J Parent Enteral Nutr* 1987; **11:** 594–7.

135. Spain DA, McClave SA, Sexton LK *et al.* Infusion protocol improves delivery of enteral tube feeding in the critical care unit. *J Parent Enteral Nutr* 1999; **23:** 288–92.

136. Pingleton SK, Hinthorn D, Lui C. Enteral nutrition in patients receiving mechanical ventilation. *Am J Med* 1986; **80:** 827–32.

137. Du Moulin GC, Paterson DG, Hedley-White J, Lisbon A. Aspiration of gastric bacteria in antacid-treated patients: a frequent cause of post-operative colonisation of the airway. *Lancet* 1982; **i:** 570–8.

138. Pollack M, Charrache P, Nieman RE, Jett MP, Reinhardt JA, Hardy PH. Factors affecting colonisation and antibiotic resistance patterns of Gram negative bacteria in hospital patients. *Lancet* 1972; **2:** 668.

139. Kingston GW, Phang PJ, Leathley MJ. Increased incidence of nosocomial pneumonias in mechanically ventilated patients with subclinical aspiration. *Am J Surg* 1991; **161:** 589–92.

140. Pingleton SK. Enteral nutrition as a risk factor for nosocomial pneumonia. *Eur J Clin Microbiol Infect Dis* 1989; **8:** 51–5.

141. Casewell MW, Cooper JE, Webster M. Enteral feeds contaminated with *Enterobacter cloacae* as a cause of septicaemia. *Br Med J* 1981; **282:** 973.

142. Levy J, Van Laethem Y, Verhaegen G. Contaminated enteral nutrition solutions as a cause of nosocomial bloodstream infection: a study using plasmid fingerprinting. *J Parent Enteral Nutr* 1989; **13:** 228–34.

143. Pottecher B, Goetch ML, Jacquemaire MA, Reeb E, Lavillaureix J. Enterocolites infectieuse chez des malades de reanimation alimentes pai, sonde naso-gastrique. *Ann Anesth Fr* 1979; **20:** 595.

144. Anderton A. Microbiological aspects of the preparation and administration of nasogastric and nasoenteric tube feeds in hospitals: a review. *Hum Nutr* 1983; **37A:** 426–40.

145. Hostetler C, Lipman TO, Geraghty M, Parker RH. Bacterial safety of reconstituted continuous drip tube feeding. *J Parent Enteral Nutr* 1982; **6:** 232–5.

146. Perez SK, Brandt K. Enteral feeding contamination: comparison of diluents and feeding bag usage. *J Parent Enteral Nutr* 1989; **13:** 306–8.

147. Anderton A. The potential of *Escherichia coli* in enteral feeds to cause food poisoning: a study under simulated ward conditions. *J Hosp Infect* 1984; **5:** 155–63.

148. Heyland D, Bradley C, Mandell LA. Effect of acidified enteral feedings on gastric colonization in the critically ill patient. *Crit Care Med* 1992; **20:** 1388–94.

149. Anderton A, Aidoo KE. The effect of handling procedures on microbial contamination of enteral feeds. *J Hosp Infect* 1988; **11:** 364–72.

150. Van Alsenoy L, De Leeuw I, Delvigne C, Van De Woude M. Ascending contamination of a jejunostomy feeding reservoir. *Clin Nutr* 1985; **4:** 95–8.

151. Crocker KS, Krey SH, Markovic M, Steffee WP. Microbial growth in clinically used enteral delivery systems. *Am J Infect Control* 1986; **14:** 250–6.

152. Payne-James JJ, Bray J, Rana S, McSwiggan D, Silk DBA. Retrograde contamination of enteral feed delivery systems. *J Parent Enteral Nutr* 1992; **16:** 369–73.

153. McKinlay J, Anderton A, Wood W, Gould IM. Endogenous bacterial contamination of enteral tube feeding systems during administration of feeds to hospital patients. *J Hum Nutr Dietet* 1995; **8:** 3–8.

154. Beattie TK, Anderton A. Enteral feeding tube guidewire – another factor in the retrograde contamination of enteral feeding systems. *J Hum Nutr Dietet* 1998; **11:** 85–93.

155. Wagner DR, Elmore MF, Knoll DM. Evaluation of closed vs open systems for the delivery of peptide-based enteral diets. *J Parent Enteral Nutr* 1994; **18:** 453–7.

156. Vaughan A, Manore M, Winston D. Bacterial safety of a closed administration system for enteral nutrition solutions. *J Am Dietet Assoc* 1988; **88:** 35–7.

157. Navajas MFC, Chacon DJ, Solvas JFG, Vargas RG. Bacterial contamination of enteral feeds as a possible risk of nosocomial infection. *J Hosp Infect* 1992; **21:** 111–20.

158. Keohane PP, Attrill H, Bones BIM, Silk DBA. A controlled trial of aseptic enteral diet preparation: significant effects on bacterial contamination and nitrogen balance. *Clin Nutr* 1983; **2:** 119–22.

159. Rees RG, Ryan J, Attrill H, Silk DBA. Clinical evaluation of two litre prepacked enteral diet delivery system: a controlled trial. *J Parent Enteral Nutr* 1988; **12:** 274–7.

160. Anderton A. What is the HACCP (hazard analysis critical control point) approach and how can it be applied to enteral tube feeding? *J Hum Nutr Dietet* 1994; **7:** 53–60.

161. Allison SP, Walford S, Todorovic V, Elliott ET. Practical aspects of nutritional support. *Res Clin Forums* 1979; **1:** 49–57.

162. Ciocon JO, Galindo-Ciocon DJ, Tiessen C, Galindo D. Continuous compared with intermittent tube feeding in the elderly. *J Parent Enteral Nutr* 1992; **16:** 525–8.

163. Pinchovsky-Devin GD, Kaminski MV. Visceral protein increase associated with interrupted versus continuous enteral hyperalimentation. *J Parent Enteral Nutr* 1985; **9:** 474–6.

164. Bonten MJM, Gaillard CA, van Tiel FH *et al.* Continuous enteral feeding counteracts preventive measures for gastric colonisation intensive care unit patients. *Crit Care Med* 1994; **22:** 939–44.

165. Adams GF, Guest D, Ciraulo DL *et al.* Maximizing tolerance of enteral nutrition in severely injured trauma patients: a comparison of enteral feedings by means of percutaneous endoscopic gastrostomy versus percutaneous endoscopic gastrojejunostomy. *J Trauma* 2000; **48:** 459–65.

166. Moncure M, Samaha E, Moncure K *et al.* Jejunostomy tube feedings should not be stopped in the perioperative patient. *J Parent Enteral Nutr* 1999; **23:** 356–9.

167. Keohane PP, Attrill H, Love M, Frost P, Silk DBA. Relation between osmolality of diet and gastrointestinal side effects in enteral nutrition. *Br Med J* 1984; **228:** 678–80.

168. Rees RG, Keohane PP, Grimble GK *et al.* Elemental diet administered nasogastrically without starter regimens to patients with inflammatory bowel disease. *J Parent Enteral Nutr* 1986; **10:** 258–62.

169. Dietscher JE, Foulks CJ, Waits M. Accuracy of enteral pumps: in vitro performance. *J Parent Enteral Nutr* 1994; **18:** 359–61.

170. McClave SA, Snider HL, Lowen CC *et al.* Use of residual volume as a marker for enteral feeding intolerance: prospective blinded comparison with physical examination and radiographic findings. *J Parent Enteral Nutr* 1992; **16:** 99–105.

171. Payne-James JJ, Rees RG, Newton MA, Silk DBA. Acute respiratory failure in association with hypophosphataemia after refeeding in anorexia nervosa. *J Clin Gastroenterol* 1988; **3:** 67–8.

172. Grimble GK, West MFE, Acuti ABC *et al.* Assessment of an automated chemiluminescence nitrogen analyzer for routine use in clinical nutrition. *J Parent Enteral Nutr* 1988; **12:** 100–6.

18

Enteral diets: clinical uses and formulation

David B A Silk

Introduction

A visit to an exhibition of enteral nutrition products may suggest that this had become a complex and difficult area of clinical nutrition. Not only might the array of different nasoenteric, percutaneous endoscopic gastrostomy and other feeding tubes confuse and the different types of diet reservoirs and feeding pumps mystify but the huge array of enteral diets would be enough to convince the novice in the field of their inadequacies. In fact, enteral nutrition is a simple subspeciality of clinical nutrition. It is cost effective and a physiological means of providing nutritional support and the side-effects, when they occur, are less serious and clinically limiting than those that can complicate parenteral nutrition.

This chapter will deal with the way in which physiological and metabolic research have been applied to the formulation of enteral diets and, importantly, how the correct clinical choice of diet can be made. The discussion will emphasise practicality and simplicity, assuming that the decision has been made that the patient requires nutrition support, either because of pre-existing malnutrition or because nutrition status should be maintained and that the most appropriate route for feeding is enteral.

Methods of administering enteral nutrition

Enteral diets can be administered by tube feeding, as a drink or as oral supplements which may be liquids, semisolid or solid. Although the palatability of these products continues to improve, interpatient differences in taste perception may be modulated by the underlying disease[1] and coexistent micronutrient deficiency.[2] Different products must therefore be presented at different times during the course of illness. As described previously (Chapter 16), enteral feeds can now be administered as sip feeds or via feeding tubes, positioned into different sites of the gastrointestinal tract.

The impact of oral supplements in nutritional treatment of patients should not be underestimated since they have been shown to confer clinical benefit following orthopaedic surgery,[3] in elderly patients[4] and following elective moderate to major gastrointestinal surgery.[5] It is likely in the future that oral sip feeding and drink feeding will assume an increasing role in enteral nutrition.

Initial patient assessment

Having decided to attempt to feed a patient enterally, several further decisions should be made (Table 18.1). The route and technique must be chosen. Nutrition requirements must be assessed (Chs 17 and 20) and an appropriate enteral diet chosen. The need for this to be done within the context of a multidisciplinary team approach has been discussed.[6] It is important to emphasise that nutrition support is but one link in the chain of therapy and that the views of ward staff and primary care physicians or surgeons are important because they will define the nature of the underlying disease process which has led to the current clinical status of the patient.

Table 18.1 – Clinical factors influencing the choice of enteral diets

- Nutrition intake of patient
- Nutrition requirements
- Impairment of gastrointestinal function:
    Nutrient malabsorption
    Failure of motility
- Presence of cardiopulmonary, liver or renal failure
- Presence of critical illness, major trauma, sepsis or multiple organ failure

Types of enteral diet available

Before discussing factors which influence enteral diet choice, it is necessary to consider the types available, which are detailed in Table 18.2.

Polymeric diets

These are the most commonly prescribed and contain protein, carbohydrate and fat in the form of whole-protein, partially digested starch and triglycerides, respectively, together with electrolytes, minerals, trace elements, haematinics and vitamins. They are used as the sole source of nutrition intake for patients with normal or near normal gastrointestinal function. Some, but not all, will contain a fibre source. Usually these diets are available in liquid form.

Predigested chemically defined elemental diets

These diets are prescribed to patients with varying degrees of nutrient malabsorption and differ from

Table 18.2 – Suggested formulation of enteral diets

		Oral dietary supplements		Polymeric enteral diets				Chemically defined elemental diet
		Nitrogen rich	Energy rich	Hypotonic 'introductory'	No major injury or sepsis	Moderate injury or sepsis	Respiratory failure	
Nitrogen	Source				Whole protein			Purified protein hydrolysate di– and tripeptides
	Concentration (g/l)	12	7.2	4.5	6	9	9	7
	% Energy	30	12	19	15	19	25	17.5
Carbohydrate	Source			Partial enzymic hydrolysate of starch				High MW starch hydrolysate polymers >10 glucose units
	Concentration (g/l)	112	267	69	125	139	112	175
	% Energy	45	71	46	50	46	30	70
Fat	Type	LCT	LCT	LCT	LCT	LCT60% MCT 40%	LCT	LCT to provide 5g/l linoleic acid
	n3:n6	5:1	5:1	5:1	5:1	5:1	5:1	
	Concentration (g/l)	100	67	23	39	47	92	12
	% Energy	25	17	35	35	35	55	12
Energy density	kcal/ml	1	1.5	0.6	1	1.2	1.5	1.2
Non-protein energy:nitrogen	kcal/g N	112:1	232:1	133:1	167:1	133:1		143:1
Trace elements	% RDA/L	100	100	67	67	67	100	100
Vitamins	% RDA/L	100	100	67	67	67	100	100
Fibre	Source			None	Multiple	Multiple		
	Concentration (g/l)				15	15		
Flavours		Multiple	Multiple					
Sodium	mmol/l							80—50

polymeric diets in that protein is replaced by partially hydrolysed protein or mixtures of free L-amino acids, and the lipid content is low and may include medium-chain triglycerides. Hitherto these diets have not contained a fibre source. They are available in both liquid and powder form.

Disease-specific diets

Cardiopulmonary diets contain an increased ratio of lipid to carbohydrate, whilst diets for patients with advanced parenchymal liver disease (with evidence of hepatic encephalopathy) contain a modified L-amino acid composition. Renal diets may contain a nitrogen source consisting of all the essential amino acids plus histidine without the non-essential amino acids.

Specialist diets

These diets include the new 'immunomodulating' formulations which are intended to improve organ function in critically ill patients. There may be nutritional additions of MCT and increased ratios of n–3:n-6 fatty acids. Significant additions of carnitine, β-carotene, nucleotides, L-arginine, L-glutamine and branched-chain amino acids may be made.

Modular diets

Modular diets are occasionally used (in less than 5% of enteral-fed patients[7]) when a particular component of the diet requires an increased intake or if a patient requires a special blend of diet.

Oral nutritional supplements

Oral nutritional supplements usually have similar composition to polymeric enteral diets and are either high in nitrogen relative to energy or vice versa. They are indicated in situations where the patient's diet is insufficient to meet requirements.

Clinical factors influencing the choice of enteral diet (Table 18.1)

Early clinical assessment can help the nutrition support team decide which category of enteral diet (Table 18.1) is likely to be most appropriate. A decision will be guided largely by the size of the gap between nutrition intake and nutrition requirements, gastrointestinal function and presence of organ failure.

Assessment of nutrition intake

The decision to institute enteral tube feeding is easiest in patients with no oral fluid or nutrient intake (e.g. gastro-oesophageal cancer or neurological dysphagia) but in other patients, formal dietary assessment may identify that intake is insufficient but could be met by oral nutritional supplements. This is an area where dietitians play an important role in decision making and the process has been eased by computer programmes that permit rapid assessments of both macro- and micro-nutrient intakes. The first edition of this book predicted that greater involvement of dietitians in bedside nutrition assessment would lead to identification of more patients requiring enteral nutrition support. Subsequent experience of screening programmes has confirmed that up to 40% of patients admitted to medical and surgical wards are malnourished[8,9] and, moreover, when enteral nutrition is instituted, nutrition status improves.[10]

Assessment of nutrition requirements

This important area of artificial nutrition support is described in detail in Chapter 9 and should guide clinical choice. Energy and nitrogen requirements are often considered together, because of the strong relationship between nitrogen and energy balance in normally nourished healthy subjects.[11,12] However, in uncomplicated starvation, relatively less nitrogen intake is required to achieve balance whilst in hyper-catabolic states relatively more is required. Normally nourished individuals of near ideal body weight do not go into positive nitrogen balance unless fed an excess of energy resulting in the gain of body fat,[11,12] but this is not the case in depleted patients. These patients are capable of retaining nitrogen if energy needs are partially[13] or only approximately matched.[14] This is an important point, as restoration of lean body mass can, at least in theory, be achieved without supplying excess energy, which may lead to respiratory and hepatic complications if a high glucose intake is given.

Energy and nitrogen requirements

Uncomplicated starvation is uncommon and patients who require nutrition support are either septic or injured or have some inflammatory process which renders them hypercatabolic. Although energy requirements are increased in these situations, earlier estimates of this erred on the side of enthusiasm. Very few uncomplicated surgical patients require more than 2000 kcal/day to achieve positive energy balance[15] whilst 35–40 kcal/kg/day is sufficient to match energy requirements of most septic patients.[16]

In contrast, nitrogen requirements have been under-estimated in the past. We have observed that where urinary nitrogen losses were approximately 15 g/day, positive nitrogen balance was only achieved when patients received a mean of 16.9 g nitrogen per day.[17] There is thus a proportionally greater need for nitrogen (cp. energy) in metabolically stressed patients following gastroenterological surgery,[18] major burns[19] or head injury.[20]

Energy requirements are best measured by indirect calorimetry which is a relatively expensive technique. Rates of O_2 and CO_2 exchange can be converted to energy expenditure using simplified formulae, with or without a correction for protein metabolism.[21,22] In the absence of this technique, energy requirements can be calculated from the Harris & Benedict equation. However, correction factors should be used with care, because they may overestimate energy expenditure in hypercatabolic patients[16] or underestimate it in burned patients.[23] Our practice is to place greater emphasis on assessing nitrogen requirements and to match those with levels of intake assessed by others.[15,16] Ideally, 24-hour nitrogen loss should be calculated. We have used a chemiluminescence technique[24] which has the advantage that losses of nitrogen in stool, stoma and fistula effluent can also be calculated. If not available, nitrogen losses can be estimated from 24-hour urinary urea nitrogen excretion.[25] In our experience, though, urea nitrogen is frequently considerably less than the assumed 80–90% of total urinary nitrogen.[24]

Practical considerations

Surveys of nutrition support practices in the UK suggest that only 37% of hospitals have a nutrition support team,[7] implying that facilities for assessing energy and nitrogen requirements are not available in most hospitals. This justifies the publication of recommendations for nitrogen and energy requirements in different subsets of patients.[26] The recommended values shown in Table 18.3 are therefore by definition 'guesstimates' based on a consensus view but will assist clinicians in diet choice.

Gastrointestinal function

The choice of enteral diet depends on the severity of the underlying illness, the presence of organ failure and the difference between intake and requirements in addition to the adequacy of gastrointestinal function. This should be confirmed not only by

Table 18.3 – Approximate energy and nitrogen requirements

	No major injury or sepsis starvation Anorexia nervosa, malnutrition due to disordered deglutition, e.g. carcinoma of oesophagus	Moderate injury or sepsis Postoperative patients, extra peritoneal sepsis, e.g. pneumonia, urological sepsis, mild to moderate trauma	Severe injury and or sepsis Burn, head injury, severe multiple trauma or sepsis
Nitrogen requirements			
g N/d	12.0	18.0	24.0
g N/kg/d	0.17	0.26	0.34
Energy requirements			
kcal/d	2000	2400	2400–3000
kcal/kg/d	28.6	34.3	34.3–42.9
Non-protein energy: N			
kcal/g	167:1	133:1	100:1–125:1
	Standard diet	Energy, nitrogen-dense diet	Stress diet

evidence of malabsorption but also from signs of disordered gastrointestinal motility. This is because the latter will often, in practice, limit the use of enteral feeding more than the former. It must be remembered that the functional absorptive capacity of the human gastrointestinal tract is large and very severe absorptive defects must exist for nutrients before these become clinically limiting, thereby influencing the choice of enteral diets.

Gastrointestinal motility

Since nutrient assimilation in man occurs mainly in the upper small intestine, intragastric nutrient administration cannot therefore be considered if gastric emptying is impaired. This is not an uncommon finding in patients requiring enteral feeding and will lead to nausea, vomiting and regurgitation and aspiration of diet and gastric atony (Table 18.4).

Table 18.4 – Patient groups and diseases associated with gastric atony

- Diabetes with neuropathy
- Hypothyroidism
- Head injuries and neurosurgical patients
- Multiple trauma
- Postabdominal surgery patients
- Intra-abdominal sepsis
- Intensive care patients on ventilators
- Some patients with neuromotor deglutition disorders
- Some patients following a cerebrovascular accident

Efficient absorption of nutrients from chyme in the upper small intestine requires a repetitive mixing action in which the mucosa dips into the chyme, minimising the diffusion barrier to absorption. This movement is accompanied by villous contractions whose propelling action aids lymphatic and blood flow to carry away the products of digestion and absorption. Interposed with these repetitive segmenting movements, there are erratic propulsive movements whereby chyme is rapidly propelled 10–30 cm distally and the segmenting process recommences.[27] Our understanding of how such complex patterns of motor activity are organised has been aided by recent technical advances that have permitted characterisation of small intestinal and colonic motility patterns in the fasting and fed state.

In the fasting state[28] small intestinal motility is characterised by a period of inactivity (phase I) followed by phase II, a period of irregular spike activity lasting, like phase I, for 30–40 min. Pressure activity increases steadily during the later half of phase II, ushering in phase III, during which there are intense repetitive high-amplitude contractions. Phase III lasts for about 4–6 min of irregular activity (phase IV) which then gives way to a new phase I. The whole cycle of activity migrates down the upper small intestine at 4–6 cm/min, slowing distally to 1–2 cm/min in the terminal ileum. This migrating motor complex (MMC) is thought to sweep debris down the small intestine and does not occur until 4–6 hours after a meal. Feeding disrupts the fasting pattern of motility by instituting irregular activity throughout the small intestine, which resembles that seen during phase II of the MMC and is therefore called 'type II activity'. Contraction frequency and speed are reduced by nutrients, thereby prolonging transit time.[29] The small intestine appears able to discriminate between different nutrients since there are qualitative differences in motor response, fat generating particularly intense non-propagating clustered contractions whose function is presumably to aid emulsification and hence absorption. In essence, therefore, the fasting function of the motility response is to propagate debris distally and the fed response is basically non-propagative in type to aid digestion and absorption of nutrients.

This analysis is relevant to enteral feeding because intraduodenal infusion of peptide and polymeric enteral diets evokes a normal postprandial motor response at enteral loads of 1.38 kcal/min or greater[30,31] whereas similar nasogastric infusions failed to evoke the same response.[32] The reason for this difference is unclear because liquids, in comparison with solids, empty rapidly from the stomach[33] and once a steady state of continuous intragastric tube feeding has been reached, the effects of nutrients on duodenal osmoreceptors and chemoreceptors during both modes of feeding should be similar. Possibly, the pyloric-brake mechanisms[34,35] delay gastric emptying during nasogastric diet infusion and this in turn leads to dilution of the feed by gastric secretions to below the critical caloric load required to activate the duodenal osmo- and chemoreceptors. The persistence of fasting small intestinal motor activity appears not to have a deleterious effect as there is no evidence of nutrient malabsorption[36] and colonic inflow volumes of fluid and electrolytes are actually less during nasogastric than nasoduodenal infusion of equivalent loads of polymeric diet.[37]

In contrast, eating food stimulates a gastrocolonic response,[38] which results in an increase in segmental colonic motor contractions.[39,40] We have shown that the normal colonic motor response to food incorporates a cephalic phase component.[41] The increase in segmental colonic contraction helps to churn and mix faeces which increase contact time of luminal contents with colonic mucosa which in turn enhances fluid and electrolyte absorption.[42] We had noted during nasogastric tube feeding that, despite normal or reduced colonic inflows of fluid and electrolytes, the majority of subjects developed diarrhoea.[32] This observation led us to conclude that the diarrhoea might be secondary to a disorder of colonic function.[32]

Subsequent studies showed that *low-load* nasogastric or nasoduodenal enteral diet infusion elicited an abnormal colonic response through:

- Failure to convert from fasting to 'fed' motor activity.[43,44]
- Rapid establishment of net water, Na+ and Cl− secretion in the ascending colon.[37]

There is a strong suspicion that these motility abnormalities which arise during enteral feeding may have clinical significance and may be related to the incidence of enteral feeding-related diarrhoea.[45] Healthy subjects will develop diarrhoea during nasogastric but not nasoduodenal feeding.[32] Although it seemed likely that VIP, neurotensin and pancreatic glucagon might be related to this, we were unable to show any causal relationship. However, PYY increased significantly during intraduodenal not intragastric feeding.[46] It should be noted that the gastrointestinal effects of PYY include reduced gastric and pancreatic secretion, delayed gastric emptying, slowing of small bowel

Table 18.5 – Causes of malabsorption

Site	Mechanism	Example
Gastric	Precipitating emptying Lack of intrinsic factor Excess acid secretion	Post-gastrectomy dumping Pernicious anaemia Zollinger–Ellison syndrome
Pancreatic	Inadequate enzyme and bicarbonate secretion	Cystic fibrosis Chronic pancreatitis Carcinoma of pancreas
Biliary	Defective micelle formation	Chronic biliary obstruction Primary biliary cirrhosis Massive ileal resection Cholestyramine
Small bowel	Loss of absorptive surface/damaged enterocyte	Coeliac disease Tropical sprue Giardiasis Small bowel resection Crohn's disease Radiation enteritis Contaminated small bowel syndrome Lymphoma
	Isolated brush border enzyme defects	Lactase insufficiency Congenital alactasia Sucrase-isomaltase deficiency Glucose-galactose malabsorption Hartnup disease
	Impaired postabsorptive fat transport	Lymphangiectasia Abetalipoproteinaemia
	Drugs	Alcohol Neomycin

transit and an increase in small and large intestinal absorption of water and electrolytes.[45,47,48]

We have hypothesised from our studies that a secretagogue is released during enteral feeding which is inhibited by PYY during intraduodenal feeding but not during intragastric feeding when there is no rise in PYY concentration; in other words, there is loss of a negative feedback loop.[45,46] The nature of this secretagogue, however, is unknown. An alternative explanation was suggested by other studies. If the enteral diet was administered orally to subjects they did not develop diarrhoea[49] nor was their colonic motor response abnormal.[50] Moreover, this was unchanged by the presence of an unused nasogastric tube *in situ*.[51] The hypothesised secretagogue may therefore be related to the cephalic phase of the colonic motor response to food (i.e. sight, taste, smell of food[48]) which is bypassed during nasogastric tube feeding.

Finally, experienced ITU nurses report that on occasions there is 'no absorption' of enteral feed, as 'unchanged' diet is observed to pass per rectum. Clearly in this situation, intraluminal digestion and absorption are grossly impaired. The previous discussion suggests that the cause for this is severely impaired small and large intestinal motility which leads to the intestines functioning as an inert or hypomotile tube. In this case, it would be logical to administer a predigested chemically defined elemental diet rather than a polymeric diet.

Nutrient malabsorption

Malabsorption is best classified by the location of the main abnormality in the digestive tract (Table 18.5) even though it is difficult to determine the quantitative effect on absorptive function. In the author's experience there are few conditions in which this is so impaired as to result in clinically significant nutrient malabsorption. In one crossover controlled clinical trial,[52] patients with moderately impaired gastrointestinal function received one of two isocaloric isonitrogenous enteral diets containing either predominantly medium-chain peptides or whole protein as the nitrogen source. Overall there was no significant difference in either stool weight, nitrogen absorption or nitrogen balance between feeding periods with the peptide- and whole protein-containing diets. The only suggestion of a nutritional advantage in administering an enteral diet whose nitrogen

source comprises oligopeptides was seen in those patients with small bowel disease.[52]

Therefore, polymeric diets should be the first choice and only a few conditions will require a predigested chemically defined elemental diet. These are listed in Table 18.6.

Table 18.6 – Indications for administering predigested chemically defined elemental diets

Disease	Mechanism
Cystic fibrosis	Exocrine pancreatic insufficiency leading to malabsorption of fat, nitrogen and carbohydrate
Cancer of pancreas	As above
Chronic biliary obstruction Primary biliary cirrhosis Cholestatic parenchymal liver disease	Obstruction to the outflow of bile leading to defective micelle formation and fat malabsorption
Nutritionally significant short bowel syndrome: • small bowel resection • Crohn's disease • radiation enteritis	Luminal and/or membrane digestion impaired and reduced absorptive area limiting nutrient assimilation
Lymphangiectasia Abetalipoproteinaemia	Impaired postabsorptive fat transport necessitating prescription of a diet containing MCT

Developing strategies

On this basis, therefore, simple strategies can be developed. Figure 18.1 describes a method for deciding whether oral dietary supplements or sip feeds or tube feeding should be used, whilst Figure 18.2 describes a strategy for choosing the type of diet for tube feeding.

Formulation of enteral diets

At a conservative estimate, there are more than 100 different enteral diets available worldwide. This sec-

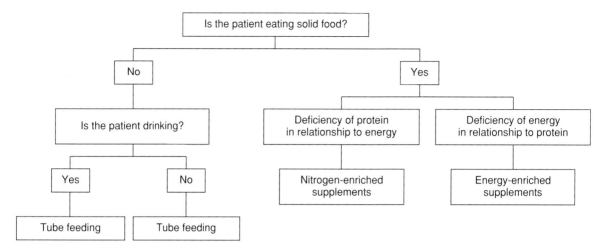

Figure 18.1 – Developing a strategy for choosing the method of administering enteral nutrition.

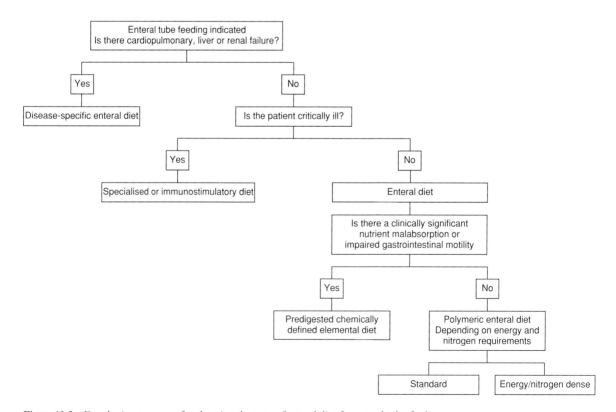

Figure 18.2 – Developing a strategy for choosing the type of enteral diet for enteral tube feeding.

tion therefore presents a personal view of enteral diet formulation in the hope that it will assist clinicians in interpreting manufacturers' claims.

Oral dietary supplements (Table 18.2)

These products are supplements which are nutritionally incomplete and because they are ingested orally, should be palatable and therefore find their way down the patient's gastrointestinal tract rather than down the hospital sluice. Geographical and ethnic differences in taste preference must be appreciated, whilst remembering that taste perception[2] is altered by underlying disease as well as antibiotic therapy.[53] Table 18.2 summarises the suggested formulation of the oral dietary supplements. They are usually marketed in 200–250 ml portions and most do not contain a fibre source. Most are lactose and gluten free and are in liquid form. Some companies are now producing oral dietary supplements in semisolid or solid form.

These supplements are usually prescribed to patients with normal or near normal gastrointestinal function. Accordingly, the nitrogen is supplied as whole protein, carbohydrate as a partial hydrolysate of starch and lipid as long-chain triglycerides (LCT).

There is now considerable discussion about the role of n-3 fatty acids in clinical nutrition since they have been shown to improve survival after burn injury and to reduce post-injury, infectious complications and immunosuppression secondary to transfusion.[54,55] Linoleic acid and other n-6 fatty acids are metabolised to form the series 2 prostanoids and series 4 leukotrienes which induce inflammation and increase suppression. In contrast, the n-3 fatty acids form series 3 prostanoids and series 5 leukotrienes which generally have anti-inflammatory properties.[56,57] Since these processes are competitive, a balanced ratio of n-6 to n-3 fatty acids is unknown but an intelligent guess suggests it might be 5:1.

The requirements for micro-nutrients (trace elements and vitamins) have been reviewed in detail in this volume (Chapter 11) and elsewhere[58] by Shenkin. Empirical considerations suggest that 25% recommended daily allowance (RDA) should be present in 250 ml of all dietary supplement (i.e. 100% RDA in 1 l) whilst nitrogen-rich dietary supplements should have an energy density of 1.0 kcal/ml and the energy-rich supplements 1.5 kcal/ml.

Polymeric diets (Table 18.2)

Polymeric diets are widely prescribed to patients requiring enteral tube feeding who have normal or near normal gastrointestinal function. The nitrogen source is thus composed of whole protein, commonly casein but sometimes mixed with soy protein. Although there is no theoretical reason why most patients receiving enteral tube feeding with a polymeric diet should not be able to absorb LCTs, some manufacturers take a view that patients who are severely stressed may not be able to completely assimilate a pure LCT fat source and accordingly have replaced proportions with MCTs. From a theoretical standpoint, MCTs may be more readily used as an energy source as, unlike LCTs, they can be transported across the mitochondrial membrane intact, a process that may be independent of carnitine (Chapter 11).

Listed in Table 18.2 are three suggested formulations for polymeric diets. Two are designed to 'match' the nutrition requirements of the first two categories of patients outlined in Table 18.3; the third is a hypotonic polymeric enteral diet. Controlled clinical trials have quite clearly shown that the incidence of gastrointestinal side-effects during the first few days of enteral tube feeding cannot be reduced by using 'starter regimens' whereby the load (concentration × rate) is incrementally increased over a 2–3-day period. This is not only so in patients with normal or near normal gastrointestinal function receiving polymeric diets[59] but also in patients with acute inflammatory bowel disease prescribed a predigested chemically defined diet.[60] The use of hypotonic polymeric diets is therefore not recommended in the introductory phase of enteral tube feeding in those patients.

The efficacy and safety of early postoperative enteral feeding following major gastrointestinal surgery have now been demonstrated.[61–64] The perception of most of the investigators performing studies of early postoperative enteral feeding has clearly been that food entry into the proximal small intestine fails to 'trigger' the digestive processes of the upper gut;[64] consequently, most have used predigested chemically defined elemental diets.[61–63,65] One trial that did specifically address the issue demonstrated equal nutritional and clinical efficacy of a polymeric and predigested chemically defined elemental diet in these patients[66] and the use of polymeric enteral diets in early postoperative enteral feeding is therefore recommended.

In contrast to enteral feeding of patients with normal or near normal gastrointestinal function, incremental increases in administered nutrient loads may be required during the first 2 days of early postoperative enteral feeding, during the period of postoperative ileus. For convenience, therefore, the formulation of low osmolality polymeric diet for introductory early postoperative enteral feeding is described in Table 18.2. It is known that gastrointestinal side-effects (abdominal distension, cramps and diarrhoea) commonly occur during days 3–5 of early post-operative feeding.[64] Experience suggests that those problems are related to a transient disturbance of gastrointestinal motility which subsequently resolves as organised peristalsis returns to the entire gut.[64] Administered nutrient loads may have to be reduced during this period, which is a further reason for proposing the formulation of a low osmolality polymeric enteral diet.

Fibre and enteral nutrition

Despite a recent review which concluded that 'very little data justify the use of fibre supplemented diets in hospitalised patients'[67] many polymeric enteral diets are supplemented with fibre. Historically, the very earliest enteral diets were designed for astronauts in space, to provide balanced nutrition and to reduce stool weight and stool frequency.[68] Subsequently it was realised that one clinical advantage of low-residue diets was that they had a low viscosity and could be administered easily through 'fine-bore' nasogastric or nasoenteric feeding tubes. Furthermore, when it became clear that there could even be a number of therapeutic advantages in administering low-residue diets[69] their widespread use became accepted without question. However, long-term enteral feeding with such diets results in clinically inconvenient consti-pation and therefore fibre-enriched enteral diets were formulated and marketed. Research has concentrated on three main topics, namely effects on bowel function, on small and large intestinal mucosal cell morphology and on mucosal barrier function.

Effect on bowel function

Constipation

Clinical studies in which fibre-free polymeric diets have been administered to normal healthy volunteers

show that compared to a self-selected diet, whole-gut transit time is prolonged and bowel frequency and mean daily stool wet weights reduced.[70,71] Although Slavin and colleagues[70] showed that the addition of large quantities (30 and 60 g/d) of soy fibre to a fibre-free polymeric enteral diet administered to normal healthy volunteers resulted in significant increases in daily wet stool weights and daily stool frequency, the results of other studies have not shown such impres-sive changes.[49,71] Thus supplementing diets with fibre derived from oat, soy polysaccharide and soy oligo-saccharide (total dietary fibre 30 g/d) had little if any impact on bowel function in normal healthy volunteers.[71]

Clinical studies generally support these findings since in two controlled studies in stable medical patients[72,73] neither the addition of 24 g/d carrot fibre nor 12.4 g/d and 38.5 g/d of soy polysaccharide fibre to fibre-free liquid formulae resulted in any significant change in the parameters of bowel function studied. In a prospective crossover study performed in 28 mentally retarded young individuals suffering from chronic constipation as a consequence of fibre-free enteral feeding, the addition of soy polysaccharide (15.6–17.4 g/d) for 2 weeks was without effect on stool weight, stool frequency or transit time.[74] In a subse-quent study from the same unit,[75] a 1-year trial in 11 mentally retarded patients showed that supplemen-tation of a fibre-free liquid diet administered via gastrostomy with 18–25 g/d soy fibre resulted in a sig-nificant increase in stool weights and bowel frequency.

Dietary fibre influences stool weights in two ways which depend on the relative rates of anaerobic fermentation in the caecum and ascending colon.[76] Rapidly fermented fibre increases faecal weight by increasing growth of the microflora,[76] which comprise 80% water, whereas poorly fermentable fibre survives to hold water[77] and it is the latter that exerts the greater stool-bulking effects.[76,78]

Since poorly fermentable fibre had no effect on bowel function, other factors may operate. The ferment-ability of fibre is known to be influenced by particle size.[79] Small particles render relatively larger surface area available to the bacterial polysaccharidase enzyme systems than larger particles.[79] Food technology demands that liquid enteral diets be supplemented by finely ground small particle-sized fibre to achieve usable solutions. It is likely therefore that particle size becomes one of the important factors that limits the efficacy of the stool-bulking property of fibre in enteral nutrition.[80]

One of the common factors in all the clinical and basic physiological studies of fibre supplementation in enteral nutrition is that single fibre sources have been employed. Colonic bacterial polysaccharide enzyme systems are substrate inducible[81] so that with time, one could anticipate that the degree of fermentability of a given fibre source would increase, thereby reducing its stool-bulking effects. We have therefore recently designed a mixed fibre source for supplementation of enteral diets[80] which comprises soluble and insoluble fibres from different sources (Table 18.2). Supplements added to a fibre-free polymeric diet significantly shortened whole-gut transit time in healthy volunteers but without effect on daily stool wet weights.[80] In separate short-term studies, supplementation of a polymeric enteral diet with this fibre source was found to alter the colonic motor response.[112] Thus while it looks likely that the demands of particle size will continue to limit the efficacy of even mixed fibre to bulk the stools of patients receiving enteral nutrition, such fibre supplements may exert other beneficial effects on gastrointestinal function.

Diarrhoea

Diarrhoea during enteral feeding remains a common problem whose causes include infected diets, lactose intolerance, concomitant antibiotic therapy, ingestion of laxatives and hypoalbuminaemia. As described above, continuous nasogastric infusion of enteral diets causes alterations in colonic motility as well as secretion of fluids and electrolytes which can be reversed if SCFA are infused into the colonic lumen.[82] Despite the lack of a cephalic phase to enteral diet infusion, there is a rationale for routine addition of fibre to polymeric enteral diets since colonic fermentation will lead to generation of SCFA. However, since concurrent antibiotic therapy may minimise colonic fermentation, this provides an explanation why clinical studies have failed to show expected benefit in prevention or treatment of enteral feeding-related diarrhoea.[83–86]

Enteral diets and epithelial cell proliferation experimental studies

The intestinal epithelium can respond to a wide variety of stimuli by altering its proliferative rates.[87] There is now a large and interesting literature on the effects of low-residue liquid enteral diets on intestinal morphology, cell turnover kinetics and function. Almost all experiments have been performed in the rat. In general, jejunal mass is maintained or increased,[88–91] the activity of brush border hydrolases maintained[88–89] or increased,[90] DNA synthesis rates maintained[88] and absorptive function maintained.[91] In sharp contrast, administration of these low-residue diets is associated with pronounced atrophy in the ileum[88–91] and colon,[88,92] compared with the feeding of a normal fibre-containing rat chow diet.

As fibre experimentally has a proliferative effect on intestinal epithelium,[93–95] its absence from liquid enteral diets has been suggested as a cause of intestinal atrophy.[91–92,96] In testing this, Ryan and colleagues showed that addition of cellulose and petroleum jelly to an oral liquid fibre-free diet resulted in significant increases in colonic weight and DNA synthesis rates compared with values seen when the fibre-free diet was fed.[92] When the same liquid polymeric diet with and without 9% added bulk was administered orally to rats for 4 weeks, however, the total weights of ileal segments were similar.[91] In one of the most comprehensive studies to date, Goodlad and colleagues[96] have studied crypt cell production rate in starved rats re-fed a liquid elemental enteral diet supplemented with very large (1:1) quantities of different fibre sources, inert bulk (kaolin), a poorly digestible fibre source (purified wood cellulose), a more readily digestible fibre source (purified wheat bran) and a soluble NSP prepared from ispaghula husk. Crypt cell production rate in the terminal ileum and colon was unaffected by the addition of inert bulk. Of the fibre sources, the most marked crypt cell production rates in terminal ileum and colon were seen when purified wheat bran was added to the diet.[96] Unfortunately the effect of soluble NSP could not be determined since not all of the diet was consumed.

One of the implications of the study of Goodlad et al.[96] is that the proliferative effect of added fibre on the distal ileum and colon is related to its digestibility and thence SCFA formation. It is of interest therefore that other research shows that intraluminal volatile fatty acids (VFAs) stimulate colonic mucosal proliferation.[97–99] Definitive proof that the trophic effects of fibre are due to the products of fibre degradation rather than fibre *per se* was gained from studies performed in germ-free rats, in whom no effect of fibre on colonocyte proliferation was seen.[100]

Of the three major SCFA liberated during colonic fibre digestion, acetate, propionate and butyrate,

butyrate is preferentially metabolised by isolated colonocytes.[101] When butyrate (20 mmol/l) was infused for 7 days into the colon of caecectomised rats fed on fibre-free elemental diets, colonic mucosal growth, as evidenced by changes in mucosal weight protein and DNA content, was stimulated as effectively as when a mixture of acetate 70 mmol/l, propionate 25 mmol/l and butyrate 20 mmol/l was infused.[102]

These experimental animal findings suggest that SCFA exert a direct trophic effect on colonic epithelium and that of the three major SCFA, butyrate has the prominent role. These findings have recently been confirmed in man;[103] *in vitro* incubation studies showed that 10 mmol/l butyrate stimulated DNA synthesis to the same extent as a SCFA mixture.

Effect of SCFA in experimental postoperative conditions

The animal studies described are interesting but may not be relevant to the human setting. For example, do starvation and parenteral nutrition cause an impairment of intestinal absorptive capacity which can be reversed by administration of luminal nutrition and, specifically, fibre? Starvation in humans is associated with marked morphological changes of the small intestinal mucosa, various degrees of villous atrophy[104–106] and reductions in the specific activity of brush border sucrase and maltase.[104] It is not clear, however, whether these changes are due to starvation *per se* or to protein deprivation. In short-term studies protein deprivation in man has been shown to result in reduced amino acid absorption rates even in the absence of demonstrable small intestinal morphological changes.[106] It is unlikely that fibre has any potential for attenuating these changes as the reintroduction of fibre-containing food for up to 29 days did not result in reversal of the morphological changes.[105]

TPN in the rat causes atrophy of the small intestinal mucosa and a significant decrease of brush border enzyme activities[107–109] but the data in man are equivocal. Here, one has to separate morphological from functional changes as it is known that the activity of the brush border enzymes tested are substrate inducible so that absence of luminal substrate would be expected to result in a lowering of specific activity. One would not, therefore, expect this situation to be influenced by dietary fibre.

Some authors have reported the development of modest changes in intestinal morphology in patients on TPN.[110–115] In one study, though, no changes were found.[116] It is interesting that there are studies that also document abnormalities of intestinal structure and function associated with enteral nutrition. Thus in normal subjects receiving oligopeptide-based and polymeric diets, intestinal morphological abnormalities developed and duodenal microsomal enzyme activities decreased compared to feeding of a home diet.[116] In one study, intestinal morphological abnormalities which were documented in patients before the institution of enteral feeding with a polymeric diet were unchanged at the end of 3 months' enteral feeding.[117] A common feature of these two studies was that the normal subjects and patients were fed fibre-free enteral diets. Clearly further studies are required to determine whether addition of fibre will reverse the enteral diet-specific effects.

Rombeau and colleagues have investigated the effects of fibre and SCFAs on colonic anastomotic integrity and on intestinal adaptation following massive small bowel resection in rats.[118–120] Following colonic anastomosis, pectin significantly enhanced colonic mucosal cell proliferation and higher pressures were required to disrupt the anastomosis in animals fed a pectin-supplemented diet.[118] Colonic infusion of SCFA also accelerated wound healing and reduced anastomotic dehiscence after colonic transsection and reanastomosis[119] whereas with pectin feeding, the suture line burst in fewer colons when tension was applied to the bowel wall.[118]

Small intestinal and colonic adaptation was significantly enhanced by pectin supplementation of an elemental diet after massive (80%) small bowel resection.[120] Interestingly, under the same experimental conditions, parenterally infused SCFA led to a significant enhancement of the adaptive response only in the jejunum and ileum and not in the colon.[121] The most recent animal studies reported by this group indicated that the trophic effects of SCFA on the colon are luminal and not parenterally mediated.[122]

The evidence therefore suggests that there could be advantages in incorporating a rapidly degradable fibre source in defined formula enteral diets. The proliferative effects of fibre are, however, related to the production of the end-products of fermentation, namely SCFA. Clinicians should be wary, therefore, of assuming that advantages of fibre-supplemented diets will accrue in patients receiving antibiotic therapy.

Fibre and gut barrier function

The barrier function of the gastrointestinal tract may be breached and allow translocation of bacteria and their products, leading to elaboration of the inflammatory response and possible multiorgan failure. This has been extensively studied in animal models and the main drivers for translocation identified as trauma, burns sepsis, mesenteric ischaemia, bacterial overgrowth, ionising radiation, chemotherapy and haemorrhagic shock.[123] The process can be nutritionally modulated as it is increased by parenteral nutrition[124–130] and by several fibre-free elemental diets[126,131–139] but some (but not all) types of fibre seem to be protective.[126,132–135,137,138,140] Whilst in man, increased intestinal permeability has been shown to be increased by multiple trauma,[141] burns,[142] major vascular[143] or gastrointestinal surgery,[144] critical illness[145] and acute liver failure,[145] this may not correlate with increased bacterial translocation,[146–151] since the key relationship is between bacterial translocation and sepsis. However, a strong association has been noted between all three in patients with acute liver failure.[152]

The animal data present a strong case for feeding trauma and major surgery patients enterally rather than parenterally[144] and the fibre enthusiast might conclude that supplemental fibre may further improve gastrointestinal barrier function. Whilst several trials have shown that enteral nutrition (cp. TPN) reduced post-surgical infectious complications,[153–156] this may be a reflection of poor TPN practice (e.g. hyperglycaemic episodes and their relationship to sepsis) rather than an intrinsic benefit of enteral feeding, as there is no evidence that enteral feeding employing fibre-free or fibre-supplemented diets influences the natural history of intestinal permeability changes in any human model of injury or trauma.[141,157] This is perhaps not surprising since in critical illness, intestinal permeability changes develop in response to splanchnic ischaemia[145] and mucosal mitochondrial dysfunction,[152] neither of which is likely to be reversed by luminal nutrition with or without SCFA.

Fibre source for polymeric enteral diets

It is more rational to consider multiple fibre sources because soluble and insoluble fibres have quite different properties. The range of fermentability which is observed in man is from <10% (e.g. cellulose[157]) to 100% (e.g. lactitol[158]) and *in vitro* fermentation studies with human stool have characterised the rapidity of this process.[159]

Poorly fermented fibre seems to have most effect on bowel and possibly gut mucosal barrier function[138,160] whilst well-fermented fibre sources (e.g. soy polysaccharide, inulin) increase colonic luminal SCFA production.[160]

Oat fibre, although poorly fermented *in vitro*,[49] failed to result in a significant increase in daily stool wet weights when used as a fibre supplement of a polymeric enteral diet administered to normal human subjects. A fibre supplement for enteral diets derived from multiple sources[80] (Table 18.2), resulted in normalisation of whole-gut transit times, but daily stool wet weights of normal subjects were not significantly different compared with when a fibre-free polymeric diet was ingested.[80] As far as the effect of fibre supplementation of enteral diets on stool weights is concerned, it looks as though particle size of the fibre is limiting rather than its fermentability.[80]

Despite the lack of evidence that bowel function during enteral feeding of polymeric enteral diets can be influenced by fibre supplementation, the experimental animal data are still persuasive. In addition, in healthy volunteers, pectin reduces the incidence of liquid stools,[161] possibly by altering the colonic motor response to enteral feeding, as we have shown for a multiple fibre source.

Whilst excessive fibre intake can reduce the bioavailability of dietary minerals,[162–164] we have shown that this was not so when loads of 15 g/l of soy polysaccharide, soy oligosaccharide or oat fibre were co-infused with an enteral diet, in healthy volunteers.[165] This is in agreement with three other clinical studies,[73,166,167] one of which demonstrated some mineral malabsorption at soy polysaccharide loads >40 g.[166] The concentration of total dietary fibre in polymeric enteral diets should not exceed 15 g/l as estimated by the AOAC method.[168]

Predigested chemically defined elemental diets

These diets are prescribed for several conditions characterised by nutrient malabsorption (see Tables 18.2 and 18.6), which is most marked in the inadequate short bowel syndrome. It is characterised by inadequate luminal and brush border membrane hydrolysis and reduced functional absorptive area.

Thus, in these patients nutrients should be provided in the form in which they are optimally absorbed in the normal setting.

The earliest elemental diets were formulated at a time when it was perceived that dietary protein was absorbed in the form of free amino acids. Consequently, the nitrogen and energy sources comprised amino acids and glucose, which were considered to be the chemically defined 'elementals' of food which could be assimilated without the necessity for pancreatic or brush border enzyme digestion in the intestine. The composition has been modified in that maltodextrins now replace glucose whilst partial enzymic hydrolysates of protein have superseded free L-amino acids in most cases. At first sight this would not seem to be a significant change. However, there are differences in the absorption of elemental and predigested hydrolysate diets, which may affect the distal small intestine and colon, thus making the definition between these two diets biologically important.

In the normally functioning human gastrointestinal tract there is no difference in the metabolic utilisation of dietary nitrogen, whether given in elemental, predigested or polymeric forms.[169] However, it is highly likely that in patients with gastrointestinal disease there may be differences in absorption of these different forms of nitrogen.

A further difference that exists between the free amino acid- and peptide-containing predigested enteral diets relates to their glutamine content. The glutamine content of the free amino acid-containing diets constitutes approximately 17% of the total amino acid composition, whereas in the diets based on the use of partial enzymic hydrolysates of whole protein, the glutamine contents are substantially less.[170] It cannot be assumed, however, that the glutamine content of the starter protein is preserved during processing of the hydrolysate and there is evidence that the glutamine residues are deaminated to glutamate,[171] bringing about an even greater discrepancy between the elemental and hydrolysate diets. Bearing in mind the current interest in glutamine, this point may be important.

The nitrogen and carbohydrate source

Elemental diets based on free amino acids still find widespread clinical usage today, particularly in patients with acute Crohn's disease.[172] However, it may be more rational to use partial hydrolysates of protein whose chain-length profile allows uptake of amino acid nitrogen via mucosal L-amino acid transporters and the di- and tripeptide transporter, PEPT1[173] (see Chapter 6). Our perfusion studies have shown that uptake of casein, ovalbumin and whey hydrolysates was faster when they comprised mainly di- and tripeptides rather than tetra- and higher peptides. Although the hydrolysates currently used in predigested enteral diets vary widely in their peptide chain length and can contain from 2% to 28% of free L-amino acids, we believe that the optimum is a mixture of di- and tripeptides.

Whereas amino acids and di/tripeptides can be absorbed at the apical brush border membrane, dietary carbohydrate requires hydrolysis to monosaccharides before uptake can occur (see Chapter 6). The carbohydrate component of all enteral diets is partially digested starch (maltodextrins) which comprise a mixture of glucose polymers of differing chain lengths. The chain-length profile can be altered during the manufacturing process either by altering the enzymes used (typically microbial a-amylase and glucoamylases) or by fractionation of the end-product by solvent extraction, chromatography or ultrafiltration. Typically, enteral maltodextrins contain approximately 50% of the glucose content as polymers containing >10 glucose molecules.[174]

We have investigated the form in which glucose is maximally absorbed by use of a human jejunal perfusion technique. These studies showed that in the absence of pancreatic secretions, uptake of glucose from fractionated high-molecular weight polymers (i.e. >10 glucose units) was poorer than from short-chain preparations. Glucose uptake from the short-chain preparations (<10 glucose units) was faster than from solutions containing the equivalent amount of free glucose. Thus, there seemed to be a kinetic advantage from the use of short-chain glucose oligomers if pancreatic function was severely impaired.[174] Predigestion of the long-chain polymer (>G10) with pancreatic juice from the perfused volunteer restored the kinetic advantage over free glucose.[175] It should be noted that the high MW fraction had a very low osmolarity and was well absorbed, even in the absence of pancreatic secretions.[175] These studies emphasise the magnitude of the hydrolytic capacity of the enterocyte brush border membrane and suggest that the osmolarity of enteral diets can be significantly reduced if a fractionated high-molecular weight maltodextrin is used.

If glucose uptake from glucose polymers is saturated (i.e. via SGLT1) then the disaccharide sucrose can be added because one of the products of its digestion by brush border sucrase-isomaltase is fructose, whose uptake is mediated by the transporter GLUT5.[176]

Lipid energy source

In the nutritionally inadequate short bowel syndrome, steatorrhoea is often very severe,[177] for several reasons which include diminished luminal bile acid concentrations due to interruption of the enterohepatic circulation of bile salts, reduced contact time between substrate and lipase enzyme systems and reductions in functional absorptive capacity of the gut mucosa. Most predigested enteral diets contain LCTs, predominantly in the form of linoleic acid in quantities thought to prevent essential fatty acid deficiency. Normally 1–4% of total energy intake in the form of linoleic acid is thought to be required for this.[178] If one makes the empirical assumption that only half the ingested LCT will be absorbed then these diets should contain sufficient quantities of an LCT source to provide approximately 5 g/l linoleic acid.

MCTs are more water soluble than LCTs and may either be absorbed intact or undergo considerably more rapid lipase hydrolysis than LCT, with subsequent direct uptake of monoglyceride and fatty acid. There is no absolute requirement for mixed micelle formation with bile acids, so there are obvious advantages to using a MCT-based lipid energy source in the predigested diets. However, clinical experience suggests that in the presence of exocrine pancreatic insufficiency, pancreatic supplements greatly enhance energy assimilation from MCT and reduce steatorrhoea.[179–180]

Sodium content

In many patients with the short bowel syndrome it is electrolyte and fluid losses which provide the greatest threat to survival. This is particularly so when the ileum and colon have been resected when large quantities of sodium, potassium, magnesium and zinc are lost in copious jejunostomy effluent.[181] Active jejunal absorption is promoted by luminal carbohydrate, bicarbonate and amino acids.[181] However, the intercellular junctions of jejunal mucosa are so leaky that active transcellular absorption is easily overwhelmed by passive secretion down a concentration gradient.[181] Thus low Na^+ drinks such as water, tea, coffee and soft drinks cause net Na^+ loss in jejunos-tomy effluent.[177,183–186] Perfusion studies in rats[187] and man[174,176] have shown that Na^+ concentration of 60–90 mmol/l is required for net Na^+ absorption in the jejunum.

Perfusion studies over 25 cm segments of jejunum in man with the amino acid-based predigested diet Vivonex or the polymeric diet Ensure (Ross Labs, Columbus, Ohio, USA) demonstrated net sodium secretion on both diets but net water secretion with Vivonex.[176] In jejunostomies, similar findings occurred with Nutranel (Roussel, Wembley, England) and Ensure.[188] All three diets had low Na^+ concentrations. It is now clear that sodium chloride absorption is the principal determinant of water absorption from polymeric diets and a major contributor in elemental diets.[176] It is therefore recommended that the Na^+ concentration of standard dilution predigested enteral diets should be in the range of 80–90 mmol/l.[177]

Trace elements and vitamins

One has to make the assumption that most patients being treated with predigested enteral diets will have malabsorption and that this is likely to affect the micro- as well as macro-nutrients. It is recommended, therefore, that more than 100% RDA for the trace elements and vitamins be contained in the diet. As outlined in Chapter 11, careful monitoring of trace element status in patients with severe malabsorption receiving nutrition support is required.

Fibre content

The impressive evidence that addition of pectin to an amino acid-based predigested enteral diet prevented the passage of liquid stools,[166] as well as other experimental data described above, constitutes sufficient evidence to recommend that future predigested enteral diets should be supplemented with pectin. None are currently available commercially.

Disease-specific enteral diets

Respiratory failure

Patients with advanced pulmonary disease or chronic obstructive pulmonary disease (COPD) have a high incidence of weight loss which is not simply due to insufficient nutrient intake. Nutrition depletion is more common in patients with emphysema than those with chronic bronchitis and decline in lung function can occur concurrently with a depletion in nutrition status and, as the disease progresses, energy requirements increase.[189–190]

Several studies have now reported poor nutrition status in patients in respiratory failure.[191,192] Importantly, improved nutrition status has been associated with more successful weaning of patients from mechanical ventilation.[193–194]

The primary defect in respiratory failure is the inability to excrete sufficient carbon dioxide (CO_2) because lung ventilation is altered in relation to perfusion, leading to hypercapnia. The goal of treatment is to decrease $PaCO_2$ and this is affected by both the amount and composition of food consumed. Initial clinical feeding studies of patients in respiratory failure[195] showed that CO_2 production and minute ventilation were higher when carbohydrate was used as the sole energy source, as compared to an energy source based on 50% carbohydrate and 50% fat. Subsequent studies have also shown that diets high in carbohydrate have resulted in respiratory failure in patients with borderline pulmonary function.[196–197]

Carbohydrate has a higher CO_2 yield/g than fat and in addition, high carbohydrate loads incur an extra penalty from the CO_2 production of lipogenesis. Thus, enteral diets which have a higher fat:carbohydrate ratio have been designed for patients in respiratory failure. In one trial,[198] patients with respiratory failure requiring ventilation received either a high-fat, low-carbohydrate enteral feed (n=9) or a standard isocaloric isonitrogenous enteral feed (n=11). During the feeding period $PaCo_2$ fell by 16% in the high-fat group but increased by 4% in the standard feed group (p=0.003) and the high-fat group spent 62 hours less time on the ventilator (p=0.006). The suggested formulation of a disease-specific diet is therefore summarised in Table 18.2. Restricted fluid intake is often a necessity in patients with pulmonary disease so the diet has a high energy density (1.5 kcal/ml).

Liver failure

Liver failure can occur in patients with acute liver disease who have no previous history of liver disease. This condition, called fulminant hepatic failure (FHF), involves massive hepatic necrosis as a consequence of

which hepatic amino acid homeostasis and albumin synthesis are markedly reduced, both factors having prognostic significance.[199] At present, most patients receive nutrition support as TPN but there is increasing use of enteral nutrition.[200–201] Clinicians are most likely to be faced with malnutrition occurring in patients with established chronic parenchymal liver disease; moreover, the incidence of infective complications in these patients appears to be related to nutrition status.[202,203] The most significant cause of this is almost certainly impaired dietary intake since intakes of protein and energy as low as 47 g/d and 1320 kcal/d respectively have been shown.[204,205]

Nutrition support in the presence of hepatic encephalopathy: the dilemma

Many patients with cirrhosis develop hepatic encephalopathy and coma at some stage during the course of their illness. This is associated with accumulation of nitrogenous compounds in blood because of defective liver metabolism and it was customary therefore to restrict protein intake. This might well exacerbate the problem in the long term, however, as protein deficiency leads to infections[206] and infection is one of the most common precipitating causes of encephalopathy.[207]

One biochemical feature of hepatic encephalopathy is that plasma concentrations of the aromatic amino acids (AAA; phenylalanine, tyrosine) and methionine and tryptophan are increased, whilst those of the branched-chain amino acids (BCAA; valine, leucine, isoleucine) are reduced. This is influenced more by endogenous protein breakdown which is quantitatively larger than dietary protein intake.[208] The explanation for reduced branched-chain amino acid concentrations is less clear. Whilst Munro suggested that hyperinsulinaemia secondary to defective hepatic clearance drove excessive BCAA into peripheral tissues,[209] this has not been confirmed by subsequent euglycaemic insulin infusion studies.[210] It is more likely that BCAA form a useful alternative energy source in patients with defective hepatic metabolism.

The relationship of the disturbed plasma amino acid profiles to the pathogenesis of hepatic encephalopathy and the development of the false neurotransmitter hypothesis has been reviewed in detail[211–214] and the rationale underlying the use of BCAA therapy in patients with hepatic encephalopathy originally proposed by Fischer *et al.*[209,215] has been fully documented.[216]

Whilst Fischer's original concept envisaged specially formulated amino acid mixtures as *primary* therapy for hepatic encephalopathy, this has been modified to safe provision of nutrition support, which does not have the expected deleterious effect on the patient's neuro-psychiatric state.[217,218] Critical analysis of therapeutic efficacy of branched-chain enriched enteral and parenteral solutions in cirrhotic patients with hepatic encephalopathy is given elsewhere.[216] In the seminal trial, a large cohort of encephalopathic patients with established cirrhosis (requiring nutrition support) received the branched-chain enriched and specially formulated enteral diet Hepatic-aid which was as effective in inducing positive nitrogen balance as an equivalent amount of protein. Encephalopathy, at the same time, was induced significantly less often during the 4 weeks of the trial.[218] The author believes that it is this trial which supports the use of specially formulated enteral diet in encephalopathic patients with established chronic parenchymal liver disease who require enteral nutrition. As outlined below, there is no indication, however, for the routine use of these diets in non-encephalopathic patients in whom the use of standard polymeric diets is indicated.[219]

Nutrition support in the absence of hepatic encephalopathy

Standard nutrition support can be used and we encourage patients to eat more normal food with or without the use of oral supplements or nasoenteral tube feeding. Two controlled clinical trials have shown that nutrition intake in hospitalised patients can be increased by means of oral supplements.[203,204] In another study, the clinical state and in-patient hospital mortality of enterally fed cirrhotic patients were both significantly better compared with those in controls who were fed the normal ward diet.[205]

Diet formulation

In these diets, the nitrogen source is provided by L-amino acids of which <50% are BCAA whilst the concentration of AAA and methionine are low. L-arginine content is high in order to enhance urea cycle activity and thus aid conversion of ammonia to urea.[220] These should contain some L-cystine and L-tyrosine as it has been shown that some patients with cirrhosis fail to retain nitrogen as a consequence of their deficiency.[221]

Since many patients will have cholestatic jaundice and be unable to assimilate LCTs, energy should comprise mainly carbohydrate whilst providing sufficient linoleic acid (ca. 4% total energy) to prevent onset of essential fatty acid deficiency.

Many patients suited to the use of this disease-specific enteral diet will have hyponatraemia, fluid retention and ascites,[222,223] and diets should thus have a low sodium content and energy density should be in the range 1.2–1.5 kcal/ml as some degree of fluid restriction may be required. Vitamins and trace elements should be present at 100% RDA 11 and if dietary intake has been very poor prior to institution of nutrition support, additional thiamine supplementation may be required in order to prevent onset of Wernicke–Korsakoff on refeeding.

Renal failure

The concepts of nutrition support in patients with acute and chronic renal failure are important and changing. Full discussions of the subject are presented in Ch 30, together with philosophies underlying diet formulation.

Specialised diets

These diets contain extra substrates which may have a beneficial impact on trauma metabolism. However, several clinical comments could be made. The first is that in the view of this author they are experimental and should be tested in adequate controlled clinical trials. Some of these specialised diets also contain more than one substrate (e.g. arginine, fish oil and nucleotides) and it is difficult to determine which is responsible for conferring clinical benefit. Clinical practice is conditioned by the universal acceptance of controlled clinical trials in which only one variable is altered (i.e. the treatment). The treatment is usually taken to mean one pharmaceutical entity and it could be argued that in the case of nutrition support itself, it is a complex mixture of macro- and micro-nutrients, all of which interact in modulating metabolism. Thus in the usually accepted sense, trials of specialised diets or immunonutrition could be considered either as administration of pharmacological agents in combination, using food as the excipient, or as a comparison of two diets which is controlled for major confounding factors. The following sections will therefore consider clinical factors.

L-*Glutamine*

This is a dispensable amino acid which is involved in many metabolic reactions and whose classification as a non essential component belies its physiologic importance. Some of the more significant functions of glutamine are as:

- Substrate for ammoniagenesis, hepatic gluconeogenesis.

- A regulator of hepatic glycogen synthesis and protein degradation.

- A precursor for synthesis of nucleotides, proteins and amino sugars.

- A significant metabolic substrate for cells of the intestinal mucosa and immune system.

The view has developed that glutamine should be considered a conditionally essential amino acid in stress starvation because its concentration in the free pool in muscle and blood is markedly reduced by major injury[224] and its consumption by the intestine increases after trauma.[225] Thus, investigators have begun to investigate the clinical efficacy of supplementing nutrition regimens with this amino acid. Initial studies were performed in patients receiving parenteral nutrition, as standard regimens contain no glutamine, and these have demonstrated changes in intestinal morphology barrier function and absorptive function when glutamine was included.[112,226] At a more clinical level, a small reduction in infectious complications and length of hospital stay was shown in one trial in bone marrow transplant patients[227] but this was not confirmed in another, similar, trial[228] nor in patients receiving treatment for haematological malignancies.[229]

Griffiths and colleagues randomised 84 critically ill patients to receive either glutamine-supplemented or glutamine-free parenteral nutrition regimens.[230] Death due to multiorgan failure and deaths in patients fed longer than 10 days were both significantly lower in the glutamine-supplemented patients and survival at 6 months was greater.[230] In contrast, a recent clinical trial of patients 'clinically accepted for parenteral nutrition' who were randomised to receive either standard TPN or a similar regime in which 3.8 g nitrogen was replaced with 20 g glutamine showed no statistically significant clinical effects.[229] Finally, in the most recent trial, Van Leeuwen and colleagues randomised 72 patients with multiple trauma (severity score 7/20) to receive glutamine-supplemented enteral nutrition or an isonitrogenous isocaloric enteral feeding regimen.

The incidence of pneumonia, bacteraemia and sepsis were all significantly lower in patients receiving glutamine-supplemented enteral nutrition.[228]

The bulk of evidence therefore points to a beneficial effect of glutamine supplementation in critically ill patients and it can be estimated that the optimum requirement for enteral feeds to meet basal and added gut requirements would be approximately 20–30 g/d.[231]

Immune *enhancing*

Immune dysfunction is associated with major injury, with trauma and sepsis or with simple malnutrition. Whilst standard enteral or parenteral nutrition support can reverse simple malnutrition,[232,233] it will not do so in the critically ill septic patient.[234,235] One new approach has been to supplement enteral diets with substrates which themselves can modulate immune responsiveness; that is, L-arginine, nucleic acids and omega-3 polyunsaturated fatty acids. L-arginine has been shown to exert an enhancing effect on immune function[236–238] as well as hormone release[236,239,240] and collagen synthesis.[236,238,241] Exogenous nucleotides may have an enhancing effect on immune function and intestinal development.[242–245] Examples of the potential benefits of omega-3 fatty acids in producing less inflammatory prostaglandins have been described earlier.[56,57]

Initial results from prospective randomised clinical trials were encouraging, since there was a significant reduction in septic complications and the length of hospital stay[246,247] but a weakness of these studies was a failure to balance nitrogen content in both control and immune-enhancing enteral diets. As a result it was not possible to exclude the possibility that the result arose because of the extra nitrogen given. More recent trials have addressed this point. A recent meta-analysis of 12 studies of Impact (which contains supplemental nucleotides, arginine and fish oil) contained 1557 critically ill subjects[248] and revealed that the diet significantly reduced infections ($p<0.006$), ventilator days ($p<0.05$) and length of hospital stay ($p<0.0002$) but not mortality. Similar results have been obtained in patients receiving surgery for colorectal, pancreatic or gastric cancer.[249] These impressive results provide solid clinical evidence to support the use of immune-enhancing diets in severely injured patients. There is no current evidence to support the *routine* use of these diets in the enteral feeding of non or relatively mildly stressed and injured patients.

Future directions

Evidence-based strategies in clinical medicine are based on efficacy and cost and should be applied to artificial nutrition support, as argued by August.[250] Unfortunately, the nutritional pharmacological approach requires the testing of multiple variables in heterogeneous groups of patients who represent poor experimental models in whom experimental end points are difficult to define. This problem has become more acute since it was described in the first edition of this book. It is therefore a sign of the maturity of nutrition support as a subspeciality that forward-looking ideas, such as the creation of specialised nutrition support outcomes research consortia,[250] are being proposed in order to determine the effectiveness of 'sophisticated, costly, and potentially hazardous nutrition support interventions'. This is a long way from the early days of research in this area when it was considered sufficient to present detailed comparisons of different diets in a single patient with inadequate short bowel syndrome.[251]

References

1. Becouvarn Y, Huerni B, Dilhuidy JM, Stockle G, Bonneteau C, Brunet R. Modification of taste in cancer patients. *Bull Cancer* 1991; **78:** 901–13.

2. Rareshide E, Amedee RG. Disorders of taste. *J LA State Med Soc* 1989; **14:** 9–11.

3. Delmi M, Rapin CH, Bengoa JM, Delmas PD, Vasey H, Bonjour JP. Dietary supplementation in elderly patients with fractured neck of femur. *Lancet* 1990; **335:** 1013–16.

4. Larsson J, Unosson M, Ek AC, Nilsson L, Thorslund S, Bjurulf P. Effect of dietary supplement on nutritional status and clinical outcome in 501 geriatric patients – a randomised study. *Clin Nutr* 1990; **9:** 179–84.

5. Rana SK, Bray J, Menzies-Gow N, Jameson J, Payne-James JJ, Frost P, Silk DBA. Short term benefits of post-operative oral dietary supplements in surgical patients. *Clin Nutr* 1992; **11:** 337–44.

6. Lennard-Jones, JE. A positive approach to nutrition. Report of a Working Party. King's Fund Centre, London, 1992.

7. Payne-James J, De Gara CJ, Grimble GK, Bray J, Silk DBA. Artificial nutrition support in hospitals in the United Kingdom, 1994: Third National survey. *Clin Nutr* 1995; **14:** 329–35.

8. Pennington CR, Powell-Tuck J, Shaffer J. Artificial nutritional support for improved patient care. *Aliment Pharmacol Therapeut* 1995; **9:** 471–81.

9. McWhirter JP, Pennington CR. Incidence and recognition of malnutrition in hospital. *Br Med J* 1994; **308:** 945–8.

10. McWhirter JP, Pennington CR. Comparison between oral and nasogastric nutritional supplements in malnourished patients. *Nutrition* 1996; **12:** 502–6.

11. Millward DJ. Human amino acid requirements. *J Nutr* 1997; **127:** 1842–6.

12. Young VR. Adult amino acid requirements: the case for a major revision in current recommendations. *J Nutr* 1994; **124:** 1517S-23S.

13. Greenberg GR, Jeejeebhoy KN. Intravenous protein sparing therapy in patients with gastrointestinal disease. *J Parent Enteral Nutr* 1979; **3:** 427–32.

14. Shaw SN, Elwyn DH, Askanazia UA, Iles M, Schwarts Y, Kinney JM. Affects of increasing nitrogen intake on nitrogen balance and energy expenditure in nutritionally depleted adults receiving parenteral nutrition. *Am J Clin Nutr* 1983; **37:** 930–40.

15. MacFie J. Active metabolic expenditure of gastroenterological surgical patients receiving intravenous nutrition. *J Parent Enteral Nutr* 1984; **8:** 371–6.

16. Jeejeebhoy KN. Energy metabolism in the critically ill. In: Garrow JS, Halliday D (eds) Substrate and energy metabolism in man. John Libby, 1985, 93–101.

17. Rees RGP, Cooper TM, Beetham R, Frost P, Silk DBA. Influence of energy and nitrogen contents of enteral diets on nitrogen balance: a double blind prospective controlled clinical trial. *Gut* 1989; **30:** 123–9.

18. Smith RC, Burkinshaw L, Hill GL. Optimal energy and nitrogen intake for gastroenterological patients requiring intravenous nutrition. *Gastroenterology* 1982; **82:** 445–52.

19. Wolfe RR, Goodenough RD, Burke JF, Wolfe M. Response of protein and urea kinetics in burn patients to different levels of protein intake. *Ann Surg* 1983; **197:** 163–71.

20. Clifton GL, Robertson CS, Grossman RG, Hodge S, Folz R, Garza C. The metabolic response to severe head injury. *J Neuro Surg* 1984; **60:** 687–96.

21. Livesey G, Elia M. Estimation of energy expenditure, net carbohydrate utilization, and net fat oxidation and synthesis by indirect calorimetry: evaluation of errors with special reference to the detailed composition of fuels. *Am J Clin Nutr* 1988; **47:** 608–28.

22. Reid CL, Carlson GL. Indirect calorimetry – a review of recent clinical applications. *Curr Opin Clin Nutr Metab Care* 1998; **1:** 281–6.

23. Yu YM, Tompkins RG, Ryan CM, Young VR. The metabolic basis of the increase of the increase in energy expenditure in severely burned patients. *J Parent Enteral Nutr* 1999; **23:** 160–8.

24. Grimble GK, Wise MFE, Acuti AB *et al.* Assesment of an automated chemiluminescence nitrogen analyser for routine use in clinical nutrition. *J Parent Enteral Nutr* 1988; **12:** 100–106.

25. Lee HA, Hartley TF. A method for determining daily nitrogen requirements. *Postgrad Med J* 1975; **51:** 441–5.

26. Jolliet P, Pichard C, Biolo G *et al.* Enteral nutrition in intensive care patients: a practical approach. Working Group on Nutrition and Metabolism, European Society of Intensive Care Medicine. *Intens Care Med* 1998; **24:** 848–59.

27. Cannon WB. The movements of the intestines studied by means of the roentgen rays. *Am J Physiol* 1902; **6:** 251–7.

28. Szurszewiski JJ. A migrating electrical complex of canine small intestine. *Am J Physiol* 1969; **217:** 1757–62.

29. Schemann M, Ehrlein HJ. Post prandial patterns of canine jejunal motility and transit of luminal contents. *Gastroenterology* 1986; **90:** 991–6.

30. Raimundo AH, Rogers J, Grimble G, Cahill E, Silk DBA. Colonic in-flow and small bowel motility during intraduodenal enteral nutrition. *Gut* 1988; **29:** A1469–A70.

31. Debongnie JC, Phillips SF. Capacity of the human colon to absorb fluid. *Gastroenterology* 1978; **74:** 698–703.

32. Raimundo AH, Rogers J, Silk DBA. Is enteral feeding related diarrhoea initiated by an abnormal colonic response to intragastric diet infusion? *Gut* 1990; **31:** A1195.

33. Cooke AR. Control of gastric emptying and motility. *Gastroenterology* 1975; **68:** 804–16.

34. Schapiro H, Woodward ER. Inhibition of gastric motility by acid in the duodenum. *J Appl Physiol* 1955; **8:** 121–7.

35. Orr WC, Cromwell MD, Lin B. Sleep and gastric function in IBS: derailing the brain–gut axis. *Gut* 1997; **41:** 390–3.

36. Kapadia SA. Fibre in enteral nutrition. MD thesis, University of Sheffield, 1993.

37. Bowling TE, Raimundo AH, Grimble GK, Silk DBA. Colonic secretory effect in response to enteral feeding in humans. *Gut* 1994; **35:** 1734–41.

38. Snape WJ Jr, Wright SH, Battle WM, Cohen S. The gastrocolic response: evidence for a neural mechanism. *Gastroenterology* 1979; **77:** 1235–40.

39. Snape WJ Jr, Matarazzo SA, Cohen S. Effect of eating and gastrointestinal hormones on human colonic myo-electrical and motor activity. *Gastroenterology* 1978; **75:** 373–8.

40. Rogers J, Henry MM, Misiewicz JJ. Increased seg-mental activity and intraluminal pressures in the sigmoid colon of patients with the irritable bowel syndrome. *Gut* 1989; **30:** 634–41.

41. Rogers J, Raimundo AH, Misiewicz JJ. Cephalic phase of colonic pressure response to food. *Gut* 1993; **34:** 537–43.

42. Read NW. Diarrhoea motrice. *Clin Gastroenterol* 1986; **15:** 657–86.

43. Raimundo AH, Jameson JS, Rogers J, Silk DBA. The effect of enteral nutrition on distal colonic motility. *Gastroenterology* 1992; **102:** A573.

44. Bowling TE, Raimundo AH, Jameson JS, Silk DBA. Suppression of colonic motility in response to enteral feeding in man. *Gastroenterology* 1993; **104(4):** A610.

45. Bowling TE, Silk DBA. Colonic responses to enteral tube feeding. *Gut* 1998; **42:** 147–51.

46. Bowling TE, Silk DBA. Hormonal response to enteral feeding and the possible role of Peptide YY in the pathogenesis of enteral feeding related diarrhoea. *Clin Nutr* 1996; **15:** 307–10.

47. Bowling TE. The Sir David Cuthbertson Medal Lecture. Enteral-feeding-related diarrhoea: proposed causes and possible solutions. *Proc Nutr Soc* 1995; **54:** 579–90.

48. Katschinski M. Nutritional implications of cephalic phase gastrointestinal responses. *Appetite* 2000; **34:** 189–96.

49. Kapadia SA, Raimundo AH, Grimble GK, Aimer P, Silk DBA. Influence of three different fiber-supplemented enteral diets on bowel function and short-chain fatty acid production. *J Parent Enteral Nutr* 1995; **19:** 63–8.

50. Duncan HD, Bowling TE, Grimble GK, Silk DBA. Effect of bolus nasogastric tube feeding on colonic water movement in humans. *Gastroenterology* 2000; **118** (suppl. 2): A770.

51. Duncan HD, Cole SJ, Bowling TE, Silk DB. Does a nasogastric tube adversely affect distal colonic motility and contribute to pathogenesis of enteral feeding related diarrhoea? *Gastroenterology* 1998; **114:** 876–7.

52. Rees RGP, Hare WR, Grimble GK, Frost P, Silk DBA. Do patients with moderately impaired gastro-intestinal function requiring enteral nutrition need a predigested nitrogen source? Prospective cross over controlled trial. *Gut* 1992; **23:** 877–81.

53. Walton JG, Seymour RA. Dental disorders. In: Davis DM (ed) *Textbook of drug reactions.* Oxford University Press, Oxford, 1991; 220–1.

54. Dominioni L, Stinnett JD, Fong CH *et al.* Gastrostomy feeding in normal and hypermetabolic guinea pigs. *J Burn Care Rehab* 1984; **5:** 100–5.

55. Alexander JW, Gottschlich MM. Nutritional immuno-modulation in burn patients. *Crit Care Med* 1990; **18:** S149–S153.

56. James MJ, Gibson RA, Cleland LG. Dietary poly-unsaturated fatty acids and inflammatory mediator production. *Am J Clin Nutr* 2000; **71:** 343S-8S.

57. Calder PC, Deckelbaum RJ. Dietary lipids: more than just a source of calories. *Curr Opin Clin Nutr Metab Care* 1999; **2:** 105–7.

58. Shenkin A. Micronutrients. In: Rombeau JL, Rolandelli WB (eds) *Clinical nutrition: enteral and tube feeding*. WB Saunders, Philadelphia, 1997, 96–111.

59. Keohane PP, Attrill H, Love N *et al*. Relation between osmolality of diet and gastrointestinal side effects in enteral nutrition. *Br Med J* 1984; **288:** 678–80.

60. Rees RGP, Keohane PP, Grimble GK, Frost P, Silk DBA. Tolerance of elemental diet administered with-out starter regime. *Br Med J* 1985; **290:** 1869–70.

61. Bower RH, Talamini MA, Sax HC *et al*. Postoperative enteral vs parenteral nutrition. A randomised controlled trial. *Arch Surg* 1986; **121:** 1040–5.

62. Fletcher JP, Little JM. A comparison of parenteral nutrition and early postoperative enteral feeding on the nitrogen balance after major surgery. *Surgery* 1986; **100:** 21–4.

63. Muggia-Sullam M, Bower RH, Murphy RF *et al*. Postoperative enteral versus parenteral nutritional support in gastrointestinal surgery. A matched pros-pective study. *Am J Surg* 1985; **149:** 106–12.

64. Hamadui E, Lefkowitz R, Olender L *et al*. Enteral nutrition in the early postoperative period: a new semi elemental formula versus total parenteral nutrition. *J Parent Enteral Nutr* 1990; **14:** 501–7.

65. Hayashi JT, Wolfe BM, Calvert CC. Limited efficacy of early postoperative jejunal feeding. *Am J Surg* 1985; **150:** 52–7.

66. Kemen M, Homann HH, Mumme A, Zumtobel V. Is intact protein superior for post-operative enteral nutrition than hydrolysed protein? *Clin Nutr* 1991; **10** (suppl): 37.

67. Compher C, Seto RW, Lew JI, Rombeau JL. Dietary fibre and its clinical applications to enteral nutrition. In: Rombeau JL, Rolandelli WB (eds) *Clinical nutrition: enteral and tube feeding*. WB Saunders, Philadelphia, 1997, 81–95.

68. Randall HT. Enteral nutrition tube feeding in acute and chronic illness. *J Parent Enteral Nutr* 1984; **8:** 113–36.

69. Russell RI. Elemental diets. *Gut* 1975; **16:** 68–79.

70. Slavin JL, Nelson NL, McNamara EA, Cashmere K. Bowel function of healthy men consuming liquid diets with and without dietary fibre. *J Parent Enteral Nutr* 1985; **9:** 317–21.

71. Kapadia SA, Raimundo AH, Silk DBA. The effect of a fibre free and fibre supplemented polymeric enteral diet on normal human bowel function. *Clin Nutr* 1993; **12:** 272–6.

72. Patil DH, Grimble GK, Keohane PP, Attrill H, Love M, Silk DBA. Do fibre containing enteral diets have advantages over existing low residue diets? *Clin Nutr* 1985; **4:** 67–71.

73. Heymsfield SB, Roogspisuthipong C, Evert M, Casper K, Heller P, Akrabawi SS. Fiber supplementation of enteral formulas: effects on the bioavailability of major nutrients and gastrointestinal tolerance. *J Parent Enteral Nutr* 1993; **12:** 265–73.

74. Fischer M, Adkin W, Hall L, Scaman P, Hsi S, Marlett J. The effects of dietary fibre in a liquid diet on bowel function of mentally retarded individuals. *J Ment Defic Res* 1985; **29:** 373–81.

75. Liebl BH, Fischer M, Van Calcar SC, Marlett J. Dietary fibre and long-term large bowel response in enterally nourished nonambulatory profoundly retarded youth. *J Parent Enteral Nutr* 1990; **14:** 371–5.

76. Stephen AM, Cummings JH. Mechanism of action of dietary fibre in the human colon. *Nature* 1990; **284:** 283–4.

77. Eastwood MA, Bryden WC, Tadasse K. Effect of fibre on colon function. In: Spiller GA, Kay RM (eds) *Medical aspects of dietary fibre*. Plenum Press, New York, 1980, 1–26.

78. Stephen AM. Constipation. In: Trowell H, Burkitt D, Heaton KW (eds) *Dietary fibre, fibre depleted food and disease*. Academic Press, London, 1985, 133–44.

79. Heller SN, Hackler LR, Rivers JM *et al*. Dietary fiber: the effect of particle size of wheat bran on colonic function in young adult men. *Am J Clin Nutr* 1980; **33:** 1734–44.

80. Kapadia SA, Raimundo AH, Grimble GK, Aimer P, Silk DBA. Influence of three different fiber-supplemented enteral diets on bowel function and short-chain fatty acid production. *J Parent Enteral Nutr* 1995; **19:** 63–8.

81. Salyers AA, Leedle JAZ. Carbohydrate metabolism in the human colon. In: Hentges DJ (ed) *Human intestinal microflora in health and disease*. Academic Press, New York, 1983, 129–46.

82. Bowling TE, Raimundo AH, Grimble GK, Silk DBA. Reversal of short-chain fatty acids of colonic fluid secretion induced by enteral feeding. *Lancet* 1999; **342:** 1266–8.

83. Guenter PA, Perlmutter S, Settle RG, Marino PL, DeSimone GA, Rolandelli RH. Tube feeding related diarrhoea in acutely ill patients. *J Parent Enteral Nutr* 1991; **15:** 277–8.

84. Hart GK, Dobb GJ. Effect of faecal bulking agent on diarrhoea during enteral feeding in the critically ill. *J Parent Enteral Nutr* 1988; **12:** 465–8.

85. Dobb GJ, Towler SC. Diarrhoea during enteral feeding in the critically ill: a comparison of feeds with and without fibre. *Intens Care Med* 1990; **16:** 252–5.

86. Frankfield DC, Beyer PL. Soy polysaccharide fibre; effect on diarrhoea in tube-fed, head injured patients. *Am J Clin Nutr* 1989; **50:** 533–8.

87. Wright NA, Alison M. Growth and proliferative responses of the gastrointestinal tract. In: The biology of epithelial cell population. Clarendon Press, Oxford, 1984, 743–76.

88. Morin CL, Ling V, Bourassa S. Small intestinal and colonic changes induced by a chemically defined diet. *Dig Dis Sci* 1980; **25:** 123–8.

89. Nelson NL, Carmichael HA, Russell RI, Lee FD. Small intestinal changes induced by an elemental diet in normal rats. *Clin Sci Mol Med* 1978; **55:** 509–11.

90. Young EA, Goletti LA, Winborn WB, Taylor JB, Weser E. Comparative study of nutritional adaptation to defined formula diets in rats. *Am J Clin Nutr* 1980; **33:** 2106–18.

91. Maxt DG, Cynck EV, Thompson RPH. Small intestinal response to 'elemental' and 'complete' liquid feeds in the rat: effect of dietary bulk. *Gut* 1987; **28:** 688–93.

92. Ryan GP, Dudrick SJ, Copeland EM, Johnson LR. Effects of various diets on colonic growth in rats. *Gastroenterology* 1979; **77:** 658–63.

93. Jacobs LR, Schneeman BO. Effects of dietary wheat bran on rat colonic structure and mucosal cell growth. *J Nutr* 1981; **111:** 789–803.

94. Tasman Jones C, Owen RL, Jones AL. Semipurified dietary fibre and small bowel morphometry in rats. *Dig Dis Sci* 1982; **27:** 519–24.

95. Jacobs LR, Lupton JR. Effects of dietary fibres on rat large bowel mucosal growth and cell proliferation. *Am J Physiol* 1984; **6:** 378–85.

96. Goodlad RA, Lenton W, Ghatei MA, Adrian TE, Bloom SR, Wright NA. Effects of an elemental diet, inert bulk and different types of dietary fibre on the response of the intestinal epithelium to refeeding in the rat and relationship to plasma gastrin, enteroglucagen and PYY concentrations. *Gut* 1987; **28:** 171–80.

97. Sakata T, Enghardt WV. Stimulating effect of short chain fatty acids on the epithelial cell proliferation in the rat large intestine. *Comp Biochem Physiol* 1983; **74A:** 49–62.

98. Sakata T. Short chain fatty acids as the luminal trophic factor. *Can J Anim Sci* 1984; **64:** 189–90.

99. Sakata T, Yajima T. Influence of short chain fatty acids on the epithelial cell division of digestive tract. *Am J Exp Physiol* 1984; **69:** 639–48.

100. Goodlad RA, Ratcliff B, Fordham JP, Wright NA. Does dietary fibre stimulate intestinal epithelial cell proliferation in germ free rats? *Gut* 1989; **30:** 820–5.

101. Roediger WEW. Utilization of nutrients by isolated epithelial cells of the rat colon. *Gastroenterology* 1982; **83:** 424–9.

102. Kripke SA, Fox AD, Berman JM, Settle RG, Rombeau JL. Stimulation of intestinal mucosal growth with intracolonic infusion of short-chain fatty acids. *J Parent Enteral Nutr* 1989; **13:** 109–16.

103. Sheppach W, Bartram P, Richter A. The effect of short chain fatty acids on the human colonic mucosa in vitro. *J Parent Enteral Nutr* 1992; **16:** 43–8.

104. Stanfield JP, Hult MSR, Tunnicliffe R. Intestinal biopsy in Kwashiorkor. *Lancet* 1965; **11:** 519–23.

105. Thomson TJ, Runcie J, Miller V. Treatment of obesity by total fasting for up to 249 days. *Lancet* 1996; **11:** 992–6.

106. Adibi SA, Raworth-Allen ER. Impaired jejunal absorption rates of essential amino acids induced by either dietary caloric or protein deprivation in man. *Gastroenterology* 1970; **59:** 404–13.

107. Castro GA, Copeland EM, Dudrick SJ, Johnson LR. Intestinal disaccharidase and peroxidase activities in parenterally nourished rats. *J Nutr* 1975; **105:** 776–81.

108. Levine GM, Deren JJ, Steiger E, Zinno R. Role of oral intake in maintenance of gut mass and disaccharide activity. *Gastroenterology* 1974; **67:** 975–82.

109. Johnson LR, Copeland EM, Dudrick SJ, Lichtenberger LM, Castro GA. Structural and hormonal alterations in the gastrointestinal tract of parenterally fed rats. *Gastroenterology* 1975; **68:** 1177–83.

110. Guedon C, Schmitz J, Lerebours E *et al.* Decreased brush border hydrolase activities without gross morphologic changes in human intestinal mucosa after prolonged total parenteral nutrition of adults. *Gastroenterology* 1986; **90:** 373–8.

111. Buchman AL, Mestecky J, Moukarzel A, Ament ME. Intestinal immune function is unaffected by parenteral nutrition in man. *J Am Coll Nutr* 1995; **14:** 656–61.

112. Van der Hulst RR, Van Kreel BK, Von Meyenfeldt MF *et al.* Glutamine and the preservation of gut integrity. *Lancet* 1993; **341:** 1363–5.

113. Sedman PC, MacFie J, Palmer MD, Mitchell CJ, Sagar PM. Preoperative total parenteral nutrition is not associated with mucosal atrophy or bacterial translocation in humans. *Br J Surg* 1995; **82:** 1663–7.

114. Pironi L, Paganelli GM, Miglioli M, Biasco G, Santucci R, Ruggeri E. Morphologic and cyto-proliferative patterns of duodenal mucosa in two patients after long-term total parenteral nutrition: changes with oral refeeding and relation to intestinal resection. *J Parent Enteral Nutr* 1994; **18:** 351–4.

115. Groos S, Hunfeld G, Luciano L. Morphological changes in human adult intestinal mucosa. *J Submicrosc Cytol Pathol* 1996; **28:** 61–74.

116. Hoensch HP, Steinhardt HJ, Weiss G, Hang D, Maier A, Malchon H. Effects of semisynthetic diets on xeno-biotic metabolizing enzyme activity and morphology of small intestinal mucosa in humans. *Gastroenterology* 1994; **86:** 1519–30.

117. Cummins A, Chu G, Faust L *et al.* Malabsorption and villous atrophy in patients receiving enteral feeding. *J Parent Enteral Nutr* 1995; **19:** 193–8.

118. Rolandelli RH, Koruda MJ, Settle RG, Rombeau JL. The effect of enteral feedings supplemented with pectin in the healing of colonic anastomosis in the rat. *Surgery* 1986; **99:** 703–7.

119. Rolandelli RH, Koruda MJ, Settle RG, Rombeau JL. Effects of intraluminal infusion of short-chain fatty acids on the healing of colonic anastomosis in the rat. *Surgery* 1986; **100:** 198–203.

120. Koruda MJ, Rolandelli RH, Settle RG, Saul SH, Rombeau JL. The effect of a pectin supplemented elemental diet on intestinal adaptation to massive small bowel resection. *J Parent Enteral Nutr* 1986; **10:** 343–50.

121. Koruda MJ, Rolandelli RH, Settle RG, Zimmaro DM, Rombeau JL. Effect of parenteral nutrition supplemented with short-chain fatty acids on adapta-tion to massive small bowel resection. *Gastroenterology* 1988; **95:** 715–20.

122. Frankel W, Singh A, Zang W, Bain A, Klurfeld D, Rombeau JL. Colon trophic effects of short-chain fatty acids are mediated locally. *Clin Nutr* 1992; **11:** 63.

123. Edmiston CE Jr, Condon RE. Bacterial translocation. *Surg Gynecol Obstet* 1991; **173:** 73–83.

124. Alverdy JC, Aoys E, Moss GS. Total parenteral nutrition promotes bacterial translocation from the gut. *Surgery* 1988; **104:** 185–90.

125. Shou J, Lappin J, Minnard EA, Daly JM. Total parenteral nutrition, bacterial translocation, and host immune function. *Am J Surg* 1994; **167:** 145–50.

126. Spaeth G, Berg R, Specian RD, Deitch EA. Food without fiber promotes bacterial translocation from the gut. *Surgery* 1990; **108:** 240–7.

127. Kueppers PM, Miller TA, Chen CK. Effect of total parenteral nutrition plus morphine on bacterial trans-location in rats. *Ann Surg* 1993; **217:** 286–92.

128. Spaeth G, Gottwald T, Haas W *et al.* Glutamine does not improve gut barrier function and mucosal immunity in total parenteral nutrition. *J Parent Enteral Nutr* 1993; **17:** 317–23.

129. Illig KA, Ryan CK, Hardy DJ, Rhodes J, Locke W, Sax HC. Total parenteral nutrition-induced changes in gut mucosal function: atrophy alone is not the issue. *Surgery* 1992; **112:** 631–7.

130. Helton WS, Garcia R. Oral prostaglandin E$_2$ prevents gut atrophy during intravenous feeding but not bacterial translocation. *Arch Surg* 1999; **128;** 178–84.

131. Mainous M, Xu D, Lu Q *et al.* Oral-TPN-induced bacterial translocation and impaired immune defenses are reversed by refeeding. *Surgery* 1991; **110:** 277–84.

132. Deitch EA, Xu D, Lu Q *et al.* Elemental diet-induced immune suppression is caused by both bacterial and dietary factors. *J Parent Enteral Nutr* 1993; **17:** 332–6.

133. Xu D, Qi L, Thirstrup C, Berg R, Deitch EA. Elemental diet-induced bacterial translocation and immunosuppression is not reversed by glutamine. *J Trauma* 1993; **35:** 821–4.

134. Spaeth G, Specian RD, Berg R *et al.* Bulk prevents bacterial translocation induced by the oral admini-stration of total parenteral nutrition solution. *J Parent Enteral Nutr* 1990; **14:** 442–7.

135. Haskel Y, Xu D, Lu Q. Elemental diet-induced bacterial translocation can be hormonally modulated. *Ann Surg* 1993; **217:** 634–43.

136. Jones WG II, Minei JP, Barber AE *et al.* Elemental diet promotes spontaneous bacterial translocation and alters mortality after endotoxin challenge. *Surg Forum* 1989; **40:** 20–2.

137. Barber AE, Jones WG II, Minei JP. Glutamine or fibre supplementation of a defined formula diet: impact on bacterial translocation, tissue composition and response to endotoxin. *J Parent Enteral Nutr* 1990; **14:** 335–43.

138. Alverdy JC, Aoys E, Moss GS. Effect of commercially available chemically defined liquid diets on the intestinal microflora and bacterial translocation from the gut. *J Parent Enteral Nutr* 1990; **14:** 1–6.

139. Haskel Y, Xu D, Lu Q *et al.* Bombesin protects against bacterial translocation induced by three commercially available liquid enteral diets: a prospective, random-ized, multigroup trial. *Crit Care Med* 1994; **22:** 108–13.

140. Inoue S, Epstein MD, Alexander JW *et al.* Prevention of yeast translocation across the gut by a single enteral feeding after burn injury. *J Parent Enteral Nutr* 1989; **13:** 565–71.

141. Pape HC, Dwenger A, Regel G *et al.* Increased gut permeability after multiple trauma. *Br J Surg* 1994; **81:** 850–2.

142. Ziegler TR, Smith RJ, O'Dwyer ST et al. Increased intestinal permeability associated with infection in burn patients. Arch Surg 1988; 123: 1313–39.

143. Roumen RMH, Van der Viet JA, Wevers RA et al. Intestinal permeability is increased after major vascular surgery. J Vasc Surg 1993; 17: 734–7.

144. Reynolds JV, Kanwar S, Welsh FKS et al. Does the route of feeding modify gut barrier function and clinical outcome in patients after major upper gastro-intestinal surgery? J Parent Enteral Nutr 1997; 21: 196–201.

145. Gabe SM, Patel M, Grimble GK, Williams R, Bjarnason I, Silk DBA. Intestinal permeability in critical illness and acute liver failure: the relationship with severity of illness, splanchnic ischemia and survival. Gastroenterology 1998; 114: A370.

146. Reed LL, Martin M, Manglano R et al. Bacterial translocation following abdominal trauma in humans. Circ Shock 1994; 42: 1–6.

147. Brathwaite CEM, Ross SE, Nagele R et al. Bacterial translocation occurs in humans after traumatic injury: evidence using immunofluorescence. J Trauma 1993; 34: 586–90.

148. Deitch EA. Simple intestinal obstruction causes bacterial translocation in man. Arch Surg 1989; 124: 699–701.

149. Brooks SG, May J, Sedman PC et al. Translocation of enteric bacteria in humans. Br J Surg 1993; 80: 901–2.

150. Sedman PC, MacFie J, Sagar P et al. The prevalence of gut translocation in humans. Gastroenterology 1994; 107: 643–9.

151. O'Boyle CJ, Zeigler D, Wadsworth C, Mitchell CJ, MacFie J. Clinical associations with bacterial trans-location. Clin Nutr 1997; 16: 48.

152. Gabe SM, Bjarnason I, Tolou-Ghamari Z et al. The effect of tacrolimus (FK506) on intestinal barrier function and cellular energy production in humans. Gastroenterology 1998; 115: 67–74.

153. Harrison L, Brennan MF. The role of total parenteral nutrition in cancer patients. Curr Prob Surg 1995; 32: 833–924.

154. Lundholm K, Edstrom S, Ekman L et al. A comparative study of the influence of malignant tumor on host metabolism in mice and man. Cancer 1978; 42: 453–61.

155. Brennan MF. Uncomplicated starvation versus cancer cachexia. Cancer Res 1977; 37: 2359–64.

156. DeWys WD, Begg C, Lavin PT et al. Prognostic effect of weight loss prior to chemotherapy in cancer patients. Am J Med 1980; 69: 491–7.

157. Kelleher J, Walters MP, Srinivasan TR, Hart G, Findlay JM, Losowsky MS. Degradation of cellulose within the gastrointestinal tract in man. Gut 1984; 25: 811–15.

158. Grimble GK, Patil DH, Silk DBA. Assimilation of lactitol, an 'unabsorbed' disaccharide in the normal human colon. Gut 1988; 29: 1666–71.

159. Rycroft CE, Fooks LJ, Gibson GR. Methods for assess-ing the potential of prebiotics and probiotics. Curr Opin Clin Nutr Metab Care 1999; 2: 481–4.

160. Silk DBA. Fibre and enteral nutrition. Clin Nutr 1993; 12 (suppl 1): 106–13.

161. Zimmaro DM, Rolandelli RH, Koruda MJ, Settle RG, Stein P, Rombeau JL. Isotonic tube feeding formula induces liquid stools in normal subjects: Reversal by pectin. J Parent Enteral Nutr 1989; 13: 117–23.

162. Sandstead H, Munroz JM, Jacob RA et al. Influence of dietary fibre on trace element balance. Am J Clin Nutr 1978; 31: 5180–4.

163. Drews LM, Kies C, Fox HM. Effect of dietary fiber on copper, zinc, and magnesium utilization by adolescent boys. Am J Clin Nutr 1979; 32: 1893–7.

164. Reinhold JG, Faradji B, Abadi P et al. Decreased absorption of calcium, magnesium, zinc and phosphorus by humans due to increased fibre and phosphorus consumption as wheat bread. J Nutr 1976; 106: 493–503.

165. Kapadia SA, Raimundo AH, Silk DBA. Small intestinal absorption of minerals during enteral feeding supplemented with 50 mg polysaccharide fibre. Gut 1992; 33: S58.

166. Taper LJ, Milan R, McCallister M et al. Mineral retention in young men consuming soy fibre augmented liquid formula diets. Am J Clin Nutr 1988; 48: 305–11.

167. Van Calcar SC, Liebl BH, Fischer M et al. Long term nutritional status of enterally nourished institutionalised population. J Clin Nutr 1989; 50: 381–90.

168. Prosky L, Asp NG, Scheweizer TF et al. Determination of insoluble, soluble and total dietary fibre in foods and food products: interlaboratory study. Journal of the Association of Official Analytical Chemists 1988; 71: 1017–23.

169. Moriarty KJ, Hegarty JE, Fairclough PD, Kelly MJ, Clarke MI, Dawson AM. Relative nutritional value of whole protein, hydrolysed protein and free amino acids in man. Gut 1985; 26: 694–9.

170. Kuhn KS, Stehle P, Furst P. Glutamine content of protein and peptide-based enteral products. J Parent Enteral Nutr 1996; 20: 292–5.

171. Robinson AB, Rudd CJ. Deamination of glutaminyl and asparaginyl residues in peptides and proteins. *Curr Top Cell Regul* 1974; **8**: 247–95.

172. Bowling TE, Jameson JJ, Grimble GK, Silk DBA. Enteral nutrition as a primary therapy in active Crohn's disease. *Eur J Gastroenterol Hepatol* 1993; **5**: 1–7.

173. Grimble GK. Mechanisms and regulation of peptide and amino acid transport. In: Fürst P, Young VR (eds) Proteins, peptides and amino-acids in enteral nutrition. Karger, Basel, 2000, 63–84.

174. Jones BJM, Brown B, Loran JS *et al.* Glucose absorption from starch hydrolysates in the human jejunum. *Gut* 1984; **24**: 1152–60.

175. Jones BJM, Brown B, Spiller RC, Silk DBA. Energy dense enteral feeds – the use of high molecular weight glucose polymers. *J Parent Enteral Nutr* 1981; **5**: 567.

176. Spiller RC, Jones BJM, Silk DBA. Jejunal water and electrolyte absorption from five proprietary enteral feeds in man: importance of sodium content. *Gut* 1987; **28**: 681–7.

177. Jones BJM. Nutritional management of the short bowel syndrome. *J Clin Nutr Gastroenterol* 1987; **2**: 99–103.

178. Goodgame JT, Lowry SF, Brennan MF. Essential fatty acid deficiency in total parenteral nutrition: time course of development and suggestions for therapy. *Surgery* 1978; **84**: 271–7.

179. Silk DBA. Diet formulation and choice of enteral diet. *Gut* 1986; **27**: 40–6.

180. Durie PR, Pencharz PB. Cystic fibrosis: nutrition. *Br Med Bull* 1992; **48**: 823–46.

181. Nightingale JM, Lennard-Jones JE, Walker ER, Farthing MJ. Oral salt supplements to compensate for jejunostomy losses: comparison of sodium chloride capsules, glucose electrolyte solution, and glucose polymer electrolyte solution. *Gut* 1992; **33**: 759–61.

182. Turnberg L. Cellular basis of diarrhoea. The Croonian lecture 1989. *J Roy Coll Physicians Lond* 1991; **25**: 53–62.

183. Lennard-Jones JE. Inflammatory bowel disease. In: Hill GL (ed) *Clinical surgery international*. Churchill Livingstone, Edinburgh, 1981, 267–80.

184. Newton CR, Gonvers JJ, Preston DM, McIntyre PB, Lennard-Jones JEJ. Effect of different drinks on fluid and electrolytes losses from a jejunostomy. *J Roy Soc Med* 1985; **78**: 27–34.

185. McIntyre PB. The short bowel. *Br J Surg* 1985; **72**: 27–34.

186. Newton CR, Drury P, Gonvers JJ, McIntyre PB, Preston DM, Lennard-Jones JE. Incidence and treatment of sodium depletion in ileostomists. *Scand J Gastroenterol* 1982; **17**: 159–60.

187. Lifshitz F, Wapnir RA. Oral rehydration solutions: experimental optimization of water and sodium absorption. *J Pediatr* 1985; **106**: 383–9.

188. McIntyre PB, Fitchew M, Lennard-Jones JE. Patients with a high jejunostomy do not need a special diet. *Gastroenterology* 1986; **91**: 25–33.

189. Brown SE, Light RW. What is now known about protein-energy depletion: when COPD patients are malnourished. *J Respir Dis* 1983; May: 36–50.

190. Openbrier DR, Irwin MM, Rogers RM. Nutritional status and lung function in patients with emphysema and chronic bronchitis. *Chest* 1983; **83**: 17–22.

191. Driver AG, LeBrun M. Iatrogenic malnutrition in patients receiving ventilatory support. *JAMA* 1980; **244**: 2195–6.

192. Driver AG, McAlevy MT, Smith JL. Nutritional assessment of patients with chronic obstructive pulmonary disease and acute respiratory failure. *Chest* 1982; **82**: 568–71.

193. Larca L, Greenbaum DM. Effectiveness of intensive nutritional regimens in patients who fail to wean from mechanical ventilation. *Crit Care Med* 1982; **10**: 297–300.

194. Bassili HR, Deitel M. Effect of nutritional support on weaning patients off mechanical ventilators. *J Parent Enteral Nutr* 1981; **5**: 161–3.

195. Askanazi J, Nordenstrom J, Rosenbaum SH *et al.* Nutrition for the patients with respiratory failure: glucose vs fat. *Anaesthesiology* 1981; **54**: 373–7.

196. Askanazi J, Elwyn DH, Silverberg PA *et al.* Respiratory distress secondary to a high carbohydrate load. A case report. *Surgery* 1980; **87**: 596–8.

197. Covelli HD, Black JW, Olsen MS, Beekman JF. Respiratory failure precipitated by high carbohydrate loads. *Ann Intern Med* 1981; **95**: 579–81.

198. Al-Saady NM, Blackmore CM, Bennett ED. High fat, low carbohydrate, enteral feeding lowers $PaCO_2$ and reduces the period of ventilation in artificially ventilated patients. *Intensive Care Med* 1989; **15**: 290–5.

199. O'Keefe SJD, Abraham R, El-Zayadi A, Marshall W, Davis M, Williams R. Increased plasma tyrosine concentrations in patients with cirrhosis and fulminant hepatic failure associated with increased plasma tyrosine flux and reduced hepatic oxidation capacity. *Gastroenterology* 1981; **81**: 1017–24.

200. Silk DBA. Nutritional support in liver disease. *Gut* 1991; (Sept.): S29–S33.

201. Wicks C, Somasundaran S, Bjarnason I *et al.* Comparison of enteral feeding and total parenteral nutrition after liver transplantation. *Lancet* 1994; **344**: 837–40.

202. O'Keefe SJD, El-Zayadi A, Carraher T, Davies M, Williams R. Malnutrition and immuno-competence in patients with liver disease. *Lancet* 1980; **ii:** 615–17.

203. Hirsch S, Bunout D, De la Maza P *et al*. Controlled trial of nutrition supplementation in outpatients with symptomatic alcoholic cirrhosis. *J Parent Enteral Nutr* 1993; **17:** 119–24.

204. Bunout D, Aicardi V, Hirsch S *et al*. Nutritional support in hospitalised patients with alcoholic liver disease. *Eur J Clin Nutr* 1989; **43:** 615–21.

205. Cabre E, Gonzalez-Huiz F, Abad-Lacruz A *et al*. Effect of total enteral nutrition on the short term outcome of severely malnourished cirrhotics. *Gastroenterology* 1990; **98:** 715–20.

206. Scrimshaw NS, San Giovanni JP. Synergism of nutrition, infection, and immunity: an overview. *Am J Clin Nutr* 1997; **66:** 464S–77S.

207. Lanthier PL, Morgan MY. Lactitol in the treatment of chronic hepatic encephalopathy: an open comparison with lactulose. *Gut* 1985; **26:** 415–20.

208. O'Keefe SJD, Abraham R, Zayadi A, Marshall W, Vies M, Williams R. Increased plasma tyrosine concentrations in patients with cirrhosis and fulminant hepatic failure associated with increased plasma tyrosine flux and reduced hepatic oxidation a capacity. *Gastroenterology* 1981; **81:** 1017–24.

209. Munro HN, Fernstrom JD, Wurtman RJ. Insulin, plasma, amino acid inbalance and hepatic comas. *Lancet* 1975; **ii:** 986.

210. Manchesini G, Forlani G. Effect of englycaemic insulin infusion on plasma levels or branch chain amino acids in cirrhosis. *Hepatology* 1983; **32:** 184–7.

211. Crossley IR, Wardall EN, Williams R. Biochemical mechanisms of hepatic encephalopathy. *Clin Sci* 1983; **64:** 247–52.

212. James JH, Ziparo V, Jeppsson B, Fischer JE. Hyper-aminoaemia, plasma amino acid inbalance and blood brain amino acid transport: a unified theory of portal/systemic encephalopathy. *Lancet* 1979; **ii:** 772–5.

213. McCullough AJ, Mullen KD, Tavill AS. Branched chain amino acids as nutritional therapy in liver disease: death or surfeit. *Hepatology* 1983; **3:** 269–71.

214. Fischer JE. Amino acids in hepatic coma. *Dig Dis Sci* 1982; **27:** 97–102.

215. Fischer JE, Funovics JM, Agurre A *et al*. The role of plasma amino acids in hepatic encephalopathy. *Surgery* 1975; **70:** 276–90.

216. Silk DBA. Branched chain amino acids in liver disease: fact or fantasy? *Gut* 1986; **27:** 103–10.

217. Blackburn GL, O'Keefe SJD. Editorial: nutrition in liver failure. *Gastroenterology* 1989; **97:** 1049–51.

218. Horst D, Grace ND, Conn HO *et al*. Comparison of dietary protein with an oral, branched chain enriched amino acid supplement in chronic portal systemic encephalopathy. A randomised controlled trial. *Hepatology* 1984; **4:** 279–87.

219. Silk DBA. Use of modified amino acid based enteral diets in the nutritional support of patients with porto-systemic encephalopathy: a rethink. *Nutrition* 1988; **4:** 401–3.

220. Walser M. Urea cycle disorders and other hereditary hyperammonaemic syndromes. In: Stanbury JB, Wyngaarden JB, Fredrickson DS, Goldstein JL, Brown MS (eds) The metabolic basis of inherited disease. McGraw-Hill, New York, 1982, 402–38.

221. Rudman D, Kutner M, Ansley J, Jansen R, Chipponi J, Bain RP. Hypotyrosinaemia, hypocystinamia and failure to retain nitrogen during total parenteral nutrition of cirrhotic patients. *Gastroenterology* 1981; **81:** 1025–35.

222. Epstein MD. Deranged sodium homeostasis in cirrhosis. *Gastroenterology* 1979; **76:** 622–7.

223. Lee J, Bisset GW. The secretion of neurohypophyseal hormones in man with special reference to liver disease. *Proc Roy Soc Med* **51:** 361–5.

224. Lacey JM, Wilmore DW. Is glutamine a conditionally essential amino acid? *Nutr Rev* 1990; **48:** 297–309.

225. Souba WW, Smith RJ, Wilmore DW. Glutamine metabolism by the intestinal tract. *J Parent Enteral Nutr* 1985; **3:** 608–17.

226. Tremel H, Kienle B, Weilemann LS, Stehle P, Fürst P. Glutamine dipeptide-supplemented parenteral nutrition maintains intestinal function in the critically ill. *Gastroenterology* 1994; **107:** 1595–601.

227. Schloerb PR, Amare M. Total parenteral nutrition with glutamine in bone marrow transplantation and other clinical applications (a randomised double-blind study). *J Parent Enteral Nutr* 1993; **17:** 407–13.

228. Houdijk APJ, Rijnsburger ER, Jansen J *et al*. Randomised trial of glutamine-enriched enteral nutrition on infectious morbidity in patients with multiple trauma. *Lancet* 1998; **352:** 772–6.

229. Powell-Tuck J, Jamieson CP, Bettany GE *et al*. A double blind, randomised, controlled trial of glutamine supplementation in parenteral nutrition. *Gut* 1999; **45:** 82–8.

230. Griffiths RD, Jones C, Palmer TCA. Six months outcome of critically ill patients given glutamine supplemented parenteral nutrition. *Nutrition* 1997; **13**(4): 295–301.

231. Silk DBA. Formulation of enteral diets. *Nutrition* 1999; **15:** 626–32.

232. Bower RH. Malnutrition and immune function. *Clin Appl Nutr* 1991; **1:** 15–24.

233. Cerra FB. Nutrition modulation of inflammatory and immune function. *Am J Surg* 1991; **161:** 71–6.

234. Cerra FB, McPherson JP, Konstantinides FN *et al.* Enteral nutrition does not prevent MOFS after sepsis. *Surgery* 1988; **104:** 727–33.

235. Kerver AJH, Rommes JH, Mevissen V *et al.* Prevention and colonization of infection in critically ill patients: a prospective randomized trial. *Crit Care Med* 1988; **16:** 1087–93.

236. Levenson SM. Influence of supplemental arginine and vitamin A on wound healing, the thymus and resistance to infection following injury. In: Winters RW, Greene HL (eds) Nutritional support of the seriously ill patient. Academic Press, New York, 1983, 53–62.

237. Daly JM, Reynolds J, Thom A *et al.* Immune and metabolic effects of arginine in the surgical patient. *Ann Surg* 1988; **208:** 512–23.

238. Kirk SJ, Barbul A. Role of arginine in trauma, sepsis and immunity. *J Parent Enteral Nutr* 1990; **14**(5), 226S-9S.

239. Merimee TJ, Lillicrap DA, Rabinowitz D. Effect of arginine on serum levels of human growth hormone. *Lancet* 1965; **2:** 668–70.

240. Mulloy AL, Kari FW, Visek WJ. Dietary arginine, insulin secretion, glucose tolerance and liver lipids during repletion of protein-depleted rats. *Horm Metab Res* 1982; **14:** 471–5.

241. Chyun JH, Griminger P. Improvement of nitrogen retention by arginine and glycine supplementation and its relation to collagen synthesis in traumatized mature and aged rats. *J Nutr* 1984; **114:** 1697–704.

242. Adjei AA, Takamine F, Yokoyama H *et al.* The effects of oral RNA and intraperitoneal nucleoside-nucleotide administration on methicillin-resistant staphylococcus aureus infection in mice. *J Parent Enteral Nutr* 1993; **17:** 148–52.

243. Rudolph FB, Kulkarni AD, Fanslow WC *et al.* Role of RNA as a dietary source of pyrimidines and purines in immune function. *J Parent Enteral Nutr* 1990; **6:** 45–52.

244. Grimble GK, Westwood OMR. Nucleotides and immunity. In: Gershwin ME, German B, Keen CL (eds) Nutrition and immunity. Humana Press, Totowa, NJ, 2000.

245. Carver JD, Pimental BP, Cox WI *et al.* Dietary nucleotide effects upon immune function in infants. *Pediatrics* 1991; **88:** 359–63.

246. Cerra FB, Lehmann S, Konstantinides FN *et al.* Improvement in immune function in ICU patients by enteral nutrition supplemented with arginine. RNA, and menhaden oil is independent of nitrogen balance. *Nutrition* 1991; **7:** 193–9.

247. Moore FA, Moore EE, Kudsk KA *et al.* Clinical benefits of an immune-enhancing diet for early post-injury enteral feeding. *J Trauma* 1994; **37:** 607–15.

248. Beale RJ, Bryg DJ, Bihari DJ. Immunonutrition in the critically ill: a systematic review of clinical outcome. *Crit Care Med* 1999; **27:** 2799–805.

249. Braga M, Gianotti L, Radaelli G *et al.* Perioperative immunonutrition in patients undergoing cancer surgery: results of a randomized double-blind phase 3 trial. *Arch Surg* 1999; **134:** 428–33.

250. August DA. Creation of a specialised nutrition support outcomes research consortium: if not now, when? *J Parent Enteral Nutr* 1996; **20:** 394–400.

251. Althausen TL, Uyeyama K, Simpson RG. Digestion and absorption after massive resection of the small intestine. I. utilization of food from a 'natural' versus a 'synthetic' diet and a comparison of intestinal absorption tests with nutritional balance studies in a patient with only 45 cm of small intestine. *Gastro-enterology* 1949; **12:** 795–807.

19

Complications of enteral nutrition

Jason Payne-James

Introduction

Complications of enteral tube feeding can largely be anticipated and prevented. If they occur most are capable of being solved without stopping enteral nutrition. Table 19.1 identifies the key areas of enteral nutrition-related complications. Certain complications (e.g. tube related, infective) are referred to in specific chapters and will only be referred to briefly here.

Table 19.1 – Complications of enteral nutrition

Enteral tube related	Malposition
	Displacement
	Unwanted removal
	Blockage
	Breakage/leakage
	Local complications (e.g. erosion of skin/mucosa)
Gastrointestinal	Diarrhoea
	Bloating
	Nausea
	Vomiting
	Abdominal cramps
	Regurgitation
	Pulmonary aspiration
	Constipation
	(Acute abdomen)
Metabolic/biochemical	Electrolyte excess or deficiency
	Vitamin, mineral, trace element deficiencies
	Drug interactions
Infective	Exogenous (handling/contamination)
	Endogenous (patient)

Complications of enteral tube feeding can be dependent on the underlying disease state, the access to the intestinal tract (e.g. nasoenteric versus percutaneous-gastric versus small bowel), the feeding technique (e.g. type of formula, gravity versus pump feeding) and the patient's metabolic state (e.g. anabolism, catabolism, postoperative stress). The reported frequency of these complications varies greatly. For example, tube-related complications have been reported to occur in 0–20% and gastrointestinal complications in 8–65% of patients during early postoperative feeding via a needle catheter jejunostomy (NCJ) using comparable techniques.[1-6] The pattern of complications, however, appears comparable in most reports. Gastrointestinal side-effects (including diarrhoea) are most frequent.[7] Differences in the definition of complications and in patient management may account for some variability between these reports. Diarrhoea, for example, can be defined by frequency, volume or consistency of stools or by a combination of all three.

Good protocols for enteral nutrition feeding under the supervision of nutrition support teams with detailed follow-up and monitoring will result in fewer complications.[8] Such protocols should allow for regular changes as the patient's needs alter. The latter part of this chapter identifies a number of areas of monitoring which may reduce the risk and incidence of complications and areas for prevention or management of specific complications should they arise.

Enteral tube-related complications

As discussed in detail in Chapter 17, enteral tube-related complications relate to the method of enteral access as well as to the material and diameter of the feeding tubes, but some broad principles are highlighted below. Complications occur at insertion and subsequently. The appropriate choice of tube for the patient will assist in reducing risk; for example, whether intragastric or postpyloric placement of tubes is chosen.

Pulmonary malposition of feeding tubes with subsequent intrapulmonary infusion of feed and the development of pulmonary abscesses may result from accidental tracheal intubation. Pneumothorax and intrathoracic infusion of feed have also been described as a consequence of incorrect tube insertion.[9-15] Patients on ventilators, those with altered consciousness and those with neurological diseases represent the groups predominantly at risk of misplacement. Any of the methods which can verify placement are advised. In any case, where the patient is obtunded in some way, X-ray confirmation of correct placement must be undertaken prior to commencing enteral diet infusion. Secondary displacement of the tip of the feeding tube may occur spontaneously or, for example, during withdrawal of a coexisting gastric suction tube or after chest physiotherapy. This may increase the risk of pulmonary aspiration. In all cases where displacement is suspected, check X-ray is indicated. Percutaneously placed feeding tubes (e.g. PEG, NCJ) may also displace into the abdominal cavity.

Using proper protocols and techniques, these complications are extremely rare with both PEG and NCJ.[16] However, if the clinical situation changes for un-explained reasons or complications (e.g. diarrhoea or vomiting) develop then review of such tubes, for example using contrast radiography, may be appropriate, in conjunction with clinical examination of the abdomen.

Gastrointestinal tract perforation with passage of the enteral tube into neighbouring structures[17,18] (including the cranium) has been reported. This complication is life threatening and again may occur particularly in the obtunded, unconscious individual on a ventilator. Any person placing a guidewire fine-bore feeding tube should have been trained in the technique and should not attempt the procedure without such training under supervision. Resistance to placement should never be overcome by increased pressure or boring. Reinsertion of a guidewire with the tube still *in situ* must never be undertaken. Endoscopic or fluoroscopic tube placement is the procedure of choice in unconscious patients in many units.

Inability to infuse via a tube may occur for two main reasons. The first, occlusion of the tube by feed, is most common and the second, knotting of the tube, may occur even when mechanically it appears unlikely. The first can generally be prevented by appropriate tube management protocols. The risk of tube occlusion may be avoided in most cases by the use of a low-viscosity formula. Solidification of various tube diets containing casein has, however, recently been reported in patients with raised gastric pH.[19] Feeding tubes should therefore be flushed after each meal or at least at daily intervals (although some authorities recommend 4-hourly flushing) with water but also with continuous feeding. Obstructed tubes should generally be replaced. Sriram and colleagues in a non-randomised study compared two groups to assess means of preventing tube blockage. After flushing enteral tubes with water, those in the study group received a 5 ml suspension of pancreatic enzymes with added bicarbonate, whilst the control group received none. Mean observation of the control group was 25 days, whilst that of the study group was 48. There were eight episodes of occlusion in the control group with one in the study group. The authors concluded that the use of pancreatic enzyme flushing is a reasonable approach in tube care.[20]

Knotting of a feeding tube in the stomach or the small bowel may render tube withdrawal difficult. Knotting appears to occur most frequently with weighted enteral tubes. The cause of this complication remains obscure. Should the tube become stuck it may be removed by cutting it at the lowest possible point, enabling evacuation per rectum. Alternatively, endoscopic intervention may allow successful tube removal.

Accidental feeding tube removal cannot be prevented and is a frequent and expected complication of nasoenteral tubes but rarely occurs with PEG or NCJ.[21] These routes are therefore the ones of choice following multiple removals of transnasal feeding tubes and for long-term feeding in any patient group.

Breakage and leakage of feeding tubes are nowadays rare owing to the use of softer catheter materials. If breakage occurs, per-nasal tubes should then be replaced. Following difficult primary tube placement (e.g. endoscopically aided tube placement for oeso-phageal carcinoma) replacement may be attempted over a guidewire following instillation of a lubricant (dextran, medium-chain triglycerides). This must, however, be undertaken under fluorographic control. Damage to the external parts of some tubes (e.g. PEG, NCJ) may be repaired using silicone adhesives (with silicone tubes) or solvents (with polyurethane tubes), which may be supplied by the tube manufacturer from whom advice should be sought, but simple exchange replacement may be more cost effective and quicker.

Leakage, infection and bleeding at the insertion site are minor complications in about 5% of PEGs.[22,23] It has been suggested that PEGs are potential reservoirs for methicillin-resistant *Staphylococcus aureus* colonisation.[24] If this is suspected, investigation and treatment should be undertaken under the supervision of a microbiologist. Persistent leakage along the exit stoma track of gastric or jejunal feeding tubes may indicate a distal obstruction of the intestinal tract. This will need to be investigated by appropriate clinical examination and imaging and if confirmed, treatment of the underlying problem is a priority and enteral feeding should be delayed until after the appropriate treatment.

Erosion, airway obstruction, ulceration and necrosis have all been described at different locations in association with enteral tubes. These are discussed in Chapter 17. Treatment of such complications requires removal of the feeding tube and reassessment of the best feeding method, although with appropriate care these complications should now be very rare.

Haemorrhage may complicate per-nasal feeding tube insertion in patients with liver cirrhosis and oesophageal varices.[25] Operative gastrostomy or jejunostomy have therefore been proposed for many years as the procedures of choice[26] but these patients are at increased risk from surgery. Furthermore, portosystemic shunts have reportedly developed between the intestinal tract and the abdominal wall and lead to bleeding complications at the tube insertion site.[27] Many units prefer to feed via soft fine-bore per-nasal tubes in these patients.

Parenteral nutrition can be infused enterally without major risk. In contrast, parenteral application of enteral formulae may be fatal.[28] Connectors of parenteral and enteral systems should therefore be strictly incompatible and most systems do fulfil this requirement, although systems vary from country to country.

Gastrointestinal complications

Gastrointestinal complications result from enteral feeding either performed with sub-optimal techniques (e.g. contamination, temperature) or which does not respect the patient's ability to tolerate feeding (e.g. constituent nutritive substrates, osmolarity, infusion rate, bolus versus continuous application). A recent study of 400 intensive care patients evaluated the frequency of gastrointestinal complications in critically ill patients receiving enteral nutrition.[29] The incidence of complications is listed in Table 19.2. It must be emphasised that this study was in critically ill patients and represents a 'worst-case scenario' for complications.

Table 19.2 – Incidence of gastrointestinal complications in critically ill patients

	%
High gastric residual volumes (≥200 ml 6 hourly)	39
Constipation	15.7
Diarrhoea (≥5 liquid stools 24h or ≥21 daily)	14.7
Abdominal distension	13.2
Vomiting	12.2
Regurgitation	5.5

The aetiology of enteral feed-related diarrhoea is addressed in Chapter 18. Often more than one potential cause of diarrhoea can be identified in a particular individual. For example, a patient who has undergone major surgery which required total parenteral nutrition may have some degree of mucosal atrophy and also be prescribed antibiotics. The management and treatment may need to address the underlying issues or be undertaken on a purely empirical basis. Failure of management by medical therapies means that other causes should be considered. A recent report identified the cause of death of an enterally fed patient as malnutrition caused by diarrhoea. Enteral feeding was taking place through a jejunostomy tube that had migrated anterogradely, creating an unsuspected 'short bowel'. Contrast studies would have identified the problem had they been undertaken through the jejunostomy.[30] It is likely that the presence of a nutrition team might have also avoided the fatal outcome in this particular case.

There are a number of key points to explore when diarrhoea is present. One of these is to appropriately quantify stool output. A new tabular tool has been validated which can assist this process which may be useful in some units.[31] Rapid administration of enteral formulae is a potential cause of gastrointestinal complications, including dumping and diarrhoea. This is particularly relevant with small-bowel administration of diet. Pump-controlled feeding ensures appropriateness of feed rates.

Lactose deficiency develops in the majority of the European population during the first and second decades of life unrelated to dietary lactose intake.[32,33] Thus, adults tolerate limited amounts of lactose when compared with children. Depending on the population under investigation, the prevalence of intolerance to the lactose content of one glass of milk has been reported to range from 0% to 75% (mean 19).[32] Furthermore, tolerance of lactose appears to decrease in the presence of malnutrition and gastrointestinal disease (secondary lactose intolerance).[33,34] Although most tube feeds are lactose free, it is not unknown for patients to supplement tube feeding with oral milk. It is therefore important to review the diet for presence of lactose and the patient for evidence of lactose deficiency or any other malabsorptive enteropathy.

Disturbances of lipid digestion and absorption have been reported in malnourished individuals, in patients with pancreatic and hepatobiliary disease, following gastric resection and with changes of the intestinal bacterial microflora. The underlying causes include inadequate secretion of bile and lipases as well as incomplete mechanical mixing of nutrients and these secretions. The resulting incomplete digestion and absorption may lead to diarrhoea and resultant nutritional deficits. Again, close clinical review and review of dietary components may identify a need for dietary modification.

Hypoalbuminaemia has historically received much attention as a potential cause of intolerance for enteral feeding.[35,36,37] Diarrhoea has been observed frequently in patients with albumin values below 30 g/l, in contrast to individuals with a serum albumin above 40 g/l. Results of experimental investigations have supported these clinical observations. It remains unclear, however, whether low albumin concentrations are merely indicative or a true cause of intolerance for enteral nutrition. Care should be taken in initiating enteral nutrition in individuals with serum albumin levels of less than 30 g/l but the most important aspect of care is to improve nutritional state and this may require therapeutic control of the enteral nutrition-related diarrhoea with drugs.

Various drugs in addition to antibiotics can cause diarrhoea.[38] Substances that have been implicated include antacids containing magnesium salts, digoxin, guanethidine, methyldopa, propranolol, chinidin and electrolyte concentrates. Treatment should be directed at the cause of the problem. The drugs should be reviewed or administered parenterally if required clinically.

Stool culture and endoscopy should be considered if diarrhoea does not respond to these measures after 3 days or so.[39] Pseudomembranous colitis is a complication observed with increasing frequency. The responsible organism, *Clostridium difficile*, is sensitive to antibiotic treatment (e.g. metronidazole, vancomycin). Recent studies have shown that the incidence of *Clostridium difficile*-associated diarrhoea is higher in hospitalised tube-fed patients than non-tube-fed patients and that this risk is increased in those receiving postpyloric feeding.[40]

The treatment of diarrhoea should always aim at elimination of the cause of the complication. Reduction in feeding rate, change of formula or addition of fibre may be indicated. Adequate volume replacement is mandatory and may require an intravenous line. Maintenance of fluid balance has priority over feeding.

Where the primary cause cannot be eliminated (e.g. clinically indicated antibiotics), symptomatic therapy must be used. Pharmacological agents such as loperamide or codeine phosphate should be used. Stopping enteral feeding is a last resort, because in most cases diarrhoea can be controlled.

Constipation is an increasingly recognised common complication during tube feeding. A combination of reduced mobility and inadequate fluid replacement is most commonly responsible. Thus, appropriate fluid replacement is the correct prophylactic measure (including an allowance of 800 ml/day of insensible losses in addition to measurable loss) after the initial bout of constipation has been treated by suppository or enema. The possibility of spurious diarrhoea being present as a result of constipation emphasises the need for rectal examination to be undertaken when clinically appropriate in all enterally fed patients with persistent diarrhoea.

Reflux, nausea, vomiting and aspiration

Nausea and bloating are symptoms experienced by many patients and may have no direct relevance to enteral nutrition. However, clinical review will assist in determining any link.

Pulmonary aspiration of gastric and small bowel contents is a potentially life-threatening complication of enteral nutrition; reported frequencies range from 0% to 38%.[41,42] Aspiration may occur without vomiting, subsequent to gastric and/or small bowel reflux.[43] The size of nasogastric tube can significantly alter the risk of gastro-oesophageal reflux, particularly in children, emphasising the need to choose the finest bore tube possible.[44] Patients with tracheostomy and those with neurologic deficit are at greatest risk. Aspiration was identified as the leading cause of death in 9.5% of 720 neurologic patients at autopsy. The risk of aspiration was increased by a factor of 10 in tube-fed individuals.[42,45,46] A history of recent pneumonia represents a further risk factor for aspiration and subsequent pneumonia. Feeding via a percutaneous endoscopic gastrostomy (PEG) does not necessarily diminish these risks.[47]

These observations make the case for alternative access routes for enteral alimentation in patients at risk (e.g. double-lumen gastric aspiration/jejunostomy feeding) (see Chapter 17). Additionally, the use of a prokinetic agent such as cisapride (at a dose of 10 mg 6 hourly) has been shown to be of use in the ICU by decreasing gastric residual volumes and increasing gastric emptying, thereby allowing enteral feeding.[48]

The degree of reflux depends significantly on the position of the feeding tube's tip. Using a constant infusion (120 ml/h) in healthy volunteers, reflux was observed in 6% of those with the tube tip in the duodenum, 4% with the tip near the ligament of Treitz and 0.4% with the tip *distal* to the ligament of Treitz. As the infusion rate increased, so did the incidence of reflux.[47]

For prophylaxis of aspiration, gastric feeding of unconscious patients should only be performed if a minimum of 30° elevation of thorax, head and neck can be achieved. Postpyloric feeding is preferable but the position of the tip of the tube must always be confirmed by X-ray or endoscopy. Even under these conditions, the tube may still displace into the stomach. Some units preferentially use NCJ in patients undergoing laparotomy and major abdominal surgery as this may offer protection against reflux and secondary displacement if adequately placed and checked prior to initiation of feeding.[49,50]

Clinical suspicion of pulmonary aspiration requires immediate cessation of feeding and verification by chest X-ray and arterial blood gas analysis. Treatment may require antibiotics, steroids and bronchial lavage and in some cases, ventilation may be required. This is a serious complication with a potentially fatal outcome. Pulmonary oedema, pneumonia or abscess are potential consequences of aspiration.

Other gastrointestinal complications

Data are not available on the frequency of gastrointestinal bleeding in association with tube feeding. A protective effect of tube feeding (by the raising of intragastric pH) has been suggested but remains unproven. Active gastrointestinal bleeding, however, is an accepted contraindication for enteral nutrition. Parenteral feeding, antacids and acid-blocking agents may all be needed.

Presentation of an acutely distended tender abdomen in any patient is an emergency and requires full assessment. Even in the presence of enteral feeding, a complication of enteral feeding as a cause is only one of the differential diagnoses and should not be immediately assumed to be the reason for the presenting symptoms.

Very occasionally, differential diagnosis of the acute abdomen during tube feeding requires special consideration of tube-feeding complications in addition to the more generally accepted causes. A rare syndrome of painful distension of the abdomen with fluorographic evidence of distended small and large bowel in the presence of increased or reduced peristaltic sounds and signs of hypovolaemia (tachycardia, hypotension) has been described during early postoperative feeding of elemental diet.[51] Conservative treatment is required in this situation, including temporary cessation of feeding and decompression of the gastrointestinal tract by suction. Operative decompression is only rarely indicated.

Pneumatosis intestinalis and necrotising enterocolitis are related diagnostic entities with difficult differential diagnoses and therapies.[52,53,54] The main symptom is a painful and distended abdomen during tube feeding in the early postoperative period. Plain X-ray will show air in the wall of the intestine, confirming the diagnosis. Reasons postulated for the accumulation of gas include insufficient decompression of the proximal intestinal tract, postoperative motor dysfunction and/or increased intestinal gas production due to the high carbohydrate load of the feeding formula. Enteral feeding must be stopped and proximal decompression of gut undertaken by tube. Stimulation of the intestinal motor activity may be beneficial. However, intramural gas can also be seen in 5–16% of patients with vascular or toxic bowel necrosis.[54] Intramural gas should almost always be further investigated by specialist imaging, laparoscopy or exploratory laparotomy.

Metabolic and other complications of enteral feeding

Patients requiring enteral feeding often have other underlying diseases, including diabetes mellitus, renal and hepatic insufficiency. Metabolic complications of enteral nutrition are similar to those of parenteral nutrition but are normally less severe owing to the homeostatic properties of the intestinal tract.[55] Each, however, needs to be anticipated and prevented before becoming a clinical problem.

Imbalances of volume and disturbances of the electrolyte pattern are comparatively frequent, especially in elderly patients. These risks require precise monitoring of fluid balance and of electrolytes, urea and creatinine.

The tube feeding syndrome is caused by hypertonic dehydration with elevated serum concentrations of sodium, chlorine, ammonia and chloride.[56,57,58] This complication is caused by inadequate volume replacement rather than by the use of a hyperosmotic formula. In recent years, methods for volume monitoring and replacement have been greatly improved so this syndrome should be rarely seen.

Electrolyte disturbances (see Table 19.3) are common but generally easily corrected according to standard medical regimens.

Table 19.3 – Incidence of electrolyte abnormalities in enterally fed patients[66]

	%
Hyperkalaemia	40
Hyponatraemia	31
Hypophosphataemia	30
Hyperglycaemia	29
Hyperphosphataemia	14
Hypozincaemia	11
Hypernatraemia	10
Hypokalaemia	<10
Hypomagnesaemia	<10
Hypocupraemia	<10
Hypoglycaemia	<10

Vitamin and trace element replacement require monitoring and precise substitution to avoid deficiency symptoms (see Chapter 11). In particular, the high metabolic demand for phosphorus in hypermetabolic patients (e.g. trauma, surgery, sepsis) should be considered and substituted according to the patient's need (oral supplements of 1 g/day of phosphorus are available)[59] as acute hypophosphataemia is well recognised in the severely malnourished patient being re-fed and, if unrecognised, can be fatal.[60]

Drug interactions

It is common practice to administer medications and drugs via enteral tubes, either by disconnection or via Y-connectors. This applies not only to liquid but also to solid medication in tablet form, which may be crushed. A recent randomised crossover study determined the effects of enteral feeds on ciprofloxacin absorption when given orally or via gastrostomy or jejunostomy. The study showed a 25–67% reduction in the mean bioavailability of ciprofloxacin. This reinforces the need to consider enteral nutrition as the cause of problems if a drug treatment appears not to be working or if a previously stable patient on regular medication (e.g. for hypertension or epilepsy[61,62] becomes unstable.[63] Some medications (e.g. tacrolimus) can be administered without absorption characteristics being altered.[64]

Infective complications

The infective complications of total parenteral nutrition are widely recognised and ways and means of reducing the incidence of intravenous catheter-related infection or sepsis have been well defined. The complication of infection associated with enteral nutrition has been less recognised possibly because enteral nutrition has not always been advocated as first-line nutrition support for the critically ill patient. In recent years, however, the proportion of patients being fed in intensive therapy units by enteral nutrition has increased and this has highlighted the possibility of infectious episodes in these patients being directly related to the administration of enteral diet. These issues and means of reducing the risks of clinically significant bacterial contamination problems are discussed in Chapter 17. In general, however, extra vigilance should be undertaken in the critically ill and the immunocompromised patient.

Monitoring

The key to anticipating and preventing complications is to have fixed administration protocols (which may vary from hospital to hospital and from unit to unit, dependent on the type of patient being fed). One of the most important aspects of this is to ensure appropriate monitoring of any patient on enteral feeding. The British Association for Parenteral and Enteral Nutrition has suggested guidelines for monitoring patients.[65] Table 19.4 is a modification of that and can

Table 19.4 – Monitoring enteral nutrition

Area monitored	Parameter	Frequency of monitoring	Rationale	Responsibility
Nutritional	a) Assess nutrient intake from enteral nutrition and normal diet b) Determine actual amount delivered	a) Regular diet charts – start and end of feed period and as clinically indicated b) Daily	To ensure patient receives amount of nutrient indicated and amount prescribed; if not, feeding method may be inappropriate	Dietitian (if available)
Anthropometric	a) Weight b) BMI c) Triceps skinfold thickness d) Mid-arm circumference	a) Weekly b) Start of feeding c) Monthly d) Monthly	To assess nutrition status and to assess whether nutrition goals are being met, short and long term without excess fat deposition	Nurse or dietitian
Biochemical	a) Urea and electrolytes b) Blood glucose c) Liver function tests – including plasma proteins d) Full blood count e) Phosphate f) Urine electrolytes g) Specific tests – e.g. 24h urinary nitrogen h) Vitamin and trace element/mineral status	a–e) Daily for first week of feeding; if stable, weekly or two weekly f) g) Weekly if indicated h) At start of feeding if severely malnourished and if feeding prolonged, as clinically indicated	To ensure patient is metabolically stable and not prone to potentially dangerous electrolyte or metabolic abnormalities, and to anticipate the need for change in formulation or addition of substrates in cases of deficiency	Clinician/biochemist
Clinical	a) General status (e.g. pyrexia, infection, etc.) b) Gastrointestinal function c) Tube integrity d) Pump function e) Drug chart review	a–e) Daily	To ensure patient is tolerating and benefiting from enteral nutrition and that complications are seen early and prevented	All

be adapted for local relevance, for example, in countries which do not have dietitians always available. In some units undertaking research, the measurements may be more frequent.

There will be occasions on which complications arise unexpectedly or occur but cannot be prevented due to some aspects of the patients disease or concurrent therapeutic interventions. Table 19.5 gives suggestions on the prevention or management of certain key complications. Again such suggestions may need to be adapted for local conditions and regulations.

Summary

In summary, complications may be best avoided if they are anticipated. Type and frequency of tube feeding-related complications are dependent on the underlying disease, the route of access to the gastrointestinal tract and the type of feeding formula employed. Individual assignment of feeding regimens to each patient and close monitoring are the best means of prevention, with monitoring with the assistance of specialist teams. Awareness of the existence, frequency and aetiological factors of complications represents the most important means of preventing them.

Table 19.5 – Prevention and management of key complications

Type of complication	Specific complication	Key concerns	Prevention and management
Gastrointestinal	Gastric aspiration and reflux	a) Tube position b) Gastric residual volume	a) Confirm tube position by either aspiration with syringe and pH 1–3 of aspirate or auscultation of 20–30 ml introduced into stomach or abdominal X-ray/fluoroscopy (advised for any obtunded patient but not as a routine method) b) If gastric residual volume >200 ml review regimen and assess patient's gastric emptying
	Bloating, nausea, vomiting	a) As for gastric aspiration and reflux b) Rate of administration c) Tube integrity d) Enteral feed load e) Central or iatrogenic cause	a) As for gastric aspiration and reflux b) Review rate and reduce if indicated c) Ensure tube not knotted or other problem d) Review load (rate × volume) and reduce if indicated e) Review drug therapy – antiemetic if indicated
	Diarrhoea	a) Confirm diarrhoea is present	a) Review medical history, current drug therapy (e.g. laxatives, antibiotics), review fibre intake, check for constipation, review enteral formulation, stool sample for analysis, feed sample for analysis, check tube integrity. If no specific cause prescribe antidiarrhoeal – avoid stopping enteral nutrition without good reason
Infective	Feed contamination or patient infection	a) Exogenous source b) Endogenous source	a) Review all components of enteral feed administration including sources, handlers, reservoirs, giving sets and tubes; take appropriate microbiology samples; replace components or alter practice as indicated b) Review all aspects of patient's clinical status for sources of infection – treat as appropriate
Other complications	Failure of drug therapy	a) Drug charts b) Enteral feeds	a) Review type and dose of drugs, route of administration, whether still indicated; seek specific information about interaction with enteral feeds and specific incompatibilities from manufacturers, pharmacists and dietitians and change as indicated b) As a)

References

1. Delany M, Carnevale NJ, Garvey JW, Moss CM. Postoperative nutritional support using needle catheter jejunostomy. *Ann Surg* 1977; **186:** 165–70.

2. Schattenkenk ME, Obertop H, Bruining HA, Van Royen W, Van Hauten H. Early postoperative enteral feeding by a catheter jejunostomy after 100 oesophageal resections and reconstructions for cancer. *Clin Nutr* 1984; **3:** 47–9.

3. Bodoky A, Heberer M, Iwatschenko P, Harder F. Die Katheterjejunostomie in der elektiven Abdominalchirurgic. *Chirurgie* 1985; **56:** 644–50.

4. Smith RC, Hartemink RI, Hollinshead JW, Gillett DJ. Fine bore jejunostomy feeding following major abdominal surgery: a controlled randomized clinical trial. *Br J Surg* 1985; **72:** 458–61.

5. Heberer M, Bodoky A, Iwatschenko P, Harder F. Indications for needle catheter jejunostomy in elective abdominal surgery. *Am J Surg* 1987; **153:** 545–52.

6. Daly JM, Bonau R, Stofberg P, Bloch A, Jeevanandam M, Morse M. Immediate postoperative jejunostomy feeding. *Am J Surg* 1987; **153:** 198–204.

7. Heymsfield SB, Bethel RA, Ansley JJD, Nixon DW, Rudmann D. Enteral hyperalimentation: an alternative to central venous hyperalimentation. *Ann Intern Med* 1979; **90:** 63–71.

8. Pattison D, Young A. Effect of a multi-disciplinary care team on the management of gastrostomy feeding. *J Human Nutr Dietet* 1997; **10:** 103–9.

9. Druml W, Kleinberger G, Base W, Haller JJ, Laggner A, Lenz K. Lung perforation by nasogastric feeding tubes. *Clin Nutr* 1984; **2:** 197–9.

10. Saitzberg DM, Goldstein MM, Levine GM. Feeding-tube induced pneumothorax. *J Parent Enteral Nutr* 1984; **8:** 714–16.

11. Eldar S, Meguid MM. Pneumothorax following attempted nasogastric intubation for nutritional support. *J Parent Enteral Nutr* 1984; **8:** 450–2.

12. Valentine RJ, Turner WW. Pleural complications of nasoenteric feeding tubes. *J Parent Enteral Nutr* 1985; **9:** 605–7.

13. Lipman TO, Kessler T, Arabian A. Nasopulmonary intubation with feeding tubes: case report and review of the literature. *J Parent Enteral Nutr* 1985; **9:** 618–20.

14. Olbrantz KR, Gelfand D, Choplin R, Wu WC. Pneumothorax complicating enteral feeding tube placement. *J Parent Enteral Nutr* 1985; **9:** 210–11.

15. Roubenoff R, Ravich WJ. Pneumothorax due to nasogastric feeding tubes: report of four cases, review of the literature, and recommendations for prevention. *Arch Intern Med* 1989; **149:** 184–8.

16. Blebea J, King TA. Intraperitoneal infusion as a complication of needle catheter feeding jejunostomy. *J Parent Enteral Nutr* 1985; **9:** 758–9.

17. Seebacher J, Nozik D, Mathieu A. Inadvertent intracranial introduction of a nasogastric tube: a complication of severe maxillofacial trauma. *Anaesthesia* 1975; **42:** 100–2.

18. Siegle RL, Rabinowitz JG, Sarasohn C. Intestinal perforation secondary to nasojejunal feeding tubes. *Am J Roentgenol* 1976; **126:** 1229–32.

19. Turner JS, Fyfe AR, Kaplan DK, Wardlaw AJ. Oesophageal obstruction during nasogastric feeding. *Intens Care Med* 1991; **17:** 302–3.

20. Sriram K, Jayanthi V, Lakshmi RG et al. Prophylactic locking of enteral feeding tubes with pancreatic enzymes. *J Parent Enteral Nutr* 1997; **21:** 353–6.

21. Goodman P, Levine MS, Parkman HP. Extrusion of PEG tube from the stomach with fistula formation: an unusual complication of percutaneous endoscopic gastrostomy. *Gastrointest Radiol* 1991; **16:** 286–8.

22. Jarnagin WR, Dub QY, Mulvihill J, Ridge JA, Schrock TR, Way L. The efficacy and limitations of percutaneous endoscopic gastrostomy. *Arch Surg* 1992; **127:** 261–4.

23. Gibson SE, Wenig BL, Watkins JL. Complications of percutaneous endoscopic gastrostomy in head and neck cancer patients. *Ann Otol Rhinol Laryngol* 1992; **101:** 43–50.

24. Nunley D, Berk SL. Percutaneous endoscopic gastrostomy as an unrecognized source of methicillin-resistant Staphylococcus aureus colonization. *Am J Gastroenterol* 1992; **87:** 58–61.

25. McGovern R, Barkin JS, Goldberg RI, Phillips RS. Duodenal obstruction: a complication of percutaneous endoscopic gastrostomy tube migration. *Am J Gastroenterol* 1990; **85:** 1037–8.

26. Bernard M, Forlaw L. Complications and their prevention. In: Rombeau JC, Caldwell MD (eds) Enteral and tube feeding. WB Saunders, Philadelphia, 1984, 542–69.

27. Edington H, Zajko A, Reilly JJ. Jejunal variceal hemorrhage: an unusual complication of needle catheter jejunostomy. *J Parent Enteral Nutr* 1983; **7:** 489–91.

28. Stellato TA, Danziger LIA, Nearman HS, Creger RJ. Inadvertent intravenous administration of enteral diet. *J Parent Enteral Nutr* 1984; **8:** 4.

29. Montejo JC. Enteral nutrition-related gastrointestinal complications in critically ill patients: a multicenter study. *Crit Care Med* 1999; **27:** 1447–53.

30. Prahlow JA, Barnard JJ. Jejunostomy tube failure: malnutrition caused by intraluminal antegrade jejunostomy tube migration. *Arch Phys Med Rehab* 1998; **79:** 453–5.

31. Guenter PA, Sweed MR. A valid and reliable tool to quantify stool output in tube-fed patients. *J Parent Enteral Nutr* 1998; **22:** 147–51.

32. Newcomer AD, McGill DB. Clinical importance of lactose deficiency. *N Engl J Med* 1984; **310:** 42–3.

33. Rothauve HW, Ernous D, Flatz G. Die Hdufigkeit der Laktoseintoleranz bei gesunden Erwachsenen in Deutschland. *Dsch Med Wschr* 1972; **97:** 376–8.

34. Chernoff R. Enteral feeding. *Am J Hosp Pharm* 1980; **37:** 65–74.

35. Brinson RR, Kolts ME. Hypoalbuminemia as an indicator of diarrhoeal incidence in critically ill patients. *Crit Care Med* 1987; **15:** 506–9.

36. Moss G. Postoperative ileus is an avoidable complication. *Surg Gynecol Obstet* 1979; **148:** 81–2.

37. Cobb LM, Cartmill AM, Gilsdorf RB. Early postoperative nutritional support using the serosal tunnel jejunostomy. *J Parent Enteral Nutr* 1981; **5:** 397–401.

38. Guenter PA, Settle PG, Perlmutter S, Marino L, DeSimone GA, Rolandelli RH. Tube feeding-related diarrhoea in acutely ill patients. *J Parent Enteral Nutr* 1991; **15:** 277–80.

39. Jolliet P, Pichard C, Biolo G *et al*. Enteral nutrition in intensive care patients: a practical approach. *Clin Nutr* 1999; **18:** 47–56.

40. Bliss DZ, Johnson S, Savik K *et al*. Acquisition of Clostridium difficile and Clostridium difficile-associated diarrhoea in hospitalised patients receiving tube feeding. *Ann Intern Med* 1998; **129:** 1012–19.

41. Newmark SR, Simpson MS, Beskitt MP. Home tube-feeding for long-term nutritional support. *J Parent Enteral Nutr* 1981; **5:** 76–9.

42. Winterbauer RH, Durning RB, Barron E, McFadden MC. Aspirated nasogastric feeding solution detected by glucose strips. *Ann Intern Med* 1981; **95:** 67–8.

43. Kingston GW, Phang PT, Leathley MJ. Increased incidence of nosocomial pneumonia in mechanically ventilated patients with subclinical aspiration. *Am J Surg* 1991; **161:** 589–92.

44. Noviski N, Yehuda Y, Serour F *et al*. Does the size of nasogastric tubes affect gastroesophageal reflux in children? *J Parent Enteral Nutr* 1999; **29:** 448–51.

45. Olivares L, Segovia A, Revuetta R. Tube feeding and lethal aspiration in neurological patients: a review of 720 autopsy cases. *Stroke* 1974; **5:** 654–62.

46. Spray SB, Zuidma GD, Cameron JL. Aspiration pneumonia: incidence of aspiration with endotracheal tubes. *Am J Surg* 1976; **131:** 701–3.

47. Gustke RF, Varma RR, Soergel K. II. Gastric reflux during perfusion of the proximal small bowel. *Gastroenterology* 1970; **6:** 890–5.

48. Spapen HD, Duinslaeger L, Diltoer M *et al*. Gastric emptying in critically ill patients is accelerated by adding cisapride to a standard enteral feeding protocol: results of a prospective, randomised, controlled trial. *Crit Care Med* 1995; **23:** 481–5.

49. Heberer M, Bodoky A, Iwatschenko P, Harder F. Indications for needle catheter jejunostomy in elective abdominal surgery. *Am J Surg* 1987; **153:** 545–52.

50. Weltz CR, Morris JB, Mullen J. Surgical jejunostomy in aspiration risk patients. *Ann Surg* 1992; **215:** 140–5.

51. Bruining HA, Schattenkerk ME, Obertop H, Ong G. Acute abdominal pain due to early postoperative elemental feeding by needle jejunostomy. *Surg Gynecol Obstet* 1983; **157:** 40–2.

52. Thompson JS. Pneumatosis intestinalis and needle catheter jejunostomy: a word of caution. *J Parent Enteral Nutr* 1983; **7:** 495.

53. Cogbill TH, Wolfson RH, Moore EE *et al*. Massive pneumatosis intestinalis and subcutaneous emphysema: complication of needle catheter jejunostomy. *J Parent Enteral Nutr* 1983; **7:** 171–3.

54. Berne TV, Halls JM. Intramural intestinal gas in adults. *Surg Gynecol Obstet* 1983; **156:** 479–84.

55. Sheldon GF, Baker C. Complications of nutritional support. *Crit Care Med* 1980; **8:** 35–7.

56. Telfer N, Persoff M. The effect of tube feeding in the hydration of elderly patients. *J Gerontol* 1965; **20:** 536–43.

57. Walike JW. Tube feeding syndrome in head and neck surgery. *Arch Otolaryngol* 1969; **89:** 533–6.

58. Kaminsky MV. A review of hyperosmolar hyperglycemic nonketotic dehydration (HHND): etiology, pathophysiology and prevention during intravenous hyperalimentation. *J Parent Enteral Nutr* 1978; **2:** 690–8.

59. Hayek ME, Eisenberg PG. Severe hypophosphatemia following the institution of enteral feedings. *Arch Surg* 1989; **124:** 1325–8.

60. Payne-James JJ, Rees RG, Newton MA, Silk DBA. Acute respiratory failure and hypophosphataemia in anorexia nervosa. *J Clin Nutr Gastroent* 1988; **3:** 67–8.

61. Bauer LA. Interference of oral phenytoin absorption by continuous nasogastric feedings. *Neurology* 1982; **32:** 57–62.

62. Saklad JJ, Graver RH, Sharp WP. Interaction of oral phenytoin with enteral feedings. *J Parent Enteral Nutr* 1986; **10:** 322–3.

63. Healy DP, Brodbeck MC, Clendening CE. Ciprofloxacin absorption is impaired in patients given enteral feedings orally and via gastrostomy and jejunostomy tubes. *Antimicrob Agents Chemother* 1996; **40:** 6–10.

64. Murray M, Grigan TA, Lever J *et al.* Comparison of tacrolimus absorption in transplant patients receiving continuous versus interrupted enteral nutritional feeding. *Ann Pharmacother* 1998; **32:** 633–6.

65. McAtear CA. Current perspectives on enteral nutrition in adults. BAPEN, Maidenhead, 1999.

66. Vanlandingham S, Simpson S, Daniel P, Newmark SR. Metabolic abnormalities in patients supported with enteral tube feeding. *J Parent Enteral Nutr* 1981; **5:** 322.

20

Paediatric enteral nutrition

Anita MacDonald, Chris Holden and Tracey Johnson

Introduction

Feeding children with chronic disease is a challenge to all involved in their care. They are particularly vulnerable to growth and nutritional problems during critical periods of development. Major illness, operations or trauma impose increased metabolic demands on already high energy and protein requirements. This is coupled with lower energy reserves and a changing body size and composition. It is, thus, not surprising that malnutrition complicates many childhood diseases and a proportion of children admitted to hospital have reported undernutrition.[1-5] Because malnutrition is serious and has potential long-term consequences, its prevention and treatment are important goals. Enteral tube feeding has been shown to be safe and efficacious for children and increasingly, home enteral nutrition support is used for children with chronic conditions. In 2000, in the UK, almost 3500 children less than 16 years of age were receiving home enteral tube feeding.[6] As a consequence, the development of specialised paediatric formulae and delivery equipment has become an exciting and rapidly expanding industry.

Nutritional vulnerability of infants and children

Low energy reserves

A growing child has a relatively low energy reserve.[7] The smaller the child, the shorter the period before tissue catabolism will commence: skeletal muscle proteins and, at times, visceral protein rapidly become a source of energy. The estimated body fat content of an infant weighing less than 1000 g is approximately 1% of body weight, so the baby would only survive three to four days during acute starvation. A 3.5 kg term infant would only survive 30 days under the same conditions.[8] Although data on body composition in children at various ages is limited, in a 9-year-old boy, fat provides just 13% of body mass and approximately 15-20% in adulthood, with theoretical starvation energy reserves varying from 50 to 100 days.[9]

Growth

During growth and development, an infant birth weight generally triples by 12 months of age and quadruples by three years of age. Birth length usually increases by 50% by the end of the first year of life with an approximately threefold increase by 10 years.[10] Nutritional requirements are, therefore, greater than those of adults to meet the extra requirements of growth[11] (Table 20.1). Infants during the first year require 397-481 kJ (95–115 kcal)/kg/day,[12] gradually falling to approximately 251–314 kJ (60–75 kcal)/kg/day for a 10-year-old and 126–167 kJ (30–40 kcal)/kg/day for a young adult. Newborn infants use 20–30% of their total energy intake for growth,[13] falling to 5% by one year.[14] Equally, neonatal protein requirements are almost four times higher than adults. Newborn infants require approximately 3.0 g/kg/day protein, decreasing to 1.5 g/kg/day by 10–12 months and 0.75 g/kg/day by adulthood. Essential amino acid requirements are approximately eight times higher than adults.

Table 20.1 – Nutritional requirements in children.[12]

| Age | Energy | | | | Protein g/kg/day |
| | kcals/kg/day | | kJ | | |
	Boys	Girls	Boys	Girls	
1 month	115	115	481.2	481.2	3.0
3 months	100	100	418.4	418.4	2.1
12 months	95	95	397.5	397.5	1.5
2 years	95	95	397.5	397.5	1.18
3 years	95	95	397.5	397.5	1.0
6 years	84	76	351.4	317.9	0.9
9 years	69	61	288.7	255.2	0.95

Consequences of malnutrition

The adverse effects of malnutrition are well known. In addition to disease-related morbidity, the consequences include:

Impaired brain growth and neuro-development

There is rapid brain growth and development during the first three years of life, with the brain reaching 70% of its adult size. This requires a significant number of calories and nutrients, and at birth the brain accounts for approximately two-thirds of basal metabolic rate.[14] Brain growth and development is particularly sensitive to periods of malnutrition, and absence of appropriate nutrients will have a permanent effect on brain function.[15] Trials on large numbers of preterm infants have clearly demonstrated that nutrition intervention in the early weeks has long-term benefits on mental development. They have also suggested that suboptimal neonatal nutrition may lead to permanent impairment of cognitive function, particularly in boys.[16] Even deficiency of single nutrients during early childhood has long-term effects. Deficiency of iron, for example, has been shown to lead to a decline in psychomotor development.[17]

Impaired gastrointestinal function

Malnutrition in children can result in changes to gastrointestinal function. High rates of protein synthesis and turnover in the gastrointestinal tract make it remarkably sensitive.[18] In severe cases of malnutrition there may be villous atrophy, reduced disaccharidase activity, particularly lactase,[19] pancreatic enzyme insufficiency, hypochlorhydria, and altered intestinal bacteria, which can lead to malabsorption and worsening failure to thrive.

Increased susceptibility to infection

Infections are more frequent in children with malnutrition due to immunological abnormalities. These in turn can exacerbate the effects of poor nutrition with further loss of appetite, increase metabolic rate and nutritional requirements and cause diarrhoea. Catch-up growth becomes difficult to achieve with each episode of infection leading to further deterioration in nutrition status.

Delayed wound healing

Severe malnutrition may delay wound healing and impede the immune response to localised tissue infection. There is correlation between nutrition status, body weight and rate of wound healing. Nutrition intervention must be provided early enough to prevent a decline in lean muscle mass, which can further impair wound healing.[20]

Impaired growth and delayed puberty

The early effect of undernutrition is weight loss and wasting. More prolonged malnutrition may result in growth failure. This is seen commonly in children with chronic illnesses and severe developmental delay who have longstanding nutritional inadequacies. Delayed sexual development or secondary amenorrhoea is common in anorectic girls.

Altered mood and depression

Malnourished children are less active, less exploratory, and more apathetic.[21] Chronic undernutrition is associated with increased irritability, decreased motivation and less energy available for activities such as play and rehabilitation.

Specific nutrient deficiencies

With the exception of iron deficiency, the majority of micronutrient deficiencies are rare. Children with a globally inadequate nutritional intake will often exhibit signs of iron deficiency anaemia resulting from a poor intake of iron rich foods. In a group of 63 children with failure to thrive, in addition to low energy intakes, poor growth, and wide scale developmental delay (55%), a third had iron deficiency with low dietary iron intakes.[22]

Effect on early nutrition on long-term health

There is evidence that poor growth *in utero* and in infancy are contributory factors to the development of adult diseases such as coronary artery disease, hypertension and diabetes.[23,24]

Indications for enteral feeding in paediatrics

The indications for enteral feeding can be divided into five main categories:

1. Inadequate oral intake

Decreased appetite and inadequate dietary intake is commonly reported in many diseases. Anorexia accompanies disorders such as cystic fibrosis, renal disease and cancer. Breathlessness associated with respiratory and cardiac disorders or oral facial malformations may reduce food intake. Malnutrition may also result from chronic intermittent nausea and intractable vomiting associated with several disorders and their treatments. In hospital, there may be prolonged periods of fasting for tests or procedures, meals which, if not unpalatable, are different from home and inadequate supervision of mealtimes, especially of young children and those who require help with feeding. In older children and adolescents with anorexia nervosa, enteral nutrition can play a crucial role in treatment.

2. Increased nutrition requirements

Many infants and children with chronic or severe illnesses have a high requirement of nutrients, particularly energy and protein, and especially in chronic illnesses such as liver disease, cystic fibrosis, congenital heart disease, and acute events such as extensive burns. Anorexia is frequently associated with the disease state, so children are unable to meet their nutrition requirements only by eating.

3. Swallowing dysfunction

Inability to swallow, uncoordinated swallowing and severe gastro-oesophageal reflux are appropriate indications for enteral feeding. With uncoordinated swallowing a high risk of pulmonary aspiration and pneumonia occurs.[25] This is common in children with cerebral palsy and other neuro-degenerative disorders. Severe gastro-oesophageal reflux in infancy is sometimes managed by giving continuous enteral tube feeds until there is a maturation of lower oesophageal spincter function and reflux ceases or, failing this, by performing a surgical antireflux procedure.[26] In preterm infants, in whom the suck–swallow reflex does not develop until approximately 34 weeks of gestation, enteral nutrition is often used in the interim.[10]

4. Primary disease management

Crohn's disease: enteral nutrition is commonly recommended as the first-line treatment for most children and adolescents with this disorder.[27] This approach aids healing of the mucosa, down–regulation of inflammation[28] and is as effective as high doses of steroids in inducing remission.[29,30] It also improves nutritional state. There is evidence that amino acid feeds (elemental),[31] whole protein (polymeric)[32] and protein hydrolysate (semi-elemental)[33] feeds may all be successful.

Short bowel syndrome: The provision of enteral nutrition, even in small quantities is essential to help intestinal adaptation,[34,35] after small intestinal resection.[19] Feeds are usually administered by continuous feeding. This is to reduce problems with delayed gastric emptying and aid nutrient absorption;

continuous feeding has been associated with better weight gain than intermittent bolus feeding.[36]

Inherited metabolic disease: Children with conditions such as glycogen storage disease type 1 and long chain fatty acid disorders need a reliable and constant supply of the substrate glucose overnight to prevent hypoglycaemia. In addition, enteral tube feeding may be required to administer an emergency regimen during illness to minimise metabolic decompensation and help prevent neurological complications associated with many of these metabolic disorders.

5. Disease or injury to the oesophagus

Examples in paediatrics include oesophageal injury after ingestion of caustic soda chemicals or tracheo-oesophageal fistula.

Special clinical indications for enteral feeding in paediatrics

Cerebral palsy and neuro-developmental disorders

Children with severe neurological disorders have a markedly increased risk of malnutrition. In the UK, enteral nutrition is used more commonly for cerebral palsy and other neurological disorders than for any other childhood disease.[6] Oral feeding can be a particular problem. Motor dysfunction leads to various difficulties that can affect feeding such as poor head control, trunk control, and inability to sit upright and align the bodies correctly for eating.[37] In addition, fine-motor impairment, coupled with limited mobility, makes it difficult for children to take food from their plate or dish to their mouth. Oral motor dysfunction can lead to drooling, spillage of foodstuffs, and prolonged feeding times. Some children aspirate because of gastro-oesophageal reflux or swallowing dysfunction, leading to recurrent aspiration pneumonia and chronic lung disease.[38] Further problems include low calorie density of pureed foods, lack of appetite, food aversion,[39] poor dentition,[40,41] lack of communication between carer and child,[42] and constipation, probably adversely affecting appetite, slowing gastric emptying and exacerbating gastro-oesophageal reflux.[37]

Although there are reports of nutrition defects and growth retardation in cerebral palsy, the prevalence of nutrition problems in children with neurological disorders is unknown. In a large group of children with spastic quadriplegic cerebral palsy, aged 2–18 years, linear growth, assessed by upper-arm and lower-leg lengths, was significantly reduced relative to age and sex-specific reference norms for healthy children. Weight and triceps skinfold thickness were on average about 65% of age and sex medians.[43] Poor nutrition status was evident in children as young as two to four years. In a further study mean weight for height SD scores was less than −2 in a group of children with dystonic cerebral palsy.[44] In addition, cerebral palsy children are frequently observed to have decrease in muscle strength, reducing the effectiveness of the cough reflex and predisposing to aspiration pneumonia and an increase in circulation time in the limbs,[45] resulting in cold, and cyanotic extremities.[46]

There is only limited research on the nutritional needs of these patients, and recommended nutrient intake and ideal growth expectation is poorly defined and must be approached on an individual basis.[47] Only a few studies of energy expenditure have been reported in the literature. They have all indicated that energy expenditure is lower or similar to normal, depending on whether the type of cerebral palsy is athetoid or spastic.[47–49] It is inappropriate to use dietary reference values for age, and it may be better to base nutrition requirements on height age. Vitamin, mineral and protein requirements should also be calculated for height age.

Nutritional support has been shown to improve weight. Brandt et al[50] demonstrated in 20 children with neurological impairment and dysphagia significant improvements in weight and a trend towards improved weight/height ratio in children under 4 years of age. Naurechas and Christoffel[38] demonstrated in a group of children with neurological disabilities that percentage ideal body weight for height age increased from 72.3 to 94.2%. Some improvements in height have been documented, but less commonly.[40,51] For long-term feeding, gastrostomy feeding is the method of choice for children with neurological disorders. Ten-year survival rates have been shown to be better for children fed by gastrostomy as compared with nasogastric tubes.[52] Gastrostomy tube placement was often in combination with an antireflux procedure or fundoplication. This practice has now been questioned and there are successful reports of percutaneous endoscopic gastrostomy without anti-

reflux procedure in children with major neurological impairment.[53] However, on the negative side, enteral feeding is associated with: obesity;[51] osteopaenia, due to low volume of enteral feed administered and therefore low intake of vitamins and minerals;[54] and an increase in mortality in children with less severe disabilities associated with pulmonary disease secondary to over-zealous nutrition support and aspiration after tube placement.[55]

Cystic fibrosis (CF)

Growth retardation and undernutrition remain common complications of cystic fibrosis (CF).[56–58] Relative underweight has been identified as prognostic of both severity of pulmonary disease and survival.[59,60] Lung function has been shown to correlate positively with percentage body fat and weight for height in some,[61,62] but not all studies.[63] The nutrition problems are multifactorial and include increases in intestinal losses, energy requirements and urinary glucose losses and one or more factors almost invariably coexist in combination with an inadequate energy intake. In addition, abnormal bile salt metabolism, liver disease, mucosal absorptive abnormalities and short bowel syndrome, following intestinal resection in the neonatal period, may all contribute. Murphy et al[64] have estimated that stool energy losses account for 10.6% of gross energy intake in CF patients, three times higher than normal.

Up to 5% of children with CF, less than 16 years old, are on overnight enteral tube feeding in the UK. It is recommended that enteral feeding should begin if there is no weight gain over a 3-month period, or if the patient's weight/height ratio declines to less than 85% of ideal.[65]

Although energy requirements vary according to individual needs, and there is no standard formula to estimate needs,[66] it is common practice to give 30–50% of the patient's energy requirements via the overnight enteral tube feed. Long-term enteral feeding is associated with significant improvements in height and weight,[67] increased total body nitrogen, improved strength, development of secondary sexual characteristics, and an improvement in body image. However, if pulmonary function is poor (i.e. FEV_1 less than 40% predicted) at the start of enteral feeding, there is little improvement in nutrition status.[68] In addition, meta-analysis of nutrition studies has indicated that behavioural intervention appears to be just as effective in improving weight gain as enteral feeding.[69]

A variety of feed types have been used for enteral feeding including elemental, semi-elemental, polymeric and high fat feeds. No differences in fat malabsorption, nitrogen absorption and weight gains have been observed when semi-elemental and polymeric formula with enzyme replacement therapy has been compared.[70]

Childhood malignancies

Malnutrition, both at the start and continuation of intensive chemotherapy treatment programmes is commonly seen. Although not prevalent in all paediatric cancers, the incidence is related to the type of tumour and extent of the disease and criteria used to define malnutrition.[71] It varies from 6–50%.[72] Malnutrition occurs more frequently in children diagnosed with Ewing's sarcoma, Wilms' tumour, head and neck tumours, advanced lymphomas and neuroblastoma.[73] Children often develop cachexia and worsening of nutrition status during therapy. Intensive chemotherapy used in the advanced stages of malignancies have significant gastrointestinal toxicity, causing nausea, vomiting and diarrhoea.[71] Side-effects of radiation therapy include mucositis, dysphagia and diarrhoea. Malnutrition can also develop as a result of major operative procedures to the abdomen, or irradiation to the head, neck, oesophagus, abdomen and pelvis. In addition, poor appetite, learned food aversion,[74] altered taste,[75] poor eating habits and non-compliance with dietary regimens may also contribute to poor nutrition. However, there is little evidence of increased resting energy expenditure in children with cancer, except in cases of very high tumour burden.[76] Malnourished children may have decreased tolerance to chemotherapy, increased toxic effects of chemotherapy, and impaired cellular immunity.[77]

The assessment of nutrition status in cancer children is problematic. Although weight for height is commonly used as the main index of nutrition status, it is unreliable in children with large tumour masses. Mid-upper arm circumference is a better indication of nutrition status in cancer children. Smith and co-workers demonstrated in a group of 48 children with malignant solid tumours that height for age and weight for height did not differ from controls, but mid-upper arm circumference was significantly lower.[78]

Both nasogastric and gastrostomy feeds have been shown to be safe and efficacious in this group of children. Smith et al[79] demonstrated in a small group of children with newly diagnosed malignancy that it improved nutrition status as measured by mid-upper arm circumference, was well tolerated and produced apparent increase in child play-scale scores. Aquino et al[77] demonstrated that 60% of 25 children with cancer returned to a desirable body weight after an average of almost five months on gastrostomy tube feeds. The most common complications were 38 episodes of inflammation at the gastrostomy tube site during periods of severe neutropaenia. Mathew et al[80] also showed that 82% of 33 children maintained ideal body weight with gastrostomy tube feeds, although one or more minor complications occurred in the majority of the patients. Enteral tube feeding has also shown to be effective in post bone-marrow transplant patients with adequate gastrointestinal function.[81,82] In fact, when compared with parenteral nutrition (PN), hypoalbuminaemia and biochemical selenium deficiency was worse in the PN group.[81]

There are few guidelines on the energy requirements of children with malignancies. They must be individualised, but most children gain weight and grow when energy intake meets the estimated average requirement for age. Large volumes of feed are not well tolerated, and the use of a high energy density feed (6 kJ or 1.5 kcal/ml) may be advisable.[79]

Congenital heart disease (CHD)

Infants and young children with CHD and cyanosis, pulmonary hypertension and congestive heart failure appear to have an increased prevalence of growth failure. In an early study, Mehziri & Drash[83] reported that 52% of children with CHD were below the 16th percentile for height, and 55% were below the 16th percentile for weight. More recently Rosenthal stated that 60–70% of infants hospitalised with CHD were failing to thrive; 27% were below the 3rd percentile for both.[84] Barton et al[85] reported that mean body mass index was only 80% of expected values in 8 infants with CHD.

Numerous studies have described mechanisms of growth failure in paediatric patients with CHD. Hypoxia and breathlessness may lead to feeding problems; anorexia or even venous congestion of the bowel may result in malabsorption; peripheral anoxia and acidosis may lead to inefficient utilisation of nutrients;[86] and frequent respiratory illnesses may compromise nutritional status. Furthermore, total daily energy expenditure has been found to be increased,[85] possibly due to increased oxygen consumption by a hypertrophied heart and a stimulation of metabolism due to increased catecholamine secretion. Optimising nutrition status improves surgical outcome in children with CHD and may contribute to reduced morbidity during respiratory infections.

Clinical studies have demonstrated that enteral feeds, usually supplemented to provide a calorie density of 4.2 kJ (1 kcal)/ml are associated with significant short-term increases in growth and weight.[86–88]

Choice of enteral feed

Selecting the appropriate formula for paediatric patients depends on several factors including: nutritional requirements, gastrointestinal function, underlying disease, nutrient restrictions, additional requirements, age, physical properties of the feed, availability and cost. Paediatric formulae can be divided into four main categories: polymeric, hydrolysed protein, elemental and modular feeds.

Polymeric feeds

Infants 0–12 months

Full-term infants with normal gastrointestinal function are fed either breast milk or normal infant formula during the first year of life. They have a calorie density of 2.9 kJ (0.67 kcal)/ml.

If breast milk is used for continuous enteral feeds, care must be taken to adjust for nutrient losses due to separation of the fat and adherence to the tubing. Lipid losses may be as high as 20% but is less of a problem with intermittent bolus tube feeds. Alternatively, standard infant formulae based on whey or casein dominant protein, lactose, ± maltodextrin and amylase, vegetable oil and milk fat may be used. Although all infant formulae available in the UK have to meet compositional guidelines directed by 'The Infant Formula and Follow-on Regulations 1995' (which enact EC Regulations 91/321/EC in the UK), there are subtle differences between brands with regard to the addition of novel nutrients such as nucleotides, β-carotene and long chain polyunsaturated fatty acids.

For tube-fed infants failing to thrive or infants over the age of 4 months, a high energy and nutrient intake is required. This may be difficult to achieve with breast or standard infant formula milk. It has been common

practice to add energy supplements in the form of glucose polymer and fat emulsion or a combination of both. Glucose polymers have the advantage that they have less effect on osmolality than disaccharide at the same caloric density. Fat has little influence on osmolality and long chain fat emulsions are favoured over medium chain fat emulsions because they have a lower osmotic effect on the gut and provide a source of essential fatty acids. The addition of carbohydrate and fat emulsion to infant formula has not been fully evaluated in infants. Tolerance depends upon the age of the infant and the maturity and absorptive capacity of the gut. As a guideline an additional 5 g/100 ml of glucose polymer and 1.5 g/100 ml of fat is added to infant formulae to provide approximately 420 kJ (100 kcal)/100 ml. Although commonly used, this practice has several disadvantages. Preparation errors, feed contamination and dilution of nutrient composition can occur. In infant formulae, the protein:energy ratio should be kept within a range of 7.5–12%, and probably a minimum of 9% is needed for catch up growth to occur.[89] If energy supplements are added to formulae to provide 4.2 kJ (1.0 kcal)/ml the protein:energy ratio is reduced to 5.5%. There is evidence to demonstrate that this practice may lead to low plasma urea concentrations and even adversely affect growth.[90]

Some centres increase the energy and nutrient profile of normal infant formula feeds by increasing the concentration from approximately 13 to 15% or even 17%. This involves adding more scoops of milk powder to a given volume of liquid. This also has disadvantages; it may cause confusion and lead to mistakes in feed preparation. Furthermore, the electrolyte and fat-soluble vitamin content are high, renal solute load increases and the amount of free water decreases.

Another option is the use of specially formulated high energy, nutrient dense infant formulae specially produced for infants who are failing to thrive. There are two formulae available designed for infants 0–1 year. They provide approximately 4.2 kJ (1.0 kcal)/ml, and are enriched with extra protein, vitamins and minerals (Infatrini, Cow & Gate, Nutricia Clinical, Wilts, UK; SMA High Energy; SMA Nutrition, Wyett Labs., Maidenhead, UK). They both meet the EC 1991 directive compositional guidelines for infant formula. Initial evidence suggests that these formulae are well tolerated and, when compared with energy supplemented normal infant formulae, result in better growth in boys.[90]

Children 1–6 years (8–20 kgs)

In the late 1980s, a high proportion of young children were being fed adult enteral feeds.[91] This was inappropriate and could have led to young children being fed excessive amounts of protein, sodium, potassium and other nutrients. In the UK, the first compositional guidelines were introduced for enteral feeds for the 1–6 year age group in 1988.[92] Now there are three low residue, nutritionally complete 4.2 kJ (1.0 kcal)/ml ready-to-use feeds available in the UK: Nutrini (Nutricia Clinical, Wilts, UK), Frebini (Fresenius, Birchwood, Warrington, UK) and Paediasure (Abbott, Maidenhead, UK). They are all based on caseinates, maltodextrin and vegetable oils ± added medium chain triglyceride oil (MCT) and are clinically lactose free. They are well tolerated and effective in improving nutrition status in this age group.[93,94] Their long-term use also leads to normal biochemical micronutrient profile.[95] In one study of a group of chronically disabled children who were given at least 90% of their estimated average requirements from a paediatric enteral feed, there was satisfactory growth, no significant changes in biochemistry and excellent gastrointestinal tolerance and acceptance.[94] These feeds should be administered at a rate of 85–95 ml/kg/day depending on age, weight, clinical condition and nutrition requirements.

There are two 6.3 kJ (1.5 kcal)/ml ready-to-use nutrient dense formula, Nutrini Extra (Nutricia Clinical, Wilts, UK and Paediasure Plus, Abbot, Maidenhead), is available for this age group. They are designed for young children with high-energy requirements or who can tolerate small feed volumes only.

There are now fibre-enriched formulae available for the 1–6-year-old age group, providing between 0.5 g and 0.75 g fibre/100 ml. This should provide short chain fatty acids for the colonocytes and help prevent diarrhoea and constipation.[96] Unfortunately, there is little data on fibre requirements in paediatrics to help determine ideal feed composition. In the US, it is recommended that children over 2 years should consume a minimum amount of dietary fibre equivalent to age (in grams) plus 5 g/day.[97] Initial data would suggest that the high fibre feeds are well tolerated, improve stool characteristics and reduce laxative usage. In a group of 20 developmentally disabled children, during a 2-month randomised crossover study, a high fibre feed containing 10 g/litre reduced use of laxatives and had no abnormal effect on growth or biochemistry.[98] However, there are few data on long-term iron and zinc biochemical status of children on these feeds.

Children over 6 years

There is no standard nutritionally complete, polymeric 4.2 kJ (1.0 kcal)/ml or 6.3 kJ (1.5 kcal)/ml feed for this age group. It is inappropriate to still use feeds designed for 1–6 years, as they are too high in nutrients such as vitamin D. There is, therefore, little choice but to use adult 4.2 kJ (1.0 kcal)/ml feeds for this age group, although the nutrition profile is not ideal. Protein, electrolyte, vitamin and trace mineral intake should be assessed and monitored to ensure this is not excessive. Adult feeds providing 6.3 kJ (1.5 kcal)/ml are generally high in protein and any containing over 6.5 g protein/100 ml are unsuitable for children over 6 years. Daily protein requirements of 7–14-year-old children are only between 19.7 g and 42 g daily.[12]

Protein hydrolysate formula

Children 0–2 years

The majority of tube-fed infants with protracted diarrhoea, short bowel syndrome or cow's milk protein enteropathy can tolerate extensively hydrolysed formula based on either casein (Nutramigen, Pregestimil, Bristol-Meyers, Middx, UK; Mead Johnson), whey (Peptijunior: Cow & Gate, Nutricia Clinical, Wilts, UK; Alfare: Nestlè, Surrey, UK) or soya and meat (Prejomin: Milupa; Pepdite: SHS Int. Ltd., Liverpool, UK) protein. Some of these formulae have been available for over 40 years. They contain short chain peptides and amino acids and are produced by heat treatment and/or enzymatic cleavage. It is well recognised that nitrogen is more rapidly and effectively absorbed in both the healthy and compromised bowel in the form of dipeptides and tripeptides than from free amino acids. In addition, peptides supply a reduced osmotic load. Carbohydrate is predominantly based on glucose syrup solids or glucose polymer. Pregestimil and Peptijunior contain 50% of their fat in the form of MCT (medium chain tryglycencie). Although MCT is hydrolysed faster than LCT (long chain tryglyceride), it can lead to osmotic diarrhoea, and dicarboxylic aciduria has been described in infants supplemented with MCT-rich formula without any proof of deleterious effect.[99]

Children over 2 years

There are only two protein hydrolysate formulae specifically produced for children over 2 years. They are based on hydrolysed meat and soya (peptide 1+ and MCT peptide 2+ : SHS) and are nutritionally complete. Pepdite 1+ contains 65% LCT and 35% MCT. MCT pepdite 2+ contains 17% LCT and 83% MCT. Intake of high quantities of MCT may produce abdominal distension, cramps, nausea and diarrhoea.

Elemental formula

There is only one amino acid based nutritionally complete formula designed for infants (Neocate: SHS Int. Ltd., Liverpool, UK). It provides 297 kJ (71 kcal) and 1.95 g protein per 100 ml at a 15% concentration. There is evidence to demonstrate that tolerance and growth on this formula is satisfactory. Equally, there is only one elemental formula suitable for the 1–6-year-old group (Neocate Advance: SHS). So far, there are few data to support its use. Elemental 028: SHS and Elemental 028 Extra: SHS, may be used for older children. They have a low protein content and have acceptable electrolyte, vitamin and mineral profiles. Both formulae have a high osmolality when made up to a 20% concentration and need careful introduction when given to a child.

Modular feeds

The availability and use of modular components for tube feeding has increased dramatically in recent years.[100] A modular feed is one that is based on separate protein, fat, carbohydrate, vitamin and mineral components. Alternatively modular ingredients can be added singly or in combination to nutritionally complete feeds to enhance nutrient composition. The chief advantage of a modular feed is its flexibility; individual ingredients and the quantities can be adapted to meet specific needs of an infant or child. They are used if complete specialised formulae are not tolerated, or if the fluid and nutrient requirements are changed with a varying clinical state, e.g. in renal, liver or inherited metabolic disease. Although useful, they are complex, require time-consuming preparations and are difficult to prepare. It is relatively easy to omit single nutrients such as essential fatty acids or add nutrient modules, which alter the composition of a diet so that a single nutrient may become deficient. It is essential that all patients on modular feeds or supplements be carefully monitored.

The routes of feeding

The appropriate access route for the delivery of feeds depends upon a number of factors, which include enteral feeding indications, anticipated duration of feeding, patient age, potential risks and surgical considerations.[101] Nasogastric or nasojejunal feeding are both easy to use for short-term feeding. The nasogastric route is considered if the risk of aspiration is low, whilst nasojejunal feeding may be used for children where gastric emptying is delayed or reflux is present.

Gastrostomy feeding is considered for patients who require feeding over a three-month period. Improved techniques of insertion have made this route of feeding more common in children.[31] Percutaneous endoscopic placement and fluoroscopically guided gastrostomy are newer methods.[96,102–105]

Creation of a gastrostomy may result in temporary ileus or gastrointestinal bleeding. Once a gastrostomy has been established and is mature, complications are more likely to be due to tube type and position, than the stoma itself. Leakage can occur by an enlarged stoma caused by the pivoting motion of a tube that is too stiff or large. It is essential to rule out gastric outlet obstruction as the cause of stomal leakage.

The gastrostomy tube may be improperly positioned initially or may migrate internally any time after placement. These problems are common if Foley catheters are used and less likely when an external 'bumper' is used. When the catheter migrates distally to the pylorus or duodenum, the gastric outlet may be obstructed, cause vomiting, gastro-oesophageal reflux, aspiration and/or stomal leakage.[106]

Jejunostomy feeding is considered for obstruction of the stomach, duodenum or the proximal jejunum and when delayed gastric emptying or severe reflux is present. The main routes of feeding reviewing the advantages and disadvantages of each route are described in Table 20.2.

An overview of some of the tubes available for feeding is presented in Table 20.3. There are a vast amount of enteral devices available on the market; so therefore, the list cannot be all-inclusive. The advent of portable systems has revolutionised feeding for children, enabling many who require more than 12 hours of feeding mobility, increased freedom and independence. Table 20.4 identifies the most important features of an ideal portable pump.

Table 20.2 – Enteral feeding routes.

Method	Advantages	Disadvantages
Nasogastric	• Short-term feeding	Tube re-insertion may be: • Distressing to child/family and nurse • Easily removed by child/baby • Risk of aspiration • Discomfort to nasopharynx • Psychosocial implications
Nasojejunal	• Less risk of aspiration • Short-term feeding	• Difficulty of insertion • Radiographic check of position[106a] • Risk of perforation • Abdominal pain and diarrhoea unless continuous infusion of feed • Discomfort in nasopharynx • Reflux of bile is facilitated
Gastrostomy	• Cosmetically more acceptable to some children • Easily hidden • Long-term feeding	• Increases reflux • Local skin irritation • Infection • Granulation tissue • Leakage • Gastric distension • Stoma closes within a few hours if accidentally removed
Gastrojejunal	• Facilitates placement beyond ligament of Treiz • Provides gastric decompression while feeding into jejunum	• Precipitation of bile into stomach • Regular gastric aspiration required
Jejunostomy	• Reduced risk of aspiration • Long-term feeding	• Surgical/Radiology procedure • Risk of perforation • Must be constant infusion of feed • Bacterial overgrowth • Dumping syndrome can occur

Complications of feeding

Complications lessen the effectiveness of enteral nutrition. However with a wider choice of feeds, administration techniques, and enteral feeding devices it should be possible to minimise these problems.

Gastrointestinal symptoms are the most common complications of enteral feeding. Diarrhoea will occur if the absorptive capacity of the small bowel is exceeded. Specimens of stools should be sent for culture and sensitivity to exclude an infective source. Stools for reducing substances and steatorrhoea should be reviewed and feed changes made as appropriate. Table 20.5 reviews some of the complications related to enteral feeding.[107–110]

Home enteral feeding

Training

Training of families is one of the key aspects of hospital predischarge care.[111] Carers/parents need to fully understand the procedures. Consequential problems and their management so feeds can be safely given at home. It will also maximise disease management as well as improve quality of lifestyle.[112] Adequate training may take several hours, but it is essential all training sessions are short, so a package of information is gradually given under the best learning conditions. Carers/parents should be fully aware of the teaching plan and be given checklists of areas to be discussed. Consistency of information is essential to prevent confusion and anxiety.

Table 20.3 Ideal feeding tubes and devices.[112a]

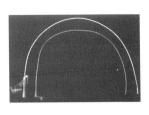 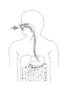

Nasogastric Tube

- **Conforms** to British Standards BS 6314 (should have a male luer and anti intravenous female connection)
- **Small FG** with a large internal diameter
- **Comfort**/cosmetically acceptable
- **Tip**: soft with no dead space; scooped end to avoid suction of the tip onto the stomach wall; aids aspiration and reduces blockage
- **Guidewires** should be stiff to ensure easy insertion; flexible to avoid damage to the tube and should not coil
- **Connectors** should be durable and fit any giving set of syringe with or without a suitable adapter
- **Radio**-paque

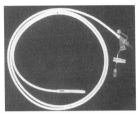 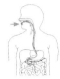

Nasojejunal Feeding Tube

- **Tube** and guidewire should be radio-paque to help confirm position
- **Biocompatible** polyurethane tube Tungsten weighted may be helpful
- **Open** distal end promotes good fluid flow
- **Comfort**/cosmetically acceptable

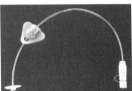

Percutaneous Endoscopic Gastrostomy Tube – (PEG Tube)

- **Bumper** bar and tube should be made of pliable, biocompatable silicone. This material easily passes down the oesophagus and helps maintain a healthy stoma
- **Bumper** bar helps to resist inadvertent removal and migration into stoma tract
- **Connections** compatible with external feeding systems to minimise separation and leakage

Gastrostomy Tube

- **Medical** grade silicone material, biocompatable and flexible for patient comfort
- **Y-Port** connector to allow easy flushing and giving of liquid medication without disconnecting feeding sets
- **Centimetre** graduations to allow assessment of potential tube migration
- **Securing** disc lifts easily for cleaning of stoma site/prevents tube migration
- **Translucent** to facilitate assessment of stoma
- **Holes** to promote airflow for a healthy stoma site
- **Gastric** balloon expands evenly to maintain a secure, comfortable fit and to minimise leakage
- **Balloon** inflation port is safely marked with the maximum balloon volume and the words 'inflation' to prevent accidental over-inflation and administration of medicines
- **Open** distal end promotes good fluid flow

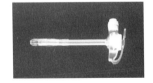

Gastrostomy Button

- **Low** profile device makes it suitable for children or adults, who may be self-conscious of standard gastrostomy tube
- **Anti-Relux** valve prevents leakage of feed when tube is not in use
- **Balloon** inflation to facilitate removal/replacement

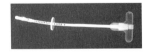

Stoma Measuring Devices for Buttons

- **Depth** of tract required is measured by a stoma measuring device
- **Measuring** device packed separately to the button to ensure correct size button is used

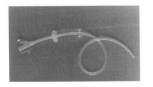

Transgastric Jejunal Feeding Tube

- **Facilitates** placement of tube beyond the ligament of Trietz for endoscopic and radiologic procedures
- **Provides** gastric decompression while simultaneously feeding into the jejunum
- **Multiple** feeding ports improve flow of feed and minimise clogging
- **Sliding** ring balloon system prevents the tube migrating and controls gastric leakage
- **Built-in** universal connectors help minimise feeding set disconnections

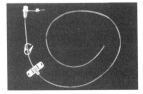

Jejunal Feeding Tube

- Flexible medical grade clear silicone to minimise site irritation
- Radiopaque allows verification of tube position

Table 20.4 – Ideal enteral feeding pump.

- Easy to operate
- Durable
- Small/lightweight
- Portable
- Accurate (5–10%) (Constant infusion available)
- Option of bolus feeding available
- Easy to clean
- Suitability of controls
- Taper proof
- Low noise level, particularly if nocturnal feeding
- Alarm : occlusion/empty and low battery
- Reliability essential

Teaching material available
- Step-by-step guides of setting up the system
- Written instructions at side of pump and also in pamphlet form
- Pamphlet information
- Training video

Purchasing
- Servicing – purchasers should identify servicing arrangements
- Information available from Medical Devices Agency
- Cost of pump and disposables to be considered

Successful training depends more on carer motivation and willingness to listen and learn than on educational ability. Education programmes should always be individualised but should include the following:

- Information about why a child requires home enteral feeding

- Safety aspects of care, including information about basic anatomy

- Psychological preparation of parent and child

- Checking tube placement and general care

- Promotion of oral feeding skills

- Hygiene: including hand-washing and cleaning surfaces for the feeds

- Preparation and storage of the feed

- Familiarisation with feeding equipment

- Advice about social and practical problems. There should always be frank discussion about problems such as the pain associated with tube insertion, potential bed wetting and frequent toilet visits overnight, and sleep disturbance

- Problem-solving advice and what to do in an emergency

- Information about how to obtain equipment and feed supplies.

- Contact information.

Information is essential to decrease anxiety and improve coping by making the procedure understandable and less frightening. There is now a selection of printed explanation booklets available on tube feeding designed for carers and children.[113–116] Information given directly to a child should be at an appropriate cognitive level to allow them to understand and use it.[117] Pictorial teaching aids are increasingly being used for non-English speaking families,[118] and those unable to understand written guidelines. Whenever possible families should also have the opportunity to talk to other children and parents who have experience of tube feeding.

The viewing of videotapes of other children, either successfully inserting nasogastric tubes or carrying out some other aspect of tube feeding, may significantly decrease distress. Research has demonstrated that coping models (children who express distress but cope adequately with the procedure) are more easily accepted by children than mastery models (children who express and successfully accomplish the task). Children and parents can also be trained in relaxation and mental imagery techniques to decrease anxiety and fear during placement of the feeding tube.[119]

A recent study on the psychological preparation of 48 children undergoing nasogastric feeding highlighted the distress experienced both by the parents and children on insertion of the tube. It concluded for younger children that if play therapists are involved in psychological preparation the tube should be inserted immediately, as delay resulted in children becoming overly upset. However parents stated that the play therapists helped their children cope with nasogastric feeding through play by providing an outlet for aggression and anger.[120]

Psychological and social implications of home feeding

Although home feeding is more cost effective than hospital based care[121] and home enteral nutrition has been shown to improve nutrition status,[122,123] the psychological and social implications of enteral feeding are rarely addressed. Results from some studies, however, do indicate that carers/parents find home enteral feeding a very stressful process.[124–126] Adams *et*

Table 20.5 – Complications of home enteral nutrition.

- Mechanical infections
- Metabolic/nutrition
- Gastrointestinal

Aspiration of feeds and/or gastric contents	<ul><li>incidence low</li><li>subclinical aspiration is probably common</li><li>risk factors include: glottis closure poor cough reflex dysphasia decreased intestinal motility, slow gastric emptying presence of nasoenteric tube neurological impairment</li></ul>

Mechanical complications

Nasogastric	<ul><li>nasopharyngeal erosions</li><li>otitis media</li><li>sinusitis</li><li>nasal cartilage erosion</li><li>oesophagitis</li><li>pneumothorax</li><li>gastric irritation from tube dislodgment</li></ul>
Nasojejunal	<ul><li>dislodgment</li><li>placement difficult</li></ul>
Gastrostomy	<ul><li>dislodgment</li><li>local erythema</li><li>infection or irritation leakage</li><li>gastric outlet obstruction</li><li>if present increases reflux</li></ul>
Gastrojejunal	<ul><li>precipitation of bile into stomach</li><li>tube requires regular gastric aspiration</li></ul>
Jejunostomy	<ul><li>risk of perforation</li><li>dumping syndrome can occur</li><li>erythema</li><li>infection</li></ul>

Microbiological problems

Feed contamination	<ul><li>common and can lead to gastroenteritis and septicaemia</li><li>manipulation of handling of feeds to be kept to a minimum[110]</li><li>strict handwashing techniques, use of disposable gloves and cleaning connections with 70% alcohol significantly reduces contamination</li></ul>
Developmental problems	<ul><li>oral feeding should be maintained if possible to prevent latter feeding problems and oral aversion</li><li>speech therapist can design and evaluate appropriate individualised oral motor stimulation programmes</li></ul>

Gastrointestinal problems

Diarrhoea	Causes include:<ul><li>improper administration of feeds/dilution</li><li>nutrient intolerance</li><li>inadequate absorption</li><li>osmotic load of feed</li><li>hyperosmolar formula, medications or additives</li><li>bacterial contamination feeds</li><li>medications</li><li>bacterial overgrowth</li></ul>

al[126] showed that caring for a child with disabilities on tube feeds is more stressful than caring for a child with disabilities alone. In particular, mothers caring for disabled children on tube feeds received less support from families, than mothers caring for children with disabilities only. Holden[124] has identified many problems with home feeding for carers. These included sleepless nights, exhaustion, lack of help, and financial problems due to loss of income and hospital visit costs. Parents/carers identified problems with rigidity of prescribed feeding regimens and lack of professional support at night when the majority of children were being given their enteral feeds.

Support services for children with disabilities on tube feeds are a problem.[45,125] There is often no specific health professional with a key responsibility for tube feeding within an area or locality. Often there are difficulties with the continuity of services for families. They may have to rely on specialist hospital staff for support, rather than local community health professionals.

The increase in children receiving home enteral feeding has important implications for health, social care and education of professionals, many of whom are experiencing difficulties in trying to provide effective support to enterally fed children and their families.[127]

Maintaining oral feeding skills

If tube feeding is only maintained for a period of less than 20 days, the majority of infants and children will return to oral feeding with the minimal of problems, particularly if non-nutritive sucking is encouraged during this time.[128] If enteral feeding is maintained for a longer time, restarting oral feeding can be very difficult. With the exception of children who do not have a safe swallow, infants and children should be encouraged to have some oral feed and take part in family mealtimes. This will enable children opportunity to learn to like different tastes and textures and to use the lips and tongue. If babies between the ages of 4 and 6 months miss out on these experiences they will have difficulty accepting them later on. Senez and co-workers[128] demonstrated in a group of 19 long-term tube-fed children, who were given regular intermittent tube feeds in combination with tactile, olfactory, and oropharyngeal cavity stimulation, that oral feeding could be successfully re-established.

References

1. Merritt RJ, Suskind RM. Nutrition survey of hospitalised pediatric patients. *Am J Clin Nutr* 1979; **32:** 1320–1325.

2. Parsons HG, Francouer TE, Howland P, Spengler RF, Pencharz PB. The nutritional status of hospitalized children. *Am J Clin Nutr* 1980; **33:** 1140–1146.

3. Cooper A, Jakobowski D, Spiker J, Floyd T, Ziegler MM, Koop E. Nutrition assessment: an integral part of the pre-operative surgical evaluation. *J Pediatr Surg* 1981; **16:** 554–561.

4. LeLeiko NS, Luder E, Fridman M, Fersel J, Benkov K. Nutrition assessment of pediatric patients admitted to an acute-care pediatric service utilizing anthropometric measurements. *J Parenter Ent Nutr* 1986; **10:** 166–168.

5. Moy RJD, Smallman S, Booth IW. Malnutrition in a UK children's hospital. *J Hum Nutr Diet* 1990; **3:** 93–100.

6. Elia M (Chairman). Report of the British Artificial Nutrition Survey August 2000. British Association of Parenteral and Enteral Nutrition, 2001. Maidenhead, Berks.

7. Heird WC, Driscoll JM, Schullinger JN. Intravenous alimentation in pediatric patients. *J Pediatr* 1972; **80:** 351–372.

8. Cockburn F, Evans J. Nutritional management of paediatric patients. *Ballière's Clin Gastroenterol* 1988; **2:** 887–904.

9. Puig M. Body composition and growth. In: Walker AW, Watkins JB (eds) *Nutrition in Pediatrics.* BC Decker, Hamilton, 1996; pp. 44–62.

10. Marian M. Pediatric nutrition support. *Nutr Clin Pract* 1993; **8:** 199–209.

11. Klein S, Klinney J, Jeejeebhoy K *et al.* Nutrition support in clinical practice: review of published data and recommendations for future research directions. *Amer J Clin Nutr* 1997; **66:** 683–706.

12. Department of Health. Dietary Reference Values for Food Energy and Nutrients for the United Kingdom. Report on Health and Social Subjects No 41 HMSO, London, 1991.

13. Barness LA, Castle JL. The term infant. In: Walker AW, Watkins JB (eds) *Nutrition in Pediatrics.* BC Decker, Hamilton, 1996; pp. 413–422.

14. Booth IW. Clinical nutrition in paediatrics. *J Singapore Paediatr Soc* 1992; **34:** 114–120.

15. MacLean WC, Lucas A. Pediatric nutrition: a distinct subspecialty? In: Walker WA, Watkins JB (eds) *Nutrition in Pediatrics.* BC Decker, Hamilton, 1997; pp. 3–6.

16. Lucas A, Morley R, Cole TJ. Randomised controlled trial of early diet in preterm babies and later intelligence quotient. *Br Med J* 1998; **317:** 1481–1487.

17. Williams J, Wolff A, Daly A, MacDonald A, Auckett A, Booth IW. Iron supplemented formula milk related to reduction in psychomotor decline in infants from inner city areas: randomised study 1999; **318:** 693–697.

18. Wheeler JE, Lukens FDW, Gyorgy P. Studies on the localisation of tagged methionine within the pancreas. *Proc Soc Exper Biol Med* 1949; **70:** 187–189.

19. Booth IW. The gastrointestinal tract. In: McLaren DS, Burman D, Belton NR, Williams AF *Textbook of Paediatric Nutrition*. Churchill Livingstone, Edinburgh, 1991; pp. 143–184.

20. Himes D. Protein-calorie malnutrition and involuntary weight loss: the role of aggressive nutrition intervention in wound healing. *Ostomy Wound Manage* 1999; **45:** 46–51.

21. Booth IW. Nutrition. In: Lissauer T, Clayden G (eds) *Illustrated textbook of paediatrics*. Mosby, London, 1997; pp. 113–122.

22. Rayner P, Rudolph MC. What do we know about children who fail to thrive? *Child Care Health Dev* 1996; **22:** 241–250.

23. Barker DJP. Mothers, babies and disease in later life. British Medical Journal Books, London, 1994.

24. Barker DJP. Fetal nutrition and cardiovascular disease in later life. *Br Med J* 1997; **53:** 96–108.

25. Zlotkin SH, Harrison D. Home pediatric enteral nutrition. In: Rombeau JL, Caldwell MD (eds) *Clinical nutrition: Enteral and Tube Feeding*. WB Saunders, Philadelphia, 1990; pp. 463–471.

26. Puntis JWL, Holden CE. Home enteral nutrition in paediatric practice. *Brit J Hos Med* 1991; **45:** 104–107.

27. Griffiths AM. Crohn's disease in adolescents. *Baillière's Clin Gastroenterol* 1998; **12:** 115–132.

28. Walker-Smith JA. Therapy of Crohn's disease in childhood. *Baillière's Clin Gastroenterol* 1997; **11:** 593–610.

29. Goulet O, Ricour C. Paediatric enteral nutrition. In: Payne-James J, Grimble G, Silk D (eds) *Artificial nutrition support in clinical practice*. Edward Arnold, London, 1995; pp. 257–270.

30. Beattie RM, Bentsen BS, MacDonald TT. Childhood Crohn's disease and the efficacy of enteral diets. *Nutrition* 1998; **14:** 345–350.

31. Cosgrove M, Jenkins HR. Experience of percutaneous endoscopic gastrostomy in children with Crohn's disease. *Arch Dis Child* 1997; **76:** 141–143.

32. Beattie RM, Schiffrin EJ, Donnet-Hughes A *et al.* Polymeric nutrition as the primary therapy in children with small bowel Crohn's disease. *Aliment Pharmacol Ther* 1994; **8:** 609–615.

33. Khoshoo V, Reifen R, Neuman MG, Griffiths A, Pencharz PB. Effect of low- and high fat, peptide-based diets on body composition and disease activity in adolescents with active Crohn's disease. *J Parent Enteral Nutr* 1996; **20:** 401–405.

34. Goulet. Short bowel syndrome in pediatric patients. *Nutrition* 1998; **14:** 784–787.

35. Murphy MS. Growth factors and the gastrointestinal tract. *Nutrition* 1998; **14:** 771–774.

36. Parker HG, Stroop S, Greene H. A controlled comparison of continuous versus intermittent feeding in the treatment of infants with intestinal disease. *J Pediatr* 1981; **99:** 360–364.

37. Stevenson RD. Feeding and nutrition in children with developmental disabilities. *Pediatr Ann* 1995; **24:** 255–259.

38. Naureckas SM, Christoffel KK. Nasogastric or gastrostomy feedings in children with neurologic disabilities. *Clin Pediat* 1994; June: 353–359.

39. Thommessen M, Heiberg A, Kase B F, Larsen S, Riis G. Feeding problems, height and weight in different groups of disabled children. *Acta Paediatr Scand* 1991; **80:** 527–533.

40. Allott L. Feeding children with special needs. In: Holden CE, MacDonald A (eds) *Nutrition and Child Health*. Baillière and Tindall, Edinburgh, 2000.

41. Shapiro BK, Green P, Krich J, Allen DA, Capute AJ. Growth of severely impaired children: neurological versus nutrition factors. *Dev Med and Child Neur* 1986; **28:** 729–733.

42. Sullivan PB, Rosenbloom L. Feeding the disabled child. MacKeith Press, London, 1996.

43. Stallings VA, Zemel BS, Davies JC, Cronk CE, Charney EB. Energy expenditure of children and adolescents with severe disabilities: a cerebral palsy model. *Am J Clin Nutr* 1996; **64:** 627–634.

44. Dahl M, Gebre-Medhin M. Feeding and nutritional problems in children with cerebral palsy and myelomeningocoele. *Acta Paediatr* 1993; **82:** 816–820.

45. Sullivan PB, Rosenbloom L. The causes of feeding difficulties in disabled children. In: Sullivan PB, Rosenbloom L (eds) *Feeding the disabled child*. Clinics in Developmental Medicine No 140. Cambridge University Press, 1996.

46. Patrick J, Boland MP, Stoski D, Murray GE. Rapid correction of wasting in children with cerebral palsy. *Dev Med Child Neur* 1986; **28:** 724–739.

47. Zemel BS, Stallings VA. Energy requirements and nutritional assessment in developmental disabilities. In: Walker WA, Watkins JB (eds) *Nutrition in Pediatrics.* BC Decker, Hamilton, 1997; pp. 169–177.

48. Berg K, Olsson T. Energy requirements of school children with cerebral palsy as determined from infirect calorimetry. *Acta Paediatr Scand* 1970; **24:** 71–80.

49. Taylor SB, Shelton JE. Calorie requirements of a spastic immobile cerebral palsy patient: a case report. *Arch Phys Med Rehabil* 1995; **76:** 281–283.

50. Brant CQ, Stanich P, Ferrara AP. Improvement of children's nutritional status after enteral feeding by PEG: an interim report. *Gastrointest Endosc* 1999; **50:** 183–188.

51. Rempel GR, Colwell SO, Nelson RP. Growth in children with cerebral palsy fed via gastrostomy. *Pediatrics* 1988; **82:** 857–861.

52. Pliopls AV, Kasnicka I, Lewis S, Moller D. Survival rates among children with severe neurologic disabilities. *South Med J* 1998; **91:** 161–172.

53. Borowitz SM, Sutphen JL, Hutcheson RL. Percutaneous endoscopic gastrostomy without an antireflux procedure in neurologically disabled children. *Clin Pediatr* (Phila) 1997; **36:** 25–29.

54. Duncan B, Barton LL, Lloyd J, Marks-Katz M. Dietary considerations in osteopenia in tube-fed non ambulatory children with cerebral palsy. *Clin Pediatr* 1999; **38:** 133–137.

55. Strauss D, Kastner T, Ashwal S, White J. Tube feeding and mortality in children with severe disabilities and mental retardation. *Pediatr* 1997; **99:** 358–362.

56. McNaughton SA, Stormont DA, Shepherd RW, Fracis PWJ, Dean B. Growth failure in cystic fibrosis. *J Paediatr Child Health* 1999; **35:** 86–92.

57. Lai HC, Kosorok MR, Sondel et al. Growth status in children with cystic fibrosis based on national cystic fibrosis patient registry data. *J Pediatr* 1998; **132:** 478–485.

58. Morrison S, Dodge JA, Cole TL et al. Height and weight in cystic fibrosis patient registry data. *J Pediatr* 1997; **77:** 497–500.

59. Sproul A, Huang N. Growth patterns in children with cystic fibrosis. *J Pediat* 1964; **65:** 664–67.

60. Kramer R, Rudeberg A, Hadorn B, Rossi E. Relative underweight in cystic fibrosis and its prognostic value. *Acta Paediatr Scand* 1978; **67:** 33–37.

61. Bogle MJ, Alford BA, Warren R, King SE. Estimating calorie needs of prepubescent children with cystic fibrosis. *Top Clin Nutr* 1990; **5:** 47–58.

62. Zemel BS, Kawchak DA, Cnaan A, Zhao H, Scanlin TF, Stallings VA. Prospective evaluation of resting energy expenditure, nutritional status, pulmonary function, and genotype in children with cystic fibrosis. *Pediat Res* 1996; **40:** 576–588.

63. Collins CE, MacDonald-Wicks L, Rowe S, O'Loughlin EV, Henry RL. Normal growth in cystic fibrosis associated with a specialised centre. *Arch Dis Child* 1999; **81:** 241–246.

64. Murphy JL, Wootton SA, Bond SA, Jackson AA. Energy content of stools in normal healthy controls and patients with cystic fibrosis. *Arch Dis Child* 1991; **66:** 495–500.

65. Ramsey BW et al. Nutrition assessment and management in cystic fibrosis: a consensus report. *Am J Clin Nutr* 1992; **55:** 108–116.

66. Reilly JJ, Evans TJ, Wilkinson J, Paton JY. Adequacy of clinical formulae for estimation of energy requirements in children with cystic fibrosis. *Arch Dis Child* 1999; **81:** 129–124.

67. Rosenfield M, Casey S, Pepe M, Ramsey BW. Nutritional effects of long-term gastrostomy feedings in children with cystic fibrosis. *J Am Diet Assoc* 1999; **99:** 191–194.

68. Walker SA, Gozal D. Pulmonary function correlates in the prediction of long-term weight gain in cystic fibrosis patients with gastrostomy tube feedings. *J Pediatr Gastroenterol Nutr* 1998; **27:** 53–56.

69. Jelalian E, Stark LJ, Reynolds L, Seifer R. Nutrition intervention for weight gain in cystic fibrosis: a meta analysis. *J Pediatr* 1998; **132:** 486–492.

70. Erskine JM, Lingard CD, Sontag MK, Accurso FJ. Enteral nutrition for patients with cystic fibrosis: comparison of a semi-elemental and non elemental formula. *J Pediatr* 1998; **132:** 265–269.

71. Yu LC. Nutrition and childhood malignancies. In: Suskind RM, Lewinter-Suskind L (eds) *Textbook of pediatric nutrition.* Raven Press, New York, 1993; pp. 417–424.

72. den Broeder E, Lippens RJJ, van't Hof MA et al. Effects of naso-gastric tube feeding on the nutritional status of children with cancer. *Eur J Clin Nutr* 1998; **52:** 494–500.

73. Tyc VL, Vallelunga L, Mahoney S, Smith BF, Mulhern RK. Nutritional and treatment related characteristics of pediatric oncology patients referred or not referred for nutritional support. *Med and Pediatr Onc* 1995; **25:** 379–388.

74. Bernstein IL. Learned taste aversion in children receiving chemotherapy. *Science* 1978; **200:** 1302–1303.

75. Wall DT, Gabriel LA. Alterations of taste in children with leukemia. *Cancer Nurs* 1983; **6:** 447–452.

76. Pencharz PB. Aggressive oral, enteral or parenteral nutrition: prescriptive decisions in children with cancer. *Int J Cancer Suppl* 1998; **11**: 73–75.

77. Aquino VM, Smyrl CB, Hagg R, McHard KM, Prestridge L, Sandler ED. Enteral nutritional support by gastrostomy tube in children with cancer. *J Pediatr* 1995; **127**: 58–62.

78. Smith DE, Stevens MCG, Booth IW. Malnutrition in children with malignant solid tumours. *J Hum Nutr Diet* 1990; **3**: 303–309.

79. Smith DE, Handy DJ, Holden CE, Stevens MCG, Booth IW. An investigation of supplementary naso-gastric feeding in malnourished children undergoing treatment for malignancy: results of a pilot study. *J Hum Nutr Diet* 1992; **5**: 85–91.

80. Mathew P, Bowman L, Williams R *et al.* Complications and effectiveness of gastrostomy feedings in pediatric cancer patients. *J Pediatr Hematol Oncol* 1996; **18**: 81–85.

81. Papadopoulou A, Williams MD, Darbyshire PJ, Booth IW. Nutritional support in children undergoing bone marrow transplantation. *Clin Nutr* 1998; **17**: 57–63.

82. Ringwald-Smith K. Enteral nutrition support in a child after bone marrow transplantation. *Nutr Clin Prac* 1995; **10**: 140–143.

83. Mehziri A, Drash A. Growth disturbance in congenital heart disease. *J Pediatr* 1962; **61**: 418–429.

84. Rosenthal A. Nutritional considerations in the prognosis and treatment of children with congenital heart disease. In: Suskind RM, Lewinter-Suskind L (eds) *Textbook of pediatric nutrition*. Raven Press, New York, 1993; pp. 383–392.

85. Barton JS, Hindmarsh, PC, Scrimgeour CM, Rennie MJ, Preece MA. Energy expenditure in congenital heart disease. *Arch Dis Child* 1994; **70**: 5–9.

86. Menon G, Poskitt EME. Why does congenital heart disease cause failure to thrive? *Arch Dis Child* 1985; **60**: 1134–1139.

87. Schwaz SM, Gewitz MH, See CC *et al.* Enteral nutrition in infants with congenital heart disease and growth failure. *Pediatr* 1990; **86**: 368–373.

88. Unger R, DeKleermaeker M, Gidding SS, Christoffel KK. Improved weight gain with dietary intervention in congenital heart disease. *AJDC* 1992; **146**: 1078–1084.

89. Shaw V, Lawson M. Clinical paediatric dietetics. Blackwell Scientific Publications, Oxford, 1994.

90. Clark S, MacDonald A, Booth IW. Abstract: Improved growth and nitrogen deficiency in infants receiving an energy-supplemented standard infant formula. Proceedings of the 2nd Annual Spring Meeting, *Roy Coll Paediat Child Health*, 1998; p. 75.

91. Dorf A. Tube feeding the young child: current practices and concerns of pediatric nutritionists. *J Am Diet Assoc* 1989; **89**: 1658–1660.

92. Russell C (Chairman). Paediatric Enteral Feeding Solutions and Systems. A report by the Joint Working Party of the Paediatric Group and Parenteral and Enteral Group of the British Dietetic Association, Birmingham BDA, 1988.

93. Finch HE, Lawson MS. Clinical trial of a paediatric enteral feed. *J Hum Nut Diets* 1993; **6**: 399–409.

94. Ramstack M, Listernick R. Safety and efficacy of a new pediatric enteral product in the young child. *J Parenter Ent Nutr* 1990; **15**: 89–92.

95. Johnston T. (1999) Personal communication.

96. Marchand, V, Baker SS, Baker RD. Enteral nutrition in the paediatric population. *Gastrointest Endosc Clin N Am* 1998; **8**: 669–703.

97. Wardley BL, Puntis JWL, Taitz LS. Handbook of child nutrition. Oxford University Press, Oxford, 1997.

98. Tolia V, Ventimiglia J, Kuhns L. Gastrointestinal intolerance of a pediatric fiber formula in developmentally disabled children. *J Am Coll Nutr* 1997; **16**: 224–228.

99. Lima LAM, Gray OP, Losty H. Excretion of dicarboxylic acids following administration with medium chain triglycerides. *J Parenter Ent Nutr* 1987; **11**: 600–601.

100. Davis A and Baker S. The use of modular nutrients in pediatrics. *J Parenter Ent Nutr* 1996; **20**: 228–236.

101. Moukarzel, AA, Reyen L, Marvin E, Ament MD. Home enteral feeding in children. In: Baker SB, Baker AD (eds) *Pediatric Enteral Nutrition*. Chapman and Hall, London, 1994.

102. Kuizon BD, Nelson PA, Salusky IB. Tube feeding in children with end stage renal disease. *Min Electrol Metab* 1997; **23**: 306–310.

103. Behrens R, Lant T, Mushchweck H, Richter T, Hofbeck M. Percutaneous endoscopic gastrostomy in children and adolescents. *J Pediatr Gastroenterol Nutr* 1997; **25(5)**: 487–891.

104. Khattak IU, Kimber C, Kiely EM, Spitz L. Percutaneous endoscopic gastrostomy in paediatric practice complications implications and outcome. *J Pediatr Surg* 1998; **33(1)**: 67–72.

105. Humphrey GM, Najmaldin A. Laparoscopic gastrostomy in children. *Pediatr Surg Int* 1997; **12(7)**: 501–504.

106. Tuchman D. Oropharyngeal and oespharyngeal complications of enteral tube feeding. In: Baker SB, Baker RD, Davis A (eds) *Pediatric Enteral Nutrition*. Chapman & Hall, London, 1994; **11**: 179–191.

106a. Pobiel RS, Bisset GS, Pobiel MS. Nasojejunal feeding tube placement in children: four-year cumulative experience. *Rad* 1994; **190(1):** 127–129.

107. Gutierrezz ED, Balfe DM. Fluoroscopically guided nasoenteric feeding tube placement: Results of a one-year study. *Radiology* 1991; **178:** 759.

108. Wheatley MJ, Wesley JR, Tkach DM, Coran AG. Long-term follow up of brain-damaged children requiring a feeding gastrostomy: Should an antireflux procedure always be performed? *J Pediatr Surg* 1991; **26:** 301–304.

109. Gauderer MWL. Percutaneous endoscopic gastrostomy: A 10-year experience with 220 children. *J Pediatr Surg* 1991; **26:** 288.

110. Patchell CJ, Anderton A, Holden C, MacDonald A, George RH, Booth IW. Reducing bacterial contamination of enteral feeds. *Arch Dis Child* 1998; **78(2):** 166–168.

111. Holden CE, MacDonald A. Nutrition support at home, emotional support and composition of feeds. *Curr Paediatr* 1997; **7:** 218–222.

112. Hill S. Home enteral nutrition in paediatrics. *Clin Nutr Update* 1998; **3:** 3, 8–10.

112a. Holden C, Johnson T, Caney D. Nutritional support for children in the community. In: Holden CE, MacDonald A (eds) *Nutrition and Child Health.* Baillière and Tindall, Edinburgh, 2000.

113. Paul L, Holden C, Smith A *et al.* Tube feeding and you. Diana, Princess of Wales Children's Hospital, Birmingham, 1998. (ISBN 0 7044 1367 1.)

114. Paul L, Holden C, Smith A *et al.* Gastrostomy feeding and you. Diana, Princess of Wales Children's Hospital NHS Trust, Birmingham, 1994. (ISBN 0 7044 1502X.)

115. Holden CE, Sexton E. Gastrostomy training package. Diana, Princess of Wales Children's Hospital, Birmingham, 1996.

116. Holden CE, Fitzpatrick G, Paul L *et al.* Gastrostomy care: a parents' guide. Diana Princess of Wales Children's Hospital NHS Trust, Birmingham, 1997.

117. Young MH. Preparation for nasogastric tube placement: psychological support. In: Baker SB, Baker RD, Davis A (eds) *Pediatric Enteral Nutrition.* Chapman & Hall, London, 1994.

118. Sexton E, Paul L, Holden C. A pictorial assisted teaching tool for families. *Pediatric Nursing* 1996; **8:** 5: 24–25.

119. Rope RN, Bush JP. Psychological preparation for pediatric oncology patients undergoing painful procedures: a methodological critique of research. *Child Health Care* 1994; **23(1):** 51–67.

120. Holden CE, MacDonald A, Ward M *et al.* Psychological preparation for nasogastric feeding in children. *Br J Nursing* 1997; **6:** 7, 376–385.

121. Colomb V, Goulet O, Ricour C. Home enteral and parenteral nutrition in children. *Ballière's Clin Gastroenterol* 1998; **12:** 877–894.

122. Kang A, Zamora SA, Scott RB, Parsons HG. Catch up growth in children treated with home enteral nutrition. *Pediatrics* 1998; **102:** 951–955.

123. Papadopoulou A, Holden CE, Paul L, Sexton E, Booth IW. The nutritional response to home enteral nutrition in childhood. *Acta Paediatr* 1995; **84:** 528–531.

124. Holden C. Enteral and parenteral feeding: Implications for homecare. MSc Thesis, Wolverhampton University, 1994.

125. Spalding K, Mc Keever P. Mothers experiences for caring for children with disabilities who require a gastrostomy tube. *J Pediatr Nursing* 1998; **13:** 234–243.

126. Adams RA, Gordon C, Spangler AA. Maternal stress in caring for children with feeding disabilities: Implications for health care providers. *J Am Diet Assoc* 1999; **99:** 962–966.

127. Townsley R, Robinson C. On line support: effective support services to disabled children who are tube fed. The Norah Fry Research Centre, University of Bristol, 1997.

128. Senez C, Guys JM, Mancini J, Paz Paredes A, Lena G, Choux M. Weaning children from tube to oral feeding. *Child's Nerv Syst* 1996; **12:** 590–594.

21

Home enteral tube feeding

Ann Micklewright and Vera E Todorovic

Home enteral tube feeding

Introduction

Enteral tube feeding has been used in a variety of forms to provide nutrition to patients unable to take sufficient food by mouth for over four hundred years.[1,2] However, it is only in the last two decades that technical innovations such as flexible fine bore nasoenteric feeding tubes and endoscopically placed gastrostomy tubes[3] have made enteral tube feeding a more acceptable modality. Development of ready-to-use complete nutrient solutions and simple administration systems, often incorporating a feeding pump, made the procedure relatively safe and easy to use. Once enteral tube feeding became well established in the hospital setting it was inevitable that patients requiring long-term enteral feeding would have the option of continuing this treatment at home.

Government policies in developed countries encourage the transfer of health care from hospital to home so that hospital beds can be made available to treat more patients. The majority of patients prefer treatment at home in familiar surroundings where they have a better chance of achieving a degree of independence and a better quality of life.

Prevalence and growth

Home enteral tube feeding began to expand rapidly in the US in the 1980s. In 1985 it was estimated that 15 000–20 000 patients (55–77 per million population) were being tube fed at home.[4] This was seen as one of the fastest growing home care therapies with a predicted annual growth rate of 25%. This prediction was sound: the prevalence is now estimated at 230 000 patients (800 per million of population). This does not include patients in home care facilities such as nursing homes who may number as many again.[5]

Similar growth rates have been demonstrated in the UK. Only 870 patients (15 per million population) were identified in 1986,[6] increasing to an estimated 2000–2500 (33–42 per million population) by 1994.[2] At the end of 1999 the British Artificial Nutrition Survey (BANS)[7] estimated that there were in excess of 15 000 patients on home enteral feeding (HETF) in the UK (220 per million population). Annual growth rate is estimated to be around 20%. Data from local centres confirm these rapid growth rates.[8,9]

Greater awareness that nutrition support has a role to play in the management of certain disorders,[10–13] the recognition that HETF can prolong life and may even improve the quality of life of certain groups,[14–16] linked with the development of safe and simple feeding procedures which have been aggressively marketed, explain in part this rapid growth in HETF.

In 1985 Wall Street analysis identified artificial nutrition as a potential area for high investment returns.[17] This prediction is upheld by the current UK expenditure in excess of £30 000 million (industry estimate) to provide nutrient solutions and disposable equipment for patients receiving HETF. The use of HETF in different countries appears to be broadly related to the overall expenditure on health (government and private) and the percentage of the gross domestic product (GDP) expended on health.[5]

Indications for home enteral feeding

Park et al[8] record their initial experience with malnourished patients with Crohn's disease and describe how over a period of 10 years their HETF service has expanded to include correction of growth retardation secondary to gastrointestinal disease, cystic fibrosis, inborn errors of metabolism, congenital heart disease, chronic renal failure, many types of neoplasia and chronic neurological diseases.

Table 21.1 lists 5465 new adult patient registrations to BANS[7] in 1999 by diagnostic group and key primary disorders. Almost 80% of all patients belonged to two diagnostic groups: disorders of the central nervous system (59%) and gastrointestinal disorders (20%). In the first group cerebrovascular accident accounted for 35% of all cases of HETF whilst in the second 5% suffered from oesophageal cancer. The main reasons patients started HETF were swallowing difficulties (73%) or to improve nutritional status (18%)

The most common diagnosis amongst 2800 children registered with BANS in 1998[7a] was cerebral palsy (19%), congenital handicap (13%) and cystic fibrosis (9%). Failure to thrive (45%) and swallowing disorders (26%) were the main reasons for commencing HETF.

Table 21.2 gives four other sources[4,18–20] which describe similar indications. Neurological disorders of swallowing included multiple sclerosis, Parkinson's

Table 21.1 – Adult HETF Patient Registrations by Diagnostic Groups and Key Diagnosis in 1999

Diagnostic Group (key primary diagnosis)	New Registrations (n=5465) %
Cardiac Disease	**3.2**
Central Nervous System	**59.4**
(Cerebrovascular Accident)	35.4
(Cerebral Palsy)	1.4
(Multiple Sclerosis)	4.2
(Cerebral trauma)	2.4
(Motor neurone disease)	5.5
(Parkinson's disease)	3.3
Renal Disease	**0.6**
Gastrointestinal disease	**24.8**
(Oesophageal cancer)	4.8
(Crohn's disease)	1.2
Respiratory disease	**2.2**
(Cystic fibrosis)	1.0
Other diseases	**9.8**

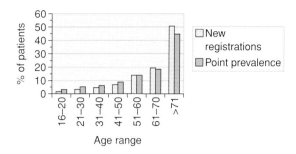

Figure 21.1 – Percentage of new registrations (n=5465) and point prevalence (n=9718) of adult patients on HETF in 1999.

disease and muscular dystrophy; malignancy was mainly of the upper gastrointestinal tract. Other indications such as failure to thrive and anorexia were associated with various conditions like inflammatory bowel disease and fistulas.

Age of patients

Figure 21.1 shows the new registrations and point prevalence of adult patients registered with BANS in 1999. Over 60% of patients at any one time were over 60 years of age. In the over 70s age range the percentage of new registrations exceeded the percentage of existing patients. This trend has been seen over four years and highlights a shift to a more elderly HETF population. This is unsurprising considering the

increasing use of this therapy to support patients who have had a cerebrovascular accident (CVA). Earlier data from the United States confirms the use of HETF for older patients: 51% patients were older than 61 years whilst 10% were more than 80 years.[20]

Between 1996 and 1998 BANS[7a] studied 14 284 patients. CVA accounted for 31% of all diagnosis and rose to over 50% in those aged over 70 years. Oesophageal cancer (32%) and multiple sclerosis (20%) were the most common diagnoses in patients aged 50–60 and 30–40 years respectively. In children, cerebral palsy accounted for 19% of the 0–15 year olds.

There is limited data about the number of children receiving HETF. Point prevalence according to BANS[7a] in 1998 was 26% of the total patient population. Earlier work by Todorovic and Micklewright[6] and Micklewright[18] suggests that about a quarter to one-third of HETF patients are children. The BANS Committee recognise that there are a significant number of children who are not registered with BANS.

Patient selection

Patients who are medically stable but unlikely to meet their nutritional needs by mouth within the foresee-

Table 21.2 – Disorders associated with home enteral tube feeding.

	Micklewright[18] %	Reitz *et al*[19] %	Nelson *et al*[20] %	Howard *et al*[4] %
Swallowing disorders	56	26	33	46
Malignancies of upper GI tract	30	30	44	40
Other conditions	14	44	23	14

able future are candidates for HETF providing they fulfil the following criteria:

- The patient has a functioning gastrointestinal (GI) tract which can be accessed by one of a number of routes.

- The patient is psychologically stable if self caring.

- The patient or relatives understand and give consent to the treatment and realise that HETF may impose major changes to their lifestyles.

- The patient or carer is capable of performing the required procedures safely.

In many situations the decision to use HETF may be clear cut, but in others, where the patient is very old or suffering from a terminal illness, the benefits must be weighed against the quality of life of the patient. Relatives anxious about the poor oral intake of a patient may agree too readily to commence HETF without regard to the additional stresses (social, emotional, financial) which long-term HETF may impose on them. Once HETF is started it is very difficult to stop.

It is of interest that only 15% of patients registered with BANS[7] were able to continue their normal activities. Figure 21.2 illustrates how dependency increases with age. 60% of these patients required total help to manage their tube feeding. This high level of dependency and the burden it places on relatives and carers needs to be taken into account when HETF is being considered.

Benefits of HETF to patients

In addition to providing the patient with adequate nutrition, HETF gives a degree of independence and allows patients to return to familiar surroundings where relationships with family and friends can be resumed. Some patients may be able to return to full time education or work.[21] HETF allows others, too disabled to return home, to exchange the acute hospital setting for the more relaxed atmosphere of the hospice or nursing home.

Puntis[22] showed improvement in the quality of life for some children (with poor appetite due to chronic disorders) and their families once HETF was started. Meal times which had once been protracted struggles,

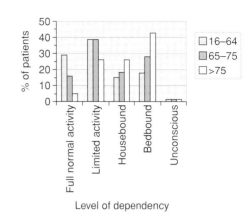

Figure 21.2 – Level of dependency of patients on HETF.[7]

sometimes dominating the life of the child and his/her parents, became more relaxed allowing the child and parents more time to concentrate on other aspects of family life.

Feeding routes (see also chap 17)

Data from the UK show that 60% of all feeding was undertaken via nasogastric tube in 1990 but by 1994 gastrostomy feeding had become more popular and was used with 71% of patients.[18] By the end of 1997 81% of adults registered with BANS[7] were being discharged with a gastrostomy, 15% with a nasogastric/enteric tube and 4% with a jejunostomy. In contrast to the adults, 54% of children were using nasogastric/enteric feeding, 45% gastrostomy and 1% jejunostomy.[7]

The choice of feeding route for HETF depends on a number of criteria: risk of aspiration, patient comfort, pathology of the gastrointestinal intestinal tract, estimated length of feeding, lifestyle of the patient, body image and competence of the patient/carer.[23]

Given these criteria, the increasing use of gastrostomy tubes, particularly with the availability of the percutaneous endoscopic gastrostomy (PEG) which can be positioned without the need for a general anaesthetic,[24] is unsurprising. These tubes are ideal for long-term feeding, being more comfortable and more discrete than nasoenteric tubes. Some children prefer a skin level device – a 'button'. This can be inserted by means of an introducer into an established gastrostomy track. Extension sets are connected to the 'button' to facilitate feeding. 'Buttons' are more discrete and allow children to undertake activities such as swimming.

Gastrostomy or jejunostomy tubes may also be placed whilst the patient is undergoing abdominal surgery. Fine needle catheter jejunostomy tubes are sometimes inserted but are prone to problems with occlusion.[23]

Nasoenteric tubes are more easily dislodged and have a greater potential for causing aspiration: 73% of the BANS[7] patients had swallowing problems so replacing these tubes would not be without difficulty. Over 50% of the UK HETF population were over 65 and only 15% of adult patients were fully independent. With such a dependent population a return to the discharging hospital may be required to repass these tubes.

Children and adolescents or their parents may prefer to pass their own nasogastric tubes. Some will do this every night and remove them in the morning before they go to school. McCrae & Hall[23] strongly advise that teaching must include the signs, symptoms, prevention and treatment of aspiration and bronchial intubation and that competency should be documented. Park[8] recommends this practice for patients with inflammatory bowel disease who have had previous gastric surgery and are unsuitable for PEG placement. Holden[9] advises against this practice when children are severely retarded with poor swallowing reflex, have severe cyanotic heart lesions or oesophageal varices and recommends X-ray confirmation of correct tube placement in these cases.

Fine bore nasoenteric tubes for long-term use are usually made from polyurethane or silicone and are passed with the aid of a guide wire. Patients who self intubate may prefer to use a fine bore polyvinyl tube without a guide-wire which is inexpensive enough to be discarded each morning.[23]

Feeds and administration methods

The patient should be well established on a feeding regimen before discharge from hospital. The type of feed chosen will depend on the patient's clinical condition, tolerance and nutritional requirements. A polymeric ready-to-use 4.2 kJ (1 kcal) or 6.3 kJ (1.5 kcal) per ml feed, available in both adult and paediatric formulation, is most commonly used.

Adult versions of these feeds are available with or without fibre. In addition to the benefits bestowed on bowel mucosa by short chain fatty acids derived from fibre, these feeds may have a potentially protective effect for multiple disease states – diverticulosis, heart disease, colon cancer and diabetes[1] – and in some instances are useful if patients are suffering from diarrhoea. Semi-elemental or elemental feeds are used for some of the small number of patients with gastrointestinal disease.

The feed may be given continuously throughout most of the day or night, or during the day time or overnight only. Nocturnal feeding is usually undertaken to supplement an inadequate oral intake. It is usual to use an energy dense feed 6.3 kJ (1.5 kcal/ml) for nocturnal feeding. Park[8] states that some patients can meet their needs by taking feeds only 4–5 nights per week and still maintain adequate nutrition.

The feed may be administered in small frequent doses (bolus feeding) using a syringe. Alternatively feed may be 'drip fed' from a 'ready-to-hang' container or reservoir (into which feed has been decanted) via a disposable plastic giving set. The feed may be 'drip fed' via gravity or with the aid of an electric feeding pump. Giving sets, reservoirs and syringes are designated for 'single use' and must be discarded after a 24-hour feeding period. Patients should be instructed to adhere to strict hygiene principles to prevent contamination of feed.[25]

Kirby[1] regards bolus feeding as a reliable method which a family member or the patient may administer at home. It frees the patient from a mechanical device and is especially beneficial for the alert active patient. It allows accurate feedings over specified time but may generate high residual volumes in the stomach. Gravity or intermittent drip feeding is not precise and, like bolus feeding, can predispose towards reflux and aspiration. Feeding pumps regulate the feed and reduce the risk of high residual volume and gastric aspiration.

Feeding pumps are now available within the UK which fulfil the criteria outlined by Park:[8] simple to use preferably without a drip stand, quiet especially for overnight feeding, practically indestructible, portable and accurate. The most common complaint is excessive noise from the rotary arm.

The choice of feeding system and method of feeding must take into account the patient's lifestyle. For instance an elderly immobile patient with low nutritional requirements may feel happier if given small frequent bolus feeds. The child who needs total nutrition could be fed throughout the day whilst at school using a back pack to hold his feeding system including a small portable pump (Fig. 21.3).

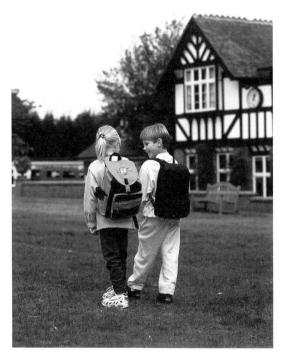

Figure 21.3 – Portable feeding system carried in back pack.

Problems and complications

Feeding tubes

According to Kirby *et al*[1] nasoenteric tubes can cause local irritation, epistaxis and sinusitis and can be easily dislodged. If the patient or relative or carer is not trained to reinsert tubes, arrangements for a designated individual to undertake this task must be made before the patient is discharged. Patients or carers need to understand that it is not a medical emergency if the tube is dislodged and that going for 24 hours without feed on a rare occasion will do no harm. Gastrostomy

feeding should be considered if nasoenteric tubes are dislodged regularly.

The most commonly reported problems with gastrostomies are: stomal leak, tube dislodgment, wound infections and excess granulation over stoma site.[8,26] Wound infections are easily treated with antibiotics. Meticulous skin care which includes cleaning the site and rotating the device daily prevents excess granulation. Chung & Schertzer[27] describe two rare complications: necrotising fasciitis and colocutaneous fistula. The first becomes evident within 3–14 days of tube placement, the second may not be detected for months, usually when the first tube is replaced.[28] When feeding comes to an end removal of the gastrostomy tube depends on the configuration of the internal retainer. Some are designed to be pulled through the stoma, others by cutting the tube at skin level and allowing the tube to pass in the stool. Stiff or rigid tubes are best removed endoscopically. When the gastrostomy is removed, either intentionally or inadvertently, there is usually prompt closure of the gastrocutaneous fistula.[1]

All tubes are likely to become blocked with residual feed or medication if correct flushing procedures are not followed. Local procedures may vary, but it is usual to flush tubes with 50 ml water after each bolus administration or, for continuous feeding, three times a day. Drinking water may be used providing the patient is not immunosuppressed.[26]

In clinical practice it is usually recommended that tubes are flushed with cooled boiled tap water provided that the patient is not immunosuppressed or fitted with a jejenostomy feeding tube; in the latter cases sterile water should be used. Additional water may be given as bolus doses if the prescribed feed is not meeting the patient's fluid requirements.

Aspiration of feed

Pulmonary aspiration is the most worrying complication of both nasogastric and gastrostomy feeding. Patients with gastro-oesophageal reflux and delayed gastric emptying are most at risk.[8] Cogen & Weinryb[29] demonstrated that 23% (109) of patients in nursing home aspirated. The only identifiable indicator of risk was that all these patients had previous histories of pneumonia.

Fay *et al*[30] described differences between long-term feeding by PEG and nasogastric feeding: within 14 days of tube placement non-fatal aspiration pneumonia occurred in 6% of patients with a PEG and 24% with a nasogastric tube. After a further 14 days the cumulative risk of aspiration by either technique was no different. Although there was a higher nasogastric tube replacement rate there was no significant difference in complications, nutrient delivery or survival in mean follow-up of 192 days with PEGs and 142 days with nasogastric tubes. This study concluded that PEGs should not be placed for those tolerating nasogastric tubes. To reduce the risk of aspiration, tube feeding should not take place with a patient in the recumbent position. The patient's bed head should be raised to an angle of 30–40 degrees during feeding and for one hour after feeding stops. Rapid bolus feeding should also be discouraged. Coben et al[31] showed that giving a bolus feed of 250 ml followed by 10 ml water over a 15 minute period caused a significant reduction in lower oesophageal pressure which was associated with free gastro-oesophageal reflux up to the sternal notch. Intermittent or continuous pump-assisted feeding or using jejunal access is recommended for high risk patients rather than rapid bolus methods.

Nutrient deficiencies

Patients whose enteral feeding is their sole source of nutrition and those non-compliant patients who do not take the full amount of the prescribed feed are at risk of developing nutritional deficiencies. Baxter[32] reported persistent mild iron deficiency anaemia in patients with oesophageal disease. Park[8] reported magnesium deficiency in a group with Crohn's disease. Ongoing biochemical monitoring is recommended for all patients on HETF.

Funding issues

In the UK feeding solutions are available on prescription via the patient's primary care physician. Disposable plastic equipment and feeding pumps are not and funding has to be found from a usually inadequate budget held by one of a number of agencies, e.g. the community nursing services, hospital dietetic or pharmacy departments. Park[8] states that a major hurdle to discharging patients is the lack of funding for disposable plastics and feeding pumps. Holden et al.[33] reported the mean time to arrange funding was 8 months (range 2 weeks–2 years). In 1998 a survey answered by 50 UK community dietitians highlights the lack of funding for equipment and inadequate provision of dietetic staff to provide satisfactory follow-up as areas of great concern (unpublished survey).

Returning the patient to the community

All centres who discharge patients into the community on HETF should have a written discharge policy and a procedure.[34] Before the decision is taken to send the patient home, the patient and his or her relatives should be made fully aware of what HETF entails. It may be useful for the patient and/or carers to have the opportunity to meet someone who is already established on HETF.[34]

Inquiries should be made about the patient's home circumstances and a home assessment should be made. The minimum standards should be: a clean sink and work area, a well placed electric point to plug in the feeding pump and a storage area for feed and equipment which is away from direct sunlight and extremes of heat.[21]

Once a discharge date has been identified the next step is to instigate a training programme. This should include the patient and a relative or carer, a community nurse if there is inadequate help at home, or nursing home staff if the patient is going to a nursing home. Training programmes should be tailored to meet the needs of the individual and sufficient time allowed for an acceptable level of competence to be achieved.

Holden[9] describes a variety of teaching programmes tailored to the needs of the individual family and child. These range from psychological preparation of the child for tube feeding, safety aspects, tube management, positioning of the child at night and recognition and management of complications. Play therapists have helped to develop an extensive play programme for preschool children. Dolls are used to demonstrate tube placement and aspiration and colouring-in books are available to explain the enteral feeding system. Older children are taught about their condition, by handling the equipment, watching videos and in some cases passing their own tubes.

Whilst training is under way, arrangements should be made for the ongoing supply of feed and equipment. Elia et al[34] describe a variety of ways this is organised in the UK. In the last few years a growing number of home care companies are providing a complete service to patients which includes training patients and carers on the use of equipment, delivery of feed and equipment, monitoring and reporting back to the discharging centre on compliance and offering a 24-hour emergency nursing service.

The patient should be provided with written information which includes details of the feeding regimen, feed administration protocol, how and when supplies will be provided, a pump manual (if a feeding pump is supplied) and contact names and telephone numbers for routine follow-up and for emergencies. Arrowsmith[21] suggests a trouble shooting guide which tells the patient:

What to do if:
- Diarrhoea, vomiting, or bloating is experienced
- The tube blocks
- The tube becomes displaced, who to contact
- Users are unable to aspirate the tube
- The PEG site is inflamed, oozing blood or pus at the exit site
- The feeding pump malfunctions
- Supplies of feed and equipment are running low.

A patients' support group such as PINNT (Patients on Intravenous and Nasogastric Nutrition Therapy PO Box 3126, Christchurch, Dorset, BH23 2XS) play an important role in providing information, auditing and improving patient care.

Follow-up and monitoring

The patient should be reviewed at regular intervals to monitor compliance with and adequacy of enteral feeding regimens. Ideally, weight, anthropometrics, full blood count, serum biochemistry and if possible micronutrient status should be recorded. In addition, for children, weight, height and head circumference should be plotted on centile charts to assess growth.[9] Patients with swallowing difficulties due to CVA should be re-assessed by a speech and language therapist to assess whether oral intake can be re-instated.

Outcome and quality of life

HETF will prolong the life of some patients, particularly those who cannot take any nourishment by mouth. Whilst it will not cure associated disease it has been shown to improve nutritional indices which indirectly may have a positive effect on clinical outcome and quality of life. For instance, nocturnal nasogastric feeding used with patients with cystic fibrosis was associated with weight gain and improved lung function;[10] HETF given for 12 months to 8 malnourished Crohn's patients had a positive effect on previously impaired linear growth and delayed sexual maturation;[35] nutritional indices such as height, weight and anthropometrics improved in a group of 17 stunted and 14 wasted children after feeding for a median duration of 15 months;[36] 19 adult patients with carcinoma of the oesophagus or tongue or oesophageal perforation who were fed for 30–435 days gained a significant amount of weight and all reported an improved quality of life.[37]

HETF appears to improve the quality of life, particularly of children. Holden et al[33] surveyed 70 families with experience of HETF. During 11 041 patient days no serious complications were seen. The nocturnal cough or chestiness noted in 10 children was attributed to occult gastro-oesophageal reflux. Sleep disturbance was common affecting 59 patients. Irrespective of these problems, parents' views were positive and advantages outweighed disadvantages; 35 children were described as being happy and active.

Michaelis et al[38] surveyed 24 carers of gastrostomy fed children about day to day problems. Problems identified were related to social functioning, recreational activities and family functioning. A positive relationship was found between problems with gastrostomy tubes and stress within the home. This study concluded that undertaking a family assessment, focusing on social and medical aspects of HETF, may maximise nutritional benefits to patients as well as improving general family functioning and reduce stress in the home.

Improvement in quality of life for adult patients is more difficult to assess as benefits bestowed by HETF may be outweighed by progressively debilitating neurological disease or terminal illness. However, Nelson et al[20] studied 53 such patients receiving HETF. They reported that the quality of life of patients receiving HETF improved for 50%, remained the same for 30% but deteriorated for the rest due to the demands of the feeding process.

The life expectancy of many patients commencing HETF is short due to underlying disease rather than complications of feeding. Weekes et al[39] and Moran and Frost[40] recorded mortality rates of 42% and 33% respectively.

Taylor and colleagues[41] followed the progress of a group of 97 patients fed by gastrostomy. At the end of 3 months 22% had died: 53% at 1 year, 65% at 1.5 years and 73% at 4 years. Those who had suffered a CVA or oesophageal malignancy had a higher mortality rate than those with neurological disorders.

BANS[7] reviewed the outcome of 8832 patients. By one year 13.6% patients had returned to full oral feeding of which 14% were patients who had suffered a CVA. Only a small percentage (1.5%) withdrew from feeding, 0.5% were in hospital and 62% continued feeding. The overall one year mortality was 22.4%, varying according to the clincal condition: 20% of all patients with a diagnosis of CVA were deceased by six months, rising to 28% at one year. Malignancies took a high toll also: oesophageal cancer (25%), oropharyngeal cancer (29.5%), gastric cancer (20%). However, 95% of the patients with cerebral palsy and 94% of those with cystic fibrosis survived for one year or more.

In the US, the Oley Foundation (1985–1990)[42] published data on 3708 patients, of whom 42% had a malignancy and 30% a neurological disorder of swallowing. Within the first year 70% of the patients with malignancy had died. By contrast, 60% of dysphagic patients survived to at least one year.

Ethical considerations

Attitudes towards prolongation of life of patients with severe and progressive disabilities vary from country to country due to different philosophical, religious and social beliefs and different national economies.[2]

HETF may be appropriate when the aim is to improve or maintain physical condition but inappropriate when the aim is palliative to provide comfort and relief of symptoms. A decision to withhold treatment is appropriate when the burden exceeds the probable benefit or it appears futile. In general treatment should not be withheld by carers on the grounds of age, lifestyle or the presence of mental or physical disability.[43]

Problems may occur in severely handicapped children in whom improved nutrition status can produce considerable benefits but may be regarded as un-

acceptably invasive by the parents. The aim of treatment should be agreed at the outset, and regular review of treatment should be undertaken to decide whether continuation is appropriate.[22] This is a sensible procedure in all circumstances when the patient's underlying condition is unlikely to improve or deteriorate and long-term feeding may be required. An initial trial of HETF is advisable for a defined period after which time it may be continued, stopped or altered as appropriate.[43]

Discussion about tube feeding often occurs after tube feedings has gone on for a time when the family and the doctor feel that further feeding is futile. Legally there is no difference between withholding and withdrawing tube feeding; however to discontinue feeding is stressful because the patient's death may be accelerated.[44]

A European perspective

The extent to which HETF is used in Europe is not accurately known since it is initiated, managed and recorded by many independent centres, public and private hospitals and commercial companies.[5] The response from key personnel in Germany, the Netherlands, Poland and Italy surveyed by the authors is shown in Table 21.3. Italy collects data relating to clinical groupings, e.g. neurological problems, but the Netherlands register patients by specialty. It is therefore difficult to determine the main indications for feeding. Three countries (Netherlands, Italy and Spain) were able to give some indication of feeding routes used, with the nasogastric route being the most common for both adults and children. Gastrostomy was the second most common feeding route.

Table 21.3 – The number of patients on HETF and national register in some European countries.

Country	National register	Number of patients receiving HETF in 1996
Germany	No	Unknown (many thousands)
Netherlands	Yes	>865
Poland	No	Unknown
Italy	No	761 (1995 data)
Spain	Yes	1193

Poland (although it is not able to estimate numbers of individuals on HETF) appears to have a structured approach with patients being cared for by their primary physicians. Training is carried out by nutrition teams who are also responsible for insertion of tubes and dealing with any complications which may arise.

The future

HETF has expanded rapidly in the US and the UK and appears to be growing in other European countries. In the future, an increasingly elderly population will place ever growing demands on national health care systems. HETF will be only one modality competing for limited finances. At present, data are unavailable to give a clear picture of the true incidence or to predict future need. In the UK the BANS register is beginning to record useful data. National HETF registers are essential to collect uniform data in relation to the incidence, clinical and cost effectiveness of this treatment in order to influence policy both at national, European and international level.

HETF in the UK has been bedevilled with funding problems ever since patients began to be discharged home in the early 1980s. This has caused problems with organisation and standardisation of care. Guidelines and standards which reflect best clinical practice, in selection, management, treatment and monitoring of patients contribute significantly to the success of HETF. These standards exist in the UK,[45,46] the US[47] and Australia.[48] Future care must be given and audited to an explicit standard in order to promote quality of care for patients and improve clinical outcomes.

References

1. Kirby DF, Delegge MH, Fleming CR. American Gastroenterological Association technical review on tube feeding for enteral nutrition. *Gastroenterology* 1995; 108; **4**: 1282–1301.

2. Elia M. Home enteral nutrition; general aspects and a comparison between the United States and Britain. *Nutrition* 1994; **10**: 2: 115–123.

3. Gauderer MWL, Ponskey JL, Izant RJ. Jr. Gastrostomy without laparotomy: a percutaneous endoscopic technique. *J Paediatr Surg* 1980; **15**: 872–875.

4. Howard L, Heaphey LL, Timchalk M. A review of the current national status of home parenteral and enteral nutrition from the consumer and provider perspective. *JPEN* 1986; **10**: 416.

5. Elia M. An international perspective on artificial nutritional support in the community. *Lancet* 1995; **345**: 1345–1349.

6. Todorovic VE, Micklewright A. Current trends in home feeding in the United Kingdom. Parenteral and Enteral Nutrition Group of the British Dietetic Association, Birmingham, UK, 1987.

7. British Artificial Nutrition Survey (BANS) *Annual Report.* PO Box 992, Maidenhead, Berks, SL6 4SH, UK (BAPEN), 1999.

7a. British Artificial Nutrition Survey (BANS) Annual Report. PO Box 922, Maidenhead, Berks, SL6 4SH, UK (BAPEN), 1997.

8. Park RH, Galloway RI, Ewing AB, MacHattie G, Davidson L. Home sweet HEN – a guide to home enteral nutrition. *Br J Clin Pract* 1992; **46**: 105–110.

9. Holden CE. Home enteral feeding. *Paediatr Nursing* 1990; July: 14–16.

10. Smith DL, Clarke JM, Stableforth DE. A nocturnal nasogastric feeding programme in cystic fibrosis adults. *J Hum Nutr Diet* 1994; **7**: 257–267.

11. Campos AC, Butters M, Meguid MM. Home enteral nutrition via gastrostomy in advanced head and neck cancer patients. *Head Neck* 1990 (Mar–April); **12**: 137–142.

12. Macdonald A, Littlewood J. Nutritional management of cystic fibrosis. Cystic Fibrosis Research Trust, Bromley, Kent, UK, 1989.

13. Rosa J, Daum F. Home nocturnal supplementary nasogastric feedings in growth retarded adolescents with Crohn's disease. *Gastroenterology* 1989; **97**: 905–910.

14. Grisel P. Identification of children with cerebral palsy unable to maintain a normal nutritional state. *Lancet* 1998; 283–285.

15. Garrington C. Fight for growth. *Clin Nutr Update* 1988; **1**: 6–7.

16. Moy RJD, Smallman S, Booth IW. Malnutrition in a UK children's hospital. *J Hum Nutr Diet* 1990; **3**: 93–100.

17. Twomey PL, Patching SC. Cost effectiveness of nutritional support. *JPEN* 1985; **9**: 3–14.

18. Micklewright A. Experience on long term home enteral nutrition in Europe. XVII ESPEN Congress, Geneva, Switzerland, 1996; pp. 131–136.

19. Reitz MV, Mattfeldt-Beman M, Ridley CM. Current practices in home nutritional support. *Nutr Supp Serv* 1988; **8**: 8.

20. Nelson JK, Palumbo PJ, O'Brien PC. Home enteral nutrition observations of a newly established programme. *Nutr Clin Pract* 1986; **1**: 193.

21. Arrowsmith HL. Discharging patients receiving enteral nutrition. *Br J Nurs* 1994: 3; **11:** 551–557.

22. Puntis JW, Holden CE. Home enteral nutrition in paediatric practice. *Br J Hosp Med* 1991; **45:** 104–107.

23. McCrae D, Hall H. Current practices for home nutrition. *J Am Dietet Assoc* 1989; **89:** 233–240.

24. Ponsky JL, Gauderer MWL, Stellato TA, Aszodi A. Percutaneous approaches to enteral alimentation. *Am J Surg* 1985; **149:** 102–105.

25. European Standard BS EN 1615. Sterile enteral feeding catheters and giving sets for single use. BSI 389 Chiswick High Street, London W4 4AL, UK, 1997.

26. Taylor S, Goodinson-McClaren S. *Nutritional Support: A team approach.* Wolfe Publishing, London, 1992.

27. Chung RS, Schertzer M. Pathogenesis of complications of percutaneous endoscopic gastrostomy: a lesson in surgical principles. *Am J Surg* 1990; **56:** 134–137.

28. Martindale RG, Witte M, Hodges G, Kelly J, Harris S, Andersen C. Necrotising fasciitis as a complication of percutaneous endoscopic gastrostomy. *JPEN* 1987; **11:** 583–585.

29. Cogen R, Weinryb J. Aspiration pneumonia in nursing home patients fed via gastrostomy tubes. *Am J Gastroenterol* 1989; **84:** 1509–1512.

30. Fay DE, Poplauskey M, Gruber M, Lance P. Long term enteral feeding: a retrospective comparison of delivery via percutaneous endoscopic gastrostomy and nasoenteric tubes. *Am J Gastroenterol* 1991; **86:** 1604–1609.

31. Coben RM, Weintraub A, DiMarino AJ Jr, Cohen S. Gastroesophageal reflux during gastrostomy feeding. *Gastroenterology* 1994; **106:** 13–18.

32. Baxter YC, Goncalves Dias MC, Maculevicius J, Faintuch J, Cecconello I, Pinotti HW. Iron deficiency anaemia in enteral nutrition: correlation with tube position. *Rev Hosp Clin Fac Med* Sao Paulo 1995 (Nov–Dec); **50:** 330–333.

33. Holden CE, Puntis JW, Charlton CP, Booth IW. Nasogastric feeding at home: acceptability and safety. *Arch Dis Child* 1991; **66:** 148–151.

34. Elia M, Cottee S, Holden C, Micklewright A, Pennington C, Plant J, Shaffer C, Wheatley C, Wood S. Enteral and parenteral nutrition in the community. BAPEN, PO Box 922, Maidenhead, UK, 1994.

35. Aiges H, Markowitz J, Rosa J, Daum F. Home nocturnal supplementary naso-gastric feeding in growth retarded adolescents with Crohn's disease. *Gastroenterology* 1989; **97:** 905–910.

36. Papadopoulou A, Holden CE, Paul L, Sexton E, Booth IW. The nutritional response to home enteral nutrition in childhood. *Acta Paediatr* 1995; **84:** 528–531.

37. Sami H, Saint-Aubert B, Szawlowski AW, Astre CH. Home enteral nutrition system: one patient, one daily ration of an 'all-in-one' sterile and modular formular in a single container. *JPEN* 1990; **14:** 173–176.

38. Michaelis CA, Warzak WJ, Stanek K, Van Riper C. Parental and professional perceptions of problems associated with long term home tube feeding. *J Am Diet Assoc* 1992; **92:** 1235–1238.

39. Weekes E, Cottee S, Elia M. Home artificial nutritional support in Cambridge health district. *Health Trends* 1992; **23:** 93–100.

40. Moran BJ, Frost RA. Percutaneous endoscopic gastrostomy in 41 patients: indications and clinical outcome. *J Royal Soc Med* 1992; **85:** 320–321.

41. Taylor CA, Larson DE, Ballard DJ, Bergstrom LR, Silverstein MD, Zinmeister AR, DiMagno EP. Predictors of outcome after percutaneous endoscopic gastrostomy: a community based study. *Mayo Clin Proc* 1992; **67:** 1042–1049.

42. Oley Foundation. First report using longitudinal data. North American home parenteral and enteral nutrition: patient registry. Annual report with outcome profiles 1985–1990. Silver Spring, MD: ASPEN, 1992.

43. Lennard-Jones JE. Ethical and legal aspects of clinical nutritional support. BAPEN, PO Box 922, Maidenhead, UK, 1998.

44. Fairman RP. Withdrawing life sustaining treatment. Lessons from Nancy Cruzan. *Arch Intern Med* 1992; **252:** 25–27.

45. Sizer T, Russell CA, Irwin S, Allison SP, Wheatley C, Whitney S, Wood S. Standards and guidelines for nutritional support of patients in hospitals. BAPEN PO Box 992, Maidenhead, Berks, SL6 4SH, UK, 1996.

46. McAtear CA, Wright C. Dietetic standards for nutritional support. Parenteral and Enteral Nutrition Group of the British Dietetic Association, Birmingham, UK, 1996.

47. ASPEN. Standards for home nutritional support. *Nutr Clin Pract* 1992; **7:** 65–6.

48. AUSPEN. Report on the ministerial working party on home enteral nutrition. Acute Health Division, Dept Human Services, Victoria, Australia, 1997.

22

Venous access for parenteral nutrition

Diane Palmer and John MacFie

Introduction

Despite the fact that parenteral nutrition is now accepted as a safe and effective therapy in the care of patients in whom enteral absorption of nutrients is insufficient, there remains controversy over the optimal means of administering this treatment. When parenteral nutrition was first established it had to be delivered through a central venous catheter and this became the standard and conventional means of venous access. In recent years there has been a revival of interest in parenteral nutrition delivered using peripheral veins. The purpose of this chapter is to outline the background to both central (CPN) and peripheral (PPN) feeding and to describe current opinion with regard to indications, techniques, materials and complications.

History of intravenous catheterisation

The description by William Harvey (1578–1657) of the continuous circulation of blood within a contained system was one of the 17th century's most significant achievements in medicine.[1] It was as a logical extension of Harvey's work that the first tentative steps into the intravenous administration of drugs and blood transfusion were made. The first documented record of an intravenous injection was by Dr Robert Boyle.[1a] He infused opium into the saphenous vein of a dog. The experiment was performed at the suggestion of Sir Christopher Wren who predicted the possibility of introducing liquids into the bloodstream with potential benefit. A quill, connected to an animal bladder which contained the drug, was used as the needle which was inserted by cut-down. Subsequent to this there were isolated accounts of attempts at intravenous therapy in both animals and man. Wine, for example, was instilled into hunting dogs using thin silver cylinders. Another 100 years or so was to pass before the full potential for intravenous therapy was realised. Following the cholera epidemic of the 1830s, O'Shaughnessy infused solutions of chlorate and nitrate into dogs, using a syringe and a silver tube.[2] One Dr Latta, a general practitioner from Scotland, made up solutions of these salts and administered them to cholera victims with considerable success.[3] In 1855 Wood developed a piston syringe with a hollow needle and similar steel needles remained in use for the best part of the next 100 years.[4] The next major advance in the hardware required for intravenous cannulation occurred in the late 1940s with the development of plastic polymers. The Rochester needle, the first plastic catheter with a needle trochar and forerunner of the modern intravenous catheter, was introduced in 1950,[5] and the prototype indwelling scalp needle appeared the same year.[6] In 1953, Seldinger published a catheter-over-wire method of intravascular catheterisation which facilitated the cannulation of veins with a relatively small needle and the replacement over this of a larger diameter plastic catheter.[7]

These advances in intravenous cannulation facilitated the use of blood transfusion and fluid replacement and encouraged the widespread adoption of various intravenous drugs. However, they all suffered from the same limitation of infusion phlebitis. This complication had been recognised for many years. Henriques and Anderson in 1913 described the association between osmolality of infusates and the risk of venous thrombosis and were amongst the first to propose the use of central veins.[8] Forssmann in 1929 described one of the first central venous cannulations in man carrying out the procedure on himself.[9] Whilst standing behind a fluoroscopic screen and looking into a mirror he threaded an oiled ureteric catheter from his cephalic vein through to the right atrium. A mere 12 years later cardiac catheterisation using lacquered silk catheters was established. These techniques did not, however, permit prolonged and safe access to the central veins. This only became a feasible proposition in 1952 following the description by a French surgeon of infraclavicular percutaneous subclavian vein cannulation.[10] This method had been used for some years in the treatment of war casualties with severe burns. It was realised that the subclavian vein although large and close to the heart was not covered anteriorly by other important structures, was superficial and therefore easily accessible and was also relatively well fixed to neighbouring structures, thereby permitting easy cannulation. Aubaniac's method was rapidly adopted by both civil and military surgeons. Indeed, it was this technique which permitted the evolution of parenteral nutrition as we know it today.

By the 1950s both glucose and protein hydrolysates solutions were available. However, both were hypertonic and rapidly resulted in infusion phlebitis if given into peripheral veins. The problem was overcome by Dudrick and colleagues[11] who adopted the technique of subclavian vein cannulation described by Aubaniac and in so doing were able to produce the first compelling evidence of successful parenteral nutrition in both animals and man (see Table 22.1).

Table 22.1 – Landmarks in the development of total parenteral nutrition.

1628	William Harvey: description of blood circulation.[1]
1654	Sir Christopher Wren. Intravenous infusion of solutions such as wine.[12a]
1712	Courten. Intravenous infusion of fat.[12b]
1831	Latta. Infusion of salt solutions to cholera patients.[3]
1855	Wood. Developed the piston syringe.[4]
1873	Hodder. Milk given intravenously to cholera patients.[12c]
1904	Friedrich. Total parenteral nutrition by subcutaneous injections of fat, peptones, glucose and salt solutions.[12d]
1913	Henriques. Intravenous infusions of beef protein hydrolysate in goats.[8]
1937	Elman. Successful intravenous infusion of protein hydrolysates in man.[12e]
1952	Aubaniac. Techniques for subclavian venous cannulation.[10]
1953	Seldinger. Described catheter over wire technique which enabled the cannulation of veins with a relatively small needle and the placement over this of a larger diameter plastic cannula.[7]
1961	Wretlind. Development of a safe intravenous fat emulsion.
1968	Dudrick. First report of long term growth and survival in puppies with intravenous feeding using central venous cannulation.[11]
1974	Solassol. Demonstrates that fat emulsions can be safely mixed crystalline amino acids and dextrose solutions.[63]
1976–84	Many studies confirm that fat emulsions have equivalent nitrogen sparing effects to glucose and are, therefore, appropriate energy source for TPN (e.g. see [58,62]).
1976–86	Stimulated by the pioneering work of Kinney with indirect calorimetry[11a] many studies confirm that few surgical patients will require more than 2000 kcals/day (e.g. see [11b,62]).

Parenteral nutrition using the central venous route (CPN)

Indications

- Patients who require long-term parenteral nutrition
- Those without adequate peripheral veins

- A small number who have specific nutrition requirements
- Many, such as those on intensive care units and the critically ill, who already have central venous access established
- Patients in whom difficulties with peripheral access are anticipated
- Those in whom peripheral parenteral nutrition (PPN) has failed
- Patients such as those with high output enterocutaneous fistulae who have large volume requirements.

CPN should be used with caution in patients with a history of major venous thrombosis of the subclavian, innominate or jugular vessels, in those who have already sustained a complication of central venous catheterisation or in whom insertion of central catheters is deemed technically difficult or dangerous. CPN should not be used as a first line approach to parenteral nutrition in otherwise uncomplicated patients in whom PPN may be a safer first option.

Some clinicians continue to advocate CPN as their preferred route of delivery for all patients requiring parenteral nutrition. They argue that modern techniques of cannulation in experienced hands are safe and the use of the central venous route precludes problems of venous access. The necessity to establish central venous access ensures that only those patients who really are in need of parenteral nutrition receive this form of treatment thereby encouraging all attempts to use the enteral route. After all, parenteral nutrition is a potentially hazardous and expensive form of treatment which should not be embarked upon unless absolutely necessary. Furthermore, the proponents of this view point to the frequent occurrence of infusion phlebitis during PPN suggesting that successful PPN is only possible in a minority of units. The counter-argument to this is that techniques that simplify the administration of parenteral nutrition such as PPN will allow patients to receive appropriate nutrition support at an earlier stage of their illness and without significant morbidity.

Central venous catheters

Catheter material

Ideally, catheters should be firm at room temperature for ease of insertion, but become soft and pliable once in the vein to minimise intimal damage. They should be of low thrombogenicity so the platelet adhesion and consequently the risk of thrombus formation is minimised. Thrombogenicity is related to the surface properties of the material employed for catheter manufacture. Catheters are produced by extrusion which inevitably results in longitudinal grooves on external surfaces. Surface irregularities can also result from addition of radiopaque material to the catheter. Surface properties of wettability, surface charge and surface tension are all also important considerations. Catheters must be inert and should not release catalysts or stabilisers locally that could induce an inflammatory reaction. The material should have properties which permit catheters to be thin-walled allowing maximum flow rates for a minimum external diameter. For prolonged use it is important that the material remains flexible and kink-resistant.

Catheters have been made from a variety of plastics including polytetrafluoroethylene (Teflon™), polyurethane, silicone elastomer, polyethylene and polyvinylchloride (PVC). The optimal material remains unknown. Polyethylene catheters have been shown to cause significantly more thrombi than the softer silicone elastomer catheters.[12] Polyurethane has the advantage over silicone of being stronger and having a greater internal diameter for the same external diameter. Platelet adherence to polyurethane appears to be less compared to polyvinyl chloride and other fluorocarbon devices.[13] The incidence of thrombosis was found to be least in association with polyurethane catheters in a post-mortem study which compared these with polyethylene and silicone elastomer.[14] The presence of catalysts and stabilisers used during the manufacture of catheters may predispose to thrombosis.[15] Bozzetti et al found venographic evidence of thrombosis in 46% of polyvinyl chloride catheters compared to 11% of silastic catheters.[16] Polyurethane may be even less thrombogenic than silicone elastomer because of its smoother surface.[17] These and other studies suggest that polyurethane is the current material of choice for catheter manufacture[18,19] although it should be noted that environmental stress cracking and calcification has been reported during long-term use.[20] It is worth stressing, however, that the perfect catheter is useless if poor technique is used and scrupulous attention to detail remains the prerequisite of good catheter care.

Catheters are now being manufactured with the specific aim of reducing line sepsis. Short-term catheters with a silver impregnated cuff have been reported as being associated with significant reductions in colonisation of catheters and associated catheter-related infections.[21] Antibiotic-coated catheters have also been shown in one randomised trial to result in significant reductions in infectious complication but have raised concern over the possibility of encouraging the growth of resistant organisms to the antibiotics employed.[22] This might be overcome by the use of antiseptic impregnated catheters and these have been shown in preliminary studies to be effective.

Catheter types

Short to medium-term parenteral nutrition (up to 3 months) is usually established using one of the many commercially available kits. These provide a needle for puncturing the vein, a guide wire which is passed down the vein and a catheter which is passed over the guide wire. There is little to choose between these kits and personal preference must dictate choice.

The catheter most frequently used for long-term and home parenteral nutrition (HPN) is the Hickman line.[23] This was a modified version of the Broviac catheter first described in the early 1970s.[24] These catheters are made of silastic and have a luer lock cap sealing the hub. Some 20–30 cm from the hub there is a small Dacron cuff, the original purpose of which was to incite a fibrous response thus stabilising the catheter. The diameter of the lumen is 1.6 mm. Hickman and Broviac catheters are passed into the superior vena cava via the subclavian vein, the proximal end being tunnelled subcutaneously in the chest wall with the exit point at a suitable location on the chest wall for patient access and dressing. One of the specific problems associated with Hickman and Broviac catheters is fracture, which could result in air embolus. The Dacron cuff on these catheters now incorporates an antimicrobial component on the presumption that this discourages bacterial migration from the hub. This thereby has a dual purpose in providing long-term securement and a barrier to catheter-related infections. There is, however, no evidence from controlled studies of significant advantage from the presence or absence of cuffs.[25] Removal of these catheters necessitates formal dissection in the operating theatre.

A later modification of the Hickman type catheter is the Groshong™ (Bard Ltd, Crawley, West Sussex, UK) which incorporates a one-way valve at the distal end. This is normally closed but will allow flow in

veins such as the cephalic, the external jugular or the saphenous with use of the Seldinger technique to pass the catheter into a major vessel. Parenteral nutrition via the femoral vein using catheters fed into the right atrium is appropriate in patients with superior vena caval obstruction but not under other circumstances.

Experience and training are essential prerequisites of central venous catheterisation whatever method is employed.[38] Morbidity related to the common complications can be minimised by careful attention to technique. Whatever method is used feeding should not be commenced until a post-insertion chest X-ray confirms that the tip of the catheter lies within the superior vena cava. The risk of venous thrombosis is considerably increased if hypertonic solutions are delivered into the subclavian or more proximal veins.[39]

Insertion of central venous catheter by radiologists using either ultrasound or fluoroscopic guidance has been advocated.[40] Time constraints on radiology departments will probably preclude this as routine practice. One study compared insertion of subclavian lines using ultrasound with conventional 'blind' techniques finding no difference in morbidity.[38]

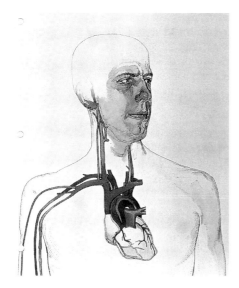

Figure 22.3 – Sites for venous access.

Complications

Complications of insertion

Complications attributable to catheter insertion occur in 3–12% of cases.[15] Whichever approach is adopted

any nearby anatomical structure is at risk. The most common following infraclavicular subclavian insertion are injury to the pleura resulting in pneumothorax and damage to the subclavian artery. A significant pneumothorax will necessitate a chest drain. Pressure on the puncture site is usually all that is required following inadvertent arterial damage. Less common complications include haemothorax, subcutaneous emphysema, subclavian haematoma, pleural effusion and hydromediastinum, brachial plexus injury, air embolism, thoracic duct damage, cardiac perforation with tamponade and perforation of the inferior vena cava or the pulmonary vessels.

Catheter-related sepsis

Infection occurs in between 3 and 14% of patients.[15] The skin is the most common source of organisms causing catheter-related infections.[41] Coagulase negative staphylococci are the bacteria most frequently isolated from catheters but in most cases this colonisation does not progress to bacteraemia. The isolation of *Staphylococcus aureus* from blood cultures is, however, strongly predictive of catheter-related bacteraemia.[42] There is a higher incidence of infection with *Corynebacterium* and *Enterococcus* species, gram negative rods and fungi in infections of tunnelled catheters compared with others but this probably reflects the decreased immune status of patients with these types of catheters.[43] *Candida* species are frequently seen. Haematogenous dissemination from other sites of infection accounts for greater than 50% of yeast infections as well as most infections due to enterococcal and gram negative organisms.[44]

A variety of hypotheses have been proposed to explain the events leading to infection of central catheters. Bacterial skin colonisation at the catheter skin interface at the time of insertion or afterwards with distal spread of the bacteria along the external catheter surface has been suggested for short-term catheters. Other studies have shown that the introduction of bacteria via the catheter hub due to frequent manipulations is another important means of access. This latter method is probably more important for long indwelling catheters. Contamination of the infusate is rare these days. Seeding of the catheter at the time of bacteraemia from a remote source can also cause catheter infection. Most now agree that infection usually arises from the catheter hub which has been found to be colonised by organisms in 70% of patients with catheter-related sepsis in one study.[28]

Catheter-related sepsis should not be diagnosed simply on the basis of a blood culture drawn through a catheter as this may reflect systemic bacteraemia. Similarly, a growth of skin commensals from the catheter tip after removal of the catheter may represent contamination during withdrawal. Diagnosis of catheter-related sepsis requires that the same organism is grown from the catheter tip as is recovered from the blood and that the clinical features of infection resolve on removal of the catheter. Removal of catheters on clinical suspicion alone results in line tip cultures being negative in 75–85% of catheters.[45] Catheter removal under these circumstances is unnecessary and an expensive waste of time. Traditional methods of diagnosing infected lines have relied upon sacrifice of the catheter and subsequent bacteriological and clinical assessment. An alternative approach is to use an endoluminal brush (FAS Medical). This device is an 8 mm long nylon-bristled, tapered brush which is passed down the catheter to its distal end and then withdrawn into a polythene sheath. The brush is sent for microbiological culture without removal of the line and simultaneous peripheral blood cultures are taken. Catheter-related sepsis is confirmed if the same microorganism is identified from endoluminal sampling and from peripheral cultures. Colonisation is presumed if only endoluminal samples are positive. A recent prospective study reported significant advantages for this method both in terms of sensitivity and specificity when compared to techniques that necessitated line removal.[46] An alternative, frequently adopted technique which also obviates the need for catheter removal depends upon comparative quantitative blood cultures. In this, blood is drawn simultaneously through the catheter and a peripheral vein. If the colony count in the catheter blood is five or more times that in the peripheral blood, catheter-related sepsis is probable.[47] Another new method for diagnosing catheter-related sepsis describes an acridine orange leucocyte cytospin test, which is reported as being both quick and sensitive.[48]

Despite this plethora of interesting developments in the diagnosis of catheter-related sepsis, most authorities continue to recommend that the present policy of changing catheters over a guide wire and of taking cultures of catheter blood and tip is a safe and effective management of suspected infection.[49] Changing over a guide wire has been shown to be safer than selecting a new insertion site unless catheter-related sepsis is confirmed.[30] Further, there is no justification for prophylactic changing of lines as is the practice in some institutions. The incidence of sepsis does not increase with duration of catheter placement and these should only be changed if a complication occurs.[30]

Venous thrombosis

Routine venography has shown that venous thrombosis complicates 45–59% of catheters but only 2.5–4.8% of patients have symptoms and clinical signs.[15] Thrombosis increases with the duration of catheterisation. Only contributing factors include the nature of the catheter and its position, venous endothelial damage during insertion of the catheter and concomitant infection. Clots form mainly in the innominate veins, the superior vena cava and the right atrium and are rare in the right ventricle. Clots in the right atrium are particularly common in neonates receiving parenteral nutrition. Catheter-related central venous thrombosis can be a devastating complication of long-term venous access.[50] Low dose warfarin is standard therapy to reduce this risk in home parenteral nutrition patients. It has been recommended that the risk of venous thrombosis can be minimised during parenteral nutrition by the use of anticoagulants.[15] However, there is a recognised morbidity associated with such treatment as well as potential problems related to stability of compounded mixtures containing both fat emulsions and heparin.[51]

Patients with clinically significant thrombosis usually present with limb swelling or with the syndrome of superior vena cava obstruction. The recommended management of unilateral limb swelling is usually to remove the catheter, instigate full anticoagulation and elevate the limb. Some have advocated that it is not necessary to remove the catheter unless it is infected, the position of its tip is unsatisfactory or its lumen is occluded.[52] The catheter can be left in place but not used until the swelling has subsided, although anticoagulation may be required for periods of up to six weeks. Clearly in patients receiving short-term parenteral nutrition this management would not be appropriate. In these patients the use of fibrinolytic therapy such as urokinase either by bolus injection or infusion remains controversial.[53] In contrast, fibrinolysis is recommended for patients with superior vena caval thrombosis particularly if the catheter remains patent.

Catheter occlusion

Catheters may be occluded by blood clot, fatty deposits or calcium salts. The use of 'all in one' mixtures containing fat, amino acids and glucose is said to be associated with a higher occlusion rate. It has been postulated that lipid particles coalesce and enlarge in these circumstances and as a result precipitate on to the catheter. Catheter occlusion is less frequent if lipid is administered separately from other nutrients.

Occlusion of catheters can be prevented by ensuring that neither blood nor nutrient solutions are allowed to stagnate within the catheter for any length of time. The use of cyclical parenteral nutrition with the catheter being locked with heparin during periods of no feeding reduces the risk of occlusion. There is also evidence that the addition of one to three units of heparin to every millilitre of infusion solution may reduce the incidence of occlusion. An early sign of impending occlusion is the inability to aspirate blood through the catheter despite satisfactory infusion of fluids. In these cases locking the catheter with a solution containing urokinase may be successful.

One recent study has shown that fibrous tissue rather than clotted material was the predominant component of sheaths found on long-term catheters.[54] Alcohol and hydrochloric acid have thus been advocated for clearing occluded catheters since clot is often not the problem. Patency was restored in 34 of 39 patients in one study using a combination of 70% ethanol and 0.1N HCL.[55] Ethanol was thought to dissolve the waxy lipid deposits and HCL dissolved mineral and drug deposits.

Peripheral parenteral nutrition (PPN)

Evolution of PPN

Peripheral parenteral nutrition is not a new concept. Indeed, all the original attempts to provide nutrients intravenously were administered into peripheral veins as there was no alternative at the time. Whilst there was some limited success with these techniques complete parenteral nutrition was not possible. It was not until Dudrick *et al* described the use of central veins for the administration of hypertonic solutions that complete parenteral nutrition became a realistic proposition.[11] Not surprisingly, CPN rapidly became established as the standard technique for parenteral nutrition and interest in PPN rapidly dwindled.

The last 20 years or so have however seen a number of research developments all of which have resulted in

modifications of technique which facilitate the use of PPN. These are summarised in Table 22.1. The first of these was the description by Schubert and Wretlind of a safe and non-toxic fat emulsion.[56] Fat emulsions are isotonic compared to plasma and can therefore be administered through a peripheral catheter. Fat emulsions have been shown to exert a protective effect on the venous endothelium.[57] The late 1970s and early 1980s saw a number of studies published all of which attested to the equivalent nitrogen sparing effects of fat versus glucose as energy sources during TPN.[58,59,60,61] Fat emulsions were no longer considered as simply a source of essential fatty acids. Today, the concomitant use of fat and glucose as energy sources together with amino acids is accepted as optimal nutrition therapy.

Another important advance was the realisation that energy and protein requirements were much lower than formerly considered necessary, thereby significantly reducing total fluid requirements – which facilitates the use of peripheral veins. During the early years of TPN, calorie intakes were frequently based on the incorrect assumption that energy and protein requirements were directly related on the basis of a 200:1 ratio. This inevitably resulted in energy intakes well in excess of 3000 kcals/day and the volumes required to administer these intakes precluded peripheral administration. There is now a wealth of data available on energy requirements based on measurements obtained by indirect calorimetry. The consensus opinion is now that very few patients will ever need in excess of 2000 (8368 kJ) kcals/day in order to achieve energy balance.[58,62] This reduces the need for large volume infusions which themselves necessitate the use of central veins.

Finally, tribute must be made to the pioneering work from Montpellier which demonstrated that fat emulsions could be safely mixed with crystalline amino acid and dextrose solutions in a single container.[63] This appreciation of the pharmaceutical considerations involved in compounding and in the compatibility of TPN constituents allowed pharmacists to provide clinicians with compounded TPN bags containing solutions which have an osmolality in the order of 300–900 mmol/L which can be safely administered by a peripheral vein. Peripheral parenteral nutrition was a feasible proposition prior to the development of compounded solutions in a single container but in practice it demanded the use of separate infusions given concurrently, using different delivery systems. These methods required considerable nursing expertise and have been shown to be associated with increased morbidity.[64]

All of these developments have facilitated the practical application of PPN in clinical practice. The cumulative effect is that PPN has now evolved as a viable alternative to CPN for many patients.

PPN: *current practice*

There is clear evidence that the use of PPN is increasing both in this country and across Europe. In a national survey of clinical nutrition in the UK in 1988, PPN had been used by 60% of all respondents.[65] PPN, however, comprised only 7% of all the parenteral nutrition given. These figures were similar when the survey was repeated in 1991 except that the number of TPN courses administered peripherally had doubled to 15%.[67] The 1994 survey reported 95% of respondents using PPN, with 18.3% completing their course with this method.[66] Clearly there has been an explosion of interest in PPN and the various techniques designed to reduce morbidity. There is now good evidence from many different centres around Europe that PPN is a viable alternative to CPN in many patient groups. It can now be considered as the first choice for parenteral nutrition in many patients.

Those unsuitable for PPN include markedly hypercatabolic patients with significantly increased energy or protein requirements. This might apply, for instance, to those with severe burns or following extensive trauma when, for whatever reason, enteral nutrition is deemed inadequate. PPN may not be appropriate in patients with substantial fluid requirements such as those with high output enterocutaneous fistulae. It is inappropriate to use PPN when patients already have an indwelling central venous catheter in which there is an available port for TPN. Obviously, PPN will not be possible in patients with poor or absent peripheral venous access. Finally, PPN cannot be considered an alternative to CPN in any patient who requires long-term (>1 month) parenteral nutrition.

It would be incorrect to conclude, however, that PPN will ever completely substitute for CPN. Figure 22.4 illustrates our indications for TPN in the last 2 years and Figure 22.5 the respective proportion of patients fed by either the peripheral or central routes. It can be seen that PPN represents a significant proportion of total feeding. The indication for feeding remains fairly

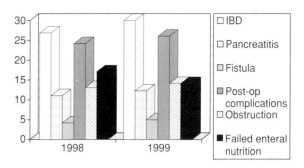

Figure 22.4 – Scarborough Hospital indications for parenteral nutrition 1998 and 1999.

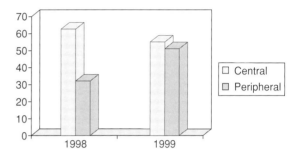

Figure 22.5 – Proportion of patients fed by peripheral and central routes in last 2 years.

constant, probably as a result of the consistent assessment criteria mediated by our nutrition team.

PPN: *limitations*

Peripheral parenteral nutrition avoids the risks of central venous catheterisation, simplifies nursing care, reduces cost and may also prevent delay in the initiation of nutrition support.[62,68,69] Despite this, there are many objections to the use of PPN. An important concern has been that insufficient calories and nitrogen can be delivered for sufficient periods of time and that it should, therefore, only be thought of as supplemental feeding. However, there is now general agreement that the protein and energy needs of the majority of patients who require parenteral nutrition will rarely exceed 0.25 g N/kg/day or 30 kcal (126 kJ)/kg/day,[62,68] which can be given in volumes of less than 3 litres/day. Such volume requirements do not preclude peripheral administration and positive energy and nitrogen balance is readily achieved with these intakes.[70] A typical regimen providing approximately 9 g of nitrogen and 1600 kcals is shown in Table 22.2.

Table 22.2 – Typical peripheral parenteral nutrition regimen.

One bag (2580 ml) contains:
Triglycerides 100 g, Phospholipids 6 g, Glycerol 11 g.
Amino acids 57 g, Nitrogen 9 g, Glucose 150 g.
Total energy 1830 kcal   From fat 1000 kcal (4.2 MJ)
   (7.7 MJ):

                     From carbohydrates 600 kcal
                     (2.5 MJ)
                     From amino acids 230 kcal
                     (1.0 MJ)
                 Non-protein energy 1600 kcal
Osmolality: 770 mosm/kg water.
pH 5.6
Electrolytes: Na 80 mmol,   K 60 mmol,   Ca 5 mmol,
                Mg 5 mmol,   P 28 mmol,   Cl 80 mmol.

A very important additional factor in the consideration of PPN as total or simply supplemental parenteral nutrition is the average duration of feeding required. The majority of hospitalised patients (>75%) in the UK with temporary intestinal failure who require parenteral nutrition receive it for less than 14 days and 50% for less than 10 days.[66] Numerous studies have demonstrated that PPN for 2 weeks is easily achievable.[71,72] Indeed, there are an increasing number of reports in which patients have been successfully fed by the peripheral route for periods up to 3 weeks or more.[64,73] Peripheral parenteral nutrition does not therefore need to be regarded simply as supplemental feeding.

Another frequently cited disadvantage of PPN is the fact that it obviously is not possible in patients with inadequate peripheral veins. In advocating CPN some authors have stated that many patients, particularly the critically ill or those referred to tertiary centres, will no longer have adequate peripheral venous access. Few prospective and randomised studies have been reported that attempted to determine what proportion of all patients who require TPN would actually be unsuitable for PPN. In one of these, patients with a wide range of acute medical and surgical gastroenterological conditions were prospectively randomised to receive either CPN or PPN.[71] Many of the patients were critically ill with exacerbations of inflammatory bowel disease, complications of acute pancreatitis or following major excisional surgery. The results demonstrated that 56% of patients randomised to PPN received their entire TPN course by this route. This finding that a large number of patients in hospital practice are suitable candidates for PPN is confirmed by others.[74] This serves to emphasise that PPN should be considered in patients who require TPN, whatever their underlying medical condition.

The most important limiting factor to PPN is the occurrence of peripheral vein thrombophlebitis (PVT). A better understanding of the aetiology of PVT and the development of techniques to minimise morbidity from this complication have dramatically altered current perceptions of PPN and its applicability to everyday practice. These are reviewed below.

Peripheral vein thrombophlebitis (PVT)

The pathogenesis and aetiology of infusion phlebitis or thrombophlebitis have been extensively reviewed elsewhere.[69] It presents to the clinician as an inflammatory response at the site of peripheral venous cannulation. Physical signs include erythema, oedema, hardness of the vein and pain. The end result of PVT is occlusion of the vein or extravasation of the infusate.

Hecker *et al* proposed that the initial event in the pathogenesis of PVT was venoconstriction at the tip of the catheter which occurred as a result of damage to the venous endothelium caused either by the catheter tip or by the infusate itself.[75] Following venoconstriction, flow is reduced such that dilution of the infusate is impaired leading to further damage. This hypothesis was extended by Payne-James who proposed that the evolution of PVT is a cycle of events incorporating endothelial damage, the release of inflammatory mediators, subsequent thrombosis and consequently further endothelial damage.[69] More recently, Everitt has questioned the importance of venoconstriction, postulating the occurrence of early and late thrombophlebitis.[76] Early PVT probably occurs as a result of venous damage created at the time of venepuncture and late PVT as a consequence of mechanical and chemical trauma causing thrombosis at the catheter tip.

A number of factors are important in the aetiology of PVT. These are summarised in Table 22.3. In essence, anything that causes endothelial damage may result in PVT. Conversely, anything that avoids or minimises endothelial damage can be expected to reduce the incidence of PVT. It is not surprising considering the complex interplay of factors involved that review of

Table 22.3 – Predisposing factors to PVT and effect of their modification.

Predisposing factor	Mode of action	Recommendation	Notes	References
bacterial colonisation	sepsis may induce inflammatory response	aseptic technique and protocols for catheter care essential	little correlation between incidence of colonisation and subsequent development of PVT. Skin commensals commonest organism	80 81
cannula size	in-dwelling cannula will inevitably cause endothelial damage.	smallest gauge cannula shortest length cannula	surface area of cannula determines extent of mechanical trauma	69 77 86
cannula material	non-flexible and rigid cannulas increase venous damage. some synthetic surfaces more prone to platelet aggregation.	polyurethane cannulas associated with significant reductions in incidence phlebitis		14
trauma at venepuncture	cannulation trauma may cause venospasm	use smallest needle possible for cannulation use largest vein possible		75 82
size of vein	larger vein permits rapid dilution infusate. larger vein permits tip of cannula to 'float' in vein minimising trauma	use largest vein possible		69 79 86
duration of infusion	continuous uninterrupted infusion will inevitably result in PVT after 4–5 days. Infusions < 12 hours rarely associated with PVT	minimise duration of infusion		78 97 64 77
osmolarity (osmolar concentration) and osmolarity rate (osmolarity★ infusion rate)	endothelial damage caused by chemical irritation	aim to use compounded solutions with osmolarity as close to 600 mosm/l as possible	major osmotic components are amino acids, glucose and electrolytes	81
pH	incidence PVT increases as pH falls parenteral nutrition solutions usually acidic (except fat)	consider buffers always incorporate fat in regimen	also consider titratable acidity	83 84
particulate matter	vary from 1 u–25 um may occur as a result of degradation of solutions during storage	consider in-line filtration		75 69
site of cannula placement	movement of cannula in vein may predispose to endothelial damage	ensure cannula fixed avoid movement across joints		69
calorie source	glucose solutions hypertonic	concomitant use of fat emulsions essential for PPN fat emulsions are isotonic and being of high energy density (9 kcals/ml) reduce total fluid requirements. May also have a direct protective effect on vein wall	recent studies suggest that glycerol may be used as a low osmolarity source of calories in place of glucose	85

the literature reveals conflicting recommendations for the reduction of phlebitis. For instance, there is no doubt that the size of the catheter, be it diameter, surface area or length, all predispose to an increased incidence of phlebitis.[69,77] This would infer that we should all use the smallest catheter possible. And yet, currently the most popular means of administering PPN is to use ultrafine long catheters. Inevitably, these have a large surface area but their use permits placement of the tip of the catheter in a large vein. Does this mean that the size of the vein and venous flow are relatively more important? Similarly, there is much evidence to show that duration of infusion is an important factor in the causation of phlebitis.[78] Despite this, many centres administer PPN on a continuous basis for reasons of medical and nursing convenience and numerous studies have reported successful PPN employing these infusion techniques.[79,86] Matters are further complicated by the many reports of successful reduction in phlebitis, or at least prolongation of catheter survival time by means of pharmaceutical manipulation (see Table 22.4). The use of glyceryl trinitrate patches, the addition of heparin or hydrocortisone to the infusate or the application of non-steroidal creams or gels have all been shown to be effective.[69] How high in importance do these rank when compared to other means of reducing phlebitis and, in this context, is their routine use, their inevitable cost and the small risk of causing complications justified?

Attempts to determine the relative importance of the various factors involved are difficult because most studies have for perfectly legitimate reasons of standardising experimental design only assessed one or possibly two independent variables. One notable exception to this was the report by Hecker in 1992 of a series of sophisticated meta analyses in which he attempted to determine the relative importance of the acidity of infusates, additive heparin and corticosteroids, topical glyceryl trinitrate, and the use of in-line filters.[75] He found that each technique significantly decreases infusion failure. Pooled odds ratios indicated that the proportions of catheters failing decreased to about 50% for steroids, 40% for both heparin and filters, 35% for neutralisation, 30% for glyceryl trinitrate and about 20% for heparin combined with steroids. Neutralisation had no additional effect over heparin plus steroids. More recent studies have confirmed the cumulative benefits from heparin and hydrocortisone but the relative importance of glyceryl trinitrate patches, in-line filtration and buffering, as independent variables, remains unclear.[74,90]

There is no doubt that the nature of the infusate influences the development of PVT. PPN is not a practicable proposition without the use of fat emulsions and it is preferable for these to be mixed with the other constituents of the feed and administered from a single container. Osmolality, osmolarity

Table 22.4 – Pharmaceutical methods of reducing PVT.

	Mode of action	Recommendation	Notes	References
glyceryl trinitrate patches	theoretically may reduce venospasm and/or promote venodilatation. May alter local prostaglandin synthesis	evidence to support routine use conflicting	cause headaches and incur additional cost	87 85
hydrocortisone	reduce inflammatory reaction	probably beneficial particularly if used in conjunction with heparin		84 89
heparin	prevents or minimises development of fibrin clot at cannula tip	probably beneficial particularly if used in conjunction with steroid	may result in instability of solutions containing fat	84 89
topical non-steroidal anti-inflammatory	reduce inflammatory reaction inhibition platelet aggregation	preliminary studies suggest significant benefit	incur additional cost	67

rate, pH, have all been shown to influence the occurrence of PVT. However, many studies have been reported that demonstrate that PPN with hyperosmolar and acidic solutions is possible suggesting that these should not be seen as major limiting factors to successful PPN.[69,91] The role of infection in the causation of PVT is less clear. Colonisation of peripheral catheter tips is common but not necessarily associated with PVT. There is no evidence to support the use of prophylactic antibiotics or creams at the insertion site. Studies have been reported which showed a significant reduction in PVT in association with aseptic technique.[92,93]

The next question is how important are these pharmaceutical considerations relative to other predisposing factors to the development of PVT. The most important of these is mechanical trauma to the vein. Trauma may occur as a consequence of the venepuncture itself, as a result of the presence of the indwelling catheter in the vein or as a consequence of the irritant effects of the infusion solutions on the vein wall. All of these may cause the release of inflammatory mediators and activation of the clotting cascade with subsequent phlebitis and thrombosis. It is important to appreciate that these changes will, ultimately, always occur in any vein subjected to the presence of an indwelling cannula. Strategies designed to reduce the incidence of phlebitis or minimise its severity must therefore address one or all of these factors. This has led to the evolution of two very different approaches to PPN administration.

PPN: methods of administration

Many now advocate the use of peripheral fine bore, sometimes termed ultrafine, catheter (usually 23 swg and of 15–20 cm in length) which have the advantage of ensuring greater dilution of nutrient solution on delivery into a vein of larger calibre and higher flow rates than in a forearm vein.[69,79,86] Further, it has been suggested that the catheter tip of the long line floats within the wider lumen thereby minimising further mechanical abrasion to the venous endothelium. Additionally, as these catheter are left in situ for as long as possible this reduces direct venous trauma from repeated venepuncture. It is recommended that these catheters are inserted into the largest available forearm vein, usually the cephalic or basilic, and that they should be fixed to minimise movement of the catheter within the vein.[69] These catheters are left in situ for as long as possible. Infusions are delivered on a continuous basis, the ultrafine gauge precluding rapid infusion rates.

The use of fine bore catheters for the delivery of PPN was first described by Kohlhardt et al in 1989. They used a catheter manufactured from silicone rubber with an external diameter of 0.6 mm (23 swg). Forty six patients were fed for a mean duration of 9 days (range 5–60) and the incidence of thrombophlebitis was 18%. The mean time to phlebitis was 7 days (range 5–19) and the daily risk of phlebitis was 0.016 episodes/patient day. The osmolarity of the solution was 1084 mosm/l and it contained heparin. Two subsequent studies in surgical patients were published by this group in which ultrafine catheters were compared to CPN.[94,95] Both confirmed long-term phlebitis-free delivery of PPN with minimal morbidity. In 1992 Madan and colleagues reported a randomised study in which a fine bore catheters (Epicutaneo Cava Vygon, Aachen, Germany) was compared to the use of a standard short Teflon catheter (Venflon) in surgical patients.[86] The median duration of feeding was 5 days in each group. Phlebitis developed in all the patients fed through the short teflon catheter but in only 2 of 27 patients fed with the ultrafine long catheter. The median life span of the ultrafine catheter was significantly greater than the teflon. Other randomised studies have also found a significant increase in phlebitis using short Teflon catheters compared to long catheters when continuous infusion without elective changes of catheter were standard practice.[90] From these studies one can conclude that ultrafine catheters provide an effective means of administering PPN which is associated with minimal morbidity.

The alternative approach to PPN administration is to minimise the duration of time for which the vein is exposed to both nutrients and the catheter. This method involves the daily rotation of venous access sites and cyclical infusion of solutions over 12-hour periods. As thrombophlebitis is, ultimately, an inevitable consequence in any vein in which there is an indwelling catheter then it is logical to interrupt the progression to phlebitis by early withdrawal of the catheter. It is interesting to note that infusion is not a prerequisite to the development of phlebitis. Studies in normal volunteers with catheters placed in forearm veins with no infusion running demonstrated that after 108 hours almost 44% of veins with catheters in place will develop phlebitis.[96] Nonetheless, the infusion itself potentiates the occurrence of phlebitis.[69] This may occur as a consequence of trauma to the endothelium from the jet of fluid emanating from the catheter as well as a consequence of chemical irritation which is determined by osmolarity, buffering pH and infusion period. It is not surprising therefore that the incidence of phlebitis can be reduced by both elective change of peripheral venous cannulas and a reduction in infusion periods. Hessov reported a negligible incidence of phlebitis during the infusion of hypocaloric solutions with infusion periods shorter than 12 hours and showed that the incidence approached 100% if infusions were continued for 4–5 days.[78] Clinical as well as experimental studies show that the risk of phlebitis increases with the length of infusion time. Dinley, in a study comparing 4 different types of catheter, showed that when these were in place for less than 12 hours phlebitis did not occur but that there was a 70% incidence when catheters were in place for more than 72 hours.[97]

Nordenstrom et al were the first to describe the technique of elective catheter change with cyclical infusion of PPN.[64] Their recommendations were to use the largest possible forearm vein, to avoid the veins on the back of the hand, to use short thin (1.0 mm diameter) plastic catheters, to complete the daily nutritional programme within 12 hours, to remove the catheter immediately after completing the infusion and to change the infusion site to the contra-lateral arm the following day. Using this method they reported an overall incidence of phlebitis of 18% with a mean duration of PPN of about 5 days. A total of 75% of their patients were successfully fed by PPN until resumption of oral nutrition. Interestingly, severe phlebitis (Maddox grade 3) rarely occurred. Other groups have also reported successful PPN using this method of administration. For example, Hill employing a solution of 640 mosm/l which provided 9 g of nitrogen and 1620 non-protein calories demonstrated that PPN administered in this way was as effective as CPN with respect to improvements in grip strength and peak expiratory flow.[98] May et al in 1996 reported the results of a prospective and randomised study in which the incidence of phlebitis was minimised in those patients who received their PPN on a cyclical basis with rotation of venous access sites when compared to groups receiving PPN as a continuous infusion with and without elective catheter changes.

To date, there has been only one prospective study reported that has compared the results of these two alternative means of PPN administration.[99] In this, surgical patients were randomly allocated to receive PPN using an ultrafine catheter (Nutriline, Vygon UK) or by the method of rotation with cyclical infusion. Both techniques permitted successful PPN

with a mean duration of feeding of 8.6 and 7.9 days in the two groups respectively. However, failures of the designated technique necessitating alternative means of feeding occurred in 9 of 24 patients with ultrafine catheters and only 2 of 26 patients with rotation. Severe phlebitis occurred in 4 patients with long catheters and in one there was a catheter-related fever. One explanation for the relatively poor results obtained in this study with ultrafine long catheters and those reported elsewhere could be that no ancillary means of reducing phlebitis were employed. In most reports of successful PPN using ultrafine catheters, management protocols have incorporated heparin, hydrocortisone, glyceryl trinitrate patches and in-line filters either alone or in combination.

The major disadvantages of administering PPN with the rotation method are that it subjects the patient to a daily venepuncture which is potentially unpleasant for the patient, time-consuming for the staff, and, there is a theoretical risk of fluid overload particularly in patients with compromised cardiovascular function from infusing daily nutrition requirements over 12 hours. Further studies are required to establish the importance of these potential problems. The advantages of this technique, however, are that it is technically simpler to establish venous access, a smaller diameter needle is used to insert the cannula which might reduce the damage to the vein wall on insertion and, as pointed out above, it may be associated with less venous morbidity related to PVT. In contrast, the use of ultrafine long catheters is convenient and minimises medical and nursing involvement, they are effective for periods up to and around 7 days in the majority of patients – which is close to the average duration of intravenous feeding in current hospital practice – and they are now well established in many centres as an effective means of providing PPN. The major drawback of using ultrafine catheters is the risk of severe phlebitis. PVT occurring in basilic or cephalic veins will usually render these veins useless for further intravenous therapy and do subject the patient to the potential complications of major venous thrombosis or catheter-related sepsis.

PPN: recommendations

The decision as to which technique of PPN administration and what additional measures should be used to reduce phlebitis will to some extent be influenced by personal preference and available facilities within any institution. Cost, convenience and complications must be considered.

All peripheral catheters should be inserted with strict attention to aseptic technique and protocols for insertion and aftercare should be as stringent as for central catheters and under the direction of the nutrition team and nutrition nurse. All catheters should be inspected at least once daily and removed if there is any suspicion of PVT. The nutrient solution must be an all-in-one mixture including a fat emulsion. Lipids reduce osmolarity and have a direct protective effect on the venous endothelium. Pharmacy support is essential to permit the provision of adequate protein, carbohydrate and fat in compounded solutions that are manipulated to be of minimal osmolarity. In-line filtration using 5 mm filters may be useful in preventing the largest microparticles from entering the venous system without cracking the lipid emulsion. The inclusion of heparin and hydrocortisone cannot be routinely recommended unless physical and chemical stability studies have been undertaken with the prescribed nutrient formulation. The evidence in favour of GTN patches and NSAID gels is unclear. Their beneficial effect in the prophylaxis of PVT may be cumulative but with improved methods of PPN administration their role may become less important. Biocompatability, clinical and structural studies suggest that polyurethane is the best material for catheters.

If the clinician opts to use ultrafine catheters, a case can be made for the routine addition of heparin and steroids to the infusate. A strong case can be made, in addition, for glyceryl trinitrate patches and in-line filters. There would appear to be little justification these days to use short Teflon catheters in preference to ultrafine catheters if the intention is to leave these in situ for as long as possible. Elective rotation of catheters and cyclical infusion is demanding on staff but does have such a negligible incidence of phlebitis that ancillary means to reduce the incidence of this complication are probably unnecessary.

By using these techniques one can anticipate phlebitis-free periods of up to a week and sometimes longer. PPN should therefore be able to fulfil the nutrition requirements of most hospitalised patients who require TPN. The next few years are likely to see further improvements in catheter materials and a better understanding of the optimal pharmaceutical means of prolonging catheter survival. Modifications of nutrient solutions may permit adjustment of osmolarity or pH with obvious spin off benefits with regards to PVT. For example, renewed interest in protein hydrolysates and dipeptides as alternative nitrogen sources may result in compounded solutions with much reduced osmolarity. Alternative methods for the commercial sterilisation of glucose and the use of triple layer bags impermeable to gases may reduce glucose oxidation and thereby diminish acidity.

Catheter care

The incidence of sepsis can be significantly reduced if catheter care is provided following strictly adhered to protocols; this applies to both central and peripheral catheters. In the case of a single lumen catheter, no solution other than the parenteral nutrition should be administered through the catheter. If a single lumen catheter offers the only available vascular access, a cyclical regimen will offer the opportunity for administration of other solutions if used carefully,[31] although this is not generally recommended. With multi-lumen catheters one lumen should be identified for parenteral nutrition and all should be handled with the same meticulous attention to aseptic technique. It is advisable to keep manipulations of the catheter to a minimum. Administration sets should be changed every 24 hours and the solution should always be administered using a volumetric pump. Connections to the venous access line should be kept to a minimum, with luer-lock connections used at all times; the recently developed closed system membrane connector could be considered where sepsis remains a problem.

Care of the catheter exit site should be regarded as one of the most important procedures associated with administration of parenteral nutrition. Most infection arises from connections in the delivery system and the catheter hub.[28] The traditional exit site dressing was dry gauze and tape, although subsequently found to be unsuitable as the tape used was frequently contaminated and the gauze easily became wet and soiled. Semipermeable, sterile, transparent dressings were then considered, having the advantage of being waterproof and providing observation of the exit site. Unfortunately these dressings were found to leave adhesive on the catheter and to retain moisture, which led to cutaneous colonisation and increased infection rates.[100] Some centres use sterile dry dressings (Primapore, Smith & Nephew UK or Mepore, Molnlycke Sweden) with a small drop of Betadine ointment covering the exit site. Manufacturers recently have claimed to produce a transparent dressing which will not leave adhesive on the catheter and will provide vapour permeability thereby reducing the incidence of moisture retention and the associated sepsis.

Regardless of type of dressing used, they all should be changed every 7 days or earlier if they become wet or their adhesive qualities appear diminished. Cannula exit sites should be cleaned with a povidone iodine solution, using non-woven gauze swabs and an aseptic technique.

Patients receiving their CPN on a cyclical regimen should have their catheters flushed after infusion with the lowest effective concentration of heparin. A solution of 10 iu/ml in a volume of 5 ml has been shown to be effective.[32] Long-term vascular access devices are prone to form fibrin build-up at the sheath. A flushing procedure incorporating a rapid pushing and pausing technique should be used in an attempt to create turbulence within the catheter.[101]

Peripheral catheters used for parenteral nutrition should have no other solutions administered through them. In the event that administration of intravenous drugs is required, alternative peripheral venous access should be found. Protocols should be established for the insertion and care of peripheral catheters. A suitable dressing should be applied which will provide security of position and comfort together with permitting easy inspection of the catheter site. Prior to insertion of a peripheral catheter, the use of local anaesthetic is recommended. The venous access site should be inspected at least twice daily; should any signs of thrombophlebitis or extravasation be observed then the catheter should be removed and an alternative access site located. When parenteral nutrition is administered via a long catheter it is important that flow is maintained at all times to prevent blockage of the narrow lumens and this necessitates the use of a volumetric infusion pump.

Nutrition teams

Multidisciplinary hospital nutrition teams provide a number of visible benefits to the administration of parenteral nutrition by whatever method this is administered.[102] They ensure that such adjuvant nutrition support is provided in the most cost effective manner and with the fewest complications.[103] The incidence of catheter-related sepsis has been reported to decrease from about 25% before the introduction of a nutrition team to between 0 and 5% after its introduction. It has been estimated that a nutrition team can save as much as £110 000–330 000 per year in a hospital feeding 300 patients per year simply by reducing the incidence of catheter-related sepsis.[104]

Nutrition teams further benefit the hospital by ensuring more uniform prescribing habits, which permits bulk ordering of feeds and accessories and helps to reduce wasting of nutrient solutions by ensuring that prescribed volumes are actually administered.[62]

To be fully effective nutrition teams should establish a hospital-wide nutrition policy and ensure that all staff can detect under-nutrition. Hospitals should have agreed protocols which identify patients who require nutrition support as well as the appropriate means of providing this support. (See chapter 14.)

Most nutrition teams should comprise a nutrition nurse specialist, a consultant clinician, a dietitian, a pharmacist, a biochemist and ideally representatives from intensive care and a speech therapist. Junior medical and nursing staff should be encouraged to attend a regular weekly meeting at which all patients receiving nutrition support are discussed. During the last 20 years the role of the nurse specialist in nutrition has evolved and developed in the UK. The role has been identified as responsible for the reduction in complications associated with the delivery of parenteral nutrition, and therefore with reducing costs. Simple, but effective policies and procedures have reduced wastage and complications, clinical education programmes have raised knowledge and reduced myths in the ward areas, whilst the scope of professional practice has seen the role expand to include responsibility for placement of IV lines, which has also been shown to reduce catheter-related sepsis and improve the quality of care.[105]

Conclusions

In marked contrast to the early years of parenteral nutrition, venous access is now rarely a limiting factor in the provision of intravenous nutrients. Most mechanical problems have been overcome and successful long-term nutrition is now an everyday reality. The majority of problems related to venous access can be minimised if not completely avoided by scrupulous attention to catheter care and this is facilitated by the use of nutrition nurses and nutrition teams. Modern techniques are such that no patient, whatever their clinical condition, need be denied adequate nutrition. The future will see more refinements of catheter materials as well as the modification of substrates which together will further minimise parenteral nutrition-related morbidity.

References

1. Harvey W. 1628. Exercitatio anatomica de motu cordis et sanguinis in animalibus. Francofurti, sumpt Guilielmi Fitzeri.

1a. Boyle R. 1659. Cited in: Lyons AS, Petrucelli RJ. Medicine an illustrated history. Abradale Press, Harry N. Abrams, Inc, New York.

2. O'Shaughnessy WB. Proposal of a new method of treating the blue epidemic cholera by the injection of highly-oxygenised salts into the venous system. *Lancet* 1831; **i**: 366–371.

3. Latta T. Relative to the treatment of cholera by the copious injection of aqueous and saline fluids into the veins. *Lancet* 1831; **ii**: 274–277.

4. Wood A. (1855). Cited in: Singer C and Underwood AE. 1962. A Short History of Medicine. Oxford University Press.

5. Massa DJ *et al*. A plastic needle. *Mayo Clinic Proceedings* 1950; **25**: 413–415.

6. Gardner LI, Murphy JT. New needle for paediatric scalp vein infusions. *Am J Dis Child* 1950; **80**: 303–304.

7. Seldinger SI. Catheter replacement of the needle in percutaneous arteriography. A new technique. *Acta Radiologica* 1953; **39**: 368–376.

8. Henriques V, Anderson AC. Uber parenterale Ernahrung durch intravenose Injektionen. *Z Physiol Chem* 1913; **88**: 257–369.

9. Forssmann W. Experiments on myself: Memoirs of a surgeon in Germany. Translated by H. Davies. 1975; New York: St. Martin's Press.

10. Aubaniac R. L'injection intraveineuse sous-claviculaire. Advantages et technique. *La Presse Medicale* 1952; **68**: 1456.

11. Dudrick S *et al*. Long-term parenteral nutrition with growth, development, and positive nitrogen balance. *Surg* 1968; **64**: 134–142.

11a. Kinney JM *et al*. A method for simultaneous measurement of gas exchange and expired radioactivity in acutely ill patients. *Metabolism* 1964; **13**: 205–211.

11b. Feurer ID *et al*. Measured and predicted resting energy expenditure in clinically stable patients. *Clin Nutr* 1984; **3**:27–34.

12. Curelaru I *et al*. Material thrombogenicity in central venous catheterisation III. A comparison between soft polyvinylchloride and soft polyurethane elastomer, long, antebrachial catheters. *Acta Anaesthesiol Scand* 1984; **28**: 204–208.

12a. Wren C. An account of the method of conveying liquors immediately into mass of blood. Phil Trans R Soc London. Cited by In Annan GL 1938. An exhibition of Books on the Growth of our Knowledge of Blood Transfusions. *Bull NY Acad Med* 1665; **15**: 623.

12b. Courten W. Experiments and observations of the effects of several sorts of poisons upon animals made at Montpellier in the years 1678 and 1679 by the William Courten. London, *Philos Trans R Soc* 27: 485–500.

12c. Hodder EM. Transfusion of milk in cholera. *Practitioner* 1873; **10**: 14–15.

12d. Friedrich PL. Die kunstliche subkutane Ernahrung in der praktischen Chirurgie. *Archiv für klin. Chirurgie* 1904; **73**: 507–516.

12e. Elman R. Amino acid content of the blood following intravenous injection of hydrolyzed casein. *Proc Soc Exp Biol Med* 1937; **37**: 437–440.

13. D'Abrera VC *et al*. The structure of intravascular devices made from a new family of polyurethanes. *Inten Ther Clin Monitor* 1988; **8**: 12.

14. Pottecher T *et al*. Thrombogenicity of central venous catheters: prospective study of polyethylene, silicone and polyurethane catheters with phlebography or post-mortem examination. *Eur J Anaesthiol* 1984; **1**: 361–365.

15. Mughal MM. Complications of intravenous feeding catheters. *Br J Surg* 1988; **76**: 15–21.

16. Bozzetti F *et al*. Subclavian venous thrombosis due to indwelling catheters: a prospective study on 52 patients. *J Parent Enter Nutr* 1983; **7**: 560–562.

17. Moran BJ, Sutton GLJ. A cuffed polyurethane catheter for long-term central venous access: a novel technique prevents early displacement. *J Parent Enter Nutr* 1990; **14**: 546–547.

18. Gaukroger PB *et al*. Infusion thrombophlebitis: a prospective comparison of Vialon and Teflon cannulae in anaesthetic and postoperative use. *Anaesth Inten Care* 1988; **16**: 265–271.

19. McKee JM *et al*. Complications of intravenous therapy: a randomised prospective study – Vialon vs Teflon. *J Intravenous Nurs* 1988; **12**: 288–295.

20. Thoma RJ. Poly(ether)urethane reactivity with metal-iron in calcification and environmental stress cracking. *J Biomaterials Applications* 1987; **1**: 449–462.

21. Maki DG *et al*. An Attachable Silver-Impregnated Cuff for Prevention of Infection with Central Venous Catheters: A Prospective Randomised Multicenter Trial. *Am J Med* 1998; **85**: 307–314.

22. Trooskin SZ *et al.* Prevention of catheter sepsis by antibiotic bonding. *Surgery* 1985; **97:** 547–551.

23. Hickman RO *et al.* A modified right atrial catheter for access to the venous system in marrow transplant recipients. *Surg Gynaecol Obst* 1979; **148:** 871–877.

24. Broviac J *et al.* A silicone rubber catheter for prolonged parenteral alimentation. *Surg Gynaecol Obst* 1973; **136:** 602–606.

25. Girvent M, Sitges-Serra A. Failure of silver impregnated subcutaneous cuffs to prevent intravascular catheter infections in cancer patients. *Ann Surg* 1995; **221:** 115–116.

26. Groeger JS *et al.* Infectious morbidity associated with long-term use of venous access devices in patients with cancer. *Ann Intern Med* 1993; **119:** 1168–1174.

27. Clark-Christoff N *et al.* Use of triple-lumen subclavian catheters for administration of total parenteral nutrition. *J Parent Enter Nutr* 1992; **16:** 403.

28. Linares J *et al.* Pathogenesis of catheter sepsis: a prospective study with quantitative and semi-quantitative cultures of catheter hub and segments. *J Clin Microbiol* 1985; **21:** 357.

29. Moro MLK *et al.* Risk factors for central venous catheter-related infections in surgical and intensive care units. *Infect Control Hosp Epidemiol* 1994; **15:** 253.

30. Savage AP *et al.* Complications and survival of multilumen central venous catheters used for total parenteral nutrition. *Br J Surg* 1993; **80:** 1287–1290.

31. Faubion WC *et al.* Total parenteral nutrition catheter sepsis: impact of the team approach. *J Parent Enter Nutr* 1986; **10:** 642–645.

32. Cottee S. Heparin lock practice in total parenteral nutrition. *Prof Nurs* 1995; **11:** 25–28.

33. Keohane PP *et al.* Effect of catheter tunnelling and a nutrition nurse on catheter sepsis during parenteral nutrition. *Lancet* 1983; **17:** 1388–1390.

34. Kowalewska-Grochowska K *et al.* Guide-wire catheter change in central venous catheter biofilm formation in a burn population. *Chest* 1991; **100:** 1090.

35. Badley AD *et al.* Comparison of the infectious risks of de novo CVP lines and replacement CVP lines [abstract J48]. Programs and Abstracts of the 34th Interscience Conference of Antimicrobial Agents and Chemotherapy. Orlando, FL 67.

36. von Meyenfeldt MM *et al.* TPN catheter sepsis: lack of effect of subcutaneous tunnelling of PVC catheters on sepsis rate. *J Parent Enter Nutr* 1980; **4:** 514–517.

37. English ICW *et al.* Percutaneous catheterisation of the internal jugular vein. *Anaes* 1969; **24:** 521–531.

38. Mansfield P *et al.* Complications and failures for subclavian vein catheterisation. *N Engl J Med* 1994; **331:** 1735–1738.

39. Kearns P, Coleman S & Wehner JH. Complications of long-arm catheters: a randomised trial of central vs peripheral tip location. *J Parent Enteral Nutr* 1995; **20:** 20–24.

40. Adam A. Insertion of long term central venous catheters: time for a new look. *BMJ* 1995; **311:** 311–342.

41. Widmer A. IV related infections. In: Wenzel RP (ed) Prevention and control of nosocomial infections. Baltimore MD: 1993; Williams & Wilkins, 556.

42. Adal KA, Farr BM. Central venous catheter-related infections: a review. *Nutr* 1996; **12:** 208–213.

43. Clark DE, Raffin TA. Infectious complications of indwelling long-term central venous catheters. *Chest* 1990; **97:** 966.

44. Hampton AA, Sheretz RJ. Vascular-access infections in hospitalised patients. *Surg Clin North Am* 1988; **68:** 57.

45. Ryan JA *et al.* Catheter complications in total parenteral nutrition. A prospective study of 200 consecutive patients. *N Engl J Med* 1974; **290:** 757–761.

46. Kite P *et al.* Evaluation of a novel endoluminal brush method for in situ diagnosis of catheter related sepsis. *J Clin Pathol* 1997; **50:** 278–282.

47. Vanhuynegem L *et al.* Detection of central venous catheter-associated sepsis. *Eur J Clin Microbiol* 1985; **4:** 46–48.

48. Tighe M *et al.* Rapid diagnosis of catheter related sepsis using the acridine orange leukocyte cytospin test and an endoluminal brush. *J Parent Enter Nutr* 1996; **20:** 215–218.

49. Rohovsky SA *et al.* Total Parenteral Nutrition. *Curr Opin Gastro* 1997; **13:** 146–152.

50. Lowell J, Bothe A. Central venous catheter related thrombosis. *Surg Oncol Clin North Am* 1995; **4:** 479–492.

51. Johnson OL *et al.* The destabilisation of parenteral feeding by heparin. *Int J Pharmac* 1989; **53:** 237–240.

52. Hurtubise MR *et al.* Restoring patency of occluded central venous catheters. *Arch Surg* 1980; **115:** 212–213.

53. Haire W, Lieberman RP. Thrombosed central venous catheters: restoring function with 6 hour low dose infusion after failure of bolus urokinase. *J Parent Enter Nutr* 1991; **16**: 129–132.

54. O'Farrell L, Griffith J, Lang C. Histologic development of the sheath that forms around long-term implanted central venous catheters. *J Parent Enter Nutr* 1996; **20**: 156–158.

55. Werlin S *et al.* Treatment of central venous catheter occlusions with ethanol and hydrochloric acid. *J Parent Enter Nutr* 1995; **19**: 416–418.

56. Schubert O, Wretlind A. Intravenous infusion of fat emulsions, phosphatides and emulsifying agents. *Acta Chir Scand* 1961; Suppl 278.

57. Hallberg D *et al.* Experimental and clinical studies with fat emulsion for intravenous nutrition. *Nutr Dieta* 1966; **8**: 245–281.

58. Jeejeebhoy KN *et al.* Metabolic studies in TPN. *J Clin Invest* 1976; **57**: 125–136.

59. Gazzaniga AB *et al.* Indirect calorimetry as a guide to calorie replacement during total parenteral nutrition. *Am J Surg* 1978; **136**: 128–133.

60. MacFie J *et al.* Glucose or fat as non-protein energy source? A controlled clinical trial in gastroenterological patients requiring intravenous nutrition. *Gastroenterology* 1981; **80**: 102–107.

61. Nordenstrom J *et al.* Nitrogen balance during total parenteral nutrition. Glucose vs fat. *Ann Surg* 1983; **197**: 27–33.

62. MacFie J Energy requirements of surgical patients during intravenous nutrition. *Ann Royal College Surg Engl* 1984; **66**: 39–42.

63. Solassol C *et al.* New techniques for long-term intravenous feeding: an artificial gut in 75 patients. *Ann Surg* 1974; **179**: 519–522.

64. Nordenstrom J *et al.* Peripheral parenteral nutrition: effect of a standardised compounded mixture on infusion phlebitis. *Br J Surg* 1991; **78**: 1391–1394.

65. Payne-James JJ *et al.* Nutritional support in hospitals in the United Kingdom: National Survey 1988. *Health Trends* 1990; **22**: 9–13.

66. Payne-James JJ *et al.* Artificial nutrition support in hospitals in the United Kingdom – 1994: Third National Survey. *Clinical Nutrition* 1995; **14**: 329–335.

67. Payne-James *et al.* Artificial nutrition support in hospitals in the United Kingdom – 1991: Second national survey. *Clin Nutr* 1992; **11**: 187–192.

68. Larsson J *et al.* Nitrogen requirements in severely injured patients. *Br J Surg* 1990; **77**: 413–416.

69. Payne-James JJ, Khawaja HT. First choice for total parenteral nutrition: the peripheral route. *J Parent Enter Nutr* 1993; **17**: 468–478.

70. MacFie J, Nordenstrom J. Full circle in parenteral nutrition. *Clin Nutr* 1992; **11**: 237–239.

71. Couse N *et al.* Total parenteral nutrition by peripheral vein – substitute or supplement to the central venous route? A prospective trial. *Clin Nutr* 1993; **12**: 213–216.

72. Everitt *et al.* Fine bore silicone rubber and polyurethane catheters for the delivery of complete intravenous nutrition via a peripheral vein. *Clin Nutr* 1993; **12**: 261–265.

73. Kerin MJ *et al.* A prospective and randomised study comparing the incidence of infusion phlebitis during continuous and cyclic peripheral parenteral nutrition. *Clin Nutr* 1991; **10**: 315–319.

74. Everitt NJ, McMahon MJ. Influence of catheter type on the occurrence of thrombophlebitis during peripheral intravenous nutrition. *J Irish Coll of Physic and Surg* 1995; **24**: 93–96.

75. Hecker JF. Potential for extending survival of peripheral intravenous infusions. *BMJ* 1992; **304**: 619–624.

76. Everitt NJ *et al.* Ultrasonographic investigation of the pathogenesis of infusion thrombophlebitis. *Br J Surg* 1997; **84**: 642–745.

77. May J *et al.* Prospective study of aetiology of infusion phlebitis and line failure during peripheral parenteral nutrition. *Br J Surg* 1996; **83**: 1091–1094.

78. Hessov I, Bjosen-Muller M. Experimental infusion thrombophlebitis. Importance of the infusion rates. *Euro J Inten Ca Med* 1976; **2**: 103–105.

79. Kohlhardt SR, Smith RC. Fine bore silicone catheters for peripheral intravenous nutrition in adults. *Br Med J* 1989; **299**: 1380–1381.

80. Payne-James JJ *et al.* Topical nonsteroidal anti-inflammatory gel for the prevention of peripheral vein thrombophlebitis. *Anaesthesia* 1992; **47**: 324–326.

81. Elliott MJ *et al.* Cannulation site survival during peripheral intravenous feeding. *Br J Parent Ther* 1984; **5**: 202–207.

82. Nitescu P *et al.* Disturbances of blood-flow velocity in the dorsal veins of the hand after vein cannulation and cannula fixation in the anaesthetized patient. *Acta Anaesthesiol Scand* 1990; **34**: 120–125.

83. Timmer JG *et al.* Peripheral venous nutrition: the equal relevance of volume load and osmolarity in relation to phlebitis. *Clin Nutr* 1991; **10**: 309–314.

84. Messing B *et al*. Peripheral venous complications of a hyperosmolar (960 mOsm) nutritive mixture: the effect of heparin and hydrocortisone. A multicentre double-blind random study in 98 patients. *Clin Nutr* 1986; **5**: 57–58.

85. Grimble GK *et al*. Total parenteral nutrition: novel substrates I. *Inten Care Clin Monitor* 1989; **2**: 12–15.

86. Madan M *et al*. Influence of catheter type on the occurrence of thrombophlebitis during peripheral intravenous nutrition. *Lancet* 1992; **339**: 101–103.

87. Wright A *et al*. Use of transdermal glyceryl trinitrate to reduce failure of intravenous infusion due to phlebitis and extravasation. *Lancet* 1985; **2**: 1148–1150.

88. Khawaja HT *et al*. Transdermal glyceryl trinitrate to allow peripheral total parenteral nutrition: a double-blind placebo controlled feasibility study. *J R Soc Med* 1991; **84**: 69–71.

89. Madan M *et al*. A randomised study of the effects of osmolality and heparin with hydrocortisone on thrombophlebitis in peripheral intravenous nutrition. *Clin Nutr* 1991; **10**: 309–314.

90. Reynolds JV *et al*. Randomised comparison of silicone versus teflon cannulas for peripheral intravenous nutrition. *Ann R Coll Surg Eng* 1995; **77**: 447–449.

91. Kane KF *et al*. High osmolality feeds do not increase the incidence of thrombophlebitis during peripheral IV nutrition. *J Parent Enter Nutr* 1995; **20**: 194–179.

92. Tomford JW *et al*. Intravenous therapy team and peripheral venous catheter-associated complications. *Arch Int Med* 1984; **144**: 1191–1194.

93. Lodge JPA *et al*. Insertion technique, the key to avoiding infusion phlebitis: a prospective clinical trial. *Br J Clin Prac* 1987; **41**: 816–819.

94. Kohlhardt SR, Smith RC, Wright CR, Sucick A. Fine-bore peripheral catheters versus venous catheters for delivery of intravenous nutrition. *Nutr* 1992; **8**: 412.

95. Kohlhardt SR *et al*. Peripheral versus central intravenous nutrition. A comparison of two delivery systems. *Br J Surg* 1994; **81**: 66–68.

96. Payne-James JJ *et al*. Development of thrombophlebitis in peripheral veins with Vialon and PTFE-teflon cannulas. Prospective randomised double blind randomised controlled trial. *Ann R Coll Surg Eng* 1991; **73**: 322–325.

97. Dinley RJ. Venous reactions related to indwelling plastic cannulae: a prospective clinical trial. *Curr Med Res Opin* 1976; **3**: 607–609.

98. Hill RL. In: Disorders of Nutrition and Metabolism in clinical surgery. GL Hill (ed) Churchill Livingstone, 1992, 131–132.

99. Palmer D *et al*. Administration of peripheral parenteral nutrition: a prospective study comparing rotation of venous access sites with ultrafine cannulas. *Clin Nutr* 1996; **15**: 311–315.

100. Conly JM *et al*. A randomised study comparing transparent and dry gauze dressings for central venous catheters. *J Infect Dis* 1989; **159**: 310–319.

101. Pennington CR *et al*. 1996. Current perspectives on parenteral nutrition in adults. British Association of Parenteral & Enteral Nutrition (BAPEN) working party recommendations.

102. Lennard-Jones JE *et al*. 1992. A positive approach to nutrition as treatment. Report of a working party, King's Fund Centre.

103. Elia MJ. Artificial nutritional support in clinical practice in Britain. *J Roy Coll Physic* 1993; **27**: 8–15.

104. Wilcock H *et al*. Artificial nutrition in the Cambridge health district with particular reference to tube feeding. *Health Trends* 1991; **23**: 93–100.

105. Hamilton H. Care improves while costs reduce. *Prof Nurse* 1993; **8**: 592–596.

23

Parenteral nutrition substrates

Peter Fürst, Katharina S Kuhn and Peter Stehle

Introduction

Few areas of medical research and development have seen such substantial and valuable progress as the recent surge of research in artificial nutrition. This is due in part to the current biochemical knowledge with regard to cellular bioenergetics and transport mechanisms and to advances in molecular biology.

One area which is applicable to clinical nutrition practice is provision of specific nutrition substrates.[1] Many investigators have proceeded on the assumption that 'tailor-made solutions' will increase the benefits of intravenous nutrition for specific patient groups. Thus, specific amino acid mixtures have been developed for treatment of renal and liver disease or to optimise the growth of young infants.[2] Other investigators still hope for benefits from solutions enriched in branched-chain amino acids.[3] Although many of these nutrition formulae are now available, they were designed to improve tolerance of nitrogen load in the presence of illness, malnutrition or organ dysfunction rather than to provide specific nutrients for individual organs or tissues.[4]

Current research directions consider individual substrates as tissue/organ-specific single nutrients as an alternative approach. Certain diseases accompanied by deficiencies, antagonisms or imbalances in a particular compartment or in various organ tissues might selectively require one or more nutrients which are appropriate for use just in that given condition to support the attenuated tissue. Administration of required substrates might thus greatly facilitate an anabolic response to a life-threatening disease.[1] The major questions are: which nutrient should be considered and in what amount should it be administered?

Great interest is being devoted to new substrates. For example, enteral and parenteral use of medium–chain triglycerides (MCT) as opposed to long–chain triglycerides (LCT), has been investigated.[5,6] New uses of n-3 fatty acids have been suggested as therapy.[7,8] Short-chain fatty acids (SCFA) may operate as true essential substrates because organ function is impaired by their absence.[9] The development of so-called 'structured lipids' is a further alternative to the MCT/LCT mixtures.[7,10–12] The technique of synthesising structural triglycerides has ushered in a new era of 'nutritional pharmacology'. The role of parenteral nucleic acids is being discussed because expression of the synthesising enzymes in the *de novo* pathway is

apparently impaired during catabolic stress.[56] Arginine is claimed to be a potent immunomodulator during episodes of stress and in particular in cancer patients.[13,14] 'Magic bullets' as integrated emulsion particles should be specifically tailored to be taken up exclusively by defined receptors, cells or tissues.[7] Supplementation with the glutamine analogues α-ketoglutarate[15] or its ornithine salt[16,17] is seen as a physiological way of providing glutamine precursors during total parenteral nutrition (TPN).

It is important to emphasise that none of the commercially available amino acid solutions contains glutamine and cystine, and only inadequate amounts of tyrosine, because these nutrients are either unstable or poorly soluble in aqueous solutions. Recent knowledge concerning the efficient utilisation of intravenously supplied di- and tripeptides[18,19] opens the possibility of substituting available amino acid solutions with glutamine, cystine and tyrosine containing stable and highly soluble short-chain peptides. Undoubtedly this new approach has introduced a new dimension, though the explosion of new information about peptide assimilation is only a prelude, prior to intravenous use of peptides in common clinical practice.[12,20,21] Taurine is postulated as an indispensable substrate during catabolic stress and uraemia. Additionally, this amine is a potent antioxidant.[12] Its intracellular transport might be improved by using synthetic taurine conjugates.[20,22]

The nutritional requirements of the catabolic patient do not differ qualitatively from those of normal subjects. All of the approximately 40–45 essential nutrients required by normal individuals must be supplied on a regular and preferably a daily basis. The *quantitative* requirements for individual nutrients, however, differ from those of normal subjects and whenever such differences have been observed, they should be seriously taken into account.[23]

In this chapter nutrition with amino acids, carbohydrates and lipids as well as the implication of novel substrates will be elaborated in relation to known nutritional deficiencies and disorders in clinical nutrition.

Historical development[18,19,24]

The first intravenous infusion is recorded as early as 1656. Sir Christopher Wren injected 'solution of nutrients' into dogs by using a goose quill attached to a pig's bladder. Wren reported to a friend that: 'The most considerable experiment I have made of late, is this, I injected wine and ale into the mass of blood of a living dog, by a vein, in good quantities, till I made it extremely drunk, but soon he pissed it out'. On page 227 of Sprat's *History of the Royal Society* this most elegant experiment of Wren is recorded as follows: '. . . by which diverse creatures were immediately infused, vomited, intoxicated, killed or revived according to the quality of the liquors injected. . .'.

William Courten from Montpellier is generally credited with being the first to give fat parenterally. These trials in the years 1678 and 1679 were discouraging but the dismal results achieved by Courten did not stop further attempts during the next 200 years, which also met with very limited success.

Interestingly, the desirability of providing carbohydrates intravenously was only recognised as late as 1848 by Claude Bernard. He demonstrated that intravenous sucrose was excreted promptly in the urine, unlike glucose which disappeared from the blood and was presumably utilised. Landerer, in 1887, proposed that 'glucose may serve as part of a regimen for artificial nutrition'.

The history of intravenous protein nutrition is closely related to the increasing knowledge in protein metabolism and absorption. In 1838, when the Dutch scientist Mulder introduced the term 'protein', at the suggestion of Berzelius, it was thought that all protein was essentially the same substance and was absorbed in intact form. This view persisted until the heterogeneity of proteins was described in the 1870s. It was then believed that proteins were absorbed as 'proteases' and 'peptones' according to the 'hypothesis of resynthesis'. As claimed by Abderhalden and others, peptones were resynthesised to proteins in the intestinal wall and subsequently absorbed into the body. Accordingly, Friedrich approached the concept of TPN by infusing a peptone solution together with fat, glucose and salt. In 1900, Otto Cohnheim showed that mucosa did not in fact synthesise proteins from peptones but broke them down by the enzyme(s) 'erepsin' into amino acids. Cohnheims's 'classical hypothesis of protein absorption' taught that intraluminal hydrolysis was complete and only free amino acids were taken up by the absorptive cells by simple diffusion. In 1904, Abderhalden and Rona injected enzymatically digested protein and in 1913 Henriques and Anderson could maintain nitrogen equilibrium in a goat by means of intravenously injected amino acids, the product of an enzymic hydrolysis as the sole intake of nitrogen.

The transposition of this basic knowledge from the 1920s to clinical practice occurred first about 15–20 years later. Elman's well-conceived and carefully conducted studies established firmly and unequivocally the great utility of parenteral protein hydrolysates and amino acids. Elman recognised the importance of preventing the nutritional deterioration of patients and of treating it if already present.

Elman used an acid hydrolysate of casein, fortified with tryptophan, methionine and some cystine. He emphasised that the injection of these amino acids must be simultaneous with the other amino acids. This was clearly a most brilliant prophecy of current so-called 'balanced amino acid solutions'.

The metabolic background to the use of parenteral amino acids in stressed patients was established by Sir David Cuthbertson, who described much of the basic knowledge about the metabolic response to trauma and injury.

There were also simultaneous developments in the provision of parenteral carbohydrate and fat. Thus, in 1915 Woodyatt and co-workers published their classical study quantitating the rate at which glucose could be infused as assessed by the appearance of glycosuria. This carefully conducted study predated the glucose clamp technique by over half a century. They showed that up to about 0.9 g/kg of glucose per hour could be infused without glucosuria and concluded that 'intravenous nutrition with glucose is, thus, proved to be a possible clinical proposition, especially at episodes of shock and in the post-operative state. . .'.

Mills in 1911 began to employ 'fat emulsions', given subcutaneously, and Marlin and Richie in 1915 injected a fat emulsion into dogs. These experiments, however, were accompanied by temperature rise and other severe complications. The dietary requirements for certain fatty acids were recognised in 1929. As a result of well-conducted studies in weanling rats, Burr and Burr coined the term 'essential fatty acids' for linoleic acid and linolenic acid because these nutrients were not synthesised by these animals but were necessary for maintenance of physiologic functions. With the advent of parenteral nutrition based on a system of continuous fat-free infusion, essential fatty acid deficiency became evident in human adults.

Finally Wretlind in Sweden undertook the challenge of developing a safe, metabolisable fat emulsion for clinical use. In 1961 he reported '. . . after a large number of trials and errors, I finally developed a method to produce suitable prepared soybean oil and eggyolk phospholipids. A fat emulsion produced from these raw materials showed no toxic or other adverse effects and provides not less than 2 kcal per ml emulsion'.

The establishment of a suitable intravenous lipid emulsion was therefore the last major stone added to the mosaic that we now know as total parenteral nutrition (TPN).

Protein nutrition substrates

The traditional classification of amino acids into essential and non-essential categories has become much modified.[24] This is because particular clinical conditions may result in certain amino acid deficiencies, antagonisms or imbalances which then cause specific changes in amino acid metabolism and requirements. Thus, some of the non-essential amino acids have to be classified as 'indispensable' or 'conditionally indispensable' substrates.

The new approach of essentiality recognised the functional and physiological properties of a given substrate under various pathological states.[9] Grimble proposes that, regardless of the definition used, a final judgement of the usefulness of an essential new substrate will be on the grounds of clinical and nutritional efficacy. According to a more general position, 'a possible and useful direction might put more emphasis on metabolic control and its regulation of tissue and organ function and nutritional status'.[25] This definition offers suggestions as to how certain metabolic characteristics shared by some substances might be used to differentiate the various nutritionally significant substrates. This would also mean that the dietary essentiality of a given substrate is dependent on the ratio of supply to demand; the distinction between 'essential' and 'non-essential' largely disappears because it is dependent on conditions.[12,25]

Histidine

In infants the evidence for a dietary histidine requirement was an early observation,[26] whereas in adults histidine was considered a dispensable amino acid. Recent studies in normal men, however, showed that long-term histidine-deficient diet (1–8 weeks) led to a significant fall in plasma histidine levels.[27] This observation raised the question as to whether, during long-term TPN, supplementation with histidine might be beneficial.

In the early 1970s, Fürst and Bergström provided the first evidence that histidine might be an indispensable amino acid in uraemia.[28] Accordingly, supplementation with histidine of tailored intravenous diets given to uraemic patients resulted in a considerably improved, even positive nitrogen balance.[29]

Serine

In healthy adults, serine can be readily synthesised from glycine and activated formaldehyde. Indeed, serine is the only non-essential amino acid which has been shown to stimulate protein synthesis *in vitro*.[30] In all clinical situations with impaired kidney function, endogenous synthesis might not cover serine requirements, resulting in low extra- and intracellular serine concentrations.[31] These findings suggest that serine may be indispensable for uraemic patients on maintenance haemodialysis and that serine depletion may be another limiting factor for protein synthesis, thereby contributing to the increased protein requirements in these patients.

Arginine

Early studies showed that it was necessary to include sufficient arginine in intravenous amino acid solutions in order to maintain urea cycle activity and prevent hyperammonaemia.[32]

Arginine may also be of significance in the critically ill because of its potential role in immunomodulation.[33,34] It is hypothesised that arginine enhances the depressed immune response of individuals suffering from injury, surgical trauma, malnutrition or sepsis. In experimental animals as well as in human studies, supplementation with arginine resulted in an improved cellular response, a decrease in trauma-induced reduction in the T-cell function and a higher phagocytosis rate.[33] Innate host cellular cytotoxicity, mediated in part by natural killer (NK) and lymphokine-activated killer (LAK) cells, is thought to play an important role in the inhibition of tumour growth and the reduction of metabolic spread. Arginine supplementation has been shown to enhance NK and LAK cytotoxicity (for references see [34]).

Interestingly, a daily supply of 30–35 g of arginine is claimed to retard tumour growth and to diminish tumour metastasis.[35] On the other hand, it has been reported that substituting ornithine for arginine in parenteral regimens will ameliorate an arginine-related increase in growth of a Ward colon tumour.[36]

When dealing with the parenteral supply of arginine it is also important to note that arginine has a specific drawback in its competition with lysine for tubular reabsorption (Fig. 23.1).[38] Thus, parenteral administration of excessive amounts of arginine may result in lysine deprivation.

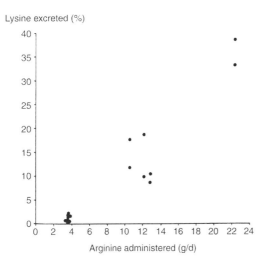

Figure 23.1 – Lysine excreted in human urine (expressed as percentage of amount infused, 2.6 g) plotted against the quantity of arginine simultaneously infused. Data adapted from Vinnars[37] with permission.

It is notable that 5 years ago, parenteral arginine was considered as a novel and valuable tool to improve immunity and to beneficially influence metabolism and pathophysiology in cancer and trauma. Remarkably, in the current literature, the intravenous arginine approach is almost absent while great emphasis is laid on enteral arginine nutrition. Presumably the reportedly highlighted drawbacks and disadvantages with large amounts of parenteral arginine have been slowly recognised and considered.

Recently, arginine was shown to be the unique substrate for the production of the biological effector molecule nitric oxide (NO). NO is formed by oxidation of one of the two identical terminal guanidino groups of L-arginine by the enzyme nitric oxide synthase (NOS). Of the three NOS isoenzymes characterised, two are constitutive, Ca^{2+} dependent

[endothelial (eNOS) and neuronal (nNOS)] and generate lower levels of NO than their inducible counterpart (iNOS). iNOS is prominent in inflammatory conditions and it is also most often implicated as the producer of NO during immune response. According to recent reports NO plays an essential role in the regulation of inflammation and immunity.[38] Interestingly, parenteral arginine may improve myocardial ischaemia in patients with obstructive coronary artery disease by producing non-stereo-specific peripheral vasodilation, thereby improving endothelium-dependent vasodilation. This effect is certainly due to stimulation of insulin-dependent NO release or non-enzymatic NO generation.[39]

Taurine

Taurine (2-aminoethanesulphonic acid) is the most abundant free amine in the intracellular compartment.[40] Low intracellular taurine concentrations in muscle are a typical feature in patients with chronic renal failure.[41] Intracellular taurine depletion might be associated with the well-known muscle fatigue in uraemia. Additional functions of intracellular taurine (e.g. stabilisation of membrane potential, promotion of calcium transport) may render this amine as a positive ionotropic and antiarrhythmic agent.

This interesting substance received very little attention until 1993, although there are numerous early indications of its clinical relevance. At present, there is some evidence that taurine might be indispensable during parenteral nutrition. We and others[42–44] found low extra- and intramuscular taurine concentrations after trauma and infection. Low taurine concentrations in plasma and platelets have been described in adults and paediatric patients receiving taurine-free TPN.[45,46] Since these patients did not receive cysteine, which is a metabolic precursor of taurine, the possibility could not be excluded that an inadequate conversion of methionine could contribute to low taurine levels. In paediatric TPN patients, low plasma taurine was accompanied with abnormal electroretinograms; addition of taurine (1.5–2.25 g/d) to the intravenous solutions restored plasma levels and normalised electroretinograms.[47] Kopple and co-workers reported that 10 mg taurine/kg body weight/day intravenously normalised plasma and blood cell taurine concentrations in long-term TPN patients.[48] Heird and colleagues have evaluated the appropriateness of a paediatric amino acid solution including taurine (0.24 g/100 g amino acids) for low birth-weight infants requiring parenteral nutrition.[49] In these patients, plasma concentrations of taurine were similar to those observed in controls fed sufficient amounts of human milk.

Low intramuscular taurine concentrations are a typical feature in chronic renal failure, probably due to impaired metabolic conversion of cysteine sulphinic acid to taurine.[41,50] Intracellular taurine depletion might be associated with the well-known muscle fatigue and arrhythmic episodes in uraemia.

Interestingly, as early as 1972 a marked increase in taurine excretion was observed after total body irradiation.[51] This finding and a profound taurine deficiency were confirmed in patients receiving intensive chemotherapy and/or radiation.[52] Experimental depletion of tissue taurine concentrations, especially in the lung, produces inflammation; administration of pro-oxidants results in severe lung oedema and interstitial fibrosis. Taurine administration ameliorates the symptoms.[53]

The potential immunomodulatory properties of taurine have been postulated, yet its precise role(s) remains to be classified. Undoubtedly, a key role of taurine in the modulation of apoptosis in a variety of cells has been demonstrated.[54] Taurine offers protection against oxidant damage in experimental lung inflammation.[55]

The underlying mechanism of taurine action may be due to its interaction with H_2O_2 and Cl^- in the myeloperoxidase reaction, thereby producing taurine chloramine, a pro-oxidant with very low reactivity, partially quenching free radical generation.[56] Actually, taurine chloramine may exert a potent anti-inflammatory effect by suppressing TNF and NO production in endotoxin and interferon-α stimulated macrophage cell lines.[57] Free crystalline taurine is available for inclusion in intravenous or enteral preparations.

However, we hypothesised that the extremely high intracellular–extracellular transmembrane gradient (250:1) might limit cellular uptake of taurine.[21] We proposed that enhanced transmembrane transport might be facilitated by binding taurine to a suitable amino acid carrier.[58] Accordingly, we synthesised three taurine conjugates, L-alanyl-taurine, L-phenylalanyl-taurine and L-tyrosyl-taurine, and investigated intestinal uptake and utilisation in a perfusion model after vascular administration.[22] Apparently, taurine conjugates are efficiently hydrolysed by membrane-bound peptidases and the liberated taurine is subse-

quently transported. Consequently, taurine conjugates may assist in the support of taurine-deficient target tissues.

Cyst(e)ine

In healthy adults, the sulphur-containing amino acid cysteine can be synthesised from methionine via the liver-specific trans-sulphuration pathway. In liver tissue of foetuses and of preterm and term infants, the activity of cystathionase, key enzyme in the trans-sulphuration pathway, has been found to be low or undetectable.[59-62] In liver disease, cysteine requirements of the body cannot be covered due to diminished trans-sulphuration capacity. In all these particular conditions, cyst(e)ine should be exogenously administered.[63,64]

Interestingly, the route of nutrient administration seems also to influence the rate of hepatic cysteine synthesis by altering the delivery of cysteine precursors to the liver. Stegink and co-workers could demonstrate in healthy men that intravenous infusion of solutions containing methionine but no cyst(e)ine resulted in depressed levels of all three forms of circulating cysteine (free cysteine, free and protein-bound cystine).[65] This result may be interpreted as saying that parenteral solutions should not only contain sufficient methionine but also additional amounts of cyst(e)ine. Presumably, such a supplementation with cyst(e)ine may be beneficial also with respect to taurine requirements during long-term TPN.

Addition of cyst(e)ine to TPN solutions is, however, problematic. At neutral or slightly alkaline pH, cysteine rapidly oxidises during heat sterilisation and storage to yield the dimer cysteine which itself is very poorly soluble (Table 23.1) and thus precipitates in the solution. Acidic conditions may lead to a reduction of the SH-group and the formation of H_2S.

There are some highly interesting studies elucidating the potential role of sulphur-containing compounds like cyst(e)ine.[66] Macrophages act as cysteine transporters under the action of inflammatory stimuli such as endotoxin and TNF. The uptake of cysteine in macrophages is competitively inhibited by glutamate.[56] During episodes of immunosuppression or in diseases with compromised immunocompetence like AIDS and malignancy, increased extra- and intracellular glutamate concentrations are observed.[67,68]

Cysteine also enhances a number of lymphocyte functions, such as cytotoxic T-cell activity.[69] A high

Table 23.1 – Chemical/physical characteristics of selected free amino acids and synthetic short-chain peptides

	Solubility (g/l H_2O at 20°C)	Stability
Cystine	0.1	yes
Cysteine-HCl	252.0	no
Bis-L-alanyl-L-cystine	>500.0	yes★
Bis-glycyl-L-cystine	541.0	yes★
Tyrosine	0.4	yes
L-Alanyl-L-tyrosine	14.0	yes
Glycyl-L-tyrosine	30.0	yes
Glutamine	36.0	yes★
L-Alanyl-L-glutamine	568.0	yes†
Glycyl-L-glutamine	154.0	yes†

★ Sterile filtration
† Heat sterilization

glutamate/cysteine ratio is associated with low share of T-helper cells.[70] N-acetyl-cysteine, reduced glutathione and cysteine inhibit the expression of the nuclear transcription factor in stimulated T-cell lines.[71,72] This observation might provide an interesting approach in the treatment of viral diseases like AIDS, since the transcription factor enhances human immuno-deficiency virus (HIV) mRNA expression. In fact, *in vitro* studies demonstrate that the stimulatory effects of TNF, induced by free radicals, on HIV replication in monocytes can be inhibited by sulphydryl compounds.[56] These basic studies indicate that treatment of inflammatory diseases and AIDS with sulphydryl compounds may be beneficial and powerful arguments have been advanced in favour of such treatment.[70,73] Clinical studies using this strategy are not yet available. One reason might be the lack of suitable preparations. The use of N-acetyl-cysteine in humans is not appropriate because of the lack of tissue acylases except in the kidney (see below).[43]

Cysteine is unstable and commercial GSH sufficiently pure for clinical use is extremely expensive. We are currently synthesising stable and highly soluble cysteine dipeptides.[12,43] The peptides are highly soluble (Table 23.1), easily available, the half-life is less than 3 minutes and the disappearance of the dipeptide is associated with simultaneous equimolar liberation of the constituent amino acids (see below).[74]

Tyrosine

The aromatic amino acid tyrosine has been traditionally considered a non-essential amino acid for adult humans. Tyrosine is synthesised exclusively from phenylalanine by hydroxylation; inclusion of tyrosine in the diet exerts a sparing effect on the dietary phenylalanine requirement.[75] However, under certain pathological conditions like classic phenylketonuria, liver and kidney disease and in premature infants, tyrosine has to be considered a conditionally indispensable amino acid. The essentiality of tyrosine is attributed to severely diminished activity of liver phenylalanine hydroxylase. In particular cases, a reduced endogenous tyrosine synthesis may also occur in full-term infants.[76]

Rudman and co-workers reported that cirrhotic patients receiving a standard TPN exhibited hypo-tyrosinaemia, hypocystinaemia and hypotaurinaemia.[63] They suggested that this resulted from impaired liver capacity to synthesise these amino acids secondary to the pathology of the disease.

Owing to its low solubility in aqueous solutions (Table 23.1), the concentration of tyrosine in amino acid preparations does not exceed 0.4-0.5 g/l, an amount which might be insufficient to cover tyrosine requirements in the above-mentioned situations. This problem can be overcome by using highly soluble and stable tyrosine-containing dipeptides (see below).

Glutamine

Glutamine is the most prevalent free proteic amino acid in the human body. In skeletal muscle, glutamine constitutes more than 60% (>19.5 mmol/l ICW) of the total free amino acid pool.[40] Glutamine not only acts as a precursor for protein synthesis but is also an important intermediate in a large number of metabolic pathways. It is a precursor that donates nitrogen for the synthesis of purines, pyrimidines, nucleotides and amino sugars. Glutamine is the most important substrate for renal ammoniagenesis and thus takes part in the regulation of the acid–base balance. As the most abundant amino acid in the bloodstream, glutamine serves as nitrogen transporter between various tissues. Owing to its diverse participation in transamination reactions, glutamine can be classified as a true regulator of amino acid homeostasis.

It is well known that glutamine represents an important metabolic fuel for the cells of the gastrointestinal tract (enterocytes, colonocytes) and many rapidly proliferating cells, including those of the immune system (for references see[12]). In addition, there is much evidence that hypercatabolic and hypermetabolic situations are accompanied by marked depressions in muscle intracellular glutamine. This has been shown to occur after elective operations, major injury, burns, infections and pancreatitis, irrespective of nutritional attempts at repletion. Reduction of the muscle free glutamine pool (about 50% of normal) thus appears to be a hallmark of the response to injury and its extent and duration are proportional to the severity of the illness.[43,77,78]

Recent studies underlined that this glutamine deprivation is mainly caused by trauma-induced alterations in the interorgan glutamine flow.[79] Muscle and, presumably, lung glutamine efflux are accelerated to provide substrate for the gut, immune cells and the kidneys,[80,81] explaining the profound decline in muscle free glutamine concentration. Two recent observations suggest that glutamine is involved in the regulation of muscle protein balance: first, the striking direct correlation between muscle glutamine and the rate of protein synthesis, and second, the positive effect of maintaining intracellular glutamine content on protein anabolic processes *in vitro*.[82,83] If maintenance of an intracellular glutamine pool promotes conservation of muscle protein, there is a theoretical case for glutamine supplements in the parenteral nutrition of stressed and malnourished patients.

Two specific chemical/physical properties hinder the inclusion of free glutamine in TPN solutions. It cannot be heat sterilised because this leaks to complete release of ammonia and formation of pyroglutamic acid.[84] Glutamine is also less soluble than the dipeptides (Table 23.1) and although solutions can be prepared by aseptic filtration and are relatively stable at 4°C (degradation $0.018 \pm 0.014\%$ per day),[85] the TPN regime will not contain more than 1.5% glutamine. Consequently, it is difficult to provide high amounts of glutamine to patients in whom the associated fluid load would be clinically unacceptable.

New substrates in protein nutrition

The obvious drawbacks of poor solubility and instability in the use of glutamine, tyrosine and cyst(e)ine as free L-amino acids have initiated an intensive research for alternative substrates which can be used as amino acid sources or amino acid precursors in parenteral nutrition.

Synthetic short-chain peptides

Owing to their high solubility in water and sufficient stability during sterilisation procedures (Table 23.1), synthetic dipeptides containing glutamine, tyrosine or cystine at the C-terminal position fulfil all chemical/ physical criteria approved by the authorities for constituents of parenteral solutions. Indeed, synthetic dipeptides might be considered as brand new candidates for parenteral nutrition. Basic studies with various synthetic glutamine-, tyrosine- and cystine-containing short-chain peptides provide convincing evidence that these new substrates are rapidly cleared from plasma after parenteral administration without being accumulated in tissues and with inconsequential losses in urine. Considerable hydrolase activity in extra-/intracellular tissue compartments[18,86–91] ensures a quantitative peptide hydrolysis, the liberated amino acids being available for protein synthesis and/or generation of energy.

Industrial production of dipeptides at a reasonable price is an essential prerequisite for implications of future dipeptide-containing solutions in clinical practice. Studies dealing with the development of novel synthesis procedures using native and/or immobilised plant proteases as biocatalysts have been undertaken.[92,93] Compared with classic synthesis methods, this biotechnological approach offers advantages, including (stereo-)selectivity of the reaction, minimal protection of functional groups and simplified purification procedures. These advantages enable increased capacity and reduced production costs.

Animal studies with glutamine or glutamine dipeptides

Basic studies with glutamine or various synthetic glutamine-containing short-chain peptides provide convincing evidence that these new substrates are rapidly cleared from plasma after parenteral administration without being accumulated in tissues and with inconsequential losses in urine. Considerable hydrolase activity in extra-/intracellular tissue compartments[86,88,89,94] ensures a quantitative peptide hydrolysis, the liberated amino acids being available for protein synthesis and/or generation of energy.

Following a bolus injection or under conditions of continuous TPN, these peptides provide glutamine for the maintenance of the intra- and/or extracellular glutamine pool.[88,95–97] Parenteral dipeptide nutrition promotes growth and nitrogen retention.[95,98,99] Intravenous provision of L-alanyl-L-glutamine (Ala-Gln) reduces muscle loss of glutamine during stress.[100] In this respect it is interesting that infusion of Ala-Gln in fasting mongrel dogs is associated with a shift of net glutamine equilibrium to glutamine utilisation in the liver. Thus, parenteral administration of Ala-Gln after fasting is not used preferentially by skeletal muscle or by gut tissues but rather predominantly by the liver.[101] Addition of Ala-Gln as a stable glutamine source or free glutamine to a standard TPN solution preserves or even enhances mucosal cellularity and function and reverses atrophy-associated gut dysfunction in parenterally fed rats with or without systemic septic complications.[95,102–112]

In isolated segments of distal ileum of piglets intravenous endotoxin infusion (50 μg/kg) was associated with increase in permeability. The endotoxin-induced permeability change could be prevented or considerably delayed by the supply of luminal glutamine.[113] Supplemental glutamine was associated with improved survival and a lower degree of bacterial translocation in experimental sepsis of gut origin.[114] In one investigation, however, the beneficial effect of parenteral glutamine nutrition on gut barrier function and mucosal immunity could not be confirmed.[115] Monosaccharide transport, water absorption and mucosal morphology were preserved with Ala-Gln enriched TPN following an experimental two-step small bowel transplantation procedure. It was concluded that glutamine is essential for physiological absorptive and barrier function of the intestinal graft.[107,116–119]

Direct intraluminal infusion of glutamine into the graft (segmental small bowel autotransplantation) improves mucosal structure and absorption of D-xylose. In this context it is notable that glutamine apparently induces heat shock protein (HSP) 70 and its RNA transcription in epithelial cells. This would mean that glutamine protects intestinal mucosa during critical illness against exogenous (chemotherapy, radiation) or endogenous (oxygen free radicals, endotoxinaemia) insults.[120] Parenteral glutamine supplementation reversed TPN-induced gut-associated lymphoid tissue (GALT) atrophy and attenuated the TPN-associated reduction of intestinal IgA. Interestingly, parenteral glutamine improved IgA-mediated protection in the upper respiratory tract.[121,122]

In a rat model of protracted peritonitis, protein synthesis in liver and skeletal muscle were improved, the morphology of the gastrointestinal tract protected and survival improved with supplemental Ala-Gln which may thus be beneficial in sepsis.[112]

Highly important reports emphasised that supplemental glutamine preserved hepatic and intestinal stores of glutathione.[123–127] The biochemical explanation for this finding rests in the fact that the highly charged glutamic acid molecule, one of the direct precursors of glutathione, is poorly transported across the cell membrane whereas glutamine is readily taken up by the cell. Glutamine is then deaminated and thus can serve as glutamic acid precursor. Furthermore, experimental feeding with glutamine resulted in a considerable increase in its gut fractional uptake and a matched increase in intestinal reduced glutathione (GSH) release.[128] This finding suggests an increased intestinal GSH production following glutamine administration.

An interesting new approach relates to the interaction between glutamine supply and endogenous arginine production. Compared with control diet, enteral glutamine enrichment resulted in higher arterial plasma concentration of citrulline and arginine in rats. It is conceivable that supplemental glutamine caused increased renal arginine production from citrulline. This observation, however, could not be confirmed in the numerous studies in which glutamine (dipeptides) were parenterally administered (see below). The question may also be raised whether this effect of enteral glutamine supplementation is beneficial considering the multiple, important biological properties of arginine.[129]

Human studies with glutamine or glutamine dipeptides

Healthy volunteers

Human studies in healthy volunteers demonstrated that Ala-Gln is readily hydrolysed after its bolus injection; the elimination half-time ranging between 3–4 min (Table 23.2).[130,131] Continuous infusion of a commercial amino acid solution supplemented with Ala-Gln or glycyl-L-glutamine (Gly-Gln) was not accompanied by any side-effects and no complaints were reported.[132,133] Infusion of the peptide-supplemented solutions resulted in a prompt increase in alanine, glutamine and glycine concentrations. During the entire infusion period, only trace

Table 23.2 – Kinetic values (± SD) for L-alanyl-L-glutamine (Ala-Gln), glycyl-L-tyrosine (Gly-Tyr) and L-alanyl-L-tyrosine (Ala-Tyr)

	Ala-Gln (n=10)★	Gly-Tyr (n=11)★	Ala-Tyr (n=7)★★
r^2	0.975 ± 0.024	0.975 ± 0.028	–
K^{el} (min^{-1})	0.185 ± 0.024	0.203 ± 0.019	–
$t_{1/2}$ (min)	3.80 ± 0.50	3.44 ± 0.32	3.30 ± 0.56
V (l)	10.52 ± 2.43	13.08 ± 2.34	5.30 ± 0.79
V' (l/kg)	0.140 ± 0.028	0.176 ± 0.032	–
Cl (l/min)	1.92 ± 0.36	2.65 ± 0.48	3.17 ± 0.53

r^2 = coefficients of determination; K^{el} = elimination rate constants; $t_{1/2}$ = elimination half-lives; V = distribution volumes; V' = coefficients of distribution; Cl = plasma clearance.
★ Data adopted from [130,132].
★★ Data adopted from [184].

amounts of the dipeptides could be measured in plasma and urinary losses of dipeptides were only about 1% of the given dose. These results indicate a nearly quantitative hydrolysis of the infused peptide and subsequent utilisation of the constituent free amino acids.

Lochs and colleagues studied the organ clearance of glutamine-containing dipeptides in postabsorptive and starved humans.[134] The clearance of Ala-Gln and Gly-Gln by the kidney was greater than those measured for the splanchnicus or skeletal muscle. Infusion of the dipeptides was associated with increased plasma concentrations and enhanced splanchnic uptake of glutamine and alanine or glycine, respectively.[134]

Clinical studies

The first clinical study with a synthetic dipeptide was performed in 1987 in patients undergoing elective resection of the colon or rectum. Infusion of Ala-Gln and Ala-Tyr supplemented TPN over 5 days resulted in an improvement of the nitrogen balance on each post-operative day compared with controls receiving iso-nitrogenous and isoenergetic TPN without peptide (Fig. 23.2).[135] The improved net nitrogen balance was associated with maintenance of the intracellular glutamine pool whereas in patients receiving the control solution, glutamine levels were markedly decreased compared to preoperative values (Fig. 23.3a). Muscle tyrosine concentrations declined without Gly-Tyr supplementation, while peptide provision enhanced intracellular values (Fig. 23.3b). The peptide was not detectable in plasma and muscle, and the plasma concentrations of the constituent amino acids

did not differ between the treatment groups. The infusion of the solutions was free of any side-effects and postoperative recovery was normal for each patient.

In good agreement with these results, intravenous supply of Ala-Gln following cholecystectomy

NITROGEN BALANCE

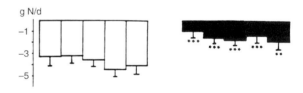

CUMULATIVE NITROGEN BALANCE

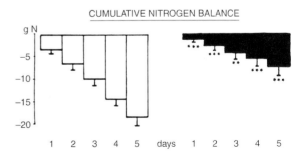

Figure 23.2 – Day-to-day and cumulative nitrogen balance (means ± SEM, n = 6) in patients after major elective surgery receiving Ala-Gln (280 mg/kg BW per day) and Gly-Tyr (50 mg/kg BW per day) supplemented (black columns) or conventional (open columns). TPN ⁎⁎⁎ p<0.001; ⁎⁎ p<0.01; see Stehle *et al.* 1989.[135]

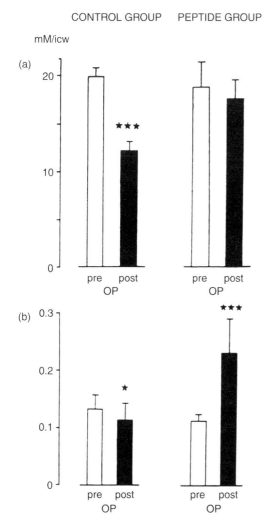

CONTROL GROUP   PETIDE GROUP

Figure 23.3 – Intracellular muscle glutamine (a) and tyrosine (b) concentrations (means ± SEM, n = 6) in control patients and in patients receiving Ala-Gln (280 mg/kg BW per day) and Gly-Tyr (50 mg/kg BW per day) supplemented TPN (peptide group). ICW = intracellular water; * p<0.05; *** p<0.001; see Stehle *et al.* 1989.[135]

preserved the intracellular glutamine pool (91% of pre-operative value) and the characteristic postoperative decline in muscle ribosomes was abolished.[136] In nutritionally depleted patients, plasma and mucosal glutamine concentrations were increased by parenteral glutamine administration.[137] It is, however, notable that glutamine concentration in the human mucosa is very low because of the ongoing enzymatic activity. Actually, critical illness *per se* is associated with slightly, but significantly increased glutamine content in the mucosa.[138]

Petersson and colleagues studied the long-term effect of postoperative TPN supplemented with Gly-Gln on protein synthesis in skeletal muscle.[139] In the glutamine group, the decrease in protein synthesis (assessed by ribosome profiles) was less pronounced compared with controls. Beneficial effects of short-term infusion of Ala-Gln on muscle protein synthesis assessed by [^{13}C]leucine incorporation were reported by Barua and colleagues in postsurgical patients receiving glutamine-free parenteral nutrition.[140] In patients undergoing major abdominal operations we were able to confirm the beneficial effects of glutamine dipeptide-supplemented TPN on nitrogen economy, lymphocyte recovery, maintenance of plasma glutamine concentration and shortened hospital stay.[141] A novel finding is the striking influence of supplemental glutamine dipeptide on cysteinyl-leukotriene (Cys-LT) metabolism. After operation the low Cys-LT concentration in isolated polymorphonuclear leucocytes was completely restored with supplemental dipeptide while remaining low with conventional TPN. Cys-LTs are potent lipid mediators. It has been emphasised that diminished release of this mediator is accompanied with an attenuated endogenous host defence.[142]

In keeping with these observations, it is of interest that in a current study of critically ill (sepsis, SIRS, sepsis syndrome) non-surviving patients revealed low LTC_4 generation while in surviving patients LTC_4 generation was normalised during convalescence. In these patients LTC_4 correlated to sepsis severity score.[143] Reduced LTC_4 generation in critically ill patients might be due to the anergic state caused by the underlying illness and/or lack of available fatty acid precursor at the site of the membrane. The likely explanation, however, is a decrease in antioxidant capacity during critical illness as intracellular stores of both glutathione and glutamine are depleted in these situations. Thus, the major question may be raised whether the combined deficiencies are intrinsically related to LTC_4-synthesising capacity of the sick cell. Indeed, we propose that the capacity of cysteinyl-leukotriene generation might be a biomarker for survival in the critically ill.[143]

In the presence of Ala-Gln, release of pro-inflammatory cytokines (IL-8, TNF-α) by polymorphonuclear leucocytes (PMN) was decreased while the ability to express the anti-inflammatory IL-10 was enhanced.[144,145] We propose that glutamine selectively influences the generation of lipid mediators and certain cytokines.

There are numerous data emphasising the immuno-stimulatory role of supplemental glutamine dipeptides.[146–148] Increased counts of circulating total lymphocytes and enhanced T-cell lymphocyte synthesis are consistently found in stressed patients following provision of glutamine or glutamine dipeptide-containing nutrition.[141,146,148]

In animal experiments it could be demonstrated that glutamine dipeptide-containing TPN may prevent trauma-related intestinal atrophy associated with glutamine-free TPN. In patients with inflammatory bowel disease and neoplastic disease, intestinal permeability could be maintained and villus height preserved with Gly-Gln supplementation.[149] In another study, Ala-Gln supplemented TPN maintained absorptive capacity (assessed by D-xylose absorption test) in the proximal portion of the small intestine in critically ill patients, compared with patients receiving conventional glutamine-free TPN.[150] As the large intestine harbours far more bacteria than the duodenum, jejunum or ileum, the maintenance of an intact colonic barrier may be crucial. The suggestion that glutamine or glutamine dipeptides exert beneficial effects on the mucosa is strongly supported by the results of a current study in which biopsies from normal human ileum, proximal colon and recto-sigmoid were incubated with glutamine, Ala-Gln and saline. Glutamine and Ala-Gln equally stimulated crypt cell proliferation and the trophic effect was mainly confined to the basal crypt compartments.[151] The link between depletion, glutamine and diminished gut function was reviewed by Soeters.[152]

In critically ill patients glutamine requirements are probably increased. This may relate to increased glutamine utilisation and requirements in tissues such as the gut mucosa and immune cells.[146,153] Provision of 20 g Ala-Gln (13 g glutamine) did not appreciably influence the intracellular muscle glutamine concentration in patients suffering from severe multiple trauma.[84] Cumulative nitrogen balance, however, was significantly better in the peptide group, the effect being greatest on days 1 and 2. Similarly, nitrogen excretion was markedly attenuated with glutamine-enriched TPN in a randomised, double-blind, controlled study in bone marrow-transplanted (BMT) patients.[147] In these patients morbidity was diminished with glutamine supplementation. Thus, the incidence of clinical infection, total and site-specific microbial colonisation and the length of hospital stay were reduced in comparison with patients receiving standard parenteral nutrition.[147]

In a similar study haematologic or solid tumour patients treated with high-dose chemotherapy and total body radiation received autologous or allogenic BMT and subsequently were treated with glutamine-supplemented TPN. There were no differences in morbidity but the length of hospital stay was reduced with glutamine supplementation.[154] In both studies glutamine-enriched parenteral feeding attenuated the expansion of extracellular and total body water.[154,155] This interesting finding suggests that provision of glutamine (dipeptide) may affect stress-induced accumulation of extracellular fluid by affecting membrane function (membrane potential) or changing the cellular hydration state.

In a fascinating hypothesis, the essential importance of cellular hydration state as a determinant of protein catabolism in health and disease has been emphasised.[156] It is postulated that an increase in cellular hydration (swelling) acts as an anabolic proliferative signal, whereas cell shrinkage is catabolic and anti-proliferative. The concentrative uptake of glutamine into muscle and liver cells would be expected to increase cellular hydration, thereby triggering a protein anabolic signal. Indeed, preparations containing glutamine dipeptides may facilitate aggressive therapeutic interventions in order to improve the cellular hydration state and subsequently modify or reverse catabolic changes.[157]

In contrast to the above-mentioned studies, in non-selected haematological patients undergoing intensive chemotherapy, no differences in neutrogenic period, fever, extra antibiotics and toxicity scores but gain in body weight were observed with Ala-Gln supplementation (40 g per day) compared with isonitrogenous control patients.[158] Thus, further studies to determine which patients may benefit from dietary glutamine (peptides) are clearly indicated in cancer chemotherapy.

In a very important prospective block-randomised double-blind study, glutamine-supplemented TPN significantly improved survival.[159] In one general intensive care unit (ICU) 84 critically ill adult patients (Apache II score ~17) received isonitrogenous and isoenergetic total parenteral nutrition with or without supplementation of glutamine in two equal groups. Survival was improved with parenteral glutamine compared to controls (24/42 versus 14/42; $p < 0.05$). This investigation clearly indicates that early glutamine-containing TPN, when used as a therapeutic measure, is beneficial after severe trauma and severe illness.

It is well known that very low birth-weight infants have sparse energy reserves at birth, an immature gastrointestinal tract and are highly susceptible to infections and feeding intolerance from enteral sources. They receive numerous medications and mechanical ventilation. All of these events are associated with metabolic stress. Indeed, in these critically ill small patients glutamine may become conditionally essential.[160,161] In current reports the beneficial effects of supplemental glutamine have been documented. Very low birth-weight (VLBW) infants receiving formula alone had a threefold higher incidence of sepsis than those receiving glutamine supplementation (0.3 g/kg) for up to 30 days. The decrease of HLA-DR T-cell subsets in glutamine-supplemented infants suggests reduced exposure to bacterial stimulation. This may be due to improved mucosal protection.[162] Interestingly glutamine supplementation with increasing amounts (0.08–0.3 g/kg) in VLBW infants resulted in differences in the rates at which certain amino acids increased from their prefeeding levels.[163] In particular, plasma concentrations of alanine, serine, threonine and the sum of non-essential amino acids were 20–30% lower in supplemented infants. These results are probably due to increased uptake of glutamine into liver and/or peripheral tissues.[164] The response of amino acids to glutamine supplementation might be interpreted as evidence of decreased tissue catabolism and enhanced gluconeogenesis.[163]

Indeed, glutamine supplementation may be of particular benefit to preterm infants receiving parenteral nutrition. Glutamine is one of the primary nutrients promoting growth; it is needed for maturation of the intestinal tract and may aid in prevention of enterocolitis.[165,166] Importantly, glutamine enhances growth, development and function of the immune system.[167] Accordingly, glutamine-supplemented premature infants at high risk for necrotising enterocolitis required fewer days on TPN, had a shorter length of time to full feeds and needed less time on the ventilator as well as revealing a tendency toward a shorter length of stay in the ICU.[168,169]

The effects of glutamine dipeptide-supplemented TPN are summarised in Table 23.3.

Table 23.3 – The effects of glutamine and glutamine dipeptide-supplemented parenteral nutrition

	Observation	Reference
Animal studies		
Intra-/extracellular glutamine pools	Maintained	Jiang et al. 1993[95]
		Lochs et al. 1988[88]
		Abumrad et al. 1989[96]
		Stehle et al. 1989[135]
		Stehle et al. 1991[97]
Growth and nitrogen retention	Supported	Jiang et al. 1993[95]
		Karner et al. 1989[99]
		Babst et al. 1993[98]
Muscle loss during stress	Reduced	Roth et al. 1988[100]
Mucosal cellularity and function	Preserved/ enhanced	Jiang et al. 1993[95]
		Yoshida et al. 1992[102]
		Tamada et al. 1992[103]
		Tamada et al. 1993[104]
		Schröder et al. 1995[107]
		Scheppach et al. 1996[108]
		Bai et al. 1996[109]
		LeLeiko and Walsh 1996[110]
		Liu et al. 1997[111]
		Naka et al. 1996[112]
Monosaccharide transport, water absorption, mucosal morphology after small bowel transplantation	Preserved	Schröder et al. 1995[107]
		Lew et al. 1996[116]
		Nemoto et al. 1996[117]
		Sasaki et al. 1996[118]
		Li et al. 1999[119]
HSP 70 expression and RNA transcription	Induced	Wischmeyer et al. 1997[120]

Hepatic, plasma and intestinal stores of GSH	Preserved	Hong et al. 1992[124]
		Harward et al. 1994[125]
		Yu et al. 1996[126]
		Denno et al. 1996[127]
		Yoshida et al. 1995[123]
TPN-induced GALT atrophy and decreased respiratory tract immunity	Reversed	Li et al. 1997[122]
		Li et al. 1998[121]
Outcome in protracted peritonitis	Improved	Naka et al. 1996[112]
Cellular hydration	Enhanced	Häussinger et al. 1993[156]
Controlled clinical trials		
Muscular glutamine concentration	Maintained	Stehle et al. 1989[135]
	Not influenced	Hammarqvist et al. 1990[136]
		Karner et al. 1989b[177]
		Fürst et al. 1990[84]
Mucosal glutamine concentration	Increased	Van der Hulst et al. 1996[137]
Nitrogen balance	Improved	Stehle et al. 1989[135]
		Fürst et al. 1990[84]
		Morlion et al. 1998[141]
Protein synthesis	Increased	Hammarqvist et al. 1990[136]
		Petersson et al. 1991[139]
		Barua et al. 1992[140]
Trauma-related intestinal atrophy	Avoided	Van der Hulst et al. 1993[149]
Weight gain in non-selected haematological patients	Improved	Van Zaanen et al. 1994[158]
Length of hospital stay	Reduced	Morlion et al. 1998[141]
		Heeneman and Deutz 1993[170]
		Schloerb and Amare 1993[154]
		Powell-Tuck 1999[171]
		Ziegler et al. 1992[147]
Survival	Improved	Griffiths et al. 1997[159]
		Ziegler et al. 1992[147]
Release of pro-inflammatory cytokines (IL-8, TNF-α)	Reduced	De Beaux et al. 1998[145]
Expression of anti-inflammatory cytokines (IL-10)	Enhanced	Morlion et al. 1997[144]
Lymphocyte proliferation	Enhanced	De Beaux et al. 1998[145]
Duration of TPN and ventilator dependency in VLBW infants	Reduced	Lacey et al. 1996[168]
Immunity	Improved	Morlion et al. 1998[141]
		Pastores et al. 1994[182]
		O'Riordain et al. 1994[148]

Cost-to-benefit ratio in clinical nutrition support with glutamine dipeptides

The reduction of hospital stay by about 5–7 days in the two BMT studies[147,170] and in surgical investigation[141,171] markedly diminished hospital costs, primarily as a function of reduced charges for room and board.[172] A decreased length of hospital stay of the magnitude seen in these studies has significant patient care and economic implications. In a standard university hospital a conservative estimate of $1000 per day and patient and 30 (BMT) patients per year would amount to a saving of $180,000 considering the observed 5.8 day average decrease of hospitalisation. Considering the abundant number of surgical patients, the savings with supplemental glutamine dipeptides are considerable, amounting to about $3000 per patient when calculating with an estimated daily cost of $490.

For glutamine recipients at the ICU the supplementation resulted in a 15% reduction of the total cost of hospital care ($6373 per patient) which, when expressed as cost per survivor, was 50% less than seen with conventional TPN ($46,403 vs $94,077). The cost of adding glutamine (dipeptides) to TPN is marginal compared with the estimated total costs at the ICU (about 0.2%) following BMT (about 2–3%) or after operations (about 4–5%).

What is the mechanism of the glutamine (dipeptide) effect?

One may speculate about the particular mechanisms underlying the effect of glutamine (dipeptides) in causing reversal of the clinical and biochemical signs of critical illness. Obviously there are distinct priorities of glutamine utilisation during stress, yet it is likely that the observed beneficial effects with supplemental glutamine (dipeptide) are interrelated.

Immune system and gastrointestinal (GI) tract may be the first priority,[173–175] improved nitrogen economy may be the next,[135,136,176] and normalisation of intracellular glutamine pools probably a third. This line of reasoning is supported by the fact that obvious beneficial effects on the immune system and GI tract can be achieved with relatively low amounts of supplemental glutamine dipeptides (10–13 g glutamine per day).[149,150] These amounts of glutamine did not appreciably influence nitrogen balance or amino acid concentrations.[149,150] Improved nitrogen balance and normalisation of the intracellular pool can be achieved in surgical patients with glutamine dipeptide supplementation,[135,136] while in severe trauma, though nitrogen balance is improved, the intracellular pool is not influenced.[84,177] Indeed, supplemental glutamine can counteract the fall in protein synthesis following surgery,[140] but an early discontinuation of the supplement results in a new fall in intracellular glutamine concentration.[178] It is likely that a replenishment of the low intracellular pool is difficult because the exogenous glutamine (dipeptide) is primarily meeting the increased demands of the immune system and GI tract.

It is conceivable that during stress and especially in critical illness, antioxidant capacity is decreased due to the formation of free radicals. As mentioned, glutamine supplementation has been shown to preserve hepatic glutathione[124] and intestinal mucosal glutathione stores.[125] In a current study, the combined therapy with vitamin E and glutamine was successful in the treatment of severe veno-occlusive disease (VOD) following BMT.[179–181] It is thus possible to assume that glutamine (dipeptide) supplementation may contribute to replenishment of depleted glutathione stores during stress and thereby counteract free radical-induced cellular injury. Indeed, these protective mechanisms combined with benefits to the immune system[146,182] may play a major role in influencing morbidity and outcome.

In conclusion, glutamine can be considered as a 'conditionally indispensable' amino acid during stress. Available data indicate that glutamine is an important amino acid in a number of clinical settings (Table 23.4). Indeed, omission of glutamine from conventional TPN and its subsequent supplementation should be considered as a replacement of a deficiency rather than a supplementation. It might thus be conceivable that the beneficial effects observed with glutamine nutrition are simply a correction of disadvantages produced by an inadequacy of conventional amino acid solutions.[159,183] The availability of stable glutamine dipeptide-containing preparations will certainly facilitate glutamine nutrition in routine clinical settings.

Table 23.4 – Patient groups that may benefit from glutamine supplementation (adapted from Ziegler et al. 1993[298])

1. Severe catabolic illness
- Burn/trauma/major operation
- Acute/chronic infection
- Bone marrow transplantation
- Other critical illness

2. Intestinal dysfunction
- Inflammatory bowel disease
- Infectious enteritis
- Intestinal immaturity or necrotising enterocolitis
- Short bowel syndrome
- Mucosal damage following chemotherapy, radiation or critical illness

3. Immunodeficiency syndromes
- Immune system dysfunction associated with critical illness or bone marrow transplantation
- AIDS (?)

4. Patients with advanced malignant disease
- Glutamine-depleted patients suffering from cancer cachexia

Other synthetic short-chain peptides

Human studies in healthy volunteers demonstrated that glycyl-L-tyrosine (Gly-Tyr) and L-alanyl-L-tyrosine (Ala-Tyr)[184] are readily hydrolysed after their bolus injection, the elimination half-lives ranging between 3.3 and 3.8 minutes (Table 23.2). Tyrosine-containing synthetic dipeptides are now commercially available and enable adequate tyrosine nutrition in clinical practice. Glycyl-L-tyrosine/L-alanyl-L-tyrosine supplementation may be of value in acute renal failure.[185] New, specialised amino acid solutions for patients with acute renal failure have been prepared to compensate for the specific amino acid abnormalities. One solution, containing both essential and non-essential amino acids, includes tyrosine (as dipeptide), serine and a reduced amount of phenylalanine. It has been shown to correct the plasma amino acid pattern and the phenylalanine/tyrosine ratio.[185]

Acute and chronic hepatic dysfunction does not affect elimination and hydrolysis of the dipeptides glycyl-L-tyrosine and L-alanyl-L-tyrosine and the constituent amino acids are released immediately. Both dipeptides may serve as parenteral tyrosine sources in liver disease. Moreover, because of its rapid hydrolysis, the use of L-alanyl-L-tyrosine, for the first time, enables a simple rapid non-isotope evaluation of tyrosine kinetics for assessment of liver function.[186]

Intravenous provision of cystine-containing peptides (bis-glycyl-cystine, bis-alanyl-cystine) results in taurine and glutathione formation. Intravenous cystine peptides are efficiently hydrolysed and subsequently provide cystine/cysteine to maintain the extracellular pool (Fig. 23.4). This might be of essential importance in situations with impaired trans-sulphuration pathway activity.[21]

N-acetylated amino acids

Early studies in experimental rats undergoing long-term TPN have clearly shown that highly soluble and stable N-acetylated amino acids, acetylcysteine, acetyl-tyrosine and acetylglutamine, are rapidly taken up and subsequently hydrolysed by acylases after their parenteral administration.[187–189] In a subsequent study in dogs, Abumrad et al observed only poor utilisation of parenterally supplied acetylglutamine associated with a large urinary excretion (38% of the amount infused).[96] Among the organs studied, only kidney cleared acetyl-glutamine to a measurable extent.

This was confirmed in healthy humans because continuous infusion of acetylglutamine,[190] acetyl-tyrosine or acetylcysteine[191] resulted in an accumulation of the respective solute in plasma whereas plasma

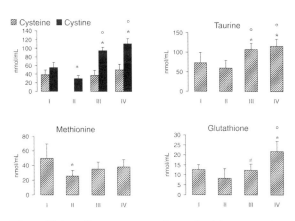

Figure 23.4 – Plasma concentrations of sulphur-containing metabolites (cysteine/cystine, methionine and taurine) in parenterally fed rats receiving: Group I: conventional TPN; Group II: methionine-deficient TPN; Group III: (Gly-Cys)₂ (359 mg/kg BW per day) supplemented TPN; Group IV: (Ala-Cys)₂ (385 mg/kg BW per day) supplemented TPN. ★ Significant vs group I, ° significant vs group II, # significant vs group IV; see[21].

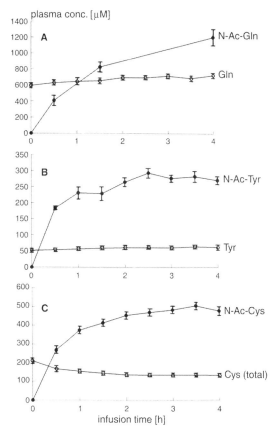

Figure 23.5 – Human plasma concentrations of acetylglutamine (AcGln), acetyltyrosine (AcTyr) and acetylcysteine (AcCys) before and during intravenous infusion of AcGln, AcTyr and AcCys, respectively. Data adopted from [239,241] with permission.

levels of the respective free amino acids were only slightly increased (Fig. 23.5). The urinary excretion rate of the acetylated amino acids approached 40–50% of the amount given. After bolus injection of acetyl-tyrosine, Druml and co-workers observed little if any hydrolysis of the acetylated amino acid.[184] Pharmaco-kinetic evaluation after intravenous supply of acetyl-cysteine in humans exhibited an elimination half-life of 2.3 hours, a value which is about 40-fold higher than those observed for cystine-containing peptides.[74]

It can be concluded that N-acetylated amino acids are poorly utilised in humans due to restricted acylase capacities.

Short-chain protein hydrolysates

Purified short-chain protein hydrolysates (>67% di- and tripeptides, <10% free amino acids) have been discussed as a low osmolality alternative to free amino acid solutions and synthetic dipeptides for peripheral parenteral nutrition.[192,193] In an enzymatically prepared short-chain casein hydrolysate, less than 10% of those amino acids which are themselves relatively insoluble or unstable (tyrosine, cystine, glutamine, tryptophan) were found to exist in free form.[194]

During intravenous infusion of a short-chain ovalbumin hydrolysate in healthy human subjects, excess peptide excretion during the infusion period accounted for only 6% of total nitrogen excretion, suggesting that a large proportion of the hydrolysate was metabolised.[195] Marked differences between infused and excreted peptide profiles indicated that utilisation of peptides from the hydrolysate was sequence specific.

Lipid nutrition substrates

Besides having direct nutritional effects, lipid infusion influences phospholipid composition of cell membranes, thereby affecting essential functions like enzyme activities, transport receptor and regulatory functions. These essential functions also relate to the formation of prostaglandins and leukotrienes. Without doubt, the nutritional and numerous structural and regulatory roles of lipids have a significant impact on major physiologic functions, including haemo-dynamics and oxygenation as well as immune status and hypermetabolism.[196–200]

Over the past 20 years, a consensus has been reached concerning the advantages of including lipid emulsions as a regular component of parenteral nutrition. Currently available intravenous emulsions consist of 10% or 20% emulsions of soybean or safflower oil.[196,197]

The aforementioned potential effects might be associated with complications. There is good evidence, however, that complications related to intravenous fat emulsions are usually due to high infusion rates that provide lipid energy in excess of resting energy expenditure. Carpentier[201] recommends a rate of triglyceride administration not exceeding 0.1 g/kg/h in hospitalised patients and 0.15 g/kg/h in home patients receiving cyclic parenteral nutrition. A more cautious tentative statement limits the infusion rates to between 0.03 and 0.05 g/kg/h.[196,202] In order to deliver adequate energy at these low rates, continuous round-the-clock infusion is required.

Parenteral administration of fat emulsions is accom-panied by increases in plasma total cholesterol and phospholipid concentrations and decreases in HDL-cholesterol while the abnormal lipoprotein fraction X is formed. Apparently these effects occur without imposing an atherogenic risk.[196,197] Interestingly, these changes are accentuated with infusion of 10% emulsions whereas administration of 20% emulsion is associated with modest changes only.[203,204] However, there is only indirect evidence that the abnormalities arising from the use of 10% emulsions are deleterious, so these observations remain a biochemical curiosity. Nevertheless, it appears sensible to reduce phospho-lipid infusion rates by replacing the 10% emulsions by 20% emulsions or by producing a 10% emulsion with reduced phospholipid content.[201]

The conventional intravenous triglyceride-based emulsions contain various amounts of oleic, linoleic and α-linolenic fatty acids. There is a growing body of evidence suggesting that a possible tailoring of the fatty acid pattern might bring about an improvement of the qualities of the emulsion. In early infancy and in some pathological conditions, transformation of linolenic acid via the intermediate τ-linolenic acid to arachidonic acid is not feasible. Thus, a new τ-linolenic acid-based triglyceride emulsion might be usefully developed in the future.[205,206]

New lipid preparations

Several new emulsions are undergoing experimental evaluation. A number of novel lipid substrates, like olive oil, medium-chain triglycerides (MCT), n-3 fatty acids, structured lipids and short-chain fatty acids (SCFA) are receiving increased attention as novel potential substrates in clinical nutrition.

Olive oil-containing lipid emulsions

Since the 1950s, there has been a growing body of evidence that the use of a Mediterranean diet is linked to a low prevalence of atherosclerosis and low incidence of coronary heart disease.[207-209] The Mediterranean diet is characterised by olive oil containing a high level of monounsaturated fatty acids (MUFA) and, thus, the consumption of this type of fat might be associated with beneficial effects related to atherosclerosis and the immune system. Clinical trials provide convincing evidence that carbohydrate-reduced, high MUFA diets can improve blood glucose and lipid profiles, minimise the amount of glucose-lowering medications required and reduce the risk of infection in patients with diabetes or other forms of hyperglycaemia (for references see [210]).

Actually, olive oil is a very old substrate in clinical nutrition now receiving a new lease of life. As outlined earlier in this chapter the first trial with parenteral fat was with olive oil in 1678–79 in Montpellier.[211] In 1869 Menzel and Perco,[212] and in 1904 Friedrich[213] concluded investigations in dogs and also in humans using subcutaneous infusion of fat; olive oil was also tried. Unfortunately, these infusions were so painful that nobody wanted to pursue this line of development in the field of clinical nutrition. The first documented report of successful total parenteral feeding including fat was provided by Helfrick and Abelson in 1944 using an olive oil-based emulsion in a 5-month-old child suffering from marasmus.[214] They were able to deliver about 130 kcal/kg/d via an ankle vein. They report that '. . . the fat pads of the cheek had returned, the ribs were less prominent, the general nutritional status was much improved and the former expression of dire misery was gone . . .'.

More than 40 years later olive oil was discovered as a suitable placebo in studies investigating the effects of fish oil since MUFA were regarded as neutral.[215,216] Interestingly, in some clinical trials reported effects were equally beneficial for the olive oil as for the test (usually fish oil) solution;[217] a subsequent letter to The Lancet is notable, stating that '. . . future studies of oil supplements should not consider olive oil as a placebo until there are more data evaluating the role of MUFA . . .'.[218]

In view of this background, the concept of an olive oil-based emulsion was recently developed. This contains 80% olive oil and 20% soybean oil, the content of egg yolk phospholipids as emulsifier being 12 g/l. The content of saturated fatty acids is 17%, of PUFA 20% and of MUFA 63%. Consequently, in comparison to soybean emulsions, the share of PUFA (n-6 fatty acids) is considerably reduced, the content of essential fatty acids is 20% and the natural content of α-tocopherol high. It is expected that the immune-suppressive effects associated with a high linoleic acid will be attenuated and the PUFA-induced oxidative stress decreased with olive oil.

The new emulsion was well tolerated by healthy volunteers. The fatty acid pattern of the olive oil emulsion is similar to human milk lipid composition[219] so it might be a more suitable lipid source for paediatric parenteral nutrition.[220] In the available clinical trials with olive oil emulsions, beneficial effects were reported.[220-222] Preterm infants revealed higher concentrations of C18:3 n-6 and C20:3 n-6 in plasma phospholipids with olive oil compared with soybean emulsions. Olive oil-based emulsions have been shown to enhance Δ-6 desaturation and elongation of linoleic acid to its more highly unsaturated metabolites.[223]

It might be pertinent to note here that olive oil emulsions do not apparently affect membrane composition. This line of reasoning could suggest that olive oil emulsions exert little effect on eicosanoid production and immune response.[224] The new lipid emulsion based on olive and soybean oil appears to be a valuable alternative for parenteral nutrition.

Medium-chain triglycerides (MCT)

MCTs were introduced more than 30 years ago as a constituent of the first 'medical food', valued because of their rapid hydrolysis and absorption in the gastrointestinal tract as well as their direct transport to the blood and liver.[225,226] Generally, MCTs contain the octanoic (73%) and decanoic (25%) acids and are derived from palm kernel or coconut oil. Pure MCT oil has an energy density of 34.7 kJ (8.3 kcal)/g.[5] Intravenous MCT emulsions are now well established in Europe and may soon be available in the USA. In early animal studies infusion of pure MCT emulsions was associated with various undesirable symptoms, including hyperketonaemia, narcosis, hyperlactacidaemia[5,225] and central nervous system toxicity.[227,228] These effects are due to the rapid hydrolysis of parenteral MCT and to the ability of the released fatty acids to cross the blood–brain barrier (in contrast to LCT). Therefore, MCT emulsions have to be administered either at very slow rates or together with LCT, which competes and thus buffers their appearance as free fatty acids in the blood.

The threshold level of competition favouring LCT over MCT has been suggested by Cotter and colleagues to yield the optimum ratio of 66–50% LCT.[229] When this concentration of 33–50% MCT was attained LCT outcompeted MCT for hydrolysis. The suggested physical mixtures of MCT and LCT were well tolerated when infused at relatively low rates.

In clinical studies, administration of an MCT/LCT mixture revealed in many cases distinct advantages over an LCT emulsion. In surgical patients the mixed emulsion produced fewer circulating triglycerides and non-esterified fatty acids than LCT, suggesting favourable utilisation.[205,230,231] The rapid plasma clearance[5,226,230,231] is associated with improved RES function[232,233] and thus results in less pulmonary sequestration of bacteria.[234,235]

n-3 fatty acids

The current interest in the use of fish and fish oils has its origin in the epidemiologic observation of lower prevalence of atherosclerosis and age-adjusted mortality in Greenland Inuit people compared with the whole Danish population.[236] The Inuits' diet contained total fat and cholesterol similar to the Danish diet but also a substantial amount of n-3 PUFA, also called n-3 fatty acids. This early study has led to an exponential increase in the number of publications on the subject of the metabolic and clinical effects of fish oil. There is the claim that n-3 fatty acids exert a protective effect in the development of cardiovascular[237] and inflammatory diseases[238,239] and the beneficial effects of fish oil supplementation in many other chronic diseases have been advocated. Some preliminary observations also suggest a potential role for fish oils in the treatment of atopic dermatitis and psoriasis.[240,241] There are also indications that premature infants have limited dietary supply of the n-3 fatty acids required for the normal composition of brain and retinal lipids.[242,243]

The biochemical basis for these proposed beneficial effects might be due to the inhibitory action of n-3 fatty acids on the cyclo-oxygenase pathway which metabolises arachidonic acid to the 2-series of prostaglandins, especially PGE_2 and PGF_{2a}, and thromboxane A_2. Eicosapentaenoic acid (EPA) is also

an excellent substrate for the enzyme 5-lipo-oxygenase. The resultant leukotriene B_5 might then exert considerably less chemotactic activity than the arachidonic acid-derived leukotriene B_4.

The major advantages of EPA- and DHA-acquired metabolites are summarised as follows.

1. EPA-derived thromboxane A_3 is less active in platelet aggregation than A_2 whereas the anti-coagulant properties and relaxation of vascular smooth muscle are preserved.

2. Leukotriene B_4 enhances chemotaxis, while others like C_4, D_4 and E_4 augment vascular permeability and contractility. EPA is converted into B_5, which has only a fraction of the activity of B_4, and platelet activating factors (PAF), resulting in decreased chemotactic migration and endothelial cell adherence. This would mean that n-3 fatty acids exert major effects on the synthesis of leukotrienes that promote inflammation.

3. Another important physiological effect of fish oils is on the immune system. Feeding with fish oils is associated with profound changes in immunoregulatory processes, including the production and release of various cytokines, interleukines and interferons. It is currently assumed that partly as a result of these changes, the natural history and progression of diseases with an inflammatory or immunologic component may be altered.

4. In addition it is demonstrated that consumption of EPA and DHA reduces serum cholesterol, LDL and triglyceride concentrations.

Several laboratories have also demonstrated that dietary pretreatment with n-3 fatty acids favourably influences pathophysiologic response to endotoxins[244,245] and exerts important modulations on eicosanoid and cytokine biology. These include inducing changes in the substrate availability for eicosanoid synthesis, altering membrane fluidity and altering the production of non-eicosanoid secondary messengers.[246] Indeed, inflammatory symptoms of rheumatoid arthritis, psoriasis, Crohn's disease and ulcerative colitis are all ameliorated by fish oil preparations, whether or not directly related to cytokine production. Consumption of EPA reduces the production of IL–1α and -β as well as TNF-α and -β in response to an endotoxin stimulus.

The anti-inflammatory effects of fish oil may also include decreased production of inflammatory substances like leukotriene B_4 and PAF, released by the action of cytokines, as well as a large reduction in cytokine-induced synthesis of prostaglandin E_2 and thromboxane B_2 in the colonic mucosa.[247,248] These findings are in line with a decrease in the arachidonic acid/EPA ratio in blood–mononuclear cell membranes as well as a decrease in neutrophil chemotaxis to leukotriene B_4.[249] The combined observations may be partly explained by the finding that leukotriene B_4 enhances blood monocyte IL-1 production after lipopolysaccharide exposure.[250]

There are few studies dealing with the effects of intravenously administered n-3 fatty acids. In our laboratory parenteral administration of a fish oil preparation (10% Omegaven, Fresenius, Germany) had no apparent influence on growth and nitrogen metabolism in catabolic rats.[251] However, TPN with fish oil resulted in a decrease of plasma free fatty acids and liver triglycerides. This is in agreement with reports that fish oil promotes fatty acid oxidation and impairs liver triglyceride synthesis. In our study,[251] fish oil feeding revealed a dose-dependent incorporation of n-3 fatty acids into tissue total lipids and phospholipids at the expense of n-6 fatty acids as early as 3–4 days after starting infusion.

The parenteral fish oil emulsion is obviously well tolerated by healthy volunteers and its prolonged infusion into postoperative patients was without complaints or side-effects.[252] In postoperative patients, treatment with fish oil-containing TPN was associated with considerable increases of EPA and DHA in leucocyte membrane phospholipids, the maximum incorporation being observed after 5 days of fish oil nutrition.[205,252,253] The leukotriene B_5 and leukotriene C_5-synthesizing capacity was also highly increased, indicating high metabolic activity of the infused EPA at the site of the 5-lipooxygenase (Fig. 23.6).[252] These results suggest immunomodulatory effects on lipid mediator generation during stress. They are also in good agreement with those in active Crohn's disease,[254] showing a marked increase in leukotriene B_5 without a decrease in leukotriene B_4, possibly due to the excessive linoleic acid content in the emulsion.

Similar results were found in patients following total oesophagus resection.[255] With fish oil emulsion an increased ratio of EPA/arachidonic acid was found in the thrombocytes accompanied by a reduced platelet aggregation, possibly due to a larger percentage of n-3 fatty acids in the phospholipids. The higher share of n-3 fatty acids might also result in an increase in the proportion of thromboxane A_3 to thromboxane A_2.

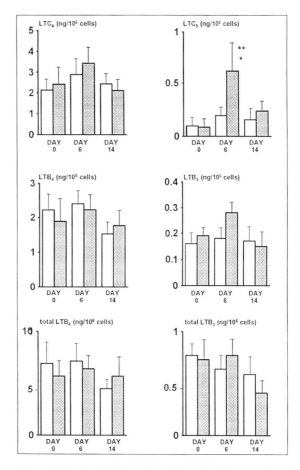

Figure 23.6 – *In vitro* leukotriene (LT)-synthesising capacity of human peripheral blood leucocytes after stimulation with the Ca^{2+}-ionophore A23187 (5 µmol/l). Patients received TPN solutions without fish oil (□, n = 10) or with fish oil (■, n = 10). Results are means ± SEM. ★ p<0.05, between groups, ★★ p<0.01, day 6 vs day 10; see 1996.[252]

The administration of fish oil emulsion might thus reduce the risk of a postoperative thrombosis.

Intravenous fish oil emulsions are also suggested as a supportive measure for adult respiratory distress syndrome patients,[256] as well as for patients undergoing chemotherapy or radiation therapy.[257] Concomitantly, n-3 fatty acid incorporation into membranes was correlated with decreased circulating TNF-α levels. Morlion and colleagues[258] speculated that lipid emulsions with an n-3 to n-6 fatty acid ratio of 1:2 would induce the highest leukotriene C_5: leukotriene C_4 ratio and exert the most favourable modulation of lipid mediator synthesis.[258]

The potential for long-chain n–3 fatty acids, when present in membrane phospholipids, to prevent cardiac arrhythmias was convincingly demonstrated in series of experiments by Leaf and colleagues[259] and was further confirmed in studies relating sudden cardiac death to dietary fish oil intake.[260,261] This may open new areas for investigation in patients suffering from myocardial infarct or benefitting from coronary revascularisation.

Structured lipids

'Structured lipids' are man-made lipids. They were synthesised originally by transesterification of mixtures of LCT and coconut oils, resulting in triglycerides with random arrangements of the fatty acids at the glycerol 1, 2 and 3 positions.[262,263]

There are studies suggesting that structured lipids are superior to the physical mixtures of MCT/LCT emulsions. In animal experiments, higher albumin concentration, nitrogen retention and growth were observed in those fed structured lipids rather than physical mixtures of MCT and LCT. A lower rate of infection and improved survival were also reported following parenteral administration of structure lipids.[263] These effects are assumed to be due to a lower production of inflammatory and immunosuppressive eicosanoids.

The value of physical combinations of emulsions or structured lipids as an energy source remains to be determined. Applied structured lipid emulsions consisting of an esterification of LCTs and MCT on the glycerol backbone are available for both preclinical and clinical studies. The structured lipid emulsion was well tolerated in healthy subjects. Also, patients undergoing major surgical procedures[264] tolerated the new emulsion without side-effects. The whole-body lipid oxidation rate was increased compared with conventional LCT-based lipid emulsions and it was associated with minor thermogenic effects[265] (Fig. 23.7). Overall nitrogen economy was not affected by the type of lipid emulsion. The positive effects with structured lipids are presumably due to their rapid plasma clearance, indicating that these energy-rich new substrates are rapidly available for oxidative processes with minimal thermic effects (energy expenditure) and thus with minor metabolic burden on the organism.[265,266]

It is claimed that parenteral administration of structured lipids improves nitrogen balance and

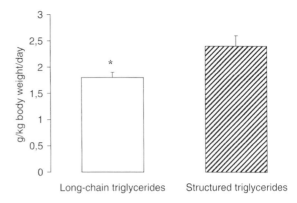

Figure 23.7 – Whole-body long-chain triglyceride and structured triglyceride oxidation in surgical patients. Results are mean ± SEM; n = 60. ⋆ p<0.01; see 1995.[265]

reduces plasma triglyceride concentrations in post-operative patients as compared with MCT/LCT emulsions[267] but the underlying mechanisms for these remarkable findings are not discussed by the authors.

Indeed, structured lipids might represent the next generation of fat emulsions that may be clinically advantageous to either LCT or physical mixtures of MCT/LCT emulsions. The decisive advancement toward better clinical efficacy might well be the modification of the LCT component with the use of n–3 fatty acids instead of the n–6 fatty acids, esterified with MCT.

Carbohydrate nutrition substrates

Glucose

Glucose is the only major nutrient to be supplied intravenously in the exact chemical form in which it is absorbed from the intestine.[268] It is considered to be an essential nutrient for central nervous tissues, erythrocytes and the kidney cortex. This particular glucose requirement is unique to humans and is about 145–160 g per day. There have been claims that injured or septic patients may require more glucose than normal subjects.[269,270] Under these conditions excessive sympathetic activity is associated with well-defined metabolic responses (i.e. considerably increased level of circulating catecholamines, resulting in an elevation of glucose and free fatty acids and a suppression of insulin). Another basic metabolic effect is the stimulation of glucagon which, with suppressed insulin levels, is of major importance in controlling hepatic gluconeogenesis. Thus, in trauma, increased gluconeogenesis and enhanced glycogenolysis result in sustained hyperglycaemia.

One might view the hypermetabolic response to injury as an effort to provide a superabundant supply of substrates from the body's own tissues under conditions where food may not be available. It is obvious that, while high circulating levels of glucose serve to fulfil the anaerobic requirement of regenerating wound tissue and to meet the obligatory glucose requirements, gluconeogenesis must persist. It is, however, remarkable that the high glucose levels which could normally suppress fatty acid oxidation in liver and muscle do not do so in trauma. In this context, one should remember that under catabolic stress glucose oxidation is diminished.[271] This implies greatly increased glycogen deposition,[272–274] enhanced thermogenesis[272,273] and extensive lipogenesis.[272,273,275,276] Consequently, under catabolic stress, large amounts of glucose may constitute a metabolic stress rather than appropriate nutrient support. For this reason, no more than 5–6 g of glucose per kg body weight should be given to hypercatabolic patients.

This finding has led to intensive searches for alternative carbohydrate fuels for intravenous nutrition.

Fructose and sorbitol

Fructose is considered by many as a good energy source. While it is true that insulin is not required for cellular fructose uptake or its initial phosphorylation, its metabolic fate is entirely dependent on insulin, in the same way as any other glycolytic intermediate.[277] Furthermore, bypassing the rate-limiting hexokinase step may lead to an accumulation of fructose-1-phosphate and to a depletion of ATP in the liver.[278,279] Lactic acidosis and hyperuricaemia may occur dependent on the rate of administration.[278,280]

On the other hand, fructose appears to represent the most powerful substrate for glycogen synthesis. The rate of liver glycogen formation from fructose has been found to be three times as high as that from glucose, whereas no significant difference in muscle glycogen synthesis was observed.[281]

Even at low insulin levels, fructose infusion results in only a moderate increase of blood glucose. A low rate of intravenous infusion of fructose is reported to be associated with nitrogen-sparing effect at insulin concentrations not exceeding the postabsorptive levels.[282]

Early technical problems in preparing parenteral nutrition (PN) solutions containing both amino acids and glucose led to a search for alternative non-reducing carbohydrates. In the 1960s, K. Lang in Germany introduced the sugar alcohol sorbitol into PN therapy.[283] Sorbitol is dehydrated in the liver to yield fructose which is then utilised via glycolysis.[284] However, sorbitol has no advantages over fructose and a considerable portion is lost in the urine.[277,285] One should keep in mind that the application of sorbitol bears the same risks as described for fructose. Thus, in patients with hereditary fructose intolerance, sorbitol infusion will result in an intracellular accumulation of fructose-1-phosphate and intracellular ATP deprivation. High concentrations of fructose-1-phosphate inhibit the activity of the glucose-generating enzymes glycogen phosphorylase and aldolase, leading to hypoglycaemia. Following some adverse incidents in clinical practice, the German authorities now deprecate the use of fructose and sorbitol in routine clinical practice.

Xylitol

Xylitol is a five-carbon polyol, a normal intermediate product in the glucuronic acid-xylulose and pentose phosphate cycles.[286] It is chiefly metabolized in the liver by insulin-dependent pathways to glucose via glucose-6-phosphate.[287] Following intravenous infusion this conversion takes place with only modest increase in blood glucose and insulin in normal[287,288] or stressed[289] conditions.

In recent studies hypocaloric administration of xylitol together with amino acids to injured patients[289] or to burned rats[290] preserved protein more efficiently than either amino acids alone or the combination of amino acids and glucose. In this context it is noteworthy that intravenously administered glucose is mainly (85%) metabolised in muscle tissue.[291] In contrast, xylitol is chiefly metabolised (80%) in the liver.[292] It is conceivable that the different organ positioning of these carbohydrates may alter in amino acid handling. Thus a recent finding by Danish investigators was that parenterally provided xylitol, independently of glucose and hormonal responses, inhibited urea synthesis and alanine metabolism.[293] This metabolic phenomenon might be theoretically beneficial as a therapeutic measure in certain catabolic conditions but the clinical implications of these findings and the long-term bio-chemical aspects of xylitol administration upon hepatic energy metabolism and whole-body nitrogen homeostasis are still not settled.[294]

Conclusion

The consensus view at present is to use glucose but a critical evaluation of the negative features is important. While we might suspect that the undesirable effects are associated with increased morbidity, there is no proof. However, excess carbohydrates are associated with pulmonary impairment due to higher CO_2 load.[295] Studies are needed to demonstrate whether or not alternative glucose substitutes, especially xylitol, are useful in certain situations. According to the literature, none of the glucose substitutes mentioned have beneficial metabolic effects superior to those of glucose.

Considering the claimed beneficial effects of xylitol and fructose, a combination of fructose, glucose and xylitol in proportions 2:2:1 and a mixture of glucose and xylitol in equal proportions have been proposed. It is assumed that by using these mixtures the infused amounts of the individual carbohydrates can be kept low, allowing an independent metabolism of the various components with sufficient energy but with fewer side-effects.[289,296,297]

References

1. Cuthbertson DP. Parenteral and enteral nutrition: whither the future. *Clin Nutr* 1982; **1:** 5–23.

2. Fürst P. Criteria underlying the formulation of amino acid regimens: established and new approaches. In: Kleinberger G, Deutsch E (eds) New aspects of clinical nutrition. Karger, Basel, 1983a, 361–76.

3. Brennan MF, Cerra F, Daly JM *et al.* Report of a research workshop: branched-chain amino acids in stress and injury. *J Parent Enteral Nutr* 1986; **10:** 446–52.

4. O'Dwyer S T, Smith RJ, Kripke SA, Settle RG, Rombeau JL. New fuels for the gut. In: Rombeau JL, Caldwell MD (eds) Clinical nutrition: enteral and tube feeding, 2nd edn. WB Saunders, Philadelphia, 540–55.

5. Bach AC, Babayan VK. Medium-chain triglycerides: an uptake. *Am J Clin Nutr* 1982; **36:** 950–62.

6. Silberman H. Total parenteral nutrition by peripheral vein: current status of fat emulsions. *Nutr Int* 1986; **2:** 145–9.

7. Wretlind A. The application of fat emulsions: history and future perspectives. In: Hartig W, Dietze G, Weiner R, Fürst P (eds) Nutrition in clinical practice. Karger, Munich, 1989, 71–6.

8. Urakaze M, Hamazaki T, Makuta M *et al.* Infusion of fish oil emulsion: effects of platelet aggregation and fatty acid composition in phospholipids of plasma, platelets, and red blood cell membranes in rabbits. *Am J Clin Nutr* 1987; **46:** 936–40.

9. Grimble GK. Essential and conditionally-essential nutrients in clinical nutrition. *Nutr Res Rev* 1993; **6:** 97–119.

10. Carpentier YA, Simoens C, Siderova V *et al.* Recent developments in lipid emulsions: relevance to intensive care. *Nutrition* 1997; **13:** 73S–78S.

11. Ekman L, Wretlind A, Moldawer LL. New developments in lipid emulsions for parenteral nutrition. *Infusionsther Klin Ern* 1987; **14** (suppl. 3): 4–8.

12. Fürst P. Old and new substrates in clinical nutrition. *J Nutr* 1998; **128:** 789–96.

13. Barbul A. The use of arginine in clinical practice. In: Cynober L (ed) Amino acid metabolism and therapy in health and nutritional disease. CRC Press, Boca Raton, 1995, 361–72.

14. Efron DT, Barbul A. Modulation of inflammation and immunity by arginine supplements. *Curr Opin Clin Nutr Met Care* 1998; **1:** 531–8.

15. Wernerman J, Hammarqvist F, Vinnars E. α-keto-glutarate and postoperative muscle catabolism. *Lancet* 1990; **335:** 701–3.

16. Leander U, Fürst P, Vesterberg K, Vinnars E. Nitrogen sparing effect of ornicetil in the immediate post-operative state. Clinical biochemistry and nitrogen balance. *Clin Nutr* 1985; **4:** 43–51.

17. Cynober L, Saizy R, Nguyen Dinh F, Lioret N, Giboudeau J. Effect of enterally administered ornithine alpha-ketoglutarate on plasma and urinary amino acid levels after burn injury. *J Trauma* 1984; **24:** 590–6.

18. Adibi SA. Experimental basis for use of peptides as substrates for parenteral nutrition: a review. *Metabolism* 1987; **36:** 1001–11.

19. Fürst P. Peptides in clinical nutrition. *Clin Nutr* 1991; **10** (suppl. 1): 19–24.

20. Fürst P, Hummel M, Pogan K, Stehle P. Potential use of dipeptides in clinical nutrition. In: Tessari P, Pittoni G, Tiengo A, Soeters PB (eds) Amino acid/protein metabolism in health and disease. Smith-Gordon, London, 1997, 237–52.

21. Fürst P, Pogan K, Hummel M, Herzog B, Stehle P. Design of parenteral synthetic dipeptides for clinical nutrition: in vitro and in vivo utilization. *Ann Nutr Metab* 1997; **41:** 10–21.

22. Hummel M, Pogan K, Stehle P, Fürst P. Intestinal taurine availability from synthetic amino acid-taurine conjugates – an in vitro perfusion study in rats. *Clin Nutr* 1997; **16:** 137–9.

23. Elwyn DH. Nutritional requirements of adult surgical patients. *Crit Care Med* 1980; **8:** 9–20.

24. Laidlaw SA, Kopple JD. Newer concepts of the indispensable amino acids. *Am J Clin Nutr* 1987; **46:** 593–605.

25. Young VE, El-Khoury AE. The notion of the nutritional essentiality of amino acids, revisited, with a note on the indispensable amino acid requirements in adults. In: Cynober L (ed) Amino acid metabolism and therapy in health and nutritional disease. CRC Press, Boca Raton, 1995, 191–232.

26. Snyderman SE. The protein and amino acid requirements of the premature infant. In: Jonxis JHP, Visser HKA, Troelstra JA (eds) Metabolic processes in the foetus and newborn infant. Kluwer, Dordrecht, 128–41.

27. Anderson HL, Cho ES, Wixom RL. Effects of long-term, low histidine diet on men. In: Fürst P, Kluthe R (eds) Histidine III. Wissenschaftliche Verlagsgesellschaft, Stuttgart, 1986, 2–25.

28. Fürst P. ¹⁵N-studies in severe renal failure. II. Evidence for the essentiality of histidine. *Scand J Clin Lab Invest* 1972; **30:** 307–12.

29. Fürst P. Amino acid metabolism in uremia. *J Am Coll Nutr* 1989; **8:** 310–23.

30. Galbraith RA, Buse MG. Effects of serine on protein synthesis and insulin receptors. *Am J Physiol* 1981; **241:** C167–71.

31. Bergström J, Alvestrand A, Fürst P. Plasma and muscle free amino acids in maintenance hemodialysis patients without protein malnutrition. *Kidney Int* 1990; **38:** 108–14.

32. Najarian N, Harper AE. A clinical study of the effect of arginine on blood ammonia. *Am J Med* 1956; **21:** 832–42.

33. Kirk SJ, Barbul A. Role of arginine in trauma, sepsis, and immunity. *J Parent Enteral Nutr* 1990; **14:** 226S–9S.

34. Evoy D, Lieberman MD, Fahey III TJ, Daly JM. Immunonutrition: the role of arginine. *Nutrition* 1998; **14:** 611–17.

35. Barbul A. Arginine and immune function. *Nutrition* 1990; **6:** 53–8.

36. Grossie VBJ. Citrulline and arginine increase the growth of the Ward colon tumor in parenterally fed rats. *Nutr Cancer* 1996; **26:** 91–7.

37. Vinnars E, Fürst P, Hallgren B, Hermansson IL, Josephson B. The nutritive effect in man of non-essential amino acids infused intravenously (together with the essential ones). I. Individual non-essential amino acids. *Acta Anaesth Scand* 1970; **14:** 147–72.

38. Albina JE. Nitric oxide regulation of inflammation and immunity. In: Cynober L, Fürst P, Lawin P (eds) Pharmacological nutrition, immune nutrition. W. Zuckerschwerdt Verlag, Munich, 1996, 21–32.

39. Quyyumi AA. Does acute improvement of endothelial dysfunction in coronary artery disease improve myocardial ischemia? A double-blind comparison of parenteral D- and L-arginine. *J Am Coll Cardiol* 1998; **32:** 904–11.

40. Bergström J, Fürst P, Noree L-O, Vinnars E. Intracellular free amino acid concentration in human muscle tissue. *J Appl Physiol* 1974; **36:** 693–7.

41. Bergström J, Alvestrand A, Fürst P, Lindholm B. Sulphur amino acids in plasma and muscle in patients with chronic renal failure: evidence for taurine depletion. *J Int Med* 1989; **226:** 189–94.

42. Askanazi J, Carpentier YA, Michelsen CB *et al.* Muscle and plasma amino acids following injury. Influence of intercurrent infection. *Ann Surg* 1980; **192:** 78–85.

43. Fürst P. New parenteral substrates in clinical nutrition. Part I. Introduction. New substrates in protein nutrition. *Eur J Clin Nutr* 1994; **48:** 607–16.

44. Pathirana C, Grimble RF. Taurine and serine supplementation modulates the metabolic response to tumor necrosis factor α in rats fed a low protein diet. *J Nutr* 1992; **122:** 1369–75.

45. Paauw JD, Davis AT. Taurine concentrations in serum of critically injured patients and age- and sex-matched healthy control subjects. *Am J Clin Nutr* 1990; **52:** 657–60.

46. Vinton NE, Laidlaw SA, Ament ME, Kopple JD. Taurine concentrations in plasma, blood cells, and urine of children undergoing long-term parenteral nutrition. *Pediat Res* 1987; **21:** 399–403.

47. Geggel HS, Ament ME, Heckenlively JR, Martin DA, Kopple BS, Kopple JD. Nutritional requirement for taurine in patients receiving long-term parenteral nutrition. *N Engl J Med* 1985; **312:** 142–6.

48. Kopple JD, Vinton NE, Laidlaw SA, Ament ME. Effect of intravenous taurine supplementation on plasma, blood cell, and urine taurine concentrations in adults undergoing long-term parenteral nutrition. *Am J Clin Nutr* 1990; **52:** 846–53.

49. Heird WC, Hay W, Helms RA, Storm MC, Kashyap S, Dell RB. Pediatric parenteral amino acid mixture in low birth weight infants. *Pediatrics* 1988; **81:** 41–50.

50. Suliman ME, Anderstam B, Bergström J. Evidence of taurine depletion and accumulation of cysteine sulfinic acid in chronic dialysis patients. *Kidney Int* 1996; **50:** 1713–17.

51. Dilley JV. The origin of urinary taurine excretion during chronic radiation injury. *Radiat Res* 1972; **50:** 191–6.

52. Desai TK, Maliakkal J, Kinzie JL, Ehrinpreis MN, Luk GD, Ceijka J. Taurine deficiency after intensive chemotherapy and/or radiation. *Am J Clin Nutr* 1992; **55:** 708–11.

53. Gordon RE, Heller RF, Heller RF. Taurine protection of lungs in hamster models of oxidant injury: a morphologic time study of paraquat and bleomycin treatment. *Adv Exp Med Biol* 1992; **315:** 319–28.

54. Neary P, Condron C, Kilbaugh T, Redmond HP, Bouchier-Hayes D. Taurine inhibits fas mediated neutrophil apoptosis. *Shock* 1997; **7:** S120.

55. Banks MA, Porter DW, Martin WG, Castranova V. Taurine protects against oxidant injury to rat alveolar pneumocytes. *Adv Exp Med Biol* 1992; **315:** 341–54.

56. Grimble RF. Nutritional antioxidants and the modulation of inflammation: theory and practice. *New Horizons* 1994; **2:** 175–85.

57. Park E, Quinn MR, Wright CE *et al*. Taurine chloramine inhibits the synthesis of nitric oxide and the release of tumor necrosis factor in activated RAW 264.7 cells. *J Leukocyte Biol* 1993; **54:** 119–24.

58. Dressel K, Stehle P, Fürst P. Novel taurine-containing substrates for clinical nutrition – in vitro evidence of hydrolysis. *Clin Nutr* 1994; **13** (suppl.1): 26 (abstract).

59. Gaull G, Sturman JA, Räihä NCR. Development of mammalian sulfur metabolism: absence of cystathionase in human fetal tissues. *Pediat Res* 1972; **6:** 538–47.

60. Snyderman SE. Recommendations for parenteral amino acid requirements. In: Winters RW, Hasselmeyer EG (eds) Intravenous nutrition in the high risk infant. John Wiley, New York, 1975, 422.

61. Sturman JA, Gaull G, Räihä NCR. Absence of cystathionase in human fetal liver. Is cystine essential? *Science* 1970; **169:** 74–5.

62. Zlotkin SH, Bryan MH, Anderson GH. Cystine supplementation to cystine-free intravenous feeding regimens in newborn infants. *Am J Clin Nutr* 1981; **34:** 914–23.

63. Rudman D, Kutner M, Ansley J, Jansen R, Chipponi JX, Bain RP. Hypotyrosinemia, hypocystinemia and failure to retain nitrogen during total parenteral nutrition of cirrhotic patients. *Gastroenterology* 1981; **81:** 1025–35.

64. Chawla RK, Lewis FW, Kutner M, Bate DM, Roy RGB, Rudman D. Plasma cysteine, cystine, and glutathione in cirrhosis. *Gastroenterol* 1984; **87:** 770–6.

65. Stegink LD, Den Besten L. Synthesis of cysteine from methionine in normal adult subjects: effect of route of alimentation. *Science* 1972; **178:** 514–16.

66. Grimble RF, Grimble GK. Immunonutrition: role of sulfur amino acids, related amino acids, and polyamines. *Nutrition* 1998; **14:** 605–10.

67. Fürst P, Bergström J, Hellström B, Kinney J. Amino acid metabolism in cancer. In: Kluthe R, Löhr GW (eds) Nutrition and metabolism. Georg Thieme Verlag, Stuttgart, 1981, 75–89.

68. Ollenschläger G, Jansen S, Schindler J, Rasokat H, Schrappe-Bächer M, Roth E. Plasma amino acid pattern of patients with HIV infection. *Clin Chem* 1988; **34:** 1787–9.

69. Dröge W, Eck HP, Gmünder H, Mihm S. Modulation of lymphocyte functions and immune responses by cysteine and cysteine derivatives. *Am J Med* 1991; **91** (suppl. 3C): 140S-4S.

70. Dröge W. Cysteine and glutathione deficiency in AIDS patients: a rationale for the treatment with N-acetyl-cysteine. *Pharmacology* 1993; **46:** 61–5.

71. Mihm S, Dröge W. Intracellular glutathione level controls DNA binding activity of NFkB like proteins. *Immunobiology* 1990; **181:** 245–7.

72. Mihm S, Ennen J, Pessagra U. Inhibition of HIV-1 replication and NFkB activity by cysteine and cysteine derivatives. *AIDS* 1991; **5:** 497–503.

73. Roederer M, Staal FJT, Elia SW, Herzenberg LA. N-acetylcysteine: potential for AIDS therapy. *Pharmacology* 1992; **46:** 121–9.

74. Stehle P, Albers S, Pollack L, Fürst P. In vivo utilization of cystine-containing synthetic short chain peptides after intravenous bolus injection in the rat. *J Nutr.* 1988; **118:** 1470–4.

75. Bässler KH. Metabolic basis for inclusion of tyrosine and cysteine in amino acid solutions. In: Hartig W, Dietze G, Weiner R, Fürst P (eds) Nutrition in clinical practice. Karger, Basel, 1989, 46–55.

76. Räihä NCR. Phenylalanine hydroxylase in human liver during development. *Pediat Res* 1973; **7:** 1–4.

77. Fürst P. Intracellular muscle free amino acids – their measurement and function. *Proc Nutr Soc* 1983b; **42:** 451–62.

78. Fürst P, Pogan K, Stehle P. Glutamine dipeptides in clinical nutrition. *Nutrition* 1997; **13:** 731–7.

79. Souba WW. Glutamine: a key substrate for the splanchnic bed. *Annu Rev Nutr* 1991; **11:** 285–308.

80. Rennie MJ, MacLennan P, Hundal HS *et al*. Skeletal muscle glutamine transport, intramuscular glutamine concentration, and muscle-protein turnover. *Metabolism* 1989; **38** (suppl. 1): 47–51.

81. Plumley DA, Souba WW, Hautamaki RD. Accelerated lung amino acid release in hyperdynamic septic surgical patients. *Arch Surg* 1990; **125:** 57–61.

82. Rennie MJ, Hundal HS, Babji P *et al*. Characteristics of a glutamine carrier in skeletal muscle have important consequences for nitrogen loss in injury, infection, and chronic disease. *Lancet* 1986; **ii:** 1008–11.

83. MacLennan P, Smith K, Weryk B, Watt PW, Rennie MJ. Inhibition of protein breakdown by glutamine in perfused rat skeletal muscle. *FEBS Lett* 1988; **237:** 133–6.

84. Fürst P, Albers S, Stehle P. Glutamine-containing dipeptides in parenteral nutrition. *J Parent Enteral Nutr* 1990; **14:** 118S-24S.

85. Grimble GK, McElroy P, Aimer P, Hardy G. The stability of L-glutamine added to TPN regimes for critically-ill patients. *Br J Intens Care* 1997; **7(4):** 126–36.

86. Stehle P, Fürst P. In vitro hydrolysis of glutamine-, tyrosine- and cystine-containing short chain peptides. *Clin Nutr* 1990; **9:** 37–8.

87. Plauth M, Kremer I, Raible A, Stehle P, Fürst P, Hartmann F. Dipeptide metabolism in the isolated perfused rat small intestine. *Clin Nutr* 1991; **10** (spec. suppl.): 25–32.

88. Lochs H, Williams PE, Morse EL, Abumrad NN, Adibi SA. Metabolism of dipeptides and their constituent amino acids by liver, gut, kidney, and muscle. *Am J Physiol* 1988; **254:** E588–E594.

89. Hundal HS, Rennie MJ. Skeletal muscle tissue contains extracellular aminopeptidase activity against Ala-Gln but no peptide transporter. *Eur J Clin Invest* 1988; **18:** 163–A34 (abstract).

90. Ahmed A, Herzog B, Stehle P, Fürst P, Rennie MJ. Skeletal muscle clearance of L-alanyl-L-glutamine: in vitro peptidase activity of rat sarcolemmal vesicles. *Clin Nutr* 1991; **10** (spec.suppl. 2): 10 (abstract).

91. Herzog B, Frey B, Stehle P, Fürst P. In vitro peptidase activity of different cell fractions of rat mucosa: kinetic studies using glutamine-containing dipeptides. *Clin Nutr* 1991; **10** (spec.suppl. 2): 32 (abstract).

92. Stehle P, Bahsitta H-P, Monter B, Fürst P. Papain-catalyzed synthesis of dipeptides. A novel approach using free amino acids as nucleophiles. *Enzyme Microb Technol* 1990; **12:** 56–60.

93. Monter B, Herzog B, Stehle P, Fürst P. Kinetically controlled synthesis of dipeptides using ficin as bio-catalyst. *Biotechnol Appl Biochem* 1991; **14:** 183–91.

94. Herzog B, Frey B, Pogan K, Stehle P, Fürst P. In vitro peptidase activity of rat mucosa cell fractions against glutamine-containing dipeptides. *J Nutr Biochem* 1996; **7:** 135–41.

95. Jiang Z-M, Wang L-J, Qi Y *et al*. Comparison of parenteral nutrition supplemented with L-glutamine or glutamine dipeptides. *J Parent Enteral Nutr* 1993; **17:** 134–41.

96. Abumrad NN, Morse EL, Lochs H, Williams PE, Adibi SA. Possible sources of glutamine for parenteral nutrition: impact on glutamine metabolism. *Am J Physiol* 1989; **257:** E228–E234.

97. Stehle P, Ratz I, Fürst P. Whole-body autoradiography in the rat after intravenous bolus injection of L-alanyl-L-[U-^{14}C]glutamine. *Ann Nutr Metab* 1991; **35:** 213–20.

98. Babst R, Hörig H, Stehle P *et al*. Glutamine peptide-supplemented long-term total parenteral nutrition: effects on intracellular and extracellular amino acid patterns, nitrogen economy, and tissue morphology in growing rats. *J Parent Enteral Nutr* 1993; **17:** 566–74.

99. Karner J, Roth E, Ollenschläger G, Fürst P, Simmel A. Glutamine-containing dipeptides as infusion substrates in the septic state. *Surgery* 1989; **106:** 893–900.

100. Roth E, Karner J, Ollenschläger G, Simmel A, Fürst P, Funovics J. Alanylglutamine reduces muscle loss of alanine and glutamine in postoperative anaesthetized dogs. *Clin Sci* 1988; **75:** 641–8.

101. Borel MJ, Williams PE, Jabbour K, Flakoll PJ. Chronic hypocaloric parenteral nutrition containing glutamine promotes hepatic rather than skeletal muscle or gut uptake of glutamine after fasting. *J Parent Enteral Nutr* 1996; **20:** 25–30.

102. Yoshida S, Leskiw MJ, Schluter MD *et al*. Effect of total parenteral nutrition, systemic sepsis, and glutamine on gut mucosa in rats. *Am J Physiol Endocrinol Metab* 1992; **263:** E368–E373.

103. Tamada H, Nezu R, Imamura I *et al*. The dipeptide alanyl-glutamine prevents intestinal mucosal atrophy in parenterally fed rats. *J Parent Enteral Nutr* 1992; **16:** 110–16.

104. Tamada H, Nezu R, Matsuo Y, Imamura I, Takagi Y and Okada A. Alanyl glutamine-enriched total parenteral nutrition restores intestinal adaptation after either proximal or distal massive resection in rats. *J Parent Enteral Nutr* 1993; **17:** 236–42.

105. Inoue Y, Grant JP, Snyder PJ. Effect of glutamine-supplemented total parenteral nutrition on recovery of the small intestine after starvation atrophy. *J Parent Enteral Nutr* 1993; **17:** 165–70.

106. Li J, Langkamp-Henken B, Suzuki K, Stahlgren LH. Glutamine prevents parenteral nutrition-induced increases in intestinal permeabiltiy. *J Parent Enteral Nutr* 1994; **18:** 303–7.

107. Schröder J, Wardelmann E, Winkler W, Fändrich F, Schweizer E, Schroeder P. Glutamine dipeptide-supplemented parenteral nutrition reverses gut atrophy, disaccharidase enzyme activity, and absorption in rats. *J Parent Enteral Nutr* 1995; **19:** 502–6.

108. Scheppach W, Dusel G, Kuhn T *et al.* Effect of L-glutamine and n-butyrate on the restitution of rat colonic mucosa after acid induced injury. *Gut* 1996; **38:** 878–85.

109. Bai M-J, Jiang Z-M, Liu Y-W, Wang W-T, Li D-M, Wilmore DW. Effects of alanyl-glutamine on gut barrier function. *Nutrition* 1996; **12:** 793–6.

110. LeLeiko NS, Walsh MJ. The role of glutamine, short-chain fatty acids, and nucleotides in intestinal adaptation to gastrointestinal disease. *Pediatr Clin North Am* 1996; **43:** 451–69.

111. Liu YW, Bai MX, Ma YX, Jiang ZM. Effects of alanyl-glutamine on intestinal adaptation and bacterial trans-location in rats after 60% intestinal resection. *Clin Nutr* 1997; **16:** 75–8.

112. Naka S, Saito H, Hashiguchi Y *et al.* Alanyl-glutamine-supplemented total parenteral nutrition improves survival and protein metabolism in rat protracted peritonitis model. *J Parent Enteral Nutr* 1996; **20:** 417–23.

113. Dugan MER, McBurney MI. Luminal glutamine perfusion alters endotoxin-related changes in ileal permeability of the piglet. *J Parent Enteral Nutr* 1995; **19:** 83–7.

114. Gianotti L, Alexander JW, Gennari R, Pyles T, Babcock GF. Oral glutamine decreases bacterial translocation and improves survival in experimental gut origin sepsis. *J Parent Enteral Nutr* 1995; **19:** 69–74.

115. Spaeth G, Gottwald T, Haas W, Holmer M. Glutamine peptide does not improve gut barrier function and mucosal immunity in total parenteral nutrition. *J Parent Enteral Nutr* 1993; **17:** 317–23.

116. Lew JI, Zhang W, Koide S, Smith RJ, Rombeau JL. Glutamine improves cold-preserved small bowel graft structure and function following ischemia and reperfusion. *Transplant Proc* 1996; **28:** 2605–6.

117. Nemoto A, Krajack A, Suzuki T *et al.* Glutamine metabolism of intestine grafts: influence of mucosal injury by prolonged preservation and transplantation. *Transplant Proc* 1996; **28:** 2545–6.

118. Sasaki K, Hirata K, Zou XM *et al.* Optimum small bowel preservation solutions and conditions: Comparison of UW solution and saline with or without glutamine. *Transplant Proc* 1996; **28:** 2620–1.

119. Li YS, Li JS, Jiang JW, Liu FN, Li N, Qin WS, Zhu H. Glycyl-glutamine-enriched long-term total parenteral nutrition attenuates bacterial translocation following small bowel transplantation in the pig. *J Surg Res* 1999; **82:** 106–11.

120. Wischmeyer PE, Musch MW, Madonna MB, Thisted R, Chang EB. Glutamine protects intestinal epithelial cells: role of inducible HSP70. *Am J Physiol* 1997; **272:** G879–G884.

121. Li J, King BK, Janu PG, Renegar KB, Kudsk KA. Glycyl-L-glutamine-enriched total parenteral nutrition maintains small intestine gut-associated lymphoid tissue and upper respiratory tract immunity. *J Parent Enteral Nutr* 1998; **22:** 31–6.

122. Li J, Kudsk KA, Janu P, Renegar KB. Effect of glutamine-enriched total parenteral nutrition on small intestinal gut-associated lymphoid tissue and upper respiratory tract immunity. *Surgery* 1997; **121:** 542–9.

123. Yoshida S, Kaibara A, Yamasaki K, Ishibashi N, Noake T, Kakegawa T. Effect of glutamine supplementation on protein metabolism and glutathione in tumor-bearing rats. *J Parent Enteral Nutr* 1995; **19:** 492–7.

124. Hong RW, Rounds JD, Helton WS, Robinson MK, Wilmore DW. Glutamine preserves liver glutathione after lethal hepatic injury. *Ann Surg* 1992; **215:** 114–19.

125. Harward TR, Coe D, Souba WW, Klingman N, Seeger JM. Glutamine preserves gut glutathione levels during intestinal ischemia/reperfusion. *J Surg Res* 1994; **56:** 351–5.

126. Yu JC, Jiang ZM, Li DM, Yang NF, Bai MX. Alanyl-glutamine preserves hepatic glutathione stores after 5-FU treatment. *Clin Nutr* 1996; **15:** 261–5.

127. Denno R, Rounds JD, Faris R, Holejko LB, Wilmore DW. Glutamine-enriched total parenteral nutrition enhances plasma glutathione in the resting state. *J Surg Res* 1996; **61:** 35–8.

128. Cao Y, Feng Z, Hoos A, Klimberg VS. Glutamine enhances gut glutathione production. *J Parent Enteral Nutr* 1998; **22:** 224–7.

129. Houdijk APJ, Van Leeuwen PAM, Teerlink T *et al.* Glutamine-enriched enteral diet increases renal arginine production. *J Parent Enteral Nutr* 1994; **18:** 422–6.

130. Albers S, Wernerman J, Stehle P, Vinnars E, Fürst P. Availability of amino acids supplied intravenously in healthy man as synthetic dipeptides: kinetic evaluation of L-alanyl-L-glutamine and glycyl-L-tyrosine. *Clin Sci* 1988; **75:** 463–8.

131. Matthews DE, Battezzati A, Fürst P. Alanylglutamine kinetics in humans. *Clin Nutr* 1993; **12:** 57–8.

132. Albers S, Wernerman J, Stehle P, Vinnars E, Fürst P. Availability of amino acids supplied by constant intravenous infusion of synthetic dipeptides in healthy man. *Clin Sci* 1989; **76:** 643–8.

133. Brandl M, Sailer D, Langer K *et al*. Parenteral nutrition with an amino acid solution containing a mixture of dipeptides in man. *Contr Infusion Ther Clin Nutr* 1987; **17:** 103–115.

134. Lochs H, Hübl W, Gasic S, Roth E, Morse EL, Adibi SA. Glycylglutamine: metabolism and effects on organ balances of amino acids in postabsorptive and starved subjects. *Am J Physiol Endocrinol Metab* 1992; **262:** E155–E160.

135. Stehle P, Ratz I, Fürst P. In vivo utilization of intravenously supplied L-alanyl-L-glutamine in various tissues of the rat. *Nutrition* 1989; **5:** 411–15.

136. Hammarqvist F, Wernerman J, Von der Decken A, Vinnars E. Alanyl-glutamine counteracts the depletion of free glutamine and the postoperative decline in protein synthesis in skeletal muscle. *Ann Surg* 1990; **212:** 637–44.

137. Van der Hulst RRWJ, Von Meyenfeldt MF, Deutz NEP, Stockbrügger RW, Soeters PB. The effect of glutamine administration on intestinal glutamine content. *J Surg Res* 1996; **61:** 30–4.

138. Ahlmann B, Ljungqvist O, Persson B, Bindslev L, Wernerman J. Intestinal amino acid content in critically ill patients. *J Parent Enteral Nutr* 1995; **19:** 272–8.

139. Petersson B, Waller S-O, Von der Decken A, Vinnars E, Wernerman J. The long-term effect of postoperative TPN supplemented with glycyl-glutamine on protein synthesis in skeletal muscle. *Clin Nutr* 1991; **10** (spec.suppl. 2): 10 (abstract).

140. Barua JM, Wilson E, Downie S, Weryk B, Cuschieri A, Rennie MJ. The effect of alanyl-glutamine peptide supplementation on muscle protein synthesis in post-surgical patients receiving glutamine-free amino acids intravenously. *Proc Nutr Soc* 1992; **51:** 104A.

141. Morlion BJ, Stehle P, Wachtler P *et al*. Total parenteral nutrition with glutamine dipeptide after major abdominal surgery – a randomized, double-blind, controlled study. *Ann Surg* 1998; **227:** 302–8.

142. Köller M, König W, Brom J *et al*. Generation of leukotriencs from human polymorphonuclear granulocytes of severely burned patients. *J Trauma* 1988; **28:** 733–40.

143. Morlion BJ, Torwesten E, Kuhn KS, Lessire H, Puchstein C, Fürst P. Cysteinyl-leucotriene generation as a biomarker for survival in the critically ill. *Crit Care Med* 1999 (in press).

144. Morlion BJ, Köller M, Wachtler P *et al*. Influence of L-alanyl-L-glutamine (ala-gln) dipeptide on the synthesis

145. De Beaux AC, O'Riordain MG, Ross JA, Jodozi L, Carter DC, Fearon KC. Glutamine supplemented total parenteral nutrition reduces blood mononuclear cell interleukin-8 release in severe acute pankreatitis. *Nutrition* 1998; **14:** 261–5.

146. Calder PC. Glutamine and the immune system. *Clin Nutr* 1994; **13:** 2–8.

147. Ziegler TR, Young LS, Benfell K *et al*. Clinical and metabolic efficacy of glutamine-supplemented parenteral nutrition after bone marrow transplantation. A randomized, double-blind, controlled study. *Ann Intern Med* 1992; **116:** 821–8.

148. O'Riordain M, Fearon KC, Ross JA *et al*. Glutamine supplemented total parenteral nutrition enhances T-lymphocyte response in surgical patients undergoing colorectal resection. *Ann Surg* 1994; **220:** 212–21.

149. Van der Hulst RRWJ, Van Kreel BK, Von Meyenfeldt MF *et al*. Glutamine and the preservation of gut integrity. *Lancet* 1993; **341:** 1363–5.

150. Tremel H, Kienle B, Weilemann LS, Stehle P, Fürst P. Glutamine dipeptide supplemented parenteral nutrition maintains intestinal function in critically ill. *Gastroenterology* 1994; **107:** 1595–601.

151. Scheppach W, Loges C, Bartram P *et al*. Effect of free glutamine and alanyl-glutamine dipeptide on mucosal proliferation of the human ileum and colon. *Gastroenterology* 1994; **107:** 429–34.

152. Soeters PB. Glutamine: the link between depletion and diminished gut function. *J Am Coll Nutr* 1996; **15:** 195–6.

153. Souba WW, Smith RJ, Wilmore DW. Glutamine metabolism by the intestinal tract. *J Parent Enteral Nutr* 1985; **9:** 608–17.

154. Schloerb PR, Amare M. Total parenteral nutrition with glutamine in bone marrow transplantation and other clinical applications (a randomized, double-blind study). *J Parent Enteral Nutr* 1993; **17:** 407–13.

155. Scheltinga MR, Young LS, Benfell K *et al*. Glutamine-enriched intravenous feedings attenuate extracellular fluid expansion after a standard stress. *Ann Surg* 1991; **214:** 385–95.

156. Häussinger D, Roth E, Lang F, Gerok W. Cellular hydration state: an important determinant of protein catabolism in health and disease. *Lancet* 1993; **341:** 1330–2.

157. Fürst P, Stehle P. Glutamine and glutamine-containing dipeptides. In: Cynober L (ed) Amino acid metabolism in health and nutritional diseases. CRC Press, Boca Raton, 1995, 373–83.

of leukotrienes and cytokines in vitro. 4th International Congress on the Immune Consequences of Trauma, Shock and Sepsis, 1997, 269–72.

158. Van Zaanen HCT, Van der Lelie J, Timmer JG, Fürst P, Sauerwein HP. Parenteral glutamine supplementation does not ameliorate chemotherapy-induced toxicity. *Cancer* 1994; **74:** 2879–84.

159. Griffiths RD, Jones C, Palmer TEA. Six-month outcome of critically ill patients given glutamine-supplemented parenteral nutrition. *Nutrition* 1997; **13:** 295–302.

160. Lacey JM, Wilmore DW. Is glutamine a conditionally essential amino acid? *Nutr Rev* 1990; **48:** 297–309.

161. Darmaun D, Roig JC, Auestad N, Sager BK, Neu J. Glutamine metabolism in very low birth weight infants. *Pediatr Res* 1997; **41:** 391–6.

162. Neu J, Roig JC, Meetze WH *et al*. Enteral glutamine supplementation for very low birth weight infants decreases morbidity. *J. Pediatr.* 1997; **131:** 691–9.

163. Roig JC, Meetze WH, Auestad N *et al*. Enteral glutamine supplementation for the very low birth-weight infant: plasma amino acid concentrations. *J Nutr* 1996; **126** (suppl): 1115S–1120S.

164. Moundras C, Remesy C, Bercovici D, Demigne C. Effect of a dietary supplementation with glutamic acid or glutamine on the splanchnic and muscle metabolism of glucogenic amino acids in the rat. *J Nutr Biochem* 1993; **4:** 222–8.

165. Souba WW, Klimberg VS, Hautamaki RD *et al*. Oral glutamine reduces bacterial translocation following abdominal radiation. *J Surg Res* 1990; **48:** 1–5.

166. Rombeau JL. A review of the effects of glutamine-enriched diets on experimentally induced enterocolitis. *J Parent Enteral Nutr* 1990; **14:** 100S–105S.

167. Newsholme EA, Newsholme P, Curi R, Challoner E, Ardawi MSM. A role for muscle in the immune system and its importance in surgery, trauma, sepsis and burns. *Nutrition* 1988; **4:** 261–8.

168. Lacey JM, Crouch JB, Benfell K *et al*. The effects of glutamine-supplemented parenteral nutrition in premature infants. *J Parent Enteral Nutr* 1996; **20:** 74–80.

169. Wilmore DW, Shabert JK. Role of glutamine in immunologic responses. *Nutrition* 1998; **14:** 618–26.

170. Heeneman S, Deutz NEP. Effects of decreased glutamine supply on gut and liver metabolism in vivo in rats. *Clin Sci* 1993; **85:** 437–44.

171. Powell-Tuck J. Total parenteral nutrition with glutamine dipeptide shortened hospital stays and improved immune status and nitrogen economy after major abdominal surgery. Commentary by J Powell-Tuck. *Gut* 1999; **44:** 155.

172. McBurney M, Young LS, Ziegler TR, Wilmore DW. A cost-evaluation of glutamine-supplemented parenteral nutrition in adult bone marrow transplantation. *J Am Diet Assoc* 1994; **94:** 1263–6.

173. Newsholme EA, Crabtree B, Ardawi MSM. Glutamine metabolism in lymphocytes: its biochemical, physiological and clinical importance. *Q J Exp Physiol* 1985; **70:** 473–89.

174. Parry-Billings M, Evans J, Calder PC, Newsholme EA. Does glutamine contribute to immunosuppression after major burns? *Lancet* 1990; **336:** 523–5.

175. Wilmore DW, Smith RJ, O'Dwyer ST, Jacobs DO, Ziegler TR, Wang X-D. The gut: a central organ after surgical stress. *Surgery* 1988; **104:** 917–23.

176. Fürst P, Albers S, Stehle P. Evidence for a nutritional need for glutamine in catabolic patients. *Kidney Int* 1989; **36** (suppl. 27): S287–S292.

177. Karner J, Roth E, Stehle P, Albers S, Fürst P. Influence of glutamine-containing dipeptides on muscle amino acid metabolism. In: Hartig W, Dietze G, Weiner R, Fürst P (eds) Nutrition in clinical practice. Karger, Basel, 1989, 56–70.

178. Petersson B, Waller S-O, Vinnars E, Wernerman J. Long-term effect of glycyl-glutamine after elective surgery on free amino acids in muscle. *J Parent Enteral Nutr* 1994; **18:** 320–5.

179. Brown SA, Goringe A, Fegan C *et al*. Parenteral glutamine protects hepatic function during bone marrow transplantation. *Bone Marrow Transplant* 1998; **22:** 281–4.

180. Goringe AP, Brown S, O'Callaghan U, Rees J, Elia M, Poynton CH. Glutamine and vitamin E in the treatment of hepatic veno-occlusive disease following high-dose chemotherapy. *Bone Marrow Transplant* 1998; **21:** 829–32.

181. Nattakom TV, Charlton A, Wilmore DW. Use of vitamin E and glutamine in the successful treatment of severe veno-occlusive disease following bone marrow transplantation. *Nutr Clin Prac* 1995; **10:** 16–18.

182. Pastores SM, Kvetan V, Katz DP. Immunomodulatory effects and therapeutic potential of glutamine in the critically ill surgical patient. *Nutrition* 1994; **10:** 385–91.

183. Fürst P, Stehle P. Are intravenous amino acid solutions unbalanced? *New Horizons* 1994; **2:** 215–23.

184. Druml W, Lochs H, Roth E, Hübl W, Balcke P, Lenz K. Utilization of tyrosine dipeptides and acetyltyrosine in normal and uremic humans. *Am J Physiol* 1991; **260:** E280–E285.

185. Druml W. Nutritional considerations in the treatment of acute renal failure in septic patients. *Nephrol Dial Transplant* 1994; **9:** S219–S223.

186. Druml W, Hübl W, Roth E, Lochs H. Utilization of tyrosine-containing dipeptides and N-acetyl-tyrosine in hepatic failure. *Hepatology* 1995; **21:** 923–8.

187. Neuhäuser-Berthold M, Wirth S, Hellmann U, Bässler KH. Utilisation of N-acetyl-L-glutamine during long-term parenteral nutrition in growing rats: significance of glutamine for weight and nitrogen balance. *Clin Nutr* 1988; **7:** 145–50.

188. Neuhäuser M, Grötz KA, Wandira JA, Bässler KH, Langer K. Utilization of methionine and N-acetyl-L-cysteine during long-term parenteral nutrition in the growing rat. *Metabolism* 1986; **35:** 869–73.

189. Neuhäuser M, Wandira JA, Göttmann U, Bässler KH, Langer K. Utilization of N-acetyl-L-tyrosine and glycyl-L-tyrosine during long-term parenteral nutrition in the growing rat. *Am J Clin Nutr* 1985; **42:** 585–96.

190. Magnusson I, Kihlberg R, Alvestrand A, Wernerman J, Ekman L, Wahren J. Utilization of intravenously administered N-acetyl-L-glutamine in humans. *Metabolism* 1989; **38** (suppl. 1): 82–8.

191. Magnusson I, Ekman L, Wangdahl M, Wahren J. N-acetyl-L-tyrosine and N-acetyl-L-cysteine as tyrosine and cysteine precursors during intravenous infusion in humans. *Metabolism* 1989; **38:** 957–61.

192. Grimble GK, Aimer PC, Morris P, Raimundo A, Weryk B, Silk DBA. Plasma amino acids and peptiduria during intravenous infusion of a short-chain ovalbumin hydrolysate, or its equivalent amino acid (AA) mixture, in man. *Proc Nutr Soc* 1992; **51:** 103A.

193. Grimble GK, Silk DA. Peptides in human nutrition. *Nutr Res Rev* 1989; **2:** 87–108.

194. Grimble GK, Rees RG, Keohane PP, Cartwright T, Desreumaux M, Silk DBA. Effect of peptide chain length on absorption of egg protein hydrolysates in the normal human jejunum. *Gastroenterology* 1987; **92:** 135–42.

195. Grimble GK, Raimundo A, Rees RG, Hunjan MK, Silk DA. Parenteral utilisation of a purified short-chain enzymic hydrolysate of ovalbumin in man. *J Parent Enteral Nutr* 1988; **12** (suppl.): 15 S.

196. Miles JM. Intravenous fat emulsions in nutritional support. *Curr Opin Gastroenterology* 1991; **7:** 306–11.

197. Carpentier YA, Van Gossum A, Dubois DY, Deckelbaum RJ. Lipid metabolism. In: Rombeau JL, Caldwell MD (eds) Clinical nutrition: parenteral nutrition, 2nd edn. WB Saunders, Philadelphia, 1993, 35–74.

198. Gottschlich MM. Selection of optimal lipid sources in enteral and parenteral nutrition. *Nutr Clin Prac* 1992; **7:** 152–65.

199. Alexander JW, Peck MD. Further prospects for adjunctive therapy: pharmacologic and nutritional approaches to immune system modulation. *Crit Care Med* 1990; **18:** S159–S164.

200. Skeie B, Askanazi J, Rothkopf MM, Goldstein S, Rosenbaum SH. Intravenous fat emulsions and lung function: a review. *Crit Care Med* 1988; **16:** 183–94.

201. Carpentier YA. Lipid emulsions. In: Fürst P (ed) New strategies in clinical nutrition. Zuckschwerdt, Munich, 1993.

202. Jensen GL, Mascioli EA, Seidner DL *et al.* Parenteral infusion of long- and medium-chain triglycerides and reticuloendothelial system function in man. *J Parent Enteral Nutr* 1990; **14:** 467–71.

203. Haumont D, Deckelbaum RJ, Richelle M *et al.* Plasma lipid and plasma lipoprotein concentrations in low birth weight infants given parenteral nutrition with twenty or ten percent lipid emulsion. *J Pediatr* 1989; **115:** 787–93.

204. Meguid MM, Kurzer M, Hayashi RJ, Akahoshi MP. Short-term effects of fat emulsion on serum lipids on postoperative patients. *J Parent Enteral Nutr* 1989; **13:** 77–80.

205. Dupont IE, Carpentier YA. Clinical use of lipid emulsions. *Curr Opin Clin Nutr Met Care* 1999, **2:** 139–45.

206. Wretlind A. Past, present and future in total parenteral nutrition. *Intake* 1990; **3:** 3–4.

207. Keys A. Coronary heart disease in seven countries. *Circulation* 1970; **41:** 1–211.

208. Nestle M. Mediteranean diets: historical and research overview. *Am J Clin Nutr* 1995; **61:** 1313S–1320S.

209. Yaqoob P, Calder PC. Cytokine production by human peripheral blood mononuclear cells: differential senstivity to glutamine availability. *Cytokine* 1998; **10:** 790–4.

210. Fürst P. Consensus roundtable on nutrition support of tube-fed patients with diabetes. *Clin Nutr* 1998a; **17** (suppl. 2): 3–6.

211. Courten W. Experiments and observations of the effects of several sorts of poisons upon animals made at Montpellier in the years 1678 and 1679 by the late William Courten. *Philos Trans R Soc London* 1712; **27:** 485–500.

212. Menzel A, Perco H. Über die Resorption von Nahrungsmitteln von Unterhaut-Zellengewebe aus Wien. *Med Wochenschr* 1869; **19:** 517.

213. Friedrich PL. Die künstliche subkutane Ernährung in der praktischen Chirugie. *Arch Klin Chir* 1904; **73:** 507–16.

214. Helfrick FW, Abelson NM. Intravenous feeding of a complete diet in a child: report of a case. *J Pediatr* 1944; **25:** 400–3.

215. Cleland LG, French JK, Betts WH, Murphy GH, Elliot MJ. Clinical and beneficial effects of dietary fish oil supplements in rheumatoid arthritis. *Journal of Rheumatology* 1988; **15**: 1471–5.

216. Virella G, Fourspring K, Hyman B *et al.* Immuno-suppressive effects of fish oil in normal human volunteers: correlation with the in vitro effects of eicopsapentaenoic acid on human lymphocytes. *Clin Immunol Immunopathol* 1991; **61**: 161–7.

217. Dehmer GJ, Popma JJ, Van den Berg EK *et al.* Reduction in the rate of early restenosis after coronary angioplasty by a diet supplemented with n-3 fatty acids. *N Engl J Med* 1988; **319**: 733–40.

218. Milner MR. Fish oil for preventing coronary restenosis. *Lancet* 1989; **i**: 693.

219. Genzel-Boroviczeny O, Wahle J, Koletzko B. Fatty acid composition of human milk during the 1st month after term and preterm delivery. *Eur J Pediatr* 1997; **156**: 142–7.

220. Koletzko B. Lipid supply and metabolism in infancy. *Curr Opin Clin Nutr Met Care* 1998; **1**: 171–7.

221. Munck A, Navarro J. Tolerance et efficacite de l'emulsion lipidique clinoleic chez l'enfant en nutrition parenteral exclusive. *Nutr Clin Metabol* 1996; **10**: 45S–47S.

222. Goulet O, De Potter S, Bereziat G *et al.* Use of a new olive oil-based emulsion in long term parenteral nutrition: a double blind randomized study in children. *Clin Nutr* 1997; **16**: 1-1.

223. Koletzko B, Göbel Y, Engelsberger I *et al.* Parenteral feeding of preterm infants with fat emulsions based on soybean and olive oils: effect on plasma phospholipid fatty acids. *Clin Nutr* 1998; **17**: S25.

224. Yaqoob P. Monounsaturated fatty acids and immune function. *Proc Nutr Soc* 1998; **57**: 511–20.

225. Bach AC, Giusard D, Debry G, Metais P. Metabolic effects following a medium chain triglycerides load in dogs. V. Influence of the perfusion rate. *Arch Physiol Biochem* 1974; **82**: 705–19.

226. Sailer D, Müller M. Medium chain triglycerides in parenteral nutrition. *J Parent Enteral Nutr* 1981; **5**: 115–19.

227. Johnson RC, Cotter R. Metabolism of medium-chain triglyceride lipid emulsion. *Nutr Int* 1986; **2**: 150–8.

228. Miles JM, Cattalani M, Sharbrough FW *et al.* Metabolic and neurological effects of an intravenous medium-chain triglyceride lipid emulsion. *J Parent Enteral Nutr* 1991; **15**: 37–41.

229. Cotter R, Taylor CA, Johnson R, Rowe B. A metabolic comparison of pure and long-chain triglyceride lipid emulsion and various medium-chain triglyceride combination emulsions in dogs. *Am J Clin Nutr* 1987; **45**: 927.

230. Crowe PJ, Dennison AR, Royle GT. A new intravenous emulsion containing medium-chain triglyceride: studies of its metabolic effects in the postoperative period compared with conventional long-chain tri-glyceride emulsion. *J Parent Enteral Nutr* 1985; **9**: 720–4.

231. Eckart J, Adolph M, Wolfram G. Elimination of parenterally administered medium chain triglycerides in intensive care patients. *J Parent Enteral Nutr* 1980; **4**: 427.

232. Meguid MM, Schimmel E, Johnson WC. Reduced metabolic complications in total parenteral nutrition: pilot study using fat to replace one-third of glucose calories. *J Parent Enteral Nutr* 1982; **6**: 304–7.

233. Sorbrado J, Moldawer LL, Pomposelli JJ *et al.* Lipid emulsions and reticuloendothelial system function in injured animal. *Am J Clin Nutr* 1985; **42**: 855–63.

234. Freidman Z, Marks KH, Maisels MJ. Effect of parenteral fat emulsion on the pulmonary and reticuloendothelial systems in the newborn infant. *Pediatrics* 1978; **61**: 694–8.

235. Lanser ME, Saba TM. Neutrophil-mediated lung local-ization of bacteria: a mechanism for pulmonary injury. *Surgery* 1982; **90**: 473–81.

236. Bang HO, Dyberg HN. The composition of food consumed by Greenland eskimos. *Acta Med Scand* 1976; **200**: 69–73.

237. Kromhout D, Bosschieter EB, Coulander CDL. The inverse relationship between fish consumption and 20-year mortality from coronary heart disease. *N Engl J Med* 1985; **312**: 1205–9.

238. Lorenz R, Weber PC, Szimnau P, Heldwein W, Strasser T, Loeschke K. Supplementation with n-3 fatty acids from fish oil in chronic inflammatory bowel disease – a randomized, placebo-controlled, double-blind cross-over trial. *J Int Med* 1989; **225** (suppl.1): 225–32.

239. Hawthorne AB, Daneshmend TK, Hawkey CJ *et al.* Treatment of ulcerative colitis with fish oil supple-mentation: a prospective 12 month randomised con-trolled trial. *Gut* 1992; **33**: 922–8.

240. Bittiner SB, Cartwright I, Tucker WFG, Bleehen SS. A double-blind, randomized placebo-controlled trial of fish oil in psoriasis. *Lancet* 1988; **1**: 378–80.

241. Bjorneboe A, Soyland E, Bjorneboe GEA *et al.* Effect of dietary supplementation with eicosapentaenoic acid in the treatment of atopic dermatitis. *Br J Dermatol* 1987; **117**: 463–9.

242. Neuringer M, Anderson GJ, Connor WE. The essentiality of n-3 fatty acids for the development and function of the retina and brain. *Annu Rev Nutr* 1988; **8**: 517–41.

243. Simonopoulos AP. Omega-3 fatty acids in growth and development and in health and disease. Part I: the role of omega-3 fatty acids in growth and development. *Nutr Today* 1988; **23:** 10–19.

244. Mascioli EA, Iwasa Y, Trimbo S. Endotoxin challenge after menhaden oil diet: effects on survival of guinea pigs. *Am J Clin Nutr* 1989; **49:** 277–82.

245. Mascioli EA, Leader L, Flores E. Enhanced survival to endotoxin in guinea pigs fed iv fish oil emulsion. *Lipids* 1988; **23:** 623–5.

246. Grimble RF. Dietary manipulation of the inflammatory response. *Proc Nutr Soc* 1992; **51:** 285–94.

247. Endres S, Ghorbani R, Kelley VE *et al.* The effect of dietary supplememtation with n-3 polyunsaturated fatty acids on the synthesis of IL-1 and TNF alpha by mononuclear cells. *N Engl J Med* 1989; **320:** 226–71.

248. Pomposelli JJ, Flores EA, Bistrian BR. Role of biochemical mediators in clinical nutrition and surgical metabolism. *J Parent Enteral Nutr* 1988; **12:** 212–18.

249. Lowry SF, Thompson WA. Nutrient modification of inflammatory mediator production. *New Horizons* 1994; **2:** 164–74.

250. Rola-Pleczynski M. Differential effects of leucotriene B4 and T4 and T8 lymphocyte phenotype and immunoregulatory functions. *J Immunol* 1985; **135:** 1357–60.

251. Nau S, Hirschmüller-Ohmes I, Sturm G, Fürst P. The influence of parenteral n-3 fatty acids on nitrogen and lipid metabolism in rats. *Am J Clin Nutr* 1993; **57** (suppl.): 821S–822S.

252. Morlion BJ, Torwesten E, Lessire A *et al.* The effect of parenteral fish oil on leucocyte membrane fatty acid composition and leucotriene-synthesizing capacity in postoperative trauma. *Metabolism* 1996; **45:** 1208–13.

253. Wachtler P, Konig W, Senkal M, Kemen M, Koller M. Influence of a total parenteral nutrition enriched with omega-3 fatty acids on leukotriene synthesis of peripheral leukocytes and systemic cytokine levels in patients with major surgery. *J Trauma* 1997; **42:** 191–8.

254. Ikehata A, Hiwatashi N, Kinouchi Y *et al.* Effect of intravenously infused eicosapentaenoic acid on the leucotriene generation in patients with active Crohn's disease. *Am J Clin Nutr* 1992; **56:** 938–42.

255. Roulet M, Frascarolo P, Pilet M, Chapuis G. Effects of intravenously infused fish oil on platelet fatty acid phospholipid composition and on platelet function in postoperative trauma. *J Parent Enteral Nutr* 1997; **21:** 296–301.

256. Zadak Z, Cervinkova Z. PUFA n-3 lipid emulsion – a promising agent in ARDS treatment [editorial]. *Nutrition* 1997; **13:** 232–3.

257. Tashiro T, Yamamori H, Hayashi N *et al.* Effects of a newly developed fat emulsion containing eicosapentaenoic acid and docosahexaenoic acid on fatty acid profiles in rats. *Nutrition* 1998; **14:** 372–5.

258. Morlion BJ, Torwesten E, Wrenger K, Puchstein C, Fürst P. What is the optimum n-3 to n-6 fatty acid (FA) ratio of parenteral lipid emulsions in postoperative trauma? *Clin Nutr* 1997; **16:** 49S (abstract).

259. Leaf A, Kang JX, Xiao Y-F, Billman GE. Dietary n-3 fatty acids in the prevention of cardiac arrhythmias. *Curr Opin Clin Nutr Met Care* 1998; **1:** 225–8.

260. Daviglus ML, Stamler J, Orencia AJ *et al.* Fish consumption and the 30-year risk of fatal myocardial infarction. *N Engl J Med* 1997; **336:** 1046–53.

261. Siscovick DS, Raghunathan TE, King I *et al.* Dietary intake and cell membrane levels of long-chain n-3 polyunsaturated fatty acids and the risk of primary cardiac arrest [see comments]. *JAMA* 1995; **274:** 1363–7.

262. Mascioli EA, Bistrian BR, Babayan VK. Medium chain triglycerides and structured lipids as unique nonglucose energy sources in hyperalimentation. *Lipids* 1987; **22:** 421–3.

263. Mok KT, Maiz A, Yamazaki K *et al.* Structured medium-chain and long-chain triglycerides emulsions are superior to physical mixtures in sparing body protein in burned rat. *Metabolism* 1984; **33:** 910–15.

264. Sandström R, Hyltander A, Körner U, Lundholm K. Structured triglycerides to postoperative patients: a safety and tolerance study. *J Parent Enteral Nutr* 1993; **17:** 153–7.

265. Sandström R, Hyltander A, Lundholm K. Structured triglycerides were well tolerated and induce increased whole body fat oxidation compared to long chain triglycerides in postoperative patients. *J Parent Enteral Nutr* 1995; **19:** 381–6.

266. Hyltander A, Sandström R, Lundholm K. Metabolic effects of structured triglycerides in humans. *Nutr Clin Prac* 1995; **10:** 91–7.

267. Kruimel JW, Naber AHJ, Van der Vliet JA, Carneheim C, Katan MB, Jansen JBMJ. Postoperative patients utilize structured triglycerides more efficiently than a physical mixture of medium- and long-chain triglycerides. *J Parent Enteral Nutr* 1997; **21:** S6.

268. Carpentier YA, Bihain BE, Rubin M *et al.* Stabilization of plasma substrate concentrations: a model for conducting metabolic studies. *Clin Nutr* 1990; **9:** 313–18.

269. Long JM, Wilmore DW, Mason AD, Pruitt BA Jr. Effect of carbohydrate and fat intake on nitrogen excretion during total intravenous feeding. *Ann Surg* 1977; **185:** 417–22.

270. Woolfson AMJ, Heatley RV, Allison SP. Insulin to inhibit protein catabolism after injury. *N Engl J Med* 1979; **300:** 14–17.

271. Shaw JH, Wolfe RR. An integrated analysis of glucose, fat and protein metabolism in severely traumatized patients. *Ann Surg* 1989; **209:** 63–72.

272. Askanazi J, Elwyn DH, Silverberg PA, Rosenbaum SH, Kinney JM. Respiratory distress secondary to a high carbohydrate load: a case report. *Surgery* 1980; **87:** 596–8.

273. Schutz Y, Acheson JK, Jequier E. Twenty-four hour energy expenditure and thermogenesis: response to progressive carbohydrate feeding in man. *Int J Obesity* 1985; **9** (suppl. 2): 111–14.

274. Wolfe RR, Durhot MS, Allsop JR, Burke JF. Glucose metabolism in severely burned patients. *Metabolism* 1979; **28:** 1031–9.

275. Acheson JK, Schutz Y, Bessard T, Ravussin E, Jequier E, Flatt JP. Nutritional influences on lipogenesis and thermogenesis after a carbohydrate meal. *Am J Physiol* 1984; **246:** E62–E70.

276. Gundemer G, Durand G, Pascal G. Relative contribution of the main tissues and organs to body fatty acid synthesis in rats. *Lipids* 1983; **18:** 223–8.

277. Woolfson AMJ. Intravenous feeding – a review of aspects of current practice. *Clin Nutr* 1985; **4:** 187–94.

278. Hultman E, Nilsson LH, Sahlin K. Adenine nucleotide content of human liver. Normal values and fructose induced depletion. *Scand J Clin Lab Invest* 1975; **35:** 245–51.

279. Mäenpää PA, Raivo KO, Kehomüki MP. Liver adenine nucleotides: fructose induced depletion and its effect on protein synthesis. *Science* 1968; **161:** 1253–6.

280. Bergström J, Hultman E, Roch-Nordlund AE. Lactic acid accumulation in connection with fructose infusion. *Acta Med Scand* 1988; **182:** 359–66.

281. Nilsson LH, Hultman E. Liver and muscle glycogen in man after glucose and fructose infusion. *Scand J Clin Lab Invest* 1974; **35:** 5–10.

282. Gelfand RA, Schwerwin RS. Nitrogen conservation in starvation revisited: protein sparing with intravenous fructose. *Metabolism* 1986; **35:** 37–44.

283. Griem W, Lang K. Versuche zur parenteralen Ernährung mit Aminosäuren-Sorbit-Lösungen. *Klin Wschr* 1960; **38:** 336–7.

284. Leuthardt F, Stuhlfauth K. Biochemische, physiologische und klinische Probleme des Fructosestoffwechsels. In: Bauer K (ed) Medizinische Grundlagenforschung Bd. III. Thieme-Verlag, Stuttgart, 1960, 417–88.

285. Bye PA. The utilization and metabolism of intravenous sorbitol. *Br J Surg* 1969; **56:** 653–7.

286. Touster O, Reynolds VH, Hutcheson RM. The reduction of L-xylulose to xylitol by guinea pig liver mitochondria. *J Biol Chem* 1960; **221:** 697–709.

287. De Kalbermatten N, Ravussin E, Maeder E, Geser C, Jequier E, Felber JP. Comparison of glucose, fructose, sorbitol and xylitol utilization in humans during insulin suppression. *Metabolism* 1980; **29:** 62–7.

288. Keller U. The sugar substitutes fructose and sorbite: an unnecessary risk in parenteral nutrition. *Schweiz Med Wochenschr* 1989; **119:** 101–6.

289. Georgieff M, Pscheidl E, Götz H et al. Untersuchungen zum Mechanismus der Reduktion der Proteinkatabolie nach Trauma und bei Sepsis durch Xylit. *Anaesthesist* 1991; **40:** 85–91.

290. Georgieff M, Pscheidl E, Moldawer LL, Bistrian BR, Blackburn GL. Mechanism of protein conservation during xylitol infusion after burn injury in rats: isotope kinetics and indirect calorimetry. *Eur J Clin Invest* 1991; **21:** 249–58.

291. Katz J, McGarry JD. The glucose paradox. Is glucose a substrate for the liver metabolism? *J Clin Invest* 1984; **74:** 1901–9.

292. Froesch ER, Zaph J, Keller U. Comparative study of the metabolism of $U^{14}C$-fructose, $U^{14}C$-sorbitol and $U^{14}C$-xylitol in the normal and in the streptozocin rat. *Eur J Clin Invest* 1971; **2:** 8–14.

293. Hansen BA, Almdal TP, Vilstrup H. Effects of xylitol versus glucose on urea synthesis and alanine metabolism in rats. *Clin Nutr* 1989; **8:** 109–12.

294. Sestoft L. An evaluation of biochemical aspects of intravenous fructose, sorbitol and xylitol administration in man. *Acta Anaesth Scand* 1985; **29:** 19–29.

295. Askanazi J, Weissman C, Rosenbaum SH, Hyman AI, Milic-Emili J, Kinney JM. Nutrition and the respiratory system. *Crit Care Med* 1982; **10:** 163–72.

296. Bässler KH. Die Rolle der Kohlenhydrate in der parenteralen Ernährung. In: Lang K, Frey R, Halmágyi M (eds) Anästhesiologie und Wiederbelebung Bd. VI. Springer-Verlag, Berlin, 1996, 20–7.

297. Bässler KH. Die künstliche Ernährung: Dosierungsrichtlinien und Nährstoffrelationen. In: Wolfram G, Eckart J, Adolph M (eds) Künstliche Ernährung (Beiträge zur Infusionstherapie, Band 25). Karger-Verlag, München, 1990, 11–18.

298. Ziegler TR, Smith RJ, Byrne TA, Wilmore DW. Potential role of glutamine supplementation in nutrition support. *Clin Nutr* 1993; **12:** S82–S90.

24

Parenteral nutrition formulation

Michael C Allwood

Historical background

Until the early 1980s, parenteral nutrition (PN) was administered using separate bottles or bags of each large-volume infusion (amino acids, glucose, saline). This required nurses to make additions to these infusions and manage co-infusion of solutions, with many changes of bottles and bags. The consequence was poor nutritional control line, infection rates often exceeding 20%.[1]

'Big Bags' allowed all daily nutrition requirements to be combined in one infusion. This could be infused at a constant rate, accurately controlled by infusion pump. The opportunity for microbial contamination during infusion was largely eliminated and, coupled with the use of central lines and protocols, infection rates were reduced to below 5%. However, to provide the daily Big Bag required for nutritional needs, the various components, often numbering in excess of 10–15 different parenterals, must be transferred under strict aseptic conditions. The need for care in compounding is essential to prevent chemical incompatibilities, leading to precipitation and/or degradation of nutrients.

In the early days following the introduction of the Big Bag system, much needed to be learnt by pharmacists about these potential risks and the fat emulsion, if prescribed, continued to be administered as a separate infusion, because it was thought that it would be rapidly broken down after addition to the complete regimen. However, research emerged to indicate that, subject to concentrations of certain electrolytes not being exceeded, it was safe to incorporate fat emulsion.[2]

A further practical development in the 1990's was the use of the multilayered bag which prevents gas transmission into the bag, thereby enhancing stability, enabling even vitamins to be added during compounding.[3] This is particularly beneficial to home patients, removing the need to make additions at home.

Research has provided a range of insights into the formulation, stability and safe administration of PN to meet nutrition requirements for both adults and children, including neonates, although some constraints still remain. This chapter reviews the current formulation and compounding of PN and highlights key issues which determine the limits of provision.

Formulation and stability

PN regimens may be compounded as either 'two-in-one' mixtures, which do not contain fat emulsion, or 'all-in-one' mixtures (AIO), in which the fat emulsion is included.

PN regimens will vary in many respects, some of which impinge on the stability and shelf-life of the final mixture. These include the volume, the proportion by volume of each infusion (in particular the amino acids and fat emulsion), the amino acid formulation (including nitrogen concentration and commercial source) and glucose concentration. Concentrations of electrolytes are also limited by the composition of the mixture, as well as the option to include fat emulsion.

Stability of intravenous lipid emulsions

It is common practice to add intravenous fat emulsions to PN mixtures. Lipid emulsions consist of two-phase systems, where one immiscible liquid is dispersed as small droplets throughout another liquid, using an emulsifying agent to stabilise the resulting emulsion. However, emulsion systems are thermodynamically unstable and therefore vulnerable to the presence of other chemical entities. The emulsifying agent used in intravenous lipid emulsions comprises lecithins (from either egg yolk or a vegetable source) which consist of phospholipids.[4] Each phospholipid has a hydrophobic fatty acid portion and a polar hydrophilic region. The ratios of these different components will influence their behaviour in emulsion stabilisation in AIO mixtures. Acidic phospholipids are those which are thought to provide interfacial binding sites for divalent ions and which have strong destabilising effects in lipid emulsions in PN mixtures.

Unfortunately, the detailed composition of phospholipids is not fully defined and varies between product batches. These variations make theoretical prediction of the interaction of lipid emulsions with other PN components, and divalent cations in particular, a complex issue, militating against theoretical predictions of AIO stability.

Emulsions are stabilised by electrostatic forces which can be divided into two different and opposing ones.[5] First, there are the destabilising attractive forces (Van der Waal's forces) between droplets which predominate over very short distances and result in droplet aggregation and may lead to droplet coalescence. The second type of force, repulsive in nature, predominates over intermediate interdroplet distances and maintains the emulsion in a stable physical form. When these latter forces are reduced, emulsion destabilisation can follow.

Mechanisms in emulsion destabilisation

Definitions for the different stages of emulsion destabilisation are shown in Figure 24.1.[5] Aggregation occurs when the electrostatic charge of each lipid droplet is minimised, such that there are no repulsive forces between droplets. These aggregates have a combined size which is greater than the majority of droplets and their natural Brownian motion is minimised so that they rise to the surface and create a 'cream' layer. Aggregation and creaming processes are reversible, as can be shown by shaking of the emulsion to restore the original emulsion state. If, however, the cream layer remains undisturbed then compaction takes place, the aggregated droplets get closer together and therefore increase the chances of coalescence – the irreversible formation of large droplets – and

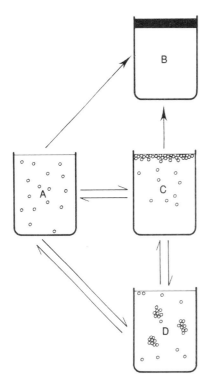

Figure 24.1 – Mechanisms of lipid emulsion instability. A = homogeneous lipid emulsion; B = cracked lipid emulsion; C = creamed lipid emulsion; D = aggregated lipid emulsion.

eventually the separation of free oil as either droplets or an oil layer. Any factor which reduces the surface charge of droplets will lead to emulsion instability.

Factors affecting emulsion stability

pH

The pH of a lipid emulsion formulation will affect the ionisation state of the hydrophilic region of the phospholipids and will thus determine the surface potential and stability of the lipid droplets. At the pH of AIO mixtures, normally between 6 and 7, the hydrophilic region is strongly charged and confers stability to the lipid emulsion. If the pH is reduced, then the hydrophilic region becomes more neutral in charge until, at a pH around 3, no charge remains and therefore no repulsive forces to droplet aggregation.[5]

Glucose

Glucose concentration can influence emulsion stability. Experience suggests that increasing the glucose concentration is likely to progressively reduce emulsion stability, although the reason remains unclear.

Amino acid source

The mixing of emulsion with amino acid solutions is beneficial to emulsion stability.[6] They enhance the mechanical barrier of the emulsifying agent by absorbing at the oil/water interface. Their strong buffering capacity minimises the potential destabilising effect of low pH caused by glucose. Specific amino acids may be involved in pH-dependent interactions with phospholipid ionic regions. By binding to the lipid emulsion droplet surface they enhance the mechanical barrier effect, as well as competing with electrolyte cations for binding sites on the emulsion droplet.[7]

Electrolytes

Cations, which have an opposite charge to the surface charge of droplets, reduce the surface potential on the droplet surface. As this surface potential falls, so do the repulsive forces between droplets. This leads to aggregation and coalescence of the lipid droplets if the surface potential falls sufficiently.

Davis[8] applied colloid theory in order to attempt quantification of the effect of cation load in any PN mixture on lipid emulsion stability. The point at which emulsion instability occurs depends on a threshold concentration of electrolytes, described by Davis as the critical aggregation number (CAN). The effect of cations depends on valency, according to the following equation, in which a, b and c represent concentrations in mmol/l of mono-, di- and trivalent cations respectively:

$$CAN \ (mmol/l) = a + 64b + 729 \ c$$

Using this equation, Burnham *et al.*[9] predicted a CAN for AIO mixtures of 130. Later work has shown this value to be very conservative and values greater than 600 have been reported for some stable PN mixtures.[2,10] The CAN approach is clearly a poor predictor of emulsion stability in AIO mixtures,[11] for both theoretical and practical reasons. The latter include its lack of consideration of pH effects or the protective influences of amino acids on emulsion stability.

Assessment of fat emulsion stability

The main criterion used to assess the physical stability of emulsions in AIO mixtures is measurement and monitoring of changes in particle size distribution of lipid droplets. Intravenous emulsions may contain droplets ranging from 10 nm up to 20 µm or more in emulsions that have started to break down. Such a wide particle size range necessitates a range of methods to determine particle size distributions, since no one measurement technique alone can cover the entire particle size distributions possible in AIO mixtures. This is illustrated in Figure 24.2. The

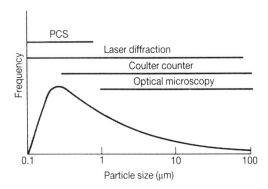

Figure 24.2 – Comparison of the particle size distribution of an intravenous lipid emulsion and the size ranges covered by various particle size analysis instruments. PCS – photon correlation spectroscopy.

problems and advantages of the use of the Coulter Counter, visual inspection, optical light microscopy and photon correlation spectroscopy methods in the analysis of emulsions in AIO mixtures have been described.[4] A combination of methods has been applied for research purposes but in practice, careful use of microscopy combined with visual checks can provide a method for routine evaluation of emulsions in PN mixtures.

Chemical stability and compatibility

Background

Because of the physicochemical complexity of PN mixtures, reactions leading to loss of nutritional efficacy or the development of potentially hazardous precipitates are possible. However, careful attention to the design of the formulation, packaging, compounding process and the subsequent storage of the mixture can minimise these changes. There follows a summary of the most important potential risks together with strategies to minimise them.

Physical incompatibility

Physical incompatibility in PN mixtures causes precipitation. Infusion of precipitates can be fatal. Therefore, prevention is vital for patient safety.

Causes of precipitation

Calcium phosphate
The commonest cause of precipitation in PN mixtures is formation of insoluble calcium phosphate. The chemistry of the reactions between calcium and phosphate ions is complex.[3] Predicting the likelihood of precipitation in particular mixtures is usually unreliable. There are, however, a number of rules to follow in order to avoid calcium phosphate precipitation.

- *pH*. Precipitation is more likely to occur at higher pH.[12] The pH of any PN mixture is governed by a number of factors but the most important variables are the amino acid infusion source and the inorganic phosphate employed. More acidic mixtures can accommodate more calcium and phosphate without exceeding the maximum solubility complex of calcium phosphate (by, for example, using potassium acid phosphate injection as the phosphate source[13]).

- *Calcium source*. More calcium can safely be added if calcium gluconate is used as calcium source, rather than the chloride salt.[12,14] However, note that calcium gluconate should be avoided in neonates and small children especially, due to its high aluminium content.[15]

- *Temperature*. Increasing temperature can lead to greater risk of precipitation if the gluconate salt is used, because raised temperature increases the dissociation reaction to release more calcium ions.[12,14]

- *Amino acid composition and concentration*. Since certain amino acids complex with calcium, more calcium and phosphate can be added to mixtures containing high concentrations of amino acids.[16,17] Amino acid composition will also therefore impact on calcium phosphate solubility.

The risk of calcium phosphate precipitation can be removed by using organic phosphate sources (such as glycerophosphate or glucose phosphate).[18] This is especially useful in neonates and small children but is usually unnecessary in adult mixtures.

Other factors, such as the order of mixing, can also be significant.[12]

Trace elements

Micro-nutrients are often added immediately before commencing infusion. It is now common practice to add them at the compounding stage. However, this introduces some risks of precipitation during storage. Two particular causes have been identified. Insoluble copper sulphide can be formed[19] by the reaction between copper ions and sulphide ions originating from hydrogen sulphide, a contaminant of amino acid mixtures containing cysteine.[20] Amino acid mixtures with relatively high amounts of cysteine/cystine may be incompatible with trace element additives after storage.[19] Secondly, insoluble iron phosphate can be formed in some mixtures containing high inorganic phosphate concentrations.[21] This reaction appears to be prevented in multilayered bags with added vitamins.

Monitoring precipitates

There are a number of methods to identify precipitation, including direct chemical analysis, particle counts, particle isolation and analysis, such as X-ray Energy Dispensive Spectorcory (EDX), and direct observation.[17,19,22]

Chemical degradation

Most ingredients in PN mixtures are remarkably stable.[3] However, some compounds may degrade rapidly, depending on many factors, in particular the nature and composition of the particular regimen, sources and chemical nature of individual infusions and additives, processing and the final container. The least stable ingredients comprise, in particular, certain vitamins. Vitamin degradation occurs during storage after compounding and administration. Ascorbic acid is the least stable ingredient, because of its reaction with dissolved oxygen.[23]

Consequently, some losses are inevitable following addition to any PN mixture and in many instances this can account for at least 50% within 24 hours. Total losses can be substantially reduced by compounding in multilayered bags, which have negligible permeability to oxygen compared with ethyl vinyl acetate (EVA) bags,[21] and removing all air from compounded bags before sealing. Some PN mixtures can be stored for extended periods of at least a month in multilayered bags and still provide sufficient ascorbate activity to meet normal nutritional needs.

Thiamine and co-carboxylase are degraded by reducing agents,[24] in particular bisulphite. So thiamine degradation in amino acid infusions containing sodium metabisulphite can be substantial.[25]

Photodegradation during administration is also significant. Vitamins A and E are the most light-sensitive compounds.[26,27] Daylight exposure during passage of the infusion through the administration set can exceed 80%.[28] However, this is caused by ultra-violet light and can be minimised by avoiding daylight and, in particular, sunlight exposure. In AIO mixtures, the fat emulsion provides some but not complete protection.[29] Covering the infusion container with a light-protecting plastic is a sensible precaution.

Drugs

Some drugs can be added to PN mixtures. For example, cimetidine and ranitidine are generally compatible in PN mixtures and cimetidine is also relatively stable.[30,31,32] Ranitidine is less stable but can be added to PN with extended shelf-lives provided a multilayered bag is used.[30]

Hydrocortisone is unstable in PN mixtures and PN mixtures with hydrocortisone should be administered within 2–3 days of compounding.

Heparin is believed to be stable in PN mixtures although there is no evidence to confirm this assumption. It should be noted that standard large molecular-weight heparins can lead to the destabilisation of fat emulsions in AIO mixtures.[5,33] However, this can be avoided by using low molecular weight heparins.[34]

Equipment and facilities

In order to compound PN formulations, the most important requirement is a suitable aseptic facility. This may comprise either a full aseptic suite, with changing rooms, Class A aseptic room with a horizontal laminar flow cabinet in which staff operate in full aseptic clothing. The alternative approach is to use aseptic isolators, which can be housed and operated within less rigorously controlled facilities, but nevertheless require appropriate clean rooms. Staff are able to work in such units without the necessity for full aseptic gowning.

The compounding of PN is a complex process. It must be designed to ensure that all the ingredients are correct, that the transfers are undertaken with no risk of microbial contamination (PN mixtures are ideal growth media for bacteria and fungi) and the techniques used minimise the risk of incompatibilities or chemical degradation. The operation of such facilities requires a number of tests and monitors, providing appropriate assurance of the quality of the finished mixture, in particular to ensure that the possibility of microbial contamination of the PN mixture during compounding is minimised, although it is impossible to completely eliminate this risk. Thus a range of routine tests and monitoring must be undertaken according to a defined protocol. Staff must also be carefully trained, their competence determined and shown to be of an acceptable standard before they are allowed to work unsupervised.

Units are subject to regular inspection by the government and standards are the same as those required in the pharmaceutical industry.

The equipment required includes the Big Bag itself, with the necessary filling lines incorporated to allow transfer of the separate large-volume infusions into the Big Bag. This may be by gravity or pumped system. Some devices for compounding can also provide measured volume transfer to allow compounding of either specific volumes from large-volume infusions or of small-volume additives using a filled syringe transfer system. Both must be operated within the aseptic facility and require considerable expertise in operation and maintenance of the equipment.

A range of plastics can be used to fabricate the bag itself, but multilayered bags are becoming increasingly popular. This not only provides a more stable mixture, in particular by reducing oxidation of key nutrients, as previously described, but also, because the film prevents air entering the contents after compounding and during storage (which can be many weeks), reduces the risk of pump alarm due to degassing of the mixture as it warms during infusion and causes 'air in line' alarming.

The most recent development is the multichambered bag (MCB), in which each large-volume component (amino acids, glucose and fat) is included in a separate compartment and these are mixed by breaking internal seals. The main compounding can therefore be undertaken without exposing infusions to risks of microbial contamination and aseptic facilities are not necessary for this process. However, micro-nutrients still need to be added aseptically.

Areas of controversy

Over the last 20 years, research and experience have shown that complete PN mixtures can be compounded and administered safely to suit most patients' requirements. The extended shelf-lives of standard regimens ensure greater cost-effectiveness in the compounding process. However, there are some groups in which the composition of the PN mixture may be restricted for pharmaceutical reasons. This is especially true for mixtures to meet the nutrition demands of neonates and small children, in particular their high demands for calcium and phosphate.

Two difficulties arise: first, ensuring that physical compatibility is maintained (organic phosphate has contributed greatly to ensuring that PN mixtures meeting these patients' requirements are safe) and second, because of the high concentrations of divalent ions, the inclusion of fat emulsion would usually be unsafe. It is therefore necessary to administer the fat emulsion as a separate infusion. The inclusion of vitamins and trace elements in PN mixtures with extended shelf-lives has also been questioned, although research has confirmed this to be a safe practice in many formulations and these safe limits have been identified.[3] However, some losses are inevitable after compounding and the current approach is to ensure that the losses can be controlled, for instance by using multilayered bags and ensuring complete removal of air after compounding and that the compounded mixture at least meets current daily needs for micro-nutrients. The possibility of degradation products influencing the stability of the PN mixture cannot, however, be ignored and some concern over possible oxalic acid residues has been raised.[35]

Recent concern has also been expressed about the possibility of lipid peroxidation in AIO mixtures during storage and administration due, for example, to trace element-mediated reactions and exposure to daylight.[36] Evidence suggests this type of reaction can occur, although the likelihood of developing clinically significant harmful changes in practice remains unconfirmed.

The compounding process is expensive, because of the need for fully validated and monitored aseptic facilities. However, the likely consequences of compromising on this asepsis in PN compounding are known from bitter experience to be fatal.[37]

Technical developments associated with facilities and bag design are contributing to a reduction in the risks associated with these processes, although this comes with some loss of flexibility in what can be compounded.

Practical applications

Patients requiring PN should always receive their feed from a Big Bag. Most patients in hospital can be accommodated using standard precompounded regimens or multichambered bags. Some minor manipulations will usually be necessary to provide micro-nutrients and possibly increases in electrolyte content.

Summary

PN mixtures are chemically complex and the possibility of reactions between different ingredients is inevitable. However, research has shown that most patient needs can be met using the Big Bag approach. The fact that the entire regimen can be combined in one infusion has

ensured that PN has become a safe and convenient system for maintaining nutrition status in patients unable to absorb all or some of their oral diet. The most important practical considerations are as follows:

- *Ensuring sterility*. Compounding must be undertaken in aseptic facilities by trained and competent staff, under the supervision of a pharmacist.

- *Avoiding physical incompatibility*. Some limitations are necessary for AIO mixtures. Limits for calcium and phosphate concentrations are necessary to prevent precipitation.

- *Vitamins* can be included during compounding but multilayered bags must be used.

- *Light protection* of the bag during administration is recommended for all PN types.

Finally, it is important that each change to a PN regimen must be considered with care and it is imperative to appreciate that minor changes, say in electrolyte content, should only be undertaken if absolutely essential. The cost of any change is not insignificant. The revision must be considered for stability, the extensive documentation for compounding must be revised (this includes worksheets, labels, etc.), the revised ingredients prepared. Daily changes are expensive in terms of both resources and time.

References

1. Maki DG. Sepsis arising from extrinsic contamination of the infusion and measures for control. In: Phillips I, Meers PD, D'Arcy PF (eds) Microbiological hazards of infusion control. MTP Press, Lancaster, 1976, 13–143.

2. Davis SS, Galloway M. Studies on fat emulsions in combined nutrition solutions. *J Clin Hosp Pharm* 1986; **11:** 33–45.

3. Allwood MC, Kearney MCJ. Compatibility and stability of additives in parenteral nutrition admixtures. *Nutrition* 1998; **14:** 697–706.

4. Washington C. The stability of intravenous fat emulsions in TPN admixtures. *Int J Pharmaceut* 1990; **66:** 1–21.

5. Barnett MI, Cosslett AG. Parenteral nutrition formulation. In: Payne-James J (ed) Artificial nutrition support in clinical practice, 1st. edn. Edward Arnold, London, 1995, 323–32.

6. Black CD, Popovich NG. A study of intravenous emulsion compatibility: effects of dextrose, amino acids and selected electrolytes. *Drug Intell Clin Pharm* 1981; **15:** 184–93.

7. Brown R, Quercia RA, Sigman R. *J Parent Enteral Nutr* 1986; **10:** 650–8.

8. Davis SS. The stability of fat emulsions for intravenous administration. In: Johnston IDA (ed) Advances in clinical nutrition. MTP Press, Lancaster, 1983, 213–39.

9. Burnham WR, Hansrani PK, Knott CE, Cook JA, Davis SS. Stability of fat emulsion based intravenous feeding mixture. *Int J Pharmaceut* 1983; **13:** 9–22.

10. Grimble GK, Rees RG, Patil DH *et al*. Administration of fat emulsions with nutritional mixtures from the 3-litre delivery system in TPN. *J Parent Enteral Nutr* 1985; **9:** 456–60.

11. Barnett MI, Cosslett AG, Duffield JR, Evans DA, Hall SB, Williams DR. Parenteral nutrition: pharmaceutical problems of compatibility and stability. *Drug Safety* 1990; **5:** 101–6.

12. Dunham B, Marcuard S, Khazanie PG, Meade G, Craft T, Nichols K. The solubility of calcium and phosphorus in neonatal parenteral nutrition solutions. *J Parent Enteral Nutr* 1991; **15:** 608–11.

13. Allwood MC. The compatibility of calcium phosphate in paediatric TPN infusions. *J Clin Hosp Pharm* 1987; **12:** 293–301.

14. Eggert ID, Rusho WJ, Mackey MW, Cahn GM. Calcium and phosphorus compatibility in parenteral nutrition solutions for neonates. *Am J Hosp Pharm* 1982; **39:** 49–54.

15. Bishop NJ, Morley R, Day JP, Lucas A. Aluminium neurotoxicity in preterm infants receiving intravenous-feeding solutions. *N Engl J Med* 1997; **336:** 1557–62.

16. Lenz GT, Mikrut BA. Calcium and phosphate solubility in neonatal parenteral nutrient solutions containing Aminosyn-PF or Trophamine. *Am J Hosp Pharm* 1988; **45:** 2367–71.

17. Poole RL, Rupp CA, Kerner JA. Calcium and phosphorus in neonatal parenteral nutrition solutions. *J Parent Enteral Nutr* 1983; **39:** 120–1.

18. Ronchera-Oms CL, Jimenez-Torres NV, Peidro J. Stability of parenteral nutrition admixtures containing organic phosphates. *Clin Nutr* 1989; **14:** 373–6.

19. Allwood MC, Martin H, Greenwood M, Maunder M. Precipitation of trace elements in parenteral nutrition mixtures. *Clin Nutr* 1998; **17:** 223–6.

20. Decsi T, Koletzko B. Hydrogen sulphide in pediatric parenteral nutrition amino acid solutions. *J Pediatr Gastroenterol* 1993; **17:** 421–3.

21. Allwood MC, Brown PW, Ghedini C, Hardy G. The stability of ascorbic acid in TPN mixtures stored in a multilayered bag. *Clin Nutr* 1992; **11:** 284–8.

22. Kaminski MV, Harris DF, Collin CF, Sommers GA. Electrolyte compatibility in a synthetic amino acid hyperalimentation solution. *Am J Hosp Pharm* 1974; **31:** 244–6.

23. Allwood MC. Factors influencing the stability of ascorbic acid in TPN infusions. *J Clin Hosp Pharm* 1984; **9:** 75–85.

24. Scheiner JM, Araujo MM, DeRitter E. Thiamine destruction by sodium bisulphite in infusion solutions. *Am J Hosp Pharm* 1981; **38:** 1911–13.

25. Kearney MCJ, Allwood MC, Neale T, Hardy G. The stability of thiamine in TPN mixtures stored in EVA and multilayered bags. *Clin Nutr* 1995; **14:** 295–301.

26. Billion-Rey F, Guillaumont M, Frederich A, Aulanger G. Stability of fat-soluble vitamins A (retinol palmitate), E (tocopherol acetate) and K (phylloqinone) in TPN at home. *J Parent Enteral Nutr* 1993; **17:** 56–60.

27. Gillis J, Jones G, Pencharz P. Delivery of vitamins A, D and E in TPN solutions. *J Parent Enteral Nutr* 1983; **7:** 11–14.

28. Shenai JP, Stahlman MT, Chytil F. Vitamin A delivery from parenteral alimentation solution. *J Pediatr* 1989; **99:** 661–4.

29. Allwood MC, Martin HJ. The photodegradation of vitamins A and E in parenteral nutrition mixtures during infusion. *Clin Nutr* 2000; **19:** 339–42.

30. Allwood MC, Martin H. Factors influencing the stability of ranitidine in TPN mixtures. *Clin Nutr* 1995; **14:** 171–6.

31. Allwood MC, Martin H. Long-term stability of cimetidine in total parenteral nutrition. *J Clin Pharm Therap* 1996; **21:** 19–21.

32. Grimble GK, Hunjan MK, Payne-James J, Silk DBA. Long-term stability of ranitidine in total parenteral nutrition solutions: effects on lipid emulsion stability. *Br J Intens Care* 1991; **1:** 32–7.

33. Johnson OL, Washington C, Davis SS, Schaupp K. The destabilisation of parenteral feeding emulsions by heparin. *Int J Pharmaceut* 1989; **53:** 237–40.

34. Durand MC, Barnett MI. Heparin in parenteral feeding: effect of heparin and low molecular weight heparin on lipid emulsions and All-in-One admixtures. *Br J Intens Care* 1992; **2:** 10–20.

35. Rockwell GF, Campfield T, Nelson BC, Uden PC. Oxalogenesis in parenteral nutrition solution components. *Nutrition* 1998; **14:** 835–9.

36. Steger PJK, Mulbach SF. Lipid peroxidation of intravenous lipid emulsions and All-in-One admixtures in TPN bags: the influence of trace elements. *J Parent Enteral Nutr* 2000; **24:** 37–41.

37. Anon. Two children die after receiving infected PN solutions. *Pharm J* 1994; **252:** 596.

25

Metabolic complications of parenteral nutrition

Anders Thorell and Jörgen Nordenström

Introduction

Total parenteral nutrition (TPN) has become a powerful therapy that can improve the recovery and survival of patients who would otherwise suffer from complications due to malnutrition during prolonged medical or surgical illness. However, the use of TPN is itself associated with adverse effects which may be of mechanical, septic, or metabolic nature in origin.

Metabolic complications may occur during TPN if nutrient intake is not adapted to the patient's requirements or the metabolic capacity for any given dietary component. Adverse metabolic effects may arise from administration of inadequate or excessive nutrients or from an inappropriate composition of nutrients. In the early days of TPN, deficiency syndromes were not uncommon, either because the administered nutrition solutions were lacking sufficient amounts of a particular substance and/or because of insufficient knowledge of the nutrition requirements of different patient groups. With the commercial intravenous products that are available today and with the better understanding of nutrition requirements of ill patients, deficiency syndromes have become rare. Metabolic complications are thus nowadays more likely to develop as a consequence of excessive rather than insufficient supply of nutrients. Although scientific data regarding nutrient requirements for various patient groups is accumulating, it may, however, be difficult to estimate needs in clinical practice, since the nutrition support may need to be regularly adjusted to the patient's metabolic profile.

Some complications affect specific organs rather than causing diffuse metabolic derangements. Organ-related complications do not usually arise from a single cause but rather from the provision of an inappropriate composition of nutrients. The liver in particular but also the kidneys are the most likely organs to be affected by this type of complication.

Criteria for diagnosing metabolic complications

Of the various metabolic complications that may occur during TPN, some are common while others are rare or only of academic interest if current recommendations of TPN formulas are followed. Some metabolic complications may be life-threatening, while others represent only benign abnormalities with little or no clinical significance. Reports which define criteria for clinically relevant metabolic complications are rare. The Veterans Affairs multicentre trial of perioperative parenteral nutritional support is a notable exception where precise definitions have been given[1] (Table 25.1). The substrates involved in the most important and most common complications are listed in this table.

Complications due to nutrient deficiencies

Sufficient amounts of calories, certain fatty acids, amino acids, vitamins and minerals in proper combinations must be administered during TPN to permit maintenance, repair and growth. Failure to administer sufficient amounts of nutrients may result in deficiency syndromes. Long-term home parenteral nutrition (HPN) has enabled previously rare nutrient deficiencies to be documented.

Patients receiving TPN are liable to develop nutrient deficiencies for several reasons. Firstly, many disease states have qualitatively and quantitatively abnormal requirements. Nutrition requirements of ill patients are not as well defined as those of healthy subjects. Recommended nutrition intake for healthy individuals may therefore not be valid for many patients. Secondly, the biosynthetic capacity to produce non-essential nutrients may be reduced in some patients with abnormal organ function which may render ordinarily non-essential nutrients to become conditionally essential. Thirdly, because parenteral nutrition solutions have anabolic properties, refeeding malnourished patients may precipitate deficiency. Micronutrients required for tissue anabolism such as potassium, phosphate and zinc are particularly relevant during attempts to correct malnutrition. Inadequate administration of nutrients may result in acute metabolic deficiencies or, if chronic, in deficiency syndromes. The most important acute deficiencies are hypoglycaemia and hypophosphataemia. Hypocalcaemia has also been reported.[2]

Acute metabolic deficiencies

Hypoglycaemia

Hypoglycaemia, although less common that hyperglycaemia (see below), is a potential life-threatening complication which must be recognised and treated

Table 25. 1 – Definition of metabolic complications.

Glucose:	
hyperglycaemia	> 16 mmol/l
hypoglycaemia	< 3 mmol/l
hyperglycaemia-ketoacidosis	> 27 mmol/l + arterial pH ≤ 7.30 + ≥ + 2 dipstick for urinary (u)-or serum (s)-ketones
Hyperosmolar hyperglycaemic non-ketosis	> 27 mmol/l + osmolarity/s > 305 m Osm/l H$_2$O + absence of ketones/u
Sodium, potassium, chloride, calcium, magnesium, phosphate	Values outside reference range
Triglyceride:	
hypertriglyceridaemia	> 150% of upper normal limit of reference measured > 8 h after lipid infusion
Urea	> twice baseline value and/or upper limit of reference
Hyperchloraemic acidosis	s-Cl > 115 mmol/l + arterial pH ≤ 7.30
Hepatic dysfunction: AST, ALT, alkaline, phosphatase, bilirubin	> twice baseline and/or > twice the upper limit of reference
Fluid overload	Clinical or X-ray findings of oedema or weight gain > 0.45 kg/d for 3 or more consecutive days
Coagulopathy: prothrombin time and/or partial thromboplastin time	> 150% of upper limit of reference

Adapted from Buzby *et al.*[1]

promptly. Rebound hypoglycaemia due to high insulin levels can occur if a high glucose infusion rate is discontinued too abruptly. A stepwise reduction of the glucose infusion rate reduces the risk of rebound hypoglycaemia. The malnourished patient is particularly likely to develop hypoglycaemia during TPN, since the pancreas has adapted to the shortage in substrates and the anabolic hormones, including insulin, might have been down-regulated. In such patients peripheral sensitivity to insulin may be increased and the risk of hypoglycaemia enhanced. Careful monitoring of glucose metabolism is therefore warranted to avoid malnutrition-associated hypoglycaemia.

Hypophosphataemia

This is a potentially dangerous complication, which has been reported to occur in less than 1% of hospitalised patients.[3] Approximately 85% of the body's phosphate content are bound to bone. Of the remaining 15%, 14% are intracellular and represent the major intracellular anion. The small proportion of phosphate that is present in plasma may therefore not be a sensitive indicator of phosphate tissue stores. During nutritional repletion, severe hypophosphataemia can develop rapidly. The provision of calories, in particular carbohydrates, stimulates insulin release and this enhances the intracellular influx of phosphate and consequently extracellular hypophosphataemia develops. Severe hypophosphataemia results in decreased respiratory,[4] cardiovascular,[5] and neuromuscular[6] function. Symptoms include paraesthesiae, muscular weakness and confusion, sometimes progressing to convulsions and coma. Even deaths have been reported.[7]

During TPN, phosphate should be added in order to avoid phosphate deficiency. The daily requirement of phosphate is approximately 20 mmol/day, and prevention of hypophosphataemia can usually be obtained by provision of about 10 mmol of phosphate/1000 kcal. Malnourished patients may require larger amounts particularly at the start of TPN.[8]

Hypocalcaemia

Hypocalcaemia has been reported to occur in 12% of critically ill patients.[9] The ionised calcium fraction should be measured in order to obtain an accurate estimate of calcium homeostasis. Free fatty acids (FFA) are carried in the circulation bound to albumin along with calcium, and variations in FFA may alter calcium binding. Increased FFA levels can therefore induce hypocalcaemia.[10] Hypocalcaemia may also occur as a consequence of insufficient calcium supply, particularly in connection with insufficient vitamin D or magnesium intakes. The administration of amino acids can furthermore induce calciuresis. Hypocalcaemia in association with an elevated serum parathyroid hormone concentration indicates that the supply of calcium should be increased.

Chronic deficiency syndromes

Deficiency syndromes encountered during long-term TPN are listed in Table 25.2. The most important deficiency syndrome is caused by lack of linoleic acid. The resulting syndrome, essential fatty acid deficiency (EFAD) may develop after a few weeks of fat-free TPN.[11] A number of trace element deficiencies have been reported during TPN, including zinc deficiency.[12] Other more rarely encountered deficiencies include those of copper,[13] chromium,[14] selenium[15] and molybdenium.[16] The great importance of an adequate trace element status is well recognised, and this has stimulated the establishment of dosage guidelines. The most common vitamin deficiencies are found within the water-soluble vitamin B family. Folic acid, thiamine and biotin are the most commonly reported vitamin deficiencies (see also Ch. 11).

Table 25.2 – Deficiency syndromes.

Nutrient	Signs and symptoms
Linoleic acid (essential fatty acid deficiency)	Dermatitis, hair loss, delayed wound healing
Zinc	Dermatitis, diarrhoea, depression
Copper	Neutropenia, anaemia
Chromium	Diabetes, neuropathy
Selenium	Myopathy
Water-soluble vitamins	Anaemia, cardiomyopathy, neuropathy, encephalopathy
Fat-soluble vitamins	Muscle weakness, haemorrhage, night blindness

Essential fatty acid deficiency (EFAD)

Linoleic acid is an essential fatty acid, which can be elongated and desaturated to form arachidonic acid,

the latter being a semi-essential fatty acid. Another fatty acid, alpha-linoleic acid, is considered as being essential in the infant. The syndrome of EFAD which is caused by lack of linoleic acid is characterised by dermatitis (scaling and dryness of the skin), hair loss and delayed wound healing.[11,17] Under normal conditions there are large stores of linoleic acid in the body, but during fat-free TPN where large amounts of glucose are given, the induction of hyperinsulinaemia will suppress the mobilisation of essential fatty acids from fat stores. Home TPN patients with short bowel syndrome have a high prevalence of biochemical EFAD.[18] Clinical signs of EFAD usually appear after 1–2 months of fat-free TPN, but biochemical evidence of EFAD may appear after a few weeks. With reduced availability of linoleic acid the same enzyme system which normally is involved in the formation of arachidonic acid will instead convert oleic acid to eicosatrienoic acid. A ratio of eicosatrienoic acid to arachidonic acid (Holman index) > 0.2 is diagnostic of EFAD.[19] A daily supply of 20–30 g of fat as long-chain fatty acid is required to prevent EFAD.

Zinc deficiency

A daily dose of about 1.5 mg zinc is required during TPN.[20] With long, (1–2 months) insufficient supplementation of zinc, a scaly and pustular rash appears, starting around the mouth and the articular prominences and subsequently over the entire body. Surgical resection of the gastrointestinal tract may result in increased losses of zinc due to reduced capacity to reabsorb endogenous secretions from the pancreas. Since 80% of all blood zinc is found in the erythrocytes, it has been suggested that patients receiving occasional infusions of fresh blood should not be at risk for developing zinc deficiency. This statement seems, however, to need further evaluation, since the relationship between serum levels of zinc and blood transfusions have been questioned.[20] Therefore, giving zinc to patients requiring long-term TPN is advisable, and has been shown to correct deficiency states.[12]

Deficiencies of other trace minerals

Copper (Cu) is an essential micronutrient and an important co-factor of several proteins and enzymes.[21] Prolonged parenteral[22] or enteral nutrition by jejunostomy[23] may cause copper deficiency in rare cases. Symptoms include haematological disturbances such as neutropaenia, anaemia or pancytopaenia.

Serum copper levels should be monitored during long-term TPN to prevent deficiencies. Chromium deficiency may also be encountered during long-term TPN and may result in impaired growth, impaired glucose metabolism, hyperglycaemia and negative nitrogen balance.[24,25] A daily supply of 10–15-μg of chromium is recommended in adults receiving TPN. Selenium is (via glutathione peroxidase) one of the key mediators in response to oxidative stress. Keshan disease is a cardiomyopathy resulting from selenium deficiency in regions of China where selenium concentration in the soil is very low. A few reports have described similar symptoms in cases of selenium deficiency during TPN.[26,27] A recommended safe and adequate range of daily intake of selenium is 50–200 μg for adults.[28] Molybdenium deficiency can cause neurological disorders but is quite rare. An intravenous daily allowance of 100–200 μg is recommended (see also ch. 11).

Vitamin deficiencies

Vitamins are essential nutrients and it is recommended that patients who require TPN for more than a week should be given water-soluble vitamins on a daily basis. In particular, supplementation of thiamine, a coenzyme necessary for oxidation of ketoacids, seems to be crucial. In recent years, there have been several reports of life-threatening complications associated with severe deficiency of thiamine (see also ch. 11).[29]

Metabolic complications from overfeeding of nutrients

Toxic effects may develop if nutrients are given in excess of the amount required to maintain metabolic homeostasis. Complications related to overfeeding are generally more difficult to prevent than deficiencies. Consequently, only by careful clinical and biochemical surveillance can such complications be prevented. The different complications that might occur are dependent on the duration of administration. Overloading of nutrients may thus result in acute metabolic disturbances, but administration of excessive amounts for long periods of time could negatively affect organ function, particularly in the liver and kidneys. Table 25.3 illustrates some of the acute metabolic complications due to overfeeding of nutrients.

Table 25.3 – Acute metabolic complications due to nutrient overloading.

Nutrient	Excess effect
Glucose	Hyperglycaemia Hyperosmolar dehydration Hypercapnia Hepatic steatosis Increased sympathetic activity Fluid retention
Fat	Hypercholesterolaemia and LPX formation★ Hypertriglyceridaemia
Amino acids	Uraemia
Calcium	Hypercalcaemia
Vitamin D	Hypercalcaemia

★ lipoprotein.

Complications associated with excessive glucose administration

Hyperglycaemia

Under normal conditions, blood glucose concentrations are tightly regulated to support a sufficient supply of carbohydrates to glucose-dependent tissues. The selection of substrates for oxidation is dependent on the availability of glucose. The normal requirement of glucose is approximately 1.4 mg/kg/min. However, at a rate of glucose infusion of 4 mg/kg/min for at least 120 min, blood glucose concentrations have been shown to be maintained at between 8 and 9 mmol/l in healthy individuals.[30] In situations of stress, such as in inflammation or after accidental or surgical trauma, the capacity to eliminate glucose from the blood is reduced due to insulin resistance,[31] and the degree of this disturbance is proportional to the severity of the underlying disease. The mechanism of this phenomenon is not fully understood, but increased concentrations of 'counter-regulatory' hormones such as glucagon, cortisol and catecholamines as well as cytokines are generally believed to be involved.[31] The risk of development of hyperglycaemia is thus high in patients with acute illness. In the veteran's study of surgical patients,[32] hyperglycaemia was defined as a blood glucose concentration above 16 mmol/l and appeared in 20% of patients. Hyperglycaemia has been shown to be an independent mortality risk factor after trauma,[33] and blood glucose concentrations above 11.1 mmol/l have been associated with 3- to 5-fold increases in the risk for mediastinitis or serious wound infection in patients undergoing thoracic surgery.[34]

The infusion of glucose at a rate which increases the plasma glucose concentration above 9 mmol/l is of no clinical benefit.[35] Conversely, this might induce metabolic side-effects such as hyperosmolar dehydration and hypophosphataemia. Excessive glucose administration may also induce fatty liver and increase catecholamine excretion in the urine. Hyperglycaemia (above 9 mmol/l) should therefore be avoided. This can be achieved either by a reduction of the glucose infusion rate, or by the administration of exogenous insulin in order to increase glucose uptake and suppress hepatic glucose production. In a study of patients undergoing elective colorectal surgery, it was found that, when total parenteral nutrition was given, it was necessary to infuse eight times more insulin to maintain normoglycaemia during TPN after operation in comparison with the preoperative situation.[36]

Hyperosmolar dehydration

D-glucose is structurally similar to mannitol and has potent osmotic diuretic properties. During infusion of large amounts of glucose, urinary sodium excretion increases which might lead to total sodium and water depletion. In severe cases, hyperosmolar hyperglycaemic non-ketotic dehydration (HHND) and coma may develop. Two mechanisms for the absence of ketoacidosis in HHND have been proposed.[37] Firstly, endogenous insulin is sufficient to maintain lipolysis at a low rate but not to prevent hyperglycaemia. Secondly, the hyperglycaemia serves to maintain adequate liver glycogen and prevents ketone body formation by a reduced β-oxidation of free fatty acids.

Hyperosmolar dehydration is avoided by infusion of glucose at a rate that does not cause significant glucosuria (or by simultaneous infusion of adequate amounts of insulin, see above). The maximum transport rate of glucose by the kidney corresponds to a plasma glucose concentration of about 14 mmol/l. If plasma glucose increases above this concentration, glucosuria will occur. The urine should therefore be regularly tested for glucose. Treatment of HHND should include careful expansion of intravascular volume to correct the water deficit and to ensure that vital organs remain perfused. The proportional losses of water exceed those of sodium, which results in hypertonic dehydration. Therefore, correction of the syndrome will ultimately require administration of hypotonic

fluids. Cardiopulmonary function needs to be reassessed repeatedly.[38]

Hypercapnia

When substrates are broken down intracellularly to produce adenosine triphosphate (ATP), formation of carbon dioxide will occur. Catabolism of carbohydrates produces more carbon dioxide per amount of energy expended for ATP generation than does lipolysis. Since the body strives for carbohydrate balance, the amount of carbohydrates utilised for oxidation is, within certain limits, proportional to the amount supplied.[39] Moreover, if carbohydrates are administered in excess, the ratio of glucose oxidation to fat oxidation continues to increase over time. Therefore, the full effect of carbohydrate overfeeding on carbon dioxide production may not be evident for several days.[40]

The body response to increased carbon dioxide production involves an increase in alveolar ventilation to expel excess carbon dioxide. The ability to increase alveolar ventilation is reduced in many patients receiving TPN and, particularly, in patients restricted to mechanical ventilation. Consequently, these patients are at risk for carbon dioxide retention if carbohydrates are given in excess.[41,42] Respiratory acidosis may occur if Pa_{CO_2} increases over 40 mmHg.[41] This, in turn, may precipitate respiratory failure in compromised patients and may necessitate mechanical ventilation or, alternatively, make weaning from mechanical ventilation more difficult or impossible.[42,43] The isocaloric substitution of part of the carbohydrate supply with fat emulsions have been shown to be associated with significant smaller increase in CO_2-production in traumatised and septic as well as in depleted patients.[44] The use of fat emulsions with concomitant monitoring of arterial blood gases, and/or respiratory quotient by indirect calorimetry, could therefore prove beneficial as a means of avoiding hypercapnia in compromised patients receiving TPN.

Hepatic steatosis

Infusions of large amounts of carbohydrates have been reported to increase the deposition of triglycerides in the liver.[45] The mechanisms behind glucose-induced hepatic steatosis are not fully understood, since *de novo* genesis of fatty acids in the liver is of minor importance in man, even during carbohydrate overfeeding.[46] If hepatic lipoprotein transport capacity is insufficient in relation to production of triglycerides from exogenous and recycled fatty acids, hepatic fat accumulation occurs. Hyperinsulinaemia is usually present in association with hepatic steatosis during carbohydrate infusion.[47]

Supplementation of infusions with lipids has been shown to reduce the incidence of carbohydrate-induced hepatic steatosis, probably by provision of choline, which is necessary for lipoprotein membrane formation.[48]

Increased sympathetic activity

Surgical stress is associated with high plasma concentrations of cortisol, glucagon and catecholamines. These hormones have counter-regulatory properties and have been proposed to be involved in the development of insulin resistance. Hypermetabolic patients with high noradrenaline excretion have been shown to respond to a glucose load with a further increase in noradrenaline excretion.[49] The sympathetic activation by hypertonic glucose infusion has been attributed to increments in plasma insulin rather than in glucose concentrations.[49,50] The observation that administration of large amounts of glucose may be associated with elevated sympathetic activity warrants some consideration. It seems reasonable to suggest that massive glucose loading (i.e. administration of calories as glucose above energy requirements) should be avoided in order not to increase the already elevated sympathetic activity observed in patients in stress. The substitution of part of the glucose calories with intravenous lipid emulsions may prevent the increased catecholamine response in such patients.[49]

Fluid retention

As indicated above, high-rate infusions of glucose, which induce hyperglycaemia, can result in water and sodium depletion. However, if hyperglycaemia is not achieved, infusion of large amounts of glucose has been shown to induce positive sodium as well as water balances.[51] Glucose-based TPN has been reported to be associated with greater water retention compared with TPN given as dual energy substrates of fat and glucose.[52] Furthermore, glutamine-supplemented intravenous feeding has been shown to attenuate fluid retention and expansion of the extracellular fluid compared to standard TPN in patients in catabolic stress.[53] These reports suggest that administration of glucose as the sole nutritional component might increase the risk of fluid retention.

Therefore, the possibility of sodium and water retention should be considered in patients with rapid weight gain (0.45 kg/d for 3 or more consecutive days; Table 25.1), particularly if large doses of glucose are given.

Complications associated with lipid emulsions

Acute side-effects of lipid emulsions are rare. Hypersensitivity reactions have been reported in a few patients following infusions of long-chain triglycerides (LCT).[54–56] Other reported acute side-effects to lipid emulsions include a rise in body temperature, chills and lower back pain. The acute effects are usually mild, are related to dosage and rate of infusion and disappear when the infusion of lipid is discontinued. Long-term administration of cottonseed-oil based fat-emulsions was associated with the occurrence of a 'fat overloading' syndrome. This syndrome consisted of fever, jaundice, anaemia, hepatosplenomegaly and blood-clotting disorders. It has been suggested that the syndrome could be explained by breaking of the lipid emulsion by antibodies formed against the emulsifier. Once the syndrome was recognised, cottonseed-oil emulsions were taken off the market.

Current lipid emulsions lack many of the toxic properties which characterised the older lipid emulsions. Today, the most commonly used lipid emulsions are composed of LCT or a combination of medium-chain triglycerides (MCT) and LCT. The long-chain fatty acids in these fat emulsions are predominantly of the Ω-6 type. Recently a number of new lipid emulsions have been introduced which have high contents of Ω-3 (fish oil) or Ω-9 (olive oil) fatty acids. In addition, a so-called structured triglyceride (STG) emulsion has been introduced where long-chain and medium-chain fatty acids have been re-esterified within a triglyceride molecule. The clinical experience with these new types of lipid emulsions is at present limited. LCT as well as MCT/LCT lipid emulsions are well tolerated but their relative merits are at present unclear. MCT-containing lipid emulsions are more readily oxidised than pure LCT emulsions. MCT lipid emulsions are therefore more prone to induce ketonaemia than those consisting of only LCT.

The most important complications during infusion of currently used lipid emulsions are caused by limitations in the capacity to metabolise intravenous fat. The development of hyperlipidaemia during lipid emulsion infusion has been associated with fat deposition in the lungs and the reticuloendothelial system,[57,58] impaired leucocyte function,[59] and bacterial defence,[60] and cholestasis.[61] Long-term administration of fat emulsions may induce a hyperactivation of the monocyte–macrophage system and the appearance of typical sea-blue histiocytes in the bone marrow.[62-63] One case of fat-overloading syndrome has been reported.[64] Some of these changes have been disputed,[65,66] and whether the infused lipid was the causative factor has been questioned.[67-69]

Hypercholesterolaemia and formation of lipoprotein X (LPX)

Hyperlipidaemia during lipid-based TPN may be considered an undesired effect. Although hypertriglyceridaemia may develop occasionally, the most common alteration of serum lipids is hypercholesterolaemia. It has been suggested that the hypercholesterolaemia is caused by excessive amounts of phospholipids (notably in 10% emulsions) which mobilise free cholesterol from extravascular tissues.[70]

The phospholipid/TG ratio is considered to be important for the formation of an abnormal lipoprotein (LPX) which has been observed during the administration of TPN containing fat.[71,72] It has been suggested that the phospholipids of artificial lipid emulsions may form single-bilayer vesicles, which extract free cholesterol from tissues and thereby produce LPX. The abnormal LPX resembles or is identical to an abnormal LDL composed of high proportions of phospholipids and free cholesterol and has a very low TG content.[72] LPX cannot serve as a precursor for other lipoproteins and is only slowly metabolised in the liver.[70] Although the clinical significance of the formation of LPX is unknown, it is therefore advisable to use lipid emulsions with low phospholipid/TG ratios (i.e. 20% rather than 10% fat emulsions).

Hypertriglyceridaemia

If the metabolic capacity to clear fat is exceeded, elevation of plasma TG levels will occur. This may be observed as 'cloudy serum'. The authors have personal experience of two patients who after several weeks of uneventful lipid infusion suddenly developed severe hypertriglyceridaemia (postprandial serum TG concentration 12–15 mmol/l). TG concentrations did not return to normal until several days after lipid admini-

stration had been stopped. In such cases of acquired lipid intolerance the administration of IV heparin (150–200 IU heparin per kg body weight per 24 h) (to increase plasma lipolytic activity) and glucose together with insulin (to increase adipose tissue LPL activity) is indicated.

Since there are great individual variations in the capacity to metabolise intravenous lipid, careful monitoring of fat tolerance should be made on a regular basis (1–2 times per week). Various methods for determining blood levels of infused fat have been suggested. These include the monitoring of plasma TG and the evaluation of plasma turbidity either by visual inspection or by measurement of light scattering index (LSI) by nephelometry. Measurement of plasma turbidity, however, has a low predictive value in assessments of TG concentration and cannot be recommended.[73] Direct measurements of TG levels should therefore be performed in order to avoid metabolic complications that may occur rarely with the use of lipid emulsions.

Complications with amino acids

Previously available crystalline amino acids carried a significant risk of development of hyperchloraemic metabolic acidosis due to their high content of free hydrochloric acid. This potential complication is rarely observed nowadays with the use of solutions containing amino acids as acetate salts. If the excretion of urea does not keep pace with the production, urea accumulates in the blood, resulting in azotaemia. In many catabolic states, as in inflammation or after trauma, stress hormones and cytokines will promote catabolism, which increases the risk of hyperaminoacidaemia. However, in such situations, the capacity of the liver, gut and other tissues to clear amino acids from the blood is usually sufficient to prevent hyperaminoacidaemia.[74] The tendency to have increased blood urea levels is greater in dehydrated patients. Elderly patients that are critically ill tend to develop azotaemia with infusion of 1.5 g protein per kilogram or more per day.[74] Measurement of blood urea nitrogen and assessment of fluid balance are thus helpful in preventing this complication.

Hypercalcaemia

This rare complication may result from infusion of excessive quantities of calcium, as a result of vitamin D toxicity[75] or might be seen in patients with malignancies and bone metastases.[76] Since calcium is bound to albumin and hypoalbuminaemia is common in many states of disease, the metabolically active serum calcium fraction may be underestimated (see above). Therefore, ionised calcium rather than the total serum calcium concentration should be measured.

Inappropriate composition of nutrients

An improper composition of various substrates often contributes to organ-specific complications. The precise aetiology of abnormalities in specific organs which may occur during TPN is often obscure and it may be impossible to single out any substrate or mechanism as being responsible. Essential fatty acid deficiency (EFAD) is an example of a complication caused by an improper composition of nutrients (resulting from continuous administration of glucose without essential fatty acids).

Hepatic dysfunction

It is well recognised that TPN, in particular if prolonged, may result in altered hepatic function tests. The abnormalities typically appear as elevated serum concentrations of alanine and aspartate amino-transferases (ALT and AST) 1–2 weeks after onset of parenteral nutrition. Histopathological changes include fatty infiltration as the initial lesion, which usually is fully reversible. With prolonged therapy, more severe alterations might appear, such as cholestasis, active chronic hepatitis, fibrosis and cirrhosis. The aetiology for the abnormalities in laboratory and histopatho-logical findings is not fully understood. It seems clear however that abnormalities are associated purely with the IV route of administration and may thus be associated with the lack of gastrointestinal stimulation in patients not receiving oral alimentation.[77,78]

A number of factors may account for TPN-induced liver changes. Hepatic dysfunction has been attributed to the use of excess glucose,[79] intravenous fat,[80] and amino acid solutions.[79] High-concentration glucose infusions increase the portal insulin : glucagon ratio and hepatic steatosis.[81] When a lipid emulsion is added to TPN infusions, the insulin : glucagon ratio falls,[82] which in turn has been shown to prevent the development of hepatic steatosis.[79] Essential fatty acids (EFAs) are required for hepatic cholesterol esterification and cholesterol synthesis. EFA deficiency may therefore contribute to hepatic steatosis by reducing the pro-

duction of lipoproteins that transport triglycerides from the liver. Other less well documented factors that may contribute to hepatic dysfunction during parenteral nutrition include tryptophane metabolites,[83] choline[84] and carnitine deficiency;[83] and increased bacterial translocation from an atrophic gut mucosa.[85]

Management of liver dysfunction during parenteral nutrition should (after exclusion of other potential causes than TPN, such as sepsis, viral or drug-induced hepatitis, and biliary obstruction) ultimately aim to have the patient eating again. If parenteral nutrition has to be continued for longer periods, and liver abnormalities persist or even worsen, the composition of the TPN solution may be changed. Administration of large amounts of calories as glucose or protein should be avoided, and lipid emulsions should be given as approximately one-third of the energy demand. However, not more than 3g/kg/day should be administered, since this has been shown to increase hepatic fat accumulation.[86] If changing to an appro-priate composition of nutrient solutions fails to improve the clinical situation, changing the time of administration by 'cyclic TPN' could be instituted. This has been shown to improve liver function tests,[87] probably by decreasing the time of persistent hyper-insulinaemia, which could induce hepatic steatosis. If liver dysfunction still persists, caloric intake should be reduced in order to avoid progressive liver disease.

Cholestasis is a less frequent complication of TPN in adults, and has been suggested to emanate from changes in bile acid composition, particularly from increases in lithocholic acid.[88] Administration of ursodeoxycholic acid[89] or S-adenosyl-L-methionine[90] might prove beneficial as therapy for TPN-induced cholestasis.

Metabolic bone disease

Long-term TPN may result in alterations of bone metabolism. Symptoms of bone disease include peri-articular bone pain. The aetiology has been attributed to a number of causes, including aluminium toxicity, an altered vitamin D sensitivity, hypercalciuria and trace element deficiency. TPN-related bone disease from casein hydrolysates is no longer seen, but the possibility of aluminium toxicity remains.[91] Most patients with TPN-related bone disease have a reduced bone mineral density.[92] Biochemical features include normal serum calcium and phosphorus levels, elevated urinary calcium excretion, PTH concen-trations in the low-to-normal range and very low serum levels of 1,25-dihydroxy vitamin D.[93] A liberal supply of calcium and phosphate will generally prevent the development of TPN-related bone disease.

The refeeding syndrome

The infusion of nutrients in severely depleted patients may be associated with clinically significant shifts in phosphorus, magnesium and potassium from extracellular to intracellular spaces. These derangements in electrolytes may cause severe cardiopulmonary and neurological complications including cardiac insufficiency, peripheral oedema, convulsions, coma and death. In the nutritionally depleted patient the stimulation of endogenous insulin secretion by glucose causes an increased tissue uptake of glucose, phosphate and water. The combination of depleted total body phosphorus stores in the malnourished patient in association with an increased cellular uptake of phosphorus during refeeding may lead to severe hypophosphataemia. Hypokalaemia and hypomagnesaemia usually develop simultaneously with the reduction of serum phosphate levels, contributing to the clinical picture of the syndrome. Approaches for the prevention and management of the refeeding syndrome (also called nutritional recovery syndrome) include supplementation of vitamins and minerals as soon as possible. Patients who habitually drink alcohol are at particular risk of being depleted of phosphate, thiamine, folate, vitamin B[6] and zinc.[94] Feeding should be initiated at 50% or less of the patient's estimated requirements and the increase in energy intake should be advanced gradually during the first days. The patient's cardiac and mineral status needs to be monitored closely.[95]

Biochemical monitoring

Measurements of various blood or urinary components are necessary for preventing metabolic complications. The time interval for such biochemical surveillance depends on the patient's clinical status (Table 25.4). In stable patients receiving long-term TPN, the time between measurements could be considerably extended.

Conclusions

Potential metabolic complications of parenteral nutrition are numerous but many have become rare as a result of better knowledge of requirements of various nutrients in different states of disease and improved nutritional preparations. In particular, deficiency syndromes have become rare. Nutrition support teams in hospitals and nutrition curricula in medical school may also be responsible for the improvements seen.[96] (see ch. 14) In recent years there has been a trend at many centres to use a limited number of standard IV nutrition (all-in-one) formulae. For the great majority of patients successful TPN is probably best achieved by use of such standard compositions.[97] Deficiency syndromes are unlikely to appear with the use of complete standard formulae, but there may be an associated increased risk of complications related to excessive nutrient supply. Only by careful clinical and

Table 25.4 – Biochemical surveillance during TPN in different patient categories.

Blood or urinary (u) parameter	TPN in intensive care patients	Patients receiving perioperative TPN	Home TPN patients
Glucose u-glucose (dipstick)	Several times daily	Daily	Twice weekly
Na, K, Cl Full blood count Creatinine, osmolarity	Daily	3 times weekly	Weekly
Triglycerides, cholesterol, albumin, urea, phosphate, liver function tests, coagulation tests	3 times weekly	Twice weekly	Twice monthly
Ca, Mg, Zn	Twice weekly	Weekly	Monthly
B[12], folic acid	–	–	Monthly

biochemical surveillance can metabolic complications be prevented.

References

1. Buzby GP, Knox LS, Crosby LO *et al.* Study protocol: a randomized clinical trial of total parenteral nutrition in malnourished patients. *Am J Clin Nutr* 1988; **47:** 366–381.

2. Zaloga GP, Chernow B. Hypocalcemia in critical illness. *JAMA* 1986; **256:** 1924–1929.

3. Bringhurst FR. Calcium and phosphate distribution, turnover, and metabolic action. In: Degroot LJ, Besser GM, Cahill GF, Marshall JC, Nelson DH, Odell WD, (eds) *Endocrinology*, 2nd edn. WB Saunders, Philadelphia, 1989; pp. 805–843.

4. Agusti AG, Torres A, Estopa R, Agusti-Vidal A. Hypophosphatemia as a cause of failed weaning: the importance of metabolic factors. *Crit Care Med* 1984; **12:** 142–143.

5. Davis SV, Olichwier KK, Chakko SC. Reversible depression of myocardial performance in hypophosphatemia. *Am J Med Sci* 1988: **295:** 183–187.

6. Brown GR, Greenwood JK. Drug- and nutrition-induced hypophosphatemia: mechanisms and relevance in the critically ill. *Ann Pharmacother* 1994; **128:** 626–632.

7. Weinsier RL, Krumdieck CL. Death resulting from overzealous total parenteral nutrition: the refeeding syndrome revisited. *Am J Clin Nutr* 1980; **34:** 393–399.

8. Thompson JS, Hodges RE. Preventing hypophosphatemia during total parenteral nutrition. *J Parent Enter Nutr* 1984; **8:** 137–139.

9. Zaloga GP, Chernow B, Cook D, Snyfer R, Clapper M, O'Brian JT. Assessment of calcium homeostasis in the critically ill patient: diagnostic pitfalls of the McLean-Hasting nomogram. *Ann Surg* 1985; **202:** 587–592.

10. Fischer JA, Blum JW, Binswanger U. Acute parathyroid hormone response to epinephrine in vivo. *J Clin Invest* 1973; **52:** 2434.

11. Wene JD, Connor WE, Den Besten L. The development of essential fatty acid deficiency in healthy man fed fat-free diets intravenously and orally. *J Clin Invest* 1975; **56:** 127–134.

12. Kay RG, Tasman-Jones C, Pybus J, Whiting R, Black H. A syndrome of acute zinc deficiency during total parenteral nutrition in man. *Ann Surg* 1976; **183:** 331–340.

13. Karpel JT, Peden VH. Copper deficiency in long-term parenteral nutrition. *J Pediatr* 1971; **80:** 32–36.

14. Brown RO, Lynn SF, Cross RE *et al.* Chromium deficiency after long-term parenteral nutrition. *Dig Dis Sci* 1986; **31:** 663–667.

15. Tsuda K, Yokoyama Y, Morita M *et al.* Selenium and chromium deficiency during long-term home total parenteral nutrition in chronic idiophatic intestinal pseudoobstruction. *Nutrition* 1998; **14:** 291–295.

16. Turnlund JR, Keyes WR, Peiffer GL, Chiang G. Molybdenium absorbtion, excretion, and retention studied with stable isotopes in young men during depletion and repletion. *Am J Clin Nutr* 1995; **61:** 1102–1109.

17. O'Neill JA Jr, Caldwell MD, Meng HC. Essential fatty acid deficiency in surgical patients. *Ann Surg* 1977; **185:** 535–542.

18. Jeppesen PB, Hoey C-E, Mortensen PB. Essential fatty acid deficiency in patients receiving home parenteral nutrition. *Am J Clin Nutr* 1998; **68:** 126–133.

19. Holman RT, Smythe L, Johnson S. Effect of sex and age on fatty acid composition of human serum lipids. *Am J Clin Nutr* 1979; **32:** 2390–2399.

20. Chen W, Chiang T-P, Chen T-C. Serum zinc and copper during long-term total parenteral nutrition. *J Formosan Med Assoc* 1991; **90:** 1075–1080.

21. Linder MC, Hazeg-Azam M. Copper biochemistry and molecular biology. *Am J Clin Nutr* 1996; **63:** 797S–811S.

22. Wasa M, Satani M, Tanano M, Nezu R, Takagi Y, Okada A. Copper deficiency with pancytopenia during total parenteral nutrition. *J Parent Enter Nutr* 1994; **18:** 190–192.

23. Camblor M, De la Cuerda C, Bretón I, Pérex-Rus G, Alvarez S, García P. Copper deficiency with pancytopenia due to enteral nutrition through jejunostomy. *Clin Nutr* 1997; **16:** 129–131.

24. Glinsmann WH, Feldman FJ, Mertz W. Plasma chromium after glucose administration. *Science* 1966; **152:** 1243–1245.

25. Jeejeebhoy KN, Chu RC, Marliss EB, Greenberg GR, Bruce-Robertson A. Chromium deficiency, glucose intolerance, neuropathy reversed by chromium supplementation, in a patient receiving long-term total parenteral nutrition. *Am J Clin Nutr* 1977; **30:** 531–538.

26. Watson RD, Cannon AD, Kurland GS, Cox KL, Frates RC. Selenium responsive myositis during prolonged home total parenteral nutrition in cystic fibrosis. *J Parent Enter Nutr* 1985; **9:** 58–60.

27. Reeves WC, Marcuard SP, Willis SE, Movahed A. Reversible cardiomyopathy due to selenium deficiency. *J Parent Enter Nutr* 1989; **13:** 663–665.

28. Diplock AT. Trace elements in human health with special reference to selenium. *Am J Clin Nutr* 1987; **45:** 1313–1322.

29. Nakasaki H, Ohta M, Soeda J, Makuuchi H, Tsuda M, Tajima T, Nitomi T, Fujii K. Clinical and biochemical aspects of thiamine treatment for metabolic acidosis during total parenteral nutrition. *Nutrition* 1997; **13:** 110–117.

30. Wolfe RR, Allsop JR, Burke JF. Glucose metabolism in man: responses to intravenous glucose infusion. *Metabolism* 1979; **28:** 210–220.

31. Thorell A, Nygren J, Ljungqvist O. Insulin resistance: a marker of surgical stress. *Curr Opin Clin Nutr Metab Care* 1999; **2:** 69–78.

32. The Veterans Affairs Total Parenteral Nutrition Cooperative Study Group (1991). Perioperative total parenteral nutrition in surgical patients. *N Engl J Med* 1991; **325:** 525–532.

33. Dunham CM, Damiano AM, Wiles CE, Cushing BM. Post-traumatic multiple organ function syndrome: infection is an uncommon antecedent risk factor. *Injury* 1995; **26:** 373–378.

34. Wallace LK, Starr NJ, Leventhal MJ, Estafanous FG. Hyperglycemia on ICU admission after CABG is associated with increased risk of mediastinitis or wound infection. *Anesthesiology* 1996; **85:** A286 (Abstract).

35. Wolfe RR. Carbohydrate metabolism and requirements. In: Rombeau JL, Caldwell MD (eds), *Parenteral Nutrition: Clinical Nutrition*, vol 2. WB Saunders, Philadelphia, 1986; pp. 53–71.

36. Brandi LS, Frediani M, Oleggini M, Mosca M, Cerri C, Boni C, Pecori N, Buzzigoli G, Ferranini E. Insulin resistance after surgery: Normalization by insulin treatment. *Clin Sci* 1990; **79:** 443–450.

37. Kaminski MV. A review of hyperosmolar hyperglycemic nonketotic dehydration (HHND): etiology, pathophysiology and prevention during intravenous hyperalimentation. *J Parent Enter Nutr* 1978; **2:** 690–698.

38. Levine SN, Sanson TH. Treatment of hyperglycemic hyperosmolar nonketotic syndrome. *Drugs* 1989; **38:** 462–472.

39. Jebb SA, Prentice AM, Goldberg GR, Murgatroyd PR, Black AE, Coward WA. Changes in macronutrient balance during over- and underfeeding assessed by 12-d continuous whole-body calorimetry. *Am J Clin Nutr* 1996; **64:** 259–266.

40. Wolfe RR, O'Donell TF Jr, Stone MD, Richman DA, Burke JF, Investigation of factors determining the optimal glucose infusion rate in total parenteral nutrition. *Metabolism* 1980; **29:** 892–900.

41. Covelli HD, Black JW, Olsen MS, Beekman JF. Respiratory failure precipitated by high carbohydrate loads. *Ann Intern Med* 1981; **85:** 579–581.

42. Aranda-Michel J, Morgan SL. Overfeeding in a patient with kwashiorkor syndrome. *Nutrition* 1996; **12:** 623–625.

43. Dark DS, Pingleton SK, Kerby GR. Hypercapnia during weaning: a complication of nutritional support. *Chest* 1985; **88:** 141–143.

44. Askanazi J, Nordenström J, Rosenbaum SH, Elwyn DH, Hyman AI, Carpentier YA, Kiney JM. Nutrition for the patient with respiratory failure: glucose vs. fat. *Anesthesiology* 1981; **54:** 373–377.

45. Kaminski DL, Adams A, Jellinek M. The effect of hyperalimentation on hepatic lipid content and lipogenic enzyme activity in rats and man. *Surgery* 1980; **88:** 93–100.

46. Aarsland A, Chinkes D, Wolfe RR. Contributions of de novo synthesis of fatty acids to total VLDL-triglyceride secretion during prolonged hyperglycemia/hyperinsulinemia in normal man. *J Clin Invest* 1996; **98:** 2008–2017.

47. Kang ES, Galloway S, Ellis J, Solomon SS, Bean W, Reger JF, Cook GA, Olson G. Hepatic steatosis during convalescence from influenza B infection in ferrets with postprandial hyperinsulinemia. *J Lab Clin Med* 1990; **116:** 335–344.

48. Shronts EP. Essential nature of choline with implications for total parenteral nutrition. *J Am Diet Assoc* 1997; **97:** 639–646, 649.

49. Nordenström J, Jeevanandam M, Elwyn DH, Carpentier YA, Askanazi J, Robin AP, Kinney JM. Increasing glucose intake during total parenteral nutrition increases norepinephrine excretion in trauma and sepsis. *Clin Physiol* 1981; **1:** 525–534.

50. Rowe JW, Young JB, Minaker KL. Effect of insulin and glucose infusion on sympathetic nervous system activity in normal man. *Diabetes* 1981; **30:** 219–225.

51. Franch G, Guirao X, Garcia-Domingo M, Gil MJ, Salas E, Sitges-Serra A. The influence of calorie source on water and sodium balances during intravenous refeeding of malnourished rabbits. *Clin Nutr* 1992; **11:** 59–61.

52. MacFie J, Smith RC, Hill GH. Glucose or fat as a non-protein energy source? A controlled trial in gastroenterological patients receiving intravenous nutrition. *Gastroenterology* 1981; **80:** 103–107.

53. Scheltinga MR, Young LS, Benfell K, Bye RL, Ziegler TR, Santos AA, Antin JH, Schloerb PR, Wilmore DW. Glutamine-enriched intravenous feedings attenuate extracellular fluid expansion after a standard stress. *Ann Surg* 1991; **214:** 385–93; discussion 393–395.

54. Kamath KR, Berry A, Cummins G. Acute hypersensitivity reaction to Intralipid. *N Engl J Med* 1981; **303**: 360.

55. Hiyama DT, Griggs B, Mittman RJ, Lacy JA, Benson DW, Bower RH. Hypersensitivity following lipid emulsion infusion in an adult patient. *J Parent Enter Nutr* 1989; **13**: 318–320.

56. Lykkelov Andersen H, Nissen I. Presumed anaphylactic shock following Lipofundin infusion. *Ugeskr Laeger* 1993; **155**: 2210–2211.

57. Friedman Z, Marks KH, Maisels J. Effect of parenteral fat emulsion on the pulmonary and reticuloendothelial systems in the newborn infant. *Pediatrics* 1978; **61**: 694–698.

58. Greene HL, Hazlett D, Demaree R. Relationship between Intralipid induced hyperlipemia and pulmonary function. *Am J Clin Nutr* 1976; **29**: 127–135.

59. Nordenström J, Jarstrand C, Wiernik A. Decreased chemotactic and random migration of leukocytes during Intralipid infusion. *Am J Clin Nutr* 1979; **32**: 2416–2422.

60. Fischer GW, Wilson SR, Hunter KW, Mease AD. Diminished bacterial defences with Intralipid. *Lancet* 1980; **2**: 1819–1820.

61. Allardyce DB. Cholestasis caused by lipid emulsions. *Surg Gynaecol Obstetr* 1982; **154**: 641–647.

62. Goulet O, Girot R, Maier-Redelsperger M, Bougle D, Virelizier JL, Ricour C. Hepatologic disorders following prolonged use of intravenous fat emulsions in children. *J Parent Enter Nutr* 1985; **18**: 284–288.

63. Bigorgne C, Le Torneau A, Messing B, Rio B, Giraud V, Molina T, Audoin J, Diebold J. Sea-blue histiocyte syndrome in bone-marrow secondary to total parenteral nutrition including fat-emulsion sources: a clino-pathological study of seven cases. *Br J Haematol* 1996; **95**: 258–262.

64. Belin RP, Bivins BA, Jona JZ. Fat overload with a 10% soybean oil emulsion. *Arch Surg* 1976; **11**: 1391–1393.

65. Palmblad J, Broström O, Lahnborg G, Udén A-M, Venizelos N. Neutrophil functions during total parenteral nutrition and Intralipid infusion. *Am J Clin Nutr* 1982; **35**: 1430–1436.

66. Schröder H, Paust H, Schmidt R. Pulmonary fat embolism after Intralipid therapy: a post-mortem artefact? *Acta Paediatr Scand* 1984; **73**: 461–464.

67. Dionigi P, Dionigi R, Prati U, Pavesi F, Jemos V, Nazari S. Effects of Intralipid on some immunologic parameters and leukocyte functions in patients with esophageal and gastric cancer. *Clin Nutr* 1985; **4**: 229–234.

68. Tulikuora I, Huikuri K. Morphological fatty changes and function of the liver, serum free fatty acids and triglycerides during parenteral nutrition. *Scand J Gastroenterol* 1982; **17**: 177–185.

69. Nordenström J, Jarstrand C, Hallberg D. Intralipid and reticuloendothelial blockade. *Lancet* 1980; **2**: 1139.

70. Untracht SH. Intravascular metabolism of an artificial transporter of triacylglycerols: alterations of serum lipoproteins resulting from total parenteral nutrition with Intralipid. *Biochim Biophys Acta* 1982; **711**: 176–192.

71. Rigaud D, Serog P, Legrand A, Cerf M, Apfelbaum M, Bonfils S. Quantification of lipoprotein X and its relationship to plasma lipid profile during different types of parenteral nutrition. *J Parent Enter Nutr* 1984; **8**: 529–534.

72. Hajri T, Férézou J, Lutton C. Effects of intravenous infusions of commercial fat emulsions (Intralipid 10 or 20%) on rat plasma lipoproteins: phospholipids in excess are the main precursors for lipoprotein X-like particles. *Biochim Biophys Acta* 1990; **1047**: 121–130.

73. Nordenström J, Thörne A, Lindholm M. Accuracy of plasma turbidity measurement for determining fat intolerance during total parenteral nutrition. *Clin Nutr* 1990; **9**: 172–175.

74. Jeevanandam M. Trauma and sepsis. In: Cynober LA (ed) *Amino acid metabolism and therapy in health and nutritional disease*. Boca Raton, FLA: London: CRC 1995: pp. 245–255.

75. Greene HL, Vitamins in total parenteral nutrition. *Drug Intell Clin Pharm* 1972; **6**: 355–360.

76. Sato K, Imaki T, Toraya S, Demura H, Tanaka M, Kasajima T, Takeuchi A, Kobayashi T. Increased 1, 25-(OH)2D2 concentration in a patient with malignancy-associated hypercalcemia receiving intravenous hyperalimentation inadvertently supplemented with vitamin D2. *Intern Med* 1993; **32**: 886–890.

77. Rager R, Finegold MJ. Cholestasis in immature newborn infants: is parenteral alimentation responsible? *J Pediatr* 1975; **86**: 264–269.

78. Nakagawa M, Hiramatsu Y, Mitsuyushi K, Yamamura M, Hioki K, Yamamoto M. Effect of various lipid emulsions on total parenteral nutrition-induced hepatosteatosis in rats. *J Parent Enter Nutr* 1991; **15**: 137–143.

79. Tulikoura I, Huikuri K. Morphological fatty changes and function of the liver, serum free fatty acid, and triglycerides during parenteral nutrition. *Scand J Gastroenterol* 1982; **17**: 177–185.

80. Allardyce DB. Cholestasis caused by lipid emulsions. *Surg Gynaecol Obstet* 1982; **154**: 641–647.

81. Li S, Nussbaum MS, Teague D, Gapen CL, Dayal R, Fisher JE. Increasing dextrose concentrations in total parenteral nutrition (TPN) causes alterations in hepatic morphology and plasma levels of insulin and glucagon in rats. *J Surg Res* 1988; **44:** 639–648.

82. Nussbaum MS, Li S, Bower RH, McFadden DW, Daual R, Fisher JE. Addition of lipid to total parenteral nutrition prevents hepatic steatosis in rats by lowering the portal venous insulin/glucagon ratio. *J Parent Enter Nutr* 1992; **16:** 106–109.

83. Grant JP, Cox CE, Kleinman LM *et al.* Serum hepatic enzyme and bilirubin elevations during total parenteral nutrition. *Surg Gynecol Obstet* 1977; **145:** 573–580.

84. Duchman AL, Dubin M, Jenda D *et al.* Lechitin increases plasma free choline and decreases hepatic steatosis in long-term parenteral nutrition patients. *Gastroenterology* 1992; **102:** 1363–1370.

85. Alverdy JC, Aoys E, Moss GS. Total parenteral nutrition promotes bacterial translocation from the gut. *Surgery* 1988; **104:** 185–190.

86. Freund U, Krausz Y, Levij IS, Eliakim M. Iatrogenic lipidosis following prolonged intravenous hyper-alimentation. *Am J Clin Nutr* 1975; **28:** 1156–1160.

87. Maini B, Blackburn GL, Bistrian BM *et al.* Cyclic hyperalimentation. An optimal technique for preservation of visceral protein. *J Surg Res* 1976; **20:** 515–525.

88. Fouin-Fortunet H, LeQuernec L, Erlinger S, Lerebours E, Colin R. Hepatic alterations during total-parenteral nutrition in patients with inflammatory bowel disease: a possible consequence of lithocholate toxicity. *Gastroenterology* 1982; **82:** 932–937.

89. Lindor KD, Burnes J. Ursodeoxycholic acid for the treatment of home parenteral nutrition–associated cholestasis. A case report. *Gastroenterology* 1991; **101:** 250–253.

90. Frezza M, Tritapepe R, Pozzato G, DiPadova C. Prevention by S-adenosyl-L-methionine of estrogene-induced hepatobiliary toxicity in susceptible women. *Am J Gastroenterol* 1988; **83:** 1098–1102.

91. Ott SM, Maloney NA, Klein GL, Alfrey AC, Ament ME, Coburn JW, Sherrard DJ. Aluminium is associated with low bone formation in patients receiving chronic parenteral nutrition. *Ann Intern Med* 1983; 910–914.

92. Harrison JE, Jeekeebhoy KN, Track NS. The effect of total parenteral nutrition (TPN) on bone mass. In: Coburn JW, Klein GL (eds) Metabolic bone disease in total parenteral nutrition. Urban Schwarzenberg, Baltimore, 1985; pp. 53–61.

93. Klein GL, Horst RL, Norman AW, Ament ME, Slatopolsky E, Coburn JE. Reduced serum levels of 1-alpha, 25-dihydroxyvitamin D during long-term parenteral nutrition. *Ann Intern Med* 1981; **94:** 638–643.

94. Cravo ML, Gloria LM, Selhub J, Nadeau MR, Camilo ME, Resende MP, Cardoso JN, Leiato CN, Mira FC. Hyperhomocysteinemia in chronic alcoholism: correlation with folate, vitamin B-12, and vitamin B-6 status. *Am J Clin Nutr* 1996; **63:** 220–224.

95. Brooks MJ, Melnik G. The refeeding syndrome: an approach to understanding its complications and preventing its occurrence. *Pharmacotherapy* 1995; **15:** 713–726.

96. ChrisAnderson D, Heimburger DC, Morgan SL, Geels WJ, Henry KL, Conner W, Hensrud DD, Thompson G, Weinsier RL. Metabolic complications of total parenteral nutrition: Effects of a Nutrition support service. *J Parent Enter Nutr* 1996; **20:** 206–210.

97. Nordenström J, Jeppson B, Lovén L, Larsson J. Peripheral parenteral nutrition: effect of a standardized compounded mixture of infusion phlebitis. *Br J Surg* 1991; **78:** 1391–1394.

26

Paediatric parenteral nutrition

John WL Puntis

Historical background

Robert Boyle published an account of his experiments with intravenous infusion of opium and sac into a dog in 1664. The animal grew fat and became the object of admiration.[1] Even then, however, parenteral nutrition was not without its complications, and the unfortunate creature was stolen.

Prompted by cholera outbreaks and insights into the pathophysiology of this disease, attempts to use intravenous therapy in human subjects were first made in the 1830s. One of the physicians involved accurately forecast that 'this . . . astonishing method of medication . . . will lead to wonderful improvements in the practice of medicine'.[2] However, technical backwardness and problems of sepsis meant that further developments were slow in coming.[3]

The first successful account of parenteral nutrition (PN) in an infant was published in 1944.[4] A mixture of 50% glucose, 10% casein hydrolysate and an olive oil/lecithin homogenate was used for five days in a child with Hirschsprung's disease, apparently to good effect. Following animal experimentation, Wilmore and Dudrick's landmark case report[5] of 1968 provided the impetus for more widespread application of total parenteral nutrition in paediatric practice.

The first patients to benefit were newborns undergoing surgery for disorders of the gastrointestinal tract. The means to provide nutrition support during gut failure transformed the prognosis of these children and quickly led to PN becoming used in an ever growing number of conditions. Premature infants now comprise the largest group of children given intravenous nutrition, yet few of the indications (although widely accepted) have been unequivocally substantiated by controlled clinical trials.[6]

Continuing improvement in the available range and quality of intravenous nutrition products, and a reduction in associated complications have ensured expansion in the use of PN over the last 30 years. For example, giving glucose as the sole carbohydrate source has removed the risk of lactic acidosis associated with the use of alcohol and fructose.[7,8] The introduction of synthetic crystalline L-amino acid solutions which replaced protein hydrolysates in the 1970s not only reduced allergic reactions but increased nitrogen retention,[9] and reduced the risks of hyperammonaemia[10] and aluminium toxicity.[11]

A greater understanding of the amino acid requirements of preterm infants has allowed specially modified solutions to be developed for this age group giving plasma amino acid profiles closer to those of breast fed infants.[12,13] New substrates such as inositol,[14] glutamine[15] and ornithine α-ketoglutarate[16] with potentially important clinical effects have been studied. The availability of well-tolerated lipid emulsions has allowed substitution of fat for glucose.[17] The combination of lipid and glucose has resulted in improved nitrogen retention compared with a high carbohydrate energy source.[18,19]

Clinical deficiency states including those related to taurine[20] and selenium[21] have been reported, whilst the hazards of over-supplying aluminium,[22,23] chromium[24] and manganese[25] have been elaborated.

Further developments in nutrition support practice include the refinement of computer assisted prescribing,[26] the creation of multi-disciplinary nutrition support teams (NST),[27] and the use of home parenteral nutrition (HPN).[28]

Special considerations in children

The limited energy reserves and the need for growth in infants and children put them at particular risk from the effects of under-nutrition. A small preterm infant of 1 kg with no more than 10 g of storage fat might survive only four days if starved, a 2 kg baby for 12 days and a 3.5 kg infant for 32 days.[29] In contrast, it has been estimated that an adult could survive for 3 months. These times are likely to be reduced when there is catabolic stress. Instituting parenteral nutrition in the small infant who cannot tolerate enteral feeds is therefore a matter of urgency.

Requirements for water, electrolytes, protein, fat and carbohydrate vary considerably with age as well as with illness. The requirement for amino acids is also qualitatively different in early infancy when histidine, taurine, cystine/cysteine, tyrosine, proline and alanine are semi-essential.

Over-supply of nutrients producing severe hyperaminoacidaemia can cause coma in the newborn[30] and irreversible brain damage.[31] In the preterm infant, immaturity of metabolic pathways may result in potentially toxic plasma concentrations of amino acids such as phenylalanine and tyrosine, although this is less likely with neonatally adapted amino acid sources.[12,13] Threonine, glycine and methionine are also poorly metabolised.

The rapidly growing brain is sensitive to periods of malnutrition as well as to metabolic insult, and accounts for around two-thirds of basal metabolic rate.[32] Caloric deprivation in the newborn period is an important determinant of subsequent brain growth.[33] Early nutritional influences appear to have profound effects on later neuro-development,[34] and malnutrition during infancy in some circumstances is known to be associated with later intellectual impairment.[35]

During the first 9 months of life immaturity of renal function means that the infant is unable to excrete inorganic solutes or hydrogen ion load efficiently. Hypernatraemia and acidosis are therefore more likely to occur over this period. In the preterm infant acidosis during PN relates in part to excess intake of choride and can be reduced by substituting acetate.[36]

Indications for parenteral nutrition

PN is indicated when malnutrition or growth failure cannot be prevented or reversed by enteral nutrition support. The principal indications are shown in Table 26.1. Ethical dilemmas may arise over children with little or no small bowel (e.g. antenatal infarction of gastroschisis) or congenital enteropathy (e.g. microvillus inclusion disease) who will never be able to tolerate full enteral feeding. Decisions regarding appropriate management should be made after careful discussion with parents and colleagues.

Sometimes PN may be the only way of maintaining an adequate nutrition intake even when the gastrointestinal tract is intact (e.g. if severe fluid restriction is necessary). When prolonged gastrointestinal failure can be predicted, as in the newborn undergoing bowel surgery, PN may be commenced in order to prevent later malnutrition. The timing and duration of such feeding must depend on the age and size (i.e. nutritional reserve) of the patient, the severity of illness and the expected duration of starvation.[29] Supervision by a multidisciplinary nutrition support team minimises inappropriate prescribing of PN.

In the premature newborn, respiratory distress syndrome, promotion of growth and prevention of

Table 26.1 – Indications for parenteral nutrition in paediatric patients.

Newborn	
Unequivocal:	Intestinal failure – functional immaturity necrotising enterocolitis short bowel
Equivocal:	Respiratory failure requiring IPPV Promotion of growth in preterm infants Prevention of necrotising enterocolitis

Older infants and children	
Intestinal failure:	Postoperative gastrointestinal surgery Short bowel Protracted diarrhoea Chronic pseudo-obstruction
Intensive care/multi-organ failure:	Hypercatabolism (e.g. extensive burns; severe trauma) Severe fluid restriction required (e.g. renal impairment; inappropriate ADH)
Exclusion of luminal nutrients:	Crohn's disease Pancreatitis

necrotising enterocolitis are relative indications for PN but there is considerable variation in nutrition support practice. For example, PN may be favoured in units where enteral feeding is seen as a major risk factor for necrotising enterocolitis[37] (NEC) and aspiration pneumonia, or when functional gastrointestinal immaturity is thought to preclude giving milk. More aggressive attempts to feed enterally are likely to be made in units where central venous catheter sepsis, cholestasis and metabolic bone disease are seen to be major problems.[38]

TPN and exclusion of enteral nutrition in infants at high risk of NEC as a prophylactic measure may in fact increase the risk of this disorder,[39] possibly as a result of atrophic changes occurring in the gastrointestinal tract. Rats denied enteral nutrients during PN rapidly develop marked atrophic changes in the bowel and pancreas.[40,41] Even volumes of enteral feed which appear to be nutritionally insignificant may play an important role in maintaining the structure and function of the gastrointestinal tract.[42] In the preterm infant, such hypocaloric enteral feeding facilitates later establishment of full enteral feeding[43,44] probably through the mediation of enteric hormones.[45] There are no data from large prospective trials which firmly establish that prophylactic use of TPN protects against NEC.

Table 26.2 – Regimen for parenteral nutrition: basic requirements of nutrients, electrolytes, minerals and vitamins. All values are given per kg body weight per day.

Patient group	Day of PN	Age (days)	Fluid (ml)	Aminoacids (g)	Carbohydrate (g)	Fat (g)	Sodium (mmol)	Potassium (mmol)	Phosphate (mmol)	Peditrace (ml)	Solivito N (ml)	Vitlipid N infant (ml)
Neonates including low birthweight	1	3	90	0.7	10	1	3	2.5	1.1	0.5	1	4
	1	4–5	120	0.7	10	1	3	2.5	1.1	1	1	4
	1	6+	150	0.7	10	1	3	2.5	1.1	1	1	4
	2	4–5	120	1.3	12	2	3	2.5	1.1	1	1	4
	2	6+	150	1.3	12	2	3	2.5	1.1	1	1	4
	3	5	120	1.7	13	3	3	2.5	1.2	1	1	4
	3	6+	150	1.7	13	3	3	2.5	1.2	1	1	4
	4+	6+	150	2.1	14	3.5	3	2.5	1.3	1	1	4
Infants 3–10 kg	1		150	0.8	10	1	3	2.5	0.5	1	1	4
	2		150	1.3	12	2	3	2.5	0.6	1	1	4
	3		150	1.7	13	2	3	2.5	0.6	1	1	4
	4+		150	2.1	14	3	3	2.5	0.7	1	1	4
10–30 kg	1–2		60	1.0	4.5	1.5	3	2.5	As req.	0.2A	1†	1†
	3+		90	2.0	7.5	2	3	2.5	As req.	0.2A	1†	1†
>30 kg	1–2		36	1.0	2	1	3	2.5	As req.	0.2A	1†	1†
	3+		60	1.5	5	2	3	2.5	As req.	0.2A	1†	1†

A = Additrace.
† Do not exceed recommended maximum dose – see manufacturer's data sheet.
Solivito, Vitlipid, Addiphos, Peditrace and Additrace are registered trade marks. All are manufactured by Pharmacia & Upjohn, Milton Keynes, UK.

Table 26.3 – System for parenteral nutrition using commercially available products. All values are given per kg body weight per day.

Patient group	Day of PN	Post-gestation (days)	Fluid (ml)	Vaminolact (ml)	Glucose 5% (ml)	Glucose 20% (ml)	Intralipid 20% (mmol)	Additional sodium (mmol)	Additional potassium
Neonate including low birthweight	1	3	90	8	47	30	5	3	2.5
	1	4–5	120	8	87	20	5	3	2.5
	1	6+	150	8	127	10	5	3	2.5
	2	4–5	120	12	68	35	5	3	2.5
	2	6+	150	12	108	25	5	3	2.5
	3	5	120	16	104	40	10	3	2.5
	3	6+	150	16	94	30	10	3	2.5
	4	6+	150	24	71	45	10	3	2.5
	5	6+	150	32	53	50	15	3	2.5
	6	6+	150	40	26	65	18	3	2.5
Infants >1 month <10 kg	1		150	8	127	10	5	3	2.5
	2		150	16	104	25	5	3	2.5
	3		150	24	71	45	10	3	2.5
	4		150	32	38	60	10	3	2.5
	5+		150	40	20	75	15	3	2.5
10–30 kg	1–2		60	14†	24	15	8	2	2
	3+		90	28†	35	20	15	1.5	1.5
>30 kg	1–2		36	14†	17	–	5	2	2
	3+		60	20†	10	20	10	1.5	1.5

Vitamins to be included as in text. Additional phosphate as in Table 26.2.
Trace elements: If weight <10 kg add Peditrace 1 ml/kg/day.
                 If weight >10 kg add Additrace 0.2 ml/kg/day.
† Vamin 9.
Vamin, Vaminolact and Intralipid are registered trade marks. All are manufactured by Pharmacia & Upjohn, Milton Keynes, UK.

Table 26.4 – Alternative system for parenteral nutrition using commercially available products. All values given per kg body weight per day.

Patient group	Day of PN	Age (days)	Fluid (ml)	Aminoplasmal Ped (ml)	Glucose 5% (ml)	Glucose 20% (ml)	Lipofundin-S 20% (ml)	Additional sodium (mmol)	Additional potassium (mmol)
Neonate including low birthweight	1	3	90	9	46	30	5	2.6	2.3
	1	4–5	120	9	86	20	5	2.6	2.3
	1	6+	150	9	126	10	5	2.6	2.3
	2	4–5	120	13	67	35	5	2.4	2.2
	2	6+	150	13	107	25	5	2.4	2.2
	3	5	120	18	102	40	10	2.2	2.0
	3	6+	150	18	92	30	10	2.2	2.0
	4	6+	150	28	68	45	10	1.8	1.8
	5	6+	150	36	49	50	15	1.4	1.6
	6	6+	150	45	21	65	18	1.0	1.4
Infants >1 month <10 kg	1		150	9	126	10	5	2.6	2.3
	2		150	18	102	25	5	2.2	2.0
	3		150	27	68	45	10	1.8	1.8
	4		150	36	34	60	10	1.4	1.6
	5+		150	45	15	75	15	1.0	1.4
10–30 kg	1–2		60	16§	20	15	8	2.1	2.0
	3+		90	36§	30	20	15	1.5	1.6
>30 kg	1–2		36	18§	17	–	5	2.1	2.0
	3+		60	27§	7	20	10	1.7	1.8

Vitamins to be included as in text. Additional phosphate as in Table 26.2.
Trace elements: If weight <10 kg add Peditrace 1 ml/kg/day
                          If weight >10 kg add Additrace 0.2 ml/kg/day
§ Aminoplasmal L5.
Aminoplasmal and Lipofundin, Braun, Bucks, UK, are registered trade marks.

Formulating feeds

Parenteral feeds can be made up using standard solutions combined to give an appropriate fluid volume (see Tables 26.2–26.4 and the appendix to this chapter). Alternatively, a more flexible approach can be used with feed prescriptions being tailored to the needs of individual patients using a computer programme[46,47] (available from Fresenius Kabi, Warrington, UK). The PN prescription can be modified to take into account the fluid and/or nutritional contribution of concurrent infusions and partial enteral feeding together with any abnormal fluid and electrolyte losses. This approach means that the planned total nutritional intake is more likely to be achieved particularly in those patients with complex fluid balance problems.[48] Each prescription is printed out (Fig. 26.1) and the computer programme also converts details of the feed into volumes of stock solutions (Fig. 26.2) producing a worksheet for the pharmacist. Feed solutions are then presented as mixtures compounded by the pharmacy department in a laminar flow work station or aseptic isolator cabinet.

Monitoring

The long list of biochemical abnormalities associated with PN is disconcerting (Table 26.5) and probably explains why published guidelines for routine monitoring often advocate frequent and comprehensive testing.[49] In fact, there has been little critical

Table 26.5 – Metabolic complications of parenteral nutrition.

Hyperglycaemia, glycosuria and osmotic diuresis
Rebound hypoglycaemia
Metabolic acidosis
Hypocalcaemia
Hypomagnesaemia
Hypophosphataemia
Hyperammonaemia
Amino acid toxicity
Hyperlipidaemia
Essential fatty acid deficiency (lipid-free infusions)
Trace metal deficiency
Trace metal overload
Aluminium overload
Hepatic dysfunction

Table 26.6 – Guidelines for monitoring stable paediatric patients during parenteral nutrition.

	Before PN	Daily	Twice weekly	Once weekly	Monthly	Six monthly
Plasma						
Na	✓		✓			
K	✓		✓			
PO₄				✓		
bilirubin	✓			✓		
Ca				✓		
Alhalic Phosphatase				✓		
glucose		✓ week 1		✓		
Cu, Zn, Se, Mn					✓	
cholesterol, triglycerides				if fat ↑ >3g/kg		✓
FBC, PT/PTT						✓
ferritin						✓
Al, Cr						✓
folate; vitamins A, E, D, B₁, B₂, B₆, B₁₂						✓
Urine						
Na	✓		✓			
K	✓		✓			
glucose		✓				
Other						
chest X ray cardiac echo ECG						✓

Continue daily glucose in the preterm infant and in infants in whom carbohydrate intake is being increased.

evaluation of the minimum necessary biochemical surveillance essential for safe PN (see also Ch. 25).

Serious, unexpected biochemical disturbance simply as a result of parenteral feeding is unusual. An appropriate monitoring regimen for paediatric patients is suggested in Table 26.6. Hypophosphataemia is a potentially serious complication usually encountered in seriously malnourished patients as part of the 'refeeding' syndrome. It is associated with reduced cellular adenosine triphosphate and red-cell 2,3-diphosphoglycerate, and encephalopathy, myocardial dysfunction and impaired neutrophil function. Slow introduction of PN with phosphate supplements particularly in severely malnourished patients prevents this condition.

Fat tolerance in the neonate should be assessed by measurement of plasma triglyceride concentrations since visual inspection for turbidity is an unreliable guide.[50] Clinical instability, extreme prematurity and organ failure necessitate closer biochemical monitoring for obvious reasons. In those patients with abnormal fluid losses, the risk of biochemical disturbance can be minimised by choosing appropriate replacement fluids (Table 26.7).

Table 26.7 – Composition of abnormal fluid losses (mmol/l).

	Na	K	Cl
Gastric	20–80	5–20	100–150
Pancreatic	120–140	5–15	90–120
Small bowel	100–140	5–15	90–130
Bile	120–140	5–15	80–120
Ileostomy	45–135	3–15	20–115
Diarrhoea	10–90	10–80	10–110

Since uncommon complications are more likely to come to light with long-term PN a wider range of investigations can be justified in this group of patients.[51] These should include 6-monthly measurements of the B-group and fat-soluble vitamins, aluminium, chromium and manganese, together with liver ultrasound (in view of the increased risk of gall stones) and electrocardiography looking for evidence of pulmonary thromboembolism.[52]

Growth, including head circumference in the infant, should be regularly monitored in hospital. There are a number of different ways of assessing nutrition status clinically,[53] such as weight-for-height as a percentage of the expected, triceps skinfold thickness (TSF) expressed as a standard deviation score, mid-arm circumference, arm muscle area,[54] and the ratio of mid-arm circumference to head circumference.[55] Knemometry may have a place in the evaluation of short-term changes in growth rate[56] and deserves further study in the preterm infant in whom accurate measurement of weight and length is fraught with difficulties.

Energy requirements

Normal energy requirements are given in Chapter 12. Pyrexia increases caloric requirements by 12% for each degree of fever above 37°C. Surgery can increase caloric needs by 20–30%, and sepsis by as much as 50%. A simple method for estimating caloric requirements in children (kcal/kg) aged 6 months to 15 years is: 95 – (3 × age in years).[57] When attempting to reverse long-term growth failure, caloric intake should be related to *expected* rather than actual weight.

Carbohydrate sources

Glucose is the carbohydrate of choice, being utilised by all cells. In the premature infant, initial infusion rates of 5–6 mg/kg/min will maintain normoglycaemia. High infusion rates may cause glycosuria, swings in plasma osmolality, and osmotic diuresis with electrolyte and water depletion. Tolerance of increasing glucose intake must be monitored by frequent blood glucose estimation and urine testing for glycosuria. Insulin infusions are rarely needed except in the extremely immature very low birthweight infant.[58]

Nitrogen sources

Protein hydrolysates have been superseded by solutions of synthetic crystalline L–amino acids[59] such as Vamin (Fresenius Kabi), based on the amino acid composition of egg protein. For efficient amino acid utilisation it is necessary to give between 22 and 32 non-nitrogen calories with each gram of amino acids.

In children, histidine, proline, tyrosine, taurine, alanine and cystine/cysteine are required during infancy, in

Vitamins and trace elements

Guidelines for vitamin and trace element intakes in infants and children receiving TPN were reviewed in 1988.[95] Debate continues regarding the optimal intake of vitamins, and supplements for PN have been reformulated.[96,97] The recomendations given in Tables 26.2–26.4 are therefore approximations.

- water-soluble vitamins should be given as Solivito N (Fresenius Kabi). When reconstituted according to the manufacturer's instructions, the dose is 1 ml/kg/day to a maximum of 10 ml.

- fat-soluble vitamins are given as Vitlipid N (Fresenius Kabi).
  - for patients under 11 years of age, the infant preparation is used in a dose of 4 ml/kg/day to a maximum of 10 ml/day.
  - for patients over 11 years of age, the adult preparation is used in a dose of 10 ml/day.
  - the vitamins are normally added to the fat emulsion. Solivito N may be added to the amino acid mix.

Preterm infants have been found to be deficient in vitamin A at birth and there is evidence that this might be implicated in chronic lung disease,[98] through the effects of retinol in modulating epithelial cell differentiation.

Understanding of trace element requirements in the preterm infant and the effect of disease states is still limited. Trace element mixtures may need to be omitted when there is impairment of renal or liver function.

- for neonates and infants under 10 kg body weight Peditrace (Fresenius Kabi) is used in a dose of 1 ml/kg/day to a maximum of 15 ml/day.

- there is no ideal trace element solution for children over 10 kg. Additrace (Fresenius Kabi) 0.2 ml/kg/day up to a maximum of 10 ml/day may be used, but since it contains no calcium and no phosphate, these should be closely monitored.

Aluminium contaminating intravenous solutions may cause bone disease,[22] encephalopathy, anaemia and cholestasis.[99] The concentration of manganese (which is secreted in bile) increases in plasma as serum bilirubin rises.[100] Newer supplements (e.g. Peditrace, Additrace, Pharmacia & Upjohn, UK) include selenium but contain less manganese and less aluminium. The latter is a significant contaminant of the older preparations, as well as being found in calcium gluconate.[23]

At present, children on total PN without selenium-containing trace element preparations for more than two weeks should have selenium supplements[101] added separately at a dose of 25 nmol/kg to a maximum of 300 nmol/day. In preterm infants and those with diarrhoea, copper and zinc intakes may need to be increased: 20 μg/kg/day is a suitable copper supplement, while additional zinc is given as zinc sulphate 4 mg/day if below 5 kg body weight, 8 mg/day if 5–10 kg, and 12 mg if above 10 kg body weight.

Techniques for administering PN

Peripheral venous access

Venous access may be from either a peripheral or central vein.[102] Hypertonic feed solutions cause thrombophlebitis in peripheral veins and the overall dextrose concentration should be no more than 12.5%. When fluid restriction is a priority, this together with time spent attempting to resite drips may contribute to inadequate energy intake. Additional hazards of peripheral infusion include extravasation injury (particularly in very small infants), and infection. The risk of phlebitis can be reduced by filtering the glucose and electrolyte mixture through a 0.22 micron pore size filter to remove particulate matter.[103] Transdermal application of glyceryl trinitrate over the infusion site has also been shown to prolong vein life in adults[104] and could be used in older children. A 0.6 mm diameter neonatal Silastic central venous catheter cut short and used as a peripheral drip appears much less likely to cause phlebitis than a teflon cannula.[105]

Central venous access

Central venous catheterisation should be used in the paediatric patient when it is anticipated that PN will be required for more than a week. The central vein may be entered directly, either surgically or percutaneously, or indirectly via a peripheral vein. The use of fine (0.6 mm external diameter) Silastic catheters such as the Vygon Epicutaneo-Cava-Catheter has found wide application in premature and older infants.[106] Insertion is performed at the bedside using a simple technique.[107] Antecubital and temporal veins are the sites of choice. Care and attention should be given to taping the catheter in place to ensure that it cannot be pulled out accidentally.

Insertion complications with this type of catheter are extremely uncommon, but position of the tip within the superior vena cava or upper right atrium must be confirmed radiologically as complications of mal-position do occur.[108,109] Rarely, even these small, soft, cannula can erode through the atrial wall causing tamponade.[110]

When it is impossible to introduce a fine Silastic catheter from a peripheral vein, a tunnelled silicone rubber catheter of the type first described by Broviac should be surgically inserted under general anaes-thesia.[111] These inert and flexible silicone rubber catheters have bore sizes ranging from 0.5 to 1.0 mm; a Dacron cuff helps fixation. The catheter was later modified by Hickman and colleagues, creating a larger lumen with a selection of diameters from 1.6 to 2.6 mm. There are now a range of radio-opaque silicone elastomer catheters of this type available.

Insertion is usually via the internal jugular vein but other sites including the femoral vein may be used.[112] The catheter tip should be in the SVC or right atrium, but not close to the tricuspid valve. Skin tunnelling does not appear to reduce the risk of catheter sepsis,[113] but helps prevent dislodgement and allows the catheter to exit at a convenient point. In a girl baby this should be away from the area of future breast development. An inter-scapular exit site may decrease the risk of catheter removal in the mobile and inquisitive toddler. Per-cutaneous placement via the subclavian vein is possible using a Seldinger technique,[114] but serious compli-cations such as pneumothorax are more likely to occur than when a direct surgical approach is employed.

Silicone elastomer catheters are still those most widely used for paediatric parenteral nutrition,[115] but a range of polyurethane catheters are also available and may be associated with a lower incidence of complications. Double- and triple-lumen catheters are not usually necessary unless additional intravenous therapies are being given. Totally implantable venous access devices with subcutaneous reservoir (e.g. Portacath, Portex Ltd, Hythe, Kent, UK) are commonly used in the treatment of oncology and cystic fibrosis patients,[116] but there is relatively little experience with them in PN. They are very expensive for short-term use and if catheter blockage occurs they are more difficult to flush than an external device.

Catheter complications

Catheter sepsis

Sepsis remains the most common and serious problem related to use of central venous catheters.[117] Catheter sepsis should be suspected in a patient with evidence of infection but with no obvious focus. In infants and children, catheter sepsis is more common than in adults and may be associated with non-specific features such as fever, unstable blood glucose, low platelet count, vomiting or diarrhoea. Other sites of possible infection such as urinary tract or CSF must always be considered. Peripheral blood cultures are nearly always positive. Whilst coagulase negative staphylococci are the most common infecting agent in adults, during long-term PN in infants Gram negative may be as common as Gram positive isolates.

Since episodes of suspected sepsis are often not related to catheter infection, it is important to try to establish a firm diagnosis before needlessly removing a catheter. Blood taken from both the catheter and a peripheral vein at the same time can be cultured and the colony count from identical blood volumes compared. A ten-fold excess in the through-line culture indicates catheter infection rather than contamination or non-catheter related bacteraemia.[118,119] The identification of organisms in a through-catheter blood sample using acridine orange is a quick, simple and sensitive test for catheter sepsis.[120]

When a child with a central venous catheter becomes acutely unwell with hypotension, shock or evidence of septic emboli, the catheter must be removed and treat-ment given with antibiotics. If the illness is less severe, a decision about maintaining central venous access must be made. For example, in a preterm infant on short-term PN it may be prudent to remove the catheter at the first suspicion of sepsis rather than await bacterial confirmation. In a child with short-bowel syndrome requiring prolonged PN, however, it is justi-fied to make every attempt to save the catheter.

Following blood cultures, PN can be continued via the catheter which is also used for giving treatment with a first line antibiotic combination of vancomycin and aztreonam until culture and sensitivities are known.

parenterally fed piglets[151] and 10 mg/kg body weight three times a day given orally has reversed cholestasis in some children on long-term PN.[152]

Particulate contamination of PN solutions

Parenteral fluids are known to contain microparticulate matter[153] derived from the packaging and administration systems and from chemical interaction between components. Clinical effects include peripheral vein thrombophlebitis[103] and pulmonary arteritis.[153,154] Attention has been drawn to the possible role of particulate contaminants acting as condensation nuclei for microthrombi which then play an important role in the pathology of adult-type respiratory distress syndrome and multiple organ failure.[155]

Quality standards for acceptable levels of particulate contamination have been set for large- and small-volume parenterals, but none exist for administration systems. In-line filtration appears to be a sensible precaution in children receiving long-term parenteral fluids, and a 0.22 micron pore size filter should be used with amino acid/dextrose solution. A 1.2 micron filter is now available for filtering lipid emulsion and may have a role in long-term PN, although the additional cost during short-term PN seem difficult to justify.

Psychosocial development

Failure to provide parenterally fed infants with some oral stimulation often leads to severe feeding difficulties and food rejection at a later stage. This can be prevented to some extent by offering comforters and, when feasible, a variety of foods of different tastes and textures. The advice of a speech and language therapist should be sought at an early stage.

The hours of isolation and separation from parents endured by young children receiving long-term PN in hospital are often associated with some degree of psycho-motor retardation. This can be minimised by encouraging parents to visit as often as possible and nominating a permanent member of staff to become the main care giver on the ward. Play and occupational therapists can provide further stimulation.

Mobility is important and can be achieved by attaching infusion pumps to the baby buggy, and by heparin-locking the central venous catheter during the day. Home PN allows children to grow and develop normally with their families,[156,157] although some may show persistent perceptual-motor deficit.[158] Other serious complications of intravenous therapy such as infection are also less common at home than in hospital.

Outcome

The technical problems providing PN, even for long periods, have to a great extent been solved. Further refinements will require careful prospective studies. The high incidence of major thromboembolic complications reported from some centres during long-term feeding is worrying and requires further investigation. Specifying the benefits of PN except for certain conditions where enteral feeding is precluded[159,160] remains problematical, not least because of the difficulty in defining 'expected outcome', particularly in the premature infant. For example, should PN prevent malnutrition, promote normal growth, or influence the underlying disease?

Although it is tempting to think that feeding practices (including the greater use of PN) must have played some role in the great improvement in prognosis over recent years for premature infants,[161] many other factors are also involved. A retrospective study in babies weighing less than 1000 g showed that male gender and chronic lung disease were associated with increased mortality, but only in those infants given PN.[162]

Finding the most rational use of PN in the paediatric population therefore constitutes a continuing clinical challenge. The importance of nutritional influences in early life on adult disease[163] and neuro-development[34] means that long-term outcome will be a key area of investigation in years to come. With moves towards early, aggressive implementation of parenteral nutrition support in the premature infant such studies are urgently needed.[164]

References

1. Boyle R. *Some Considerations Touching the Usefulness of Experimental Natural Philosophy*. Henry Hall, Printer to the University, Oxford, 1664; pp. 52–55.

2. Cosnett JE. The origins of intravenous fluid therapy. *Lancet* 1989; **1:** 768–771.

3. Wretlind A. Total parenteral nutrition. *Surg Clin North Am* 1978; **58**: 1055–1070.

4. Helfrick FW, Abelson NM. Intravenous feeding of a complete diet in a child: a report of a case. *J Pediatr* 1944; **25**: 400–403.

5. Wilmore DM, Dudrick SJ. Growth and development of an infant receiving all nutrients by vein. *J Am Med Assoc* 1968; **203**: 860–864.

6. Heird WC. Parenteral feeding. In: Sinclair JC, Bracken MB (eds) Effective care of the newborn infant. Oxford University Press, Oxford, 1992; pp. 141–160.

7. Oliva PB. Lactic acidosis. *Am J Med* 1970; **48**: 209–225.

8. Sahebjami H, Scalettar R. Effects of fructose infusion on lactate and uric acid metabolism. *Lancet* 1971; **1**: 366–369.

9. Duffy B, Gunn T, Collinge J, Pencharz P. The effect of varying protein quality and energy intake on the nitrogen metabolism of parenterally fed very low birth-weight (less than 1600g) infants. *Pediatr Res* 1981; **15**: 1040–1044.

10. Johnson JD, Albritton WL, Sunshine P. Hyper-ammonaemia accompanying parenteral nutrition in newborn infants. *J Pediatr* 1972; **81**: 154–161.

11. Heyman MB, Klein GL, Wong A *et al.* Aluminum does not accumulate in teenagers and adults on pro-longed parenteral nutrition containing free amino acids. *J Parent Enter Nutr* 1986; **10**: 86–87.

12. Puntis JWL, Ball PA, Preece MA, Green A, Brown GA, Booth IW. Egg and breast milk based nitrogen sources compared. *Arch Dis Child* 1989; **64**: 1472–1477.

13. McIntosh N, Mitchell V. A clinical trial of two amino acid solutions in neonates. *Arch Dis Child* 1990; **65**: 692–699.

14. Hallman M, Bry K, Hoppu K, Lappi M, Pohjavuori M. Inositol supplementation in premature infants with respiratory distress syndrome. *New Engl J Med* 1992; **326**: 1233–1239.

15. Lacey JM, Crouch JB, Benfell K *et al.* The effects of glutamine-supplemented parenteral nutrition in premature infants. *J Parenter Enter Nutr* 1996; **20**: 74–80.

16. Moukarzel AA, Goulet O, Salas JS *et al.* Growth retardation in children receiving long-term total parenteral nutrition: effects of ornithine α-keto-glutarate. *Am J Clin Nutr* 1994; **60**: 408–413.

17. Rubecz I, Mestyan J, Varga P, Klujber L. Energy metabolism, substrate utilisation and nitrogen balance in parenterally fed postoperative neonates and infants. *J Pediatr* 1981; **98**: 42–46.

18. Macfie J, Smith R, Hill GL. Glucose or fat as a non-protein energy source? A controlled clinical trial in gastroenterological patients requiring intravenous nutrition. *Gastroenterology* 1981; **80**: 103–107.

19. Nose O, Tipton JR, Ament ME, Yabuuchi H. Effect of the energy source on changes in energy expenditure, respiratory quotient, and nitrogen balance during total parenteral nutrition in children. *Pediatr Res* 1987; **21**: 538–541.

20. Geggel HS, Ament ME, Heckenlively JR, Martin DA, Kopple JD. Nutritional requirement for taurine in patients receiving long term parenteral nutrition. *New Engl J Med* 1985; **312**: 142–146.

21. Kelly DA, Coe AW, Shenkin A, Lake BD, Walker-Smith JA. Symptomatic selenium deficiency in a child on home parenteral nutrition. *J Pediatr Gastroent Nutr* 1988; **7**: 783–786.

22. Sedman AB, Klein GL, Merritt RJ *et al.* Evidence of aluminum loading in infants receiving intravenous therapy. *N Engl J Med* 1985; **312**: 1337–1343.

23. Bishop NJ, Morley R, Day JP, Lucas A. Aluminum neurotoxicity in preterm infants receiving intravenous-feeding solutions. *N Engl J Med* 1997; **336**: 1557–1561.

24. Fell JME, Reynolds AP, Meadows N *et al.* Manganese toxicity in children receiving long-term parenteral nutrition. *Lancet* 1996; **347**: 1218–1221.

25. Moukarzel AA, Song MK, Buchman AL *et al.* Excessive chromium intake in children receiving total parenteral nutrition. *Lancet* 1992; **339**: 385–388.

26. Gale R, Gale J, Branski D, Armon Y, Zellingher J, Roll D. An interactive microcomputer program for calculation of combined parenteral and enteral nutrition for neonates. *J Pediatr Gastroent Nutr* 1983; **2**: 653–658.

27. Puntis JWL. Establishing a nutritional support team. *Baillières Clinical Paediatrics* 1997; **5**: 177–188.

28. Meadows N. Home parenteral nutrition in children. *Baillières Clinical Paediatrics* 1997; **5**: 189–199.

29. Heird WC, Driscoll JM, Schullinger JN, Grebin B, Winters RW. Intravenous alimentation in pediatric patients. *J Pediatr* 1972; **80**: 351–372.

30. Touloukian RJ. Isosmolar coma during parenteral alimentation with protein hydrolysate in excess of 4 mg/kg/day. *J Pediatr* 1975; **86**: 270–273.

31. Olney JW, Ho OL, Rhee V. Brain damaging potential of protein hydrolysates. *New Engl J Med* 1973; **289**: 391–395.

32. Holliday MA. Metabolic rate and organ size during growth from infancy to maturity and during late gestation and early infancy. *Pediatrics* 1971; **47**: 169–179.

33. Georgieff MK, Hoffman JS, Pereira GR, Bernbaum K, Hoffman-Williamson M. Effect of neonatal caloric deprivation on head growth and 1-year developmental status in preterm infants. *J Pediatr* 1985; **107:** 581–587.

34. Morley RT, Lucas A. The influence of early diet on outcome in pre-term infants. In: Davies DP (ed) *Nutrition in Child Health.* Royal College of Physicians of London, London, 1995; pp. 67–75.

35. Stoch MB, Smythe PM. 15-year study on the effects of severe under-nutrition during infancy on subsequent physical growth and intellectual functioning. *Arch Dis Child* 1976; **51:** 327–336.

36. Peters O, Ryan S, Matthew L, Cheng K, Lunn J. Randomised controlled trial of acetate in preterm neonates receiving parenteral nutrition. *Arch Dis Child* 1997; **77:** F12–F15.

37. Eyal F, Sagi E, Arad I, Avital A. Necrotising entero-colitis in the very low birthweight infant: expressed breast milk compared with parenteral feeding. *Arch Dis Child* 1982; **57:** 274–276.

38. Glass J, Hume R, Lang MA, Forfar JO. Parenteral nutrition compared with transpyloric feeding. *Arch Dis Child* 1984; **59:** 131–135.

39. LaGamma EF, Ostertag SG, Birenbaum H. Failure of delayed oral feedings to prevent necrotising entero-colitis. *Am J Dis Child* 1985; **139:** 385–389.

40. Hughes CA, Dowling RH. Speed of onset of adaptive mucosal hypoplasia and hypofunction in the intestine of parenterally fed rats. *Clin Sci* 1980; **59:** 317–327.

41. Hughes CA, Prince A, Dowling RH. Speed of change in pancreatic mass and in intestinal bacteriology in parenterally fed rats. *Clin Sci* 1980; **59:** 329–336.

42. Hughes CA, Talbot RC, Ducker DA, Harran MJ. Total parenteral nutrition in infancy: effect on the liver and suggested pathogenesis. *Gut* 1983; **24:** 241–28.

43. Dunn L, Hulman S, Weiner J, Kleigman R. Beneficial effects of early hypocaloric enteral feeding on neonatal gastrointestinal function: preliminary report of a randomized trial. *J Pediatr* 1988; **112:** 622–629.

44. Slagel TA, Gross SJ. Effect of early enteral substrate on subsequent feeding tolerance. *J Pediatr* 1988; **113:** 526–531.

45. Lucas A, Bloom SR, Aynsley-Green A. Metabolic and endocrine effects of depriving preterm infants of enteral nutrition. *Acta Paediatr Scand* 1983; **72:** 245–249.

46. Ball PA, Candy DCA, Puntis JWL, McNeish AS. Portable bedside microcomputer system for manage-ment of parenteral nutrition in all age groups. *Arch Dis Child* 1985; **60:** 435–439.

47. Wormleighton C. Give infants IV feeds safely. *Pharmacy in Practice* 1997; May: 256–260.

48. Cade A, Thorp H, Puntis JWL. Does the computer improve nutritional support of the newborn? *Clinical Nutrition* 1997; **16:** 19–23.

49. Hughes CA. Parenteral nutrition. In: Insley J, Wood B (eds) *A Paediatric Vade-Mecum*, 10th edn. Lloyd-Luke, London, 1982; pp. 60–67.

50. Schreiner RL, Glick MR, Nordschow CD, Gresham EL. An evaluation of methods to monitor infants receiv-ing intravenous lipids. *J Pediatr* 1979; **94:** 197–200.

51. Bisset WM, Stapleford P, Long S, Chamberlain A, Sokel B, Milla PJ. Home parenteral nutrition in chronic intestinal failure. *Arch Dis Child* 1992; **67:** 109–114.

52. Pollard AJ, Sreeram N, Wright JG, Beath SV, Booth IW, Kelly DA. ECG and echocardiographic diagnosis of pulmonary thromboembolism associated with central venous lines. *Arch Dis Child* 1995; **73:** 147–140.

53. Smith DE, Booth IW. Nutritional assessment of children: guidelines on collecting and interpreting anthropometric data. *J Hum Nutr Dietet* 1989; **2:** 217–224.

54. Tanner JM, Frisancho A. New norms of upper limb fat and muscle areas for assessment of nutritional status. *Am J Clin Nutr* 1981; **34:** 2540–2545.

55. Sasanow SR, Georgieff MK, Pereira GR. Mid-arm circumference and mid-arm/head circumference ratios: standard curves for anthropometric assessment of neonatal nutritional status. *J Pediatr* 1986; **109:** 311–315.

56. Wales JKH, Milner RDG. Knemometry in assessment of linear growth. *Arch Dis Child* 1987; **62:** 166–171.

57. Weil WB, Balie MD. Fluid and electrolyte metabolism in infants and children: a unified approach. Grune & Stratton, New York, 1977; p. 33.

58. Binder ND, Raschko PK, Benda CI, Reynolds JW. Insulin infusion with parenteral nutrition in extremely low birthweight infants with hyperglycaemia. *J Pediatr* 1989; **14:** 273–280.

59. Zlotkin SH, Stallings VA, Pencharz PB. Total parenteral nutrition in children. *Pediatr Clin N Am* 1985; **32:** 381–400.

60. Rigo J, Senterre J, Putet G, Salle B. A new amino acid solution specially adapted to preterm infants. *Clin Nutr* 1987; **6:** 105–109.

61. Pohlandt F, Wagner M, Rhein R, Obladen M. A new amino acid solution for the parenteral nutrition of preterm and term neonates, and infants. *Infusiontherapie* 1990; **17:** 40–46.

62. Burger U, Wolf H, Bauer M. Development of a pediatric amino acid solution for premature and full-term newborn infants based on phamacokinetic considerations. *Infusiontherapie* 1978; **5:** 254–260.

63. Heird WC, Dell RB, Helms RA *et al.* Amino acid mixture designed to maintain normal plasma amino acid patterns in infants and children requiring parenteral nutrition. *Pediatrics* 1987; **80:** 401–408.

64. Van Goudoever JB, Sulkers EJ, Timmerman M *et al.* Amino acid solutions for premature neonates during the first week of life: the role of N-acetyl-L-cysteine and N-acetyl-L-tyrosine. *J Parent Ent Nutr* 1994; **18:** 404–408.

65. Macfie J, Holmfield JH, King RF, Hill GL. Effect of the energy source on changes in energy expenditure and respiratory quotient during total parenteral nutrition. *J Parent Enter Nutr* 1983; **7:** 1–5.

66. Tulikoura I, Huikuri K. Morphological fatty changes and function of the liver, serum free fatty acids, and triglycerides during parenteral nutrition. *Scand J Gastroenterol* 1992; **17:** 177–185.

67. Lima LAM, Murphy JF, Stansbie D, Rowlandson P, Gray OP. Neonatal parenteral nutrition with a fat emulsion containing medium chain triglycerides. *Acta Paediatr Scand* 1988; **77:** 332–339.

68. Shenna AT, Bryan MH, Angel A. The effect of gestational age on Intralipid tolerance in newborn infants. *J Pediatr* 1977; **91:** 134–137.

69. Andrew G, Chan G, Schiff D. Lipid metabolism in the neonate. I: The effects of Intralipid infusion on plasma triglyceride and free fatty acid concentrations in the neonate. *J Pediatr* 1976; **88:** 273–278.

70. Olegard R, Gustafson A, Kjellmer I, Victorin L. Nutrition in low-birth-weight infants. III: lipolysis and free fatty acid elimination after intravenous administration of fat emulsion. *Acta Paediatr Scand* 1975; **64:** 745–751.

71. Dhanireddy R, Hamosh M, Sivasubramanian KN, Chowdhry P, Scanlon JW, Hamosh P. Post-heparin lipolytic activity and Intralipid clearance in very low birthweight infants. *J Pediatr* 1981; **98:** 617–622.

72. Coran AG, Edward B, Zaleska R. The value of heparin in the hyperalimentation of infants and children with a fat emulsion. *J Pediatr Surg* 1974; **9:** 725–732.

73. Palmblad J. Intravenous lipid emulsions and host defense: a critical review. *Clin Nutr* 1991; **10:** 303–308.

74. Chawla RK, Berry CJ, Kutner MH, Rudman D. Plasma concentrations of transsulfuration pathway products during nasoenteral and intravenous hyperalimentation of malnourished patients. *Am J Clin Nutr* 1985; **42:** 577–584.

75. Penn D, Schmidt-Sommerfeld E, Pascu F. Decreased carnitine concentrations in newborn infants receiving total parenteral nutrition. *Early Hum Dev* 1979; **4:** 23–28.

76. Helms RA, Whitington PF, Mauer EC, Catarau EM, Chistensen ML, Borum PR. Enhanced lipid utilization in infants receiving oral L-carnitine during long-term parenteral nutrition. *J Pediatr* 1986; **109:** 984–988.

77. Starisnsky R, Shatrir E. Displacement of albumin-bound bilirubin by free fatty acids: implications for neonatal hyperbilirubinaemia. *Clin Chim Acta* 1970; **29:** 311–318.

78. Brans YW, Ritter DA, Kenny JD, Andrew DS, Dutton EB, Carrillo DW. Influence of intravenous fat emulsion on serum bilirubin in very low birthweight neonates. *Arch Dis Child* 1987; **62:** 156–160.

79. Pereira GR, Fox WWE, Stanley CA, Baker L, Schwartz JG. Decreased oxygenation and hyperlipidaemia during intravenous fat infusions in premature infants. *Pediatrics* 1980; **66:** 26–30.

80. Lloyd TR, Boucek MM. Effect of Intralipid on the neonatal pulmonary bed: an echocardiographic study. *J Pediatr* 1986; **108:** 130–133.

81. Prasertsom W, Phillipos EZ, Van Aerde JE, Robertson M. Pulmonary vascular resistance during lipid infusion in neonates. *Arch Dis Child* 1996; **74:** F95–F98.

82. Puntis JWL, Rushton DI. Pulmonary intravascular lipid in neonatal necropsy specimens. *Arch Dis Child* 1991; **66:** 26–28.

83. Murphy S, Craig DQM, Murphy A. An investigation into the physical stability of a neonatal parenteral nutrition formulation. *Acta Paediatr* 1996; **85:** 1483–1486.

84. Cooke RWI. Factors associated with chronic lung disease in preterm infants. *Arch Dis Child* 1991; **66:** 776–779.

85. Pitkanen O, Hallman M, Andresson S. Generation of free radicals in lipid emulsion used in parenteral nutrition. *Pediatr Res* 1991; **29:** 56–59.

86. Hagemen JR, McCullock K, Gora P, Olsen EK, Pachman L, Hunt CE. Intralipid alterations in pulmonary prostaglandin metabolism and gas exchange. *Crit Care Med* 1983; **11:** 794–798.

87. Hammerman C, Aramburo MJ. Decreased lipid intake reduces morbidity in sick premature neonates. *J Pediatr* 1988; **113:** 1083–1088.

88. Gilbertson M, Kovar IZ, Cox DJ, Crowe L, Palmer NT. Introduction of intravenous lipid administration on the first day of life in the very low birthweight neonate. *J Pediatr* 1991; **119:** 615–623.

89. Alwaidh MH, Bowden L, Shaw B, Ryan SW. Randomised trial of effect of delayed intravenous lipid administration on chronic lung disease in preterm neonates. *J Pediatr Gastroent Nutr* 1996; **22:** 303–306.

90. Koo WWK, Tsang RC, Succop P, Krug-Wispe SK, Babcock D, Oestreich AE. Minimal vitamin D and high calcium and phosphorus needs of preterm infants receiving parenetral nutrition. *J Pediatr Gastroenterol Nutr* 1989; **8:** 225–233.

91. Poole RL, Rupp CA, Kerner JA. Calcium and phosphorus in neonatal parenteral nutrition solutions. *J Parenter Enter Nutr* 1983; **7:** 358–360.

92. Pelegano JF, Rowe JC, Carey DE *et al.* Effect of calcium/phosphorus ratio on mineral retention in parenterally fed premature infants. *J Pediatr Gastroent Nutr* 1991; **12:** 351–355.

93. Hanning RFM, Atkinson SA, Whyte RK. Efficacy of calcium glycerophosphate vs conventional mineral salts for total parenteral nutrition in low-birth-weight infants: a randomized clinical trial. *Am J Clin Nutr* 1991; **54:** 903–908.

94. MacMahon P, Mayne PD, Blair M, Pope C, Kovar IZ. Calcium and phosphorus solubility in neonatal intravenous feeding solutions. *Arch Dis Child* 1990; **65:** 352–353.

95. Greene HL, Hambidge KM, Schanler R, Tsang RC. Guidelines for the use of vitamins, trace elements, calcium, magnesium and phosphorus in infants and children receiving total parenteral nutrition: a report of the Subcommittee on Pediatric Parenteral Nutrient Requirements from the Committee on Clinical Practice Issues of the American Society for Clinical Nutrition. *Am J Clin Nutr* 1988; **48:** 1324–1342.

96. Moore MC, Greene HL, Phillips B *et al.* Evaluation of a pediatric multiple vitamin preparation for total parenteral nutrition in infants and children. I: Blood levels of water-soluble vitamins. *Pediatrics* 1986; **77:** 539–547.

97. Greene HL, Courtney Moore ME, Phillips B *et al.* Evaluation of a pediatric multiple vitamin preparation for total parenteral nutrition. II: Blood levels of vitamins A, D and E. *Pediatrics* 1986; **77:** 539–547.

98. Shenai JP, Kennedy KA, Chytil F, Stahlman MT. Clinical trial of vitamin A supplementation in infants susceptible to bronchopulmonary dysplasia. *J Pediatr* 1987; **111:** 269–277.

99. Klein GL. Aluminium in parenteral products: medical perspective on large and small volume parenterals. *J Parent Sci Tech* 1989; **43:** 120–124.

100. Hambidge KM, Sokol RJ, Fidanza FJ, Goodall MA. Plasma manganese concentrations in infants and children receiving parenteral nutrition. *J Parent Enter Nutr* 1989; **13:** 168–171.

101. von Stockhausen HB. Selenium in total parenteral nutrition. *Biol Trace Elem Res* 1988; **15:** 147–155.

102. Goutail-Flaud MF, Sfez M, Berg A *et al.* Central venous catheter-related complications in newborns and infants: a 587–case survey. *J Pediatr Surg* 1991; **26:** 645–650.

103. Falchuk KH, Peterson L, McNeil BJ. Microparticulate induced phlebitis. *New Engl J Med* 1985; **312:** 78–82.

104. Khwaja HT, Williams JD, Weaver PC. Transdermal glyceryl trinitrate to allow peripheral total parenteral nutrition: a double blind placebo controlled feasibility study. *J Roy Soc Med* 1991; **84:** 69–72.

105. Madan M, Alexander DJ, McMahon MJ. Influence of catheter type on occurrence of thrombophlebitis during peripheral intravenous nutrition. *Lancet* 1992; **339:** 101–103.

106. Puntis JWL. Percutaneous insertion of central venous feeding catheters: the first choice in paediatric parenteral nutrition. *Intens Ther Clin Monit* 1987; **8:** 7–10.

107. Shaw JCL. Parenteral nutrition in the management of sick, low birthweight infants. *Pediat Clin North Am* 1973; **20:** 333–358.

108. Rushforth A, Green MA, Levene MI, Puntis JWL. Subdural fat emulsion complicating parenteral nutrition. *Arch Dis Child* 1991; **66:** 1350–1351.

109. Rubin S, Hewson P, Roberton NRC. Pulmonary complications of total parenteral nutrition in a neonate. *J Roy Soc Med* 1986; **79:** 545–547.

110. Cade A, Puntis JWL. Cardiac tamponade in a neonate. *Clin Nutr* 1997; **16:** 19–23.

111. Broviac JW, Cole JJ, Scribner BH. A silicone rubber atrial catheter for prolonged parenteral alimentation. *Surg Gynecol Obstet* 1973; **136:** 602–606.

112. Jewett TC. Techniques with catheters and complications of total parenteral nutrition. In: Lebenthal E (ed) *Total Parenteral Nutrition*. Raven Press, New York, 1986; pp. 185–206.

113. Keohane PP, Attrill H, Northover J, Jones BJM, Cribb A, Frost P. Effect of catheter tunnelling and a nutrition nurse on catheter sepsis during parental nutrition. *Lancet* 1983; **2:** 1388–1390.

114. Eichelberger MR, Rous PG, Hoelzer DG, Garcia VF, Everett Koop C. Percutaneous subclavian venous catheters in neonates and children. *J Pediatr Surg* 1981; **16:** 547–553.

115. Editorial: Central venous access in children. *Lancet* 1991; **338:** 1301–1302.

116. Essex-Cater A, Gilbert J, Robinson T, Littlewood JM. Totally implantable venous access systems in paediatric practice. *Arch Dis Child* 1989; **64:** 119–123.

117. Decker DM. Central venous catheter infections. *Pediatr Clin N Am* 1988; **35:** 579–612.

118. Raucher HS, Hyatt AC, Barzilai A *et al*. Quantitative blood cultures in the evaluation of septicaemia in children with Broviac catheters. *J Pediatr* 1984; **104:** 29–33.

119. Fan ST, Teoh-Chan CH, Lau KF. Evaluation of central venous catheter sepsis by differential quantitative blood cultures. *Eur J Clin Microbiol Infect Dis* 1989; **8:** 142–144.

120. Rushforth JA, Hoy C, Kite P, Puntis JWL. Rapid diagnosis of central venous catheter infection. *Lancet* 1993; **342:** 402–403.

121. Yao JDC, Arkin CF, Karchmer AW. Vancomycin stability in heparin and total parenteral nutrition solutions: a novel approach to therapy of central venous catheter-related infections. *J Parent Enter Nutr* 1992; **16:** 268–274.

122. Goulet O, Larchet M, Gaillard JL *et al*. Catheter-related sepsis during long-term parenteral nutrition in paediatric gastroenterology patients: a study of 185 consecutive central venous catheters. *Clin Nutr* 1990; **9:** 73–78.

123. Flynn PM, Shenep JL, Stokes DC, Barrett FF. *In situ* management of confirmed central venous catheter-related bacteraemia. *Pediatr Infect Dis J* 1987; **6:** 729–734.

124. Puntis JWL, Holden CE, Smallman S, Finkel Y, George RH, Booth IW. Staff training: a key factor in reducing intravascular catheter sepsis. *Arch Dis Child* 1991; **66:** 335–337.

125. Winthrop AL, Wesson DE. Urokinase in the treatment of occluded central venous catheters in children. *J Pediatr Surg* 1984; **19:** 536–538.

126. Haire WD, Lieberman RP. Thrombosed central venous catheters: restoring function with a 6–hour urokinase infusion after failure of bolus urokinase. *J Parent Enter Nutr* 1991; **16:** 129–132.

127. Pennington CR, Pithie AD. Ethanol lock in the management of catheter occlusion. *J Parent Enter Nutr* 1987; **11:** 507–508.

128. Duffy LF, Kerzner B, Gebus V. Treatment of central venous catheter occlusions with hydrochloric acid. *J Pediatr* 1989; **114:** 1102–1104.

129. Sandilands D. The disappearing feeding line: some recent experiences. *Intens Ther Clin Monit* 1989; **9:** 209.

130. Mocellin R. Transluminal extraction of catheter fragments from the heart and pulmonary artery in children. *Zeit Kinderchir* 1987; **42:** 343–345.

131. Gladman G, Sinha Λ, Sims DG, Chiswick ML. Staphylococcus epidermidis and retention of neonatal percutaneous central venous catheters. *Arch Dis Child* 1990; **65:** 234–235.

132. Dollery CM, Sullivan ID, Bauraind O, Bull C, Milla PJ. Thrombosis and embolism in long-term central venous access for parenteral nutrition. *Lancet* 1994; **344:** 1043–1045.

133. Auty B. Choice of instrumentation for controlled IV infusion. *Intens Ther Clin Monit* 1989; **10:** 117–122.

134. Auty B. Advances in infusion pump design. In: Rennie M (ed) *Intensive Care Britain 1991*. Greycoat Publishing, London, 1992; pp. 95–102.

135. Infusion equipment. In: Rennie M (ed) *Intensive Care Britain 1991*. Greycoat Publishing, London, 1992; pp. 138–143.

136. Merritt RJ. Cholestasis associated with total parenteral nutrition. *J Pediatr Gastroent Nutr* 1985; **5:** 9–22.

137. Beale EF, Nelson RM, Bucciarelli RL, Donnelly WH, Eitzman DV. Intrahepatic cholestasis associated with parenteral nutrition in premature infants. *Pediatrics* 1979; **64:** 342–347.

138. Pereira GR, Sherman MS, DiGiacomo J, Ziegler M, Roth K, Jacobowski D. Hyperalimentation-induced cholestasis. *Am J Dis Child* 1981; **135:** 842–845.

139. Dunn L, Hulman S, Weiner S, Kliegman R. Beneficial effects of early hypocaloric enteral feeding on neonatal gastrointestinal function: preliminary report of a randomised trial. *J Pediatr* 1988; **112:** 622–629.

140. Wolf A, Pohlandt F. Bacterial infection: the main cause of acute cholestasis in newborn infants receiving short-term parenteral nutrition. *J Pediatr Gastroent Nutr* 1989; **8:** 297–303.

141. Clayton PT, Bowron A, Mills KA, Massoud A, Casteels M, Milla PJ. Phytosterolemia in children with parenteral nutrition-associated cholestatic liver disease. *Gastroenterology* 1993; **105:** 1806–1813.

142. Cooper A, Betts JM, Pereira GR, Ziegler MM. Taurine deficiency in severe hepatic dysfunction complicating total parenteral nutrition. *J Pediatr Surg* 1984; **19:** 462–465.

143. Farrell MK, Balistreri WF, Suchy FJ. Serum sulfated lithocholate as an indicator of cholestasis during parenteral nutrition in infants and children. *J Parent Enter Nutr* 1982; **6:** 30–33.

144. Fouin-Fortunet, Le Quernec L, Erlinger S, Lerebours E, Colin R. Hepatic alterations during total parenteral nutrition in patients with inflammatory bowel disease: a possible consequence of lithocholate toxicity. *Gastroentrology* 1982; **82:** 832–837.

145. Dorvil NP, Yousef IM, Tuchweber B, Roy CC. Taurine prevents cholestasis induced by lithocholic acid sulfate in guinea pigs. *Am J Clin Nutr* 1983; **37:** 221–232.

146. Belli DC, Fournier L-A, Lepage G, Yousef IM, Roy CC. The influence of taurine on the bile acid maximum secretory rate in the guinea pig. *Pediatr Res* 1988; **24:** 34–37.

147. Guertin F, Roy CC, Lepage G, Perea A, Giguere R, Yousef I, Tuchweber B. Effect of taurine on total parenteral nutrition-associated cholestasis. *J Parent Enter Nutr* 1991; **15:** 247–251.

148. Thornton L, Griffin E. Evaluation of a taurine containing amino acid solution in parenteral nutrition. *Arch Dis Child* 1991; **66:** 21–25.

149. Mashako MNL, Cezard J-P, Boige N, Chayvialle JA, Bernard C, Navarro J. The effect of artificial feeding on cholestasis, gall-bladder sludge and lithiasis in infants: correlation with plasma cholecystokinin levels. *Clin Nutr* 1991; **10:** 320–327.

150. Rintala RJ, Lindahl H, Pohjavuori M. Total parenteral nutrition-associated cholestasis in surgical neonates may be reversed by intravenous cholecystokin: a preliminary report. *J Pediatr Surg* 1995; **30:** 827–830.

151. Duerksen DR, Van Aerde JE, Gramich L *et al.* Intravenous ursodeoxycholic acid reduces cholestasis in parenterally fed newborn piglets. *Gastroenterology* 1996; **111:** 1111–1117.

152. Spagnuolo MI, Iorio R, Vegnente A, Guarino A. Ursodeoxycholic acid for treatment of cholestasis in children on long-term total parenteral nutrition: a pilot study. *Gastroenterology* 1996; **111:** 716–719.

153. Puntis JWL, Wilkins KM, Ball PA, Rushton DI, Booth IW. Hazards of parenteral therapy: do particles count? *Arch Dis Child* 1992; **67:** 1475–1477.

154. Garvan JM, Gunner BA. The harmful effects of particles in intravenous fluids. *Med J Aust* 1964; **11:** 1–5.

155. Kirkpatrick CJ. Aspects of the pathogenesis of multiple organ failure. *EEC Internat* 1990; **2:** 177–182.

156. Armanath RP, Fleming CR, Perrault J. Home parenteral nutrition in chronic intestinal disease: its effect on growth and development. *J Pediatr Gastroentrol Nutr* 1987; **6:** 89–95.

157. Ralson CW, O'Connor MJ, Ameny M, Berquist W, Parmalee AH. Somatic growth and developmental functioning in children receiving prolonged home parenteral nutrition. *J Pediatr* 1984; **105:** 842–846.

158. O'Connor MJ, Ralston CW, Ament ME. Intellectual and perceptual-motor performance of children receiving prolonged home total parenteral nutrition. *Pediatrics* 1988; **81:** 231–236.

159. Wilmore DW. Factors correlating with a successful outcome following extensive intestinal resection in newborn infants. *J Pediatr* 1972; **80:** 88–95.

160. Goulet OJ, Revillon Y, Jan D *et al.* Neonatal short bowel syndrome. *J Pediatr* 1991; **119:** 18–23.

161. Georgieff MK, Mills MM, Lindeke L, Iverson S, Johnson DE, Thompson TR. Changes in nutritional management and outcome of very-low-birthweight infants. *Am J Dis Child* 1989; **143:** 82–85.

162. Unger A, Goetzman BW, Chan C, Lyons AB, Miller MF. Nutritional practice and outcome of extremely premature infants. *Am J Dis Child* 1986; **140:** 1027–1033.

163. Barker DJP, Osmond C. Infant mortality, childhood nutrition, and ischaemic heart disease in England and Wales. *Lancet* 1986; **1:** 1077–1081.

164. Heird WC, Gomez MR. Parenteral nutrition. In: Tsang RC, Lucas A, Uauy R, Zlotkin S (eds) *Nutritional Needs of the Preterm Infant.* Williams and Wilkins, London, 1993; pp. 225–242.

27

Home parenteral nutrition

Barry Jones

Introduction

Provision of parenteral nutrition at home Home Parenteral Nutrition (HPN) allows release from the hospital environment for those patients unable to gain their independence through adequate gastrointestinal function. The sole indications for HPN are partial or complete intestinal failure such that nutritional needs, including electrolytes and water, can only be satisfied by partial or total PN. HPN is a versatile therapy. Short-term release from hospital increases the flexibility of other treatments such as chemotherapy, or surgery to reconstitute bowel continuity. Medium-term HPN provides time for the adaptive response to occur in those with short bowel syndrome (SBS). Long-term HPN is the only choice for those whose absorptive capacity will never return. Although small bowel transplantation is becoming a more successful treatment in children in whom HPN may be limited by hepatic complications and vascular access, survival rates in adults are not yet good enough to present a routine alternative to HPN.[1]

HPN remains a complex, dangerous and expensive therapy. It follows that the provision of HPN must be based on proper indications and provided by an efficient and effective team in partnership with patient and carers. The risks of complications must not outweigh the benefits and the costs of HPN should be less than continuing in-patient care.

Historical aspects

It was not long after the first attempts to parenterally feed in-patients that the technique was extended to out-patients. Initially, the multi-bottle systems were cumbersome and impractical. In the 1970s, cyclical feeding with diurnal catheter heparin locking became the norm. By 1986, 90% of European patients were receiving 'All-in-One' solutions of up to 3 l/day. This development was a prerequisite for overnight cyclical feeding or ambulant (portable) systems and gave patients the freedom to return to normal daily activities, work and travel.[2] Subsequent developments have focused on:

- Refining venous access.
- The impact of novel substrates on gut adaptation.
- Long-term nutrient deficiency and excess.
- HPN-related liver disease and metabolic bone disorders.

- Extending HPN to all those who might benefit.
- Ethical considerations.
- Patient support groups.

Epidemiology and indications

The incidence and prevalence of HPN have increased greatly. Major differences have been identified in the incidence and prevalence of HPN in different countries (Table 27.1), and even in the distribution of HPN within individual countries.

Table 27.1 – Prevalence of HPN in different countries: 1997[★]

Country	Point prevalence/million
USA	30–40[†]
Denmark	12.7
Scotland	10[‡]
UK	3.7
The Netherlands	3.7
France	3.6
Belgium	3.0
Poland	1.1
Spain	0.65

★ Derived from ESPEN Home Artificial Nutrition Group survey.[6] Data limited to above European countries by incomplete reporting.
† Usually quoted as a yearly prevalence of 120/million. Point prevalence estimated by Howard.[5]
‡ Personal communication, C.R. Pennington, Scottish Managed Clinical Network.

Between 1989 and 1992, Medicare funded HPN in the USA rose from 4500 to 10 000 patients per year but these represented only a small proportion of the total of 40 000 at that time. By contrast, in the UK yearly prevalence rates rose from 232 in 1996 to 317 in 1999. When expressed in terms of the population served, there are staggering differences between the USA and UK. Thus the yearly USA prevalence rose from 80/million in 1987 to 120/million by 1992, cancer and HIV representing 75% of the growth. In the UK, prevalence was only 2/million in 1993, rising to 3.7/million in 1997 and 8/million in 1998.[3]

Hospital cost shifting towards cheaper home-based care, increased numbers of homecare companies, smaller hospitals feeding small numbers of HPN patients, the influence of insurance companies and poor patient selection have been suggested as causes.[4,5]

In Canada and Europe, the increase in expertise and experience of established centres, the good overall survival rates of HPN in non-malignant, non-AIDS diseases and the cost effectiveness of HPN compared to in-patient care have been offset by careful patient selection and financial restrictions.

Cancer is the predominant indication for HPN in the USA and Europe as a whole (Fig. 27.1a), but is the least common in Canada, Ireland, Denmark and the UK (Fig. 27.1b). By comparison, Crohn's disease is the most frequent indication for HPN in the UK and Canada. There are clear differences in the approach to HPN in the care of cancer patients in the USA (40%), France (27%), Germany (78%), Sweden (80%) and Holland (60%) compared to the UK (5%).[4,6] Mesenteric infarction, scleroderma and other malabsorption syndromes, radiation enteritis and pseudo-obstruction (neuropathic, myopathic and mitochondrial) comprise the remainder.[7] In the USA, the contribution of cancer rose from 16% to 39% in 1991. Recent data points to a fall in AIDS patients, reflecting improvements in the treatment of AIDS.[6] Otherwise, the common indications for HPN remain stable. It could be argued that national and international reporting systems have led to more HPN being reported but it has proved very difficult to obtain complete national data on HPN patients.

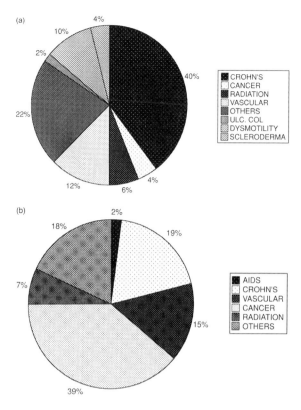

Figure 27.1 – Indications for HPN in the UK, 1998 (a) and in Europe, 1997 (b).

Practical considerations

The insertion of a cuffed, tunnelled Hickman or Broviac style catheter must be performed by an experienced operator under sterile conditions. Silicone rubber or polyurethane catheters are preferred over polyvinylchloride lines, which are associated with a higher incidence of central vein thrombosis.[8,9] The siting of the exit point must take account of handedness, adequate neck flexion, stomas and fistulae, hirsute and sweaty areas and the neckline, especially in women. Tunnelled femoral lines should only be used as a last resort. The Dacron cuff should be placed close to the exit point so that fibroblastic activity can lead to fixation of the line and sealing of the tunnel.

A dry non-occlusive dressing changed every 48 hours is preferred except when showering, bathing or swimming, when an occlusive transparent dressing can be used. Such dressings have been associated with increased sepsis and are best avoided in the immuno-suppressed and febrile, or when the site is moist. The line should be dedicated to HPN alone and must have NO taps. Multilumen lines are also best avoided for long-term HPN but may offer advantages in the short term with concurrent chemotherapy. The use of closed Luer lock devices with a self-sealing membrane allows access to the catheter whilst maintaining a closed system. Although they save nursing and HPN patient time, they do not obviate the need for strict asepsis.

The use of antiseptic spray or solutions to sterilise the catheter hub and connections as well as the skin are essential.[9] Alcohol should be avoided on polyurethane tubes.

Route of administration

The predominant administration route remains a catheter with an external section. Subcutaneous ports were used by only 9% of HPN patients in 1999[7] and are preferred by some patients because of the freedom to swim and bath. When sepsis occurs, removal of the implanted port and line is mandatory.

Pumps

All patients should be protected during infusion by a suitable pump with appropriate warning devices. The pumps should also be as light and robust as possible. Commercial companies supplying the HPN feed and pump should provide an efficient breakdown service. An easily portable stand suitable for use around the home is available from the British patients' organisation PINNT (Patients on Intravenous and Nasogastric Nutritional Therapy, PO Box 3126, Christchurch, Dorset, BH23 2XS). An ambulatory system, which fits into a small backpack, allows patients to continue feeding away from home.

Complications of home parenteral nutrition

HPN shares all the complications of PN as discussed in Chapter 25. However, the long-term nature of HPN brings specific problems. These can limit the success of HPN, impact on quality of life and prognosis for survival. HPN patients also have to cope with the natural history of their underlying disease and its complications.

HPN complications can be divided into the following categories (Table 27.2):

- Line related.
- HPN feed related.
- Underlying disease related.
- Associated drug therapies.

Catheter-related sepsis

This remains the commonest complication of HPN but affects some patients more than others, particularly smokers[10] and intravenous drug misusers.[11] Prerequisites for an independent sepsis-free existence are good eye–hand coordination, motivation, social

Table 27.2 – Complications of HPN

Line-related complications (see elsewhere)

HPN feed-related complications
Central vein thrombosis
Macro- and micro-nutrient excess
Macro- and micro-nutrient deficiency
Hepatobiliary dysfunction:
    Steatosis
    Fibrosis or cirrhosis
    Calculous or acalculous cholecystitis
    Cholestasis
Metabolic bone disorders related to underlying disease:
    Pre-existing osteomalacia
    Secondary or tertiary hyperparathyroidism
    Osteoporosis
Metabolic bone disorder related to HPN:
    Vitamin D-induced osteomalacia
    Aluminium induced
    Excess phosphate
    Magnesium or calcium deficiency with secondary
      hyperparathyroidism
    Osteoporosis
    Vitamin K deficiency
Psychological
Ethical

Underlying disease-related complications
Short bowel syndrome related:
    Water, electrolyte and divalent cation losses
    Inappropriate fluid replacement
    Renal impairment
    Gastrointestinal acid–base losses
    Blind loop syndrome/bacterial overgrowth
Fistulae
Obstruction
Intercurrent surgery
Natural history of disease, e.g. cancer, HIV

Associated drug therapy
Corticosteroids and immunosuppressants
Opiates – intravenous drug misuse carries adverse prognosis
HRT
Octreotide
Antibiotics
Proton pump inhibitors

circumstances or community support and proper training for patients and carers. Meticulous attention to asepsis is required, particularly with regard to the catheter hub as described elsewhere. In patients who suffer repeated infections, the use of antibiotic locks with vancomycin 50 mg or taurolin, a non-toxic antimicrobial, can be effective.[12] Observation of the patient in the home whilst setting up or disconnecting from the feeding line can be invaluable. Telemedicine may have a valuable role in overcoming technical problems and providing psychological support.

The treatment of line and insertion site sepsis is referred to in Chapter 29.

Line or hub fracture

These should always be dealt with urgently by the patient and the line clamped before seeking help from the patient's support centre. Line repair prevents unnecessary line replacement but carries a risk of infection. Line fracture almost always occurs outside the tunnel but the trend to clear and sample blocked lines with fine brushes might increase the risk of perforation within the tunnel. Patients travelling abroad should be trained in repair techniques and carry a repair kit.

Tunnel swelling

Tunnel swelling during feeding is usually a sign of occlusive fibrotic or thrombotic sleeve formation over the catheter tip and extending back to the venous entry point. This can be difficult to solve.[13] Tunnel swelling with tenderness, rising temperature or exudate should lead to line removal, microbiological assessment, drainage of the tunnel abscess and antibiotics.

Central vein thrombosis (CVT)

CVT is a major threat to HPN patients.[14] Many of the patients on HPN have an underlying prothrombotic tendency as a result of inflammatory bowel disease, neoplastic disease or the cause of spontaneous mesenteric vascular occlusion. Superimposed on these factors are the specific risks of malnutrition such as essential fatty acid deficiency and hyperhomocysteinaemia.[15] Finally, HPN may also promote CVT through malpositioning of the catheter tip, catheter sepsis or high concentrations of glucose.[16,17] Many units advise long-term anticoagulation but the risks of heparin (osteoporosis and alopecia) make oral anticoagulation preferable. The absorption of warfarin occurs early in the small bowel but unpredictable gastric emptying and small bowel transit make for difficult control. Many patients also ingest variable amounts of vitamin K in their normal diet and receive HPN solutions containing vitamin K rendering anticoagulation difficult. Use of a vitamin K-free preparation avoids this problem. Another approach is to use low-dose warfarin in HPN patients with no pro-

thrombotic history.[18] As little as 1 mg/day may be sufficient to protect from CVT.

The ideal HPN prescription

HPN is provided exclusively by 'All-in-One Bags', although additional bags of saline may be required when travelling in hot climates. Many factors must be taken into account in each individual case. A balance must be struck between conflicting variables. Prescribing for HPN patients must aim to avoid:

- Instability and incompatibilities.
- Thrombogenesis.
- Line occlusion.
- Hepatobiliary and metabolic bone disorders.
- Inadequate or excessive fluid intake.
- Nutrient deficiency or excess.

Lipid promotes line occlusion but protects against major vein thrombosis associated with high concentrations of glucose. No more than 1 g lipid/kg/day is recommended to avoid hepatic complications.[19] Any reduction in lipid energy supply must not be offset by an increase in glucose content in excess of oxidative capacity or lead to inadequate overall energy intake. Since HPN bags are usually supplied fortnightly, nutrient interactions and instability must be avoided. The practice of using some lipid-free bags each week could theoretically lead to lipid- and glucose-related complications. The use of compartmentalised bags can significantly enhance the shelf-life of HPN feeds and reduce the need for additions by the patient.

Close monitoring of micronutrients allows detection of unusual complications but nutrition status is best assessed by weighing and subjective clinical assessment.[20] Selenium deficiency was identified as causing a painful skeletal myopathy at a time when negligble selenium was included in HPN.[21] Selenium-related fatal cardiomyopathy on HPN has also been reported.[22] At least 100 μg of selenium should be supplied daily.[23] More recently, neurological symptoms attributable to manganese deposition in the basal ganglia and high serum manganese levels have been described.[24] At St Mark's Hospital Intestinal Failure Unit, micronutrient deficiencies were identified in 33% on HPN but serious sequelae are uncommon.[25] Of those deficiencies identified, iron, folate, biotin and vitamin A deficiency were clinically evident. Biotin deficiency was associated with dry eyes, angular cheilitis and hair loss.

Hepatobiliary complications of long-term HPN

HPN is frequently associated with hepatobiliary complications. Italian experience indicates hepatic dysfunction in 57% and gallstones in 11%.[26] Cholestasis predominates in infants and children, steatosis and fibrosis in adults and biliary sludge is common in all age groups. Most patients on HPN have a minor degree of liver function test abnormality but some go on to develop serious, life-threatening problems, particularly in children.

Factors associated with hepatobiliary dysfunction in HPN are:

- Associated diagnoses often related to the primary diagnosis leading to HPN, e.g. primary sclerosing cholangitis and inflammatory bowel disease, gallstones and previous ileal resection for Crohn's disease, ongoing sepsis.

- Complications of short bowel syndrome.

- Nutrient excess or deficiency.

- Concomitant drugs, e.g. octreotide-related gallstones.

- Lack of enteral stimulation.

- Disturbances of bile acid metabolism.

Steatosis and steatohepatitis

It has long been known that glucose excess leads to steatosis. True **hyperalimentation** is now rare although the term lives on in North American literature. Steatosis occurs within a few days of starting PN and is a benign, reversible and non-progressive condition[27] occurring in 40%.[28] Impaired triglyceride excretion may contribute, as may essential fatty acid, carnitine and choline deficiency. Mild right upper quadrant tenderness due to hepatic enlargement is the only clinical manifestation. By contrast, steatohepatitis is associated with necro-inflammatory changes similar to those of the NASH (non-alcoholic steatohepatitis) syndrome.

Intrahepatic cholestasis

Intrahepatic cholestasis was first reported in 1971 and is a particular threat in infants and children but also has become recognised as a major problem in adults on HPN. In children, cholestasis can progress to cirrhosis rapidly. Up to 25% of HPN patients developed cholestasis in the European 1997 survey.[28] Messing's group reports 26% involvement at 2 years and 50% at 6 years, accounting for 22% HPN mortality in 90 HPN patients between 1985 and 1996.[19] The median age was 45 years (6–77). Indications for HPN differed from those in the UK, with mesenteric infarction (35%) and radiation enteritis (27%) predominating over Crohn's disease (10%). Cancer and HIV patients were excluded. HPN feeds comprised 20% fat emulsions containing n-6 rich long-chain triglyceride. Chronic cholestasis developed in 58 (65%) after a median of 6 months and 37 (45%) developed complicated HPN-related liver disease after 17 months. The histological findings were very similar to those of NASH syndrome, with fat deposition, ductular proliferation, portal inflammation, and bridging fibrosis which can evolve into cirrhosis. Microsteatosis and phospholipidosis require specific stains to avoid underestimation of these findings. Factors correlating with the development of HPN liver disease were chronic cholestasis or parenteral lipid intake of >1 g/kg/day. Chronic cholestasis was also associated with a bowel remnant <50 cm. The association with lipid in excess of 1 g/kg/day means that adult HPN patients should receive less than the commonly used 500 ml of 20% Intralipid/day. Excess carbohydrate was not a factor, as their patients received only 88±13% of basal energy expenditure from non-protein. Complicated liver disease can therefore occur despite hypocaloric HPN.

The accumulation of toxic bile acids such as glycolithocholic acid has led to treatment with ursodeoxycholic acid and taurine-enriched HPN, both of which have been shown to improve outcome. The absorption of ursodeoxycholic acid must be very suspect in those with interrupted enterohepatic bile acids circulation due to ileal resection. Antibiotic therapy with metronidazole or gentamicin has also proved of value, perhaps because of small bowel bacterial overgrowth or translocation of bacterial toxins into the portal circulation. For some, liver and small bowel transplantation may be the only option, particularly in children. The International Registry of Intestinal Transplantation reports 48% of the 260 combined liver–intestinal transplants were performed for severe liver disease on HPN.[29]

Biliary sludge and stones

HPN is frequently associated with abnormal gallbladder dilatation, acalculous cholecystitis, biliary sludge and gallstones. Development of sludge in 50%

of patients after 4–6 weeks of TPN has been demonstrated[19] and almost 100% after 6 weeks. Interestingly, the sludge disappeared 4 weeks after the withdrawal of HPN in all cases. The development of sludge is independent of calorie source. The role of ongoing enteral intake is critical in determining gall bladder function.

Most patients in the UK and in Europe are able to take some oral intake which may explain anecdotal evidence of the declining incidence of biliary problems in HPN patients in recent years. No controlled trials of HPN with and without enteral intake have been performed, although such a trial would be difficult to justify. There is, however, good evidence of the beneficial effect of cholecystokinin–octapeptide daily.[30] Ursodeoxycholic acid may also be protective but again there are no controlled trials in this field.

When HPN patients develop symptomatic gallstones, cholecystectomy can be very difficult in those who have undergone many previous laparotomies. Cholestatic HPN patients may need to have copper and manganese removed from their feeds, since these metals are excreted in bile.

Bone disorders and HPN

These can be a major cause of morbidity during HPN.[31,32] Pre-existing secondary hyperparathyroidism due to excessive calcium and magnesium losses compounded by vitamin D deficient osteomalacia may already coexist with osteoporosis. Attempts to correct these problems can often be frustrated by worsening bone symptoms as HPN becomes established and nutritional state improves. This has long been known as the 'paradox of rickets' in which the symptoms do not occur unless the patient is gaining weight and actively growing. The pain and tenderness of this condition in HPN are located in periarticular areas, which is atypical for symptomatic osteomalacia. It was recognised as long ago as 1981 that the pain of symptomatic bone disease settled with the withdrawal of TPN.[32a] This paradox has been the subject of much unresolved debate.

In the 1980s, aluminium toxicity was implicated, particularly in North America, but this theory was challenged by the Toronto group led by Jeejeebhoy.[33] He suggested that the extremely debilitating slow-onset bony pains experienced by their patients after 0.75–15.5 years of vitamin D-supplemented HPN might be due to vitamin D-induced osteomalacia

which recovered with the withdrawal of vitamin D. This disorder is characterised by:

- Osteomalacia, fractures and bone pain.

- A histological picture of inadequate bone mineralisation, increase in osteoid and reduced tetracycline uptake.

- Intermittent hypercalcaemia, hypercalcuria, loss of skeletal calcium.

- Low levels of parathyroid hormone (PTH).

- Low 1,25-dihydroxyvitamin D and normal plasma 25-hydroxyvitamin D.

The Toronto unit went on to show that their patients recovered clinically with up to 4.5 years of no vitamin D supplements. Calcium, phosphate and 25-hydroxyvitamin D did not change but spinal bone density, 1,25-dihydroxy vitamin D and parathormone levels normalised. It is postulated that in the absence of enteral calcium absorption, infusion of calcium and phosphorus in HPN renders the physiological role of vitamin D redundant.[34] However, not all patients develop this syndrome whilst receiving vitamin D. Jeejeebhoy recommends that vitamin D should be withdrawn if PTH and 1,25-dihydroxy vitamin levels fall with normal 25-hydroxy vitamin D levels.[34]

Recently, it has been suggested that a typical cyclical overnight HPN feeding pattern might suppress parathormone secretion which is mainly released at night (J. Shaffer, Personal communication).

Italian experience differs from the Canadian group, with no evidence of vitamin D induced bone disease.[35] This group undertook a longitudinal study of patients fed by HPN for <4 months and another group fed for >12 months. Bone turnover was initially hyperkinetic. After 6 months, these patients had normal bone resorption but normal to high bone formation. At a later stage beyond 1 year, resorption remained normal but bone formation had declined to low or low–normal rates. These findings were independent of concurrent steroid usage.

Osteoporosis

Many patients will also develop severe debilitating osteoporosis. Bone demineralisation occurred in 57% in an Italian study.[26] All parts of the skeleton are affected including the mandible, although Danish patients had similar dental and periodontal states as age-matched controls.[36] Previous steroid treatment, smoking, prolonged inactivity, hypogonadism in both sexes, excessive losses of calcium and magnesium all contribute to this problem. Magnesium deficiency inhibits parathormone secretion, thereby inhibiting calcium absorption from the gut, and requires energetic replacement. All patients entering an HPN programme should have their bone density assessed with dual spectrum densitometry (DEXA scanning). Steroid therapy should be minimised or withdrawn whenever possible. Smoking should be actively discouraged. Low-impact exercise can be promoted as energy and lean body mass return with nutritional repletion. Hormone replacement therapy should be advised for postmenopausal women and should be given as patches or depot injection to bypass un-predictable intestinal absorption. Raloxifene should be considered in those who cannot tolerate conventional HRT. Amenorrhoea usually resolves, often after many months, with increase in weight and resolution of the metabolic response to injury and sepsis. Apart from adequate replacement of calcium and magnesium and the above measures, more aggressive treatment may be required.[37] Bisphosphonates administered orally have variable absorption and are often poorly tolerated in HPN patients. In this situation, pamidronate 30–60 mg/month can be given intramuscularly[37] and is used for this purpose at Hope Hospital Intestinal Failure Unit (Salford, UK) (J. Shaffer, personal communication). Calcitonin is beneficial in sarcoidosis but has not been formally evaluated in HPN,[37] but this author has used nasal calcitonin to good effect.

Recent interest has centred on the role of vitamin K in bone metabolism. Chronic vitamin K deficiency may be implicated in osteoporosis in Crohn's disease. This situation could be exacerbated by the need to exclude vitamin K from HPN solutions in those maintained on warfarin which, unlike heparin, is not thought to promote osteoporosis. It may be necessary, in the future, to include small amounts of vitamin K in HPN and to adjust warfarin dosage accordingly.

Other causes of HPN-related bone disease are less well established. Copper, zinc and manganese deficiency states have been reported but do not conform to the pattern of HPN bone disorders in which no evidence of deficiency of these elements could be identified. Vanadium is of particular interest because of its ability to suppress PTH secretion.[37]

Elements which could be present in toxic concentrations in HPN fluids include cadmium, lead, mercury, strontium and aluminium. However, none of these have ever been found to be present in toxic amounts in **modern** HPN solutions.[37] When casein hydrolysates were used as a nitrogen source, aluminium was demonstrated to be present in increased amounts. Aluminium has been located at the ossification front of HPN patients' bones.[38] The substitution of amino acids for casein hydrolysates has led to a marked reduction in aluminium concentration in HPN solutions. The similarities between the osteomalacic form of renal dialysis bone disease are worth noting. Both are associated with painful metabolic bone disease characterised by normal or low levels of PTH; low serum 1,25-dihydroxy-vitamin D; a tendency towards hypercalcaemia; and stainable aluminium which interferes with the deposition of tetracycline and calcium at the ossification front. Aluminium can also inhibit PTH release. Both the renal and HPN aluminium-related bone disorders are now rare.

In summary, metabolic bone disease is a complex but common problem in HPN and can significantly detract from the quality of life achievable with long-term HPN.

Areas of controversy

Teams, specialist centres and small units

An absolute prerequisite for an HPN service is a properly constituted and functioning multidisciplinary nutrition support team (NST). Such a team must already have demonstrated its ability to provide in-patient parenteral nutrition to a high standard with minimal complications and to be competent in enteral feeding which can complement or obviate HPN in many cases. In the UK, the implementation of the 1992 King's Fund recommendation that all acute hospitals should have a functioning team had not been taken up by more than 41% in 1999.[7] In France, HPN is confined to 14 'approved' centres with a surprising degree of follow-up in primary care.[6] In Denmark, there is only one centre to which all patients are referred. In the UK, there are two nationally funded intestinal failure units subserving only 50% of the total HPN workload. The remainder is provided in up to 50 other centres.[3] Many of these care for no more than one or two patients sporadically. There is good evidence that such small centres have a worse record of complications than the larger centres where expertise and staffing ratios can be optimised.[7a] To date, only Scotland has attempted to rationalise this problem by setting up a managed clinical network involving all units providing HPN services. This network is supported at a national level and coordinated from a major centre. Inequity of access is thereby avoided. Common standards of care, audit, research and economies of scale can be addressed throughout the network. In the rest of the UK, there is evidence of inequity of access to HPN, the prevalence of which varies from region to region from 0 to 36/million.[3] This would suggest that not all patients who might benefit from HPN are being offered it. This might explain the poor representation of cancer as an indication for HPN in the UK. It is clear that both financial and structural organisation must be optimised for the adequate provision of HPN.

Quality of life, outcome and cost-effectiveness

The evidence base for HPN relies on the definition of intestinal failure as a condition incompatible with normal life span or quality. By definition, such patients would not survive without support so controlled clinical trials with a no HPN treatment arm are almost impossible to undertake.

Outcome depends on diagnosis.[5] BANS data for 1999 shows 76% continued to receive HPN at 1 year, 14% returned to oral intake and 7% died. Survival was best in Crohn's (96% at 1 year) and worst in cancer (35%).[7] Mortality rates in a European multicentre survey were Crohn's (4%), vascular diseases (13%) and radiation enteritis (21%), compared to cancer (74%). Interestingly, mortality in AIDS fell from 88% in 1993 to 34% in 1997.[6] Death on HPN is rarely HPN treatment related,[39] accounting for no more than 5% of deaths. The high mortality of cancer patients on HPN with survivals of only 4 months[5] pose difficult ethical dilemmas.[6] Many HPN patients return to oral intake or enteral nutrition. One year after starting HPN, BANS data records 14% as having returned to oral nutrition.[7] The highest rate of discontinuation of HPN is in Crohn's disease – 52%.[6]

HPN-related complication rates fall with experience. In Scotland, the major HPN centre in Dundee recorded a complication rate of 1 in 3.4 treatment years,[40] similar to those of the most experienced units in the UK. In the author's unit, with only 1000 patient weeks of experience, we recorded a line complication rate, including infection, of 1 in 1.93 treatment years.[41] The greater complication rates noted in small units in previous years will hopefully

decline with developments such as the Scottish Managed Clinical Network and 'hub and spoke' centres in the rest of the UK. However, the path to becoming an established HPN centre is not easy.[42,43]

Quality of life issues are of fundamental importance in assessing the value of HPN. Distinction should be drawn between malignant and non-malignant indications for HPN.[4,44,45] Functional data from The British Artificial Nutrition Survey (BANS)[7] shows that 99% of patients were outside hospital after 1 year of HPN. Very few were bed-bound (4.5% of patients >65 years) or housebound (3% of patients 16–64 years; 9% of 65–75 years). A minority required some help (14%) or total help (7%) with their HPN and 97.9% were in their own home after 1 year. Full activity was achieved in 70.4% of adults aged 16–64 years and in 36.4% aged 65–75. Formal assessment of qualify of life in British patients with benign disease has shown worse scores than for normals and that younger patients did better than older ones. Narcotic addiction scored badly. The majority felt too ill to work.[46] Another study found disappointing scores compared to patients with short bowel syndrome patients not on HPN.[47] These findings may reflect the greater degree of bowel symptomatology in the HPN group and do not accord with the experience of many other units.[46]

For patients with malignant conditions, the picture is both very different and controversial.[48] In the early days of HPN in the UK, it was felt that HPN should be used only in exceptional circumstances for malignancy.[49] Since then, the divergence of practice between the UK and Canada[39] on the one hand and the USA and mainland Europe on the other hand suggests that both extremes could be moderated. Howard alludes to the perverse incentives that have influenced HPN practice in the USA.[5] Most cancer patients on HPN are dead within 6 months to 1 year.[6,49–52] Adult cancer patients have the same rehospitalisation rates for HPN complications as radiation enteritis and Crohn's disease, but four times as many for the underlying disease.[51] Quality of life in those surviving >3 months is better than those surviving <3 months and in those with a Karnofsky score of >50% on starting HPN.[45] Use of HPN in those with high small bowel obstruction is potentially beneficial and can be combined with a drainage gastrostomy. Most patients so treated die at home, often within 2 months. Many will be young women with gynaecological cancers.[53] However, the treatment is regarded to be of benefit by the patients, their families and their medical carers.[53–55] Five-year survival of 'non-terminal' cancer was surprisingly high in the Mayo clinic series at 38%.[56] Whether short-term TPN or HPN is beneficial for transient intestinal failure during chemoradiotherapy remains controversial.[57]

Cost benefits of HPN

A number of studies attest to the cost-effectiveness of HPN when compared to in-patient costs.[2,46,58] Annual costs of adult HPN have been estimated at $150 000–$250 000 in the USA and £55 000 in the UK, representing 25–50% of in-hospital costs. Cost–utility appraisals in adults have shown the cost of one quality adjusted year to be £69 000 in the UK in 1995.[59] HPN is therefore a relatively cost-effective treatment.

Summary and key points

HPN is an established cost-effective treatment for intestinal failure. HPN should be provided by centres with adequate experience and an effective multi-disciplinary nutrition team. Avoidance of catheter-related sepsis, central vein thrombosis, metabolic bone disease and hepatobiliary complications permits an improved quality of life and prolonged survival. The implications of national differences in indications for HPN require further study, particularly with regard to cancer. Equity of access to HPN depends on improvement in organisation at a national level.

References

1. Messing B. Home parenteral nutrition. In: *Artificial Nutrition Support in Clinical Practice*, 1st edition. Arnold, London, 1995; pp 365–79.

2. Messing B, Landais P, Goldfarb B *et al*. Home parenteral nutrition for adults. Results of a multicentre survey in France. *Presse Med* 1988; **17:** 845–9.

3. Elia M, Russell C, Shaffer J *et al. Report of the British Artificial Nutrition Survey August 1999.* British Association of Parenteral and Enteral Nutrition, 1999.

4. Messing B, Lemann M, Landais P *et al*. Prognosis of patients with nonmalignant chronic intestinal failure receiving long-term home parenteral nutrition. *Gastroenterology* 1995; **108:** 1005–8.

5. Howard L. Home parenteral nutrition: a transatlantic view. *Clin Nutr* 1999; **18:** 131–3.

6. Van Gossum A, Bakker H, Bozzetti F *et al*. Home parenteral nutrition in adults: a European multicentre survey in 1997. *Clin Nutr* 1999; **18:** 135–40.

7. Elia M, Russell CA, Stratton RJ *et al. Trends in Home Artificial Nutrition Support in the UK during 1996–1999. A report by the British Artificial Nutrition Survey (BANS).* The British Association for Parenteral and Enteral Nutrition.

7a. Mughal M, Irving MH. Home PN in the United Kingdom and Ireland. *Lancet* 1986; **328:** 383–6.

8. Beau P, Matrat S. A comparative study of polyurethane and silicone cuffed-catheters in long term home parenteral nutrition patients. *Clin Nutr* 1999; **18:** 175–7.

9. Maroulis J, Kalfarentzos F. Complications of parenteral nutrition at the end of the century. *Clin Nutr* 2000; **19:** 295–304.

10. O'Keefe SJ, Burnes JU, Thompson RL. Recurrent sepsis in home parenteral nutrition patients: an analysis of risk factors. *J Parent Enteral Nutr* 1994; **18:** 256–63.

11. Richards DM, Scott NA, Shaffer JL, Irving MH. Opiate and sedative dependence predicts a poor outcome for patients receiving home parenteral nutrition. *J Parent Enteral Nutr* 1997; **21:** 336–8.

12. Pennington CR. Parenteral nutrition: the management of complications. *Clin Nutr* 1991; **10:** 133–7.

13. Ghosh A, Griffiths DM. Sleeve thrombus fibrosis causing neck pain. *J Parent Enteral Nutr* 2000; **24:** 180–2.

14. Dollery CM, Sullivan ID, Bauraind O, Bull C, Milla P. Thrombosis and embolism in long term central venous access for parenteral nutrition. *Lancet* 1994; **344:** 1043–5.

15. Compher CW, Kinosian B, Evans-stoner N, Huzineec J, Buzby GP. Hyperhomocysteinemia is associated with venous thrombosis in patients with short bowel syndrome. *J Parent Enteral Nutr* 2001; **25:** 1–8.

16. Beers TR, Burnes J, Fleming CR. Superior vena caval obstruction with gut failure receiving home parenteral nutrition. *J Parent Enteral Nutr* 1990; **14:** 474–9.

17. Bozzetti F, Seapra D, Terno G. Subclavian thrombosis due to indwelling catheters. A prospective study on 52 patients. *J Parent Enteral Nutr* 1983; **7:** 560–2.

18. Veerabagu MP, Tuttle-Newhall J, Maliakkal R, Champagne C, Mascioli EA. Warfarin and reduced venous thrombosis in home total parenteral nutrition patients. *Nutrition* 1995; **11:** 142–4.

19. Cavicchi M, Beau P, Crenn P, Degott C, Messing B. Prevalence of liver disease and contributing factors in patients receiving home parenteral nutrition for permanent intestinal failure. *Ann Intern Med* 2000; **132:** 525–32.

20. Egger NG, Carlson GL, Shaffer JL. Nutritional status and assessment of patients on home parenteral nutrition: anthropomometry, bioelectric impedance, or clinical judgement? *Nutrition* 1999; **15**: 1–6.

21. Mansell PI, Rawlings J, Allison SP, Shenkin A, Compton G, Beck S *et al*. Reversal of a skeletal myopathy with selenium supplementation in a patient on HPN. *Clin Nutr* 1987; **6**: 179–83.

22. Quercia RA, Korn S, O'Neill D *et al*. Selenium deficiency and fatal cardiomyopathy in a patient receiving long-term home parenteral nutrition. *Clin Pharmacol* 1984; **3**: 531–5.

23. Rannem T, Ladefoged K, Hylander E, Hegnhoj J, Jarnum S. Selenium depletion in patients on home parenteral nutrition. *Biol Trace Elem Res* 1993; **39**: 81–90.

24. Reynolds N, Blumsohn A, Baxter JP, Houston G, Pennington CR. Manganese requirement and toxicity in patients on home parenteral nutrition. *Clin Nutr* 1998; **17**: 227–30.

25. Forbes GM, Forbes A. Micronutrient status in patients receiving home parenteral nutrition. *Nutrition* 1997; **13**: 941–4.

26. Pironi L, Migliou M, Ruggeri E, Longo N, Surian I, Masselli S *et al*. Home parenteral nutrition for the management of chronic intestinal failure: A 34 patient–year experience. *Ital J Gastroenterol* 1993; **25**: 411–18.

27. Angelico M, Guardia D. Review article: hepatobiliary complications associated with total parenteral nutrition. *Aliment Pharmacol Ther* 2000; **14**: 54–7.

28. Shaffer J and ESPEN-HAN Group. A European survey on the management of metabolic complications in home parenteral nutrition. *Clin Nutr* 1997; **16**(suppl 2): 79.

29. Grant D. Intestinal transplantation: 1997 report of the International Registry. Intestinal Transplant Registry. *Transplantation* 1997; **67**: 1061–4.

30. Sitzman JV, Pitt HA, Steinhorn PA, Pasha ZR, Sanders RC. Cholecystokinin prevents parenteral nutrition induced biliary sludge in humans. *Surg Gynecol Obstet* 1990; **170**: 25–31.

31. Jeejeebhoy KN. Metabolic bone disease and total parenteral nutrition: a progress report. *Am J Clin Nutr* 1998; **67**: 186–7.

32. Klein GL. Metabolic bone disease of total parenteral nutrition. *Nutrition* 1998; **14**: 149–52.

32a. Klein GL, Horst RL, Norman AW, Ament ME, Slatapolsky E, Coburn JW. Reduced levels of 1,25-dihydroxyvitamin D during long term total parenteral nutrition. *Ann Int Med* 1981; **84**: 638–43.

33. Jeejeebhoy KN, Shike M, Sturtridge W *et al*. TPN bone disease at Toronto. In: Coburn JW, Klein GL (eds) *Metabolic Bone Disease in Total Parenteral Nutrition*. Urban and Schwarzenberg, Baltimore, 1985; pp 19–29.

34. Verhage AH, Cheong WK, Allard JP, Jeejeebhoy KN. Increase in lumbar spine bone mineral content in-patients on long-term parenteral nutrition without vitamin D supplementation. *J Parent Enteral Nutr* 1995; **19**: 431–6.

35. Pironi L, Zolezzi C, Ruggeri E, Paganelli F, Pizzoferrato A, Miglioli M. Bone turnover in short term and long term home parenteral nutrition for benign disease. *Nutrition* 2000; **16**: 272–7.

36. Von Wowern N, Klausen B, Hylander E. Bone loss and oral state in patients on home parenteral nutrition. *J Parent Enteral Nutr* 1996; **20**: 105–9.

37. Buchman AL, Moukarzel A. Metabolic bone disease associated with total parenteral nutrition. *Clin Nutr* 2000; **19**: 217–31.

38. Klein GL, Alfrey AC, Miller NL *et al*. Aluminium loading during total parenteral nutrition. *Am J Clin Nutr* 1982; **35**: 1425–9.

39. Howard L, Ament M, Fleming CR, Shike M, Steiger E. Current use and clinical outcome of home parenteral nutrition therapies in the United States. *Gastroenterology* 1995; **109**: 355–65.

40. Johnson DA, Pennington CR. Home parenteral nutrition in Tayside. *Scott Med J* 1993; **38**: 110–11.

41. Ransford RAJ, Jones BJM. A thousand weeks of home parenteral nutrition at a district general hospital in the UK. *Br J Intensive Care* 2000; **10**: 150–4.

42. Burgess P, Irving MH. Problems and organisation of a home parenteral nutrition service. *Baillière's Clin Gastroenterol* 1988; **2**: 905–14.

43. Jones BJM. Taking the tube home. *Nurs Times* 1998; **94**: 67–8.

44. Howard L, Heaphey L, Fleming CR, Lininger L, Steiger E. Four years of north American home parenteral nutrition outcome data and their implications for patient management. *J Parent Enteral Nutr* 1991; **15**: 384–93.

45. Cozzaglio L, Balzola F, Deciccio M *et al*. Outcome of cancer patients receiving home parenteral nutrition. Italian Society of Parenteral and Enteral Nutrition. *J Parent Enteral Nutr* 1997; **21**: 339–42.

46. Richards DM, Irving MH. Assessing the quality of life of patients with intestinal failure on home parenteral nutrition. *Gut* 1997; **40**: 218–22.

47. Jeppesen PB, Langholz E, Mortensen PB. Quality of life in patients receiving home parenteral nutrition. *Gut* 1999; **44**: 844–52.

48. Sharp JW, Roncagli T. Home parenteral nutrition in advanced cancer. *Cancer* 1993; *Pract* **1:** 119–24.

49. Stokes MA, Irving MH. Mortality in patients on home parenteral nutrition. *J Parent Enteral Nutr* 1989; **13:** 172–5.

50. Balzola F, Gallitelli L, Palmo A *et al.* Home parenteral nutrition (HPN) in adult patients: data from the Italian register. *Riv Ital Nutr Parenterale Enterale* 1992; **10:** 93–101.

51. Howard L. Home parenteral nutrition in patients with a cancer diagnosis. *J Parent Enteral Nutr* 1992; **16**(suppl): P93S–99S.

52. Jeppesen PB, Staun M, Mortensen PB. Adult patients receiving home parenteral nutrition in Denmark from 1991 to 1996: who will benefit from intestinal transplantation? *Scand J Gastroenterol* 1998; **33:** 839–46.

53. King LA, Carson LF, Konstantinides N *et al.* Outcome assessment of home parenteral nutrition in patients with gynaecologic malignancies: what have we learned in a decade of experience? *Gynecol Oncol* 1993; **51:** 377–82.

54. August DA, Thorn D, Fisher RL, Welchek CM. Home parenteral nutrition for patients with inoperable malignant bowel obstruction. *J Parent Enteral Nutr* 1991; **15:** 323–7.

55. Kirita T, Mabuchi G, Seshimo A *et al.* Evaluation of loco-regional cancer chemotherapy with assistance of home parenteral nutrition. *Gan To Kagaku Ryoho* 1992; **19**(suppl): 1709–12.

56. Scolapio JS, Fleming CR, Kelly DG, Wick DM, Zinsmeister AR. Survival of home parenteral nutrition-treated patients: 20 years of experience at the Mayo Clinic. *Clin Proc Mayo Clin* 1999; **74:** 217–22.

57. Klein S, Kinney J, Jeejeebhoy K *et al.* Nutrition support in clinical practice: review of published data and recommendations for future research directions. *J Parent Enteral Nutr* **21:** 133–56.

58. Detsky A, McLaughlin JR, Abrams H. A cost utility analysis of the HPN program at Toronto General Hospital 1970–1982. *J Parent Enteral Nutr* 1986; **10:** 49–57.

59. Puntis JW. The economics of home parenteral nutrition. *Nutrition* 1998; **14:** 809–12.

28

Nutrition and liver disease

Claire Wicks

Historical background

Patients with liver disease have presented nutritional problems since the condition was first recognised. In early descriptions patients were often portrayed as being 'sickly looking' with jaundiced skin, hollowed cheeks and wasted limbs. It is from such accounts that the first understanding of the importance of nutrition in the treatment of liver disease started to evolve. The many functions of the liver that are now understood were still largely unknown and the mechanisms by which these patients became malnourished and wasted, were similarly unknown.

Around 400 BC Hippocrates described the condition we now recognise as cirrhosis of the liver. He also stressed the importance of nutrition in the treatment of disease and believed that most diseases could be attributed to poor digestion. The first proper description of cirrhosis was probably given by John Browne in 1685 but it was Laennec (1781–1826) who first suggested the use of the word 'cirrhosis' to describe the diseased liver. Derived from the Greek word $K\iota\rho\rho\omega\sigma\iota\sigma$, meaning dead or damaged cells, it aptly describes the cirrhotic liver and for many years the term 'Laennec's cirrhosis' was used to define the micronodular cirrhosis typically seen in patients with chronic alcoholic liver disease.

Our knowledge of the influence of a malfunctioning liver on the nutritional state of the body is surprisingly small, as is our ability to effectively use nutritional intervention in the treatment of some of the consequences of liver disease.

In the early part of this century, interest in the role of nutrition in liver disease focused primarily on the notion that fundamental dietary constituents could modify or protect against acute experimental liver injury in animals. As more data accumulated, it became apparent that a combination of adequate body protein stores and energy (supplied principally in the form of carbohydrates) could serve to both protect and promote repair, following liver injury.[1] The extension of these approaches to the nutritional management of acute or chronic liver diseases in humans soon followed. It was considered that recovery from acute viral hepatitis could often be enhanced by a high fat diet,[2] whilst the outcome of chronic liver disease could be benefited by the supplemental supply of essential nutrients, in particular protein and B vitamins.[3]

As recently as the 1960s it was still widely accepted that malnutrition was largely responsible for the liver damage seen in alcoholism[4] and in malnourished populations. The terms 'nutritional' or 'dietary' liver injury and 'nutritional cirrhosis' were generally used. The belief that malnutrition was the cause of liver damage stemmed from:

- The high incidence of cirrhosis and primary hepatocellular carcinoma in malnourished populations

- The coexistence of malnutrition and liver damage in alcoholics

- The results of experiments in animals fed nutritionally deficient diets.

This belief was partly reinforced by the finding that fatty liver is associated with protein–energy malnutrition (PEM) in young children,[5] but it is rarely seen in children over the age of 10 or in adults, and that on refeeding a balanced diet, the liver returns to normal and there is no evidence of permanent liver damage or the development of cirrhosis.[6,7]

In industrialised countries, where malnutrition due to the unavailability of food is rare, the cause of liver disease was still often attributed to dietary deficiencies. Gradually it has become clear that, if malnutrition is not the primary cause but rather a consequence of liver disease, then some other factor must be responsible for the high incidence of unexplained cirrhosis in the poorer countries of the world. Viral hepatitis is common in Asia and Africa. Cirrhosis in the Bantu people is now largely attributed to excessive intake of alcohol and iron and/or unknown toxins present in native concoctions. Naturally occurring hepatotoxins have been identified in foods,[8] e.g. *mycetesmus choleriformis* poisoning from various species of mushroom[9] and pyrrolizidine alkaloids which are found in over 2000 species of plants in many parts of the world and are found in Jamaican 'bush teas'.[10,11] The contamination by mycotoxins, e.g. aflatoxin, of cheap (and frequently mouldy) foods in poverty stricken areas is common. The consumption of these toxins via the food supply may underlie the development of liver disease in many cases in these countries. Today, it is accepted that (apart from in kwashiorkor) malnutrition is not a primary causative factor in the development of liver disease but it will almost certainly contribute to morbidity and mortality.

Theoretical problems and benefits of support

Abnormalities in protein and energy metabolism occur frequently in chronic liver disease and may lead to 'constitutive' malnutrition even if the diet is generally adequate. Since many of the complications of liver disease (e.g. encephalopathy, sepsis and immunosuppression) are associated with concurrent negative nitrogen balance, nutritional therapy has been promoted as a means to correct malnutrition and thereby improve the clinical outcomes of patients with chronic liver disease. Unfortunately, the potential benefits of aggressive nutrition therapy in these patients remains a largely unproven and highly controversial area of clinical hepatology. These controversies persist for a number of reasons, which include: inadequately controlled studies, significant heterogeneity in the nutritional status of the patients with liver disease, the lack of an optimal reference standard for evaluating nutritional efficacy and an incomplete understanding of the pathophysiological processes responsible for the malnourished status of these patients.

The reported prevalence of PEM in chronic liver disease ranges widely, from 0–100% of the populations studied.[12–16] Much of this variation is probably explained by differences in the methods of assessment applied, the reference populations used, and the aetiology of the liver diseases in the patients studied. For example, Bunout et al.[14] and Mills et al.[15] compared their anthropometric values in patients with standards derived from a survey of military personnel in Turkey, Greece and Italy in 1961 for the design of protective clothing, whereas the reference standards used by Simko et al.[13] were derived from 20 non-alcoholics attending (for unstated reasons) a medical centre. Also, whereas the anthropometric measurements were carried out by a single observer in each of the studies by Simko et al.,[13] Bunout et al.[14] and Mills et al.,[15] the results of Mendenhall et al.[16] were obtained by at least six different investigators in different centres with no reported assessment of inter-observer variability. Furthermore, body weight was used as a nutritional index in these and other studies[17] whether or not patients had ascites, but only Mendenhall et al.[16] attempted to correct for this by estimating the weight of ascitic fluid (although it is not clear how this was done). Serum albumin was also used in the assessment of nutritional status in most of these studies even though this parameter is affected by the presence of ascites and the synthetic function of the liver.

Much of the evidence for malnutrition in liver disease has come from these and other studies on hospitalised patients with alcoholic liver disease. The Veterans Administration (VA) co-operative study on alcoholic hepatitis found that malnutrition was frequent and correlated with poor dietary intake and severity of liver dysfunction.[16] In hospitalised patients with less severe disease, evidence of protein malnutrition has been reported in 30–40% of cases.[12,13,18,19] Nevertheless, the available information suggests that malnutrition is also common in patients with other liver disorders, with reports of allergy to skin hypersensitivity tests in 60%, weight loss greater than 20% of the predicted value in 14%,[20] and deficiencies in fat soluble vitamins occurring in 40%.[12] In the latter study, dietary intake was found to be adequate and the vitamin deficiencies were reportedly not attributable to the mild to moderate steatorrhoea occurring in 50% of the patients. In a study by Morgan,[19] which included clinical grading of malnutrition, several anthropometric measurements, creatinine/height indices and assessment of dietary intakes found that 40% of patients with primary biliary cirrhosis (PBC) and 12% with chronic hepatitis were malnourished. Dietary intake, which is often affected by the nausea and anorexia accompanying liver diseases of any aetiology, was found to be within the normal range and was unrelated to the degree of malnutrition. Similar results were found by Wicks et al.[21] in a study of 80 patients with PBC, where 33% had some degree of malnutrition. These various studies suggest that the prevalence of malnutrition in liver disease is high, but that factors other than diminished dietary intake are involved and that variations with the aetiology of the disease may occur.

Several studies have examined the role of malnutrition as an independent risk factor for predicting clinical outcome in patients with chronic liver disease,[16,22–27] but it has been difficult to demonstrate a clear causal relationship between malnutrition and reduced survival in these patients, since there are usually multiple pathophysiological processes occurring simultaneously. Nutrition status was first used as a prognostic factor in the Child–Turcotte classification for estimating mortality in patients undergoing portacaval shunt surgery.[22] Qiao and co-workers,[27] in their epidemiological study, stressed the importance of malnutrition as a prognostic factor in non-surgical patients with liver disease. It has also been reported that patients with ascites treated by placement of a peritoneal venous shunt showed improved nutritional status and immune responsiveness as the ascitic fluid decreased,[24,25] and that evidence of malnutrition predicted altered immunity, greater susceptibility to infection, and increased mortality in hospitalised cirrhotic patients with ascites.[20,23,26]

Despite this it is only quite recently that any clinical value of nutritional intervention, in terms of altering the morbidity and mortality of these patients, has been demonstrated.[28,29] Two short-term studies suggest that nutrition intervention has a beneficial effect on morbidity and mortality. In the first, a significant improvement in mortality was seen in hospitalised, severely malnourished cirrhotics who were enterally fed.[30] In the second, Reilly and co-workers[31] demonstrated an improved nitrogen balance when post-transplant patients were given parenteral nutrition (PN) support. They noted that both duration of intubation and length of time under intensive care were reduced, and they attributed this to the improved nutrition status.

The pathogenesis of malnutrition in liver disease is unquestionably multifactorial, with several of the causes listed in Table 28.1 occurring, with varying degrees of severity, in an individual patient at any one time. A poor dietary intake would undoubtedly be an important risk factor for the development of mal-

Table 28.1 – Causes of malnutrition in liver disease.

1. *DECREASED ORAL INTAKE*
   (a) Anorexia, nausea, vomiting
   (b) Unpalatable diets
   (c) Purgation
   (d) Hospitalisation related

2. *IMPAIRED NUTRIENT DIGESTION AND ABSORPTION*
   (a) Pancreatic and bile salt deficiency
   (b) Enteropathy

3. *INCREASED ENERGY REQUIREMENTS*
   (a) Complications, e.g. ascites, infection
   (b) Energy cost of alcohol metabolism

4. *INCREASED PROTEIN LOSS*
   (a) Ascites
   (b) Impaired renal function
   (c) Intestinal bleeding
   (d) Gut fragility (protein-losing enteropathy)

5. *INCREASED PROTEIN BREAKDOWN*

6. *DECREASED PROTEIN SYNTHESIS*

nutrition in both hospitalised and out-patients with liver disease. The same can be said of the well recognised problems of impaired digestion, malabsorption and decreased hepatic storage. The instigation of early, aggressive nutrition support may well minimise the effects of the first three factors listed in Table 28.1.

Practical applications

Despite an adequate or good dietary intake and improved nutrient absorption, malnutrition may still be a problem in the cirrhotic patient. There is evidence to suggest that accelerated protein breakdown and poor protein synthesis are further contributory factors.[32] Early tracer studies utilising (^{14}C)tyrosine suggested that protein turnover was increased in cirrhotic patients, although an increase in protein breakdown was only seen in fulminant hepatic failure.[33,34] It should be stressed that the majority of protein kinetic studies have been performed during clinically stable periods when poor nutrition status is less likely to have been a problem. Abnormalities in protein metabolism certainly occur during periods of decompensation when poor nutrition intake,[35] diminished activity[36] and intercurrent illnesses[37] are more common. Additionally, episodes of acute tissue injury where the release of monocyte-derived cytokines occur may have an effect on protein metabolism.[38,39]

In summary, no consensus of opinion has been reached, but, the above evidence indicates that protein breakdown is increased in cirrhosis. Furthermore, this may occur in association with decreased protein synthesis and increased nitrogen loss. All of these factors indicate that severe protein restriction in patients with liver disease will do more harm than good; hence, such restrictive diets should be avoided. As a general guideline, protein requirements for patients with cirrhosis range between 0.8 g/kg and 1.2 g/kg 'dry' body weight. However, in a stress situation, e.g. alcoholic hepatitis or decompensated cirrhosis, requirements may be increased to 1.5–2.0 g/kg/day.

Energy expenditure, requirements and substrate utilisation

Disturbances in energy expenditure in patients with liver cirrhosis are not clearly understood.[40] Most studies using indirect calorimetry to measure energy expenditure have found no difference between cirrhotics and controls. The only exception is one study by Green and colleagues[41] which demonstrated an increased absolute energy expenditure in patients with primary biliary cirrhosis. However, three studies found an increase in energy expenditure[42–44] when results were expressed per unit of lean body mass (determined by urinary creatinine excretion). In primary biliary cirrhosis[41] and alcoholic hepatitis,[43] energy expenditure increases with worsening liver function. In contrast, energy expenditure decreases with the worsening function in alcoholic and post hepatic cirrhosis.[44] Therefore, if urinary creatinine excretion reflects total lean body mass, it appears that cirrhotics have increased resting energy expenditure, which correlates inconsistently with the severity of liver dysfunction and is dependent on the aetiology of liver disease. In addition, energy expenditure following glucose infusion[45] or a test meal is increased, indicating that diet-induced thermogenesis may be abnormally increased in cirrhosis.

There are inherent difficulties in the measurement of both lean body mass and energy expenditure which are compounded by differences within patient populations, such as sex, and type and stage of disease. These difficulties have been highlighted in a study of 123 patients being evaluated for liver transplantation.[46] In this heterogeneous group of patients, a wide range of energy expenditure was found with 18% of patients being hypermetabolic, 51% normometabolic and 31% hypometabolic. Energy expenditure correlated with fat free body mass rather than the type, duration or severity of liver disease. This suggests that hypermetabolism (whilst present in a proportion of patients) is not a constant feature of cirrhosis and maybe influenced more by extrahepatic than hepatic factors.

As a general guideline, 30–35 kcal/kg 'dry' body weight would seem appropriate for the maintenance of most patients with stable cirrhosis, whereas those with decompensated liver disease may require up to 45 kcal/kg 'dry' body weight.

Accurate calculation of a 'dry' body weight in patients with ascites and/or peripheral oedema is not possible but the following gives a very rough guide for the estimation of dry body weight.

- Guide for assessing weight of ascites
  Minimal   2.2 kg
  Moderate 6.0 kg
  Severe   14.0 kg

- Guide for assessing weight of peripheral oedema
  Mild   1.0 kg
  Moderate 5.0 kg
  Severe   10.0 kg

Regardless of the rate of energy expenditure, there is also a change in the preferred fuel substrate in cirrhotic patients when compared to normal controls. All of the studies shown in Table 28.2 reported a decrease in the respiratory quotient (RQ) after an overnight fast. This indicates that cirrhotics obtain approximately 75% of their calories from fat after an overnight fast compared to 35% for controls who would take approximately 48–72 hours of starvation to obtain the low RQ levels obtained after only 12–18 hours in cirrhotics.[44,46–49] This demonstrates the importance of frequent feeding and the avoidance of relatively short periods of starvation, an approach confirmed in a study where nitrogen balance was assessed in a group of cirrhotic patients who were fed the same amount of energy distributed over different time intervals.[50] Patients receiving a late evening snack were able to maintain a greater positive nitrogen balance than those that did not. Again, these studies were all carried out in stable cirrhotics, and account needs to be taken of evidence showing that the presence of either sepsis[51,52] or ascites[53] increases demands for energy.

Table 28.2 – Respiratory quotients in cirrhotic patients.

Study	Year	Cirrhotics (n)	Controls (n)
Owen et al.[47]	1983	0.74 ± 0.02 (9)	0.85 ± 0.02 (10)
Mullen et al.[48]	1986	0.75 ± 0.01 (6)	0.84 ± 0.03 (6)
Merli et al.[49]	1990	0.78 ± 0.04 (25)	0.87 ± 0.05 (10)
Schneeweiss et al.[44]	1990	0.72 ± 0.01 (22)	0.84 ± 0.01 (20)
Muller et al.[46]	1992	0.73 ± 0.02 (123)	0.83 ± 0.01 (30)

All respiratory quotients are corrected for urinary nitrogen excretion.
The results from the cirrhotics are significantly less than controls in all studies.

Assessment of nutrition status in liver disease

In view of the reported prevalence and risks associated with malnutrition in patients with liver disease, the ability to accurately assess and monitor nutrition status in this group is essential. Despite this, many of the traditional indices used in the assessment of nutrition status are frequently affected by the presence of liver disease. Deficiencies in specific nutrients may be masked by the effects of hepatic inflammation and, conversely, abnormalities caused primarily by liver injury may suggest depletion of body stores of a nutrient. An example of this situation exists when low levels of circulating proteins (such as albumin) are found in a patient with liver disease. The abnormality may be caused by a decrease in the intrinsic hepatic capacity for protein synthesis due to the liver disease, and not necessarily reflect visceral protein depletion. The four usual circulating plasma proteins utilised to monitor visceral protein stores (albumin, transferrin, prealbumin and retinol binding protein) are synthesised largely by liver cells. In one study, the circulating levels of these proteins did not correlate with the severity of malnutrition assessed by anthropometric methods but did correlate with the extent of liver injury.[54] It is likely that a combination of poor hepatic function and malnutrition may explain the hypoproteinaemia seen in advanced liver disease. In view of this, caution must be exercised when interpreting individual components of a nutrition assessment in patients with liver dysfunction and it is important to bear in mind the limitations of nutrition assessment imposed by the presence of liver disease.

Nutrition assessment should always include a complete dietary history, physical examination and evaluation of fat and protein stores. Such assessments are usually most accurately performed by an experienced dietitian. An appraisal of the patient's pre-admission nutrition intake for energy and nitrogen should highlight any pre-existing nutrition problems and emphasise any requirement for early supplementation of the diet. Continued assessment of oral intake during hospitalisation is important to monitor efficacy of any nutrition therapy and detect early deterioration in nutrition state. This can be done using standard food record charts which can be completed by the patient, relative or nurse. Whoever completes the chart must be made aware of the importance of accuracy and detail to ensure a correct and valuable assessment. From this macro- and micronutrient intakes can be assessed using a computer dietary analysis programme and the results compared with dietary reference values.[55]

Pronounced muscle wasting and loss of subcutaneous fat are obvious on physical examination but inter-observer variation and the inability to quantitate the losses can be problematic. Fat stores can be evaluated and quantified using upper arm anthropometry, whilst the somatic protein compartment can be assessed by the measurement of the mid-arm muscle circumference. Body weight may still be a useful marker but care must be taken as this measurement can provide erroneous results due to the presence of oedema (which may not be clinically apparent). The result is a potential underestimation of the severity of protein and fat losses.[56–58]

Nitrogen balance, plasma urea nitrogen, serum alpha-amino nitrogen and plasma amino acids are all markers that have been advocated in the assessment of protein nutrition status. In liver disease these indices are unreliable as impaired urea synthesis and intra- and extracellular accumulation of ammonia may considerably underestimate a negative or positive nitrogen balance and amino acid concentrations can alter dramatically in the presence of liver disease. In a recent study using a rat model it was reported that depressed amino acid concentrations were dependent on a decreased oral dietary intake, regardless of the presence of liver disease, whilst elevated concentrations of the aromatic amino acids were primarily determined by the severity of the liver injury.[59]

Assessment of body stores of micronutrients will also be affected by the presence of liver disease, in particular the fat soluble vitamins. Low vitamin A serum concentrations may be seen despite normal hepatic stores if hepatic synthesis of retinol-binding protein is impaired.[60] Vitamin E is transported in plasma bound to lipoproteins and normal or elevated serum concentrations of vitamin E can be found in hyperlipidaemia, such as that which occurs in cholestatic liver disease, despite subnormal vitamin E stores.[61,62]

New and more sophisticated techniques of measuring body composition are being developed. Such techniques include dual-energy X-ray absorptiometry (DEXA) and bioelectrical impedance analysis (BIA). DEXA was initially developed for the precise measurement of total bone mineral content but its ability to identify soft tissue and categorise it as fat or lean mass has created a potential use in determining the body composition of individuals. The initial drawbacks of this method are the need for expensive equipment and the high cost of performing the measurement. In addition, the technique has not been validated for many disease states.[63] A study by Wicks et al.[21] has demonstrated a good correlation between

DEXA and upper arm anthropometry in patients with primary biliary cirrhosis. BIA is a more convenient method of assessing body composition. This technique has been validated in many clinical settings but in liver disease its accuracy is poor due to varying states of hydration.[64,65]

Complications of liver disease and the nutrition implications

Ascites

For patients with ascites a low sodium diet should be instigated whether it be via the oral, nasogastric or intravenous route. The level of sodium restriction is dependent on the individual as these diets are generally unpalatable and frequently go uneaten. On the other hand an abdomen tense with ascites is uncomfortable and is frequently the cause of anorexia so should not go untreated. A sodium intake of around 40 mmol per day should be aimed for in the presence of gross ascites, 40–60 mmol in moderate ascites and 60–100 mmol in mild ascites. Good education and support with regular follow-up from an experienced dietitian is essential for the success of this difficult dietary restriction.

Encephalopathy

The nutritional management of encephalopathy is often controversial with some believing that protein should be withdrawn totally for the first 24–48 hours of treatment and then slowly reintroduced up to a maximum of 40 g per day. As discussed earlier in this chapter withdrawal of protein may be detrimental to the liver patient where requirements may be increased and synthesis decreased thus making the above practice both unsuitable and unsafe.

During periods of acute decompensation of liver disease and grade IV encephalopathy the patients should have their full protein requirements met via either a nasogastric or intravenous feed; restriction of protein is not recommended.

In the chronically encephalopathic patient some restriction of protein intake may be warranted. This should only be instigated after all other possible causes of encephalopathy have been investigated and either eliminated or treated. The nutrition status and dietary intake of the patient should be reviewed regularly and the restriction removed as soon as possible to prevent the development of protein energy malnutrition. If protein intake is distributed evenly throughout the day it is rarely necessary to reduce intake below 1 g/kg body weight.

The efficacy of branched-chain amino acids (BCAA) to reduce encephalopathy remains unclear. Many studies have been published on the use of BCAA supplemented feeds but results are often conflicting and no definite conclusions have been drawn as to the benefits concerning morbidity. However, it is thought that, by supplementing with BCAA, more nitrogen can be given to the patient without precipitating or worsening encephalopathy, but until further studies are done their use is probably not justified.

Jaundice and steatorrhoea

A patient with jaundice does not automatically require fat restriction, as is often mistakenly believed. The only time fat should be restricted is for the symptomatic relief from steatorrhoea. In this case the aim of the dietary treatment is to alleviate the diarrhoea and thereby maintain nutrition status by reducing malabsorption. It is not possible to specify a level of restriction as individuals vary in their ability to tolerate fat. Advice should therefore be given on an individual basis after taking a careful and detailed dietary history. Follow-up is also important to check the suitability of the level of restriction imposed. It is important to note that if fat is restricted energy intake will be reduced; patients must be advised on other suitable foods with which they can make up this deficit. This is most significant if the patient was underweight at presentation. Increasing both complex and refined carbohydrate in the diet will suffice but may make the diet bulky which is undesirable in the anorexic patient. The use of medium chain triglycerides (MCT) as a useful source of energy may be warranted in this situation. MCT is partially water soluble so does not require bile for emulsification therefore making it available to the cholestatic patient. In addition, it will improve the range and palatability of meals and variety of cooking methods.

Intramuscular injection of fat-soluble vitamins should be given regularly to all individuals with cholestasis, unless there is evidence that they are able to adequately absorb their oral intake. Calcium supplements may be required if cholestasis is prolonged. For patients who do not suffer from steatorrhoea fat provides a palatable and concentrated source of energy which should not be restricted unless absolutely necessary.

Acute liver failure

Acute liver failure is a rare disorder in which massive liver cell necrosis is rapidly followed by dysfunction in other systems – notably cardiovascular disturbance, marked coagulopathy, renal failure and cerebral oedema. In 1970 Trey and Davidson introduced the term fulminant hepatic failure (FHF) to describe patients without previous liver disease who have rapidly progressive liver failure with the onset of encephalopathy within eight weeks of the appearance of symptoms.[66] In the UK paracetamol hepatotoxicity following overdose is still the most common cause of FHF. Other aetiological factors include viral hepatitis and other drug-induced hepatic necrosis.

In 1973 the mortality rate in this group of patients was 80%, but over the last 20–25 years there has been a steady improvement in survival, with good survival rates now being achieved in some aetiological groups treated in specialist centres. With such improved prognosis due to better intensive care support, clearly the provision of good nutrition for these patients is of vital importance for hepatocyte regeneration and for the function of other organs and systems to be adequately maintained. The maintenance of a good nutrition state is also important because liver transplantation has become a viable clinical management option in these cases.[31,57,67]

Most patients are in good nutrition state prior to the onset of FHF but they rapidly become catabolic and develop protein–calorie malnutrition with muscle wasting becoming apparent within 7–10 days of the onset of liver failure. A major problem with these patients is how best to determine their nutrient requirements. Estimations of energy requirements can be made using tables to predict basal metabolic rate, which can then be adjusted to take account of the altered demands of the stressed or septic patient. The accuracy of these tables when applied to FHF is questionable but they remain useful in the absence of a suitable alternative.

The provision of nutrition support for these very unstable patients is also a challenge, because of problems with venous access, sepsis, deteriorating renal function and rapid haemodynamic changes. The enteral route for nutrition support should be used wherever possible. Where gastric emptying is delayed the use of a prokinetic agent may be all that is required in order to maintain enteral feeding. A standard whole protein, isotonic feed is suitable for the patient who does not require a fluid restriction. If fluid intake needs to be restricted, a high protein, high energy feed may be used in order to meet nutrition requirements.

Total parenteral nutrition (TPN) may be required if the enteral route cannot be maintained and this can be provided by the central or peripheral route. Energy should be provided from both fat[68] and carbohydrate sources. As haemodialysis is often required to combat the renal failure that occurs in many FHF patients and it has been shown that this leads to losses of up to 21% of the amino acids administered in parenteral feeding solutions,[69] care must be taken that adequate amounts of nitrogen are provided and that a low protein regimen is not administered despite encephalopathy.

Once patients are on the road to full recovery there is rarely a need for any dietary restriction. The aim at this stage is to restore good nutritional status using basic healthy eating principles.

Liver transplantation

There are significant nutrition differences between patients with acute and chronic liver disease presenting for transplant surgery. The majority of patients waiting for a transplant have chronic end-stage liver disease with the likelihood of poor nutrition status associated with advanced disease, as discussed earlier in this chapter. In contrast, patients with acute liver failure do not present with the wasting associated with chronic disease, but instead they are generally severely catabolic and often septic with a rapidly deteriorating nutrition state as reserves become depleted.

The relationship between malnutrition and patient survival following liver transplantation was evaluated by Shaw and co-workers.[70] The preoperative records of 160 adult liver transplant patients were retrospectively reviewed for the purposes of identifying characteristics that would predict survival within six months after surgery. The malnutrition score was based on general assessment of nutrition status and was one of six variables found to be highly correlated with patient survival. A randomised prospective study by Reilly et al.[31] evaluated the benefits of nutrition

49. Merli M, Riggio O, Romiti A *et al.* Basal energy production rate and substrate use in stable cirrhotic patients. *Hepatology* 1990; **12:** 106–112.

50. Swart GR, Zillikens MC, van Vuure JK *et al.* Effect of a late evening meal on nitrogen balance in patients with cirrhosis of the liver. *Br Med J* 1989; **299:** 1202–1203.

51. Cerra FB, Hirsch J, Mullen KD *et al.* The effect of stress level, amino acid formula and nitrogen retention in traumatic and septic stress. *Ann Surg* 1987; **205:** 282–287.

52. Novel O, Bernuau J, Rueff B *et al.* Hypoglycaemia. A common complication of septicemia in cirrhosis. *Arch Intern Med* 1981; **141:** 1477–1478.

53. Dolz C, Raurich JM, Ibanez J *et al.* Ascites increases the resting energy expenditure in liver cirrhosis. *Gastroenterology* 1991; **100:** 738–744.

54. Merli M, Romiti A, Riggio O *et al.* Optimal nutritional indexes in chronic liver disease. *JPEN* 1987; **11:** 130S–134S.

55. Department of Health. Dietary reference values for food, energy and nutrients for the United Kingdom. Her Majesty's Stationery Office (Reports on health and social subjects; 41), London, 1991.

56. Heymsfield SB, Casper K. Anthropometric assessment of the adult hospitalized patient. *JPEN* 1987; **11:** 36S–41S.

57. Shronts EP, Teasley KM, Thoele SL *et al.* Nutritional support of the adult liver transplant candidate. *J Am Diet Assoc* 1987; **87:** 441–451.

58. Shronts EP. Nutritional assessment of adults with end-stage hepatic failure. *Nutr Clin Pract* 1988; **3:** 113–119.

59. Benjamin IS, Engelbrecht G, Saunders S *et al.* Amino acid imbalance following portal diversion in the rat. *J Hepatol* 1988; **7:** 208–214.

60. Leo MA, Lieber CS. Hepatic vitamin A depletion in alcoholic liver injury. *N Engl J Med* 1982; **307:** 597–601.

61. Sokol RJ, Heubi JE, Iannoccone S *et al.* Vitamin E deficiency with normal serum vitamin E concentrations in children with liver disease. *N Engl J Med* 1984; **310:** 1209–1212.

62. Munoz SJ, Heubi J, Maddrey WC. Status of lipid soluble vitamins in primary sclerosing cholangitis. *Gastroenterology* 1989; **96:** A636.

63. Roubenoff R, Kehayias JJ, Dawson-Hughes B *et al.* Use of dual-energy x-ray absorptiometry in body-composition studies: not yet a 'gold standard'. *Am J Clin Nutr* 1993; **58:** 589–591.

64. McCullough AJ, Mullen KD, Kalhan SC. Measurements of total body and extracellular water in cirrhotic patients with and without ascites. *Hepatology* 1991; **14:** 1102–1111.

65. Zillikens MC, Van den Berg JW, Wilson JHP *et al.* Whole-body and segmental bioelectrical-impedance analysis in patients with cirrhosis of the liver: changes after treatment of ascites. *Am J Clin Nutr* 1992; **55:** 621–625.

66. Trey C, Davidson C. The management of fulminant hepatic failure. Grune and Stratton, New York, 1970, pp. 282–298

67. Hehir DJ, Jenkins RL, Bistrian BR *et al.* Nutrition in patients undergoing orthotopic liver transplant. *JPEN* 1985; **9:** 695–700.

68. Forbes A, Wicks C, Marshall W *et al.* Nutritional support in fulminant hepatic failure: The safety of lipid solutions. *Gut* 1987; **28:** 1347–1348.

69. Davies SP, Reaveley DA, Brown EA *et al.* Amino acid clearances and daily losses in patients with acute renal failure treated by continuous arteriovenous hemo-dialysis. *Crit Care Med* 1991; **19:** 1510–1515.

70. Shaw BW, Wood WP, Gordon RD *et al.* Influence of selected patient variables and operative blood loss on six-month survival following liver transplantation. *Semin Liver Dis* 1985; **5:** 385–393.

71. Oates JA, Wood AJJ. Cyclosporine. *N Engl J Med* 1989; **321:** 1725–1738.

72. Hasse JM. Nutritional implications of liver transplanta-tion. *Henry Ford Hosp Med J* 1990; **38:** 235–240.

73. Carroll PB, Boschero AC, Li MY *et al.* Effect of the immunosuppressant FK506 on glucose-induced insulin secretion from adult rat islet of Langerhans. *Transplantation* 1991; **51:** 275–278.

29

Nutrition support in trauma and sepsis

Jukka Takala, Raili Suojaranta-Ylinen and Otto Pitkänen

Historical background

Nutrition is essential in the treatment of patients with severe trauma and infection. The main goal of nutritional support is to minimise the loss of protein and energy; replacement of nutrient losses is usually not possible in the acute phase of the illness. Gastrointestinal dysfunction, loss of appetite and the consequent reduced food intake with concomitant increased requirement of nutrients are common problems after extensive surgery, in severe infections and after injury. Under these circumstances, insufficient nutrient intake will rapidly lead to nutritional depletion, which can markedly interfere with the recovery and rehabilitation.

If sufficient enteral intake of nutrients is not possible, all or part of the nutrition can be given intravenously. Before the development of total parenteral nutrition in the 1960s, patients who, for a prolonged period could not be fed enterally due to a postoperative complication, trauma or sepsis, died as a consequence of malnutrition.

Increased energy expenditure and catabolic loss of nitrogen following accidental and surgical trauma were observed in the 1930s,[1] and clinicians have long recognised the association between weight loss and morbidity.[2,3] The loss of energy and nitrogen that occurs during the acute phase of the illness cannot be replaced until convalescence starts, and nutritional and functional recovery may take weeks, even months.

By means of total parenteral nutrition, large intakes of energy and amino acids could be given in the acute phase of the disease. Clinicians and researchers were tempted to believe that it would be advantageous to give nutrients in excess of losses in hypermetabolic and hypercatabolic patients. The very large energy intakes were abandoned due to obvious disadvantages and side-effects; large loads of glucose were poorly tolerated and severe hyperglycaemia and hyperosmotic states were common.[4] The large glucose loads were also associated with liver dysfunction, which at least in part was due to accumulation of fat and glycogen.[5] High carbohydrate intakes were also shown to increase CO_2-production with a consequent increase in ventilatory demand.[6] The development of modern fat emulsions made the use of more balanced diets possible and helped to avoid excessive carbohydrate intake. The most severe adverse effects of nutrition support have become rare, once the goal of nutrition therapy in the acutely ill surgical and infected patients has been changed: reduction of excessive losses of nutrients has replaced the unsuccessful attempts to reverse the metabolic response to injury and infection. In addition, estimates of raised resting energy expenditure (REE) following injury have been revised downwards.

Enteral feeding techniques and preparations have markedly developed during the last two decades.[7] The majority of patients requiring nutrition support due to infection or injury can currently be fed enterally. Enteral nutrition is likely to be beneficial even if the nutritional needs cannot be fully met, since gastrointestinal function and mucosal integrity may be better preserved although parenteral nutrition retains its significant role (see Chapter 42).[8]

Many nutrients have properties beyond their direct nutritional effects and these are of potential therapeutic value in the severely injured or infected patient. Depletion of the intracellular glutamine pool may be one of the key elements of sustained nitrogen loss and catabolism; arginine and glutamine may be important for the immune system; the branched-chain and aromatic amino acids may interact with neurotransmission; lipids interact with e.g. prostaglandin and leukotriene metabolism and cell membranes. These pharmacological effects of nutrients may have great impact on nutrition management of the injured and infected patient in the future.

Theoretical problems and benefits of support

The metabolic response to trauma and sepsis is characterised by hypermetabolism and increased tissue catabolism.[1,2,9] These reactions are probably a result of evolution and are aimed at assuring the availability of endogenous nutrients, when the dietary requirements are high and the individual is unable to obtain exogenous nutrients. The fasting patient with trauma or sepsis is usually both hyperglycaemic and hyperinsulinaemic and there is very little ketogenesis.[4,10] The injured tissue utilises large amounts of glucose via glycolysis,[11] and one of the goals of the hyperglycaemia is to provide substrates for the traumatised tissue even if nutritive capillary blood flow is impaired by the tissue injury.

Despite the hyperglycaemia fat oxidation is the prevailing source of energy, except in the injured tissue and the brain.[6,11,12] The catabolism of body proteins provides amino acids for gluconeogenesis, which remains increased even if large amounts of glucose are given.[9,13] It has been speculated that muscle protein catabolism especially may be necessary to provide energy for the peripheral tissues. This is unlikely, since even in severe catabolism the oxidation of protein rarely exceeds 30% of energy expenditure and the rest is mostly obtained from fat oxidation.[14] Rather, muscle protein catabolism is aimed at providing substrates for gluconeogenesis, and thereby guaranteeing sufficient amounts of glucose for the injured tissue and the brain in the immediate post-traumatic period, while the injured individual is unable to eat or to obtain food. In addition to increased proteolysis, protein synthesis is also increased in infection and after injury.[15] Since protein synthesis increases less than proteolysis, the net effect is the loss of protein and nitrogen. Nevertheless, it has been suggested that the increased protein turnover *per se* is necessary for the synthesis of acute phase proteins and repair of tissue injury.

These characteristic metabolic changes are mediated by increased activity of the sympathetic nervous system, increased levels of epinephrine, cortisol and glucagon, and the activation of inflammatory reaction cascades. Recent studies indicate that cytokines have a central role both in triggering and modifying the hypermetabolic and hypercatabolic response to injury and infection.[16]

The traditional ebb or shock-phase after severe injury has been shortened or practically eliminated as a result of advanced support of vital functions and the flow-phase starts promptly after adequate primary resuscitation.[17] During the flow-phase energy expenditure is increased and tissue energy stores are mobilised.[18] Even though both anabolic and catabolic processes are activated, the net result is the loss of body protein and fat, while the total body water and especially its extracellular compartment are expanded.[19] If the post-operative or post-traumatic recovery is uncomplicated, nutritional support is rarely a major problem. On the other hand, if serious complications develop and the patient has severe infections and needs repeated operations, the hypermetabolic flow-phase and the net loss of protein and tissue energy stores can be prolonged for several weeks or even months. Under these circumstances, appropriate nutrition support becomes vital for survival.

The endocrine response to trauma and infection depends on the severity of the insult and can be markedly modified by early fluid resuscitation.[19] Sepsis tends to magnify and prolong the endocrine response to injury. Afferent nerve stimuli from the injured tissues stimulate the release of antidiuretic hormone, adrenocorticotropic hormone, norepinephrine and cortisol. Increased aldosterone release promotes sodium retention and potassium excretion in the kidney. In addition to the effects of the tissue injury itself, intravascular volume depletion induces and modifies the hormonal changes. Reduced renal perfusion due to hypovolaemia activates the renin–angiotensin system, which increases the release of aldosterone. The osmoreceptors in the hypothalamus and the portal system and the intrathoracic volume receptors mediate the release of antidiuretic hormone. The antidiuretic hormone increases distal tubular reabsorption of water and, together with the sodium retention promoted by aldosterone, facilitates maintenance and expansion of circulating blood volume.[19] Increased production of lactate is the inevitable consequence of inadequate tissue perfusion and hypoxia. Systemic lactic acidosis is a sign of severe perfusion failure and necessitates prompt intervention to correct tissue hypoxia.

In addition to absolute fluid losses following haemorrhage or gastrointestinal losses, blood volume and the functional interstitial fluid volume (i.e. the compartment in rapid equilibrium with plasma) commonly decreases as the result of endothelial and capillary leak.[16,20] This is characteristic of severe infections and septic shock and may also be a consequence of severe prolonged hypovolaemic shock. Recent studies strongly suggest that cytokines, especially tumour necrosis factor (TNF), are important inducers of the capillary leak in severe sepsis and shock.[16]

TNF is capable of reproducing many of the metabolic and endocrinological changes that are characteristic of injury and sepsis. It causes anorexia, increased whole body protein catabolism, hypermetabolism, fever, shock and tissue injury. TNF induces a variety of secondary mediators, including other cytokines (e.g. interleukins -1, -6, and -8, various growth factors), hormones (e.g. cortisol, glucagon, epinephrine, norepinephrine), eicosanoids, acute phase proteins and nitric oxide. The metabolic and immunological interactions between these various mediators are obviously complex; it is evident that there is no single common pathway of reactions in the response to injury and infection.[16]

Practical applications

The characteristic changes in substrate metabolism in trauma and sepsis depend on the severity of disease and the clinical status of a patient. Assessment of the severity of disease and injury has been attempted in order to facilitate interpretation of data from various studies. The Injury Severity Score and the sepsis score of Elebute and co-workers in 1983 [21] are examples of useful scoring systems.

Resting energy expenditure (REE) increases only moderately even after major elective surgical procedures:[22] after total hip replacement and major abdominal surgery by up to +10%;[17,23,24] after coronary artery bypass surgery, the increase may be somewhat higher.[25] After severe injury and in sepsis, the REE ranges from 110 to 140% of the predicted REE.[26-28]

The severity of injury or infection is also reflected in the nitrogen balance. The daily nitrogen balance for a 70 kg man during 5% glucose infusion is approximately −3 g in normal subjects, −6±1 g in malnourished patients, −7±2 g after total hip replacement, −11±6 g in sepsis, and −18±6 g after severe injury.[18] Isolated severe head injury induces marked nitrogen loss; protein conservation has not been achieved by increasing caloric intake up to and beyond twice the basal energy expenditure.[29] Spinal cord injury induces extensive muscle wasting and negative nitrogen balance despite feeding for several weeks.[30]

Substrate utilisation in trauma and sepsis

Proteolysis for energy production by oxidation of amino acids has been recognised since Cuthbertson's observations[1] as characteristics of serious injury and infection. The net nitrogen loss contributes to weakness, loss of immunocompetence, hypoalbuminaemia and failure to heal wounds. Gluconeogenesis is increased and, paradoxically, administration of glucose fails to reduce the excessive gluconeogenesis.[4] Fasting blood glucose and insulin levels are increased in septic patients compared to normals, and there is net release of glucose from the splanchnic circulation. During glucose infusion in normals, there is a consistent reversal of hepatic glucose output to a net uptake. In septic patients, continued hepatic release of glucose into the circulation is evident, despite high arterial glucose levels. Glucose released from the liver is derived by breakdown of hepatic glycogen as well as by gluconeogenesis from amino acids, lactate, pyruvate and glycerol.[31] Insulin and elevated blood glucose levels oppose the action of epinephrine and glucagon on hepatic gluconeogenesis. After major trauma and in sepsis, the insulin/glucagon ratio is low, which favours the conversion of amino acids to glucose.[32] Energy is largely derived from fat[33] and the increased protein catabolism provides precursors for enhanced hepatic gluconeogenesis. The fuel utilisation during glucose-based parenteral nutrition in hypermetabolic patients with injury and sepsis is markedly different from nutritionally depleted patients.[18] The depleted patients readily shift to glucose oxidation whereas, in hypermetabolic patients, net fat oxidation continues despite administration of glucose in excess of energy expenditure. The excess glucose is apparently converted to glycogen while fat stores are utilised partially to meet energy needs. This strongly suggests that the septic and injured patient preferentially utilises endogenous fat as energy source. Also the utilisation of exogenous fat is highly enhanced in septic patients as compared to healthy subjects and non-depleted cancer patients, and lipolysis cannot be inhibited significantly by glucose infusion.[34] Lipolysis, assessed by measurement of glycerol turnover, is increased two to threefold in septic and injured patients, and cannot be suppressed by hypercaloric, glucose-based TPN.[35]

Peripheral energy substrate exchange in patients with sepsis and trauma is characterised by highly elevated peripheral glucose uptake, production of lactate and release of amino acids.[36] Total peripheral release rate of amino acids is increased three-fold; in addition, leucine, valine, isoleucine, asparagine, aspartate and glutamic acid can be oxidised locally. Glucose oxidation is reduced in sepsis, and fat oxidation continues despite infusion of glucose in excess of the energy expenditure.[6,12] The extent of these changes seems to be related to the severity of sepsis. Fat utilisation may become impaired in sepsis at a stage at which signs of impaired oxidative metabolism and major metabolic abnormalities also develop.[37]

The contribution of glucose and fat to the energy content of TPN has little or no effect on whole-body protein synthesis, breakdown, or net synthesis in a wide range of glucose to lipid ratios.[38] In patients with infection or trauma, enteral feeding with either carbohydrate or a fat-based diet mainly modifies the oxidation rate of carbohydrate.[39]

42. Arnold J, Shipley KA, Scott NA, Little RA, Irving MH. Lipid infusion increases oxygen consumption similarly in septic and nonseptic patients. *Am J Clin Nutr* 1991; **53:** 143–148.

43. Gil KM, Askanazi J, Elwyn DH, Gump FE, Kinney JM. Energy expenditure after infusion of glucose-based total parenteral nutrition. *Am J Physiol* 1987; **253:** E135–E141.

44. Askanazi J, Carpentier YA, Michelsen CB, *et al.* Muscle and plasma amino acids following injury; influence of intercurrent infection. *Ann Surg* 1980; **192(1):** 78–85.

45. Smith RJ. Glutamine metabolism and its physiologic importance. *J Parenter Enter Nutr* 1990; **14(4):** 40S–44S.

46. Hall JC, Heel K, McCauley R. Glutamine. *Br J Surg* 1996; **83:** 305–312.

47. Lochs H, Hubl W. Metabolic basis for selecting glutamine-containing substrates for parenteral nutrition. *J Parenter Enter Nutr* 1990; **14(4):** 114S–117S.

48. Newsholme EA, Parry-Billings M. Properties of glutamine release from muscle and its importance for the immune system. *J Parenter Enter Nutr* 1990; **14:** 63–67S.

49. Häussinger D. Glutamine and hepatic metabolism. In: Kinney JM, Tucker HN (eds) *Organ metabolism and nutrition: Ideas for future critical care.* Raven Press, New York, 1994: pp. 315–329.

50. Neptune EM. Respiration and oxidation of various substrates by ileum in vitro. *Am J Physiol* 1965; **209:** 329–332.

51. McAnena OJ, Moore FA, Moore EE, Jones TN, Parsons P. Selective uptake of glutamine in the gastro-intestinal tract: confirmation in a human study. *Br J Surg* 1991; **78:** 480–482.

52. Ahlman B, Ljungqvist O, Persson P, Bindslev L, Wernerman J. Intestinal amino acid content in critically ill patients. *J Parenter Enter Nutr* 1995; **19:** 272–278.

53. van der Hulst RRWJ, von Meyenfeldt MF, Deutz NEP, Soeter PB. Glutamine extraction by the gut and the effect of nutritional depletion. *Ann Surg* (in press).

54. van der Hulst RRWJ, van Kreel BK, von Meyenfeldt MF, *et al.* Glutamine and the preservation of gut integrity. *Lancet* 1993; **341:** 1363–1365.

55. Tremel H, Kienle B, Weilemann LS, Stehle P. Glutamine dipeptide-supplemented parenteral nutrition maintains intestinal function in the critically ill. *Gastroenterology* 1994; **107:** 1595–1601.

56. Ziegler TR, Young LS, Benfell K, *et al.* Clinical and metabolic efficacy of glutamine supplemented parenteral nutrition after bone marrow transplantation. *Ann Intern Med* 1992; **112:** 821–828.

57. Griffiths RD, Jones C, Palmer TEA. Outcome and cost of intensive care patients given glutamine-supplemented nutrition. *Clin Nutr* 1996; **15: suppl1:** 20.

58. Gennari R, Alexander JW, Eaves-Pyles T. Effect of different combinations of dietary additives on bacterial translocation and survival in gut-derived sepsis. *J Parenter Enter Nutr* 1995; **19:** 319–325.

59. Von Meyenfeldt MF, Soeters PB, Vente JP, *et al.* Effect of branched-chain amino acid enrichment of total parenteral nutrition on nitrogen sparing and clinical outcome of sepsis and trauma: a prospective randomized double blind trial. *Br J Surg* 1990; **77:** 924–929.

60. Woolfson AMJ, Heatley RV, Allison SP. Insulin to inhibit protein catabolism after injury. *New Engl J Med* 1979; **300(1):** 14–17.

61. Takala J, Ruoleone E, Webster NR *et al.* Increased mortality associated with growth hormone treatment in critically ill adults. *N Engl J Med* 1999; **391:** 785–792.

62. Calloway DH, Spector H. Nitrogen and energy balance as related to caloric and protein intake in active young men. *Am J Clin Nutr* 1955; **2:** 405–412.

63. Munro HN. Regulation of protein metabolism. In: Munro HN, Allison JB (eds) *Mammalian protein metabolism.* Academic Press, New York, 1964: pp. 381–481.

64. Larsson J, Mårtenson J, Vinnars E. Nitrogen requirements in hypermetabolic patients. *Clin Nutr* 1984; **4(Special suppl):** O.4.

65. Wilmore D.W. Glutamine and the gut. *Gastroenterology* 1994; **107:** 1885–1886.

66. Stehle P, Zander J, Mertes N, *et al.* Effect of parenteral glutamine peptide supplements on muscle glutamine loss and nitrogen balance after major surgery. *Lancet* 1989; **1:** 231–233.

30

Nutrition support in renal disease

Giuliano Brunori

Background

Patients suffering from acute or chronic renal failure will present with catabolic illnesses requiring nutrition support.

Acute renal failure (ARF) can be defined as an acute and marked reduction in glomerular filtration rate (GFR). Metabolic waste products accumulate in association with an inability to regulate mineral and water balance. This may develop during shock, sepsis, trauma, and medical therapy. Nutrition support is needed in these cases. Conversely, there are some other cases of ARF in which the patient is not catabolic and nutrition support is not required. These may include the use of nephrotoxic drugs (e.g. radio-contrast agents, non-steroidal anti-inflammatory drugs) and obstruction of the urinary tract.

Patients with chronic renal failure (CRF), either during the conservative period or during the dialytic period (haemodialysis or peritoneal dialysis), may also be unable to meet nutrition requirements orally because of nausea, anorexia or vomiting, or when they sustain intercurrent illnesses. Such illnesses include infection, or cardiovascular disease and peritonitis. Artificial nutrition techniques (enteral or intravenous) may be required.

When patients with acute renal failure or chronic renal failure need nutrition support, the dosage and composition of the nutrients must be modified to take into account the metabolic derangement associated with impaired or absent renal function and the nutritional limitations imposed by renal failure, dialysis and associated illness.

Uraemic patients treated with low-protein diets, supplemented with a high percentage of essential amino acids together with adequate calories, showed a clinical improvement of uraemic symptoms and a stabilisation or decrease in blood urea concentration.[1,2] These observations form part of the basic principles of nutrition support in renal disease.

Recently, there has been an increased interest in the nutrition therapy of patients with acute or chronic renal failure. This is a consequence of the observations that patients with renal failure may be malnourished[3,4] and that the mortality rate of patients with ARF has not improved substantially in 30 years.[5]

Several factors may induce the catabolic process in uraemia. Plasma concentrations of catabolic hormones are frequently elevated; these include cortisol, epinephrine and catecholamine. Parathyroid hormone is another potentially catabolic hormone which is often increased in acute and chronic renal failure.[6] Cytokines and monokines, interleukin 1 (IL-1) or tumour necrosis factor, are reported to be increased in severe sepsis and other catabolic conditions that may be present in septic ARF patients.[7,8]

Frequently, the patient loses nutrients in fistulae and during haemodialysis or peritoneal dialysis. Dialysis itself can be catabolic (due to release of IL-1, or loss of amino acids or proteins). Additionally, blood sampling, gastrointestinal bleeding and blood sequestration in the haemodialyser are other factors which may increase malnutrition and wasting.

In the era before dialysis, nutrition therapy was often used to reduce uraemia and water and electrolyte abnormalities. Anabolic steroids and low protein diets were recommended until renal function recovered. The maintenance of a good nutrition status was a secondary aim. Now that dialysis is readily available for the control of uraemia, fluid balance and electrolyte abnormalities, and modern techniques of nutrition therapy have been developed, the achievement of a good nutrition status has become a primary goal.

Enteral nutrition, when feasible, offers some advantages over parenteral nutrition (PN). These include lower cost, safety and convenience for both the patient and the health care team. In patients with renal failure, water restriction is often necessary and enteral formulations can be more concentrated, giving a smaller water load. Additionally, the gastrointestinal barrier in patients with renal failure is operative during enteral feeding and can play an important role in the excretion of excess minerals or other impurities, which are not readily excreted in the urine.

Nitrogen (N) balance

Patients with ARF or CRF may maintain neutral nitrogen and caloric balance. They are also able to maintain a neutral water, electrolyte and acid–base balance. Usually, these patients do not present with catabolic underlying illnesses.

If these patients do develop a severe illness, they become more catabolic and undergo marked protein breakdown and water retention, with disorders of electrolyte and acid–base balance. Since amino acid efflux from skeletal muscle and consequent urea-genesis occurs at an unusual rate during many critical illnesses, blood urea nitrogen (BUN) may rise rapidly even if exogenous proteins are not administered. Severe protein breakdown in muscle or liver may accelerate the rise in plasma levels of potassium, phosphorus and nitrogenous metabolites, including creatinine and urate. Metabolic acidosis, often presenting with an elevated anion gap, has been recently identified in humans as a cause of muscle proteolysis. The abnormal turnover of proteins during metabolic acidosis is thought to be a consequence of the stimulation of branched-chain amino acid oxidation in skeletal muscle.[9,10] Nitrogen balance can improve substantially when acidosis is corrected in patients with chronic uraemia.[11]

Malnutrition may thus develop very quickly. Malnutrition is well recognised as a risk factor for death particularly for uraemic patients.[12] In the severely ill patients with ARF, net protein breakdown can induce a loss of 4% per day of the total non-collagen protein mass.[13] Highly catabolic patients become malnourished more rapidly than unstressed patients, so nutrition supplements may alter outcome at a relatively early stage in the catabolic process.

Urea is the major nitrogenous product of protein and amino acid degradation. Therefore, the urea nitrogen appearance (UNA) can be used to estimate the total nitrogen balance.[14,15] The UNA is the sum of the urea nitrogen that accumulates in all body fluids and the output of urea nitrogen in urine and in dialysate. The UNA may be employed to estimate the magnitude of net protein breakdown and (by comparing the patient's intake to the UNA), to estimate nitrogen or protein balance. The UNA is calculated as follows:

UNA (g/day) = urinary urea nitrogen (g/day) + dialysate urea nitrogen (g/day) + change in body urea nitrogen (g/day)

Change in body urea nitrogen (g/day)
= $(SUN_f - SUN_i) \times BW_i \times (0.60\ l/kg) + (BW_f - BW)$
$\times SUN_f \times (1.0\ l/kg)$

In the second formula, i and f refer to initial and final values, obtained during the period of observation; SUN is the serum urea nitrogen (expressed in g/l/day); BW is the body weight (expressed in kg). The fractional body water (normally estimated as 0.60

of body weight) may be increased in lean or oedematous patients and may be decreased in children and obese patients. The factor 1.0 (l/kg) is the estimated fractional volume of distribution of urea in the weight that is gained or lost during the measurements. If the patient is treated by haemodialysis or intermittent peritoneal dialysis, to circumvent the difficulty and inaccuracy in the measurement of urea nitrogen in the dialysate, the UNA is best measured during an interdialytic interval and then normalised for a 24-hour period.

The total nitrogen output can be estimated from the UNA as follows:

Total nitrogen output = 0.97 UNA (g/day) + 1.93

In this formula 1.93 is the sum (in grams) of nitrogen losses in compound or by routes not covered by the first formula (e.g. urate, creatinine, stool or vomiting).

The formula cannot be applied for patients with large losses of proteins (e.g. patients with nephrotic syndrome) or with severe acidosis.

Nutrition management of renal failure

In the 1960s, low protein diets were introduced for the treatment of patients with chronic renal disease to prevent uraemic toxicity. These diets were advocated by some clinicians for the treatment of patients with ARF. The low nitrogen intake (i.e. about 0.20–0.35 g of amino acids or protein/kg/day) was used to reduce uraemic toxicity and to decrease the need for dialysis. The diet was believed to reduce the UNA, the accumulation of nitrogenous metabolites and the degree of protein breakdown.[16] Subsequent studies however showed that a low protein diet did not provide adequate protein nutrition for many patients with renal failure.

Recently, a very low protein diet supplemented with ketoacid salts of five essential amino acids and the other four essential L-amino acids (threonine, lysine, histidine, tryptophan) has been administered in patients with advanced renal failure.[17] Protein restriction has been advocated for slowing the progression of renal failure and deferring dialysis. This diet, in conjunction with blood pressure control and frequent follow-ups, seems to reduce the progression of renal failure and prevent malnutrition. Furthermore, elderly and very elderly patients (at present, the groups of patients with the higher rate of acceptance in dialysis) can accept this diet more easily than adult or young patients and this can postpone the need for dialysis.

Dialysis is used to control azotaemia, fluid status and electrolyte abnormalities. Even patients with severe circulatory shock may be treated with continuous venous–venous haemofiltration. Thus nutrition therapy has moved away from its first aim: from prevention of uraemic symptoms to maintenance of good nutrition status.

A number of investigators have examined formulations for the treatment of patients with ARF. A solution of pure crystalline essential L-amino acids (in amounts designed to meet or exceed the minimum daily requirement) together with hypertonic glucose was administered to a patient with ARF and severe abdominal injuries.[18] Stabilisation or reduction of serum use nitrogen (SUN), improved wound healing and weight gain in the patient was reported. Ten patients with acute renal failure were treated with the same formulation.[19] A greater than 50% reduction of blood urea nitrogen (BUN) was described, eliminating or decreasing significantly the need for dialysis. Decreased serum potassium and phosphate and positive nitrogen balance were often observed.

In a prospective double-blind study, 53 patients with acute renal failure were randomly assigned to receive infusions of either an average of 16 g/day of essential amino acids and hypertonic glucose or hypertonic glucose alone.[20] The two solutions provided 5966 and 6866 kJ/day (1426 and 1641 kcal/day), respectively. The authors observed a significantly greater incidence of recovery of renal function in the 28 patients receiving the essential amino acids and glucose, although the overall hospital mortality rate was not different between the two groups. In patients with more severe renal failure, indicated by the need for dialysis, and in those with serious complications (pneumonia or generalised sepsis), the hospital survival rate was greater in those who were treated with essential amino acids and glucose.

A non-randomised retrospective comparison of 129 postoperative patients with ARF,[21] showed that 63 patients treated with a fibrin hydrolysate and hypertonic glucose had a survival rate of 54%. The other 66 patients (hypertonic glucose alone) had a survival rate of 30%.

A retrospective comparison in patients with no complications showed there was no difference in survival between the group treated with hypertonic glucose and a mixture of essential and non-essential amino acids and the group treated with hypertonic glucose alone.[22] In those patients with three or more complications (or with peritonitis) there was a significantly greater survival in the patients treated with hypertonic glucose and amino acids as compared with those receiving hypertonic glucose alone.

Improved morbidity and mortality was reported in patients with ARF given PN with amino acids and glucose compared with patients treated with glucose alone.[23] However, the study was neither randomised nor prospective.

Eleven patients were randomly assigned to receive intravenous solutions of 17.5% essential L-amino acids and 47% dextrose and 9 patients to receive infusions of 47% glucose alone;[24] the rate of increase in SUN was significantly lower in the first group. The rates of recovery of renal function or survival were no different between the groups.

In a prospective study, 30 patients with ARF were randomised in three different TPN formulations: hypertonic glucose alone; hypertonic glucose plus 21 g/day of essential amino acids; and hypertonic glucose plus 21 g/day of essential amino acids and 21 g/day of non-essential amino acids.[25] The mean energy intake was similar in all the three groups (9623–11 297 kJ – 2300–2700 kcal/day). In this study, 13 out of 30 patients recovered renal function and 11 survived. There was no significant difference in survival between the three treatment groups, so the outcome was influenced by the underlying disease. The highest mortality (83%) was observed in patients with shock or sepsis. Nitrogen balances in the three groups were not significantly different. The patients receiving 21 g/day of the essential amino acids tended to have a greater recovery of renal function and survival. On average, the patients receiving a higher calorie intake (167 kJ; 40 kcal/kg/day) had a higher survival rate than those who received a lower calorie intake (139 kJ; 32 kcal/kg/day). It is possible that the greater energy intake in the patients who survived may reflect their greater tolerance for water and, hence, healthier state rather than a positive survival effect of higher energy intakes.

Based on these results, a second study was carried out in 11 patients with ARF,[26] designed to ascertain whether higher nitrogen intakes might maintain more positive nitrogen balance. The patients were randomly assigned to receive PN as hypertonic glucose plus 21 g/day of essential amino acids (group A) or as hypertonic glucose plus essential and non-essential amino acids in equal amounts (group B). The second formulation was an attempt to infuse a quantity of amino acid nitrogen equal to the UNA. The results indicated that nitrogen balances were similar in both groups, although nitrogen intake was five times higher in group B, and the essential amino acid intake in group A was about twice as great as in group B. Indeed, the UNA fell significantly in the patients receiving the essential amino acids formulation and tended to rise in the group B.

In a recent review the benefits, risks and uncertainties regarding PN in ARF were considered.[27] The authors concluded that protein and non-protein calories given must meet the patient's calculated resting energy expenditure (REE) using these equations.[28]

REE (men) = 66.5 + (13.7 × weight, kg) + (5.0 × height, cm) − (6.8 × age, yrs)
REE (women) = 655 + (9.6 × weight, kg) + (1.7 × height, cm) − (4.7 × age, yrs)

The value obtained is then multiplied by a stress factor for the increased energy expenditure associated with different clinical conditions.[29] Lipids can be used to provide up to 30% of total calories; protein requirements should be calculated by estimating the nitrogen losses from UNA and calculated non-urea nitrogen.

Patients (including those not treated by dialysis and those on maintenance haemodialysis or peritoneal dialysis) who develop an intercurrent illness that precludes oral intake may be treated with the same enteral or parenteral nutrition therapy used for patients with ARF. Usually, patients with CRF are able to maintain a neutral nitrogen balance with an intake of 0.55–0.60 g/kg/day of protein and 146 kJ (35 kcal)/kg/day energy.[30,31] However during a severe, superimposed catabolic illness the energy and nitrogen needs are clearly greater and seem to be similar to those of patients with severe catabolic illness without renal failure.

Experimental studies

In experimental studies in rats with mercuric chloride-induced acute tubular necrosis (ATN), a rapid increase in the synthesis of protein, nucleic acids and phospholipids in renal tissue was observed.[32,33] In animals or in patients with ARF the low plasma amino acid concentrations may enhance the need for nutrients to support the increased synthesis in the affected kidney.[25,34] In another report the intracellular leucine in regenerating tubular cells was 17% below normal.[35] The same group showed that nutrition therapy with essential amino acids and glucose in rats with ATN increased the rate of new cell membrane formation and either decreased severity or enhanced recovery of renal function.[35,36]

Several other experimental studies in rats suggest that amino acid or protein intake may increase the susceptibility of the kidney to ARF induced by ischaemia or nephrotoxic drugs.[37,38] The severity and the incidence of ARF induced by these agents seem to be increased by the nutrients. The type of amino acids may influence the risk of ARF. Among the amino acids, D-serine, DL-methionine, L-lysine seem to be particularly nephrotoxic,[39] whereas glycine may have a protective effect in a rat model.[40]

Clinical management of nutrition therapy

The optimal nutrition therapy for patients with ARF or CRF and superimposed severe illness is still not clear from the available research findings. The following approach to nutrition management is based upon the published literature[41] and the author's own experience.

The nutrition intake for patients with ARF should depend on the individual's nutrition status, catabolic rate as estimated by UNA, residual renal function and need for dialysis. Nutrients should be administered as needed, and the development of fluid or electrolyte disorders or accumulation of waste products should be prevented by adjusting the intensity of dialysis. Evidence in stressed, catabolic non-uraemic patients indicates that a higher intake of proteins or of purified essential and non-essential amino acids (e.g. 1.5–2.0 g/kg/day) may promote more positive nitrogen balance. However, generation of urea and probably other potentially toxic nitrogenous metabolites may increase substantially. For patients with ARF or with CRF and superimposed severe illness who are intolerant of the accumulation of nitrogenous metabolites, administration of essential amino acids may have certain advantages. Research suggests that lower quantities of essential amino acids alone are utilised more efficiently and may produce less UNA for the same degree of nitrogen balance than mixtures containing higher quantities of essential and non-essential amino acids.

Patients who are severely malnourished may be given a higher intake of protein or essential and non-essential amino acids and dialysed as needed. On the other hand, patients who are entering the recovery phase of ARF may be given high calorie formulae and small quantities of water, electrolyte and essential amino acids in order to avoid or delay the need for dialysis.

When dialysis is not used the intake of fluid should be about 400 ml higher than total output. This practice takes into account the water production of metabolism and the insensible losses; the fluid intake may be higher in a patient with high fever. Patients must be monitored each day, with assessment of the oedema status and body weight.

Patients with ARF or CRF and marked catabolism usually require frequent dialysis in order to control plasma osmolality, extracellular fluid volume, acid-aemia, uraemia and electrolyte disorders. The potential loss of nutrients during treatment into the dialysate must be taken into consideration. About 6–10 g of free amino acids, 2–3 g of bound amino acids and (with glucose-free dialysate) 10–25 g of glucose are removed during a typical dialysis cycle. In markedly hyperglycaemic patients, glucose losses may increase by several hundred grams during a single treatment.

The nitrogen intake may be tailored to the UNA. If the patient has a low UNA (i.e. equal to or less than 4–5 g nitrogen/day), and there is no evidence of mal-nutrition, a low oral, enteral or intravenous nitrogen intake may be prescribed. The diet should provide 0.10–0.30 g/kg/day of miscellaneous protein and 10–20 g per day of essential amino acids or ketoacids. If the patient cannot be fed enterally, intravenous infusion of the nine essential amino acids (0.30–0.50 g/kg/day), with or without arginine may be employed. No more than 30–40 g/day of the essential amino acids must be prescribed because greater amounts may cause severe amino acid imbalance. Unless the patient is very catabolic, this protocol should maintain an acceptably low rate of accumulation of nitrogen metabolites and a neutral or mildly to moderately negative nitrogen balance, so that the need for dialysis is minimised. Very low doses of essential amino acids are not given for more than three weeks.

In a patient with residual renal function, who is minimally catabolic, it is possible to use the same diet as for non-dialysed patients with CRF: 0.55–0.60 g/kg desirable body weight (based on the Metropolitan height and weight tables) of primary high biological value protein or about 0.28 g protein/kg/day supplemented with 6–10 g/day of essential amino acids or 0.28 g/kg of a mixture of essential amino acids and ketoacids. This diet can be used until the patient recovers normal renal function. If patients cannot be fed enterally, they may be given 0.55–0.60 g/kg/day of essential and non-essential amino acids intravenously. For a patient who is more catabolic and has higher levels of UNA (greater than 5 g nitrogen/day), who is wasted and needs regular dialysis, the daily intake of protein or amino acids may be 1.0–1.2 g/kg/day (when treated by haemodialysis) or 1.2–1.5 g/kg/day (when treated by intermittent or continuous peritoneal dialysis).

For these levels of amino acid intake, both essential and non-essential amino acids should be used. It is possible that solutions with a higher ratio of essential to non-essential amino acids may be more anabolic than preparations with a 1:1 ratio and may be safer than high doses of essential amino acids alone (i.e., more than 30–40 g/day).[42] However, amino acid solutions containing a higher proportion of the branched-chain amino acids, and particularly leucine, appear to be more anabolic.[43] In fact, a key role in glucose metabolism is played by the branched-chain amino acids, because they may be oxidised in muscle as a primary energy source.[44,45] Protein turnover seems to be regulated by branched-chain amino acids and a deficit of these amino acids can contribute to altered protein metabolism in stressed patients.[46,47]

The optimal energy intake for patients with renal failure is not well defined. Stressed, catabolic patients with ARF are usually in negative energy and nitrogen balance. It has been suggested that these patients may benefit from a greater energy intake to reduce protein wasting and improve mortality. As indicated above, this question has not been examined in a prospective randomised manner, and so the data are inconclusive.

The estimated energy requirements for patients with ARF or CRF and catabolic stress are usually between 146 and 209 kJ (35 and 50 kcal)/kg/day. The higher intake is used for those patients who have a higher UNA or are more sick. Larger doses are not used because no significant advantages have been shown in administering more calories to catabolic patients. Indeed, high glucose levels can induce fatty liver and functional liver damage,[48] and high calorie intakes can lead to hyperlipidaemia and obesity. Moreover, large amounts of fluid are necessary for the administration of nutrients and the water load to the patient may be increased significantly. In addition, the greater carbon load from these high-energy intakes generates more carbon dioxide.[49] This can promote hypercapnia and may precipitate respiratory failure or prevent weaning from ventilators if pulmonary function is impaired.[50] In patients who have marginally impaired respiratory function or who are being removed from mechanical ventilator support, the carbon load may be gradually reduced to decrease the tendency for hypercapnia. This may be accomplished by increasing the proportion of calories provided from fat.

Patients receiving PN for more than 5–7 days should have a daily minimum of 50–100 g of lipids. The lipids should preferably be given daily, but not less than twice weekly, to prevent essential fatty acid (EFA) deficiency and to provide a balanced energy mix. The metabolic benefits of lipids are optimised by the continuous infusion of fat emulsion. Many researchers routinely provide about 20–30% of total calories each day from fat,[50,51] which is similar to the recommendations for diets of normal individuals. Fat administration is preferred since energy metabolism is thought to depend on fat oxidation and fatty acid turnover is increased.[52]

Minerals, trace elements and vitamin requirements

The intake of sodium, potassium, phosphorus, magnesium, calcium and trace elements should be carefully monitored to prevent accumulation or deficits. Patients with renal failure cannot regulate mineral levels by urinary excretion and this increases the risk of developing clinically hazardous blood or tissue levels. Electrolyte levels are controlled by haemodialysis or continuous arteriovenous haemofiltration. Serum electrolyte levels at the onset of nutrition therapy are often altered and a change of formulation may be necessitated.

Serum potassium and phosphorus can fall rapidly after the initiation of PN. The administration of glucose or amino acids causes the entry of these elements into the cell. Hence, patients who have hyperkalaemia or hyperphosphataemia at the onset of PN are given a nutrition formulation containing little or no potassium or phosphate. The patients must be closely monitored because they may develop low serum levels of these elements after 1–3 days and require addition of these elements to the infusion.

The intracellular shift of phosphate may induce in septic patients a transient but severe hypophosphataemia.[53] Patients with chronic alcoholism or intravenous drug abusers often develop hypophosphataemia, because of nutritional deficiencies and depletion of the body phosphate pool. Hypophosphataemia can impair leucocyte function, enhances the risk of rhabdomyolysis and causes other disorders, such as respiratory arrest, coma and death.

The urinary phosphate excretion is impaired in patients with a severe decrease in renal function. Because the reduction in plasma phosphate levels by haemodialysis is small, patients with renal failure may present with hyperphosphataemia. This may result from an excessive intake of phosphate or from muscle catabolism. Hyperphosphataemia may enhance secondary hyperparathyroidism and may induce a precipitation of calcium phosphate crystal in soft tissue. Treatment with phosphate binders is necessary: calcium carbonate, calcium citrate, aluminium hydroxide or other formulations available may be used.[54] In patients with CRF, bone toxicity, anaemia, dementia or myopathy have been observed after long-term use of aluminium carbonate or hydroxide. These side-effects are not observed in the short term.

Hypomagnesaemia may occur in some patients with renal failure. Magnesium salt should be added to nutrition formulae used for tube feeding to avoid hypomagnesaemia. Conversely, magnesium is primarily excreted in the urine and great care should be taken in oliguric or anuric patients to prevent hypermagnesaemia.

Hypocalcaemia may occur in some patients with ARF or CRF. These patients should be given supplements of basic calcium salts (as calcium carbonate, calcium citrate or calcium gluconate). Dialysis does not induce calcium losses, because the dialysate contains calcium ions. In patients with CRF, supplements of vitamin D may be given to facilitate intestinal uptake of calcium. This supplementation should be done only in patients without elevated serum phosphorus or calcium concentrations.

Patients with ARF or CRF usually present with metabolic acidosis. Bicarbonate may be given, but in severe cases the best treatment is haemodialysis. Bicarbonate dialysis is preferred to acetate dialysis in patients with hypotension or unstable circulatory volume because bicarbonate may protect against hypotension more than acetate.[55,56] Sodium bicarbonate may be added to the tube feeding formulae or may be infused intravenously to ensure plasma bicarbonate concentrations of at least 20 mmol/l, if frequent dialysis is not needed for the treatment of these patients.

In catabolic patients with ARF or CRF, the quantity of minerals that is both required or tolerated for enteral feeding varies greatly between individuals. These supplements per day are recommended in patients who have normal plasma concentrations: sodium 40–50 mmol/l; potassium 40–60 mmol/l; phosphorus 200–400 mg; calcium 800 mg; magnesium 100 mg. Frequent monitoring of the serum concentrations of these minerals must be done and the intake adjusted to prevent deficits or accumulation.

In patients with renal failure the nutrition requirements for trace elements are not well established. In patients with ARF of less than 3 weeks' duration, trace element supplements are probably not needed with the exception of iron and zinc. Iron is given at a dose of 10 mg/day for men and women, increased to 18 mg/day for menstruating women. If the serum iron level is very low, the supplement may be increased to 60 mg/day or greater. About 15 mg/day of zinc should be given.

The vitamin requirements for patients with ARF have not been well defined. Vitamin A is probably best avoided for the first two weeks because in chronic renal failure its levels are elevated. It is also unlikely that a deficiency of this fat-soluble vitamin will occur in patients treated with PN for only a few days to weeks.

Vitamin D stores should not become depleted during the first few days of artificial nutrition in patients with ARF. The turnover of 1,25-dihydroxicholecalciferol, its most active analogue, is much faster. Since this analogue is primarily produced by the kidney, it may be needed for patients with ARF. In patients with CRF or in maintenance dialysis, the use of vitamin D prevents secondary hyperparathyroidism. Hypocalcaemia in patients with ARF or CRF may be an indication for administering both enteral calcium and vitamin D.

Vitamin K supplements should be given routinely to patients with ARF receiving PN, particularly if they receive antibiotics that may suppress the intestinal growth of bacteria that synthesise vitamin K.[57]

Vitamin B_6 deficiency may be prevented or corrected by 10 mg/day of pyridoxine hydrochloride (i.e. 8.2 mg/day of pyridoxine).[58] Not more than 60–100 mg/day of ascorbic acid should be given to the patients with ARF because of the risk of increased oxalate production and elevated serum oxalate levels.[59]

Method of administration

Whenever possible, patients should be fed orally. If they do not eat adequately, they may be offered liquid formula diets, or tube or enterostomy feeding. Many commercially available enteral formulae can be employed for patients with ARF or CRF. The use of these formulae offers many advantages: they are relatively inexpensive, since they are premixed, readily available and administration is simple. However, there are some disadvantages. The calorie/nitrogen ratio is often low; the contents of certain minerals (in particular phosphorus, potassium, magnesium and trace elements) are excessive; and the contents of vitamins A and C may be excessive. Patients with ARF or CRF and superimposed severe illness often do not have well-functioning gastrointestinal tracts and PN may be the preferred technique for providing an adequate nutrient intake.

Peripheral or partial parenteral nutrition (PPN – see Chapter 22) may be advantageous for patients who are able to receive part of their daily nutrition needs through the gastrointestinal tract. These patients may receive adequate nutrition by a combination of enteral and PPN. In these patients, as much of the essential nutrients as feasible, including the carbohydrates, should be administered via the enteral route. An 8.5–10% amino acid solution or a 20% lipid emulsion may be infused intravenously. Because these infusions are not hypertonic, it is not necessary to infuse the nutrients through a central vein. PN is needed in the more catabolic patients with ARF or CRF because these patients usually have sustained surgical or other trauma to the abdomen, often associated with severe infection. Chapter 22 describes techniques for administration of PN and potential complications during this treatment.

Continuous arteriovenous haemofiltration (CAVH) can be used to control salt and water balance and uraemia in patients receiving PN.[60] This treatment is particularly useful for patients with excessive body water or fluid intolerance or who are receiving large volumes of intravenous infusions. If the patients are hypercatabolic, CAVH may be inadequate to control uraemia and haemodialysis is often required.

It seems clear that the hypercatabolic status of patients with ARF or CRF and superimposed severe illness impairs their ability to utilise the nutrients given. Anabolic agents that are being evaluated or have been investigated for stressed patients include insulin,[61] growth hormone or insulin-like growth factor-1,[62–64] and inhibitors of glucocorticoids.[65]

Recently, numerous studies have been carried out in malnourished uraemic patients using recombinant human growth hormone (rhGH) or IGF-1, alone or together. In patients with CRF, hormonal disorders are frequently observed. In particular, the anabolic response in uraemic patients may be impaired. The use of rhGH or IGF-1 can overcome this problem.

A strong anabolic response during treatment with rhGH has been reported in severely malnourished MHD patients.[62] The response was concomitant with a sustained increase in IGF-1. In two patients, who presented during the study period with an acute illness, the nitrogen balance was moderately positive and serum IGF-1 slightly increased.

Ten stable adult patients, treated with continuous ambulatory peritoneal dialysis (CAPD), have been evaluated to determine the short-term effects and safety of rhGH on urea kinetics and commonly measured biochemical parameters.[63] The authors reported a net decrease in total urea nitrogen excretion, and this is consistent with an anabolic effect.

Another study evaluated the anabolic effect of rhGH combined with intradialytic parenteral nutrition (IDPN) in seven malnourished MHD patients.[64] The nutrition therapy (glucose 60%, essential amino acid 8.5% and Intralipid (Clintec, Deerfield IL)) delivered 75 kJ (18 kcal), 0.69 g of protein/kg body weight and 50 g of fat during each dialysis. After 6 weeks of treatment, rhGH was added. The authors reported an increase in serum albumin concentration and IGF-1, and a decrease in intradialytic urea.

In the absence of a larger randomised population, and with a very different treatment schedule, these data should be considered as preliminary and in need of confirmation.

Conclusions

The altered metabolic and physiological status and frequent occurrence of hypercatabolism in patients with ARF or CRF and superimposed severe illness complicate their nutrition management. The hypermetabolic response can be tolerated in the short term, but a longer period of hypercatabolism depletes body proteins and fuel, and patients become malnourished and susceptible to complications. Malnutrition seems to be implicated in multiple organ failure, cellular metabolism being limited by fuel deficiency in organ structure, function and energy production.[51]

It is of value to monitor the patient's UNA to assess the level of catabolism. In patients with normal metabolism a protein-restricted diet can be used to avoid dialysis and to prevent uraemic symptoms. In hypercatabolic patients more complete nutrition support is required and early dialysis must be started. If possible the gastrointestinal tract should be used for nutrition. Sometimes patients may be given only a fraction of their required nutritional intake via the gastrointestinal tract, the remainder of their nutrients being received by peripheral venous infusion. Patients who are given partial or total PN must be carefully monitored for signs of fluid or electrolyte and other metabolic disorders.[66]

Further studies are needed to understand the mechanism(s) responsible for the increased susceptibility to protein catabolism in these patients. Moreover, prospective randomised studies are necessary to evaluate the benefit of nutrition support and to understand the potential role of anabolic agents to prevent the hypercatabolic status of stressed patients with ARF or CRF.

References

1. Giordano C. Use of exogenous and endogenous urea for protein synthesis in normal and uremic subjects. *J Lab Clin Med* 1963; **62:** 231–246.

2. Giovannetti S, Maggiore Q. A low nitrogen diet with proteins of high biological value for severe chronic uremia. *Lancet* 1964; **1**: 1000–1003.

3. Cianciaruso B, Brunori G, Kopple JD *et al.* Cross-sectional comparison of malnutrition in continuous ambulatory peritoneal dialysis and hemodialysis patients. *Am J Kidney Dis* 1995; **26**: 475–486.

4. Bergstrom J, Furst P, Alvestrand A, and Lindholm B. Protein and energy intake, nitrogen balance and nitrogen losses in patients treated with continuous ambulatory peritoneal dialysis. *Kidney Int* 1993; **44**: 1048–1057.

5. Chew SL, Lins RL, Daelemans R, De Broe ME. Outcome in acute renal failure. *Nephrol Dial Transplant* 1993; **8**: 101–107.

6. Kopple JD, Cianciaruso B, Massry SG. Does para-thyroid hormone cause protein wasting? *Contrib Nephrol* 1980; **20**: 138–144.

7. Fong Y, Lowry SF, Cerami A. Cachectin/TNF: a macrophage protein that induces cachexia and shock. *J Parent Enter Nutr* 1988; **12 (suppl 6)**: S72–S77.

8. Hakim RM, Wingard RL, Parker RA. Effect of the dialysis membrane in the treatment of patients with acute renal failure. *N Eng J Med* 1994; **331**: 1338–1342.

9. Reaich D, Channon SM, Scrimgeour CM *et al.* Correction of acidosis in human with CRF decreases protein degradation and amino acid oxidation. *Am J Physiol* 1993; **265**: E230–E235.

10. Garibotto G, Russo R, Sofia A *et al.* Skeletal muscle protein synthesis and degradation in patients with chronic renal failure. *Kidney Int* 1994; **45**: 1432–1439.

11. Papadoyannakis NJ, Stefanidis CJ, McGeown M. The effect of correction of metabolic acidosis on nitrogen and potassium balance of patients with chronic renal failure. *Am J Clin Nutr* 1984; **40**: 623–627.

12. Lowrie EG, Lew NL. Death risk in hemodialysis patients: the predictive value of commonly measured variables and an evaluation of death rate differences between facilities. *Am J Kidney Dis* 1990; **5**: 458–482.

13. Chill G. Starvation in man. *N Eng J Med* 1970; **282**: 668–678.

14. Maroni B, Steinman T, Mitch WE. A method for estimating nitrogen intake of patients with chronic renal failure. *Kidney Int* 1985; **27**: 58–65.

15. Bergstrom J, Lindholm B. Nutrition and adequacy of dialysis. How do hemodialysis and CAPD compare? *Kidney Int* 1993; **43 (suppl. 40)**: S39–S50.

16. Berlyne G, Bazzard F, Booth E *et al.* The dietary treat-ment of acute renal failure. *Q J Med* 1967; **141**: 59–68.

17. Coresh J, Walser M, Hill S. Survival on dialysis among chronic renal failure patients treated with a supple-mented low-protein diet before dialysis. *J Am Soc Nephrol* 1995; **6**: 1379–1385.

18. Wilmore DW, Dudrick SJ. Treatment of acute renal failure with intravenous essential L-amino acids. *Arch Surg* 1969; **99**: 669–673.

19. Dudrick SJ, Steiger E, Long J. Renal failure in surgical patients: Treatment with intravenous essential amino acids and hypertonic glucose. *Surgery* 1970; **68**: 180–186.

20. Abel RM, Beck CH jr, Abbott WM *et al.* Improved survival from acute renal failure after treatment with intravenous essential L-amino acids and glucose: Results of a prospective, double-blind study. *N Eng J Med* 1973; **288**: 695–699.

21. Baek SM, Makaboli GG, Bryan-Brown CW *et al.* The influence of parenteral nutrition on the course of acute renal failure. *Surg Gynecol Obstet* 1975; **141**: 405–412.

22. McMurray SD, Luft FC, Maxwell DR *et al.* Prevailing patterns and predictor variables in patients with acute tubular necrosis. *Arch Inter Med* 1978; **138**: 950–958.

23. Milligan S, Luft FC, McMurray S *et al.* Intra-abdominal infection and acute renal failure. *Arch Surg* 1978; **113**: 467–474.

24. Leonard CD, Luke RG, Siegel RR. Parenteral essential amino acids in acute renal failure. *Urology* 1975; **6**: 154–157.

25. Feinstein E, Blumenkrantz M, Healy H *et al.* Clinical and metabolic responses to parenteral nutrition in acute renal failure. A controlled double-blind study. *Medicine* 1981; **60**: 124–137.

26. Feinstein E, Kopple JD, Healy H *et al.* Total parenteral nutrition with high or low nitrogen intake in patients with acute renal failure. *Kidney Int* 1983; **26 (suppl 16)**: S319–S323.

27. Sponsel H, Conger JD. Is parenteral nutrition therapy of value in acute renal failure patients? *Am J Kidney Dis* 1995; **25**: 96–102.

28. Harris J, Benedict F. A biometric study of basal metabolism in man. Carnegie Institute, Washington, D.C.; 1919; Publ. No 279.

29. Wilmore D. The metabolic management of the critically ill. Plenum Medical Book, New York, 1977.

30. Monteon F, Laidlow S, Shaib J *et al.* Energy expenditure in patients with chronic renal failure. *Kidney Int* 1986; **30**: 714–747.

31. Kopple JD, Monteon F, Shaib J. Effect of energy intake on nitrogen metabolism in nondialyzed patients with chronic renal failure. *Kidney Int* 1986; **29**: 734–742.

32. Cuppage F, Chiga M, Tate A. Cell cycle studies in the regenerating rat nephron following injury with mercuric chloride. *Lab Invest* 1972; **26**: 122–125.

33. Nicholls D, Ng K. Regeneration of renal proximal tubules after mercuric chloride injury is accompanied by increasing binding of aminoacyltransfer ribonucleic acid. *Biochem J* 1976; **160**: 357–365.

34. Flugel-Link R, Salusky I, Jones M *et al*. Enhanced muscle protein degradation and urea nitrogen appearance (UNA) in rats with acute renal failure. *Am J Physiol* 1983; **244**: E615–E23.

35. Tobak F. Amino acid enhancement of renal generation after acute tubular necrosis. *Kidney Int* 1977; **12**: 193–198.

36. Tobak F, Dodd R, Maier E *et al*. Amino acid enhancement of renal protein synthesis during regeneration after acute tubular necrosis. *Clin Res* 1979; **27**: 432A.

37. Andrews P, Bates S. Dietary protein prior to renal ischemia dramatically affects postischemic kidney function. *Kidney Int* 1987; **32 (suppl 22)**: S76–S80.

38. Malis E, Racusen C, Solez K *et al*. Nephrotoxicity of lysine and of a single dose of aminoglycoside in rats given lysine. *J Lab Clin Med* 1984; **1023**: 660–676.

39. Kaltenbach J, Ganote C, Carone E. Renal tubular necrosis induced by compounds structurally related to D-serine. *J Exp Mol Pathol* 1979; **30**: 209–214.

40. Gabbai F, Pederson O, Blantz R. Protective effect of glycine infusion in a single nephron model of acute renal failure. *Kidney Int* 1989; **35**: 406 (Abstr).

41. Kopple JD. The nutritional management of the patients with acute renal failure. *J Parenter Enter Nutr* 1996; **20**: 3–12.

42. Motil KJ, Harmon WE, Grupe WE. Complications of essential amino acid hyperalimentation in children with acute renal failure. *J Parent Enter Nutr* 1980; **4**: 32–36.

43. Buse M, Reid S. Leucine. A possible regulator of protein turnover in muscle. *J Clin Invest* 1975; **56**: 1250–1253.

44. Felig P. The glucose-alanine cycle. *Metabolism* 1973; **22**: 179–207.

45. Beisel WR, Wannemacher RW. Gluconeogenesis, ureagenesis and ketogenesis during sepsis. *J Parent Nutr* 1980; **4**: 277–285.

46. Hasselgren PO, Almersjo O, Gustavsonn B *et al*. Aminoacid incorporation into liver proteins during short-term ligation of the hepatic artery in the dog. *Eur Surg Res* 1979; **11**: 366–371.

47. Freund HR, James JH, Fisher JE. Nitrogen-sparing mechanism of singly administered branched-chain amino acids in the injured rat. *Surgery* 1981; **90**: 237–243.

48. Wolfe RR, O'Donnell TF, Stone MD. Investigation of factors determining the optimal glucose infusion rate in total parenteral nutrition. *Metabolism* 1980; **29**: 892–900.

49. Askanazi J, Rosenbaum SH, Hyman AL *et al*. Respiratory changes induced by the large glucose loads of total parenteral nutrition. *J Am Med Assoc* 1980; **243**: 1444–1448.

50. Al-Saady NM, Blackmore CM, Bennet ED. High fat, low carbohydrate, enteral feeding lowers $PaCO_2$ and reduces the period of ventilation in artificially ventilated patients. *Intensive Care Med* 1989; **15**: 290–295.

51. Cerra FB. Hypermetabolism, organ failure and metabolic support. *Surgery* 1987; **101**: 1–14.

52. Cerra FB, Alden PA, Negro F *et al*. Sepsis and exogenous lipid metabolism. *J Parent Nutr* 1988; **12 (suppl 6)**: S63–S68.

53. Kuretin P, Kouba J. Profound hypophosphatemia in the course of acute renal failure. *Am J Kidney Dis* 1987; **10**: 346–349.

54. Makoff R. The value of calcium carbonate in treating acidosis, phosphate retention and hypocalcemia. *Nephrol News Issue* 1991; **5**: 16–19.

55. Leenen FH, Buda AJ, Smith DL *et al*. Hemodynamic changes during acetate and bicarbonate hemodialysis. *Artif Organs* 1984; **8**: 411–417.

56. Maeda K, Fujita Y, Shinzato T *et al*. Mechanism of dialysis-induced hypotension. *Trans Am Soc Artif Organs* 1989; **35**: 245–247.

57. Udall J. Human sources and absorption of vitamin K in relation to anticoagulant stability. *J Am Med Assoc* 1965; **194**: 127–131.

58. Kopple JD, Mercurio K, Blumenkrantz M *et al*. Daily requirement for pyridoxine supplements in chronic renal failure. *Kidney Int* 1981; **19**: 694–704.

59. Pru C, Eaton J, Kjellstrand C. Vitamin C intoxication and hyperoxalemia in chronic hemodialysis patients. *Nephron* 1985; **39**: 112–116.

60. Monson P, Mehta RL Nutritional consideration in continuous renal replacement therapies. *Semin Dialysis* 1996; **9**: 152–160.

61. Woolfson AMJ, Heatley RV and Allison SP. Insulin to inhibit protein catabolism after injury. *N Eng J Med* 1979; **300**: 14–19.

62. Kopple JD. The rationale for the use of growth hormone or insulin-like growth factor 1 in adult patients with renal failure. *Miner Electrolyte Metab* 1992; **18**: 269–275.

63. Ikizler TA, Wingard RL, Breyer JA *et al*. Short-term effects of recombinant human growth hormone and intradialytic parenteral nutrition in malnourished haemodialysis patients. *Am J Kidney Dis* 1993; **21**: 527–534.

64. Schulman G, Wingard RL, Hutchison RL *et al*. The effects of recombinant human growth hormone and intradialytic parenteral nutrition in malnourished haemodialysis patients. *Am J Kidney Dis* 1993; **21:** 527–534.

65. Schaefer RM, Tescher M, Riegel W *et al*. Reduced protein catabolism by the antiglucocorticoid RU 38486 in acutely uremic rats. *Kidney Int* 1989; **36 (suppl 27):** S208–S211.

66. Inadomi DW, Kopple JD. Fluid and electrolyte disorders in total parenteral nutrition. In: Maxwell M, Kleeman C, Narins R (eds) *Clinical Disorders of Fluid and Electrolyte Metabolism*, 4th edn. McGraw-Hill, New York, 1987; pp. 945–966.

31

Nutrition support in respiratory disease

Thomas W. Felbinger, Ulrich Suchner, Klaus Peter and Jeffrey Askanazi

Respiratory failure includes a wide variety of diseases, ranging from the malnourished patient with chronic obstructive pulmonary disease to the well-nourished but hypercatabolic patient with adult respiratory distress syndrome (ARDS). Nutrition is an important issue in patients with acute or chronic respiratory disease. Respiratory failure, in particular if complicated by ventilator dependency, may lead to inadequate oral intake and consequently cause malnutrition. However both malnutrition and overfeeding can impair respiratory function. In patients with compromised respiratory muscle function assessment of nutrition status in addition to intensive and specialised nutrition support is essential for improving outcome.

Effects of respiratory disease on nutrition status

Patients with chronic obstructive lung disease have long been recognised as having the potential to develop malnutrition. Emaciation with emphysema was reported as early as 1898.[1] Change in body composition was discussed in chronic lung disease in which 'thinness' was a prominent feature.[2] Filley and colleagues described the clinical subtypes of chronic obstructive bronchopulmonary disease (COPD) as 'pink puffers' (PP) and 'blue bloaters' (BB). The former group was characterised by a thin appearance and a history of 'major weight loss'.[3]

Up to 25% of out-patients with stable COPD are malnourished (defined as > 15% weight loss), while COPD patients requiring admission to hospital show signs of malnutrition in up to 50% of cases.[4,5] When acute respiratory failure complicates the clinical course, severe malnutrition is observed in 60% of cases.[6,7] Decreases in body weight, in triceps skinfold thickness, forearm circumference, creatinine-height index, total lymphocyte count, serum transferrin and retinol-binding protein have all been observed in such patients.

Reduced oral food intake is observed to occur in COPD patients and may result from a series of psychological and physiological factors.[8] Taste perception may be altered by chronic mouth breathing. Appetite may be reduced by depression which may accompany COPD. Dyspnoea increases fatigue during meals leading to reduced eating time. The resulting

reduced oral intake is also diminished by aerophagia which leads to discomfort and gastric distension. Food intake is further hindered by reliance on oxygen when the patient has to choose between using an oxygen mask and food intake. The use of pharmaceutical agents such as antibiotics may cause gastrointestinal disturbances, while chronic steroid intake and long-lasting infections may induce a prolonged catabolic state, which increases metabolic rates and substrate requirements.[5]

The increased work of breathing in COPD requires a higher energy expenditure.[9–11] Both 'pink puffer' and 'blue bloater' have increases in basal metabolic rate and oxygen consumption (VO_2). Moreover, during exercise, the PP group show a greater increase in VO_2.[3]

It has been shown that the increased workload of the respiratory musculature is accompanied by diminished muscle efficiency resulting in increases in the energy cost of breathing.[12] Thus the patient with respiratory impairment has increased energy requirements with decreased caloric intake, causing muscle wasting.

In 487 COPD patients severity of pulmonary disease was related to weight loss over a 4-year period of evaluation.[13] Of particular interest was the finding that body weight also correlated with the FEV_1. Patients with the highest degree of airway obstruction showed the most severe nutritional depletion.[14]

Vendenburgh et al.[15] examined weight loss accompanying COPD in 71 patients over a 7-year period. All patients had established COPD but no other known pulmonary pathology. 29 patients with comparable lung disease but no weight loss were also followed. COPD patients with weight loss were found to have a significantly lower survival rate than COPD patients without weight loss (49% vs 76%). Patients who lost weight were found to have reduced caloric intake, which was in most instances below their estimated requirements. This is even more striking if we account for the fact that energy expenditure is often underestimated in COPD patients when using standardised formulae such as Harris–Benedict.

The detection and treatment of malnutrition directly affects patients' outcome. Several studies have shown that hospital stay is prolonged in malnourished patients compared with normally nourished surgical patients.[16,17] Pingleton et al. showed that malnourished patients requiring mechanical ventilation had a higher mortality than ventilated patients with a normal nutrition status.[18]

Effects of malnutrition and refeeding on respiratory system

Malnutrition has been shown to have an adverse effect on clinical outcome.[19] The impact of protein/energy deficiency on lung function has been studied in both laboratory and clinical environments. Severe protein/energy deficiency has adverse effects in the absence or presence of primary pulmonary disease but in patients with reduced pulmonary function the effects are worsened. The relationship of malnutrition to the development of chronic lung disease has been addressed in a number of studies. Nutrition status and the respiratory system interact at the level of central ventilatory drive, respiratory muscle function, lung parenchyma and cellular metabolism. As a consequence the increased effort of breathing and impaired gas exchange may lead to respiratory failure. Both malnutrition and overfeeding have a negative impact on patients with pulmonary disease.

Central ventilatory drive

Arterial $PaCO_2$ is controlled within a narrow range by the matching of alveolar ventilation and CO_2 production derived from cellular metabolism. $PaCO_2$ via its effect at the brain stem is a major control of central ventilatory drive through changes in pH of the cerebrospinal fluid. Nutrition intake and nutrition status affect ventilatory drive by multiple mechanisms.[20] Nutrition factors influencing the metabolic rate result in changes of tidal volume, VCO_2, VO_2 and the pattern of breathing via a direct central effect of increasing metabolic rate.[21] A decrease of metabolic rate like that seen in starvation depresses hypoxic ventilatory response but this reverses after refeeding.[20,22] In contrast overfeeding and exercise may increase metabolic rate and ventilatory drive.[23,24] Increased CO_2 production such as that seen in the hypermetabolism that accompanies chronic respiratory disease results in a higher demand for alveolar gas exchange. If the situation is complicated by impaired respiratory muscle performance in association with the increased work of breathing, elevation of alveolar partial pressure of CO_2 occurs, increasing the risk of the need for artificial ventilation. Increased dead space contributes further to

higher ventilatory demand in order to maintain normal $PaCO_2$. Independent of the metabolic rate, a high protein load during isocaloric parenteral nutrition has also been shown to enhance ventilatory response to carbon dioxide.[21] A partial explanation of this phenomenon is the specific thermodynamic effect of protein. But increased ventilatory drive is not fully explained by the increase of VO_2 during protein load. The relationship between minute ventilation and $PaCO_2$ during inhalation of CO_2 has been shown to shift leftwards indicating an increased ventilatory sensitivity to CO_2.[21] The hypothesis has been put forward that certain amino acids may affect neurotransmission.[25] Serotonin does act as a potent inhibitor of the ventilatory response. The amino acid tryptophan is precursor of serotonin synthesis. Tryptophan competes with phenylalanine and tyrosin as well as with the branched-chain amino acids (BCAA) valin, leucine and isoleucine in using the same transport mechanism for crossing the blood–brain barrier. Increased BCAA administration may result in decreased serotonin concentration in CNS leading to increased ventilatory drive.[26,27] The increased ventilatory drive may become a therapeutical tool in sleep apnoea syndrome or during weaning from artificial ventilation[25,28,29] but may also lead to respiratory muscle fatigue in patients with chronic respiratory disease.

Respiratory muscle function

The function of respiratory muscles is profoundly disturbed as nutrition status declines.[30] Respiratory muscle strength is closely associated with body weight and lean body mass in patients with COPD.[31,32] There is linear correlation between loss of body weight and decrease of diaphragm muscle mass.[33] The loss of muscle strength and endurance is equally distributed between inspiratory and expiratory muscles and may be measured by reduction of maximal voluntary ventilation and vital capacity. The principal mechanical abnormality in airway obstruction is hyper-inflation of the lungs which shortens the inspiratory muscle contraction. Decrease of diaphragm contractility results in reduction of vital capacity.[34] Malnutrition results in both increased muscle fatiguability and an altered pattern of muscle contraction and relaxation which is reversible by nutrition supplementation.[35] Respiratory muscle failure in malnourished patients might occur because muscle glycogen and amino acids are depleted while energy needs are increased due to enhanced work of breathing. Felig & Wahren[36] have shown that work in a selected group of skeletal muscles depletes glycogen not only from the working muscle, but from resting muscle groups as well. Thus, glycogen stores are mobilised on a whole-body basis for use by the working muscle. This global utilisation of muscle glycogen does not spare the respiratory musculature. Therefore, starvation or stress depletes respiratory muscles of fuel stores which leads to decreased ventilatory endurance.[37,38]

Increase of airway obstruction appears to be associated with decreased amounts of phosphocreatine in intercostal muscles.[39] In the absence of an available fuel source, working muscle has the capacity to utilise intracellular amino acids for fuel. This eventual breakdown of muscle protein progressively weakens the muscles as contractile fibre proteins are consumed. Studies in malnourished COPD patients have shown that diminished protein synthesis contributes to airway obstruction and alveolar dysfunction.[40] With weakening and diminished endurance of the respiratory musculature, alveolar hypoventilation ensues. Thereby the availability of functional airway becomes reduced, increasing the physiological shunt. Since anatomical dead space remains unchanged, the efficiency of ventilation has to be diminished. As a consequence inefficient ventilation performance increases the work of breathing and thereby enhances muscle energy demands. The increased need for fuel in the absence of an available fuel source leads to rapid muscle depletion of glycogen. In ventilator dependent patients this can lead to prolonged failure to wean.

A decline in minute ventilation, tidal volume and respiratory rate will reduce total lung expansion. As lung segments must be expanded periodically to prevent atelectasis, it is conceivable that the reduction in lung expansion predisposes to pulmonary infection and ongoing lung inflammation. This perpetuates the vicious cycle of abnormal lung response to infection and injury, and may constitute permanent lung damage. Since malnourished individuals are known to have deficiencies in cellular and humoral immunity, they may be prone to pulmonary infections which are particularly severe. Despite this hypothesis there are only limited data on improving pulmonary function after refeeding of malnourished patients. After two weeks of refeeding COPD patients demonstrated increase of transdiaphragmatic pressures by 41%.[41] These results were confirmed in patients with anorexia nervosa and with cystic fibrosis.[42,43]

The imbalance of electrolytes and trace elements that may be seen in malnourished patients may contribute to decreased respiratory muscle function.[44,45] In particular low serum phosphate levels reduce creatine phosphates and 2,3-DPG causing muscle weakness, hemolytic anemia and leucocyte dysfunction. Failure to wean patients with severe hypomagmesemia from the ventilator has been reported.[45,46] Hypomagnesemia, and hypermagnesemia and hypokalemia may be important reasons for respiratory muscle weakness.[47,48]

Improved intracellular electrolyte levels during refeeding may also contribute to early improvement of muscle strength and endurance even when a substantial improvement in body composition is not measurable.[49]

Lung parenchyma

Parenchymal effects of malnutrition include structural changes, abnormal alveolar defence mechanisms, altered microcirculation due to abnormal eicosanoid metabolism as well as changes in intercellular lung water content.

Structural changes

The discrimination between the disease-specific impact of malnutrition alone and the interactions between malnutrition and other effects on pulmonary organ structure has not been assessed in humans. The physicians of the famous Warsaw Ghetto studies described a series of clinical events which was termed hunger disease. Weight loss greater than 50% of pre-internment weight was associated with three progressive degrees of illness: fat depletion, withering and terminal cachexia.[50] Post-mortem observations on starvation victims revealed a striking incidence of emphysema in young adult individuals without known risk factors.[51] Stein & Fenigstein stated that of 370 cases, where a detailed lung study was conducted, 50 (13.8%) revealed emphysema.[52] Twenty of these cases were patients under 40 years of age. The pathologists stated: 'Although the changes were present mostly in young adults they resembled those of emphysema of old age'. Histology was performed in five of these cases and each of these showed emphysematous changes.

Advanced hunger disease was characterised by decreases in diaphragmatic excursion, minute ventilation, respiratory rate and the depth of ventilation. There was an increased incidence of bronchitis, pneumonia and tuberculosis. The classic study of Keys[53] in which subjects underwent a 24-week period of semistarvation reaffirms these findings in relation to decreased minute ventilation, tidal volume and respiratory rate coincident with malnutrition. It was also demonstrated in this investigation that these subjects exhibited diminished respiratory efficiency during work. These studies of essentially normal individuals subjected to a spectrum of malnutrition from fasting to death by starvation provide the foundation for the study of malnutrition and chronic lung disease. When starvation is allowed to continue, malnutrition leads to an increased incidence of pulmonary infections and eventually to the premature development of chronic lung disease.

The reported alterations in the lung's injury and repair process in malnourished patients pose a serious threat to the lung cellular structure. By disrupting the balance of protein breakdown and synthesis, such changes have the potential to induce chronic lung disease.

The lung matrix is a dynamic structure constantly undergoing removal and replacement of elastin and collagen. Proteinases and collagenases remove damaged elastin, fibronectin and collagen. This proteolytic activity is kept in check by counterbalance systems such as the antiproteinase α_1-antitrypsin. This balance ensures that only a graded amount of tissue breakdown occurs. Elastin and collagen synthesis is then promptly activated to restore the structural integrity. In malnutrition, both sides of this equation may be abnormal. Neutrophil migration and elastase activity is increased, resulting in an increase of proteolytic activity. The circulating antiproteinases are depleted. As recognised with other circulating proteins during starvation, this is probably due to their utilisation as fuel sources. Instead of a graded, controlled removal of damaged matrix, unopposed destructive activity ensues. Normally, such enhanced destruction would be matched by increased synthesis of elastin, collagen and the other elements of the lung matrix. However, in malnutrition protein synthesis and fibril cross-linking are impaired, resulting in a weakened and structurally abnormal lung matrix.[54]

The skeletal muscle is the principal site of free intracellular glutamine. The critically ill patient with respiratory insufficiency shows a combination of malnutrition with decreased glutamine stores and increased demand of glutamine during catabolic states. This gains more importance as glutamine not only preserves the function of the gut. There is also evidence that endothelial cells of the lung have a high capacity for glutamine utilisation.[55]

The abnormalities in injury and repair do not fully explain the changes in lung mechanics observed in malnutrition. Sahebjami[56,57] and others have described changes in surface recoil in malnourished laboratory animals. Lung pressure–volume curves become abnormal during malnutrition and are restored after refeeding. This is apparently related to a decrease in the production of pulmonary surfactant, which has been shown to decline with malnutrition. The synthesis of surfactant, dipalmitoyl phosphatidylcholine, is markedly influenced by nutrition status.[58] After application of palmitinic acid the synthesis of surfactant was shown to have increased.[59]

Pulmonary immune response

In addition to the direct effects of malnutrition on lung mechanics, malnutrition has profound effects on both the cellular and humoral arms of the immune system. Malnourished individuals have a higher incidence of spontaneous and postoperative infections and are considered to be compromised hosts.[58,60] This may be due to a decrease in the number of alveolar macrophages and lung phagocytic activity as well as diminished IGA synthesis and complement levels.[60-62] Pulmonary clearance of bacteria was found to be severely impaired in starvation. Bacterial adherence to respiratory epithelium was found to be increased in malnourished patients, suggesting a link between nutrition status and the degree of bacterial colonisation.[63] Refeeding of malnourished patients led to restoration of absolute lymphocyte number within one week whereas the phagocytic activity needed about three weeks to return to normal levels.[64]

The cyclo-oxygenase pathway converts eicosanoids to prostaglandins whereas the lipo-oxygenase pathway produces leukotrienes. The products of fatty acid metabolism are potent modulators of inflammation throughout the body. The thromboxanes and leukotrienes B_4 and C_4, D_4, and E_4 are powerful pro-inflammatory agents. PGE_2 and prostacyclin, on the other hand, are anti-inflammatory. The availability of linoleic acid plays a key role in the production of these substances. It has been demonstrated that administration of linoleic acid resulted in an increased production of PGE_2 and prostaglandin metabolites. Such linoleic acid supplementation would exert an anti-inflammatory effect provided that it did not result in additional production of the pro-inflammatory prostaglandins and leukotrienes. Dosages must be large enough to stimulate PGE_2 and prostacyclin but less than that required to produce thromboxane.

Fatty acids other than linoleic acid may play a role as immune modulators. Linolenic acid is an essential fatty acid because of its extensive incorporation into membranes of the neonate. It is structurally distinct from linoleic acid predominantly because of the existence of double bond 3 carbons from the N–terminal, n–3. When linolenic acid is substituted for linoleic, eicosapentanoic acid is formed instead of arachidonic. The resulting prostaglandins and leukotrienes are chemically different from those derived from linoleic acid. Linolenate-derived prostaglandins are designated by the subset 3 and leukotrienes by the subset 5. Remarkably, the slight difference in structure of linoleic and linolenic acid metabolites affects their role in inflammation. For example, thromboxanes A_3 and PGE_3 are patho-physiologically less active and leukotriene B_5 is markedly less chemotactic than its arachidonic acid counterpart, B_4. However, prostazyklin, PGE_2 is equipotent to PGE_3 prostacyclin (PGI_2) is equipotent to PGI_3. Thus, the net effect of substituting linolenic acid for linoleic appears to strongly favour an anti-inflammatory effect. This work has important implications for the interaction between malnutrition and chronic lung disease.

Altered microcirculation and interstitial lung water content

The initial data on worsening of pulmonary gas exchange after lipid infusion were interpreted as mechanical obstruction of the pulmonary micro-circulation by lipid aggregates.[65,66] Whereas this may rarely occur, the more accepted mechanism is the effect of eicosanoid metabolites on bronchial smooth muscle, vascular tone and pulmonary secretions in addition to their immunological influence in the lung. For example, prostaglandins PGD_2 and $PGF_{2\alpha}$ and leukotrienes C_4, D_4, and E_4 are potent broncho-constrictors and may worsen COPD.

Protein deficiency as a consequence of malnutrition may result in low serum albumin levels with decreased colloid osmotic pressure. The accordingly increased interstitial lung water impairs pulmonary gas exchange contributing to the development of respiratory failure.[67,68]

Cellular metabolism

In order to reduce catabolism during starvation glycogen and fat is used as primary fuel. During prolonged malnutrition down-regulation of all aspects of cellular metabolism is the favoured mechanism for preventing protein degradation. However a protein loss cannot be prevented completely and may be substantial during starvation despite all efforts to reduce metabolic rate. After preferential use of labile proteins, muscle protein (including respiratory muscles) is metabolised for providing fuel effecting respiratory function.[69] A study of prolonged fasting in normal volunteers[70] examined the physiological effects produced by a restricted diet that resulted in a 10% weight loss. In that experiment, basal metabolic rate declined by 15–20%. Oxygen consumption declined by a mean of 18% and minute ventilation by 12%. The minute volume decrease was produced by reductions of both respiratory rate and tidal volume. This was not accompanied by a rise in $PaCO_2$, however, suggesting that ventilatory drive was adjusted based on CO_2 production rather than O_2 consumption.

It has long been shown that the metabolic rate, and therefore the respiratory demand, increases during carbohydrate and protein intake.[71] During refeeding it has to be recalled that excessive carbohydrate loads as major fuel sources produce larger amounts of CO_2 compared to a mixed nutrient intake containing balanced amounts of carbohydrates (50%) and lipids (50%). This is based on the different O_2 content of the oxidising substrates leading to a different respiratory quotient. Oxidation of 1010 kcal (4226 kJ) carbo-hydrates (250 g) produces 54 litres CO_2 more than oxidation of 1010 kcal lipids (107 g). Applying 1010 kcal of carbohydrates within 8 hours increases CO_2 production to a 30% higher degree compared to lipid application with the same caloric content.[72] As a consequence there is an increase in the work of breathing. To maintain pCO_2 levels an increase of carbon dioxide production by 30% leads to an increase of alveolar ventilation by 30%. Thus, CO_2 production and ventilatory work are closely related. High carbohydrate loads would therefore appear to be inappropriate for patients at risk of pulmonary decompensation. If increasing CO_2 production cannot be compensated for by increase of alveolar ventilation acute respiratory failure may develop. Optimising CO_2 production is essential in patients who do encounter threatening respiratory failure and the respiratory quotient therefore should be an important parameter to monitor.

110. Schols AM, Soeters PB, Mostert R, Pluymers RJ, Wouters EF. Physiologic effects of nutritional support and anabolic steroids in patients with chronic obstructive pulmonary disease. A placebo-controlled randomized trial. *Am J Respir Crit Care Med* 1995; **152:** 1268–1274.

111. Burdet L, Muralt B, Schutz Y, Pichard C, Fitting J.-W. Administration of growth hormone to underweight patients with chronic obstructive pulmonary disease. *Am J Respir Crit Care Med* 1997; **156:** 1800–1806.

112. Pichard C, Kyle U, Chevrolet JC *et al.* Lack of effects of recombinant growth hormone on muscle function in patients requiring prolonged mechanical ventilation: A prospective, randomized, controlled study. *Crit Care Med* 1996; **24:** 403–413.

113. Roth E, Valentini L, Semsroth M *et al.* Resistance of nitrogen metabolism to growth hormone treatment in the early phase after injury of patients with multiple injuries. *J Trauma* 1995; **1:** 136–141.

32

Nutrition and inflammatory bowel disease

Miquel A Gassull and Fernando Fernández-Bañares

Background

The term inflammatory bowel disease (IBD) includes ulcerative colitis and Crohn's disease (granulomatous enteritis). In both diseases there is inflammation and ulceration of the mucosa with different patterns and degrees of severity. In ulcerative colitis the inflammatory response includes only the mucosa and submucosa, whereas in Crohn's disease the whole thickness of the bowel wall, from mucosa to serosa, is involved. In addition, granulomata in the submucosa are found in about 60% of cases of Crohn's disease.[1] The aetiology is unknown, although in both diseases there is a familial pattern suggesting a genetic basis. Various genes have been implicated in the pathogenesis of IBD, but genetic markers of the major histocompatibility complexes are not consistently associated.[2] The pathogenesis of IBD may be the result of either an anomalous or exaggerated immune response to intestinal alimentary, bacterial or autoantigens, or a normal response to persistent stimuli,[3] which triggers the release of inflammatory mediators (e.g. cytokines, eicosanoids) responsible for the clinical and histological manifestations of the disease.[4]

Ulcerative colitis and Crohn's disease are diagnosed by a set of clinical, endoscopic and histologic characteristics.[1,3] In ulcerative colitis only the colon is involved and colectomy, either with permanent ileostomy or an ileo-anal pouch anastomosis, is considered to be a curative procedure; however, these patients frequently develop complications of the ileo-anal reservoir or have the inconvenience of a permanent ileostomy. In contrast, Crohn's disease may involve any part of the gastrointestinal (GI) tract, often two or more segments at the same time. Following resection of an involved segment, Crohn's disease may recur at any level of the GI tract; thus, unlike ulcerative colitis, surgery cannot be seen as a curative therapeutic approach. Crohn's disease often also involves the anal and perianal region.

The management of both diseases include steroids and salicylates, but is often complex. Despite the differences, there is a group of patients sharing features of both diseases, and in 15% of cases a clear cut diagnosis cannot be established.[5] The length of the bowel involved may not correlate with the severity of the inflammatory activity. Inflammation may be severe in patients with disease confined to a short length of the bowel, whereas some individuals with extensive disease and malnutrition may only show a mild inflammatory activity. Moreover, the patterns of clinical onset and evolution, especially in

Crohn's disease, may vary in different patients, even in those with the same anatomical distribution of the disease.

Therefore, the different patterns of clinical presentation and evolution and in the absence of established aetiological agents or definitive genetic markers, there is the possibility that what is named ulcerative colitis and Crohn's disease may include a spectrum of disease with different aetiologies and a common clinical presentation.

Protein–energy malnutrition (PEM) is common in GI and liver disease, and is frequently associated with active ulcerative colitis and Crohn's disease.[6–11] In addition, in both diseases, changes in the status of micronutrients, some of them involved in important metabolic pathways, have also been described.[9–13] As a consequence, patients with both active ulcerative colitis and Crohn's disease may suffer the additional consequences of these nutritional deficits, which may negatively influence their clinical outcome. In recent years data supporting the hypothesis that nutritional derangement might have some influence in the pathophysiological mechanisms involved in the inflammatory process have been published. For this reason it has been suggested that artificial nutrition, in addition to the supply of energy and nitrogen, might exert a therapeutic effect.

The possible influence of the altered nutrition status in the pathophysiology of IBD and the role of nutrition support in its treatment, in view of the existing data, will be analysed. Also, guidelines for the nutritional management of patients with acute attacks of ulcerative colitis and Crohn's disease, based upon the current knowledge, will be provided.

Nutrition status in IBD

Protein–energy malnutrition, micronutrient deficiency, growth and sexual retardation are often associated with both ulcerative colitis and Crohn's disease.[6–13] In this section, the mechanisms and consequences of PEM and micronutrient deficiency will be described separately.

PEM in IBD

Nutritional deficits are frequently observed in IBD, mainly in Crohn's disease patients with extensive involvement of the small bowel. These may manifest as weight loss, growth retardation and delayed sexual maturation, anaemia, asthenia, osteopenia, diarrhoea, oedema, muscle cramps, impaired cellular immunity and poor wound healing.

The prevalence of PEM in IBD in the literature ranges from 20 to 85%.[6–11] This wide range is due to the fact that most series group together ulcerative colitis, Crohn's disease, hospitalised and ambulatory patients. This results in a mixture of different disease processes, inflammatory activities and organ involvement (small or/and large bowel). In a prospective study, performed in adult patients with moderate–severe active IBD, at hospital admission, the overall prevalence of PEM in IBD was 85%.[7] In the ambulatory patient in clinical remission, this figure is very much lower, but it has been described that multiple nutritional and functional deficits may persist, especially in patients with long-standing Crohn's disease, mainly if they are receiving continuous steroid therapy.[13] PEM in children with IBD may lead to growth retardation and delayed sexual maturation; it is considered that irrespective of steroid use, around 20–30% of children have abnormally short stature as adults.[14–17]

Various factors are involved in the aetiology of malnutrition in IBD. The most important mechanisms are: poor nutrient intake, increased metabolism, increased intestinal protein losses and malabsorption.

Nutrient intake

Poor nutrient intake is common in IBD since anorexia, nausea and vomiting, fear of diarrhoea, abdominal pain or discomfort, and/or medical restrictions on some foods are frequent in the acute attacks of either ulcerative colitis and Crohn's disease. In addition, in Crohn's disease up to 33% of cases may have upper GI tract (oesophagus, stomach and duodenum) involvement,[18] and 34% suffer one or more episodes of intestinal obstruction during the course of the disease.[19] Some drugs used in the treatment of active IBD may induce gastric upset (sulphasalazine, metronidazole, 5-ASA).[20,21] All these factors negatively influence food intake.

The possibility that alimentary antigens might act as triggering factors for the inflammatory response in IBD, and the fact that diarrhoea is the most prominent feature in both ulcerative colitis and Crohn's disease, has for many years prompted the use of 'therapeutic' fasting, together with intravenous steroids and fluids, in the treatment of the acute attacks of both diseases in order to achieve bowel rest. The consequence of this therapeutic approach was the deterioration of the nutrition status.[22] A study assessing the level of food ingestion in hospitalised active IBD patients showed that 44% of the theoretical daily food ingestion was never eaten, because of therapeutic fasting and anorexia.[23] In another paper, studying patients with Crohn's disease without extensive small bowel involvement but with recent weight loss, this was largely the consequence of a decrease in energy and protein intake, and was not related to an increased energy loss.[24] The reasons for this decreased food intake were poor and decreased appetite and little pleasure related to eating. In particular, decreased food intake was reinforced by attendants' and physicians' advice: in almost one-third of the patients a reduction in food intake could be related to an inadequate restricted diet which prescribed a reduction of fat- and fibre-rich foods. The authors were unable to find any relationship between weight loss or nutrition status and disease activity at the time when it was recorded. Therefore, close attention to the diet may be crucial in these patients to prevent malnutrition. This may be achieved by offering palatable energy- and protein-rich foods which do not exacerbate the disease or symptoms of obstruction.

It has been recently shown that prednisone treatment in Crohn's disease patients stimulates food intake and promotes an overall positive energy balance despite large faecal nutrient losses.[25]

Increased metabolism

Reports on energy metabolism in patients with IBD have been contradictory. Resting metabolic rate has been found to be increased,[26] normal,[27] or even reduced[28] in Crohn's disease patients compared to healthy control subjects. This may be partly due to the fact that patients with different disease extent, inflammatory activity and nutrition status were included together. Crohn's disease patients with fever or with very active disease have been known to have a 10–20% increase in resting energy expenditure (REE) (D Rigaud, unpublished observations, 1993; mentioned in reference 24). One possible explanation proposed for the finding of normal REE despite inflammatory processes would be that patients had increased energy expenditure for each unit of free fatty mass (FFM), but low lean body mass.[24] In that study, REE/FFM was higher in patients who had lost weight and had active disease than in those patients with stable weight and quiescent disease, or than in healthy subjects. In addition, it has been shown that REE/FFM is linked to Crohn's disease activity index (CDAI).[24]

In ulcerative colitis it was shown that the energy expenditure was 19% higher than that which could be predicted for healthy adults using the Harris-Benedict equation.[29] Inflammation, as any hypercatabolic process, increases protein degradation through the action of inflammatory mediators causing a negative nitrogen (N) balance.[30] In adults and children with active IBD on artificial nutrition, an increase of both protein synthesis and degradation as disease activity becomes more severe has been demonstrated.[31,32] Moreover, deficiency of some vitamins, minerals and trace elements, which occurs in IBD (see below), negatively influences the synthesis and function of enzymes and other proteins.

Increased intestinal blood and protein losses

Increased blood and protein losses through the inflamed bowel is another contributory factor in the development of PEM.[33] Protein losses parallel the degree of inflammation of the intestinal mucosa and the quantification of this phenomenon has been used as an index of disease activity.[34] Moreover, the possible existence of small intestinal bacterial overgrowth,[35] the changes in the intercellular tight junctions of the mucosal epithelium[36] and the difficulties in the lymphatic drainage[37] may contribute to the negative N balance.

Malabsorption

When Crohn's disease involves the small intestine, malabsorption of various nutrients may occur.[1] This may be an important contributing factor for the development of PEM in such situations. However, the inflamed mucosa is seldom the primary cause of gross nutrient malabsorption in Crohn's disease, except when the disease involves a very extensive area of the small intestine or successive surgical resections resulted in short bowel. Nutrient malabsorption is more often secondary to bile acid malabsorption or small intestine bacterial overgrowth.[35,38] Bile-salt malabsorption often occurs when the terminal ileum is extensively diseased or when the terminal ileum and the right colon has been resected. In such a situation, bile-salt producing diarrhoea results in diminished bile-salt pool, abnormal micellar solubilisation and fat malabsorption.[38] Bacterial overgrowth occurs in 30% of patients with Crohn's disease,[39] secondary to

strictures in the small bowel or to the resection of the ileo-caecal valve. In addition to an increased consumption of vitamin B_{12}, small intestine bacterial overgrowth deranges carbohydrate and protein absorption and bile-salt metabolism.[35]

In summary, PEM in IBD is caused by the association of several factors: the severity of the inflammatory process (increased energy requirements, increased protein breakdown, increased intestinal protein losses); the location of the disease itself (malabsorption); and finally, insufficient nutrient ingestion either related to the disease itself (anorexia), the effect of drugs (gastric upset) or iatrogenic (therapeutic fasting). In Table 32.1, the different factors contributing to the development of PEM in ulcerative colitis and Crohn's disease are summarised. Two factors, seldom mentioned, may be relevant regarding the severity of malnutrition: the time elapsed since the onset of the disease, which usually is longer in Crohn's disease, and

Table 32.1 – Pathophysiological factors contributing to the development of protein–energy malnutrition in IBD.

	Ulcerative colitis	Crohn's disease
Poor nutrient intake		
● Anorexia	+	+
● Inadequate diets	+	+
● Therapeutic fasting	+	+
● Intestinal obstruction	−	+
● Drug-induced gastric upset (Salazopyrine,5-ASA)	+	+
● Metallic taste (metronidazole)	−	+
Increased metabolism		
● Mucosal inflammation and ulceration	+	+
● Septic complications	+	+
● Steroid treatment	+	+
Increased intestinal protein losses		
● Mucosal inflammation	+	+
● Fistulas	−	+
● Poor lymphatic drainage	−	+
Nutrient malabsorption		
● Diarrhoea	−	+
● Mucosal inflammation	−	+
● Previous intestinal resections	−	+
● Small intestine bacterial overgrowth	−	+
● Poor lymphatic drainage	−	+
● Bile salt malabsorption	−	+
● Treatment with cholestyramine	−	+

the acuteness of the attack, which is usually greater in ulcerative colitis. These factors are related to the type of PEM developed which is predominantly marasmatic, or mixed in Crohn's disease and hypo-albuminaemic (kwashiorkor-like) in ulcerative colitis.[7]

Micronutrient deficiency

Micronutrient deficiency, as well as its possible role in the pathogenesis of IBD, has been poorly documented in the literature. The main problems in interpreting the results reported on micronutrient status in hospitalised and ambulatory patients, are:

- the lack of reference values in healthy individuals obtained in the areas where the results are reported

- the lack of agreement about the type of sample to be analysed for a particular micronutrient (whole blood, plasma, urine, tissue)

- the concept of subclinical deficiency or inadequacy for a given nutrient.[40]

This last concept may be of importance in IBD, since in disease states such as ulcerative colitis and Crohn's disease, clinically apparent vitamin or trace element deficiency (except for iron and folate) seldom appears. However, micronutrient inadequacies might play an important role in relevant metabolic pathways in the pathogenesis of IBD.

Vitamins

It is well recognised that patients on sulphasalazine can develop folate deficiency.[41] Also, vitamin B_{12} malabsorption-related megaloblastic anaemia may appear in patients with ileal Crohn's disease, ileal resection or small intestine bacterial overgrowth.[35,39] Although the inadequate levels of some vitamins in general hospital patients has been described,[42,43] this aspect has seldom been studied in IBD, and most reports deal only with the status of particular vitamins such as vitamins A,[44,45] K,[46] D[47,48] and C.[49] There are few series in the literature reporting the simultaneous status of a wide range of vitamins, in relation to the segments of the bowel involved (extensive colitis vs. ileal/ileocaecal).[12,13,50] In one study,[12] plasma or blood levels of biotin, folate, beta-carotene and vitamins A, C and B_1 were reported to be significantly lower in both extensive colitis and ileal/ileocolonic disease as compared to those in healthy controls. Moreover, ileal and/or ileo-caecal involvement were specifically associated to low levels

of vitamin B_{12}, whereas low levels of riboflavin were additionally seen in acute colitis. Although no patient showed clear clinical signs of vitamin deficiency, $> 40\%$ of patients were at risk of developing hypo-vitaminosis (defined as plasma levels of a particular vitamin below the 15th percentile of healthy controls) in both acute colitis and in patients with small intestinal involvement for vitamins A, beta-carotene, folate, biotin, vitamin C and thiamin. A weak correlation between protein–energy nutritional parameters and vitamin values was found.

However, a recent study evaluated the status of multiple vitamins in patients with long-standing Crohn's disease currently in remission.[13] Serum concentrations of beta-carotene, vitamin C, vitamin E and vitamin D were lower in Crohn's disease patients than in age- and sex-matched healthy control subjects, in spite of the fact that daily nutrient intakes were similar between both groups. The proportion of patients with biochemical indexes below the 15th percentile of control subjects was around 40–50% for vitamin E and C, and was 90% for beta-carotene. Therefore, vitamin inadequacies are frequent even in quiescent disease, which may be due to impaired absorption of nutrients (e.g. with small bowel resection or mucosal damage). On the other hand, a significant correlation between serum vitamin D concentrations and the degree of osteopaenia was observed; in fact, levels of vitamin D were correlated with total-body bone fracture risk in patients with long-standing Crohn's disease.[51]

Interpreting vitamin status in IBD is difficult. Low values of vitamin A and E in Crohn's disease involving the small intestine could be attributed to fat malabsorption. However, gross malabsorption is not a frequent finding in unresected Crohn's patients and cannot explain the finding of low plasma vitamin A values in acute colitis (where malabsorption is not expected). Protein losses of visceral proteins, such as prealbumin and retinol binding protein, through the inflamed mucosa, may account for low plasma vitamin A levels, since it circulates in blood bound to these proteins. Thus, low levels of plasma vitamin A reported in the literature[12,44,45] may not reflect the true status of the body stores. Tocopherol circulates in blood bound to lipoproteins, and elevated or low serum lipids result in similar changes in serum vitamin E.[52] The tocopherol/cholesterol ratio is considered a good index of vitamin E status in situations causing hyperlipidaemia,[53–55] but not in hypolipidaemia.[56] The low plasma tocopherol levels found in acute colitis and

Crohn's disease, although they could be explained by the low cholesterol values, do not rule out the existence of inappropriate tissue vitamin E levels in IBD.

Biotin deficiency is extremely rare and recently has been described in patients on long-term total parenteral nutrition (TPN).[57] The possible role of diarrhoea and/or antibiotics producing changes in the biotin forming intestinal microflora is still to be explored.

The pathophysiological and clinical implications of suboptimal vitamin status found in acute IBD are unknown. However, some vitamin–dependent enzyme systems are presumably altered in these patients. Low folate levels were associated to epithelial dysplasia in ulcerative colitis,[58] and low biotin levels were associated with a diminished natural-killer cyto-toxicity of mononuclear cells in Crohn's disease.[59] Inappropriate levels of antioxidant vitamins (beta-carotene, vitamins A, E and C) as well as biotin and vitamin B_2, involved in the scavenging of reactive oxygen radicals and in the polyunsaturated fatty acid biosynthesis, may be of pathobiological importance in the future.

Minerals and trace elements

Iron deficiency, due to blood loss[60] and hypomagnes-aemia[13,61] has been described in active and inactive IBD. Zinc[13,45,62–68] and selenium[13,68–73] status have been studied in Crohn's disease, and less often in ulcerative colitis.[62,68,72–75] Copper, chromium, molybdenum and manganese status in IBD have very seldom been reported.[62,68,73,76]

The interest in evaluating zinc status in Crohn's disease relates to its role in growth retardation[67] and because overt zinc deficiency associated with TPN can occur. Low zinc levels have been found in plasma, hair and urine in active Crohn's disease,[13,62–68] related to plasma albumin levels and disease activity. Zinc plasma levels were also lower in ulcerative colitis,[68] but unlike Crohn's disease these values were unrelated to both serum albumin and disease activity. However, they were positively correlated with low plasma vitamin A levels, probably because the negative effect of zinc deficiency upon the hepatic synthesis of retinol-binding protein.[77] This would be a contributive factor in maintaining low plasma vitamin A levels in ulcerative colitis.

It is difficult to assess the total-body zinc status in acute IBD. The alternatives to the assessment of plasma zinc-dependent enzymes activity (e.g. alkaline phosphatase), which have been used for confirming true zinc deficiency,[78] are the measurement of hair or urinary zinc[79] or the leucocyte zinc content,[71] techniques which are not readily available. Unfortunately, plasma alkaline phosphatase activity cannot be of help in assessing zinc deficiency in IBD since mild increases of this enzyme are common in these patients.[80]

The significance of serum zinc concentrations in the assessment of zinc status is a controversial matter and 60–70% of the circulating zinc is considered exchangeable since it is loosely bound to albumin and is delivered to the metabolically active tissues.[70] Supporting this concept, a correlation between serum and ileal mucosa zinc levels in patients with and without IBD has been reported,[81] as have low mucosa zinc levels in active colitis.[82] In addition, some studies on zinc kinetics have shown low serum levels in relation to an accelerated zinc clearance from the circulation in active Crohn's disease, which correlated positively with the severity of the disease.[83] This suggests an increased zinc turnover at the inflamed tissue. Further arguments suggesting increased requirements of zinc in IBD would be the finding of low levels of zinc-dependent proteins (superoxide dismutase and metalothionein) in the intestinal mucosa of both ulcerative colitis and Crohn's disease.[82,84,85] In this sense, serum zinc concentrations may still provide enough information about zinc status. In addition, in IBD, after both parenteral and enteral nutrition, serum zinc failed to increase in spite of a significant rise in serum albumin concentration.[68,72,86] It has been suggested that rapid anabolism, in the absence of adequate supply, may result in profound falls in serum zinc levels in patients with acute IBD.[86,87]

Other factors may explain increased zinc needs in IBD. Oxidative stress in the inflamed mucosa, as shown in Crohn's disease and ulcerative colitis,[88] might account for increased zinc requirements, since it acts as cofactor of the scavenger enzyme superoxide dismutase, which recently has been shown to be decreased in the neutrophils and in the mucosal biopsies of patients with IBD.[84,85] In addition, zinc is involved in the cell-mediated immunity response in the inflamed mucosa.[89]

Serum selenium is low in IBD patients with severe attacks, associated malnutrition and/or long-standing disease, and tends to increase in patients on either nutrition support or prednisone therapy.[13,68–71,73] Glutathione peroxidase is a selenium-dependent enzyme with antioxidant functions which activity has been found to be decreased in plasma of patients with both ulcerative colitis and Crohn's disease.[13,82] However, overt symptoms of deficiency, including myopathy and cardiomyopathy, are rare.

As previously mentioned, changes in micronutrient status may not only have nutritional importance but influence some of the processes involved in inflammation and tissue damage. In addition to the anti-oxidant vitamins, copper and zinc are necessary for the polyunsaturated fatty acid biosynthesis, and a high Cu/Zn ratio might contribute to an abnormal arachidonate and eicosanoid synthesis in IBD.[90] Otherwise, copper, zinc and selenium may be involved in the processes of reactive oxygen radicals formation and scavenging.[91,92] In this sense all therapeutic manoeuvres intended to support patients with IBD nutritionally should take these aspects into account.

The consequences of PEM and micronutrient deficiency in IBD are the same as in any malnourished patient and are listed in Table 32.2.

Table 32.2 – Consequences of protein–energy mal-nutrition in IBD.

- Immunosuppression (septic episodes)
- Growth retardation and delayed sexual maturation (children)
- Taste alterations
- Anaemia
- Weight loss, asthenia
- Osteopenia
- Delayed healing of fistulas and poor wound healing
- Deficient plasma transport of drugs
- Increased surgical risk
- Delay in achieving remission
- Intestinal villous atrophy (diarrhoea and malabsorption)
- Increased mortality and morbidity
- Increased oxygen-free radicals production
- Impaired cellular immunity

Artificial nutrition support in IBD

In previous sections, the rationale for nutritionally supporting patients with active IBD has been provided. Artificial nutrition now has a well-recognised role as adjuvant treatment in IBD.[93]

Total parenteral nutrition

The advent of TPN gave a means of preventing and treating PEM associated to IBD. It also allowed patients to be 'enterally fasted' so 'bowel rest', one of the cornerstones of the treatment, could be achieved.[22,94,95] Various studies have been published on the effect of TPN in IBD. Interpreting these data is often difficult since some of them are retrospective[22,94-104] or non-controlled.[105-107] Patients with both ulcerative colitis and Crohn's disease involving different segments of the bowel and various degrees of severity and complications are studied together.[22,94,96,97,100,103,105,106] Otherwise, the concepts of drug resistance or failure to medical therapy are not always well defined. Taken together, the controlled and uncontrolled studies indicate that 40–80% (mean 64%) of patients with acute Crohn's disease refractory to medical management respond symptomatically enough to be declared in remission after 2–3 weeks of TPN. Relapse rates range from 28 to 85% after 1 year.[108]

If TPN does have a beneficial effect on Crohn's disease, the reason remains unclear. The initial hypothesis was that bowel rest was important. However, the available data suggest that this is not a significant factor. A prospective, controlled trial in patients with Crohn's disease unresponsive to other medical treatment did not support a role for bowel rest in Crohn's disease.[109] Patients were on steroids and either TPN plus bowel rest, enteral formula diet, or ad libitum oral food plus peripheral parenteral nutrition. Disease activity (CDAI) significantly decreased in all treatment groups, with remission rates of 71, 58 and 60% respectively. The nutrition status did not change in any group. After a year follow-up, there were no differences in the relapse rates among the groups. These results are in accordance with an earlier work of Lochs *et al.*[110] and suggest that 'bowel rest' does not influence clinical outcome in active Crohn's disease. On the other hand, there have been no prospective, randomised, controlled clinical trials comparing TPN with steroids for Crohn's disease.

In contrast, TPN has no therapeutic effect in ulcerative colitis, in which gold standard therapy is steroids. In addition, data suggest that 'bowel rest' does not influence outcome in active ulcerative colitis. In 1980, Dickinson *et al.*[111] reported the first prospective controlled trial comparing the effect of TPN plus steroids vs steroids alone in severe acute colitis (ulcerative colitis and Crohn's disease) to evaluate the effect of nutrition support and 'bowel rest'. No beneficial effect was observed since colectomy was necessary between 32 and 50% in both groups, the rate being higher when only patients with ulcerative colitis were considered. The authors conclude that 'bowel rest' does not have a therapeutic role in acute colitis. A further controlled study by McIntyre et al.[112] also showed no benefit of 'bowel rest' in two groups of severe acute colitis on full steroid therapy when given TPN plus 'bowel rest' or oral diet. There were no differences in the number of patients requiring surgical treatment or in mortality rates between the groups studied. Various concepts in this last study are worth mentioning. First, no patient with Crohn's colitis on either treatment required surgical treatment, whereas in ulcerative colitis 60 and 40% of the cases required colectomy in TPN and oral diet groups respectively. Second, serum albumin increased significantly at the 7th day only in the oral diet group, and this finding was unrelated with the number of units of intravenous albumin administered. However, the number of patients with total colitis was greater in the TPN as compared to the oral diet groups (17 vs 8). This might account for the quicker increase in serum albumin concentrations in the oral diet group as well as for the rate of surgical treatment needed in the TPN group.

From the data described, despite the methodological defects of some studies, some aspects deserve evaluation. First, in Crohn's disease irrespective of the location 'bowel rest' makes little difference even when complications such as fistula or inflammatory mass are present.[109] Second, in severe ulcerative colitis, TPN and 'bowel rest' do not influence clinical outcome.[111,112] Third, ulcerative and Crohn's colitis have a clearly different outcome (surgical treatment being more often required in the former), irrespective of adding TPN and 'bowel rest' to steroid treatment. Data related to side-effects due to catheter insertion, sepsis, hepatic and metabolic complications of TPN are described in the above (controlled, uncontrolled and retrospective) series, but it is difficult to ascertain the true incidence of complications since this information is not always provided. The impact of nutrition support on both complications of surgery and nutrition status is seldom included in studies.

In spite of the absence of primary objective therapeutic effects in ulcerative colitis, TPN is often indicated in severe attacks of colitis when surgical treatment is envisaged in a short-term period. This is because TPN has been proven to promote weight gain and partially restore respiratory and peripheral skeletal muscle function in malnourished IBD patients.[113] However, some data[6,7] suggest that total enteral nutrition (TEN), but not hospital diet plus oral supplements, also prevents nutritional derangement in patients with acute attacks of ulcerative colitis. Moreover, TEN, unlike oral diet, was associated with significant increments in mid-arm muscle circumference and significant lower requirements of intravenous albumin infusions. In a recent prospective controlled trial,[114] the effect of adding TPN plus 'bowel rest' or TEN, with similar caloric and nitrogen distribution and contents, to steroid therapy in severe acute ulcerative colitis was compared. Remission was achieved in 54 and 50% in TEN and TPN groups respectively. Forty-five and 50% of patients in each group required colectomy for similar reasons. Postoperative infections and nutrition support-related complications were significantly more frequent in the TPN than in the TEN group. These results suggest that TEN, despite the fact that it neither influences clinical outcome nor avoids surgery, should be utilised in patients with severe ulcerative colitis, since it is well tolerated and associated with a lower rate of septic complications of surgery than TPN. An additional point is that TEN is an easy method to secure an adequate nutrient intake in these patients, who often need to be encouraged to eat.[23] In this sense, it has been shown that rises in the levels of interleukin-1, a feature in IBD, decreases food motivation in these patients (Kent et al. 1992, personal communication).

Enteral nutrition

The need to withhold nutrients from the intestine to achieve clinical remission in acute Crohn's disease has been questioned,[109,110] prompting the use of the enteral instead of parenteral route in Crohn's disease. The interest in the enteral route has been also related to the simplicity of its use, the lower rate of complications inherent to the technique and the cheaper price of the enteral formulas as compared to TPN. Moreover, the presence of nutrients in the gut may exert beneficial effects upon the functional intestinal barrier,[115] might produce fewer metabolic demands[116] and favours an enhanced protein synthesis.[117] Likewise, the reduced immunological competence associated with undernutrition in Crohn's disease patients improves by short-term nutritional treatment using enteral formula diets.[118] A theoretical inconvenience for using the enteral route in Crohn's disease is the possible antigenic effects of dietary proteins as triggers of the inflammatory response in the bowel. For this reason, elemental (amino acid-based) enteral diets have been used.[119] However, data do not support the hypothesis that the primary therapeutic effect of enteral diets in Crohn's disease was due to the composition of the nitrogen source, since whole-protein-based diets seem to be as effective as amino acid- or peptide-based diets, as mentioned below.

A large number of studies have compared the effectiveness of TEN and steroids as primary therapy for active Crohn's disease.[119–128] Three meta-analyses of the randomised controlled trials have reached the same conclusion: standard steroid treatment is better than any type of enteral nutrition.[129–131] In spite of that, the overall remission rates by intention-to-treat after enteral nutrition were of 60%, which is a figure substantially higher than the reported placebo responses of 20–30%,[132,133] suggesting that enteral nutrition may be an effective therapy. This suggestion has to be taken with some caution since there are no studies directly comparing enteral nutrition with placebo therapy for active Crohn's disease. However, the hypothetical composition of a placebo diet for Crohn's disease is unknown and ethical permission to undertake such a study is unlikely to be forthcoming.

Few studies have evaluated the long-term remission rates after enteral nutrition as compared to steroids. In three studies the length of follow-up was 2–3 months;[119–121] the remission rate after enteral nutrition ranged from 41 to 73%, while after steroids it varied from 70 to 100%. Two other studies evaluated the 1-year remission rates. The first study compared an amino acid-based diet with prednisolone;[125] at 1 year, remission was maintained in only one of the 11 enteral diet-treated patients (9%) compared with six of the 19 prednisolone-treated patients (32%) ($P < 0.05$). The second study evaluated a whole protein-based diet as compared to prednisone.[126] At 1 year, remission rates were 33% for the steroid group and 58% for the enteral diet group, without significant differences in the cumulative relapse probability. The results with the amino acid-based diet in the first study are not in agreement with data of uncontrolled studies in large series of patients with very long follow-up.[134] In that study, the cumulative probability of maintaining remission for 113 patients with active Crohn's disease treated with an amino acid-based diet was retrospectively assessed. The probability of maintaining remission after 1, 3 and 5 years was 55%, 38% and 33% respectively. There were no significant differences

when remission rates of patients treated with the enteral diet were compared to a group of patients of similar characteristics treated with prednisolone during the same period of time in which the study was performed. Therefore, although data are scarce and mainly retrospective, current evidence suggests that there are not clinically relevant differences in long-term remissions after therapy with steroids or enteral diets.

Recent studies performed in children with Crohn's disease, suggest that enteral nutrition does not seem more efficacious in paediatric than adult populations.[135] When comparing the outcomes in the Canadian Paediatric Collaborative Trial[127] and the adult European Collaborative Crohn's disease study,[122] it seems likely that the higher remission overall rate with enteral nutrition in the paediatric study (75%) versus the adult study (53%) reflects differences in the nature of patients randomised rather than an inherent difference in responsiveness of childhood Crohn's disease.[135] This was mainly due to the absence of patients with disease confined to the colon in the paediatric study (22% in the adult trial), and the inclusion of a greater number of patients in relapse in the adult study. In this sense, the remission rate of patients with disease in relapse treated with enteral nutrition in the paediatric trial was of 50%, similar to the figure in the adult study.

On the other hand, there were not significant differences in the use of amino acid-, peptide- or whole-protein-based diets in the above mentioned meta-analyses. Therefore, based on current evidence, the type of enteral diet used is not important.

In the meta-analyses, patients who withdrew from the studies because of intolerance to the diets were considered to be treatment failures on the intention-to-treat analysis. In addition, some of the subgroup analysis included few patients. So, the comparison between amino acid-based diets and steroids only included three studies with a total number of assigned patients of 81, and there were not significant differences between both groups. Likewise, it was not possible to compare whole-protein-based diets with steroids since only one study (including 32 patients) has been published.[126,129] Therefore, results of large series of patients treated with enteral nutrition in uncontrolled trials may be relevant. In fact, the analyses of the remission rates excluding patients withdrawn by lack of compliance due to either diet unpalatability or intolerance to the enteral-tube of all uncontrolled and controlled trials yields interesting findings.[136] Sixteen studies, including 549 compliant adult patients with active Crohn's disease (at least 15 patients in each study treated with enteral nutrition), assessed the effect of amino acid-based diets administered by at least 2 weeks on the induction of clinical remission. The end-point of these studies was the remission rate, which ranged from 42 to 100%, with a mean value of 79%. On the other hand, 124 compliant adult patients included in ten studies received whole-protein-based diets, the mean remission rate being 70% (range 36–90%). These data greatly reinforce the suggestion that enteral nutrition may be an effective therapy when it is well-tolerated and should promote the performance of further controlled studies in active Crohn's disease.

One fact seldom taken into account when comparing the therapeutic effect of diets in Crohn's disease is the possible differences in their fat composition. The possible role of fatty acids and their derivatives (i.e. the eicosanoids) in mediating the inflammatory processes has been emphasised.[137–139] It could be hypothesised that quantitative or qualitative changes in the administered fat (unsaturated vs monounsaturated vs polyunsaturated), may modify eicosanoid synthesis and some immunomodulatory mechanisms, which may influence disease outcome. The number of patients in the different trials comparing enteral nutrition formulas with various amounts of fat is too small to draw definite conclusions about the effect of dietary fat content on disease activity. However, it has been hypothesised that low fat diets (0.6–3% of total calories) may be associated with a favourable outcome, with remission rates of 60–100%.[140,141] In contrast, intermediate or high fat diets (20–36% of total calories) produce controversial results in the enteral feeding trials, with remission rates between 36 and 92%, being lower for the diets with the highest amount of fat.[140,141]

In addition to the quantity, differences in the type of fat among diets may be of importance. It has been hypothesised that clinical remission achieved using amino acid-based diets might be induced by the absence of enough substrate for n-6 derived eicosanoid synthesis (Figs 32.1 and 32.2).[140] In fact, experimental work has shown that the administration of either low fat diets,[142] or diets with low essential fatty acid contents[143] have an immunomodulatory effect in animal models. Moreover, essential fatty acid deficiency diminishes acute inflammation[144] and improves the colitis induced in the rat.[145] Conversely,

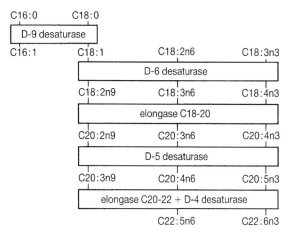

Figure 32.1 – Polyunsaturated fatty acid synthesis (PUFA). PUFA of the different series (n-3, n-6, n-9, n-7) are synthesised by alternative desaturations (addition of a double bound) and elongations (addition of two C atoms). Each series produces their own long-chain PUFA from their own precursors and are not interchangeable in vivo. The precursors of the n-3 and n-6 series are essential fatty acids (linoleic and linolenic acids respectively).

high fat diets containing linoleic acid might be detrimental;[146] and, in contrast, high fat diets containing monounsaturated fatty acids as the predominant fat may be more favourable,[126,147] since they may diminish the availability of eicosanoid polyunsaturated precursors.

Current practice in the nutritional management in IBD

Ulcerative colitis

There are two main indications for artificial nutrition support in ulcerative colitis:

- acute severe attacks
- chronic continuous bouts.

Both situations lead to PEM and nutrition support has to be used as adjuvant therapy to the standard medical treatment. In addition, patients with severe acute ulcerative colitis may require surgical treatment which further worsens nutrition status. When calculating

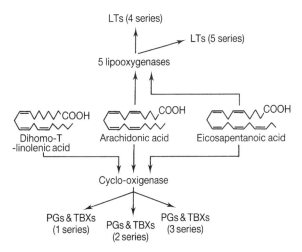

Figure 32.2 – Eicosanoid (prostaglandin, leukotriene and thromboxane) synthesis from long-chain PUFA of the n-6 (di-homo-gamma-linolenic and arachidonic acids) and n-3 (eicosa-pentanoic acid) series.

nutritional requirements for these patients, two aspects have to be taken into account. First, acute colitis is a hypermetabolic state and, second, if the patient is already malnourished they not only have to be nutritionally maintained but replenished.

TPN is the technique of choice in cases of toxic megacolon, intestinal obstruction, paralytic ileus, intestinal perforation, or massive colonic bleeding. In the remaining situations, either TPN or TEN can be used since both have shown to be nutritionally effective and neither prevents surgical treatment when necessary. However, enteral diets are well tolerated by these patients and are associated with fewer post-operative complications. In addition, TEN is cheaper than TPN.

It has to be taken into account that thrombo-embolic disease, which may complicate ulcerative colitis, occurs more often in patients on TPN.[114] Also, catheter sepsis may worsen the course of the disease, and complications such as liver function derangement have been reported to be more frequent in parenterally than in enterally fed IBD patients.[148–150]

Crohn's disease

In Crohn's disease, enteral nutrition is the choice. It is indicated for the treatment of marked mal-nutrition in long-standing disease and to prevent growth retardation in children and adolescents. Moreover, amino acid-based, peptide-based, whole-protein-based diets have shown to be effective in inducing remission. We and others have hypo-thesised that low-fat diets or those containing monounsaturated fatty acids appear to be those with primary therapeutic effect.

TEN should be indicated as primary therapy in active Crohn's disease, mainly in patients in whom steroid therapy is contraindicated, i.e. in the activity bouts of children and adolescents who are growing and of adults with osteopaenia and risk of bone fracture. Further studies are needed to define other possible indications of enteral nutrition. However, it has to be taken into account that 20–30% of patients treated with steroids develop steroid dependence, requiring the administration of strong immunosuppressive drugs such as azathioprine or 6-mercaptopurine to maintain remission and withdraw steroids. Thus, although enteral nutrition therapy seems to be less effective than steroid therapy, it would be indicated in some situations considered to have a better response to the diet, such as initial bouts, ileocolonic disease and mild to moderate clinical activity, with the finality of retarding or avoiding the administration of steroids and their adverse events.

This nutritional approach can be used in patients with either an incomplete obstructive, inflammatory or fistulous (excluding mid-jejunal fistulas) pattern of the disease, even in cases with inflammatory abdominal mass. When occlusion is complete or there are mid-jejunal fistulas, TPN has to be used. Patients with complicated Crohn's disease may need long-term home enteral nutrition to maintain their energy requirements. In such circumstances, the insertion of a percutaneous endoscopic gastrostomy should be considered. In all cases, prior to performing these procedures, a careful endoscopic and histological study should be performed in order to rule out the possibility of gastric involvement by the disease to avoid the risk of a permanent fistulous tract develop-ing if this procedure is carried out on a diseased gastric wall.

Administration technique and monitoring

Administration and monitoring of TPN in IBD do not differ markedly to that in other disease states. TEN should be continuously infused (20–22 hours per day) with the aid of a peristaltic pump through a fine-bore feeding tube in the stomach, since the pylorus regulates the delivery of nutrient to the intestine.[151] Recent reports show that, in healthy subjects, duodenal infusion of enteral diets slows gastric emptying, increases pancreatic secretion and favours gastro-esophageal reflux.[152]

Although some authors have recommended that starter regimens are not used in enterally fed IBD patients,[153] it is advisable to use them in these cases because diarrhoea is a predominant feature of the disease, and may be the major drawback of this therapy. In most cases both full diet volume and strength can be achieved by 3 days.

Both TEN administration and tolerance have to be closely monitored. The appearance or worsening of diarrhoea needs a careful evaluation. This is particularly important in ulcerative colitis patients with prominent rectal symptoms, in whom the repeated passage of blood and mucus, without real faecal content, can be misinterpreted as intolerance to enteral feeding. These patients respond to topic anti-inflammatory treatment without withdrawing enteral feeding.

Difficulties in interpreting diet tolerance may also arise in patients with bacterial overgrowth associated to Crohn's disease. Diarrhoea in these cases may not be due to either inflammation or improper use of TEN but to bacterial fermentation of carbohydrates and hydroxylation of fats of the diet. Metronidazole can prevent the appearance of such phenomenon.

Complications of enteral nutrition have been recently reviewed.[154] Patients with Crohn's disease with wide intestinal resections have to be treated nutritionally and pharmacologically as a short bowel syndrome.

Future trends in artificial nutrition for IBD

The future of artificial nutrition in IBD relies on the use of new nutritional substrates with possible relevance in the metabolism and pathophysiology of the disease.

n-3 fatty acids (marine oils)

The use of long-chain n-3 polyunsaturated fatty acids has been proposed as primary therapy in IBD since they are precursors of eicosanoid with markedly attenuated proinflammatory activity (Fig. 32.2). In addition, n-3 fatty acids may suppress the synthesis of proinflammatory cytokines, including interleukin-1α and tumour necrosis factor-α.[139] To our knowledge, ten trials have been published in both active and inactive ulcerative colitis (seven of them controlled) showing conflicting results.[155–164] The major criticisms to these trials are:

1. most of them are cross-over studies, a design which may not be reliable in a disease that spontaneously changes with time

2. the placebo oils used (linoleic and oleic acids) are not real placebos, but active substances.

On the other hand, two placebo-controlled trials evaluating the role of fish oil for maintaining remission in Crohn's disease have also provided conflicting results. In the first study,[165] Belluzzi et al. randomised 78 patients to receive 2.7 g of an enteric-coated fish oil or placebo. After 1 year of treatment, 59% of patients in the fish oil group remained in remission as compared to 26% in the placebo group. On the other hand, Lorenz-Meyer et al.[166] randomised 204 patients to 2.6 g of n-3 fatty acids as an ethyl ester fish oil concentrate and found no differences in the 1-year remission rate between groups (30% in each group). Disagreement between these two studies may be due to differences in the patients included. In Belluzzi's study, patients who had some laboratory evidence of inflammation and were in clinical remission for fewer than 24 months before the study were included. Patients with these characteristics had a 75% greater risk of relapse than those who have been in remission longer and have normal laboratory results. In addition, the coated fish-oil preparation was associated to few gastric side-effects and the level of compliance was high. The unpleasant taste of other fish-oil preparations is unacceptable to many patients.

Short chain fatty acids (SCFA)

The role of short chain fatty acids as essential fuel for the colonic epithelium has been stressed in the past few years.[167] Short chain fatty acids are generated in the colon by bacterial fermentation of non-absorbed carbohydrates, such as dietary fibre or resistant starches. It was proposed that ulcerative colitis is an energy-deficient state of the colonic mucosa, since reduced SCFA oxidation by colonocytes from patients with ulcerative colitis was observed.[168] It was originally suggested that there might exist a deficiency of SCFA production in these patients. However, reduced, normal or increased levels of SCFA have been found in stool samples of ulcerative colitis patients, suggesting that the problem was a decreased uptake or oxidation of butyrate by colonocytes.[169] Nevertheless, topical SCFA preparations have been used to treat patients with distal ulcerative colitis, being the rationale that higher physiological luminal SCFA concentrations may be able to overcome the postulated metabolic defect in the colonocytes. Results of uncontrolled and controlled trials have been reviewed recently,[169] supporting a role of SCFA irrigation, either as a mixture or as a butyrate monotherapy, in the treatment of mild to moderate distal ulcerative colitis, mainly in patients with a relatively short current episode of colitis (< 6 months) and in those who complied with the enema protocol. On the other hand, recent studies have shown that butyrate may modulate the expression of pro-inflammatory cytokines (tumour necrosis factor, interleukin-8, interleukin-6) by inhibiting the transcription factor NF-κB,[170–172] suggesting that butyrate is a factor by which the luminal contents of the colon may modulate the epithelial immune response.

The possible therapeutic role of fermentable dietary fibre (the main source of SCFA) in enteral feeding formulas and TPN solutions needs to be further explored in patients with colitis.[173–175] However, a recent multicentre open-label study assessed the efficacy of an oral preparation of fermentable fibre containing *Plantago ovata* seeds as compared to the standard therapy with mesalamine to maintain remission in ulcerative colitis.[176] The 1-year relapse rates were similar between both groups (40% for *Plantago ovata* and 35% for mesalamine). The administration of *Plantago ovata* was associated with an increase in the faecal concentrations of butyrate. Further studies are needed to confirm these promising results.

Structured lipids

These compounds would allow the administration, either enterally or parenterally, of different types of fatty acids in a single triglyceride molecule. That means that short, medium and long chain fatty acids could be administered together without the problems inherent to osmolality or stability of the solutions. In this sense, formulas for different metabolic or pathophysiological situations might be designed in the future.[175]

Glutamine

Glutamine has multiple effects on the structure and function of the GI tract, and its effects on improving morbidity and mortality in animal models of GI damage has led to a series of studies in man, which have produced variable results.[177]

A recent study has shown that the colonic mucosa metabolic flux of glutamine was reduced in both ulcerative colitis and Crohn's colitis compared with healthy controls.[178] These changes were more marked in moderate to severe active disease. On the other hand, there were no differences in the glutamine flux in the ileal mucosa between healthy controls and patients with either ulcerative colitis or Crohn's colitis. Authors concluded that the changes observed in colonic mucosal metabolism of glutamine in inflammatory bowel disease are secondary to the inflammatory process and are not indicative of a primary metabolic disorder of the mucosa. However, studies on experimental colitis have shown that glutamine enemas attenuate mucosal injury,[179] and that a glutamine-supplemented elemental diet prevents colonic damage and modulates the inflammatory activity of interleukin-8 and tumour necrosis factor-α.[180] Thus, glutamine might have an anti-inflammatory effect although data in humans with inflammatory bowel disease are scarce. To our knowledge, only one study has assessed the anti-inflammatory effect of glutamine in humans. In a pilot study, glutamine suppositories were administered to patients with chronic pouchitis after ileal pouch–anal anastomosis.[181] Resolution of symptoms was observed in six of ten patients. Further studies of the effect of glutamine supplementation are needed, as well as additional research to define its mechanism of action.

Micronutrients

Micronutrient enriched-diets have to be investigated since some of these elements (Zn, Se, vitamins A, E, C, biotin, etc.) may have implications in the pathophysiology of the disease (see above), and their contents in the present formula-diets may be insufficient.[68,182]

References

1. Kornbloth A, Sachar DB, Salomon P. Crohn's disease. In: Feldman M, Scharschmidpt B, Sleisenger MH (eds) *Sleisenger and Fordtram Gastrointestinal and Liver Disease*. WB Saunders Co, Philadelphia, 1998; pp. 1708–1734.

2. Sartor RB. Pathogenesis and immune mechanisms of chronic inflammatory bowel disease. *Am J Gastroenterol* 1997; **92:** 5S–11S.

3. Podolsky DK. Inflammatory bowel disease (Part 1). *N Engl J Med* 1991; **325:** 928–937.

4. Fiocchi C. Immunology of inflammatory bowel disease. *Curr Opin Gastroenterol* 1991; **7:** 654–661.

5. Kirsner JB, Shorer RG. Recent developments in 'non-specific' inflammatory bowel disease. *N Engl J Med* 1982; **306:** 775–786.

6. Abad A, Cabré E, Giné JJ, Dolz C, González-Huix F, Xiol X, Gassull MA. Total enteral nutrition in inflammatory bowel disease. *J Clin Nutr Gastroenterol* 1986; **1:** 1–8.

7. Gassull MA, Abad A, Cabré E, González-Huix F, Giné JJ, Dolz C. Enteral nutrition in inflammatory bowel disease. *Gut* 1986; **27 (S1):** 76–80.

8. Harries A, Jones L, Heatley RV, Rhodes J. Malnutrition in inflammatory bowel disease. An anthropometric study. *Hum Nutr Clin Nutr* 1982; **36C:** 307–313.

9. Heatley RV. Nutritional implications of inflammatory bowel disease. *Scand J Gastroenterol* 1984; **19:** 995–998.

10. Rosenberg IH, Bengoa JM, Sitrin MD. Nutritional aspects of inflammatory bowel disease. *Ann Rev Nutr* 1985; **5:** 463–484.

11. Gee MI, Grace MGA, Wensel RH, Sherbaniuk R, Thompson ABR. Protein–energy malnutrition in gastroenterology outpatients: Increased risk in Crohn's disease. *J Am Diet Assoc* 1985; **85:** 1466–1474.

12. Fernández-Bañares F, Abad-Lacruz A, Xiol X *et al.* Vitamin status in patients with inflammatory bowel disease. *Am J Gastroenterol* 1989; **84:** 744–748.

13. Geerling BJ, Badart-Smook A, Stockbrügger RW, Brummer RJM. Comprehensive nutritional status in patients with long-standing Crohn's disease currently in remission. *Am J Clin Nutr* 1998; **67:** 919–926.

14. Kirshner BS, Voinchet O, Rosenberg IH. Growth retardation in inflammatory bowel disease. *Gastroenterology* 1978; **75:** 504–511.

15. Burbige EJ, Huang SH, Bayless TM. Clinical manifestations of Crohn's disease in children and adolescents. *Pediatrics* 1975; **55:** 866–871.

16. McCafferty TD, Nasr K, Lawrence AH, Kirsner JB. Severe growth retardation in children with inflammatory bowel disease. *J Pediatr* 1970; **45:** 386–393.

17. Seidman E. Nutritional therapy for Crohn's disease: lessons from the St. Justine Hospital experience. *Inflam Bowel Dis* 1997; **3:** 49–53.

18. Danesh BJZ, Park RHR, Upadhyay R, Howatson A, Lee F, Russell RI. How useful are upper gastro-intestinal biopsies in patients with Crohn's disease? *Gut* 1988; **29:** A703.

19. Farmer RG, Hawk WA, Turnbull RB. Clinical patterns in Crohn's disease: A statistical study of 615 cases. *Gastroenterology* 1975; **68:** 627–635.

20. Singleton JW, Law DH, Kelley ML, Mekhjian HS, Sturdevant RAL. National Cooperative Crohn's disease study: adverse reactions to drugs. *Gastroenterology* 1979; **77:** 870–882.

21. Riley SA, Mani V, Goodman MJ, Herd ME, Dutt S, Turnberg LA. Comparison of delayed-release 5-aminosalicylic acid (mesalazine) and sulfasalazine as maintenance treatment for patients with ulcerative colitis. *Gastroenterology* 1988; **94:** 1383–1389.

22. Mullen JL, Hargrove WC, Dudrick SJ, Fitts WT, Rosato EF. Ten years experience with intravenous hyperalimentation and inflammatory bowel disease. *Ann Surg* 1978; **187:** 523–528.

23. Gassull MA, Cabré E, Vilar L, Montserrat A. Nivel de ingesta alimentaria y su posible papel en el desarrollo de malnutrición calórico-proteica en pacientes gastro-enterológicos hospitalizados. *Med Clin (Barc)* 1985; **85:** 85–87.

24. Rigaud D, Angel LA, Cerf M *et al.* Mechanisms of decreased food intake during weith loss in adult Crohn's disease patients without obvious mal-absorption. *Am J Clin Nutr* 1994; **60:** 775–781.

25. Mingrone G, Benedetti G, Capristo E, De Gaetano A, Greco AV, Tataranni PA, Gasbarrini G. Twenty-four-hour energy balance in Crohn's disease patients: metabolic implications of steroid treatment. *Am J Clin Nutr* 1998; **67:** 118–123.

26. Kushner FS, Schoeller DA. Resting and total energy expenditure in patients with inflammatory bowel disease. *Am J Clin Nutr* 1991; **53:** 161–165.

27. Stokes MA, Hill GL. Total energy expenditure in patients with Crohn's disease: measurement by the combined body scan technique. *J Parenter Enteral Nutr* 1993; **17:** 3–7.

28. Chan ATH, Fleming R, O'Fallon WM, Huitzenga KA. Estimated versus measured basal energy require-ments in patients with Crohn's disease. *Gastroenterology* 1986; **91:** 75–78.

29. Klein S, Meyers S, O'Sullivan P, Barton D, Lleliko N, Janowitz HD. The metabolic impact of active ulcerative colitis. Energy expenditure and nitrogen balance. *J Clin Gastroenterol* 1988; **10:** 34–40.

30. Hartig W, Matkowitz R, Faust H. Post-aggression metabolism: hormonal and metabolic aspects. *J Clin Nutr Gastroenterol* 1986; **1:** 255–260.

31. Powell-Tuck J, Garlick PJ, Lennard-Jones JE, Waterlow JC. Rates of whole body protein synthesis and break-down increase with the severity of inflammatory bowel disease. *Gut* 1984; **25**: 460–464.

32. Thomas AG, Miller V, Yaylor F, Maycock P, Scrimgeour CM, Rennie MJ. Whole body protein turnover in childhood Crohn's disease. *Gut* 1992; **33**: 675–677.

33. Steinfeld JL, Davidson JD, Gordon RS Jr, Greene FE. The mechanism of hypoproteinemia in patients with regional enteritis and ulcerative colitis. *Am J Med* 1960; **29**: 405–415.

34. Crama-Bohbouth G, Peña AS, Biemond J *et al.* Are activity indices helpful in assessing active intestinal inflammation in Crohn's disease? *Gut* 1989; **30**: 1236–1240.

35. King CE, Toskes PP. Small intestine bacterial overgrowth. *Gastroenterology* 1979; **76**: 1035–1055.

36. Bjarnason I, O'Morain C, Levi AJ, Peters TJ. Absorption of 5-chromium-labelled ethylendiaminetetraacetate in inflammatory bowel disease. *Gastroenterology* 1983; **85**: 318–322.

37. Kovi J, Duong HD, Hoand CT. Ultrastructure of intestinal lymphatics in Crohn's disease. *Am J Clin Pathol* 1981; **76**: 385–394.

38. Hoffmann AF, Poley JR. Role of bile acid malabsorption in pathogenesis of diarrhoea and steatorrhoea in patients with ileal resection. *Gastroenterology* 1972; **62**: 918–932.

39. Farivar S, Fromm H, Schindler D, McJunkin B, Schmidt F. Tests of bile acid and vitamin B_{12} metabolism in ileal Crohn's disease. *Am J Clin Pathol* 1980; **73**: 69–74.

40. Pietrzik K. Concept of borderline vitamin deficiency. *Int J Vit Nutr Res* 1985; **27**: 61–73.

41. Hoffbrand AV, Stewart JS, Booth CC, Mollin DL. Folate deficiency in Crohn's disease: incidence, pathogenesis, and treatment. *Br Med J* 1968; **2**: 71–75.

42. Leevy CM, Cardi L, Frank O *et al.* Incidence and significance of hypovitaminosis in a randomly selected municipal hospital population. *Am J Clin Nutr* 1965; **17**: 259–271.

43. Lemoine A, Le Devehat C, Codaccioni JL, Monges A, Bermond P, Salkeld RM. Vitamin B_1, B_2, B_6 and C status in hospital inpatients. *Am J Clin Nutr* 1980; **33**: 2595–2600.

44. Imes S, Pinchbeck B, Dinwoodie A, Walker K, Thompson ABR. Vitamin A status in 137 patients with Crohn's disease. *Digestion* 1987; **37**: 166–170.

45. Schoelmerich MS, Becher MS, Hoppe-Seyler P *et al.* Zinc and vitamin A deficiency in patients with Crohn's disease is correlated with activity but not with localization or extent of the disease. *Hepatogastroenterology* 1985; **32**: 34–38.

46. Krasiski SD, Russell RM, Furie BC *et al.* The prevalence of vitamin K deficiency in chronic gastrointestinal disorders. *Am J Clin Nutr* 1985; **41**: 639–643.

47. Driscoll RH, Meredith SC, Sitrin M, Rosenberg IH. Vitamin D deficiency and bone disease in patients with Crohn's disease. *Gastroenterology* 1982; **83**: 1252–1258.

48. Harries AD, Brown R, Heatley RV, Williams LA, Woohead S, Rhodes J. Vitamin D status in Crohn's disease: Association with nutrition and disease activity. *Gut* 1985; **26**: 1197–1203.

49. Gerson CD, Fabry EM. Ascorbic acid deficiency and fistula formation in regional enteritis. *Gastroenterology* 1974; **64**: 907–912.

50. Kuroki F, Iida M, Tominaga M, Matsumoto T, Hirakawa K, Sugiyama S, Fujishima M. Multiple vitamin status in Crohn's disease. Correlation with disease activity. *Dig Dis Sci* 1993; **38**: 1614–1618.

51. Schoon EJ, van Nunen AB, Heidental G *et al.* Low body fat and risk for osteoporosis in Crohn's disease. *Gut* 1996; **39 (suppl)**: A958.

52. Horwitt MK, Harvey CC, Dahm CH Jr, Searcy MT. Relationship between tocopherol and serum lipid levels for determination of nutritional adequacy. *Ann NY Acad Sci* 1972; **203**: 223–236.

53. Sokol RJ, Heubi JE, Iannaccone ST, Bove KE, Balistreri WF. Vitamin E deficiency with normal serum vitamin E concentration in children with chronic cholestasis. *N Engl J Med* 1984; **310**: 1209–1212.

54. Sokol RJ, Balistreri WF, Hoofnagle JH, Jones EA. Vitamin E deficiency in adults with chronic liver disease. *Am J Clin Nutr* 1985; **41**: 66–72.

55. Thurnham DI, Davies JA, Crump BJ, Situnayake RD, Davis M. The use of different lipids to express serum tocopherol: lipid ratios for the measurement of vitamin E status. *Ann Clin Biochem* 1986; **23**: 514–520.

56. Sokol RJ. Assessing vitamin E status in childhood cholestasis. *J Pediatr Gastroenterol Nutr* 1987; **6**: 10–13.

57. Mock DM, DeLorimer AA, Liebman WM, Sweetman L. Biotin deficiency: an unusual complication of parenteral alimentation. *N Engl J Med* 1981; **304**: 820–823.

58. Lashner BA, Heidenreich PA, Su GL, Kane SV, Hanauer SB. Effect of folate supplementation on the incidence of dysplasia and cancer in chronic ulcerative colitis. A case–control study. *Gastroenterology* 1989; **97**: 255–259.

59. Okabe N, Urabe K, Fujita K, Yamamoto T, Yao T. Biotin effects in Crohn's disease. *Dig Dis Sci* 1988; **33:** 1495–1501.

60. Barr M, Delava S, Zetterstrom R. Studies of the anaemia in ulcerative colitis with special reference to the iron metabolism. *Acata Pediatr* 1975; **44:** 62–72.

61. Valentin N, Nielsen OV, Olesen KH. Muscle cell electrolytes in ulcerative colitis and Crohn's disease. *Digestion* 1975; **13:** 284–290.

62. Penny WJ, Mayberry JF, Agget PJ, Gilbert JO, Newcombe RG, Rhodes J. Relationship between trace elements, sugar consumption, and taste in Crohn's disease. *Gut* 1983; **24:** 288–292.

63. McClain C, Soutor C, Zieve L. Zinc deficiency: a complication of Crohn's disease. *Gastroenterology* 1980; **78:** 272–279.

64. Solomons NW, Rosenberg IH, Sandstead HH, Vo-Khactu KP. Zinc deficiency in Crohn's disease. *Digestion* 1977; **16:** 87–95.

65. Fleming CR, Huizenga KA, McCall JT, Gildea J, Dennis R. Zinc nutrition in Crohn's disease. *Dig Dis Sci* 1981; **26:** 865–870.

66. Valberg LS, Flanagan PR, Kertesz A, Bondy DC. Zinc absorption in inflammatory bowel disease. *Dig Dis Sci* 1986; **31:** 724–731.

67. Nishi Y, Lifshitz F, Bayne MA, Daum F, Silverberg M, Aiges H. Zinc status and its relation to growth retardation in children with chronic inflammatory bowel disease. *Am J Clin Nutr* 1980; **33:** 2613–2621.

68. Fernández-Bañares F, Mingorance MD, Esteve M *et al.* Serum zinc, copper, and selenium levels in inflammatory bowel disease: Effect of total enteral nutrition on trace element status. *Am J Gastroenterol* 1990; **85:** 1584–1589.

69. Jacobson S, Plantin LO. Concentration of selenium in plasma and erythrocytes during total parenteral nutrition in Crohn's disease. *Gut* 1985; **26:** 50–54.

70. Loeschke K, König A, Haeberlin ST, Lux F. Low blood selenium concentration in Crohn's disease (letter). *Ann Intern Med* 1987; **106:** 908.

71. Hinks LJ, Inwards KD, Lloyd B, Clayton B. Reduced concentrations of selenium in mild Crohn's disease. *J Clin Pathol* 1988; **41:** 198–201.

72. Porschen R, Fischer Ch, Purrmann J, Wesch H, Wienbeck M. Urinary excretion and plasma concentrations of trace elements in Crohn's disease (CD): zinc and selenium deficiency is not compensated by treatment with an elemental diet (abstract). *Gastroenterology* 1989; **96:** A396.

73. Ringstad J, Kildebo S, Tomassen Y. Serum selenium, copper, and zinc concentrations in Crohn's disease and ulcerative colitis. *Scand J Gastroenetrol* 1993; **28:** 605–608.

74. Dronfield MW, Malone JDG, Langman MJS. Zinc in ulcerative colitis: a therapeutic trial and report on plasma levels. *Gut* 1977; **18:** 33–36.

75. Mills PR, Fell GS. Zinc and inflammatory bowel disease (letter). *Am J Clin Nutr* 1979; **32:** 2172–2173.

76. Cabré E, Fernández-Bañares F, Esteve M, Gassull MA. Micronutrients in inflammatory bowel disease. *J Clin Nutr Gastroenterol* 1989; **4:** 100–102.

77. Smith JE, Brown ED, Smith JD Jr. The effect of zinc deficiency on the metabolism of retinol-binding in the rat. *J Lab Clin Med* 1974; **84:** 692–697.

78. Hendricks KM, Walker WA. Zinc deficiency in inflammatory bowel disease. *Nutr Rev* 1988; **46:** 401–408.

79. Solomons NW. On the assessment of zinc and copper nutriture in man. *Am J Clin Nutr* 1979; **32:** 856–871.

80. Dew MJ, Thompson H, Allan RN. The spectrum of hepatic dysfunction on inflammatory bowel disease. *Q J Med* 1979; **48:** 113–117.

81. Clarkson JP, Elmes ME. Correlation of plasma zinc and ileal enterocyte zinc in man. *Ann Nutr Metab* 1987; **31:** 259–264.

82. Sturniolo GC, Mestriner C, Lecis PE *et al.* Altered plasma and mucosal concentrations of trace elements and antioxidants in active ulcerative colitis. *Scand J Gastroenterol* 1998; **33:** 644–669.

83. Nakamura T, Higashi A, Takano S, Akagi M, Matsuda I. Zinc clearance correlates with clinical severity of Crohn's disease. A kinetic study. *Dig Dis Sci* 1988; **33:** 1520–1524.

84. Mulder TPJ, Verspaget HW, Janssens AR, de Bruin PAF, Peña AS, Lamers CBHW. Decrease in two intestinal copper/zinc containing proteins with anti-oxidant function in inflammatory bowel disease. *Gut* 1991; **32:** 1146–1150.

85. Lih Brody L, Powell SR, Collier KP *et al.* Increased oxidative stress and decreased antioxidant defenses in mucosa of inflammatory bowel disease. *Dig Dis Sci* 1996; **41:** 2078–2086.

86. Main ANH, Hall MJ, Russell RI, Fell GS, Mills PR, Shenkin A. Clinical experience of zinc supplementation during intravenous nutrition in Crohn's disease: value of serum and urine measurements. *Gut* 1982; **23:** 984–991.

87. Kay RG, Tasman-Jones C, Pybus J, Whiting R, Black H. A syndrome of acute zinc deficiency during total parenteral alimentation in man. *Ann Surg* 1976; **183:** 331–340.

88. Grisham MB, Granger DN. Neotrophil-mediated mucosal injury. Role of reactive oxygen metabolites. *Dig Dis Sci* 1988; **33 (suppl):** 6S–15S.

89. Kruse-Jarres JD. The significance of zinc for humoral and cellular immunity. *J Trace Elem Electrolytes Health Dis* 1989; **3:** 1–8.

90. Cunnane SC. Differential regulation of essential fatty acid metabolism to the prostaglandins: Possible basis for the interaction of zinc and copper in biological systems. *Prog Lipid Res* 1982; **21:** 73–90.

91. Samuni A, Chevion M, Czapski G. Unusual copper-induced sensitization of the biological damage due to superoxide radicals. *J Biol Chem* 1981; **256:** 12632–12635.

92. Blake DR, Allen RE, Lunee J. Free radicals in biological systems – a review orientated to inflammatory processes. *Br Med Bull* 1987; **43:** 371–385.

93. Fernández-Bañares F, Gassull MA. Revisión y consenso en terapia nutricional: Nutrición en la Enfermedad Inflamatoria Intestinal. *Nutr Hosp* 1999; **16 (Suppl 2):** 71–80.

94. Fischer JE, Foster GS, Abel RM, Abbott WM, Ryan JA. Hyperalimentation as primary therapy in inflammatory bowel disease. *Am J Surg* 1973; **125:** 165–175.

95. Vogel CM, Corwin TR, Baue AE. Intravenous hyperalimentation in the treatment of inflammatory diseases of the bowel. *Arch Surg* 1974; **108:** 460–467.

96. Reilly J, Ryan JA, Strole W, Fischer JE. Hyperalimentation in inflammatory bowel disease. *Am J Surg* 1976; **131:** 192–200.

97. Driscoll RH, Rosenberg IH. Total parenteral nutrition in inflammatory bowel disease. *Med Clin North Am* 1978; **62:** 185–201.

98. Strobel CT, Byrne WJ, Ament ME. Home parenteral nutrition in children with Crohn's disease: An effective management alternative. *Gastroenterology* 1979; **77:** 272–279.

99. Bos LP, Weterman IT. Total parenteral nutrition in Crohn's disease. *World J Surg* 1980; **4:** 163–166.

100. Seashore JH, Hillemeier AC, Grybosji JD. Total parenteral nutrition in the management of inflammatory bowel disease in children: a limited role. *Am J Surg* 1982; **143:** 504–507.

101. Shiloni E, Freund HR. Total parenteral nutrition in Crohn's disease. Is it a primary or supportive mode of therapy? *Dis Colon Rectum* 1983; **26:** 275–278.

102. Ostro MJ, Greenberger GR, Jeejeebhoy KN. Total parenteral nutrition and complete bowel rest in the management of Crohn's disease. *J Parenter Enteral Nutr* 1985; **9:** 280–287.

103. Harford FJ, Fazio VW. Total parenteral nutrition as primary treatment for inflammatory disease of the bowel. *Dis Col Rect* 1978; **21:** 555–557.

104. Milewski PJ, Irving MH. Parenteral nutrition in Crohn's disease. *Dis Col Rect* 1980; **23:** 395–400.

105. Elson CO, Layden TJ, Nemchausky BA, Rosenberg JL, Rosenberg IH. An evaluation of total parenteral nutrition in the management of inflammatory bowel disease. *Dig Dis Sci* 1980; **25:** 42–48.

106. Muller JM, Keller HW, Erasmi H, Pichlmaier H. Total parenteral nutrition as the sole therapy in Crohn's disease – a prospective study. *Br J Surg* 1983; **70:** 40–43.

107. Hanauer SB, Sitrin MD, Bengoa JM, Newcomb SA, Kirsner JB. Long-term follow-up of patients with Crohn's disease treated by supportive total parenteral nutrition. *Gastroenterology* 1984; **86:** A1106.

108. Dieleman LA, Heizer WD. Nutritional issues in inflammatory bowel disease. *Gastroenterol Clin N Am* 1998; **27:** 435–451.

109. Greenberg GR, Fleming CR, Jeejeebhoy KN, Rosenberg IH, Sales D, Tremaine WJ. Controlled trial of bowel rest and nutritional support in the management of Crohn's disease. *Gut* 1988; **29:** 1309–1315.

110. Lochs H, Meryn S, Marosi L, Ferenci P, Hortnag H. Has total bowel rest a beneficial effect in the treatment of Crohn's disease? *Clin Nutr* 1983; **2:** 61–64.

111. Dickinson RJ, Ashton MG, Axon ATR, Smith RC, Yeung CK, Hill GL. Controlled trial of intravenous hyperalimentation and total bowel rest as an adjunct to the routine therapy of acute colitis. *Gastroenterology* 1980; **79:** 1199–1204.

112. McIntyre PB, Powell-Tuck J, Wood SR *et al.* Controlled trial of bowel rest in the treatment of severe acute colitis. *Gut* 1986; **27:** 481–485.

113. Christie PM, Hill GL. Effect of intravenous nutrition on nutrition and function in acute attacks of inflammatory bowel disease. *Gastroenterology* 1990; **99:** 730–736.

114. González-Huix F, Fernández-Bañares F, Esteve M *et al.* Enteral versus parenteral nutrition as adjunct therapy in acute ulcerative colitis. *Am J Gastroenterol* 1993; **88:** 227–232.

115. Dowling RH. Small bowel adaptation and its regulation. *Scand J Gastroenterol* 1982; **17 (suppl 74):** 53–74.

116. Mochizuki H, Trocki O, Dominioni L, Brackett KA, Joffe SN, Alexander JW. Mechanism of prevention of postburn hypermetabolism and catabolism by early enteral feeding. *Ann Surg* 1984; **200:** 297–310.

117. Petterson VM, Moore EE, Jones TN et al. Total enteral nutrition versus total parenteral nutrition after major injury: attenuation of hepatic protein repriorization. Surgery 1988; 104: 199–207.

118. Harries AD, Danis VA, Heatley RV. Influence of the nutritional status on immune functions in patients with Crohn's disease. Gut 1984; 25: 465–472.

119. O'Moráin C, Segal AW, Levi AJ. Elemental diet as primary treatment of acute Crohn's disease: a controlled study. Br Med J 1984; 288: 1859–1862.

120. Seidman EG, Bouthillier L, Weber AM, Roy CC, Morin CL. Elemental diet versus prednisone as primary treatment of Crohn's disease. Gastroenterology 1986; 90: A1625.

121. Malchow H, Steinhartdt HJ, Lorenz-Meyer H et al. Feasibility and effectiveness of a defined-formula diet regimen in treating active Crohn's disease. European Cooperative Crohn's disease study III. Scand J Gastroenterol 1990; 25: 235–244.

122. Lochs H, Steinhardt HJ, Klaus-Wentz B et al. Comparison of enteral nutrition and drug treatment in active Crohn's disease. Results of the European Cooperative Crohn's disease study IV. Gastroenterology 1991; 101: 881–888.

123. Sanderson IR, Udeen S, Davies PSW et al. Remission induced by an elemental diet in small bowel Crohn's disease. Arch Dis Child 1987; 61: 123–127.

124. Lindor JD, Fleming CR, Burnes JU et al. A randomized prospective trial comparing a defined formula diet, corticosteroids, and a defined formula diet plus corticosteroids in active Crohn's disease. Mayo Clin Proc 1992; 67: 328–333.

125. Gorard DA, Hunt JB, Payne-James JJ et al. Initial response and subsequent course of Crohn's disease treated with elemental diet or prednisolone. Gut 1993; 34: 1198–1202.

126. González-Huix F, de Leon R, Fernández-Bañares F et al. Polymeric enteral diets as primary treatment of active Crohn's disease. A prospective steroid controlled trial. Gut 1993; 34: 778–782.

127. Seidman E, Griffiths A, Jones A et al. Semi-elemental diet vs prednisone in pediatric Crohn's disease. Gastroenterology 1993; 104: A778.

128. Ruuska T, Savilahti E, Mäki M, Örmälä T, Visakorpi JK. Exclusive whole protein enteral diet versus prednisolone in the treatment of acute Crohn's disease in children. J Pediatr Gastroenter Nutr 1994; 19: 175–180.

129. Fernández-Bañares F, Cabré E, Esteve-Comas M, Gassull MA. How effective is enteral nutrition in inducing clinical remission in active Crohn's disease? A meta-analysis of the randomized clinical trials. J Parenter Enteral Nutr 1995; 19: 356–363.

130. Griffiths AM, Ohlsson A, Sherman PM et al. Meta-analysis of enteral nutrition as a primary treatment of active Crohn's disease. Gastroenterology 1995; 108: 1056–1067.

131. Messori A, Trallori G, D'albasio G, Milla M, Vannozzi G, Pacini F. Defined-formula diets versus steroids in the treatment of active Crohn's disease: a meta-analysis. Scand J Gastroenterol 1996; 31: 267–272.

132. Summers RW, Switz DM, Sessions JT Jr et al. National cooperative Crohn's disease study: results of drug treatment. Gastroenterology 1979; 77: 847–869.

133. Singleton JW, Hanauer SB, Gitnick GL et al. Pentasa Crohn's disease study group. Gastroenterology 1993; 104: 1293–1301.

134. Teahon K, Bjarnason I, Pearson M, Levi AJ. Ten years' experience with an elemental diet in the management of Crohn's disease. Gut 1990; 31: 1133–1137.

135. Griffiths AM. Inflammatory bowel disease. Nutrition 1998; 14: 788–791.

136. Gassull MA. Diet or steroids. In: Jewell DP, Mortensen N, Warren BF (eds) Questions and Uncertainties about Inflammatory Bowel Disease. Oxford Academic Press, Oxford, 2001 (in press).

137. Strasser T, Fischer S, Weber PC. Leukotriene B5 is formed in human neutrophils after dietary supplementation with eicosapentaenoic acid. Proc Natl Acad Sci USA 1985; 82: 1540–1543.

138. Lee TH, Hoover RL, Williams JD et al. Effect of dietary enrichment with eicosapentaenoic and docosahexaenoic acids on in vitro neutrophil and monocyte leukotriene generation and neutrophil function. N Engl J Med 1985; 312: 1217–1224.

139. Endres S, Ghorbani R, Kelley VE et al. The effect of dietary supplementation with n-3 polyunsaturated fatty acids on the synthesis of interleukin-1 and tumor necrosis factor by mononuclear cells. N Engl J Med 1989; 320: 265–271.

140. Fernández-Bañares F, Cabré E, González-Huix F, Gassull MA. Enteral nutrition as primary therapy in Crohn's disease. Gut 1994; 25: S55–59.

141. Middleton SJ, Rucker JT, Kirby GA, Riordan AM, Hunter JO. Long-chain triglycerides reduce the efficacy of enteral feeds in patients with active Crohn's disease. Clin Nutr 1995; 14: 229–236.

142. Morrow WJW, Homsy J, Swanson CA et al. Dietary fat influences the expression of autoimmune disease in MLR 1pr/1pr mice. Immunology 1986; 89: 439–443.

143. Schreiner GF, Flye W, Brunt E et al. Essential fatty acid depletion of renal allografts and prevention of rejection. Science 1988; 240: 1032–1033.

144. Denko CW. Modification of adjuvant inflammation in rats deficient in essential fatty acids. *Agents Actions* 1976; **65:** 636–641.

145. Lohoues MJ, Russo P, Gurbindo C, Roy C, Levy E, Lepage G, Seidman E. Essential fatty acid deficiency improves the course of experimental colitis in the rat: possible role of dietary immunomodulation. *Gastroenterology* 1992; **102:** A655.

146. Giaffer MH, North G, Holdsworth CD. Controlled trial of polymeric versus elemental diet in treatment of active Crohn's disease. *Lancet* 1990; **335:** 816–819.

147. Park RHR, Galloway A, Danesh BJZ, Russell RI. Double-blind controlled trial of elemental and polymeric diets as primary therapy in active Crohn's disease. *Eur J Gastroenterol Hepatol* 1991; **3:** 483–490.

148. Dolz C, Xiol X, Abad A *et al*. Changes in liver function tests in patients with inflammatory bowel disease on enteral nutrition. *J Parenter Enteral Nutr* 1989; **13:** 401–405.

149. Abad-Lacruz A, González-Huix F, Esteve M *et al*. Liver function tests abnormalities in patients with inflammatory bowel disease receiving artificial nutrition: a prospective randomized study of total enteral nutrition vs total parenteral nutrition. *J Parenter Enteral Nutr* 1990; **14:** 618–621.

150. Bengoa JM, Hannauer SB, Sitrin MD *et al*. Pattern and prognosis of liver function test abnormalities during parenteral nutrition in inflammatory bowel disease. *Hepatology* 1985; **5:** 79–84.

151. Silk DBA. Enteral nutrition: the future. *J Clin Nutr Gastroenterol* 1986; **1:** 91–96.

152. Holtmann G, Kelly DG, DiMagno EP. What is the preferred site of enteral nutrition in humans with a normal gut? *Gastroenterology* 1992; **102:** A558.

153. Rees RGP, Keohane PP, Grimble GK, Frost PG, Attrill H, Silk DBA. Elemental diet administered naso-gastrically without starter regimens to patients with inflammatory bowel disease. *J Parenter Enteral Nutr* 1986; **10:** 258–262.

154. Cabré E, Gassull MA. Complications of enteral feeding. *Nutrition* 1993; **9:** 1–9.

155. Lorenz R, Weber PC, Szimnau P, Heldwein W, Strasser T, Loeschke F. Supplementation with n-3 fatty acids from fish oil in chronic inflammatory bowel disease – a randomized, placebo-controlled, double-blind cross-over trial. *J Intern Med* 1989; **225 (suppl. 1):** 225–232.

156. Hawthorne AB, Daneshmen TK, Hawkey CJ, Shaheen MZ, Edwards TJ, Filipowicz BL, Everitt SJ. Fish oil in ulcerative colitis: Final results of a controlled clinical trials. *Gastroenterology* 1990; **98:** A174.

157. Tobin A, Suzuki Y, O'Morain CO. Controlled double blind cross over study of eicosapentaenoic acid (EPA) in chronic ulcerative colitis (UC). *Gastroenterology* 1990; **98:** A207.

158. Hillier K, Jewell R, Dorrell L, Smith CL. Incorporation of fatty acids from fish oil and olive oil into colonic mucosal lipids and effects upon eicosanoid synthesis in inflammatory bowel disease. *Gut* 1991; **32:** 1151–1155.

159. Stenson WF, Cort D, Rodgers J, Burakoff R, DeSchryver-Kecskemeti K, Gramlich TR, Beeken W. Dietary supplementation with fish oil in ulcerative colitis. *Ann Intern Med* 1992; **116:** 609–614.

160. Aslan A, Triadafilopoulos G. Fish oil fatty acid supplementation in active ulcerative colitis: a double-blind, placebo-controlled, crossover study. *Am J Gastroenterol* 1992; **87:** 432–437.

161. Greenfield SM, Green AT, Teare JP, Punchard NA, Thompson RPH. Final results of a controlled trial of fatty acid supplementation in maintenance treatment of ulcerative colitis. *Gastroenterology* 1992; **102:** A631.

162. McCall TB, O'Leary D, Bloomfield J, O'Morain C. Therapeutic potential of fish oil in the treatment of ulcerative colitis. *Aliment Pharmacol Ther* 1989; **3:** 415–424.

163. Salomon P, Kornbluth AA, Janowitz HD. Treatment of ulcerative colitis with fish oil n3-omega-fatty acid: an open trial. *J Clin Gastroenterol* 1990; **12:** 157–161.

164. Salomon P, Kornbluth A, Janowitz HD. Maintenance of remission in ulcerative colitis using fish oil omega-3 fatty acid. *Gastroenterology* 1990; **98:** A201.

165. Belluzzi A, Brignola C, Campieri M, Pera A, Boschi S, Miglioli M. Effect of an enteric-coated fish-oil preparation on relapses in Crohn's disease. *N Engl J Med* 1996; **334:** 1557–1560.

166. Lorenz Meyer H, Bauer P, Nicolay C *et al*. German Crohn's disease study group. Omega-3-fatty acid and low carbohydrate diet for maintenance of remission in Crohn's disease. A randomized controlled multicenter trial. *Scand J Gastroenterol* 1996; **31:** 778–785.

167. Palacio JC, Rolandelli RH, Settle RG, Rombreau JL. Dietary fiber's physiologic effects and potential applications to enteral nutrition. In: Rombeau JL, Caldwell MD (eds) *Enteral and Tube Feeding*, 2nd edn. WB Saunders Co, Philadelphia, 1990; pp. 556–574.

168. Roediger WEW. The colonic epithelium in ulcerative colitis: an energy-deficient disease. *Lancet* 1980; **2:** 712–715.

169. Kim Y. Short chain fatty acids in ulcerative colitis. *Nutr Rev* 1998; **56:** 17–24.

170. Wu GD, Huang N, Wen XM *et al.* Induction of IKB-beta expression by sodium butyrate inhibits transcriptional activation of the interleukin 8 gene. *Gastroenterology* 1997; **112:** A1121.

171. Chevassus P, France PB, Nancey S, Bienvenu J, Andre F, Descos L, Flourie B. Butyrate strongly inhibits the in vitro stimulated release of inflammatory cytokines and cytokines involved in the Th1/Th2 balance. *Gastroenterology* 1999, **116:** A680.

172. Luhrs H, Schauber J, Boxberger F *et al.* Butyrate-mediated inhibition of nuclear factor Kappa B activation. *Gastroenterology* 1999; **116:** A563.

173. Rolandelli RH, Saul SH, Settle RG *et al.* Comparison of parenteral nutrition and enteral feeding with pectin in experimental colitis in the rat. *Am J Clin Nutr* 1988; **47:** 715–719.

174. Palacio JC, Barbera CF, DePaula JA *et al.* Fermentable fiber stimulates colonic mucosal cell proliferation in an experimental model of mucosal ulcerative colitis. *Surg Forum* 1989; **40:** 13–18.

175. Koruda MJ, Rolandelli RH, Bliss DZ *et al.* Parenteral nutrition supplemented with short-chain fatty acids. Effect on the small bowel mucosa in normal rats. *Am J Clin Nutr* 1990, **51:** 685–691.

176. Fernández-Bañares F, Hinojosa J, Sánchez-Lombraña JL *et al.* Randomized clinical trial of Plantago ovata seeds (dietary fiber) as compared with mesalamine in maintaining remission in ulcerative colitis. *Am J Gastroenterol* 1999; **94:** 427–433.

177. Elia M, Lunn PG. The use of glutamine in the treatment of gastrointestinal disorders in man. *Nutrition* 1997; **13:** 743–747.

178. Duffy MM, Regan MC, Ravichandran P, O'Keane C, Harrington MG, Fitzpatrick JM, O'Connell PR. Mucosal metabolism in ulcerative colitis and Crohn's disease. *Dis Colon Rectum* 1998; **41:** 1399–1405.

179. Kaya E, Gür ES, Ozgüç H, Bayer A, Tokyay R. L-glutamine enemas attenuate mucosal injury in experimental colitis. *Dis Colon Rectum* 1999; **42:** 1209–1215.

180. Ameho CK, Adjei AA, Harrison EK *et al.* Prophylactic effect of dietary glutamine supplementation on interleukin 8 and tumour necrosis factor alpha production in trinitrobenzene sulphonic acid induced colitis. *Gut* 1997; **41:** 487–493.

181. Wischmeyer P, Pemberton JH, Philips SF. Chronic pouchitis after ileal pouch-anal anastomosis: responses to butyrate and glutamine suppositories in a pilot study. *Mayo Clin Proc* 1993; **68:** 978.

182. Abad-Lacruz A, Fernández-Bañares F, Cabré E *et al.* The effect of total enteral nutrition on the vitamin status of malnourished patients with inflammatory bowel disease. *Int J Vit Nutr Res* 1988; **58:** 428–435.

33

Nutrition support during the acute care of moderately or severely burned patients

John J Cunningham, Kathy Prelack, Robert Sheridan and
John P Remensnyder

Introduction

The acute care of massively burned patients has evolved to include a series of specific components:

- Effective management of the fluid and electrolyte shifts immediately following injury

- Debridement of burn eschar

- The use of skin substitutes for the temporary coverage of healing skin or excised wound areas (e.g. xenograft or synthetics)

- Autografting from unburned donor sites for the permanent closure of excised wounds

- Nutrition support to ensure donor site and graft healing.

As a result, survival rates have greatly increased for those sustaining full thickness (sometimes termed third degree) burns encompassing more than half of the total body surface area (BSA).

Nutrition support during the acute care period (i.e. until substantial wound closure and autografting are completed) must be designed to meet the unique metabolic demands of severe burn trauma. Chapter 1 outlines the physiological responses to trauma and excellent reviews of strategies for surgical and nutritional management specific to massive burn injury are available elsewhere.[1-3] Energy requirements are increased during the hypermetabolic phase of trauma – the 'flow phase' described by Cuthbertson[4] for trauma. For burns, this appears to begin approximately 36–48 hours after injury. Thereafter, wound healing is directly dependent on a net anabolic state characterised by positive nitrogen balance in the face of ongoing metabolic responses to trauma. Electrolyte concentrations are labile and may be altered by fluid management or antibiotic treatment. Correction of these shifts is especially critical in the cases of potassium, sodium, calcium and phosphorus which may present life-threatening deficiencies. Correction of magnesium deficit is important as an adjunct to improve management of potassium and calcium status. The provision of nutrition must, however, be structured to accommodate the schedule of life-saving surgical procedures.

The initiation of formal, non-volitional nutrition support is required for those patients presenting with moderate to severe burn injury. These injuries are defined here as involving more than 30% of the body surface area burned (BSAB). Children are correspondingly classified as moderate at 25% BSAB and infants at 20% BSAB owing to their higher normal surface-to-volume proportions. The BSAB percentage is determined by standard mapping of body regions described elsewhere.[2,5]

Monitoring the progress of nutrition support poses a challenge in moderate and severe burns. The traditional indices such as body weight, anthropometrics, total body water, rapid turnover proteins (e.g. transferrin, retinol binding protein, prealbumin), or urinary metabolites (e.g. creatinine) do not accurately reflect body composition or nutrient stores during acute burn trauma.

From the outset it is important to emphasise that injured young children, and especially infants, present unique nutritional demands and these needs are less well characterised by clinical research. The literature on nutrition support for severe burns is based primarily on studies of adults and extrapolation must be done with caution for those younger than 6 years. For example, Table 33.1 illustrates the very high energy requirements of moderately to severely burned infants or children as well as the corresponding differences in the appropriate energy:nitrogen ratios that are recommended. Our own experience from over a decade and that of others provides an empirical basis for recommendations in these cases.

Nutrients provided at the levels described in Table 33.1 are sufficient to maintain adequate body weight while promoting anabolic healing of both the autografted primary wound and the donor areas, as is documented by outcome data.[6] Generally, weight loss is expected following a severe burn injury and muscle mass will not be maintained while on strict bed-rest. Maintaining body weight at or above 90% of ideal (IBW) will represent a departure from the normal growth curve in the cases of young infants or toddlers.

Enteral nutrition support should be provided whenever feasible. Several factors may preclude full utilisation of the enteral route, necessitating parenteral nutrition (PN). These factors include poor gastric emptying, severe ileus, abdominal distension and the practice of repeatedly withholding gastric feedings to accommodate the overall surgical excision/grafting schedule. Impaired gastrointestinal motility following trauma or surgery is primarily due to gastric atony while the remaining portion of the gut continues the function.[7] This notion has fostered the practice of

Table 33.1 – Approximations of energy and protein (amino acids) goals for infants, children, adolescents and adults during acute recovery from moderate to severe burns.

Age (years)	Ideal weight (IBW) (kg)	Body surface area (BSA) (m²)	Energy goal (kcal/day)	Protein goal (g/day)	Ratio★ (kcal/gN)
0.25–1.5	5–10	0.27–0.47	100 × kg	3 × kg	200
1.5–3.0	11–15	0.48–0.65	90 × kg	3 × kg	185
3–6	15–20	0.65–0.80	80 × kg	3 × kg	165
6–10	21–30	0.80–1.00	70 × kg	2.5 × kg	175
10–12	31–40	1.0–1.3	1000 +(40 × kg)	2.5 × kg	170
12–14	41–50	1.3–1.5	1000 +(35 × kg)	2.5 × kg	140
15–18	50–70	1.5–1.7	45 × kg	2.5 × kg	110
Adults	50–75	1.5–2.0	40 × kg	2.5 × kg	100

Note: An *individual's* energy goal is more precisely calculated by the nutrition support staff from the IBW (or the BSA).
★ Subtract 25 for the *non-protein* cal:N ratio, if used.

bypassing the stomach when providing enteral tube feeding. Newly developed techniques for transpyloric feeding tube placement at the bedside using fluoroscopy or pH guided wires permit greater ease in achieving such access (see ch 17). Modern solutions for overcoming frequent interruption of feedings for surgical interventions include shortening of fasting times preoperatively and perioperative jejunal feedings combined with gastric decompression.[8,9] However, the disadvantages of transpyloric feedings are the additional surgical procedure and the risk of tube dislodgement. Also, the normal regulatory capacity of the stomach is lost and that may contribute to feeding intolerance. In our unit, the coincident administration of nasogastric feeding as tolerated and PN permits optimal nutrient intake during periods of transition towards full enteral feeding.

Diarrhoea and constipation may influence the course of enteral support (see chs 18 and 19). While diarrhoea has often been viewed as a complication of nutrient density (osmolality) other possibilities including enteral administration of medications and micronutrient supplementation must be considered. Constipation is a frequently overlooked side-effect of opiate narcotics. Close monitoring of bowel patterns and implementation of a bowel medication regime are important in assuring continued tolerance to enteral nutrition. In our experience, sepsis may also induce an ileus or impair intestinal absorption. The use of either central vein parenteral nutrition (CPN) or peripheral parenteral nutrition (PPN) is indicated in these instances.

Fluid requirements and resuscitation

A detailed presentation of fluid requirements and management is beyond the scope of this chapter and is well treated elsewhere.[2,5,10] The guiding principle in fluid therapy is to establish and maintain adequate urine output, often estimated as an hourly rate of 30–50 ml in adults or 1 ml per kg in children. In the absence of renal impairment, fluid provision in the early course of moderate or severe BSAB injury should almost always exceed normal maintenance levels. In instances of unresponsive oliguria or anuria in severely burned children, peritoneal dialysis has been successfully employed at our Institute using intermittent exchanges of 2–4% glucose dialysis mixtures with 45–90 minute dwellings.[10] Controversies remaining with respect to fluid resuscitation include the role of colloid, the differences between children and adults and the influence of inhalation injury or delayed resuscitation on fluid requirements. Regardless of the formula and protocol chosen to initiate resuscitation, subsequent fluid administration is best guided by regular reassessment of resuscitation end points, rather than textbook predictions.

Vasoactive mediators released from injured tissue cause a diffuse capillary leak shortly after a major burn, with extravasation of both crystalloid and colloid for the first 18–24 h after burning. This pathophysiology explains the enormous volume requirements seen in such patients and is the reason that most protocols withhold colloid until 24 hours after the injury.[11] Children are thought to require fluid in excess of that predicted by several common formulae.[12,13] In toddlers and older children whose renal concentrating abilities are more mature, targeting urine flow of 0.5–1 ml/kg/h results in overall fluid requirements much closer to that of the adult and less overall oedema. Patients with inhalation injury have volume requirements greater than that predicted by standard formulae,[14] possibly secondary to the release of vaso-active mediators from injured pulmonary tissue.

Several schemes have been proposed for the initiation of immediate fluid therapy.[2,5] The Parkland method can be used to calculate requirements as:

$$4 \text{ ml} \times \text{weight(kg)} \times \%\text{BSAB}.$$

Others use 2 ml × weight(kg) × %BSAB plus 2000 ml.

For children, an alternative to the Parkland formula has been proposed by Herrin and Crawford[10] as:

$$(2 \text{ ml} \times \text{IBW(kg)} \times \% \text{ BSAB}) + (1500 \text{ ml} \times \text{BSAB (m2)}).$$

The large number of fluid resuscitation formulae in common usage reflects the clinical reality that no one formula accurately predicts fluid requirements in every patient. Because of wide inter-individual variability, no formula can replace a physician at the bedside who frequently reassesses the patient's physiology throughout the resuscitative period.

During the first 24 hours, Ringers Lactate is the primary resuscitative fluid. Because children less than 20 kg can develop hypoglycaemia if glucose is not administered, Ringers Lactate or half normal saline with 5% dextrose at a maintenance rate is given along with a reduced amount of Ringers Lactate: (3 ml × weight(kg) × %burn over 24 hours). Dextrose containing fluid should not be given as the primary resuscitative fluid as hyperglycaemia and osmotic diuresis will result. One half of the calculated 24-h total is given during the first 8 hours after injury and the calculated rate to deliver that volume is based on the time of injury, not on the time that vascular access is achieved. During this first 24-h period it is critical to adjust the Ringers Lactate infusion rate up or down in 10% increments every hour based on age-specific resuscitation end points including urine output, sensorium, base deficit, filling pressures, pulse and blood pressure.

The importance of an hourly bedside evaluation during this period cannot be overemphasised.

During the second 24-h period the diffuse capillary leak which characterises the first 18–24 h abates. Colloid infusions are advised as colloid will now remain intravascular. Ringers Lactate with added albumin is administered by infusion at a dose based on burn size. At this phase, as the diffuse capillary leak seals, crystalloid requirements markedly diminish and transeschar free water loss has a major influence on serum electrolyte concentrations unless an aqueous topical antimicrobial such as 0.5% silver nitrate solution is used. In the former situation free water administration is required and in the latter case transeschar leeching of sodium (estimated as 350 mEq Na × BSA(m²) over 24 hours) demands continued administration of isotonic crystalloid. There is major morbidity associated with aberrations of serum sodium, so diligent electrolyte monitoring during this period is important.

Hypertonic saline (250–300 mmol/l) resuscitation has been used to minimise fluid shifts from plasma into interstitial spaces.[2] It is, therefore, of maximal benefit when initiated early. The initiation of formal nutrition support during this resuscitation phase has not been shown to impart direct benefit. The early use of the enteral route, however, has been suggested to maintain the barrier function of the intestinal mucosa and reduce bacterial translocation from the intestine which may result in sepsis.

Fluid balance during the acute care stage varies according to the medical and surgical needs of the individual patient. Routine monitoring of total daily inputs and daily urinary outputs (the so-called 'Is and Os') generally shows a positive balance in the order of 1500–2000 ml × BSA(m²) or 50–75 ml × weight(kg). This 'positive' volume is not an accurate reflection of fluid retention. Rather, the fluid 'gap' approximates the sum of appreciable extra-cellular fluid (ECF) losses through open wounds into dressings and some degree of oedema. Clinical oedema is common but is not responsive to albumin replacement infusions in the early acute phase. Heightened catabolism of infused albumin is a phenomenon often reported but, as yet, unexplained.

Fluid resuscitation generally perturbs plasma electrolyte concentrations, both because of the volumes infused and because the infused solutions lack several minerals. Although initiation and gradual advancement of feedings may take place during the resuscitative phase, hypomagnesaemia, hypophosphataemia, hypocalcaemia (specifically a low ionised calcium) are likely to be problematic until full nutrition support is achieved. Close monitoring and supplementation are in order. Magnesium balance can affect potassium requirements.[15] Hypophosphataemia is an especially common phenomenon among burn patients as a consequence of glucose administration.[16,17] These mineral imbalances are not necessarily reversed with the institution of nutrition support, and frequently require additional supplementation. Since virtually all patients require potassium supplementation before nutrition support, the risk of hypophosphataemia can be minimised by the delivery of half of the potassium as potassium–phosphate.

Setting energy goals

Energy expenditure for an individual patient can be measured directly at the bedside, but more often it is predicted from formulae based on the body surface area (BSA)[18] or the ideal body weight (IBW),[5] in some instances including the BSAB directly as an additional factor.[19–21] Several commonly applied formulae are listed in Table 33.2. All targets for energy are estimated on the basis of a predicted normal expenditure per unit BSA or IBW to which an increment accounting for the hypermetabolism of injury is added. The use of estimates based on IBW offers the simplicity of prediction in the absence of any measurement and avoids the issue of oedema from fluid resuscitation. Computation of BSA requires weight (or IBW) and a measured or estimated height. For infants or young children, one can presume that the height is appropriate for weight so that BSA can be derived from weight alone (see nomogram, Fig. 33.1). Errors of estimation will be in proportion to the degree of under- or over-weight prior to injury. If IBW is to be employed, the 50th percentile weight-for-age is used as the IBW. Ranges for IBW and BSA for infants and children are approximated in Table 33.1. Weights from preburn history or family paediatric records may also be useful as a guide in decisions to substitute the 75th or 90th percentile weight for the IBW. It is our practice to use the appropriate IBW (i.e. 50th, 75th or 90th percentile) rather than BSA in estimating energy targets for all of our paediatric patients. This ensures that errors of estimation are over-estimates rather than under-estimates in children small for age, whether or not undernutrition is suspected.

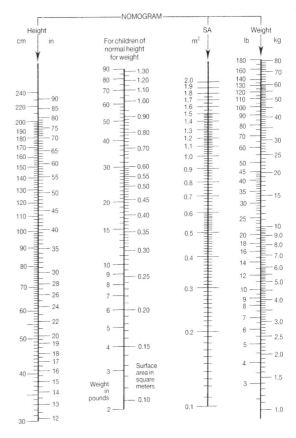

Figure 33.1 – Nomogram for approximating body surface area (BSA). Reproduced with permission from West.[42]

In our acute care ward, the energy goal (kcal or kJ) during the healing phase following moderate to severe burns is termed metabolic energy expenditure (MEE) to distinguish it from the normal metabolic state of resting energy expenditure (REE, also referred to as basal metabolic rate or BMR). MEE incorporates non-standard conditions such as temperature, medications, bedside procedures, continuous feedings, that all modify individual needs. MEE is estimated as:

$$MEE = (1.7 - 2) \times \text{predicted REE}$$

This represents an extrapolation from our published measurements of MEE for adults,[22] our experience with children younger than three years of age[6,23] and a review of the data of others as summarised in Table 33.3.[23] There is substantial agreement that the MEE reaches a plateau for burns with BSAB of 50–95% BSAB. The maximum elevation of MEE only infrequently or transiently exceeds twice the predicted normal REE.

Table 31.2 – Predictions of energy needs in severe burns.

Reference	Equation (kcal)	kcal/day for 50% burn★
Adults		
4	2 × predicted REE	3200
7	2000 × BSA	3800
11	(25 × kg)+(40 × %BSAB)	3750
12	RMR × 1.2 × injury factor	
(8)	(Burn factor = 1.7–2.0)	3700
Children		
13§	Age 0–1: REE +(15 × %BSAB)	(200–600) + 750
	Age 1–3: REE +(25 × %BSAB)	(550–950) + 1250
	Age 4–15: REE +(40 × %BSAB)	(1000–1700) + 2000
14	(1800 × BSA) + (2200 × %BSAB(m²))‡	800–2800‡
4	2 × predicted REE:	
	Age 0–1	450–1200
	Age 1–3	1200–2000
	Age 4–15	2000–3400

★BSA = body surface area; BSAB = body surface area burned as % or m²; calculation assumes BSA = 1.9 m² (adult) or 1.4 m² (child) or 0.4 m² (infant).
§ Reported for %BSAB below 50% (mean = 16%) in 30 children aged 0.5–15 years (mean 4.1) using regression analysis of kcal fed versus weight loss.
‡ Revised downwards in 1989 to approx 1.6 × RMR (see reference 15).

Bedside indirect calorimetry can be used to quantify MEE more precisely. However, this provides merely a glimpse of daily MEE under conditions of measurement that are usually the most restful for the patient. Therefore, we apply a factor of 1.3 as a multiplier to a measured MEE to account for additional stress-related expenditures during dressing changes, physical therapy, etc. In our practice we do not use an additional multiplier for 'activity' during acute care since increases in activity usually coincide with decreases in stress expenditure as the course of healing progresses.

Setting protein goals

Protein requirements are known to be increased by severe burn trauma. Two components contribute to the elevated protein need. Metabolic turnover of the protein pool is increased, including both the rate of protein synthesis and the rate of protein catabolism. Secondly, a redistribution of body protein occurs from peripheral locations, primarily skeletal muscle, to visceral compartments. The magnitude of this amino nitrogen requirement has been less well characterised than energy needs, largely due to the difficulty in estimating nitrogen losses through open wounds, including urea, ammonia, amino acids and some proteins. The literature on nitrogen balance in moderate to severe burns is not complete but, somewhat paradoxically, the amount of protein that should be provided is closely agreed upon (Table 33.4). Of the formulae used to calculate protein targets, only one incorporates %BSAB as a factor. The energy:N ratios of nutrition support formulations in common use by practitioners primarily differ because of MEE estimates rather than the protein goal.

The provision of protein (or amino acids in CPN or PPN) at 2.5 g/kg IBW, or 3 g/kg IBW for infants and children below 20 kg, is sufficient to promote wound healing. Enteral nutrition offers an opportunity for increased protein intake; however, very high protein diets are known to decrease appetite. The nasogastric tube feedings discussed below have been selected for energy:N ratios close to those in Table 33.1. Most deliver adequate energy in fluid volumes of 0.8–1 ml/kcal. Commercially available 'high nitrogen' formulations are useful for older children, adolescents or adults but not for infants, toddlers and younger children whose target energy:N ratios are elevated. Excessive N may be detrimental to any patient and should not exceed 4 g/kg daily.

Table 31.3 – Measured metabolic energy expenditure of burned adults.

Adults¶	N	% BSAB (range)	DPB	Factor (kcal)	MEE (kcal/day)★
Cope *et al.*	11	(20–68)	1–80	$1.3–1.7 \times nl/m^2$	2850–3750
Birke *et al.*	8	57 (20–85)	1–10	$1.5–2 \times HBEE$	2500–3300
Epstein *et al.*	6/17	44/24†	1–5	$225 ml O_2/m_2/min$	3000–3050
Harrison *et al.*	13‡	65 (40–91)	1–10	$1600/m^2/day$	2720 ± 300
Roe & Kinney	1	50	1–11		3400–4000
Roe *et al.*	2	50	10, 13	$2, 1.25 \times nl$	2900, 2350
Gump *et al.*	8	43 (25–60)	6–26	$170 ± 93 ml O_2/m^2$	2300 ± 1250
Gump & Kinney	8	(35–90)	1–14 8–12 (peak)	325–500 ml/min	2275–3500 3500
Neeley *et al.*	7	46 (36–75)	Periodic	$70 W/m^2$ covered $105 W/m^2$ open	2660§ 3975
Zawacki *et al.*	12	40 (17–68)	3–20	$1.5 \times nl/m^2$	3300
Wilmore *et al.*	20	45 (7–84)	6–10	$67 ± 3/m^2/h$	2900–3200
Arturson	16	43 (13–66)	0–35	$35–55 kcal/m^2/h$	1600–2500
Bartlett *et al.*	15	46 (20–70)	1–55	$1.5–2 \times nl/m^2$	2700–5000
Aulick *et al.*	20	44 (10–86)	8–22	$40–90/m^2/h$	1800–4000
Saffle *et al.*	28	35 (3–80)	2 × weekly	$1.4–2.0 \times HBEE$	2500 ± 550
Turner *et al.*	35	34 (10–75)	15 (1–64)	$1.7 \times HBEE − 900$	2160 ± 640
Ireton *et al.*	17	43 (26–79)	2–26	$1.5 \times HBEE$	2500 ± 566
Ireton-Jones *et al.*	20	50 (31–74)	7–99		1000–5000
Shane *et al.* (Maximum)	21 (17)	31 (21–81)	2–26	$HBEE \times af \times if$ admit: discharge:	2640 ± 670 2370 ± 515 (3100 ± 650)
Rutan *et al.*	7 6	67 ± 6 55 ± 3	4–20 4–20	$1300/m^2/day$ $1500/m^2/day$	2600 ± 200 3000 ± 400
Serog *et al.*	24	40 ± 3	2–3	1160/BSAB/day	2640 ± 100
Matsuda *et al.*	28	29 (8–58)	Unknown	30–35 kcal/kg/day	2100–2500
Wolfe *et al.*	18‡	(60–90)	9–48	$1.23 \times HBEE$	2100
Yu *et al.*	12	36 (10–60)	8–50	31 ± 2.4/kg/day	2200 ± 175
Cunningham *et al.* (Maximum)	87 (28)	64 (30–98)	4–150 (4–28)	HBEE, BSAB, DPB	2530 ± 567 (2960 ± 600)
Belcher *et al.*	12	21 (15–45)	6–10	$1200 kcal/m^2/day$	2280
Allard *et al.*	23	39 (7–90)	Periodic	HBEE, BSAB, CI, T, DPB	2220 ± 59
Allard *et al.*	10	49 (30–90)	25 ±4	HBEE, BSAB, CI, T, DPB	2537 ± 86

nl = normal energy expenditure; W = watts; HBEE = Harris–Benedict equation expenditure; MEE = metabolic energy expenditure; DPB = day postburn when measurements taken; CI = caloric intake; af and if are factors for the prediction (see reference 12); T = temperature in centigrade.
★ Assume $1.9 m^2$ and 70 kg. Values in final column calculated by the present author.
† Burn index = (% third degree + % second degree) ÷ 2.
‡ Studies included children.
§ Calculated as 1 W = 0.83 kcal/h.
¶ See reference 18 for details.

Parenteral nutrition formulation

Total PN delivered through a central vein (TPN) can sustain healing even in burns in excess of 95% BSA.

With respect to energy, it is vital to choose a reasonable target since the choice has a profound influence on the volume of formulation required. By virtue of metabolic limitations to the utilisation of continuously infused substrates, TPN will fall short of delivery of the desired energy targets in a relationship generally

Table 33.4 – Predictions of protein need in severe burns.

Reference	Formula	Amount (g/day)
Adults		
1.7 m² BSA		
7	94 g × BSA(m²)	160
4	2.5 g × IBW	175
20	(1 g × kg)+(3 g × %BSAB)	220 (50% BSAB)
21	20–25 gN × BSA(m²)	210–260
Children		
4	2.5 g × IBW (> 20 kg)	50–140
	3 gm × IBW (< 20 kg)	20–60
22	134 g × BSA(m²)	45–200
23	0.4–0.5 gN × kg	20–150

inverse to the age of the patient (see Table 33.5). These limitations include the finite capacities for glucose oxidation[24] (even when glucose can be cleared from plasma with exogenous insulin) and triglyceride clearance and the frequency of surgical procedures

during which intravenous lipid emulsion is not infused. There is some comfort in the knowledge that MEE predictions usually overestimate actual expenditure. As noted, this is the case even for twice predicted REE which is one of the lowest MEE predictors used in severe burns. Coordination with the anaesthesia service enables infusion of the PN solution during the surgical procedures. This is especially important when the early excision and grafting of large areas may occupy several surgical days during the first two weeks of acute care.

Two components of TPN are routinely employed for nutrition support. A crystalloid 'hyperal' solution (hyperalimentation: a clinically used term for parenteral water soluble mixtures) provides dextrose, amino acids, minerals and vitamins and is continuously infused. 'Hyperal' solutions can be formulated in a standardised composition and are referred to as PN solutions in the remainder of this text. Our specific standard TPN solution is outlined in Table 33.6. Sodium and potassium may be increased when indicated. Vitamins and minerals are adjusted to the

Table 33.5 – Rates of infusion for standard CPN formulation⋆ and intravenous lipid emulsion (20%) and the energy deficit that remains to achieve twice REE.

IBW (kg)	CPN infusion			20% Lipid (ml/h)	Total energy		Deficit (2 × REE)	
	(ml/h)	(total ml)	(kcal/kg)		(kcal)	(kcal/kg)	(kcal)	(kcal/kg)
5	8	190	37	1.5	260	52	240	48
6	10	240	39	2	340	57	260	43
7	12	300	42	2	400	57	300	49
8	14	340	42	3	500	62	300	37
9	16	390	42	3	550	61	350	39
10	17	410	40	4	600	60	400	40
11	18	430	38	4	620	56	480	44
12	20	480	39	5	720	60	480	40
13	22	530	40	5	770	59	530	41
14	24	600	42	5	840	60	560	40
15	25	625	41	6	915	61	585	39
16	26	630	39	6	930	58	670	42
17	28	670	39	7	1000	59	700	41
18	30	720	39	7	1050	58	750	42
19	32	770	40	8	1170	62	730	38
20	34	816	40	9	1230	61	770	39
21–30	1.5 × kg	750–1080	35	10	(35 × kg)+500		200–750	10–25
31–40	1.5 × kg	1120–1440	35	10	(35 × kg)+500		150–200	5 × kg+500
41–50	1.5 × kg	1475–1800	35	10	(35 × kg)+500		400–500	10
Teen	1.5 × kg	1800–2500	35	10	(35 × kg)+500		250–0	0–3
Adult	1.5 × kg	1800–2500	35	0–5	(35 × kg)+(0–250)		250–0	0–5

Note: Infusion rates should not be increased by more than 10% without consultation.
⋆ CPN is 20% dextrose with 7.4% amino acids and provides 0.98 kcal/ml.

Table 33.6 – Composition of crystalloid central parenteral nutrition (CPN) solutions.

	Standard	Alt-A (per litre)	Alt-B
Energy (kcal)	986	760	540
Nitrogen (g)	11.7	9.5	7.8
Osmolality (mmol)	1950	1450	1175
Formulation:			
Dextrose (g)	200	150	100
Amino acid (g) (as Novamine)	74	60	50
Potassium (mEq)	30	20	20
Sodium (mEq)	30	20	20
Magnesium (mEq) (as sulphate)	18	12	12
Calcium (mEq)	13	9	9
Chloride (mEq)	26	18	18
Acetate (mEq)	86	65	65
Phosphorus (mM)	13	9	9
Ascorbic acid (mg)	500	500	500

Additives:
Vitamins (per litre):   5 ml of standard intravenous vitamin preparation 10 ml daily maximum (i.e. none in third litre, if used)
Trace elements (per day): 6 ml standard parenteral mixture to provide Zn, Cu, Mn, Cr

American Medical Association (AMA) guidelines for parenteral delivery, with vitamin C raised to 500 mg/l. Electrolytes and additives are 50% higher than in alternative formulations shown in Table 33.6 because of the 'fluid restriction' volumes employed for nutrition support in our routine practice. The TPN solutions are formulated to restore electrolytes to a stable and nearly normal concentration in most cases. The exceptions are potassium and ionised calcium which require precise management and supplementation in response to their labile shifts. The concentration of magnesium in our PN solution is higher than routinely found in continuous infusions. This is a result of observations of frequent sustained hypomagnesaemia during PN and the 'magnesium wasting' urinary losses when aminoglycoside antibiotics are used.[15] When patients are enterally nourished a magnesium supplement may also be needed. Since Mg absorption is estimated to be 40–50%, daily Mg need can be calculated from Table 33.5 using the recommended PN infusion volume multiplied by 0.036 mEq.

The TPN composition used in our practice for burned patients differs from other routinely used parenteral mixtures by its 'fluid restriction' composition and relatively high amino acid concentration. Recent studies support targeting energy:N at 100:1 for trauma patients. As a result, while 'textbook' PN typically delivers 150:1, the ratio of our PN solution is significantly lower at approximately 85:1. Thus, when the protein goal is met by the rates suggested in Table 33.5, the energy goals (see Table 33.1) are not. Additional energy is needed, provided via tube feeding or infused as an intravenous lipid emulsion.

Fat is an important source of both energy and cell membrane components in critical illness. It is frequently used to make up the difference between the estimated energy requirements and the tolerated carbohydrate. Short and medium chain fatty acids are used as energy sources and long chain fatty acids are important in cell membrane formation. Current consensus clinical practice is to administer no more than 60% of total calories as fat. Although disputed, there exist data to suggest that the long chain fatty acids in parenteral lipid formulations may exacerbate pulmonary dysfunction and increase oxygen consumption in patients with sepsis-induced respiratory failure.[25] Therefore, enteral triglyceride is preferred whenever possible. When the provision of enteral tube feeding is not possible, the intravenous infusion of lipid should be considered. While the manufacturers suggest that the daily total lipid infusion should not exceed 4 g/kg for infants or children and 2.5 g/kg for adolescents (and in no case should lipid kilocalories exceed 60% of the total), the approach in an ICU setting should be more cautious. The rates in Table 33.5 conform to these more stringent guidelines. A visual lipaemia check is performed every 24 hours. Lipid is stopped when lipaemia is evident and restarted at a lower rate when lipaemia has resolved. The known stimulation of lipoprotein lipase by heparin affords the opportunity to increase lipid clearance but we do not routinely employ this option.

The intravenous infusion of dextrose in TPN outlined above approximates to 5–6 mg/kg of IBW each minute and is well tolerated by ventilator-dependent patients. Blood glucose should remain in the 'fed' range of 5.5–8 mmol (100–150 mg/dl) without exogenous insulin. Should hyperglycaemia result from any PN infusion, a choice between the risk of development of fatty liver[24] and the benefit from positive nitrogen balance must be made according to the overall patient management plan. Liver function tests are recommended on a regular basis. Very infrequently a young patient will exhibit hyper-glycaemia at the suggested TPN infusion rate. Insulin is not recommended as an additive since the increased clearance of glucose from plasma that follows exogenous insulin is not associated with a substantial increase in glucose oxidation, but rather increases the risk of fat deposition in the liver.[24] A reduction in the dextrose content of TPN without a change in the rate of PN infusion will decrease the glucose load without compromising amino acid delivery. For a patient already receiving the 10% dextrose formulation (Alt-B), a reduction of the infusion rate to correct hyperglycaemia is warranted. This may require co-incident infusion of a 10% amino acid solution should the duration of insulin resistance be prolonged. The standard PN formulation can be delivered at a rate exceeding that recommended, provided that plasma glucose remains below 150 mg/dl, in order to increase nutrient delivery when energy delivery from intralipid is problematic. We do not exceed 110% of the recom-mended rate without a specific nutrition consult.

TPN for infants and young children

For infants and children younger than approximately 6 years (IBW of less than 20 kg) the standard PN formulation (Table 33.6) is infused at an hourly rate of 1.75 ml/kg (42 ml/kg daily total) as shown in Table 33.5. This delivers glucose at 5.8 mg/kg/min and amino acids at 3 gm/kg daily. This rate of dextrose infusion should not be supplemented by dextrose in saline solutions due to potential adverse effects of the increased glucose load. If this formulation is not avail-able but desired, a 0.23% saline solution without added dextrose can be made from 0.45% saline and sterile water in equal volumes. Note that the standard TPN is designed as a 'fluid restriction' formulation and specifically not to deliver the total fluid requirement of the patient. Additional saline infusions are expected to be routinely used with the advantage that the potassium content of the saline solution may be adjusted according to need. As noted, the TPN infusion rate may be increased according to patient tolerance with consultation.

As an alternative, a 10% dextrose formulation can be prepared to contain 0.54 kcal (2.26 kJ)/ml (Alt-B in Table 33.6). The recommended infusion rate for this solution is 1.5 times the rate listed for the standard PN

in Table 33.5. This results in 25% less dextrose (4.4 mg/kg/min) but continues to provide 3 g amino acids per kg IBW daily. Electrolytes are decreased by 50% in this alternative formulation to compensate for the increased rate of infusion. In essence, free water is added and the amino acids are decreased to 5%.

TPN in older children, adolescents and adults

The standard formulation (Table 33.6) is delivered as TPN at an hourly rate of 1.5 ml/kg (36 ml/kg daily total) for children over 6 years of age and adolescents. This provides glucose at a rate of 5.3 mg/kg/min and amino acids at 2.5 gm/kg daily when infused at the rates in Table 33.5. When dextrose is not tolerated at this rate, the ALt-A solution can be used at an hourly rate of 1.75 ml/kg (42 ml/kg daily) to deliver amino acids at 2.5 g/kg daily with dextrose at 4.2 mg/kg/min.

The column labelled 'Deficit' in Table 33.5 high-lights the concern for energy balance in the younger patients. Adolescents and adults are expected to do quite well with little or no intravenous lipid or supplementary tube feeding. Generally, the younger the child, the greater the need for either higher rates of lipid infusion or nasogastric feeding. Severely burned infants (for whom twice the BMR is expected to be the normal preburn oral intake) often receive substantially less than their calorie goal on PN. Adequate graft healing will occur, nevertheless, if the amino acid component is fully delivered (Cunningham et al 1990);[26] that is, lipid infusion is desirable for calories but is sometimes omitted whereas the glucose/amino acid PN solution is con-sidered obligatory.

Enteral nutrition support

The area of enteral nutrition support for severely burned children attracts intensive research. Specialised formulations containing amino acids, peptides and other nutrients as 'immune modulators' in trauma are under development and/or in clinical trials. The role of nutrients in maintaining gut mucosal integrity and reducing the uptake of pathogenic bacteria and toxins is another area of intense interest.

The generalisation that 'when the gut works use it' does not fully apply to severely burned patients for several reasons. Ventilator-assisted breathing is usually required early in care. Preoperative fasting, even for a few hours, is an unaffordable luxury from the nutrition standpoint. Also, progressively longer post-operative ileus is seen with successive surgeries. Enteral tube feeding, even when delivering at a low rate, appears to aid in maintaining integrity and barrier function and thereby minimises invasion by gut microorganisms such as candida. Therefore, enteral nutrition is important as a component of the feeding strategy as soon as is feasible, especially in units where duodenal placements can be established.

In burns exceeding 30% of the total surface area, the feeding of liquid diets by nasogastric tube, or by nasoduodenal tube when ileus is present or gastric residuals are continually high, can be achieved in many instances. Conditions that should be considered when assessing the feasibility of the early use of this preferred route include:

- The risk of aspiration injury
- Bowel motility
- The extent of the energy deficit with TPN (Table 33.5)
- The surgical schedule.

A partial or total transition from TPN to enteral feeding should be made as soon as tolerated. After auto-graft closure of the majority of wounds it may be appropriate to revise the estimates of energy and protein needs for individual patients to promote this transition. However, a transition to enteral feeding during early care with substantial ungrafted wounds should use the same targets as for TPN (Table 33.1). When an oral diet is introduced a transitional feeding plan is implemented to encourage a patient's appetite while maintaining adequate nutrition. Based on the patient's oral intake, a gradual progression to overnight infusion of tube feeding is made. Subsequently, once the patient meets 85% of the established goal on a consistent basis, tube feedings may be discontinued. Feeding success should be judged by the achievement of protein targets; therefore, a careful count of oral protein is required, including good assessment of the portion sizes actually consumed. Menus can be coded by portion size to facilitate this count for the nursing staff. Using energy to calculate deficits and tube feeding rates is less reliable.

Commercial formulations with reasonable osmolalities are very well tolerated. These should be selected for energy:N ratios such as are listed in Table 33.1. Premature infant formulations for those younger than 2 years, normal paediatric mixtures for children and high nitrogen products for adolescents or adults are appropriate (Table 33.7). Modular components such as egg powder, casein, oil and either glucose polymers or the equivalent maltodextrin can be used to formulate enteral tube feeding liquids. When done, total osmolality and electrolyte concentrations must be monitored. Vitamins and non-electrolyte minerals should also be adjusted.

Nasogastric or nasoduodenal tube feeding should be infused at an hourly rate calculated to deliver the protein goal. Most commercially available products such as those in Table 33.7 provide 1–1.5 kcal (4.2–6.3 kJ)/ml at isotonic strength (300–500 mmol/l). In general, most standard products may be initiated at full strength. In situations of prolonged malnutrition or demonstrated intolerance, the rate of infusion and strength of formulation are advanced in steps of 2–4 hours. Prolonged use of paediatric electrolytes for infants is to be avoided since no protein is supplied and the osmolality is as great as that of elemental intraduodenal options such as Pregestimil (Ross Laboratories, Columbus, OH, USA) or Alimentum (Mead Johnson Nutritionals, Evansville, IN, USA).

Nutritional immunomodulation in burns

A therapeutic manoeuvre of great potential utility and ongoing research consists of supplementing conditionally essential nutrients, defined as those that become essential only during periods of intense physiological stress.[27,28] There are data to suggest that glutamine, arginine and ω-3 fatty acids may fit this definition in certain subsets of the seriously injured.

The non-essential amino acid, glutamine, which comprises approximately 6% of mixed whole protein, is unique among amino acids in that it is a favoured fuel of rapidly dividing cells,[29] such as enterocytes and immune cells, and is an important intermediary allowing for accelerated gluconeogenesis from skeletal muscle protein during stress states.[30] Glutamine also

Table 33.7 – Representative commercial enteral feedings.

Product	Energy		Osmolality (mosm/kg)	Protein		Na	K	Fe (mg/l)	RSL‡ (mosm/kg)
	(kcal/l)	(kcal : N)		(g/l)	en%	(mEq/l)			
0–2 years									
Enfamil-Premie 24 (MJ)	800	210★	300	24	12	13	22	1.2†	150§
Prosobee (MJ) intraduodenal	670	165	200	25	13	13	20	13	125§
Alimentum (R)	670	230★	370	18	11	13	20	12	125§
Pregestimil (MJ)	670	220★	350	18	11	13	18	12	125§
1–6 years									
Pediasure (R)	1000	225★	300	28	12	16	33	14	200
Newtrition (KMI) intraduodenal as above	1200	175	310	36	14	26	26	14	320
7 years to adult									
Osmolite-HN (R)	1000	140‖	300	44	17	40	40	13	375
Newtrition-HN (KMI)	1200	150	310	60	20	26	26	14	450
Traumacal (MJ) intraduodenal	1500	116¶	490	83	22	51	36	9	620
Vital-HN (R) fibre-containing	1000	150	450	42	17	20	34	12	320
Jevity (R)	1000	150	310	44	17	36	36	13	375
Replete (R)	1000	100	300	63	25	22	40	18	390

★ Denotes formulations containing energy:N ratios matching goals (Table 33.1).
† Low iron content should be considered when used.
‡ RSL = renal solute load = (grams protein/0.175 + mmol Na + K + Cl) per litre.
§ For infants where urine concentration capacity is a concern, the alternative calculation of 'potential RSL' = RSL + mmol P may be more appropriate (see reference 26).
‖ Appropriate energy:N ratio for 7–12 year olds (Table 33.1).
¶ Appropriate energy:N ratio for adolescents and adults (Table 33.1).
MJ = Mead Johnson Nutritionals, Evansville, IN.
R = Ross Laboratories, Columbus, OH.
KMI = Knight Medical Inc., Cambridge, MA.

may enhance intracellular repletion of glutathione, an important scavenger of reactive oxygen species.[31] Glutamine levels have been demonstrated to be profoundly decreased after thermal injury and this may explain in part the impaired cellular immunity seen in burn patients.[32] Animal and limited clinical data[33] support the supposition that supplemental glutamine may improve outcome in acute illness, probably through diminishing skeletal muscle catabolism and thereby maintaining intracellular glutamine levels by providing a 'preferred substrate' for gut and immune cells.[33,34] Glutamine is not provided in standard commercial nutrition support preparations in significant quantity because of its relatively short shelf-life, although it can be provided as an inexpensive supplement to enteral feeding. Ongoing work will clarify for

us if supplemental glutamine should be administered to burn patients.

Arginine has an important role in the urea cycle and in the generation of nitric oxide and is required to maintain immune cell competence.[35] Early animal data suggests that arginine supplementation may improve immune function in stressed states and recent studies in burn patients suggest that supplies of this important amino acid may be inadequate in the physiologically stressed state.[36] Work is ongoing to determine if clinical outcomes will be favourably affected by supplemental arginine.

Ω-3 long chain fatty acids play a particularly important role in the function of immunocompetent cell membranes.[37] There are some animal data to suggest that supplementation with these unique fatty acids may improve immune function in sepsis. Limited human data are consistent with this thinking,[38] and work is ongoing to determine if clinical outcomes will be improved with this therapy.

Anabolic agents in burns

Another area of intense interest and ongoing research centres on the possibility that administering anabolic agents to burn patients might improve protein accretion and wound healing. Systemically administered recombinant human growth hormone, the beta-agonist clenbuterol and anabolic steroids are most representative of this effort.

Recently made available by recombinant technology, human growth hormone has been actively explored as an adjunct to protein supplementation in an effort to improve nitrogen accretion in critically ill patients.[39] Although its use has been associated with improved protein accretion and more rapid healing of donor sites in burned children, the cost of treatment, as well as the common side-effects of hyperglycaemia and fluid retention, have resulted in less than widespread acceptance in critical care units. However, this therapy does show real promise. Early work with insulin-like growth factor-1 (IGF-1), the effect of much of the positive effects of growth hormone, is also exciting and may lead to useful therapies in selected patients.[40]

Anabolic steroids, although abused in athletic circles, have been used in nonsurgical catabolic disorders and may play a role in critically ill surgical patients in the future.[41] Although the experience with this therapy in burn patients is limited, trials are ongoing.

Administration of the beta-agonist agent, clenbuterol, is associated with enhanced protein accretion in animals. Trial use has occurred in small numbers of critically ill patients with encouraging pilot data being generated. However, the potential side-effects of this agent must be considered when planning therapy. Data are currently not sufficient to support the routine use of anabolic agents in critically ill patients.

Acknowledgement

The authors gratefully acknowledge the contributions of Paul Harmatz, M.D. and John Udall Jr., M.D., Ph.D. that have been carried over from the corresponding chapter in the first edition.

References

1. Burke JF. *Surgical Physiology*. WB Saunders, Philadelphia, 1983.

2. Martyn JA, Szyfelbein SK. Pathophysiology and management of burn trauma in children. *Semin Anesth* 1984; **III:** 75–87.

3. Molnar JA, Wolfe RR, Burke JF. Metabolism and nutritional therapy in thermal injury. In: Schneider HA, Anderson CE, Coursin DB (eds) *Nutritional Support in Medical Practice*, 2nd edn. Harper & Row, Philadelphia, 1983.

4. Cuthbertson DP. Observations on the disturbance of metabolism produced by injury to the limbs. *Quart J Med* 1932; **1:** 233–246.

5. McManus WF, Pruitt BA. Thermal injuries. In: Moore EE, Mattox KL, Feliciano DV (eds), *Trauma*, 2nd edn. Appleton & Lange, Norwalk, CT: 1991, ch. 47.

6. Prelack K, Cunningham JJ, Sheridan R, Tompkins RG. Energy and protein provisions for thermally injured children revisited: An outcome-based approach for determining requirements. *J Burn Care Rehabil* 1997; **18:** 177–181.

7. Wells C, Rawlinson K, Tinckler L, Jones H, Saunders J. Ileus and postoperative intestinal motility. *Lancet* July 16, 1961; pp. 136–137.

8. Hu O, Ho ST, Wang JJ, Ho, W, Wang AJ, Lin CY. Evaluation of gastric emptying in severe burn-injured patients. *Crit Care Med* 1993; **21(4):** 527–531.

9. Jenkins ME, Gottschlich MM, and Warden GD. Enteral feedings during operative procedures in thermal injuries. *J Burn Care Rehabil* 1994; **15:** 199–205.

10. Herrin JT, Crawford JD. The seriously burned child. In: Smith CA (ed) *The Critically Ill Child*. WB Saunders, Philadelphia, 1972; pp. 46–61.

11. Goodwin CW, Dorethy J, Lam V, Pruitt BA, Jr. Randomized trial of efficacy of crystalloid and colloid resuscitation on hemodynamic response and lung water following thermal injury. *Ann Surg* 1983; **197:** 520–531.

12. Merrell SW, Saffle JR, Sullivan JJ, Navar PD, Kravitz M, Warden GD. Fluid resuscitation in thermally injured children. *Am J Surg* 1986; **152:** 664–669.

13. Graves TA, Cioffi WG, McManus WF, Mason AD, Jr., Pruitt BA, Jr. Fluid resuscitation of infants and children with massive thermal injury. *J Trauma* 1988; **28:** 1656–1659.

14. Navar PD, Saffle JR, Warden GD. Effect of inhalation injury on fluid resuscitation requirements after thermal injury. *Am J Surg* 1985; **150**: 716–720.

15. Cunningham JJ, Anbar RA, Crawford JD. Hypomagnesemia: a multifactorial complication of the treatment of patients with severe burns. *J Parent Enter Nutr* 1987; **11**: 364–367.

16. Mozingo DW, Cioffi WG, Mason AD Jr, Milner EA, McManus WF, Pruitt BA Jr. Initiation of continuous enteral feeding induces hypophosphatemia in thermally injured patients. Proceedings of the 35th World Congress of Surgery/International Society Surgical Week. 22–27 August 1993.

17. Hayek ME, Eisenberg PG. Severe hypophosphatemia following the institution of enteral feedings. *Arch Surg* 1989; **124**: 1325–1328.

18. Wilmore DW. Nutrition and metabolism following thermal injury. *Clin Plast Surg* 1974; **1**: 603–619.

19. Souba WW, Bessey PQ. Nutritional support of the trauma patient. *Infect Surg* 1984; 727–738.

20. Turner WW, Ireton CS, Hunt JL, Baxter CR. Predicting energy expenditures in burned patients. *J Trauma* 1985; **25**: 11–16.

21. Allard JP, Pichard C, Hoshino E, *et al*. Validation of a new formula for calculating the energy requirements of burned patients. *J Parent Enter Nutr* 1990; **14**: 115–118.

22. Cunningham JJ, Hegarty MT, Meara PA, Burke JF. Measured and predicted calorie requirements of adults during recovery from severe burn trauma. *Am J Clin Nutr* 1989; **49**: 404–408.

23. Cunningham JJ, Lydon ML, Russell WE. Calorie and protein provision during recovery from severe burns in infants and young children. *Am J Clin Nutr* 1990; **51**: 553–557.

24. Burke JF, Wolfe RR, Mullany CJ, Mathews DE, Bier DM. Glucose requirements following burn injury. *Ann Surg* 1979; **190**: 274–285.

25. Chassard D, Guiraud M, Gauthier J, Gelas P, Berrada KR, Bouletreau P. Effects of intravenous medium-chain triglycerides on pulmonary gas exchanges in mechanically ventilated patients. *Crit Care Med* 1994; **22**: 248–251.

26. Cunningham JJ. Factors contributing to increased energy expenditure in thermal injury: a review of studies employing indirect calorimetry. *J Parent Enter Nutr* 1990; **14**: 649–656.

27. Alexander JW, Peck MD. Future prospects for adjunctive therapy: pharmacological and nutritional approaches to immune system modulation. *Crit Care Med* 1990; **18**: S159–164.

28. Meyer NA, Muller MJ, Herndon DN. Nutrient support of the healing wound. *New Horizons* 1994; **2**: 202–214.

29. Souba WW. Glutamine: a key substrate for the splanchnic bed. *Ann Rev Nutr* 1991; **11**: 285–308.

30. Souba WW, Austgen TR. Interorgan glutamine flow following surgery and infection. *J Parent Ent Nutr* 1990; **14**: 90S–93S.

31. Harward TR, Coe D, Souba WW, Klingman N, Seeger JM. Glutamine preserves gut glutathione levels during intestinal ischemia/reperfusion. *J Surg Res* 1994; **56**: 351–355.

32. Newsholme EA. Biochemical control logic and the metabolism of glutamine. *Nutrition* 1994; **10**: 178–179.

33. Souba WW. Total parenteral nutrition with glutamine in bone marrow transplantation and other clinical applications. *J Parent Ent Nutr* 1995; **17**: 403–Oct.

34. O'Riordain MG, Fearon KC, Ross JA, *et al*. Glutamine-supplemented total parenteral nutrition enhances T-lymphocyte response in surgical patients undergoing colorectal resection. *Ann Surg* 1994; **220**: 212–221.

35. Daly JM, Reynolds J, Thom A, *et al*. Immune and metabolic effects of arginine in the surgical patient. *Ann Surg* 1988; **208**: 512–523.

36. Yu YM, Sheridan RL, Burke JF, Chapman TE, Tompkins RG, Young VR. Kinetics of plasma arginine and leucine in pediatric burn patients. *Am J Clin Nutr* 1996; **64**: 60–66.

37. Barton RG, Wells CL, Carlson A, Singh R, Sullivan JJ, Cerra FB. Dietary omega-3 fatty acids decrease mortality and Kupffer cell prostaglandin E2 production in a rat model of chronic sepsis. *J Trauma* 1991; **31**: 768–773.

38. Alexander JW, Gottschlich MM. Nutritional immunomodulation in burn patients. *Crit Care Med* 1990; **18**: S149–153.

39. Gilpin DA, Barrow RE, Rutan RL, Broemeling L, Herndon DN. Recombinant human growth hormone accelerates wound healing in children with large cutaneous burns. *Ann Surg* 1994; **220**: 19–24.

40. Cioffi WG, Gore DC, Rue LW, 3rd, *et al*. Insulin-like growth factor-1 lowers protein oxidation in patients with thermal injury. *Ann Surg* 1994; **220**: 310–316.

41. Hollyoak MA, Muller MJ, Meyers NA, Williams WG, Barrow RE, Herndon DN. Beneficial wound healing and metabolic effects of clenbuterol in burned and nonburned rats. *J Burn Care Rehab* 1995; **16**: 233–240.

42. West CD, Boyd NA. In: Winklestein J (ed) *The Harriot Lane Handbook*, 7th edn. Yearbook Medical Publishers, 1975.

34

Nutrition support for the intensive care unit

Jan Wernerman

Historical background

Intensive care medicine has developed as a specialty in its own right in the last 30 years or so. Ventilator treatment (in the modern sense) developed as a therapeutic answer to the effects of poliomyelitis. As the beneficial effects of close monitoring of patients with acute myocardial infarction were demonstrated, coronary care units became established. The technical development of haemodialysis made such treatment accessible not only to patients with chronic renal failure, but also to critically ill patients with acute renal failure. Concurrently, pharmacological treatment has revolutionised intensive therapy. The therapeutic arsenal of potent loop diuretics, inotropic drugs and modern antibiotics has dramatically improved outcome. In addition, artificial nutrition has emerged as a mainstay in treatment, by preventing patients from starving to death while other treatment of the underlying disease is being undertaken.

In the 30 years that intensive care has existed management of clinical problems has altered dramatically. This may explain some of the conflicting data in the literature.

The management of patients treated in an intensive care unit (ICU) is very variable both geographically and over time, and the use of nutrition support is no exception.

The geographical differences in the use of nutrition support (e.g. a predominance of enteral feeding in France, whilst parenteral nutrition is more frequently used in Scandinavia and Germany) has been dependent, to some extent, on the local skills available. When a new route of administration has been tried, the frequency of complications has sometimes increased, negatively influencing the willingness to continue a new regimen. Usually experience and technical skill in combination with metabolic knowledge has made one regimen superior to any alternative. For these reasons, well-planned studies comparing different techniques for nutrient administration are very scarce, although in the literature there are a fair number of controlled studies comparing enteral and parenteral nutrition. When these studies were reviewed in a meta-analysis no difference in objective outcome measures could be discovered.[1] The studies involved not only ICU patients, but also patients in departments of gastroenterology, neurosurgery, oncology and haematology. The authors concluded a superiority for enteral nutrition in 30% of the studies, a superiority for parenteral nutrition in 20% and no difference in 50%. In no case was there any difference in mortality or morbidity that influenced hospital stay.

Before parenteral nutrition became available in the early 1960s, the patient in need of nutrition support could only be fed by the enteral route. In cases without access to the gastrointestinal tract, starvation was the only alternative. Energy sources such as alcohol and sugars were used, sometimes in combination with protein hydrolysates. Around 1960, however, crystalline amino acid solutions and fat emulsions were introduced and for the first time a complete intravenous nutrition was made available.[2] Very soon Sir David Cuthbertson's observations in the 1920s that, despite a complete and balanced nutrition, nitrogen balance in well-nourished critically ill patients cannot be achieved, were confirmed.[3] At the same time the use of indirect calorimetry demonstrated that critically ill patients had a drastically increased energy expenditure, suggesting that caloric requirements were very high.[4] Similarly high resting energy expenditure was seen in patients with severe infection without effective antibiotic treatment and in patients with extensive burns. Overenthusiasm for the, at the time, new and effective possibility to nourish patients created the concept of 'hyperalimentation' to supply patients with sufficient nutrition. However, this pattern has changed dramatically and nowadays, with modern therapeutic regimens, an energy expenditure of more than 50% above the estimated basal resting energy expenditure is very rarely seen.[5] Consequently, during the last 10–20 years critically ill patients have sometimes been dangerously over-fed. This over-feeding applies both to energy and nitrogen supply, and the adverse effects may outweigh the beneficial ones. Over-feeding results in an increased CO_2 production with a larger respiratory burden upon the patient, which may cause difficulties in weaning the patient off the ventilator.[6-7] In addition a higher than necessary caloric load causes fever and results in fat deposition.[8]

It is highly unlikely that controlled randomised trials comparing nutrition to semistarvation in ICU patients will ever achieve ethical permission. Two months of total starvation will kill most people, and in critical illness this period is shorter because of the elevated requirements for a number of nutrients. Malnutrition undoubtedly contributes to mortality and is not specifically related to critical illness.[9] Furthermore malnourished individuals are more prone to develop complications.[10]

Preventing the development of malnutrition during the course of critical illness is therefore a major therapeutic goal in the ICU. Whether this goal is best achieved by conventional nutrition therapies is still open to debate, and there are studies pointing out that side-effects of nutrition can outweigh the benefits if nutrition support is not handled properly.[10–11] Enteral nutrition is sometimes reported to be superior to parenteral nutrition in ICU patients. However, most often such reports are not well controlled and the composition of nutrition administered by the different routes is not comparable. It has even been suggested that parenteral nutrition may be hazardous for the patients. It is obvious that the most ill patients are given parenteral nutrition, while those who are better can be fed enterally. Since it is extremely difficult to overfeed patients enterally, these patients are spared all the complications related to overfeeding in addition to the hazards related to intravenous catheters. In general enterally fed patients tend to have a better prognosis and an enteral regimen is less likely to cause adverse effects. However, when parenteral nutrition is totally banned, some patients will definitely be starved or semi-starved. This is unacceptable and therefore a combination of enteral and parenteral nutrition should be given in cases when enteral nutrition alone is not sufficient. Each patient should be guaranteed nutrition support that is adequate, effective and safe.

Theoretical problems and benefit of therapy

Critically ill patients in an ICU are a very hetero-geneous group with respect to illness, age and nutrition status. One way of considering nutrition support for such a group of patients would be to separate the different organ systems and/or the underlying diseases and to describe support in a continuous spectrum of patients (from almost healthy individuals to the critically ill) in respect of each particular organ system. In this chapter, the general treatment of critical illness is discussed and emphasis is put on close monitoring of the nutrition support and how to avoid the possible adverse effects. In addition, new strategies in nutrition support of the critically ill are outlined.

At the cellular level there are some differences between the metabolic response to elective surgical trauma and to critical illness irrespective of the under-lying disease.[12] The main difference is the time over

which such metabolic alterations persist. Earlier chapters detail the metabolic effects and the response of the different organ systems to injury. In general, although peripheral tissues are depleted after injury, the possibility of lipogenesis and fat deposition still exists[13] and conventional nutrition, by supplying adequate amounts of calories and protein, will not impede the production and outflow of substrates from the periphery.[14] An accumulation of fat is observed in parallel to the depletion of protein and of amino acids which are exported by the bloodstream from peripheral tissues, in particular from skeletal muscle.[15] Estimates of body composition in critical illness show an overall loss of protein and a gain of fat when conventional nutrition is given (Fig. 34.1).[8] This pattern is present also at the tissue level in skeletal muscle.[16]

The relative proportion of exported amino acids from muscle during critical illness does not differ from that seen in the basal postabsorptive state, but the total export of amino acids is enhanced two- or three-fold.[12] In parallel with this elevated export, the intra-cellular level of free amino acids in muscle changes,[17] particularly for glutamine which decreases to 10–25% of values seen in normal individuals (Fig. 34.2).[18–19] Total muscle protein content also diminishes over time,[16] a depletion which amounts to approximately 10% per week (Fig. 34.3) ultimately giving a picture similar to that seen in protein malnutrition. Muscle

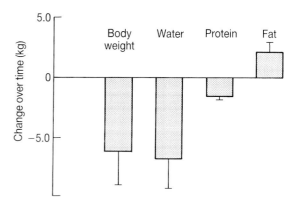

Figure 34.1 – Body composition of critically ill patients immediately after resuscitation and 10 days later. All subjects received 150% or more of energy expenditure and 0.2 g N/kg BW/day of a conventional amino acid solution. After resuscitation the fluid overload was reduced and the patients lost weight in parallel. The protein content decreased while the fat content increased in these patients, indicating that the nutrition support merely stimulated lipogenesis and did not prevent the loss of body proteins. Data from Streat *et al.*[8]

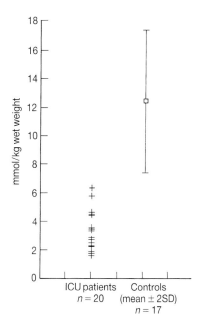

Figure 34.2 – Glutamine is the most abundant free amino acid in muscle tissue. In healthy individuals the concentration varies widely, but a 95% confidence interval covers the range between 8 and 18 mmol/kg BW in muscle. Critically ill patients, however, show very low values distinctly outside the confidence interval of normal subjects. Muscle glutamine may be a good measure of the metabolic strain upon muscle in critical illness. Data from Gamrin *et al.*[19]

protein synthesis is extremely variable but the average is low compared to controls (Fig. 34.4),[20] while muscle protein breakdown is markedly elevated,[21–23] resulting in this net loss of muscle proteins. When skeletal muscle proteins are severely depleted, a similar effect is eventually seen also in cardiac muscle. Regardless of whether parenteral or enteral nutrition is given, this can still be seen today, as long as the metabolic alterations associated with trauma or critical illness persist. Severe protein malnutrition is often linked to failure of various organs. Multi-organ failure is still a poorly characterised clinical entity.[24]

The mechanisms underlying the peripheral protein loss are not well understood.[25–26] Stress hormones and cytokines are most certainly involved in those processes. Immobilisation is another contributing factor particularly when muscle relaxing agents are used. Early in the course of immobilisation protein catabolism is marginal and muscle protein depletion in response to immobilisation alone is not very fast.[27–28] It is possible that immobilisation is more detrimental when combined with other protein catabolic stimuli

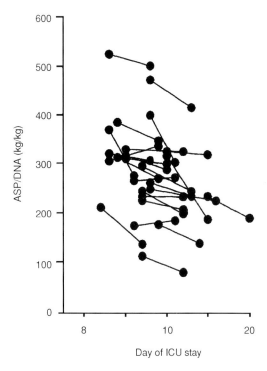

Figure 34.3 – The protein content in skeletal muscle decreases over time in critically ill patients. The decrease of alkali soluble proteins (ASP) per DNA is approximately 10%/week during the initial 30 days of ICU stay. The patients were fed conventional nutrition equal to 100–120% of their resting energy expenditure. The two biopsies were taken 5–7 days apart. Data from Gamrin *et al.*[16]

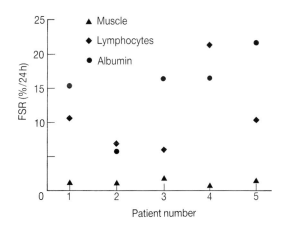

Figure 34.4 – Protein synthesis rate in various tissues in critically ill patients and compared to a 95% confidence interval of normal subjects. Muscle protein synthesis (1.49 ± 0.16%/day) is depressed, while fractional synthesis rate of albumin (12.81 + 1.23%/day) and of proteins measured *in vivo* in lymphocytes (11.10 + 1.82%/day) is increased. Data from Essén *et al.*[20]

in the ICU patients than in otherwise healthy individuals. The oxidative stress causes a change in the redox status of muscle, the concentration of glutathione decreases and more glutathione appears in the oxidised form, which is difficult to normalise in a state of metabolic stress.[29] During the development of critical illness there may be individual differences, but later on the pattern of change is fairly uniform. The rationale for the peripheral protein loss is not yet clear but an appealing hypothesis is that central organs and cell systems have priority for substrates used in energy production and proteins synthesis.[30-31] Although the splanchnic area is the target of the substrate export from the periphery, there are several indices that the supply of substrates may be inadequate. The intestinal mucosa exhibits atrophy and the absorptive capacity is lowered.[32] The glutamine content is not different from normal and it is linked to the plasma glutamine concentration.[33] The signs of depletion in the intestinal mucosa are less pronounced when enteral feed is given. In immunocompetent cells the metabolism is enhanced and the substrate uptake is particularly high in the spleen.[34] The connection between nutrition and immune function is obvious, but the mechanisms are still rather obscure.

A better knowledge of the underlying pathophysiology of the metabolic alterations seen in critical illness is essential to enable the value of nutrition support in the ICU to be optimised. Nutrition can be adjusted to the needs of the specific patient. As part of nutrition support, specific substrates may be used in order to improve the efficacy of the treatment. Presently, however, there are very few studies showing effects upon mortality/morbidity in critical illness.[9-11,35] The shortage of conclusive data in support of nutrition in ICU is explained by the heterogeneity of the patients which makes the detection of beneficial effects unlikely unless large patient populations are used. There are two ways out of this methodological dilemma. The first is to define a group of patients with a mortality high enough and in whom metabolic treatment with specific substrates is likely to be effective. It is also important to determine if nutrition is likely to influence mortality during the ICU stay or if a longer follow-up period is necessary to evaluate the effect. Short-term mortality and morbidity is normally determined by the underlying pathology that made ICU care necessary from the start. The second approach is to define a goal of therapy biochemically. The difficulty here is to define biochemical parameters which are likely to be indicative of a clinically relevant effect. For many patient groups the most widely used

biochemical parameter is the nitrogen balance. However, critical illness introduces several difficulties in the interpretation of nitrogen balance results (e.g. how to include the provision of blood products given to the patient in the nitrogen economy) which for practical purposes make nitrogen economy calculations an unsatisfactory measure of nutritional effects.[36]

Quantitative estimates of protein metabolism in the whole body by amino acid flux measurements represent another way of assessing important metabolic events. Unfortunately, these measurements suffer from methodological shortcomings which become more pronounced in states of critical illness.[37] The labelled amino acids used in such experiments are not distributed uniformly throughout the body, because there appear to be several subcompartments that lay open to question the validity of the 'steady state' needed for the calculations. In addition, the intracellular compartmentation of the free amino acid pool leads to great difficulties in determining labelled amino acid enrichment in the immediate precursor pool for protein synthesis, the amino-acyl-tRNAs.[38-39] The difficulties in interpreting such results make questionable the use of whole-body flux measurements of labelled amino acids for assessing the effect of nutrition support. The best choice is to find biochemical parameters that correlate with relevant clinical effects, i.e. to focus on changes in the content of protein, nucleic acids, and/or amino acids in specific tissues and organs.[40-41] Thus the effect of treatment should be defined as an effect on such parameters. Concurrently the relevance of the biochemical parameter(s) chosen must be substantiated by correlating them with clinical events.

Practical applications

Energy supply

Energy need should be estimated by measurement of energy expenditure by indirect calorimetry. In a healthy population only 50% of the individuals have a resting energy expenditure that is within ±10% of the predicted value according to Harris & Benedict.[5] In critical illness the scatter is far more pronounced. Published estimates with various correction factors are potentially a dangerous way of estimating the caloric need of an individual patient.

Although the resting energy expenditure may be estimated by indirect calorimetry, the amount of caloric supply needed is sometimes controversial. Both fat and carbohydrate should be used for energy supply. Carbohydrate is best given as glucose, although other sugars are reported to make patients less prone to develop hyperglycaemia in isocaloric amounts. The tendency for critically ill patients to develop hyperglycaemia occasionally limits the amount of glucose given. It has been demonstrated that a blood sugar of less than 10 mmol/l is associated with fewer infections of clinical importance in ICU patients.[42] It is therefore recommended that the glucose level is kept below 10–12 mmol/l either by administration of insulin or by reduction of the infused amount of carbohydrate.

The provision of fat emulsion intravenously has a longer tradition in Europe than in the USA. Some adverse effects related to overdosage have been reported but in general modern fat emulsions are well tolerated by critically ill patients. The rate of plasma clearance is faster than in healthy volunteers or patients undergoing elective surgery.[43] The clinical significance of this finding, however, is unclear. Fat particles given are initially metabolised by the action of endothelial lipoprotein lipase to triglycerides, and then into free fatty acids and glycerol. The activity of lipoprotein lipase is highly susceptible to heparin (even in low doses) often given to patients as prophylaxis against thromboembolism.[44] Although this alters the activity of lipoprotein lipase, utilisation of the fat emulsion seems to be very little affected. In the individual cells the free fatty acids are transported into the mithchondria for beta-oxidation. This transport is carnitine-dependent, and states of carnitine deficiency have been described in critically ill patients.[45] Some critically ill patients may therefore require carnitine supplementation.

However, identifying carnitine deficiency may be difficult as plasma levels give very little information about the actual carnitine status. Long chain fatty acids in a fat emulsion can be replaced by medium chain triglycerides (MCTs), which do not require carnitine for transport into the mitochondria.[46] Products consisting of a mixture of MCTs and long chain triglycerides, or as structured triglycerides with both types of fatty acids, are now commercially available. They can be used in critically ill patients because of this theoretical advantage.[47] Faster oxidation is seen with MCT; however, this results in a higher metabolic burden if the fat emulsion is infused too rapidly.[48] The place for medium chain fatty acids in the nutrition support of the critically ill patient is not yet established. The possible advantage must be compared with

the risks of overloading the patient. The relatively short time during which this new emulsion has been available means that indications and margins of safety may not yet be clear in the clinical situation.

The same considerations apply to enteral support. Beneficial effects of n-3 fatty acids contained in formulae for enteral use have been reported from animal studies.[49] Positive results are also reported from enteral use of a formula enriched with n-3 fatty acids, nucleotides and arginine in critically ill patients.[50] In ICU patients a few large studies have compared such an enriched formula to an ordinary formula. Tendencies towards a possible positive effect upon infections and ICU stay are reported, but so far these effects are not accompanied by shorter hospital stay or lower mortality except when retrospective subgroups are designed.[51–52] These formulae are interesting and such results should stimulate further research concerning both the theoretical background and the indications for clinical use which are necessary before any recommendation may be given.

Nitrogen supply

The appropriate nitrogen source for nutrition support in the ICU excites many opinions. The same problem applies to the quantity of nitrogen given as well as the quality (amino acid composition) of the nutrient. The composition of cristalline amino acid solutions used for intravenous support varies widely between manufacturers. Most often the composition is chosen to mimic the amino acid profile of a high-quality protein. For pharmaceutical reasons, the content of tyrosine and cysteine is generally low because of poor solubility, and glutamine has been lacking because of poor stability in aqueous solution. These shortcomings have been in part overcome by the use of dipeptides. The instability of glutamine in solution can also be overcome by manufactoring amino acid solutions locally,[53] thus avoiding the problem of instability related to prolonged storage. Another way of overcoming this problem in the case of glutamine may be to provide alpha-ketoglutarate,[54] the corresponding carbon skeleton, which is stable in aqueous solution.

A balanced amino acid solution contains all the essential as well as non-essential amino acids in amounts sufficient to provide for the minimal physiological requirements. However, minimal requirements are defined for *healthy* individuals, and not for those who are critically ill. It is not at all obvious that these requirements will remain the same throughout the period of critical illness. Indeed, some amino acids (such as tyrosine, cysteine and glutamine) that are non-essential in healthy subjects become more or less essential in disease. The quantitative requirements of some amino acids (e.g. cysteine, glutamine and perhaps arginine) seem to be very different in critical illness. The role of the branched-chain amino acids (BCAAs) has been debated, and very conflicting results are reported. However, a number of well-controlled studies, including critically ill patients with clear end-points, failed to demonstrate any beneficial effects attributable to higher intakes of BCAA.[55]

The dosage of nutrients containing nitrogen is a controversial matter. In the traumatised or septic state, nutrition regimens containing calories but without amino acids or protein do not lead to the kind of metabolic adaptation seen in total starvation or in cases of low protein intake.[56] However, when the nutrition intake is increased the losses increase in parallel. The traditional view was that, although the losses increased, at least a small portion of the nitrogen was retained in the body and even a marginal nitrogen saving may be important for the critically ill patient. Well-controlled studies do not support this hypothesis. An amino acid intake above 0.10–0.15 gN/kg/day does not improve nitrogen economy,[57] and a high nitrogen intake leads to a metabolic burden (Fig. 34.5). When amino acids or proteins are metabolised there is an obligatory heat production of around 30% of the caloric content of the amino acid intake.[58] A high amino acid intake is accompanied by significant heat production.[7] This results in an elevated body temperature sometimes misinterpreted as fever caused by infection, and, even worse, treated with antibiotics. It is important to emphasise, therefore, that there is no scientific evidence that an amino acid intake above 0.10–0.15 gN/kg/day has any beneficial effect that can outweigh the potentially adverse effects.

The future

Glutamine

The dependence on glutamine as an oxidative substrate in mucosal cells and in lymphocytes becomes critical in severe illness.[59] The peripheral tissues export large amounts of glutamine (approximately a third of the total efflux). The absence of glutamine in conventional amino acid solutions becomes problematic when the demand is very high, as in critical illness. There are convincing data showing that a glutamine-

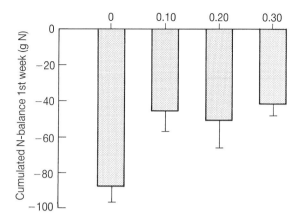

Figure 34.5 – Cumulative nitrogen balance over 8 days in critically ill patients with multiple fractures or burns. Patients received approximately 150% of their resting energy expenditure and in addition they were randomised to receive various amounts of amino acid corresponding to 0, 0.10, 0.20, or 0.30 gN/kg BW/day. Subjects who received 0.10 gN/kg BW/day had much better nitrogen economy than those who did not receive any amino acid solution. However larger amounts of amino acids did not improve the nitrogen balance. Data from Larsson et al.[57]

containing amino acid solution produces a better nitrogen economy in postoperative patients.[60–61] There are also reports of a preserved gastrointestinal morphology and function,[32,62] and an improved lymphocyte function.[63] The low level of muscle glutamine in critical illness (see Fig. 34.2) is a highly reproducible sign of both muscle protein depletion and of protein malnutrition.[18–19] A further drop of glutamine is prevented by glutamine therapy,[64] but a pre-existing low level is not easily repleted. Alpha-ketoglutarate, on the other hand, does seem to have an effect on the muscle glutamine content,[65] and may therefore be a more appropriate substrate in some situations. In long-staying ICU patients a decrease in mortality in patients given glutamine-containing parenteral nutrition is reported when the follow-up period is extended to 6 months.[35] This is a reasonable evaluation of treatment as glutamine supplementation is most likely to have effects for patients staying a very long time in the ICU and for patients during the convalescence and rehabilitation period. In haematological patients given parenteral nutrition containing glutamine, shorter hospital stay and fewer infections are reported following bone marrow transplant.[66]

The dosage of glutamine required is not yet settled. Should the supply be that of a high-quality protein or should the amino acid composition mimic that of the flux from the peripheral tissues? The latter seems to give the best results in critical illness in terms of restoring amino acid metabolism. If pharmacological doses of glutamine are used, on the other hand, metabolic difficulties and subsequent adverse effects may occur. Since ammonia is produced by glutamine metabolism in the splanchnic tissues, the liver must be functioning well enough to handle such a load if a rise in the ammonia levels in the systemic circulation is to be avoided. For nutrition by the enteral route glutamine supplementation may also be beneficial although no data demonstrating effects on mortality or hospital stay are presently available. Nevertheless fewer infections,[67] in particular abdominal abscesses[68,69] are reported in trauma patients.

Arginine

Arginine is an amino acid associated with beneficial effects on the immune system.[70] The effects of arginine in experimental animals and in *in vitro* systems are well documented. So far, however, no results are available for critically ill human subjects. Studies involving formulas enriched with n-3 fatty acids, nucleotides, arginine and sometimes glutamine are at hand,[51-52,68-69] but the contributions of different compounds in the formulae cannot be isolated.

Growth hormone

Adjuvant therapies in addition to conventional nutrition have been suggested, of which growth hormone is the most investigated. Such therapy was tried many years ago in animals,[71] and its introduction into clinical practice was delayed until recombinant human growth hormone (hGH) became available. Provision of GH in a supraphysiological dose results in a definite improvement of nitrogen economy in critical illness as well as in the postoperative state.[72-74] In burned children an improvement of wound healing and a shorter hospital stay is also reported.[75] For hGH, as for glutamine, the positive effect on nitrogen economy may be considered. In the case of hGH there are indications that the glutamine content in skeletal muscle is preserved.[73] This, however, could be the result of a decrease in glutamine export to glutamine-dependent tissues,[74] thus perhaps withholding an important substrate. As a result, muscle tissue may be preserved at the expense of more critical tissues. In that case a combination therapy of hGH and glutamine/alpha-ketoglutarate may be the best and safest metabolic support for the patient. Recently a

large multicentre study turned out to show an increase in mortality when ICU patients received pharmacological doses of hGH. The interpretation of this investigation is not conclusive presently, but the use of hGH outside strict endocrinological indications cannot be advocated at this time.

Conclusion

Nutrition support in the ICU deals with a very heterogenous group of patients. All patients should be guaranteed the amount of nutrition that prevents an accelerated depletion and which, therefore, gives the patient as long a time as possible to receive therapy for the underlying pathology without malnutrition intervening. To achieve this nutrition goal a combination of enteral and parenteral nutrition is often necessary. All patients should receive enteral nutrition if possible but, when such support is inefficient, parenteral administration should be added. Complications related to feeding are unacceptable and close metabolic monitoring of these patients is mandatory. ICU patients are particulary susceptible to complications related to overfeeding and that makes a personally tailored nutrition regimen for each patient desirable. The nutrition required should be assessed daily to determine that the prescribed amounts are administered.

The new substrates described, and which now appear in commercially available products, are all basically 'endogenous' in character. This fact makes it unlikely that short-term outcome for ICU patients will change dramatically. This is also a strong argument why clinicians should take all possible measures to try to tailor the nutrition to be as 'physiologic' as possible for individual patients within the ICU setting.

In the meantime, the following summary lists the key actions that may be taken to optimise nutrition in the ICU setting.

Practical guide for ICU nutrition

- Measure basal energy expenditure using indirect calorimetry. If not possible or if equipment is not available, estimate using the Harris and Benedict formula.
- Give the measured basal energy expenditure, preferably as enteral nutrition.
- Make a daily record of the amount of nutrition given.

- If necessary give parenteral nutrition to achieve the caloric goal. Give at least 30%, but not more than 60%, of non-protein calories as an LCT fat-emulsion, the rest as glucose. Give a balanced amino acid solution if possible containing glutamine (0.10–0.15 gN/kg/day).

- Administer nutrition continuously as a complete nutrient solution over 18–24 hours.

- Monitor regularly the levels of blood glucose, serum urea and triglycerides. Make repeated estimates of resting energy expenditure.

- – Blood glucose > 10 mmol/l: Give insulin in parallel or reduce the amount of glucose, but not to less than 2 g/kg/day. Ensure that blood glucose remains below 12 mmol/l.

  – Triglycerides > 5 mmol/l: Monitor regularly. If stable, accept if below 10 mmol/l. If higher or rising, reduce the amount of lipid or consider an MCT-containing emulsion.

  – Urea > 20 mmol/l: If stable, take no action. If rising progressively, lower amino acid support to 0.10 gN/kg/day. If volume problems ensue due to low urinary output (or if urea > 40 mmol/l), use haemofiltration/haemodialysis.

- Re-evaluate the nutrition regimen frequently:

  – Is the enteral route used properly?

  – Is fever a sign of over-feeding? (Remember nitrogen 'intake' in the form of resorption of haematomas or intestinal blood.)

  – Closely observe fluid balance. Weigh the patient regularly to prevent fluid overload. Bear in mind possible osmotic overload: patients with cardiac insufficiency are particularly susceptible.

References

1. Dunham M. Enteral nutrition does not decrease SIRS, MODS and mortality. *Shock* 1997; **7 (suppl 1):** 147.

2. Wretlind A. Parenteral nutrition. *Surg Clin N Am* 1978; **58:** 1055–1070.

3. Cuthbertson DP. The distribution of nitrogen and sulphur in the urine during conditions of increased catabolism. *Biochem J* 1931; **25:** 236–244.

4. Kinney JM, Long CL, Duke JH. Energy demands in the surgical patient. I: Body fluid replacement in the surgical patient. In: Foc CL, Nathas GG (eds) *Body Fluid Replacement in the Surgical Patient.* Grune & Stratton, New York, 1970; pp. 296–300.

5. Foster GD, Knox LS, Dempsey DT, Mullen JI. Caloric requirements in total parenteral nutrition. *J Am Coll Nutr* 1987; **6:** 231–254.

6. Carlsson M, Burgerman R. Overestimation of caloric demand in a long-term critically ill patient. *Clin Nutr* 1985; **4:** 91–93.

7. Henneberg S, Sjölin J, Stjernström H. Overfeeding as a cause of fever in intensive care patients. *Clin Nutr* 1991; **10:** 266–271.

8. Streat SJ, Beddoe AH, Hill GL. Aggressive nutritional support does not prevent protein loss despite fat gain in septic intensive care patients. *J Trauma* 1987; **27:** 262–266.

9. Mullen JL, Buzby GP. Nutritional assessment support and outcome in surgical patients. In: Kleinberger G, Deutsch E (eds) *New Aspects of Clinical Nutrition.* Karger, Basel, 1983; pp. 114–127.

10. The Veteran Affairs Total Parenteral Nutrition Cooperative Study Group. Perioperative total parenteral nutrition in surgical patients. *New Engl J Med* 1991; **325:** 525–532.

11. Sandström R, Drott C, Hyltaander A *et al.* The effect of postoperative intravenous feeding (TPN) on outcome following major surgery evaluated in a randomized study. *Ann Surg* 1993; **217:** 185–195.

12. Clowes GHA, Randell HT, Chu CJ. Amino acid and energy metabolism in septic and traumatized patients. *J Parent Enter Nutr* 1980; **4:** 195–203.

13. Nordenström J. Utilization of exogenous and endogenous lipids for energy production during parenteral nutrition. *Acta Chir Scand* 1982; **suppl 510:** 1–79.

14. Vinnars E, Holmström B, Schildt B, Odebäck A-C, Fürst P. Metabolic effects of four intravenous nutritional regimens in patients undergoing elective surgery. II: Muscle amino acids and energy-rich phosphates. *Clin Nutr* 1983; **2:** 3–11.

15. Wernerman J, Vinnars E. The effect of trauma and surgery on interorgan fluxes of amino acids. *Clin Sci* 1987; **73:** 129–133.

16. Gamrin L, Essén P, Andersson K, Hultman E, Nilsson E, Wernerman J. Longitudinal changes of biochemical parameter in muscle during critical illness. *Metabolism* 1997; **46:** 756–762.

17. Vinnars E, Bergström J, Fürst P. Influence of the post-operative state on the intracellular free amino acids in human muscle tissue. *Ann Surg* 1975; **182:** 665–671.

18. Roth E, Funovic J, Mühlbacker F *et al.* Metabolic disorders in severe abdominal sepsis: glutamine deficiency in skeletal muscle. *Clin Nutr* 1982; **1:** 25–42.

19. Gamrin L, Essén P, Forsberg A-M, Hultman E, Wernerman J. A descriptive study of skeletal muscle metabolism in critcally ill patients: Free amino acids, energy-rich phosphates, protein, nucleic acids, fat, water, and electrolytes. *Crit Care Med* 1996; **24:** 575–583.

20. Essén P, McNurlan MA, Gamrin L *et al*. Tissue protein synthesis in the critically ill patient.*Crit Care Med* 1998; **26:** 92–100.

21. Sjölin J, Stjernström H, Friman G, Larsson J, Wahren J. Total and net muscle protein breakdown in infection determined by amino acid effluxes. *Am J Physiol* 1990; **258:** E856–E863.

22. Tiao G, Hobler S, Wang JJ *et al*. Sepsis is associated with increased mRNAs of the ubiquitin-proteasome proteolytic pathway in human skeletal muscle. *J Clin Invest* 1997; **99:** 163–168.

23. Mansoor O, Beaufrere B, Boirie Y *et al*. Increased mRNA levels for components of lysosomal Ca$_{2+}$ activated and ATP-ubiquitin-dependent proteolytic pathways in skeletal muscle from head trauma patients. *Proc Natl Acad Sci USA* 1996; **93:** 2714–2718.

24. Border JR. Sepsis, multi system organ failure, and the macrophage. *Arch Surg* 1988; **123:** 285–286.

25. Wilmore DW. Are the metabolic alterations associated with critical illness related to the hormonal environment? *Clin Nutr* 1986; **5:** 9–19.

26. Tracy KJ. TNF and other cytokines in the metabolism of septic shock and cachexia. *Clin Nutr* 1992; **11:** 1–11.

27. Schoenheyder F, Heilskov NSC, Olesen K. Isotopic studies on the mechanism of negative nitrogen balance produced by immobilisation. *Scand J Clin Lab Invest* 1954; **6:** 178–188.

28. Gamrin L, Berg HE, Essén P *et al*. The effect of unloading on protein synthesis in human skeletal muscle. *Acta Physiol Scand* 1998; **163:** 369–377.

29. Hammarqvist F, Luo J-L, Andersson K, Cotgreave IA, Wernerman J. Skeletal muscle glutathion is depleted in critically ill patients. *Crit Care Med* 1997; **25:** 78–84.

30. Souba WW, Smith RJ, Wilmore DW. Glutamine metabolism in the intestinal tract. *J Parent Enter Nutr* 1985; **9:** 608–617.

31. Newsholme E, Crabtree B, Ardawi MSM. Glutamine metabolism in lymphocytes: its biochemical, physiological and clinical importance. *Quart J Exper Physiol* 1985; **70:** 473–489.

32. van der Hulst RRWJ, van Kreel BK, von Meyenfeldt MF *et al*. The role of parenteral glutamine administration in preserving gut integrity. *Lancet* 1993; **334:** 1363–1365.

33. Ahlman B, Ljungqvist O, Persson B, Bindslev L, Wernerman J. Intestinal amino acid content in critically ill patients. *J Parent Enter Nutr* 1995; **19:** 272–278.

34. Deutz NEP, Reijven PA, Athanasas G, Soeters PB. Post-operative changes in hepatic intestinal, splenic and muscle fluxes of amino acids and ammonia in pigs. *Clin Sci* 1992; **83:** 607–614.

35. Griffith RD, Jones C, Palmer TEA. Six-month outcome of critically ill patients given glutamine supplemented parenteral nutrition. *Nutrition* 1997; **13:** 295–302.

36. Nordenström J, Askanazi J, Elwyn DH *et al*. Nitrogen balance during total parenteral nutrition: glucose *vs* fat. *Ann Surg* 1983; **197:** 27–33.

37. Garlick PJ, Fern EB. Whole-body protein turnover: theoretical considerations. In: Garrow JS, Halliday D (eds) *Substrate and Energy Metabolism in Man*. John Libbey, London, 1985; pp. 7–15.

38. Garlick PJ, Heys S, McNurlan MA, Wernerman J. Organ-specific measurements of protein turnover in man. *Proc Nutr Soc* 1991; **50:** 217–225.

39. Ljungqvist OH, Persson M, Ford GC, Nair KS. Functional heterogeneity of leucine pools in human skeletal muscle. *Am J Physiol* 1997; **273:** E564–E570.

40. Forsberg AM, Nilsson E, Wernerman J, Bergström J, Hultman E. Muscle composition in relation to age and sex. *Clin Sci* 1991; **81:** 249–256.

41. Bergström J, Fürst P, Norée L-O, Vinnars E. Intracellular free amino acid concentrations in human muscle tissue. *J Appl Physiol* 1974; **36:** 693–697.

42. Bistrian BR. Trends in nutrition research: lipids. *16th Clinical Congress, ASPEN* 1992; 141–143.

43. Lindholm M, Rössner S. Rate of elimination of the intralipid fat emulsion from the circulation in intensive care patients. *J Crit Care Med* 1982; **10:** 740–746.

44. Persson E, Nordenström J, Hagenfeldt L, Nilsson-Ehle P. Plasma lipolytic activity after subcutaneous administration of heparin and a low molecular weight heparin fragment. *Thromb Res* 1987; **46:** 697–704.

45. Bremer J. Carnitine: metabolism and function. *Physiol Rev* 1983; **63:** 1420–1480.

46. Dawes RFH, Royle GT, Dennison AR, Crowe PJ, Ball M. Metabolic studies of a lipid containing medium chain triglyceride in perioperative and total parenteral nutrition infusions. *World J Surg* 1986; **10:** 38–46.

47. Eckar J, Adolph M, van den Muhlen U, Naab V. Fat emulsion containing medium chain triglycerides in parenteral nutrition of intensive care patients. *J Parent Enter Nutr* 1980; **4:** 350–366.

48. Scheig R. Hepatic metabolism of medium chain fatty acids. In: Senior JR (ed) *Medium Chain Triglycerides*. University Press, Philadelphia, 1969; pp. 39–49.

49. Spielmann D. Metabolism of unsaturated fatty acids. Role of n-3 and n-6 fatty acids in clinical nutrition. In: Kinney JM, Borum P (eds) *Perspectives in Clinical Nutrition*. Urbaan & Schwarzenberg, Baltimore, 1989; pp. 351–378.

50. Gottschlich MM, Jenkins M, Warden GD *et al*. Differential effects of three enteral dietary regimens on selected outcome variables in burn patients. *J Parent Enter Nutr* 1989; **14**: 225–236.

51. Bower R, Cerra F, Bershadsky B. Early enteral administration of a formula (impact) supplemented with arginine, nucleotides, fish oil in intensive care unit patients: results of a multi-center prospective, randomized clinical trial. *Crit Care Med* 1995; **23**: 436–449.

52. Atkinson S, Seifferet E, Bihari D. A prospective randomized double-blind clinical trial of enteral immunonutrition in the critically ill. *Crit Care Med* 1998; **26**: 1164–1172.

53. Khan K, Hardy G, McElroy B, Elia M. The stability of L-glutamine in total parenteral nutrition solutions. *Clin Nutr* 1991; **10**: 193–198.

54. Wernerman J, Hammarquist F, Vinnars E. Alpha-ketoglutarate and postoperative muscle catabolism. *Lancet* 1990; **335**: 701–703.

55. Brennan MF, Cerra FB, Daly JM *et al*. Report of a research workshop: branched-chain amino acids in stress and injury. *J Parent Enter Nutr* 1986; **10**: 446–452.

56. Ewerth S, Allgén L-G, Fürst P *et al*. Metabolic effects of four intravenous regimens after elective surgery. I: Clinical data and biochemistry. *Clin Nutr* 1983; **1**: 313–324.

57. Larsson J, Lennmarken C, Mårtensson J, Sandstedt S, Vinnars E. Nitrogen requirements in every injured patient. *Br J Surg* 1990; **77**: 413–416.

58. Thörne A, Wahren J. Diet-induced thermogenesis in well-trained subjects. *Clin Physiol* 1989; **9**: 295–305.

59. Newsholme EA, Newsholme P, Curi R, Crabtree B, Ardawi MSM. Glutamine metabolism in different tissues: its physiological and pathological importance. In: Kinney JM, Borum PR (eds) *Perspectives in Clinical Nutrition*. Urban & Schwarzenberg, Baltimore, 1989; pp. 71–97.

60. Stehle P, Mertes N, Puchstein C, Zander J, Albers S, Lawin P. Effect of parenteral glutamine peptide supplements on muscle glutamine loss and nitrogen balance after major surgery. *Lancet* 1989; **i**: 231–233.

61. Hammarqvist F, Wernerman J, Ali MR, von der Decken A, Vinnars E. Addition of glutamine to total parenteral nutrition after elective abdominal surgery spares free glutamine in muscle, counteracts the fall in muscle protein synthesis, and improves nitrogen balance. *Ann Surg* 1989; **209**: 455–461.

62. Tremel H, Kienle B, Weilemann LS, Stehle P, Fürst P. Glutamine dipeptide-supplemented parenteral nutrition maintains intestinal function in the critically ill. *Gastroenterology* 1994; **107**: 1595–1601.

63. O'Riordan MG, Fearon KC, Ross JA. Glutamine supplemented total parenteral nutrition enhances T-lymphocyte response in surgical patients undergoing colorectal resection. *Ann Surg* 1994; **220**: 212–221.

64. Karner J, Roth E. Alanyl-glutamine infusions to patients with acute pancreatitis. *Clin Nutr* 1990; **9**: 43–44.

65. Petersson B, Gamrin L, Hammarqvist F, Vinnars E, Wernerman J. Alpha-ketoglutarate given together with TPN improves the glutamine levels in skeletal muscle of critically ill patients. *Clin Nutr* 1992; **11** (suppl) (abstract): 26.

66. Ziegler TR, Young LS, Benefell K *et al*. Clinical and metabolic efficacy of glutamine-supplemented parenteral nutrition after bone marrow transplantation. *Ann Intern Med* 1992; **116**: 821–828.

67. Houdijk APJ, Rijnsburger ER, Jansen J *et al*. Randomized trial of glutamine-enriched enteral nutrition on infectious morbidity in patients with multiple trauma. *Lancet* 1998; **352**: 752–757.

68. Moore FA, Moore EE, Kudsk KA, Brown RO, Bower RH, Koruda MJ. Clinical benefits of an immune-enhancing diet for early postinjury enteral feeding. *J Trauma* 1994; **37**: 607–615.

69. Kudsk KA, Minard G, Croce MA *et al*. A randomized trial of isonitrogenous enteral diets after severe trauma – An immune-enhancing diet reduces septic complications, *Ann Surg* 1996; **224**: 531–540.

70. Daly JM, Reynolds J, Thorn A *et al*. Immune and metabolic effects of arginine on the surgical patient. *Ann Surg* 1988; **208**: 512–522.

71. Cuthbertson DP, Shaw GB, Young FG. The anterior pituitary gland and protein metabolism. II: The influence of anterior pituitary extract on the metabolic response in the rat to injury. *J Endocrinol* 1941; **12**: 574–581.

72. Ziegler TR, Young LS, Ferrari-Baliviera E, Demling RH, Wilmorre DW. Use of human growth hormone combines with nutritional support in a critical care unit. *J Parent Enter Nutr* 1990; **12**: 574–581.

73. Hammarqvist F, Strömberg C, von der Decken A, Vinnars E, Wernerman J. Biosynthetic growth hormone preserves both muscle protein synthesis, the decrease in muscle free glutamine and improves whole body nitrogen economy postoperatively. *Ann Surg* 1992; **216**: 184–191.

74. Mjaaland M, Unneberg K, Larsson J, Nilsson L, Revhaug A. Growth hormone after gastrointestinal surgery: attenuated forearm glutamine, alanine, 3-methylhistidine and total amino acid efflux in patients treated with total parenteral nutrition. *Ann Surg* 1993; **217**: 413–422.

75. Herndon DN, Barrow RE, Kunkel KR, Broemeling L, Rutan RL. Effects of recombinant human growth hormone on donor site healing in severely burnt children. *Ann Surg* 1990; **212**: 424–431.

35

Nutrition support for the surgical patient

Karel WE Hulsewé, Maarten F von Meyenfeldt and Peter B Soeters

Historical background

More than 50 years ago the relationship between pre-operative weight loss and postoperative complications was documented for the first time.[1] Studley observed, in a series of 50 consecutive patients undergoing elective surgery for peptic ulcer disease, that a pre-operative weight loss of over 20% was associated with an operative mortality of 33%, while mortality in patients who had suffered less than 20% weight loss was 3.5%. Other factors such as age, impaired cardio-pulmonary function, type of surgery, duration of the surgical procedure and the surgeon performing the operation were not associated with outcome. From his observations, Studley found 'reason to believe that more patients will be saved, provided efforts are concentrated on the preoperative preparation of those who have lost a good deal of weight'. At about the same time, Sir David Cuthbertson started his studies on the effects of trauma on protein homeostasis in which he described the muscle as the prime source of the increased nitrogen losses he observed in the post-injury state.[2] This has provided the basis for our understanding of the relationship between surgical trauma and the development of depletion. Appreciation of the practical implications of this understanding led to numerous efforts to develop artificial nutrition formulae for either enteral or parenteral administration. The first report of successful short-term total parenteral nutrition (TPN) was published by Helfrick and Abelson.[3] Dudrick and co-workers popularised the method by the demonstration that puppies could grow normally solely with TPN.[4–6] Only after the development of a safe fat emulsion by Wretlind[7] did long-term TPN become even safer, leading to an unabashed enthusiasm for the use of this new therapy. Initial enthusiasm was, as with many new therapies, uncritical. Since then, interest in the field of nutrition and metabolism has increased considerably, leading to clearer definitions of the indications for the use of artificial nutrition. Research has included further definitions of nutrition depletion, and of its effects on outcome of surgery. Developments are rapid, and while nutrition depletion is still being defined and the clinical benefits of artificial nutrition support are still being demonstrated, new tools become available to manipulate metabolic processes.[8,9a,9b]

In this chapter the term 'malnutrition' is purpose-fully avoided because nutrition depletion may be caused by factors other than starvation or an un-balanced diet, including alterations in intermediary metabolism resulting in energy losses and changes in protein homeostasis. Although it is acknowledged that malnutrition has different causes, the term inappropriately focuses on nutrition, ignoring the important contribution that altered intermediary metabolism has on the development of this condition. We therefore prefer to employ the term 'depletion'.

Theoretical benefits of nutrition support

In order to establish the theoretical basis for the value of perioperative nutrition support, a number of factors must be considered.

As expected, depletion is associated with changes in body composition. Depending on the causes, decrements in lean body mass and fat mass are found. Usually both compartments are affected. It is very important, however, to realise that in contrast to glucose and fat, no inert protein stores exist. This implies that loss of protein mass (i.e. lean body mass) leads to loss of organ function. Indeed it has been observed that nutrition depletion causes loss of organ function even before structural changes can be detected. In malnourished but also in fasted subjects, in whom no changes in body composition could be found, changes in force frequency characteristics and recovery from fatigue by the adductor pollicis muscle are observed.[10] Similarly other organs can also be expected to suffer from loss of organ function as a consequence of depletion.

The wasting of muscle is associated with an increase in muscle fatiguability as a result of loss of primarily type II fibres leading to a decreased muscle function.[11] Respiratory muscle function is also affected. Patients with a decreased fat-free mass show impaired inspiratory and expiratory ventilatory function, most clearly visible in the parameters assessing maximal power output of respiratory muscles: VO_2 max and maximal inspiratory and expiratory mouth pressures.[12] Nutritionally depleted patients also show loss of cardiac function with bradycardia, low systolic and diastolic blood pressures, low central venous pressure and reduced cardiac output.[13] The effect of depletion on the gastrointestinal tract has been the subject of several recent investigations. Loss of body weight is associated with loss of mucosal architecture as characterised by decreased villus height and crypt depth, and with brush-border enzyme deficiencies and impaired barrier function.[46] The presence of depletion has furthermore been shown to affect immune function, resulting in an impaired response to skin testing[14] as well as other derangements in the immune response.[14a,14b]

Surgical risk

Since weight loss was implicated as the major risk factor for the development of postoperative complications,[1] surgery has benefited from the availability of prophylactic antibiotics, infusion fluids, knowledge of physiology and pathophysiology of respiratory and circulatory function, anaesthetic techniques and many other developments. This has led to a well-documented decrease in morbidity and mortality of surgical therapy (for example in fistula and stomach surgery).[15] Of course, it is less certain that the relationship between the presence of depletion and the outcome of surgery is still as clear as it was 50 years ago. Although several prospective studies have shown that nutritionally depleted patients are more prone to the development of complications after major surgery, none of these studies analysed other well-accepted surgical risk factors as co-factors, thus leaving uncertain the true contribution of depletion to the development of complications.

The issue of surgical risk is further complicated by the absence of a commonly accepted definition of depletion. Values of parameters used to describe depletion are often considered to be abnormal if these values are associated with an increased incidence of complications after major surgery. Thus, generally accepted parameters for nutrition assessment (total protein, transferrin, albumin and pre-albumin, either alone[16] or in nutritional indices[17-22]), parameters identifying muscle mass and fat stores, creatinine–height index, muscle function tests, immunological status, and weight and weight loss,[16,23,24] all show a significant correlation with postoperative morbidity and mortality, and are therefore often used to calculate the risk for development of postoperative complications.[15a,16,18-22,24-32]

A further complication is that some of the parameters previously used to identify impaired 'nutrition status' are actually indicative of the presence of metabolic stress.[33]

This emphasis on the role of 'nutrition status' parameters as risk indicators has distracted attention from the roles that disease- and surgery-related factors have in the development of postoperative outcome. We have recently analysed the additional risk caused by suboptimal nutrition status,[34] and have related the outcome of surgery not only to the presence of nutrition depletion but also to other well-accepted surgical risk factors, such as patient-related factors (age[35,36] and coexisting diseases), type and extent of the surgical procedure (perioperative blood loss and transfusion,[37,38] duration of surgical procedure), skill of the surgeon[24] and the disease itself. Virtually all parameters in Meijerink's study were, in a monofactorial analysis (ANOVA and chi-squared), significantly correlated with outcome. However, a multiple logistic regression analysis with complication rate as a dependent factor, revealed perioperative blood loss as the most important factor associated with the development of postoperative complications. Age, in addition, significantly correlated with the occurrence of postoperative complications. When a complication occurred, percentage ideal weight (PIW) and duration of operation were associated with the severity of the complication. The results of this study suggest that the extent of a surgical procedure, as reflected by blood loss and duration of the procedure, and age are associated with the development of postoperative complications. Separate from these factors, parameters of nutrition status, as reflected by weight loss and PIW, are associated with the severity of the effects of the occurring complication. This analysis which is supported by findings of Giner et al.[38a] in British hospitals, confirms the observation by Studley[1] and re-establishes the presence of nutrition depletion as an independent determinant of the development of serious complications after major abdominal surgery.

Nutrition support and correction of nutrition depletion

The attractiveness of the association of nutrition depletion with postoperative complications has always been the suggestion that an impaired nutrition status can be treated, in contrast to many other risk factors. Nutrition support has indeed been shown to reduce weight loss, improve nitrogen balance and serum protein parameters.[39-41] There is clinical evidence that nutrition support restores tissue function. This is supported by observations of impaired skeletal muscle force and decreased fatiguability.[42] Some reports suggest an improvement of ventilatory function as a result of nutritional intervention.[43] The same observation has been made with regard to cardiac function.[44] Improvement of gastrointestinal tract function by nutrition support has been claimed,[45-47] but is still the subject of further study. The capability of nutrition support to restore skin test anergy, presumably equivalent to improved immune function, has long been known. These observations have led to high expectations of the ability of nutritional intervention to decrease morbidity and mortality from surgical therapy. However, it has been difficult to prove that clinical outcome, determined by so many factors, is indeed improved by nutritional intervention.

Practical applications

Identification of population at risk

The first requirement for any therapy to succeed is to define the patient group likely to benefit from the intervention. A number of studies investigating effects of nutritional interventions on postoperative outcome, however, have failed to do this. As many trials have included well nourished or only moderately malnourished patients clinical benefits could not be detected[48] or even worse, an increase in the incidence of complications, due to the nutritional intervention, was found.[49] A large Swedish study investigating the effects of postoperative parenteral nutrition[48] confirmed the fact that well nourished patients can tolerate a surgical trauma easily without oral intake for up to 9–14 days. The time during which an insufficient oral intake can be tolerated without ill effects, however, may be shorter in the critically ill, severely injured trauma victims and in patients who are nutritionally depleted prior to surgery. In contrast to acute illness and trauma, nutrition depletion can be treated before the surgical intervention. Large studies such as the Veteran's Administration trial[49] and the Maastricht trial[50] have shown that malnourished individuals benefit from preoperative nutritional interventions: the incidence of postoperative (septic) complications was reduced in the treated groups. Recently this has been confirmed by Bozetti and coworkers[50a] who demonstrated improved outcomes in depleted cancer patients undergoing surgery after preoperative total parenteral nutrition for 10 days. The assessment of nutrition status, however, is far from easy. Many of the parameters used are associated with nutritional state but can be influenced to a large extent by other factors which are not nutritionally related. Furthermore, we are still not certain how functional deficits result from nutrition depletion, and consequently which functional deficits are important to describe while assessing nutrition status. Therefore, current measures circumscribe, rather than indicate nutrition status.

Beside the severely traumatised or depleted patients, there are a number of specific surgical diseases that benefit from nutritional therapy. These illnesses comprise diseases which either improve by withholding normal enteral nutrition, or which include malabsorption that if left untreated would lead to depletion. Examples are (small) intestinal fistulas, active Crohn's disease, pancreatitis or pancreatic fistulas, chyle leakage, high output stoma's and short bowel syndrome. Other chapters in this book deal with these conditions in more detail.

In summary, current evidence suggests that well nourished individuals can sustain an average surgical trauma without nutrition during 10 days without ill effects. Malnourished individuals, or patients who have sustained a serious trauma or who are seriously ill cannot tolerate the abstinence of nutrition for such long times and should be fed earlier.

As explained in Chapter 10, depletion is not easy to measure. In clinical practice involuntary weight loss of more than 10% in the last 6 months or a body weight of less than 95% of the ideal body weight are frequently used as indications for preoperative nutritional interventions. Finally, certain surgical diseases can benefit from artificial nutrition if there is an indication for 'bowel rest' or if the condition has led to malabsorption.

Pre- versus postoperative nutrition

The important metabolic effects of (surgical) trauma are discussed in Chapter 1. The difference between the patient who is in a stable condition, but suffers from the effects of chronic derangements in energy and protein balance in combination with mild changes in intermediary metabolism leading to nutrition depletion, and the patient who has undergone a major surgical procedure, is profound. In the immediate postoperative period a loss of cellular protein, gain in extracellular fluid, decrease in plasma protein concentrations and impaired immune function may be observed. The surgical trauma being a limited insult allows for a fairly rapid restoration of intermediary metabolism to normal, in contrast to the septic condition where the derangements often carry a more severe and prolonged character. From the latter condition we know that it is unresponsive to nutritional intervention.[51] Based on these observations preoperative nutrition support may be expected to restore deficiencies more efficiently than in the postoperative situation, provided the patient is in a stable condition and not suffering from sepsis, necrosis or bowel obstruction. This is illustrated by several studies which were recently reviewed by Waitzberg et al.[51a] showing that there is no place for routine postoperative parenteral nutrition. Early postoperative enteral nutrition, on the other hand, appears to have beneficial effects in the early postoperative period as will be discussed in the next paragraph.

Current evidence suggests that preoperative nutrition can indeed improve surgical outcome in malnourished individuals provided that they are adequately fed for at least 7–10 days.[49,50] Shorter interventions have not been able to demonstrate any effects.

The nature of the illness naturally dictates whether the surgery can be postponed for this period. A total gastric outlet obstruction, for example, carries a high risk for aspiration with consequently serious pulmonary complications, and surgical intervention for patients with this condition should therefore not be delayed despite the potentially beneficial effects of preoperative nutrition.

There is increasing evidence that high risk surgical patients benefit from early postoperative enteral nutritional interventions: positive results have been claimed for immunocompetence, wound healing and septic morbidity.[52,53] The results of early postoperative parenteral nutrition have been more confusing.[48,54,55] Therefore, as soon as the patient has been stabilised artificial enteral nutrition should be started, preferably within 24 h. If the enteral route will not be available for more than 1 week, early administration of TPN should be considered.

Enteral or parenteral nutrition? (see also Chapter 42)

Each route of administration of artificial nutrition is accompanied by different complications, as discussed in previous chapters. The nature of the complications which can be caused by enteral nutrition are generally less severe than the potential complications caused by the more invasive parenteral administration of nutrients. Furthermore, the effects of nutrition on organ systems, in particular the gastrointestinal tract, differ.[56]

The intestine has many different functions which explain the important consequences of intestinal organ failure. The gut absorbs nutrients, is metabolically active, secretes a variety of products, produces several hormones and forms a (microbiological) barrier between the environment and the body. Moreover, the intestine is the largest immunological organ: it contains approximately 50% of all reticuloendothelial and other immune cells and it produces the largest amount of antibodies (mainly IgA).[57] During the last 2 decades much research has been dedicated to the role of the gut during illness in general and to the relation between bacterial translocation and the development of multi-organ failure (MOF) in particular.[55,58–63]

In contrast to standard parenteral nutrition, enteral feeding prevents the development of mucosal atrophy, stimulates intestinal perfusion, preserves normal gut flora, maintains the absorptive[64] and barrier functions, and several studies suggest an improvement in gut immune function,[65] Tagaki et al.[65a] described a decrease in endotoxin translocation and modulation of the systemic cytokine response resulting in lower immunosuppressive IL-6 and IL-10 levels in patients receiving enteral nutrition as opposed to parenteral nutrition after thoracic esofagectomy. Furthermore, enteral nutrition has been described to result in amelioration of wound healing[55] and a decrease in septic morbidity. Clinical trials have shown that in contrast to parenteral nutrition, early administration of enteral nutrition (within 24 h postoperatively) decreased the incidence of septic complications.[66,67] A meta-analysis confirmed the reduction in septic morbidity rates in patients fed via the enteral route compared to TPN, even when catheter sepsis was excluded from the analysis.[53] Moreover, in the post-operative situation similar results were found.[52] Therefore, a general consensus exists that, whenever possible, artificial nutrition should be delivered by the enteral route. However, a disadvantage of enteral nutrition is that the amount of nutrition administered frequently does not meet the calculated requirements; this is in contrast to parenteral nutrition, which generally leads to fewer problems in this respect. Therefore, if enteral nutrition cannot be administered in sufficient amounts, a combination with parenteral nutrition is a good alternative.

Pharmaconutrition

Administration of a balanced nutritional regimen has been proven adequate as a treatment for pure mal-nutrition. In practice, however, most patients lose body cell mass not only due to a decreased intake, but also because of changes in host metabolism as a consequence of the presence of disease. Feeding a patient can at best result in a quenched catabolic response but cannot reverse it into an anabolic state. Therefore, in addition to supplementation of nutritional deficiencies, much attention has been paid recently to influencing metabolic responses to disease by the administration of specific nutrients or hormones. Some relevant examples will be discussed.

Glutamine

Glutamine is the most abundant free amino acid in the body. It plays an important role as a carrier for inter-organ nitrogen transport, acid base homeostasis, nucleic acid synthesis, fuel for fast replicating cells such as enterocytes, lymphocytes and fibroblasts, and it plays a role in the antioxidant defence by influencing glutathione synthesis.[68-71] Normally, glutamine is produced in sufficient quantities (mainly by the muscle). Under certain circumstances such as nutrition depletion or severe stress, glutamine concentrations in plasma as well as in target organs fall,[47] possibly because the endogenous capacity to produce glutamine falls short of the amounts required for organ systems such as the immune system and the gut.

It has only recently been possible to add glutamine to parenteral nutrition in the form of a dipeptide.[72] Most studies evaluating the efficacy of glutamine enrichment of nutritional regimens have concentrated on the main glutamine-consuming organs, i.e. the gut and immune system. Van der Hulst et al demonstrated that glutamine-enriched parenteral nutrition maintains the mucosal architecture and the intestinal barrier function in contrast to glutamine-free, TPN.[58] Clinical benefits on outcome have been shown by Ziegler et al,[73] who demonstrated that addition of glutamine leads to a decrease in septic complications and a decrease in hospital stay for patients having undergone a bone marrow transplant. Morlion and coworkers[73a] also found a decrease in hospital stay in patients receiving glutamine enriched total parenteral nutrition after elective abdominal surgery. This was accompanied by a quicker recovery of lymphocytes and an improved granulocyte function postoperatively. The indications for the administration of glutamine in clinical practice remain to be clarified further. Neither theoretical arguments nor experimental evidence justify the routine use of glutamine in all patients. At present, only in selected patient groups, e.g. bone marrow transplant[73] and short-bowel patients,[74] nutritionally depleted[46,47,58] and possibly also critically ill patients,[75]

does an indication for addition of glutamine to TPN exist. Furthermore enteral nutrition enriched with glutamine decreased infection rates in trauma patients as described by Houdijk et al.[75a]

Arginine

Arginine is considered a non essential amino acid as it is produced mainly by the kidneys. It is an essential component for the synthesis of polyamines, nucleic acids and it is also a direct precursor for nitric oxide synthesis.[76] Furthermore, arginine stimulates the secretion of several hormones such as growth hormone, prolactin, glucagon and insulin. These effects are possibly an explanation for the positive effects of arginine administration on the nitrogen balance and the immune response. Supplementation of arginine in healthy humans has been demonstrated to improve wound healing.[76] However, only one clinical study investigating the effects of arginine alone in postoperative patients has been performed showing an enhanced lymphocyte response in vitro.[30] Moreover, clinical studies have shown benefits in enhancing the immune response in postoperative patients.[77]

n–3 fatty acids

In our normal diet most unsaturated fatty acids consist of n-6 fatty acids. These nutrients play important roles in the structural and functional integrity of the cell membrane, as a precursor for eicosanoid synthesis and in the intercellular signal transduction.[78] It is possible to influence these functions by replacing the n-6 fatty acids by the n-3 variants, which are present in high concentrations in fish oil. The products of the eicosanoid synthesis with n-3 fatty acids are significantly less potent than if n-6 fatty acids are used as precursor. This implies that the inflammatory response could be influenced by the use of these fatty acids. In vitro and in vivo experiments have indeed shown that proinflammatory cytokines such as TNF are secreted in lower amounts after stimulation with lipopolysaccharide. Recently clinical effects have been observed in patients with active Crohn's disease: intake of capsules with fish oil led to a significant decrease in the incidence of exacerbations.[79] Studies in which the effect of n-3 fatty acids alone on postoperative outcome has been studied have not yet been published.

In the past few years several studies employing an enteral diet enriched with specific nutrients such as arginine, n-3 fatty acids, RNA, selenium and vitamins

C and E have been published claiming improvements in immunological parameters and clinical outcome.[59,79a,80-85] These diets are not primarily aimed to correct nutritional deficiencies but to manipulate the (postoperative) immune response. Recently these studies were summarized in a meta-analysis by Heys *et al.*[85] They showed that the use of these nutritional regimens in cancer patients undergoing surgery decrease the total incidence of infections and shorten hospital stay. Mortality, however was not affected significantly by these interventions. These multimodality treatments, however, permit no conclusions with regard to the effects of the different components separately.

In conclusion, it appears to be feasible to modulate metabolic and inflammatory responses with specific nutrients. The clinical relevance of these interventions for the surgical patient, however, remains to be further elucidated in well carried out clinical trials.

The future

Developments in relation to perioperative nutrition will concentrate on two issues.

- A further characterisation of the cellular and tissue functional defects associated with nutrition depletion. Correlating these functional defects with outcome of surgical treatment may point to the most crucial functional defects: these may include disturbances in intracellular energy metabolism, impaired energy or nitrogen transfer between organ systems leading to defective functioning of what turns out to be a crucial organ. The gut may prove to play that central role. Such knowledge will improve the techniques to identify depleted patients.

- A further improvement of the composition of artificial nutrition. Knowledge of the defects in intermediary metabolism will provide tools to manipulate specific metabolic processes, presumably leading to improvements of several of the derangements. Such manipulations may include substrate alterations (e.g. deletion or extra administration of specific nutrients such as amino acids, fat components) or manipulation in the processes that induce altered intermediary metabolism: hormones and/or cytokines. Properly designed clinical trials, however, will remain necessary to establish the clinical benefit of these manipulations. Improved international cooperation is necessary to obtain a

sufficient pace for these developments, especially with regard to the performance of clinical trials, where the number of participating patients needed to prove the manipulations of metabolic support being effective will increase. Much may be learned in this respect from trial organisations in the field of clinical oncology.

References

1. Studley HO. Percentage weight loss, a basic indicator of surgical risk in patients with chronic peptic ulcer. *JAMA* 1936; **106:** 458–460.

2. Cuthbertson DP. Second annual Jonathan E. Rhoads Lecture. The metabolic response to injury and its nutritional implications: retrospect and prospect. *J Parenter Enteral Nutr* 1979; **3:** 108–129.

3. Helfrick FW, Abelson NM. Intravenous feeding of a complete diet in a child: report of a case. *J Pediat* 1944; **23:** 400–403.

4. Dudrick SJ, Rhoads JE, Vars HM. Growth of puppies receiving all nutritional requirements by vein. *Fortschr Parent Ernähr* 1967; **2:** 16–18.

5. Dudrick SJ, Wilmore DW, Vars HM, Rhoads JE. Long-term total parenteral nutrition with growth, development, and positive nitrogen balance. *Surgery* 1968; **64:** 134–142.

6. Wilmore DW, Dudrick SJ. Growth and development of an infant receiving all nutrients exclusively by vein. *JAMA* 1968; **203:** 860–864.

7. Wretlind A. Development of fat emulsions. *J Parenter Enteral Nutr* 1981; **5:** 230–235.

8. Jacobs DO, Evans DA, Mealy K, O'Dwyer ST, Smith RJ, Wilmore DW. Combined effects of glutamine and epidermal growth factor on the rat intestine. *Surgery* 1988; **104:** 358–364.

9. Stehle P, Zander J, Mertes N, Albers S, Puchstein C, Lawin P, Furst P. Effect of parenteral glutamine peptide supplements on muscle glutamine loss and nitrogen balance after major surgery. *Lancet* 1989; **1:** 231–233.

9a. Lin E, Kotani JG, Lowry SF. Nutrition modulation of immunity and the inflammatory response. *Nutrition* 1998; **14:** 545–550.

9b. Pointing GA, Halliday D, Teale JD, Sim AJW. Postoperative positive nitrogen balance with intravenous hyponutrition and growth hormone. *Lancet* 1988: 438–440.

10. Jeejeebhoy KN. Assessment of nutritional status. In: Rombeau JL, Caldwell MD (eds) *Clinical nutrition: enteral and tube feeding*, 2nd edn. WB Saunders, Philadelphia, 1990; pp 118–126.

11. Russell DM, Walker PM, Leiter LA *et al*. Metabolic and structural changes in skeletal muscle during hypocaloric dieting. *Am J Clin Nutr* 1984; **39**: 503–513.

12. Schols AM, Mostert R, Soeters PB, Wouters EF. Body composition and exercise performance in patients with chronic obstructive pulmonary disease. *Thorax* 1991; **46**: 695–699.

13. Abel RM, Grimes JB, Alonso D, Alonso M, Gay WA Jr. Adverse hemodynamic and ultrastructural changes in dog hearts subjected to protein-calorie malnutrition. *Am Heart J* 1979; **97**: 733–744.

14. Superina R, Meakins JL. Delayed hypersensitivity, anergy, and the surgical patient. *J Surg Res* 1984; **37**: 151–174.

14a. Rikimaru T, Taniguchi K, Yartey JE, Kennedy DO, Nkrumah FK. Humoral and cell-mediated immunity in malnourished children in Ghana. *Eur J Clin Nutr* 1998; **52**: 344–350.

14b. Chandra RK. Nutrition and the immune system: an introduction. *Am J Clin Nutr* 1997; **66**: 460S–463S.

15. Rinsema W. Gastro-intestinal fistulas: management and results of treatment. Thesis, Maastricht University, 1992; (ISBN 90-5291-073-1).

15a. Mullen JL. Complications of total parenteral nutrition in the cancer patient. *Cancer Treat Rep* 1981; **65 (suppl 5):** 107–113.

16. Hickman DM, Miller RA, Rombeau JL, Twomey PL, Frey CF. Serum albumin and body weight as predictors of postoperative course in colorectal cancer. *J Parenter Enteral Nutr* 1980; **4**: 314–316.

17. Harvey KB, Moldawer LL, Bistrian BR, Blackburn GL. Biological measures for the formulation of a hospital prognostic index. *Am J Clin Nutr* 1981; **34**: 2013–2022.

18. Klidjian AM, Foster KJ, Kammerling RM, Cooper A, Karran SJ. Relation of anthropometric and dynamometric variables to serious postoperative complications. *Br Med J* 1980; **281**: 899–901.

19. Mullen JL, Buzby GP, Waldman MT, Gertner MH, Hobbs CL, Rosato EF. Prediction of operative morbidity and mortality by preoperative nutritional assessment. *Surg Forum* 1979; **30**: 80–82.

20. Mullen JL, Gertner MH, Buzby GP, Goodhart GL, Rosato EF. Implications of malnutrition in the surgical patient. *Arch Surg* 1979; **114**: 121–125.

21. Dionigi R, Cremaschi RE, Jemos V, Dominioni L, Monico R. Nutritional assessment and severity of illness classification systems: a critical review on their clinical relevance. *World J Surg* 1986; **10**: 2–11.

22. Detsky AS, Baker JP, Mendelson RA, Wolman SL, Wesson DE, Jeejeebhoy KN. Evaluating the accuracy of nutritional assessment techniques applied to hospitalized patients: methodology and comparisons. *J Parenter Enteral Nutr* 1984; **8**: 153–159.

23. Windsor JA, Hill GL. Weight loss with physiologic impairment. A basic indicator of surgical risk. *Ann Surg* 1988; **207**: 290–296.

24. Warnold I, Lundholm K. Clinical significance of preoperative nutritional status in 215 noncancer patients. *Ann Surg* 1984; **199**: 299–305.

25. DeMatteis R, Hermann RE. Supplementary parenteral nutrition in patients with malignant disease. Guidelines to patient selection. *Cleve Clin Q* 1973; **40**: 139–145.

26. Nordenstrom J, Carpentier YA, Askanazi J *et al*. Metabolic utilization of intravenous fat emulsion during total parenteral nutrition. *Ann Surg* 1982; **196**: 221–231.

27. Forse RA, Christou N, Meakins JL, MacLean LD, Shizgal HM. Reliability of skin testing as a measure of nutritional state. *Arch Surg* 1981; **116**: 1284–1288.

28. Collins JP, McCarthy ID, Hill GL. Assessment of protein nutrition in surgical patients – the value of anthropometrics. *Am J Clin Nutr* 1979; **32**: 1527–1530.

29. Muller JM, Keller HW, Brenner U, Walter M, Holzmuller W. Indications and effects of preoperative parenteral nutrition. *World J Surg* 1986; **10**: 53–63.

30. Daly JM, Reynolds J, Thom A, Kinsley L, Dietrick-Gallagher M, Shou J, Ruggieri B. Immune and metabolic effects of arginine in the surgical patient. *Ann Surg* 1988; **208**: 512–521.

31. Bellantone R, Doglietto GB, Bossola M, Pacelli F, Negro F, Sofo L, Crucitti F. Preoperative parenteral nutrition in the high risk surgical patient. *J Parenter Enter Nutr* 1988; **12**: 195–197.

32. de la Hunt MN, McDonald PJ, Karran SJ. Anthropometric nutritional assessment is of value in colorectal patients. *Dis Colon Rectum* 1984; **27**: 296–298.

33. Klein S. The myth of serum albumin as a measure of nutritional status. *Gastroenterology* 1990; **99**: 1845–1851.

34. Meijerink WJHJ. Perioperative nutrition in GI cancer patients. Thesis, Maastricht University, 1992;

35. Harbrecht PJ, Garrison RN, Fry DE. Role of infection in increased mortality associated with age in laparotomy. *Am Surg* 1983; **49**: 173–178.

36. Starker PM, LaSala PA, Askanazi J, Gump FE, Forse RA, Kinney JM. The response to TPN. A form of nutritional assessment. *Ann Surg* 1983; **198**: 720–724.

37. Norwegian Gastro-Intestinal Group (NORGAS) Infectious problems after elective surgery of the alimentary tract: the influence of perioperative factors. *Curr Med Res Opin* 1988; **11**: 179–195.

38. Szczepanski KP, Skaarup P, Stear-Johansen T. Pleuropulmonary complications following major surgery (thoracic surgery excluded). *Acta Chir Scand* 1973; **139**: 425–430.

38a. Giner M, Laviano A, Meguid MM, Gleason JR. In 1995 a correlation between malnutrition and poor outcome in critically ill patients still exists. *Nutrition* 1996; **12**: 23–29.

39. Heatley V, Lewis MH, Williams RHP. Perioperative intravenous feeding: a controlled trial. *Postgrad Med J* 1979; **55**: 541–545.

40. Collins JP, Hill GL, Oxby CB. Intravenous amino acids and intravenous hyperalimentation as protein sparing therapy after major surgery. *Lancet* 1978; **5**: 788–790.

41. Holter AR, Fischer JE. The effects of perioperative hyperalimentation on complications in patients with carcinoma and weight loss. *J Surg Res* 1977; **23**: 31–34.

42. Russell DM, Leiter LA, Whitwell J. Skeletal muscle function during hypocaloric diets and fasting: a comparison with standard nutritional assessment parameters. *Am J Clin Nutr* 1983; **37**: 133–138.

43. Schols AM, Soeters PB, Mostert R, Pluymers RJ, Wouters EF. Physiologic effects of nutritional support and anabolic steroids in patients with chronic obstructive pulmonary disease. A placebo-controlled randomized trial. *Am J Respir Crit Care Med* 1995; **152**: 1268–1274.

44. Abel RM, Fischer JE, Buckley MJ. Malnutrition in cardiac patients: results of a prospective randomised evaluation of early postoperative total parenteral nutrition (TPN). *Acta Chir Scand* 1976; **466**: 77.

45. Souba WW, Klimberg VS, Plumley DA, Salloum RM, Flynn TC, Bland KI, Copeland EM. The role of glutamine in maintaining a healthy gut and supporting the metabolic response to injury and infection. *J Surg Res* 1990; **48**: 383–391.

46. van der Hulst RRWJ, Deutz NEP, Meyenfeldt von MF, Elbers JMH, Stockbrügger RW. Decrease of mucosal glutamine concentration in the nutritionally depleted patient. *Clin Nutr* 1994; **13**: 228–233.

47. van der Hulst RRWJ, Deutz NEP, von Meyenfeldt MF, Elbers JMH, Stockbrügger RW, Soeters PB. Nutritional depletion and mucosal glutamine concentration. *Clin Nutr* 1994; **13**: 228–233.

47a. van der Hulst RR, Meyenfeldt von MF, Tiebosch A, Buurman WA, Soeters PB. Glutamine and intestinal immune cells in humans. *JPEN* 1997; **21**(6): 310–315.

48. Sandstrom R, Drott C, Hyltander A, Arfvidsson B, Schersten T, Wickstrom I, Lundholm K. The effect of postoperative intravenous feeding (TPN) on outcome following major surgery evaluated in a randomized study. *Ann Surg* 1993; **217**: 185–195.

49. The Veterans Affairs Total Parenteral Nutrition Cooperative Study Group. Perioperative total parenteral nutrition in surgical patients. *N Engl J Med* 1991; **325**: 525–532.

50. von Meyenfeldt MF, Meijerink WJHJ, Rouflart MMJ, Buil-Maassen MTHJ, Soeters PB. Perioperative nutritional support: a randomised clinical trial. *Clin Nutr* 1992; **11**: 180–186.

50a. Bozetti F, Gavazzi C, Miceli R, Rossi N, Mariani L, Cozzaglio L, Bonfanti G, Piacenza S. Perioperative total parenteral nutrition in malnourished, gastrointestinal cancer patients: a randomized clinical trial. *J Parenter Enteral Nutr* 2000; **24**: 7–14.

51. von Meyenfeldt MF, Soeters PB, Vente JP *et al*. Effect of branched chain amino acid enrichment of total parenteral nutrition on nitrogen sparing and clinical outcome of sepsis and trauma: a prospective randomized double blind trial. *Br J Surg* 1990; **77**: 924–929.

51a. Waitzverg DL, Plopper C, Terra RM. Postoperative total parenteral nutrition. *World J Surg* 1999; **23**: 560–564.

52. Beier-Holgersen R, Boesby S. Influence of postoperative enteral nutrition on postsurgical infections. *Gut* 1996; **39**: 833–835.

53. Moore FA, Feliciano DV, Andrassy RJ *et al*. Early enteral feeding, compared with parenteral, reduces postoperative septic complications. The results of a meta-analysis. *Ann Surg* 1992; **216**: 172–183.

54. Brennan MF, Pisters PW, Posner M, Quesada O, Shike M. A prospective randomized trial of total parenteral nutrition after major pancreatic resection for malignancy. *Ann Surg* 1994; **220**: 436–441.

55. Law NW, Ellis H. The effect of parenteral nutrition on the healing of abdominal wall wounds and colonic anastomoses in protein-malnourished rats. *Surgery* 1990; **107**: 449–454.

56. Munro HN. Differences in metabolic handling of orally versus parenterally administered nutrients. In: Green M, Greene HL (eds) *The role of the gastrointestinal tract in nutrient delivery*. Academic Press, London, 1984; pp. 183–198.

57. Brandtzaeg P, Halstensen TS, Kett K *et al*. Immunobiology and immunopathology of human gut mucosa: humoral immunity and intraepithelial lymphocytes. *Gastroenterology* 1989; **97**: 1562–1584.

58. van der Hulst RRWJ, van Kreel BK, Meyenfeldt von MF, Brummer RJ, Arends JW, Deutz NEP, Soeters PB. Glutamine and the preservation of gut integrity. *Lancet* 1993; **341:** 1363–1365.

59. Gianotti L, Alexander JW, Nelson JL, Fukushima R, Pyles T, Chalk CL. Role of early enteral feeding and acute starvation on postburn bacterial translocation and host defense: prospective, randomized trials. *Crit Care Med* 1994; **22:** 265–272.

60. Sedman PC, Macfie J, Sagar P, Mitchell CJ, May J, Mancey Jones B, Johnstone D. The prevalence of gut translocation in humans. *Gastroenterology* 1994; **107:** 643–649.

61. Alexander JW. New data on enteral feeding, selected nutrients, microbial translocation, and postsurgical sepsis. *J Crit Care Nutr* 1995; **2:** 14–19.

62. Hadfield RJ, Sinclair DG, Houldsworth PE, Evans TW. Effects of enteral and parenteral nutrition on gut mucosal permeability in the critically ill. *Am J Respir Crit Care Med* 1995; **152:** 1545–1548.

63. Reynolds JV. Gut barrier function in the surgical patient. *Br J Surg* 1996; **83:** 1668–1669.

64. Suchner U, Senftleben U, Eckart T et al. Enteral versus parenteral nutrition: effects on gastrointestinal function and metabolism. *Nutrition* 1996; **12:** 13–22.

65. Li J, Kudsk KA, Gocinski B, Dent D, Glezer J, Langkamp Henken B. Effects of parenteral and enteral nutrition on gut-associated lymphoid tissue. *J Trauma* 1995; **39:** 44–51.

65a. Takagi K, Yamamori H, Toyoda Y, Nakajima N, Tashiro T. Modulating effects of the feed route on stress response and enotoxin translocation in severely stressed patients receiving thoracic esophagectomy. *Nutrition* 2000; **16:** 355–360.

66. Kudsk KA, Croce MA, Fabian TC et al. Enteral versus parenteral feeding. Effects on septic morbidity after blunt and penetrating abdominal trauma. *Ann Surg* 1992; **215:** 503–511.

67. Moore FA, Moore EE, Jones TN, McCroskey BL, Peterson VM. TEN versus TPN following major abdominal trauma: reduced septic morbidity. *J Trauma* 1989; **29:** 916–922.

68. Newsholme EA, Parry Billings M. Properties of glutamine release from muscle and its importance for the immune system. *J Parenter Enteral Nutr* 1990; **14:** 63S–67S.

69. Souba WW, Herskowitz K, Salloum RM, Chen MK, Austgen TR. Gut glutamine metabolism. *J Parenter Enteral Nutr* 1990; **14:** 45S–50S.

70. Smith RJ. Glutamine metabolism and its physiologic importance. *J Parenter Enteral Nutr* 1990; **14:** 40S–44S.

71. Hong RW, Helton WS, Rounds JD, Wilmore DW. Glutamine-supplemented TPN preserves hepatic glutathione and improves survival following chemotherapy. *Surg Forum* 1990; **41:** 9–11.

72. Furst P, Albers S, Stehle P. Glutamine-containing dipeptides in parenteral nutrition. *J Parenter Enteral Nutr* 1990; **14:** 118S–124S.

73. Ziegler TR, Young LS, Benfell K et al. Clinical and metabolic efficacy of glutamine-supplemented parenteral nutrition after bone marrow transplantation. A randomized, double-blind, controlled study. *Ann Intern Med* 1992; **116:** 821–828.

73a. Morlion BJ, Stehle P, Wachtler P, Siedhoff HP, Koller M, Konig W, Furst P, Puchstein C. Total parenteral nutrition with glutamine dipeptide after major abdominal surgery: a randomized, double-blind, controlled study. *Ann Surg* 1998; **227:** 302–308.

74. Byrne TA, Persinger RL, Young LS, Ziegler TR, Wilmore DW. A new treatment for patients with short-bowel syndrome. Growth hormone, glutamine, and a modified diet. *Ann Surg* 1995; **222:** 243–254.

75. Griffiths RD, Palmer TEA, Jones C. Parenteral glutamine supply in intensive care patients. *Nutrition* 1996; **12:** S73–S75.

75a. Houdijk APJ, Rijnsburger ER, Jansen J, Wesdorp RIC, Wesis JK, McCamish MA, Teerlink T, Meeuwissen SGM, Haarman HJthM, Thijs LG, Leeuwen van PAM. Randomised trial of glutamine-enriched enteral nutrition on infectious morbidity in patients with multiple trauma. *Lancet* 1998; **352:** 772–776.

76. Barbul A, Lazarou SA, Efron DT, Wasserkrug HL, Efron G. Arginine enhances wound healing and lymphocyte immune responses in humans. *Surgery* 1990; **108:** 331–336.

77. Daly JM, Copeland EM III. Use of parenteral nutrition in the patient with cancer [letter]. *Surgery* 1985; **97:** 756–758.

78. Kinsella JE, Lokesh B. Dietary lipids, eicosanoids, and the immune system. *Crit Care Med* 1990; **18:** S94–S113.

79. Belluzzi A, Brignola C, Campieri M, Pera A, Boschi S, Miglioli M. Effect of an enteric-coated fish-oil preparation on relapses in Crohn's disease. *N Engl J Med* 1996; **334:** 1557–1560 (abstract).

79a. Daly JM, Leiberman MD, Goldfine J, Shou J, Weintraub F, Rosato EF, Lavin P. Enteral nutrition with supplemental arginine, RNA, and omega-3 fatty acids in patients after operation: immunologic, metabolic, and clinical outcome. *Surgery* 1992; **112:** 56–67.

80. Daly JM, Weintraub FN, Shou J, Rosato EF, Lucia M. Enteral nutrition during multimodality therapy in upper gastrointestinal cancer patients. *Ann Surg* 1995; **221:** 327–338.

81. Bower RH, Cerra FB, Bershadsky B, Licari JJ, Joyt DB, Jensen GL, Van Buren CT, Rothkopf MM, Daly JM, Adelsberg BR. Early enteral administration of a formula (Impact) supplemented with arginine, nucleotides, and fish oil in intensive care unit patients: results of a multicenter, prospective, randomized, clinical trial. *Crit Care Med* 1995; **23:** 436–449.

82. Braga M, Gianotti L, Cestari A, Vignali A, Pellegatta F, Dolci A, Di Carlo V. Gut function and immune and inflammatory responses in patients perioperatively fed with supplemented enteral formulas. *Arch Surg* 1996; **131:** 1257–1264.

83. Braga M, Gianotti L, Radaelli G, Vignali A, Mari G, Gentilini O, Di Carlo V. Perioperative immuno-nutrition in patients undergoing cancer surgery. *Arch Surg* 1999; **134:** 428–433.

84. Gianotti L, Alexandra JW, Nelson JL, Fukushima R, Pyles T, Chalk CL. Role of early enteral feeding and acute starvation on postburn bacterial translocation and host defense: prospective, randomized trials. *Crit Care Med* 1994; **22:** 265–272.

85. Heys SD, Walker LG, Smith I, Eremin O. Enteral nutritional supplementation with key nutrients in patients with critical illness and cancer; a meta-analysis of randomized controlled clinical trials. *Ann Surg* 1999; **229:** 467–477.

36

Nutrition support in human immunodeficiency virus infection

Derek C Macallan, Jacqui Cotton and George E Griffin

Background and historical perspective

HIV and the acquired immunodeficiency syndrome

The Acquired Immune Deficiency Syndrome (AIDS) was first identified in cohorts of homosexual men in New York City and Los Angeles in 1981.[1,2,3,4] The syndrome has been shown to be due to infection with the Human Immunodeficiency Virus (HIV), a retrovirus.[5]

Infection with the virus, usually by sexual transmission or parenteral inoculation, is followed after some months by seroconversion, at which time the infected individual makes specific antibody responses to viral glycoprotein antigens; this may be accompanied by a glandular fever-like illness and is referred to as Seroconversion or stage I disease.[6] Individuals may then remain clinically well for several years following seroconversion (stage II disease). If HIV infection proceeds untreated a constitutional syndrome may develop which is characterised by symptoms such as fever, night sweats or weight loss.

After a period of time, often of the order of about 10 years, virtually all untreated HIV-infected individuals develop immunodeficiency, primarily due to depletion in the number of CD4 positive 'helper' T-cells. Such depletion results in loss of the ability to mount specific immune responses to antigens and thus renders the individual susceptible to opportunistic infections, particularly those caused by viruses, protozoa and fungi. In addition, susceptibility to malignancies such as lymphoma and Kaposi's sarcoma (KS) is greatly increased; such heightened susceptibility may be related to tumour-inducing viruses such as Epstein–Barr Virus (EBV) and HHV8 or Kaposi's sarcoma associated virus. As clinical HIV disease progresses the development of AIDS, or stage IV disease, is defined by the occurrence of an opportunistic infection, an HIV-associated malignancy, or substantial weight loss.[6] The course of clinical disease following HIV infection is, however, very variable; some individuals develop a rapidly progressive disease whilst others, termed long-term non-progressors, do not show signs of immunodeficiency even after many years of infection, although it is now thought that even such non-progressors will eventually develop clinical immunodeficiency.

Antiretroviral treatment

The clinical 'face' of HIV has been radically altered in the last few years by the introduction of potent antiretroviral drugs which are able to block the cycle of infection of and multiplication within T-lymphocytes. The impact of such therapies is demonstrated by dramatic reduction in the level of circulating viral particles, the 'viral load' which reflects the rate of infection, destruction and re-infection of CD4 positive lymphocytes. Such treatment, commonly referred to as highly-active antiretroviral therapy (HAART), is usually associated with a marked increase in the number of circulating CD4 cells, even in late stage disease, and has resulted in recovery of immune protection against pathogenic organisms and reduced mortality in patients with HIV infection.

Whether such therapies will ever be able to completely eradicate HIV infection has not yet been established. At the time of writing, the emergence of viral resistance to such drugs is a formidable obstacle. The rate of development of such resistance can be reduced by the use of combination treatments and by changing treatment at the first signs of viral load rebound. Combination treatments generally necessitate a major pill-burden and gastrointestinal side-effects are frequent; both these factors may have deleterious effects on nutrition state as described below. However, the dramatic effect of HAART on patient well-being is very clear and has been reflected by a major shift in HIV care from inpatient treatment of opportunistic infections to outpatient management of antiretroviral therapy.[7]

Wasting in AIDS

Early experience of the clinical progression of HIV infection and AIDS revealed that wasting and weight loss were important features of this disease and weight loss was included in the widely-adopted clinical classification of HIV infection produced by the Centre for Disease Control (CDC).[6] The wasting and weight loss that occur during HIV infection are closely associated with disease progression[8] and may be of enormous magnitude.[9,10]

Wasting has a major impact on morbidity and mortality. Early studies showed that timing of death from AIDS correlated well with the decline of nutrition status, particularly progressive depletion of body cell mass.[11] The impact of nutrition state, and particularly loss of the lean mass compartment, on survival was elegantly shown by Suttmann et al who demonstrated an independent effect of loss of body cell mass on survival.[12] More recently the CPCRA (Community Programs for Clinical Research in AIDS) demonstrated that a weight-losing trend predicts subsequent mortality and susceptibility to opportunistic infections.[13] Thus there does appear to be evidence that impaired nutrition state adversely influences disease progression and this observation has under-girded the supposition that improving nutrition state may improve clinical outcome.

The impact of HAART on wasting and metabolism in HIV

Patients who have lost weight frequently experience weight recovery when they commence HAART; such weight gain is often associated with improved clinical well-being.[14–17] Thus the first goal of therapy, in virological, immunological and nutritional terms is to achieve effective viral control with antiretroviral treatment. Despite such virological control, most studies still include a number of individuals who fail to gain weight or still continue to lose weight. For example, in a large study of patients commencing treatment with indinavir, after a median of 176 days on treatment, body weight had increased in 119 out of 160 patients (74.4%), had not changed in 13 (8.1%) and had fallen in 28 (17.5%), relative to baseline.[18] Overall, the response of cohorts of patients commencing antiretroviral therapy is quite variable; one study of a cohort of patients starting a new protease inhibitor-based antiretroviral regimen demonstrated no change in weight trend of the group as a whole.[19]

Thus it appears that even in the era of active antiretroviral therapy, wasting does continue to remain a clinical problem, albeit far less commonly than in earlier years. Wasting may become more frequent once again if viral resistance to antiretroviral drugs becomes an increasing clinical problem.

Lipid abnormalities and antiretroviral treatment

Even when HAART does restore body mass, not all metabolic abnormalities are reversed. Recently a new constellation of metabolic abnormalities have been recognised in treated HIV patients, which have been collectively termed 'lipodystrophy'.[20] The features of this syndrome include the redistribution of body fat away from subcutaneous areas, particularly facial fat deposits, with a concurrent accumulation of fat in the

visceral compartment or in the dorsocervical fat pad.[21–23] As a consequence, abdominal swelling may develop whilst peripheral tissues such as limbs and face become grossly wasted. At the same time, plasma triglycerides are often grossly increased, sometimes dramatically to levels at which pancreatitis is likely.[24,25] In addition there are reports of premature atherosclerosis in individuals on HAART.[26–30]

Thus it appears that, although antiretroviral treatment does result in clinical improvement in an overall nutrition state, not all metabolic abnormalities are reversed and patients on therapy may still require further investigation and management of metabolic syndromes.

AIDS in developing countries

In the setting of developing countries, antiretroviral therapy is rarely available in a consistent way because of its cost. In Africa, the cardinal feature of AIDS is tissue wasting and this has led to the description 'Slim Disease' being applied.[31] Such wasting was originally thought to be the consequence of malabsorption due to the high prevalence of enteropathogens, particularly enteric coccidia such as cryptosporidiosis and isosporiasis in the African setting.[32] However it is now well recognised that other chronic opportunistic infections, particularly tuberculosis, may be of great aetiological significance[33] and such co-infection may compound the metabolic and nutritional effects of HIV infection.[34]

The primary focus of this chapter is to assess critically the pathophysiological mechanisms of weight loss in HIV infection and to discuss nutrition support of adults with HIV infection and AIDS. The implications of paediatric HIV infection for nutrition and the implications of AIDS for feeding and nutrition in the developing world are subjects of immense importance but will only be touched upon briefly in this chapter. The chapter will focus on wasting rather than other metabolic and nutritional complications of HIV infection, such as 'lipodystrophy', despite their major clinical importance, since such abnormalities rarely require 'nutrition support' and since the implications of lipodystrophy for nutrition support remain unclear at present.

Pathophysiology of weight loss

AIDS is not a single disease in the sense that the clinical syndrome consists of a variety of substantially different clinical events and complications super-imposed on a common background of immuno-deficiency. For this reason, weight loss is often multifactorial, even within individual patients, and may occur for completely different reasons in different individuals.[35] Potential causes of weight loss are summarised in Figure 36.1.

Patterns of weight loss

When weight loss does occur in HIV infected individuals it may occur in a number of ways. Opportunistic infections, such as pneumocystis carinii pneumonia (PCP), are frequently associated with rapid weight loss, whilst chronic gastrointestinal disease or gut dysfunction are more associated with chronic progressive patterns of weight loss.[36]

Gastrointestinal involvement in HIV infection

Gastrointestinal disease is common in HIV infected subjects. Conditions which commonly affect the gastrointestinal tract are shown in Figure 36.1. Diarrhoea is the commonest symptom and failure to identify an opportunistic enteropathogen is not unusual in these circumstances.[37,38] The common endpoint of several of these processes affecting the small intestine is malabsorption. Malabsorption of fat is very common and can be detected in stage II, III, and IV disease.[39,40] It is at least partly due to jejunal villous atrophy,[37,38,41,42] as shown in Figure 36.2. A

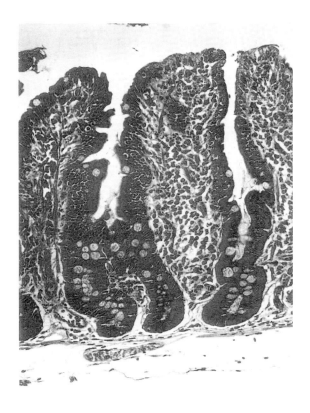

Figure 36.2 – Jejunal biopsy from an asymptomatic HIV antibody positive subject showing partial villous atrophy and crypt hyperplasia. ×80 magnification.

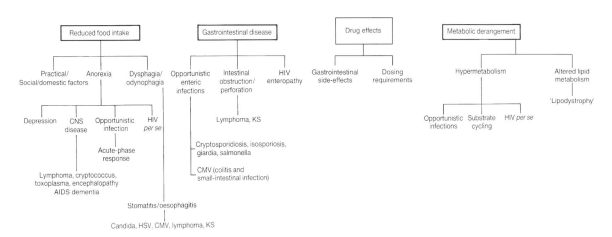

Figure 36.1 – Potential causes of weight loss in HIV infection. HSV = Herpes simplex virus, CMV = Cytomegalovirus, KS = Kaposi's sarcoma.

direct effect of HIV infection on the gut is likely as HIV genomic DNA has been detected in and live virus recovered from intestinal biopsies of patients with HIV infection.[43] The evolution of partial villous atrophy under such conditions is not yet understood but is likely to result from the release of mediators such as cytokines from HIV-infected reticuloendothelial cells. When patients with disordered gastrointestinal function are effectively treated with HAART, indices of gastrointestinal function usually improve and this is at least partially responsible for the weight gain frequently seen in patients commencing therapy.

Energy balance

Energy balance is the ultimate determinant of weight gain or loss. Negative energy balance drives wasting and this is almost always the consequence of reduced energy intake rather than excessive energy expenditure. Despite this, alterations in energy expenditure have been identified.

Resting energy expenditure (REE) is elevated in both stage II and stage IV HIV infection.[44-47] Although there is considerable disparity between studies, the consensus seems to be that HIV infection *per se* raises REE by about 10% in clinically well individuals with further elevation in the presence of secondary infection (Fig. 36.3).

Such elevation of REE may partly be a direct effect of the viral pathology itself as there is an association between viral load and elevation of REE.[48] However considerable heterogeneity exists in terms of energy expenditure.[49] In individuals with primarily gastrointestinal disease and a malnutrition-type response, REE may be reduced and thus it may be very difficult to predict REE in individuals with HIV infection. These findings have important implications for the determination of macronutrient requirements for people with HIV infection and AIDS.

Although studies of REE have helped define the metabolic effects of HIV infection, REE does not solely determine energy expenditure. Studies of total energy expenditure (TEE) using doubly-labelled water ($^2H_2$ ^{18}O) have demonstrated that TEE is relatively low in weight-losing individuals, primarily because such weight loss commonly coincides with being clinically unwell and activity levels are markedly reduced (Fig. 36.4a).[50] The reason such weight-losing individuals are in negative energy balance is because they are unable to maintain an adequate food intake, energy intake values being dramatically reduced during such weight loss phases (Fig. 36.4b). Such phases frequently correlate with secondary infection; similar findings have been made during such infections (see Fig. 36.3b). Thus reduced energy intake is the primary determinant of weight loss or gain in HIV infection (Fig. 36.5).[51]

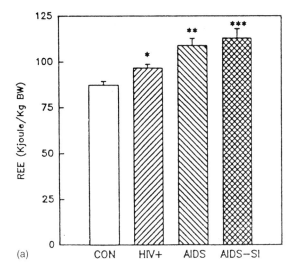

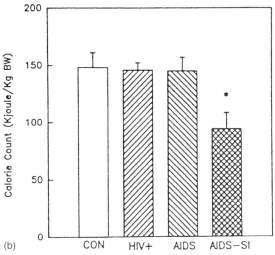

Figure 36.3 – Resting Energy Expenditure (a) and energy intake (b) in HIV infection. Subjects with asymptomatic HIV infection (HIV+), AIDS and AIDS with secondary infection (AIDS-SI), compared with a control group (CON). Results are normalised for body weight and shown as mean ± SE. (a) ★ P<0.025 vs control; ★★ P< 0.0001 vs control, P<0.025 vs HIV+; ★★★ P<0.0001 vs control, P<0.01 vs HIV+. (b) ★ P<0.02 vs control, HIV+, and AIDS groups. From Grunfeld *et al.*[56]

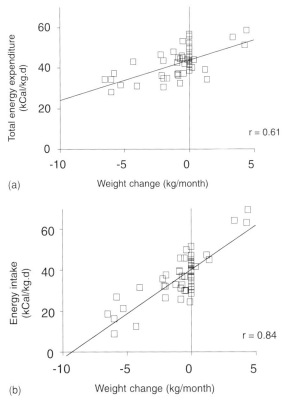

(a)

(b)

Figure 36.4 – Total energy expenditure (a) and energy intake (b) in HIV-infected men according to rate of weight loss or gain (n=51). Weight loss is explained by reduced intake not accelerated expenditure. From Macallan *et al.*[50]

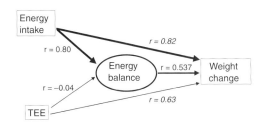

Figure 36.5 – Predictors of energy balance and weight change. Relationship of energy intake and total energy expenditure (TEE) with energy balance and weight change in a cohort of HIV infected men at various stages in their illness. Values represent path coefficients. Energy intake is the strongest predictor of energy balance and weight change. From Sheehan *et al.*[51]

HAART and energy metabolism

The impact of HAART on energy expenditure remains unclear. The association between viral load and resting energy expenditure (REE) suggests that

viral infection itself may be instrumental in the increased REE commonly seen in HIV infection. From this it might have been expected that reducing viral load with therapy would impact negatively on REE. However some studies of REE in patients have failed to demonstrate an association between viral load and REE, e.g. Grinspoon *et al.*[52] A multivariate analysis has suggested that HAART may have a two-component effect, the reduction in viral load reducing REE whilst the therapy itself independently increases REE.[53] There are, as yet, no data on total energy expenditure (TEE) in HAART but it might be expected that increased well-being would result in increased activity with a consequent increase in TEE. Failure to regain weight with HAART is probably the consequence of inadequate energy intake just as wasting in untreated HIV infection is commonly the consequence of reduced food intake.[50]

Fat metabolism

Fat metabolism is markedly deranged in HIV infection. In the era before the widespread use of anti-retroviral drugs, it was known that increased circulating plasma triglyceride levels were often seen in HIV infection. The increase was primarily due to an increased VLDL and this was closely related to increased *de novo* lipid synthesis in the liver.[54,55] In addition, there was evidence of reduced triglyceride clearance due to impaired tissue utilisation of fats.[56] Such phenomena may be related to the action of pro-inflammatory cytokines, such as TNF and alpha-interferon, and an association between alpha-interferon levels and triglycerides has been demonstrated in AIDS patients.[57]

More recently, dramatic changes have been observed in lipid metabolism with fat redistribution and hyperlipidaemia, so-called 'lipodystrophy', as described above. The relative contributions of drug therapy and HIV infection to this phenomenon remain contentious. Initially it was thought that such hyperlipidaemia and fat redistribution were specific to a single class of drug, the protease inhibitors. It has now become apparent in individuals on other classes of therapy and similar anthropometric changes have been reported in patients not receiving antiretroviral therapy.[58]

To date, the role for dietary intervention and exercise in lipodystrophy remains unclear. The hyperlipidaemias often seen as part of this lipodystrophy syndrome have implications for nutrition support. As part of routine management of hyperlipidaemia, individuals are conventionally advised on a lipid lowering diet. This advice would, amongst other changes, include a reduction in the total amount of dietary fat, a reduction in refined carbohydrates and a reduction in the amount of alcohol consumed. A reduction in all of these dietary components could subsequently lead to a reduction in energy intake. Indeed, in the HIV patient this may lead to a conflict in dietary goals. It may become difficult for a patient to maintain an adequate energy intake to prevent weight loss whilst following a lipid lowering dietary regimen. Nutrition support in these incidences needs to be a compromise worked out on an individual basis. Changes to the diet may be suggested to bring diet in line with a lipid lowering protocol, but different strategies will need to be utilised to preserve energy intake. In some cases it may prove very difficult to follow a regimen with a strict fat restriction.

Body composition and protein synthesis

Weight loss experienced by HIV-infected subjects consists of both fat and lean tissue. In studies in non-infected subjects, the proportion of fat or lean tissue loss experienced as a result of reduced food intake alone has previously been shown to be dependent on initial body composition; fatter individuals lose proportionately more fat.[15a] During the course of severe infection, however, this balance is perturbed and there is a disproportionate loss of protein. The same phenomenon may apply in HIV infection; for example, in a study in HIV-related cytomegalovirus (CMV) infection, weight loss consisted of 60% lean tissue, far more than would have been predicted.[59] In animal models of infection and during severe infection in humans, the normal anabolic response to nutrition in muscle and the accretion of body protein appears to be impaired, so-called 'anabolic block'.[60,61]

Our measurements of whole body protein metabolism in HIV infection showed an increase in protein turnover in patients with stage IV disease (AIDS), consistent with the changes seen in other infective situations.[62] Several other studies have subsequently confirmed this observation. However, we were unable to demonstrate a quantitative reduction in the utilisation of protein for protein synthesis on feeding or 'anabolic block', despite being able to demonstrate that this was the case in tuberculosis;[63] such an observation suggests that the anabolic response to feeding is usually intact in HIV infection.[62] However, there may still be redirection of protein synthesis away from structural proteins towards shorter lived proteins, such as acute phase proteins.

The implication of such observations for nutrition support is that, even during opportunistic infections, nutrients, particularly proteins, may still be utilised; maintenance of adequate intake of substrates remains the priority in such patients.

Rationale for nutrition support in HIV infection

Energy and macronutrients

It is undoubtedly true that weight loss is a major contributor to morbidity in HIV infection. Loss of protein in particular is likely to be important in terms of fatigability, malaise, poor wound healing and delayed recovery from infection. Improved supply, absorption and utilisation of macronutrients in wasted patients would therefore be expected to reduce morbidity, ameliorate weight loss and improve body composition and might also be expected to have an impact on mortality.

Malnutrition in other clinical situations has been shown to have a deleterious effect on immune function. For example, type IV immune responses, exemplified by delayed hypersensitivity skin reactions to both new and recall antigens, have been shown to be reduced in malnourished children.[64] In addition, several other indices of immune function, such as the proportion of helper to suppressor cells,[65] the activity of the complement pathway[66–68] and acute phase protein synthesis[69] are reduced by malnutrition. Furthermore, the integrity of mucosal barriers, such as the intestine and respiratory tract, may be deleteriously affected by protein-energy malnutrition.[70] Although such immune deficits have been ascribed to macronutrient deficiency, lack of specific nutrients or micronutrients may also contribute as these play key roles in metabolic pathways important in immune function. For example glutamine is an important substrate for lymphocyte- and enterocyte metabolism and may become 'conditionally essential' in inflammatory states.

Some authors have suggested that malnutrition itself may be the cause of death in some patients with AIDS; certainly nutrition parameters correlate with disease progression and thus with timing of death[9,11] but cause and effect is not clear. Given that malnutrition impairs immune function and that AIDS is primarily a disease due to impaired immune function, it seems reasonable to suppose that improved nutrition status may ameliorate the loss of immune function resulting from HIV infection. In addition, as malnutrition is known to be a major risk factor for the development of clinical infection in non-HIV-infected humans, it is likely that malnutrition may exacerbate clinical progression of HIV infection. There is thus a strong case for the likely benefit of nutrition support in HIV infection.

If malnutrition does accelerate the progress of HIV infection, it might be argued that improving nutrition state may improve clinical outcome. Although this appears to be implicitly true from the above evidence, it has been much harder to demonstrate such an effect at the clinical level. There is a wide literature addressing this question but much of the data are difficult to interpret, either as a result of having poor or absent controls or having inappropriate outcome measures. There are many difficulties assessing the effect of nutritional intervention on HIV because nutrition status is so inextricably linked with clinical status and because it is neither practical nor ethical to have a control group in nutrition studies. In addition, other factors, such as the presence or absence of opportunistic infections, the impact of drug treatment, and environmental, social and psychological factors may have a dramatic effect on clinical outcome. It is quite possible that even if a particular nutritional intervention had a major effect, it might not be apparent in the presence of so many other confounding factors.

One area however, where nutritional intervention can be shown to be of clear benefit is in severe malnutrition or wasting. Here provision of adequate nutrition may have a dramatic effect on survival. For example, in one study of severely malnourished patients receiving TPN, survival was extended to 211 days compared to 57 days in those not receiving TPN.[71] Similarly, studies of percutaneous endoscopic gastrostomy (PEG) feeding in malnourished patients have demonstrated a trend towards improved survival (210 versus 109 days).[72] Several other studies have demonstrated the importance of nutrition support in severe wasting.

Micronutrients

The impact of micronutrients on HIV disease progression has also been an area of great interest. Several studies have shown an association of disease progression with poor micronutrient status. For example,

Baum et al[73] showed an association between declining plasma vitamin A or B_{12} levels and reduced CD4 counts; conversely they found that normalisation of vitamin B_{12} or zinc status was associated with an increase in CD4 count. However there are considerable difficulties in interpreting plasma vitamin levels, particularly since they are affected by the acute phase response and susceptible to changes in binding proteins. Similarly there are difficulties in interpreting the impact on clinical outcome when surrogate markers such as CD4 count are used as indices of efficacy. Some investigators have chosen to look at micronutrient intake rather than plasma levels. For example, Tang et al[74] demonstrated that high intakes of vitamin C, vitamin B1 or niacin were associated with a reduced relative risk of disease progression whereas high intakes of zinc were associated with an increased risk of disease progression. Vitamin A intake appeared to have a U-shaped relationship with outcome; both very high and very low intakes were associated with poorer outcome.[74] It has been suggested that large doses of vitamin A or beta-carotene may have beneficial virological and immunological effects but this has not been borne out in randomised studies.[75,76]

In gastrointestinal disease, micronutrient absorption may be compromised. Infection with *Cryptosporidia* or *Isospora* and other conditions which affect the terminal ileum may impair vitamin B_{12} absorption.[77] Since vitamin B_{12} deficiency may cause neuropathy, supplementation under these conditions is likely to prevent such a complication which, in the clinical situation, may be difficult to distinguish from drug-induced or HIV-related neuropathy. Other B group vitamins may be important, such as thiamine, deficiency of which has been demonstrated in AIDS[78] and possibly B_6[79] but there is no evidence that very large doses of such vitamins are beneficial and they may indeed be harmful. Folate absorption is reduced in HIV infection, probably as a non-specific effect of enteropathy,[80] but levels in serum and erythrocytes have not been consistently reduced.[81,82]

In terms of trace elements, selenium deficiency has been described as a cause of cardiomyopathy and ostemalacia and may be clinically important.[83] Zinc deficiency has been described in adult AIDS patients[84] but such cases are not representative of all AIDS patients where cohort studies have found zinc levels to be within the normal range.[85]

Certainly it does appear that some individuals with HIV infection develop moderate to severe micronutrient deficiency and that this impacts on their clinical state; such patients should clearly receive adequate vitamin supplementation. Extrapolating such selective use of vitamin supplements to universal supplementation for all HIV infected individuals is a strategy which is more difficult to justify from the available evidence. However large clinical studies designed to prove the value of universal supplementation are almost impossible to perform in the current changing clinical climate and are unlikely to be forthcoming. Micronutrients, of course, are normally ingested with macronutrients as part of food; weight loss, indicative, by definition, of macronutrient deficiency, is therefore likely to be a useful marker of risk of micronutrient deficiency. Thus, it seems appropriate to target weight-losing patients for micronutrient supplementation.

Micronutrients and mother-to-child transmission of HIV infection

One area of particular interest in terms of the place of micronutrients in HIV disease is their potential role in modifying mother-to-child transmission of HIV around the time of childbirth. This is particularly pertinent in developing world settings where vertical transmission is a common mode of transmission and where such interventions may potentially be affordable, particularly compared to very expensive antiretroviral therapy. A recent study from Africa showed that vitamin A deficiency was very common among pregnant women and that the degree of deficiency correlated strongly with the risk of transmission from mother to baby (Fig. 36.6).[86] Similar results were observed in a similar study in two metropolitan areas in the US.[87] These observations have given rise to several interventional trials the results of which are still awaited. One trial has now published the results of pregnancy outcome (but not HIV transmission which requires a longer follow-up period).[88] Groups received

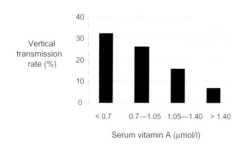

Figure 36.6 – Vitamin A status and risk of mother-to-child transmission of HIV. From Semba *et al.*[86]

multivitamin supplementation and/or vitamin A supplementation. Surprisingly, vitamin A supplementation appeared to have no impact on pregnancy outcome whereas multivitamin supplementation did have a major impact in terms of fetal death, low birthweight, preterm birth and low weight-for-age. Hopefully the role and relative contributions of different vitamin supplementation strategies (multivitamin, vitamin A etc) should become clearer as several studies in the developing world reach completion over the next few years.

Nutrition support – practical application

Guidelines

Figures 36.7–36.9 summarise our approach to nutrition support.

General considerations

Nutrition support in HIV infection should be tailored to individual requirements because of the variety of pathophysiological processes that may contribute to weight loss and malnutrition. Different strategies will be required at different clinical stages of disease and according to the differing complications which may arise.

Practical and financial factors need to be considered to ensure that the patient is able to maintain an adequate supply and intake of appropriate foods. Treatment with antiviral drugs may result in weight gain and improvement in nutrition status and effective antiretroviral therapy is the cornerstone of both clinical and nutrition therapy. Prompt investigation and treatment of opportunistic infections helps ameliorate weight lost during such episodes. Weight loss may precede specific symptoms and signs of secondary infection[36] and therefore should be carefully investigated.

Asymptomatic HIV infection

In uncomplicated phases, individuals can maintain energy balance via the oral route[89,90] but the combination of malabsorption, which may be asymptomatic, and raised resting energy expenditure may mean that macronutrient requirements are higher than would be predicted from body composition.[35] Such metabolic changes may occur early in the disease and for this reason dietetic assessment should be offered to individuals with asymptomatic HIV infection. In addition, establishment of good nutrition status in early asymptomatic disease may delay disease progression and should ameliorate the effects of subsequent metabolic challenges.

After a diagnosis of HIV infection has been made, individuals often become more conscious of their diet and try to adopt a 'healthy' diet.[91] 'Healthy Eating' guidelines however have been formulated primarily for an overweight, Western population with long life-expectancy in the developed world in order to reduce the risks particularly of coronary artery disease. Such guidelines are not necessarily appropriate in HIV infection and appropriate dietary education is an important part of the management of HIV infection.

Diet in symptom-control

Nutrition therapy may have aims other than purely nutritional goals. For example, manipulation of the diet may ameliorate symptoms. Diarrhoea may be related to fat malabsorption and thus symptoms may be improved by a reduction in dietary fat; lactase deficiency causing lactose intolerance may be ameliorated by a lactose-free diet. Similarly, local pain in the mouth or odynophagia are suitable targets for dietary modification in addition to specific therapy. Such symptom-relieving measures should not be forgotten as potential targets of dietary manipulation.

Diet and drug therapy

In the era of HAART, patients face the additional challenge of adjusting their diets to fit with the timing and dietary guidelines associated with their specific drug combination. These guidelines are given in order to both optimise absorption and increase tolerability of the medications (Table 36.1). For example, one of the nucleoside drugs, didanosine requires that it be taken one hour before food and at least two hours after food. Within the protease inhibitor group it is recommended that indinavir should be taken with a low fat meal or without food, unless it is taken in combination with ritonavir. The other drugs in this class, however, should all be taken with food.

Patients are rarely on a combination of less than three drugs and they may have to make significant alterations to their habitual diet patterns in order to meet the requirements of their drug regimen. This can prove difficult for certain individuals and may result in

Table 36.1 – Dietary recommendations for taking various antiretroviral drugs.

Nucleoside analogues

Didanosine	Take on an empty stomach
Lamivudine	Preferably taken without food
Stavudine	Taken 1 hour before food or with a light meal

Non-nucleoside reverse transcriptase inhibitors

Efavirenz	Avoid high fat meals

Protease inhibitors

Indinavir	Take on an empty stomach, 1 hour before or 2 hours after a meal
Nelfinavir	Take with a meal or light snack
Ritonavir	Take with a meal
Saquinavir	Take within 2 hours after a full meal

problems meeting their energy and macronutrient requirements. They may thus need specific dietary advice and counselling on the best way of fitting a well balanced diet around their specific drug regimen. Other individuals may find this alteration of lifestyle so difficult that it may lead to reduced adherence with their drug treatment and consequent loss of efficacy of antiretroviral therapy.

Side-effect management

The antiretroviral medications may cause unpleasant side-effects, particularly in the early weeks of starting a new regimen. Common complaints include nausea, vomiting, abdominal discomfort and diarrhoea. Nutrition support is often required for a short time to help with symptom management and to prevent reduced dietary intakes.

Food hygiene

Food hygiene is important, particularly in patients with advanced immunosuppression. Such patients are vulnerable to gastrointestinal pathogens such as *Salmonella* sp., *Cryptosporidium* sp. and *Isospora* sp. In some circumstances it may be advisable to boil drinking water, and patients should be reminded to wash fresh fruit and vegetables and avoid raw or rare meat, fish and eggs. The key issue here, as in many other aspects of HIV nutrition, is one of patient education.

Dietary supplementation

Where food intake is markedly reduced, the first line approach to nutrition support often includes the use of energy-rich supplements. The most commonly used products include Ensure Plus (Abbott, Maidenhead, UK), Entera (Fresenius, Birchwood, UK), and Fortisip (Nutricia Clinical, Wilts, UK), which are nutritionally complete and provide 1.5 kcal/ml. Other products now available offer more choice to patients; these include 'juice-like' supplements, including Fortijuce (Nutricia Chemical, Wilts, UK), Provide Extra (Fresenius, Birchwood, UK) and Enlive (Abbott, Maidenhead, UK), and a yoghurt drink product, Fortifresh (Nutricia Chemical, Wilts, UK). Some supplements have a high energy content but the fats they contain may not be well absorbed; such malabsorption may cause diarrhoea or may be asymptomatic, resulting in overestimation of true caloric intake. Energy and/or nitrogen intake can be increased by the use of incomplete supplements such as Maxijul (SHS) and Calsip (Fresenius) for carbohydrate and Maxipro (SHS) powder for protein. Such supplements, however, should be seen as an adjunct to, not a replacement for, oral food intake.

Specialised diets

Because problems with nutrient absorption occur in HIV infection, normal foodstuffs and standard supplements may not be well tolerated. In these circumstances, predigested formulae such as Peptamen Nestlè Clinical, Surrey, UK (Nerlle), Perative (Abbott) or elemental formulae such as Emsogen (SHS) and E-028 (SHS) may achieve greater absorption of protein substrates. They should probably be reserved for those with demonstrable malabsorption and continuing weight loss, in which situations they may be beneficial.[92] Acceptability is the major problem with these diets and thus they are usually given by enteral tube.

Similarly, fat absorption may be improved by the use of preparations rich in medium-chain triglycerides (MCT), e.g. Peptamen Nestlè Clinical, Surrey, UK (Natts), Nutrison MCT (Nutricia). Such feeds have been shown to be beneficial for some individuals both in terms of weight gain and improvement in diarrhoea.[92]

Enteral nutrition

Enteral nutrition using liquid feeds should be considered where adequate nutritional intake cannot be achieved orally. Nasogastric fine-bore feeding (NG) tubes are an effective way of delivering nutrients to the stomach but are not well-tolerated for long periods. Percutaneous endoscopically-placed gastrostomy feeding (PEG) tubes are better tolerated than nasogastric tubes. Although they have a somewhat higher risk of infection and complications than NG tubes,[93] the risk appears to be no higher in HIV-positive individuals than in similar HIV-negative patients.[94] Where enteral nutrition is likely to be required for a prolonged period (more than 4 weeks) PEG tubes are probably preferable. They often allow the administration of greater caloric intakes than could be achieved orally and may be very effective in repleting body tissue.[72,93–95] The administration of liquid feeds via PEG gastrostomy does not, of course, mean that patients cannot also eat food orally. Psychological factors, such as motivation and acceptability, should be carefully considered before commencing therapy; they may be as important as physiological factors in determining the success of PEG feeding.

Standard enteral feeds may be used in most individuals requiring enteral tube feeding but the considerations relating to fat and lactose content above should be noted. Rate of administration should meet fluid and nutrition requirements; although HIV infection does increase resting metabolic rate, in an unwell patient whose activity levels are low, requirements are not much in excess of calculated resting metabolic rate (RMR) and the temptation to feed excessively should be avoided.

Parenteral nutrition

Parenteral nutrition should be considered as a therapeutic option in intestinal failure or when enteral nutrition fails to meet requirements and cannot be envisaged to do so. There is a reluctance to commence patients with AIDS on total parenteral nutrition (TPN) for a variety of reasons, not least decisions regarding the appropriateness of nutrition intervention in late-stage disease. Such decisions may be influenced by changing options for effective antiretroviral therapy. Infection rates associated with central venous catheterisation in HIV infection are probably higher than in other groups although reported infection rates in AIDS patients of the order of 0.12 per 100 catheter days are not dissimilar to rates in similar patient groups receiving home TPN.[96] The aim of TPN is to meet nutrition and fluid requirements; hyperalimentation is unlikely to be of benefit. Standard regimens with trace element and vitamin supplements should be given as no definite benefit has been demonstrated with specialised TPN regimens.

TPN improves nutrition state.[97] Although it stimulates whole body protein synthesis,[62] the response in terms of repletion of lean tissue may be impaired in patients with active opportunistic infection.[97] In severe macronutrient deficiency, quality of life may be improved[98,99] and survival extended.[71]

Micronutrients

Definitive guidelines are currently not available for requirements of vitamins and micronutrients under conditions of increased metabolic need such as infection. A well balanced diet probably provides adequate vitamins and trace elements. The dietitians in the HIV/AIDS (DHIVA) group of the British Dietetic Association recommend a balanced diet as being the best way to provide adequate micronutrients. They suggest taking a multivitamin and mineral tablet daily to provide an additional 1–2 times the Daily Recommended Value, DRV. We do not routinely prescribe such supplements although many of our patients do choose to take multivitamins. Excessive doses, for example of vitamin B_6 or zinc, may be harmful and should be discouraged. However, specific deficiencies may arise in the context of generalised malnutrition or malabsorption particularly with diarrhoea and clinicians should be aware of this possibility. A standard dose of a vitamin/mineral supplement should be recommended in this situation or if dietary intake is poor. Gastrointestinal disease, particularly infection of the terminal ileum with coccidial enteropathogens, may reduce absorption of vitamin B_{12} which is absorbed in this area complexed with intrinsic factor.[100] In these patients parenteral vitamin B_{12} (hydroxocobalamin), which is inexpensive, should be given regularly.

Drugs

Appetite stimulants

Anorexia is an important cause of energy and protein deficit in HIV infection. Megestrol acetate (Megace, Bristol-Myers, UK), a progestogen with anabolic effects, has been successfully used to improve appetite and achieve weight gain in HIV infection[101] but most of the tissue gain is fat rather than lean tissue.[102] Side-effects include urticaria, thrombophlebitis and feminis with impotence. Diabetes mellitus has also been described[103] and plasma glucose should be monitored in subjects receiving megestrol.

The canniboid dronabinol has also been advocated for use as an appetite stimulant in HIV infection. It

increases perceived appetite but this does not appear to translate into increased food intake and weight gain.[104,105] Other drugs, such as pizotifen, hydrazine and glucocorticoids have been used as appetite stimulants in anorexia associated with malignant disease and may be considered in HIV infection. Depression is a common cause of anorexia and anti-depressant drugs may improve appetite in affected individuals.

Anabolic drugs

There is an extensive literature on the use of anabolic agents in HIV wasting which is beyond the scope of this chapter. Recombinant human growth hormone (rhGH) is a highly potent anabolic agent both in short-term metabolic studies[106] and in more prolonged clinical use.[107] Even in the presence of opportunistic infection it is effective in redirecting protein metabolism towards protein synthesis[108] although muscle protein responsiveness does appear to decline with more advanced disease.[109] Other anabolic agents such as nandrolone and oxandrolone also appear to be effective.[102] An alternative approach is to combine megestrol acetate, for its appetite-stimulating effects, with testosterone, for its androgenic and anabolic effects. Testosterone should certainly be considered in male patients with biochemical evidence of hypogonadism.

Pancreatic enzymes

Exocrine pancreatic insufficiency has not been shown to be a major clinical problem in HIV infection[110] and therefore pancreatic enzyme supplementation is not routinely indicated.

Paediatric HIV infection

Nutrition is of paramount importance to the child with HIV infection. The clinical presentation of HIV-related malnutrition is different in children to that in adults; failure to thrive, growth impairment and developmental retardation are major consequences of HIV infection in children.[111,112] Wasting is only seen in more severe disease. Caloric requirements may be higher than in non-infected children particularly during 'catch-up' growth following treatment of opportunistic infections. As with adult HIV infection, the clinical picture has been dramatically altered by the advent of potent antiretroviral drugs. Despite the

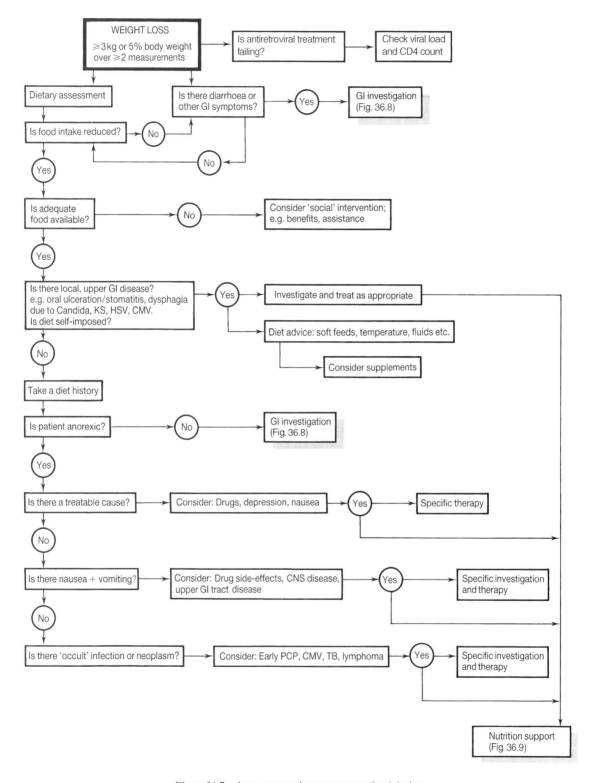

Figure 36.7 – Assessment and management of weight loss.

availability of such treatment, nutrition support may be indicated.

Children are more susceptible to micronutrient deficiency than adults and clinically significant deficiency of folate,[113] causing neurological symptoms, selenium,[83] causing cardiomyopathy, zinc,[114] with acrodermatitis enteropathica, and iron[115] have been described. Deficiency is more likely where diarrhoeal

disease is part of the clinical picture. Supplementation at least up to recommended levels of intake is likely to be beneficial and but there is no evidence that it is helpful to exceed this at present. Gut dysfunction is common in children with HIV infection and may be manifest as lactose intolerance.[116,117]

General principles of nutrition support in children should be applied; details are dealt with elsewhere

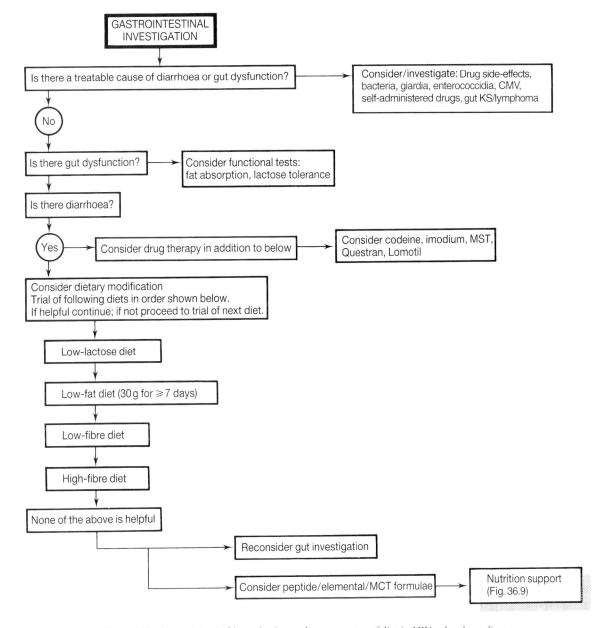

Figure 36.8 – Gastrointestinal investigation and management of diet in HIV-related gut disease.

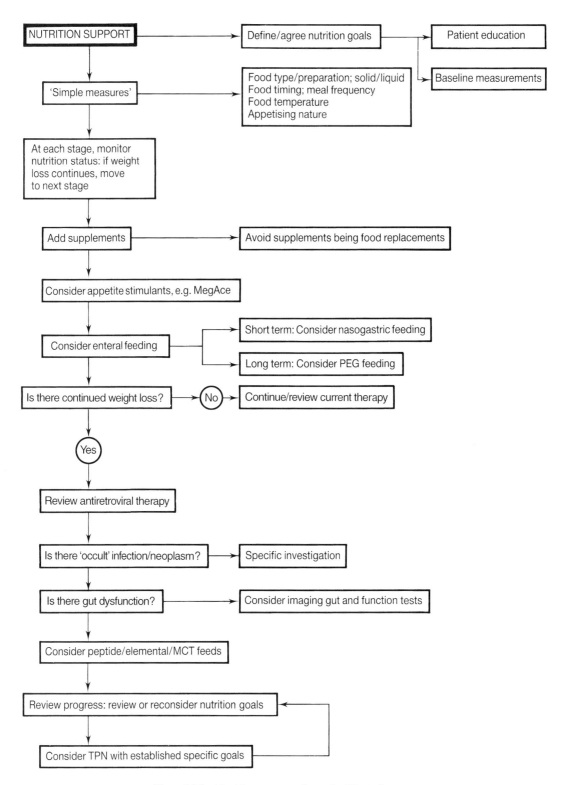

Figure 36.9 – Nutrition support scheme for HIV infection.

(Chs. 20 and 26). Specific aspects of paediatric HIV infection are beyond the scope of this chapter but are reviewed elsewhere.[112]

Breast-feeding

Breast-feeding has been shown to be a possible route of transmission of HIV infection to the neonate.[118,119] In countries with an adequate supply of safe water and good supply of appropriate formula feeds, breast-feeding is therefore strongly discouraged for HIV-positive mothers.[120] However, in many developing regions of the world, such requirements are not met and food and water-borne enteric infections are a major cause of mortality. Breast-feeding is highly protective against early childhood mortality and morbidity in such settings, not to mention its psychological and social benefits. The potential risks of contracting HIV need to be weighed against the risks associated with not breast-feeding.[121,122] Appropriate advice in this context will depend heavily on local factors and is likely to change as new information becomes available.

Current World Health Organisation advice includes the following statement:

'When children born to women living with HIV can be ensured uninterrupted access to nutritionally adequate breast-milk substitutes that are safely prepared and fed to them, they are at less risk of illness and death if they are not breast-fed. However, when these conditions are not fulfilled, in particular in an environment where infectious diseases and malnutrition are the primary causes of death during infancy, artificial feeding substantially increases children's risk of illness and death.'

(A Policy Statement developed collaboratively by UNAIDS, UNICEF and WHO; April 1999 – available on the UNAIDS website, http://www.unaids.org).

Their recommendations also emphasise the importance of informed choice and access to HIV counselling and testing.

Summary and future perspectives

Remarkable advances have been made in the last 10 years towards understanding, managing and treating HIV infection although, at present, no definitive curative treatment is yet available. Similarly, we now have a far greater understanding of the disturbances of metabolism and nutrition that occur during the course of HIV infection although novel and unexpected complications, such as 'lipodystrophy', continue to arise. The basis of nutrition support however remains the same: the disease-specific and patient-specific application of standard nutritional principles, maintenance of adequate energy and protein intake being a priority. Further progress will depend upon the execution of well-designed clinical trials of differing nutrition strategies. The place of anabolic therapies and pharmacological agents such as growth hormone needs further clarification.

Education is central in the application of nutrition support. This applies firstly to health care professionals who must be shown the value of dietetic manipulation and the importance of good nutrition to clinical outcome. It also applies to patients with HIV infection who need to understand the rationale of the nutrition therapy they are being recommended. Nutrition education is also an important component of empowering patients to influence the course of their illness.

Improved nutrition management needs to progress hand-in-hand with improved antiretroviral and drug therapy. Very rapid progress has occurred in recent years. Approaches to nutrition support will need to be continually updated to keep pace with the changing clinical environment.

References

1. Gottlieb MS, Schroff R, Schanker HM *et al.* Pneumocystis carinii pneumonia and mucosal candidiasis in previously healthy homosexual men: evidence of a new acquired cellular immunodeficiency. *N Engl J Med* 1981; **305**: 1425–1431.

2. Masur H, Michelis MA, Greene JB *et al.* An outbreak of community acquired Pneumocystis carinii pneumonia: initial manifestation of cellular immune dysfunction. *N Engl J Med* 1981; **305**: 1431–1438.

3. Siegal FP, Lopez C, Hammer GS *et al.* Severe acquired immunodeficiency in male homosexuals manifested by chronic perianal ulcerative herpes simplex lesions. *N Engl J Med* 1981; **305**: 1439–1444.

4. Gottlieb MS, Groopman JE, Weinstein WM, Fahey JL, Detel R. The Acquired Immunodeficiency Syndrome. *Ann Int Med* 1983; **99**: 208–220.

5. Gallo RC, Salahuddin SZ, Popovic M *et al.* Frequent detection and isolation of cytopathic retroviruses (HTLV-III) from patients with AIDS and at risk for AIDS. *Science* 1984; **224**: 500–503.

6. Centers for Disease Control. Revision of the CDC case surveillance definition for acquired immuno-deficiency syndrome. *MMWR CDC Surveill Summ* 1987; **36(suppl 1S)**: 3S–14S.

7. Palella FJJ, Delaney KM, Moorman AC *et al*. Declining morbidity and mortality among patients with advanced human immunodeficiency virus infection. HIV Outpatient Study Investigators [see comments]. *N Engl J Med* 1998; **338**: 853–860.

8. Hoover DR, Graham NMH, Palenicek JG, Bacellar H, Saah AJ. Weight changes in HIV-1 seropositive and seronegative homosexual men. *Nutr Res* 1992; **12**: 297–305.

9. Kotler DP, Tierney AR, Wang J, Pierson RN. Magnitude of body-cell-mass depletion and the timing of death from wasting in AIDS. *Am J Clin Nutr* 1989a; **50**: 444–447.

10. Kotler DP, Wang J, Pierson RN. Body composition studies in patients with the acquired immunodeficiency syndrome. *Am J Clin Nutr* 1985; **42**: 1255–1265.

11. Chlebowski RT, Grosvenor MB, Bernhard NH, Morales LS, Bulcavage LM. Nutritional status, gastrointestinal dysfunction, and survival in patients with AIDS. *Am J Gastroenterol* 1989; **84**: 1288–1293.

12. Suttmann U, Ockenga J, Selberg O, Hoogestraat L, Deicher H, Muller MJ. Incidence and prognostic value of malnutrition and wasting in Human Immunodeficiency Virus-infected outpatients. *J Acquir Immune Defic Syndr* 1995; **8**: 239–246.

13. Wheeler DA, Gibert CL, Launer CA *et al*. Weight loss as a predictor of survival and disease progression in HIV infection. Terry Beirn Community Programs for Clinical Research on AIDS. *J Acquir Immune Defic Syndr* 1998; **18**: 80–85.

14. Teixeira A, Leu JC, Honderlick P, Trylesinski A, Zucman D. Variation in body weight and plasma viral load in HIV patients treated with tritherapy including a protease inhibitor. *Nutrition* 1997; **13**: 269.

15. Force G, Jockey C, Tugler MH, Khayat G, Champetier de Ribes D. Characteristics of change in body composition with efficiency of antiretroviral treatment in AIDS patients. *Nutrition* 1997; **13**: 290.

15a. Forbes GB. Lean body mass–body fat interrelationships in humans. *Nutr Rev* 1987; **45**: 225–231.

16. Silva M, Skolnik PR, Gorbach SL *et al*. The effect of protease inhibitors on weight and body composition in HIV-infected patients. *AIDS* 1998; **12**: 1645–1651.

17. Stricker RB, Goldberg B. Weight gain associated with protease inhibitor therapy in HIV-infected patients. *Res Virol* 1998; **149**: 123–126.

18. Carbonnel F, Maslo C, Beaugerie L *et al*. Effect of indinavir on HIV-related wasting. *AIDS* 1998; **12**: 1777–1784.

19. Schwenk A, Kremer G, Cornely O, Diehl V, Salzberger B, Fatkenheuer G. Body weight changes with protease inhibitor treatment of HIV infection. *Nutrition* 1999; **15**: 453–457.

20. Carr A, Samaras K, Burton S *et al*. A syndrome of peripheral lipodystrophy, hyperlipidaemia and insulin resistance in patients receiving HIV protease inhibitors. *AIDS* 1998; **12**: F51–58.

21. Miller KD, Jones E, Yanovski JA, Shankar R, Feuerstein I, Falloon J. Visceral abdominal fat accumulation associated with use of indinavir. *Lancet* 1998; **351**: 871–875.

22. Lo JC, Mulligan K, Tai VW, Algren H, Schambelan M. 'Buffalo hump' in men with HIV-1 infection. *Lancet* 1998; **351**: 867–870.

23. Carr A, Samaras K, Chisholm DJ, Cooper DA. Pathogenesis of HIV-1-protease inhibitor-associated peripheral lipodystrophy, hyperlipidaemia, and insulin resistance. *Lancet* 1998; **351**: 1881–1883.

24. Sullivan AK, Feher MD, Nelson MR, Gazzard BG. Marked hypertriglyceridaemia associated with ritonavir therapy [letter]. *AIDS* 1998; **12**: 1393–1394.

25. Henry K, Melroe H, Huebesch J, Hermundson J, Simpson J. Atorvastatin and gemfibrozil for protease-inhibitor-related lipid abnormalities [letter]. *Lancet* 1998; **352**: 1031–1032.

26. Gallet B, Pulik M, Genet P, Chedin P, Hiltgen M. Vascular complications associated with use of HIV protease inhibitors. *Lancet* 1998; **351**: 1958–1959.

27. Laurence, J. Vascular complications associated with use of HIV protease inhibitors. *Lancet* 1998; **351**: 1960.

28. Vittecoq D, Escaut L, Monsuez JJ. Vascular complications associated with use of HIV protease inhibitors. *Lancet* 1998; **351**: 1959.

29. Behrens G, Schmidt H, Meyer D, Stoll M, Schmidt RE. Vascular complications associated with use of HIV protease inhibitors. *Lancet* 1998; **351**: 1958.

30. Henry K, Melroe H, Huebsch J, Hermundson J, Levine C, Swensen L, Daley J. Severe premature coronary artery disease with protease inhibitors. *Lancet* 1998; **351**: 1328.

31. Serwadda D, Sewankambo NK, Carswell JW *et al*. Slim disease: a new disease in Uganda and its association with HTLV-III infection. *Lancet* 1985; **2**: 849–852.

32. Sewankambo NK, Mugerwa RD, Goodgame R *et al*. Enteropathic AIDS in Uganda. An endoscopic, histological and microbiological study. *AIDS* 1987; **1**: 9–13.

33. Lucas SB, De Cock KM, Hounnou A *et al*. Contribution of tuberculosis to slim disease in Africa. *Br Med J* 1994; **308**: 1531–1533.

34. Macallan DC. Malnutrition in tuberculosis. *Diagnostic Microbiol Infect Dis* 1999; **34**: 153–157.

35. Grunfeld C, Feingold KR. Metabolic disturbances and wasting in the Acquired Immunodeficiency Syndrome. *N Engl J Med* 1992; **327**: 329–337.

36. Macallan DC, Noble C, Baldwin C, Foskett M, McManus T, Griffin GE. Prospective analysis of patterns of weight change in stage IV human immunodeficiency virus infection. *Am J Clin Nutr* 1993; **58**: 417–424.

37. Kotler DP, Gaetz HP, Lange M, Klein EB, Holt PR. Enteropathy associated with the Acquired Immunodeficiency Syndrome. *Ann Int Med* 1984; **101**: 421–428.

38. Kotler DP, Francisco A, Clayton F, Scholes JV, Orenstein JM. Small intestinal injury and parasitic diseases in AIDS. *Ann Int Med* 1990; 113, 444–449.

39. Kapembwa MS, Fleming SC, Griffin GE, Caun K, Pinching AJ, Harris JRW. Fat absorption and exocrine pancreatic function in Human Immunodeficiency Virus infection. *Quart J Med* 1990; **74**: 49–56.

40. Gillin JS, Shike M, Alcock N et al. Malabsorption and mucosal abnormalities of the small intestine in the Acquired Immunodeficiency Syndrome. *Ann Int Med* 1985; **102**: 619–622.

41. Miller ARO, Griffin GE, Batman PA et al. Jejunal mucosal architecture and fat absorption in male homosexuals infected with Human Immunodeficiency Virus. *Q J Med* 1988; **69**: 1009–1019.

42. Batman PA, Miller ARO, Forster SM, Harris JRW, Pinching AJ, Griffin GE. Jejunal enteropathy associated with human immunodeficiency virus infection: quantitative histology. *J Clin Pathol* 1992; **42**: 275–281.

43. Nelson JA, Wiley CA, Reynolds-Kohler C, Reese CE, Margaretten W, Levy JA. Human Immunodeficiency Virus detected in bowel epithelium from patients with gastrointestinal symptoms. *Lancet* 1988; **1**: 259–262.

44. Hommes MJT, Romijn JA, Godfried MH et al. Increased Resting Energy Expenditure in Human Immunodeficiency Virus-infected men. *Metabolism* 1990; **39**: 1186–1190.

45. Melchior JC, Salmon D, Rigaud D et al. Resting energy expenditure is increased in stable, malnourished HIV-infected patients. *Am J Clin Nutr* 1991; **53**: 437–441.

46. Hommes MJT, Romijn JA, Endert E, Sauerwein HP. Resting energy expenditure and substrate oxidation in human immunodeficiency virus (HIV)-infected asymptomatic men: HIV affects host metabolism in the early asymptomatic stage. *Am J Clin Nutr* 1991; **54**: 311–315.

47. Grunfeld C, Pang M, Doerrler W, Shigenaga JK, Jensen P, Feingold KR. Lipids, lipoproteins, triglyceride clearance, and cytokines in Human Immunodeficiency Virus infection and the Acquired Immunodeficiency Syndrome. *J Clin Endocrinol Metab* 1992; **74**: 1045–1052.

48. Mulligan K, Tai VW, Schambelan M. Energy expenditure in Human Immunodeficiency Virus infection. *N Engl J Med* 1997; **336**: 70–71.

49. Schwenk A, Hoffer-Belitz E, Jung B et al. Resting energy expenditure, weight loss and altered body composition in HIV infection. *Nutrition* 1996; **12**(9): 595–601.

50. Macallan DC, Noble C, Baldwin C et al. Energy expenditure and wasting in Human Immunodeficiency Virus infection. *N Engl J Med* 1995; **333**: 83–88.

51. Sheehan LA, Macallan DC, Griffin GE. Determinants of energy intake and energy expenditure in HIV and AIDS. *Nutrition* 1999 (in press).

52. Grinspoon S, Corcoran C, Miller K et al. Determinants of increased energy expenditure in HIV-infected women. *Am J Clin Nutr* 1998; **68**: 720–725.

53. Shevitz AH, Knox TA, Spiegelman D, Roubenoff R, Gorbach SL, Skolnik PR. Elevated resting energy expenditure among HIV-seropositive persons receiving highly active antiretroviral therapy [In Process Citation]. *AIDS* 1999; **13**: 1351–1357.

54. Grunfeld C, Kotler DP, Hamadeh R, Tierney AR, Wang J, Pierson RN. Hypertriglyceridemia in the Acquired Immunodeficiency Syndrome. *Am J Med* 1989; **86**: 27–31.

55. Hommes MJT, Romijn JA, Endert E, Schattenkerk JKME, Sauerwein HP. Basal fuel homeostasis in symptomatic human immunodeficiency virus infection. *Clin Sci* 1991; **80**: 359–365.

56. Grunfeld C, Pang M, Shimizu L, Shigenaga JK, Jensen P, Feingold KR. Resting energy expenditure, caloric intake, short-term weight change in human immunodeficiency virus infection and the acquired immunodeficiency syndrome. *Am J Clin Nutr* 1992; **55**: 455–460.

57. Grunfeld C, Kotler DP, Shigenaga JK et al. Circulating interferon-α levels and hypertriglyceridemia in the acquired immunodeficiency syndrome. *Am J Med* 1991; **90**: 154–162.

58. Engelson ES, Kotler DP, Tan Y et al. Fat distribution in HIV-infected patients reporting truncal enlargement quantified by whole-body magnetic resonance imaging. *Am J Clin Nutr* 1999; **69**: 1162–1169.

59. Kotler DP, Tierney AR, Altilio D, Wang J, Pierson RN. Body mass repletion during ganciclovir treatment of cytomegalovirus infections in patients with acquired immunodeficiency syndrome. *Arch Intern Med* 1989; **149**: 901–905.

60. Ash SA, Griffin GE. Effect of parenteral nutrition on protein turnover in endotoxaemic rats. *Clin Sci* 1989; **76**: 659–666.

61. Streat SJ, Beddoe AH, Hill GL. Aggressive nutritional support does not prevent protein loss despite fat gain in septic intensive care patients. *J Trauma* 1987; **27**: 262–266.

62. Macallan DC, McNurlan MA, Milne E, Calder AG, Garlick PJ, Griffin GE. Whole body protein turnover from leucine kinetics and the response to nutrition in Human Immunodeficiency Virus infection. *Am J Clin Nutr* 1995; **61**: 818–826.

63. Macallan DC, McNurlan MA, Kurpad AV *et al*. Whole body protein metabolism in human pulmonary tuberculosis and undernutrition: Evidence for anabolic block in tuberculosis. *Clin Sci* 1998; **94**(3): 321–331.

64. Chandra RK. Nutrition and immunity: lessons from the past and new insights into the future. *Am J Clin Nutr* 1991; **53**: 1087–2101.

65. Chandra RK, Gupta S, Singh H. Inducer and suppressor T cell subsets in protein-energy malnutrition. *Nutr Res* 1982; **2**: 21–26.

66. Chandra RK. Serum complement and immuno-conglutininin malnutrition. *Arch Dis Child* 1975; **50**: 225–229.

67. Srisinha S, Edelman R, Suskind RM, Charupatana C, Olson RE. Complement and C3 proactivator levels in children with protein-energy malnutrition and effect of dietary treatment. *Lancet* 1975; **1**: 1016–1120.

68. Haller L, Zubler RH, Lambert PH. Plasma levels of complement components and complement hemolytic activity in protein-energy malnutrition. *Clin Exp Immunol* 1978; **34**: 248–254.

69. Doherty JF, Golden MHN, Raynes J, Griffin GE, McAdam K. Acute-phase protein response is impaired in severely malnourished. *Clin Sci* 1993; **84**: 169–175.

70. Chandra RK, Gupta SP. Increased bacterial adherence to respiratory and buccal epithelial cells in protein-energy malnutrition. *Immunol Infect Dis* 1991; **1**: 55–57.

71. Melchior JC, Gelas P, Carbonnel F *et al*. Improved survival by home Total Parenteral Nutrition in AIDS patients: Follow up of a controlled randomized prospective trial. *Nutrition* 1997; **13**: 272 (Abstract).

72. Crotty B, McDonald J, Mijch AM, Smallwood RA. Percutaneous endoscopic gastrostomy feeding in AIDS. *J Gastroenterol Hepatol* 1998; **13**: 371–375.

73. Baum MK, Shor-Posner G, Lu Y *et al*. Micronutrients and HIV-1 disease progression. *AIDS* 1995; **9**: 1051–1056.

74. Tang AM, Graham NMH, Kirby AJ, McCall LD, Willett WC, Saah AJ. Dietary micronutrient intake and risk of progression to Acquired Immunodeficiency Syndrome (AIDS) in Human Immunodeficiency Virus type 1 (HIV-1)-infected homosexual men. *Am J Epidemiol* 1993; **138**: 937–951.

75. Humphrey JH, Quinn T, Fine D *et al*. Short-term effects of large-dose vitamin A supplementation on viral load and immune response in HIV-infected women. *J Acquir Immune Defic Syndr Hum Retrovirol* 1999; **20**: 44–51.

76. Coodley GO, Coodley MK, Lusk R *et al*. Beta-carotene in HIV infection: an extended evaluation. *AIDS* 1996; **10**: 967–973.

77. Kapembwa MS, Bridges C, Joseph AE, Fleming SC, Batman P, Griffin GE. Ileal and jejunal absorptive function in patients with AIDS and enterococcidial infection. *J Infect* 1990; **21**: 43–53.

78. Butterworth RF, Gaudreau C, Vincelette J, Bourgault AM, Lamothe F, Nutini AM. Thiamine deficiency in AIDS. *Lancet* 1991; **338**: 1086 (letter).

79. Baum MK, Mantero-Atienza E, Shor-Posner G *et al*. Association of vitamin B6 status with parameters of immune function in early HIV-1 infection. *J Acquir Immune Defic Syndr* 1991; **4**: 1122–1132.

80. Revell P, O'Doherty MJ, Tang A, Savidge GF. Folic acid absorption in patients infected with the Human Immunodeficiency Virus. *J Int Med* 1991; **230**: 227–231.

81. Herbert V, Jacobson J, Colman N *et al*. Negative folate balance in AIDS. *FASEB J* 1989; **3**: A1278 (abstract).

82. Beach RS, Mantero-Atienza E, Eisdorfer C, Fordyce-Baum MK. Altered folate metabolism in early HIV infection. *J Am Med Assoc* 1988; **259**: 519 (letter).

83. Kavanaugh-McHugh AL, Ruff A, Perlman E, Hutton N, Modlin J, Rowe S. Selenium deficiency and cardio-myopathy in Acquired Immunodeficiency Syndrome. *J Parenteral Enteral Nutr* 1991; **15**: 347–349.

84. Fabris N, Mocchegiani E, Galli M, Irato L, Lazzarin A, Moroni M. AIDS, zinc deficiency and thymic hormone failure. *J Am Med Assoc* 1988; **259**: 839–840.

85. Falutz J, Tsoukas C, Gold P. Zinc as a cofactor in Human Immunodeficiency Virus induced immuno-suppression. *J Am Med Assoc* 1988; **259**: 2850–2851.

86. Semba RD, Miotti PG, Chiphangwi JD *et al*. Maternal vitamin A deficiency and mother-to-child transmission of HIV-1 [see comments]. *Lancet* 1994; **343**: 1593–1597.

87. Greenberg BL, Semba RD, Vink PE *et al*. Vitamin A deficiency and maternal-infant transmissions of HIV in two metropolitan areas in the United States. *AIDS* 1997; **11**: 325–332.

88. Fawzi WW, Msamanga GI, Spiegelman D *et al.* Randomised trial of effects of vitamin supplements on pregnancy outcomes and T cell counts in HIV-1-infected women in Tanzania [see comments]. *Lancet* 1998; **351**: 1477–1482.

89. Kotler DP, Tierney AR, Brenner SK, Couture S, Wang J, Pierson RN. Preservation of short-term energy balance in clinically stable patients with AIDS. *Am J Clin Nutr* 1990; **51**: 7–13.

90. Foskett M, Kapembwa MS, Sedgwick P, Griffin GE. Prospective study of food intake and nutitional status in HIV infection. *J Hum Nutr Diet* 1991; **4**: 149–154.

91. Summerbell CD, Gazzard BG, Catalan J. The nutritional knowledge, attitudes, beliefs and practices of male HIV positive homosexuals. *Int Conf AIDS* 1991; **7**: W.D.4209.

92. Voss T, Rowe B, Graf L, Keye, C, Beal J. Management of HIV-related weight loss and diarrhoea with an enteral formula containing whey peptides and medium-chain triglycerides. Proc VII *Int Conf AIDS* 1991; W.B.2165.

93. Cappell MS, Godil A. A multicenter case-controlled study of percutaneous endoscopic gastrostomy in HIV-seropositive patients. *Am J Gastroenterol* 1993; **88**: 2059–2066.

94. Ockenga J, Suttmann U, Selberg O *et al.* Percutaneous endoscopic gastrostomy in AIDS and control patients: risks and outcome. *Am J Gastroenterol* 1996; **91**: 1817–1822.

95. Kotler DP, Tierney AR, Ferraro R *et al.* Enteral alimentation and repletion of body cell mass in malnourished patients with acquired immunodeficiency syndrome. *Am J Clin Nutr* 1991; 53: 149–154.

96. Singer P, Rothkopf MM, Kvetan V, Kirvela O, Gaare J, Askanazi J. Risks and benefits of home parenteral nutrition in the Acquired Immunodeficiency Syndrome. *J Parenteral Enteral Nutr* 1992; **15**: 75–79.

97. Kotler DP, Tierney AR, Culpepper-Morgan JA, Wang J, Pierson RN. Effect of home total parenteral nutrition on body composition in patients with Acquired Immunodeficiency Syndrome. *J Parenteral Enteral Nutr* 1990; **14**: 454–458.

98. Cimoch PJ, Friedberg G, Jackowski J, Reiter WM. Supplemental parenteral nutrition in patients with AIDS and protein-calorie malnutrition. VIth International Conference on AIDS 1990; Th.B. 387, p218.

99. Peck K, Howes G, Robinson V, George R. Total Parenteral Nutrition in palliation of AIDS. *Int Conf AIDS* 1991; 1, M.D.4182 (abstract).

100. Kapembwa MS, Bridges C, Joseph AEA, Fleming SC, Batman PA, Griffin GE. Ileal and jejunal absorptive function in patients with AIDS and enterococcidial infection. *J Infect* 1990; **21**: 43–53.

101. Von Roenn JH, Murphy RL, Weber KM, Williams LM, Weitzman SA. Megestrol acetate for treatment of cachexia associated with Human Immunodeficiency Virus (HIV) infection. *Ann Int Med* 1988; **109**: 840–841.

102. Muurahainen N, Mulligan K. Clinical trials update in human immunodeficiency virus wasting. *Semin Oncol* 1998; **25**: 104–111.

103. Henry K, Rathgaber S, Sullivan C, McCabe K. Diabetes mellitus induced by megestrol acetate in a patient with AIDS and cachexia. *Ann Int Med* 1992; **116**: 53–54.

104. Beal JE, Olson R, Lefkowitz L *et al.* Long-term efficacy and safety of dronabinol for acquired immuno-deficiency syndrome-associated anorexia. *J Pain Symptom Manage* 1997; **14**: 7–14.

105. Beal JE, Olson R, Laubenstein L *et al.* Dronabinol as a treatment for anorexia associated with weight loss in patients with AIDS. *J Pain Symptom Manage* 1995; **10**: 89–97.

106. Mulligan K, Grunfeld C, Hellerstein MK, Neese RA, Schambelan M. Anabolic effects of recombinant human growth hormone in patients with wasting associated with human immunodeficiency virus infection. *J Clin Endocrinol Metab* 1993; **77**: 956–962.

107. Mulligan K, Tai VW, Schambelan M. Use of growth hormone and other anabolic agents in AIDS wasting. *J Parenter Enteral Nutr* 1999; **23**(6 Suppl): S202–S209.

108. Paton NIJ, Newton PJ, Sharpstone DR *et al.* Short-term growth hormone administration at the time of opportunistic infections in HIV-positive patients. *AIDS* 1999; **13**(10): 1195–1202.

109. McNurlan MA, Garlick PJ, Steigbigel RT *et al.* Responsiveness of muscle protein synthesis to growth hormone administration in HIV-infected individuals declines with severity of disease. *J Clin Invest* 1997; **100**: 2125–2132.

110. Kapembwa MS, Fleming SC, Griffin GE, Caun K, Pinching AJ, Harris JRW. Fat absorption and exocrine pancreatic function in Human Immunodeficiency Virus infection. *Q J Med* 1990; **74**: 49–56.

111. Henderson RA, Talusan K, Hutton N, Yolken RH, Caballero B. Resting energy expenditure and body composition in children with HIV infection. *J Acquir Immune Defic Syndr Hum Retrovirol* 1998; **19**: 150–157.

112. Miller TL. Nutritional assessment and its clinical application in children infected with the human immunodeficiency virus [editorial; comment] [see comments]. *J Pediatr* 1996; **129**: 633–636.

113. Smith I, Howells DW, Kendall B, Levinsky R, Hyland K. Folate deficiency and demyelination in AIDS. *Lancet* 1987; **2**: 215.

114. Tong TK, Andrew LR, Albert A, Mickell JJ. Childhood Acquired Immune Deficiency Syndrome manifesting as acrodermatitis enteropathica. *J Pediatr* 1986; **108**: 426–428.

115. Nicholas SW, Leung J, Fennoy I. Guidelines for nutritional support of HIV-infected children. *J Pediatr* 1991; **119**: S59–S62.

116. Miller TL, Orav EJ, Martin SR, Cooper ER, McIntosh K, Winter HS. Malnutrition and carbohydrate malabsorption in children with vertically transmitted human immunodeficiency virus 1 infection. *Gastroenterology* 1991; **100**: 1296–1302.

117. Yolken RH, Hart W, Oung I, Shiff C, Greenson J, Perman JA. Gastrointestinal dysfunction and disaccharide intolerance in children infected with human immunodeficiency virus. *J Pediatr* 1992; **118**: 359–363.

118. Thiry L, Sprecher-Goldberger S, Jonckheer T *et al.* Isolation of AIDS virus from cell-free breast milk of three healthy virus carriers. *Lancet* 1985; **2**: 891–892.

119. Van de Perre P, Simonon A, Msellati P *et al.* Postnatal transmission of Human Immunodeficiency Virus Type 1 from mother to infant. *N Engl J Med* 1991; **325**: 593–598.

120. Joint United Nations programme on HIV/AIDS (UNAIDS) HIV and infant feeding: an interim statement. *Wkly Epidemiol Rec* 1996; **71**: 289–291.

121. Nicoll A, Newell ML, Van Praag E, Van de Perre P, Peckham C. Infant feeding policy and practice in the presence of HIV-1 infection [editorial]. *AIDS* 1995; **9**: 107–119.

122. IAS Panel Members. IAS position paper on prevention of HIV-1 mother-to-child transmission. *AIDS* 1999; **13**: IAS Newsletter 5–IAS Newsletter 9.

37

Nutrition support in patients with cancer

Federico Bozzetti

History

Although it has been known since the beginning of the history of medicine that cachexia is often associated with malignant disease, it was only at the start of the century that the first investigations on nitrogen balance in cancer patients began to be published.[1,2,3]

However, the problem became truly focused in 1932, when S. Warren determined that cachexia played a major role in the death of cancer patients.

The first systematic attempts at feeding cancer patients parenterally or enterally date back to the period 1949–1956 by Waddell and Grillo,[4] Bolker,[5] Pareira et al.,[6,7] Terepka and Waterhouse[8] and subsequently Watkin and Steinfeld.[9]

It is noteworthy that some controversial issues still surrounding the role of nutrition support in cancer patients had already been partially recognized at that time, i.e. the possible stimulation of tumour growth by TPN or EN, the poorer response of cancer patients versus non-cancer patients in terms of nutritional benefit, the conditioning effect of the malignant disease on the metabolic response to the nutrition support, and so forth.

Some of these issues are still being debated and investigated, and some hypotheses have been tested in clinical trials.

The first modern paper specifically dealing with TPN in cancer patients can probably be attributed to Schwartz et al.[10]

Cancer cachexia

Definition

Cancer cachexia is a syndrome that occurs during the terminal course of the disease in approximately 70% of cancer patients, but it is also sometimes evident at clinical presentation. The syndrome is characterised by asthenia, anorexia, weight loss with depletion and alterations in body compartments, possible disturbances in water and electrolyte metabolism and the progressive impairment of vital functions.

The clinical appearance of patients affected by cancer cachexia is characteristic: they have pale and atrophic skin and emaciated faces, and suffer from severe skeletal muscle wasting and a considerable loss of subcutaneous fat stores, sometimes hidden by the presence of oedema.

Specific investigations on the composition of the body compartments of cancer patients have frequently demonstrated a state of anaemia with potassium deficiency, hyperhydration with normal distribution of the volume of intra- and extracellular water, depletion of muscular mass and fat stores and a relative sparing of the overall protein content. Unlike patients with simple anorexia nervosa in whom weight loss is due to a more or less proportional decrease in the size of all organs, patients with malignant cachexia have an increase in the size of the liver, kidney and spleen, as well as significant involvement of other parenchyma.

According to a recent proposal,[11] the emaciation of cancer patients would be more properly defined as 'wasting', which involves a decrease in both body cell mass and weight that is usually associated with poor dietary intake, as opposed to cachexia, which is a decrease in body cell mass even in the presence of stable or increasing weight.

Prevalence

The prevalence and severity of wasting are not directly related to calorie intake, histological variety or type of tumour spread; nor are they related to tumour size, since wasting may be present even when the tumour represents less than 0.01% of the total body weight.[12]

Several investigations have demonstrated that cachexia represents a major problem at least in terms of prevalence:

1) Patients with malignant tumours have the highest prevalence of malnutrition of any segment of the hospitalised population.[13] In some cancer patients, weight loss may be the most frequent presenting symptom,[14] and up to 66% of patients develop inanition during the course of their disease.[13,15] A weight loss greater than 10% of the pre-illness body weight may occur in up to 45% of hospitalised adult cancer patients.[16] The prevalence of malnutrition in different cancer populations is shown in Table 37.1.

2) A relationship exists between weight loss and tumour type. In a study of the Eastern Cooperative Oncology Group (ECOG) involving 3047 patients with 11 different tumour types, DeWys et al.[15]

Table 37.1 – Incidence of malnutrition in cancers of different sites.

Reference	Tumour type or site	Incidence of malnutrition
Issell et al.[17]	Lung (squamous cell)	50%
	Breast	36%
	Sarcoma	39%
	Colon	54%
	Prostate	56%
	Lung (small cell)	60%
	Lung	61%
	Pancreas	83%
DeWys et al.[15]	Gastric	83%
Samuels et al.[18]	Testicular cancer	25%
Nixon et al.[19]	Colorectal cancer	60%
Popp et al.[20]	Diffuse lymphoma	55%
Shamberger et al.[21]	Sarcoma	66%
Goodwin & Torres[22]	Head and neck cancer	72%
Clamon et al.[23]	Lung (small cell)	about 50%
Rickard et al.[24]	Neuroblastoma	56%
Bashir et al.[25]	Bronchial carcinoma	66%
	Breast	9%
	Rectum	40%
Larrea et al.[26]	Oesophagus	79%
Tan et al.[27]	General cancer population	63%
Bozzetti et al.[28]	General cancer population	– 60%

found that patients with favourable subtypes of non-Hodgkin's lymphomas, breast cancer, acute non-lymphocytic leukaemia and sarcomas had the lowest prevalence of weight loss (31–41%), while patients with unfavourable non-Hodgkin's lymphoma, colon cancer, prostate cancer and lung cancer had a 48–61% prevalence of weight loss. Finally, patients with pancreatic or gastric cancer had the highest prevalence of weight loss (83–87%). Several studies have reported that patients with upper gastrointestinal malignancy and especially cancer of the oesophagus are frequently affected by malnutrition,[29,29a,30,31,32] whereas 43–61% of patients with lung cancer have weight loss, depending on the state of the disease.[33] In the ECOG study,[15] a positive relationship was also demonstrated between the above-mentioned types of cancer and the prevalence and severity of weight loss.

As regards studies in children with cancer, The most significant data concerning children were collected in a collaborative paediatric study.[34] A deterioration in the nutrition status, determined by the ratio of weight and height compared to an age-adjusted standard (50th percentile for a normal population for each sex), was reported in 23–30% of the children involved in the study. Unlike the situation in adults, this worsened status did not correlate with tumour type, with performance status, nor, due to the small numbers in the subgroups with regional or metastatic disease, with stage of disease.

Aetiology and pathogenesis

Our understanding of the aetiopathogenesis of cancer wasting is limited and based more on the knowledge of abnormalities in nutrition behaviour and metabolic patterns than on the identification of specific mediators. Three theories have been put forth over time:

- Metabolic competition
- Malnutrition
- Alterations of metabolic pathways.

Metabolic competition theory

The time-honoured metabolic competition theory suggests that neoplastic cells compete with host tissues for amino acids, functioning thereby as 'nitrogen trap'. This may be true in experimental tumours, where neoplastic tissue accounts for a very high percentage of the carcass weight, but it is unlikely to be a mechanism in human tumours, where the common experience is the opposite: there are cases of cachectic patients with tumours of only a few grams, and also patients who have huge abdominal masses, but who are otherwise relatively fit.

Hypophagia and anorexia

The second theory cites undernutrition as the main cause underlying the development of cancer wasting.

The reason for the reduced intake of nutrients in patients with lesions of the upper digestive tract is clear. However, regardless of the tumour's location, anorexia is the most common cause of hypophagia and usually consists of a loss of appetite and/or a feeling of early satiety. Anorexia is often a presenting symptom of malignancy; abnormalities of food intake and feeding patterns occur in over 50% of newly diagnosed cancer patients.[35]

A study carried out by the Istituto Nazionale Tumori, in Milan involving 186 cancer patients showed that the prevalence of subjective anorexia ranged from 33 to 40% of patients (depending on the type and site of the tumour), and that most of the nutritionally related variables were significantly worse in anorectic patients than in non-anorectic patients.[36]

The mechanisms involved in the onset of anorexia are poorly understood. Older studies supported the role of intermediate metabolites (lactate, ketones, low molecular weight peptides, oligonucleotides) coupled with a state of relative hypoinsulinism. More recently, however, several authors have postulated the existence of an amino acid imbalance with accumulation of tryptophan and serotonin in the brain[37] and the possible role of cytokines.

Hypophagia has also been related to the presence of dysgeusia.[38] The diminished ability to perceive sweet flavours has been linked to anorexia, whereas the decrease in the threshold for bitter flavours has been linked to an aversion to meats rich in bitter substrates (amino acids, purines, polypeptides). Dysosmia is also related to aversion to foods.

In underfed patients there are secondary changes in the digestive tract, such as a decrease in secretions and atrophy of the mucosa and musculature,[39] which may be responsible for the feeling of fullness and delayed emptying, the defective digestion and the poor absorption of nutrients.

Finally, particularly in children, anorexia may be the consequence of a learned food aversion.[40]

Metabolic abnormalities

Energy expenditure
Studies in laboratory animals have demonstrated that

Table 37.2 – Studies on resting metabolic expenditure in cancer patients.

Year	Authors	No. of patients	Type of tumour	% Hypermetabolic patients (REE ≥ 110% PEE)
1869–1924	(several)	34	Leukaemia	97
1914	Wallersteiner[47a]	33	Gastric carcinoma	45
1924	Minot & Means[46]	71	Leukaemia	86
1950	Silver et al.[47]	41	Leukaemia/lymphoma	100
		23	Carcinoma	91
1951	Waterhouse[48]	5	Leukaemia/lymphoma	5
1956	Terepka[8]	12	Solid tumours	67
1965	Watkin[9]	4	Solid tumours	75
1978	Warnold et al.[49]	10	Miscellaneous	80
1980	Bozzetti et al.[28]	65	Miscellaneous	58
1980	Burke et al.[50]	42	Gastrointestinal tumours	↑ in males
1982	Long et al.[51]	16	Miscellaneous	0
1980	Knox et al.[52]	200	Miscellaneous	63
1982	MacFie et al.[42]	43	Gastrointestinal tumours	↑
1984	Dempsey et al.[53]	173	Gastrointestinal tumours	54
1984	Dempsey et al.[53]	73	Colorectal carcinoma	30
1983	Axelrod et al.[54]	5	Carcinoma of the lung	100★
1984	Shike et al.[55]	31	Lung cancer	100
1984	Russel et al.[56]	31	Carcinoma of the lung	100
1986a	Hansell et al.[57]	24	Colorectal carcinoma	0
1986b	Hansell et al.[57a]	98	Miscellaneous	0
1988	Shaw et al.[58]	7	Sarcoma	100★
1988	Nixon et al.[59]	83	Colon and lung carcinoma	0★
1988	Fearon et al.[60]	58	Colon and lung carcinoma	0★
1990	Merli et al.[61]	–	Hepatocarcinoma	–

★ referred to a control group.
REE = resting energy expenditure; predicted energy expenditure.

tumour transplants cause an increase in the energy expenditure of the host, which is high even before the tumour is palpable. Brooks et al.[41] have reported a 40% increase in energy expenditure in rats transplanted with a human hypernephroma.

In humans, this issue has been the subject of numerous debates, mainly because of a lack of an appropriate standard of reference and the disparity of the patients investigated in terms of tumour type, stage and nutrition status.

It is now generally accepted, on the basis of many European studies,[42–44] that many cancer patients are mildly hypermetabolic, with an excess energy expenditure ranging between 138 and 289 kcal (577–1209 kJ)/day. If not compensated by an increased calorie intake, this excess expenditure can cause a loss of body fat from 0.5–1 kg to 1.1–2.3 kg of muscular mass per month. Some studies have correlated hypermetabolism with deterioration in the nutrition status[28] and with tumour size.[62] Data on the prevalence and

severity of hypermetabolism are reported in Tables 37.2 and 37.3.

Falconer et al.[63] have reported that patients with pancreatic cancer had an increased resting energy expenditure (REE) as compared with controls, and that it was significantly greater in those patients with an acute phase response.

The finding that despite hypophagia and weight loss many cancer patients have a mildly increased or even normal energy expenditure suggests a defective adaptation to starvation.

In fact, under conditions of chronic fasting, normal subjects who begin a regimen that burns off fat have a decrease in oxygen consumption due to a reduction in ATP requirements. This occurs because the synthesis of glycogen, fatty acids and triglycerides due to the transitory excess of nutrients decreases. Production of carbon dioxide increases, and the respiratory quotient falls to 0.7. The causes of this increased or at least dis-

Table 37.3 – Resting metabolic expenditure and type of tumour.

Site/type	No. of patients	% patients with increase in MB	Median increase of MB	Authors
Lung	5	100	–	Axelrod et al.[54]
	31	100	31%	Shike et al.[55]
	22	0	–	Fearon et al.[60]
	38	0	–	Nixon et al.[59]
Leukaemia	133	74	35%	Grafe[64]
				Gunderson[65]
				Boothby-Sandiford[66]
Lymphoma	18	–	22%	Bozzetti et al.[28]
Sarcoma	9	–	14–18%	–
– localised	4	–	33–41%	Shaw et al.[58]
– metastatic	7	100	35%	–
Gastric carcinoma	28	40	10%	Dempsey et al.[53]
	7	–	20%	Bozzetti et al.[28]
Colorectal carcinoma	73	22	20%	Muller et al.[67]
	24	0	–	Hansell et al.[57]
	16	–	28%	Bozzetti et al.[28]
	38	0	–	Fearon et al.[60]
	45	0	–	Nixon et al.[59]
Gastrointestinal carcinoma	42	–	↑ in males	Burke et al.[50]
– local	24	–	4%	–
– metastatic	19	–	8%	MacFie et al.[42]

proportionate energy expenditure are not understood, but it is unlikely that they are directly related to tumour cell metabolism.

Biochemical aberrations involving the metabolism of carbohydrates, lipids and proteins have all been suggested as possible causes of the change in energy expenditure. It is known that tumours can increase production of lactic acid through anaerobic glycolysis. The lactic acid is then converted to glucose through the utilization of fatty acids, to the detriment of the host's organs (liver or kidney). Since this cycle involves a net loss of 4 ATP/mol of glucose formed (2 ATP formed by anaerobic glycolysis and 6 consumed by the synthesis of lactate into glucose), it has been hypothesised that this energy depletion is a cause of the change in energy expenditure. In fact, a correlation has been observed between an increase in energy expenditure, and the activity of the Cori cycle, metabolism and glucose oxidation. However, in human tumours, (which never exceed 4–5% of the total body weight), this increase in energy expenditure cannot exceed 10% of the host's total caloric expenditure.

Furthermore, even if 15% of the total production of lactate were oxidised, the resulting production of ATP would compensate for the caloric deficiency of the conversion of 85% of the lactate into glucose. Finally, the blocking of this cycle due to inhibition of phosphoenolpyruvatocarboxykinase by tryptophan, hydrazine sulphate or 2-3 pyrimidine dihydroxide has not been effective in either laboratory or clinical experiments. Considering the increase in the metabolism of glucose not only in terms of the increase in the Cori cycle but also in terms of increased gluconeogenesis by glycerol and the amino acids, some authors have reached the conclusion that the Cori cycle is responsible for at least 87% of the increase in energy expenditure. Another hypothesis states that hypermetabolism may be related to the dissociation of oxidative phosphorylation (documented by *in vitro*, but not *in vivo*, studies). Activation of futile cycles has also been suggested as a possible cause.

A further explanation for the alteration in energy expenditure is based on the observation that cancer patients tend to oxidise a higher quantity of non-essential fatty acids (NEFA) in comparison to control subjects even in the presence of other energy substrates. This indirectly implies a channelling of carbohydrate intermediates towards lipogenesis before

oxidation, which represents a costly metabolism in terms of the consumption of ATP.

It has also been reported that protein turnover can account for up to 50% of the REE, with the liver usually accounting for 20-25% of the overall oxygen consumption. Investigations in humans have shown that while the synthesis of muscle protein is diminished in cancer patients, the hepatic synthesis of secretory proteins, acute phase reactants, fibrinogen, glycoproteins and immunoglobulins can be increased.

However, although studies with leucine have shown a 50-70% increase in the leucine flux in advanced cancer patients, a recent study did not substantiate the relationship between the whole body protein turnover rate and the REE.

Carbohydrate metabolism
The main alterations in carbohydrate metabolism identified in older studies included decreased glucose tolerance, which occurred in up to 60% of tumour-bearing patients[68] and normal or increased fasting blood glucose. Subsequent studies have determined that fasting serum insulin is normal or decreased and that there is a reduced response to both endogenous and exogenous insulin. Gluconeogenesis from several precursors (lactate, alanine, glycerol) has been reported to be increased,[69] as have total glucose production, turnover and recycling. The outpouring of lactic acid by some tumours leads to an increase in the conversion of lactate to glucose by the liver. This process is energy-consuming, as already mentioned, because the conversion of 2 mol of lactate to glucose requires 6 mol of ATP, while only 2 mol of ATP are recovered in the conversion of glucose back to lactate. While the Cori cycle normally accounts for 20% of glucose turnover, it is increased to 50% in cachectic cancer patients and accounts for disposal of 60% of the lactate produced.[70] Cancer patients also have an increased glucose flux, which could consume up to 40% of the carbohydrates ingested and may contribute to the weight loss.[72]

There is some evidence that a disproportionate requirement of glucose by the tumour accounts for the increase in glucose turnover and consumption. In perfusion experiments Norton et al.[62] determined that glucose uptake by tumour tissue in patients with soft tissue sarcomas corresponded to approximately 160 mg/min. This is equal to approximately 230 g of glucose/day when uptake remains constant for 24 hours. Glucose uptake is proportional to tumour size and corresponds to approximately 1.4 g/day/g of tumour. This value corresponds fairly well with the increase in glucose metabolism (170 g/24 h) observed by Holroyde and Reichard.[72]

Glucose is usually metabolised by cancer tissue through anaerobic glycolysis, which persists in environments that are rich in oxygen due to the peculiar distribution and concentration of the intracellular enzymes that control metabolism.

Therefore, it would seem that the tumour forces the host to expand the glucose pool through the increase in turnover and recycling and hepatic gluconeogenesis. In fact, studies in hepatic cell culture from tumour-bearing subjects have demonstrated a dose-related increase in glucose synthesis from physiological concentrations of lactate and alanine (and a further increase in the presence of an excess of precursor), which probably takes place through a mechanism of induction of the gluconeogenic enzymes.[73] The main abnormalities of carbohydrate metabolism are summarised in Table 37.4.

Lipid metabolism
There is an overall depletion of fat stores and lipid content in muscle samples. The rates of depletion are homogeneous, as suggested by the relative increase in fractions (phospholipid and free cholesterol) of PUFA and an increased oleic-to-stearic acid ratio in red blood cells and plasma lipids.[74]

Table 37.4 – Metabolic abnormalities in the cancer patient.

Carbohydrate
- Increased gluconeogenesis from amino acids, lactate and glycerol
- Increased glucose disappearance and recycling
- Insulin resistance

Lipid
- Increased lipolysis
- Increased glycerol and fatty acid turnover
- Lipid oxidation non-inhibited by glucose
- Decreased lipogenesis
- Decreased lipoprotein lipase activity
- Variable increase in NEFA and lipid

Protein metabolism
- Increased muscle protein catabolism
- Increased whole-body protein turnover
- Increased liver protein synthesis
- Decreased muscle protein synthesis

There is an increased oxidation of fat[63] which is proportional to the stage of disease and the severity of the malnutrition[75] and an increased rate of removal of infused lipids from the blood.[76] It is interesting that the administration of glucose fails to inhibit fat mobilisation and oxidation, as usually occurs in normal subjects.[77] Other studies have reported an impaired oxidation of intravenously-infused triglycerides.[78] Consequently, some patients exhibit a clear state of hyperlipidaemia, and, especially if undernourished, have a decrease in plasma lipoprotein-lipase. The elevated plasma lipid level may be immunosuppressive, and thereby affect ultimate survival.[79]

Cancer patients with weight loss have an increased glycerol and fatty acid turnover compared with normal subjects or cancer patients without weight loss.[80] Some studies have reported elevated plasma levels of NEFA,[81] while others have reported normal levels.[82] The main abnormalities of lipid metabolism are summarised in Table 37.4.

Protein metabolism
Abnormalities of protein metabolism in cancer patients are shown in Table 37.4 and include: nitrogen depletion in the host, changes in hepatic and muscular protein turnover, an increase of gluconeogenesis from amino acids and anomalous patterns of plasma amino acids. Investigations on protein kinetics have given conflicting results. Whole-body protein turnover has been reported as being not significantly different from control[83,84] or even increased.[85–91]

The discrepancy in absolute values may reflect methodological differences whilst the differences between cancer patients and controls may be related to the type of cancer population and choice of controls. The exceptionally high protein turnover rate found in some patients with hepatocellular carcinoma has been demonstrated to be a consequence of elevated endogenous protein breakdown and oxidation of amino acids.[92]

Protein metabolism in muscle
Few studies have focused on protein kinetics in skeletal muscle, and only Emery *et al.*[83] and Shaw *et al.*[91] have combined the evaluation of both whole body and skeletal muscle protein metabolism. Comparing a heterogeneous group of well-nourished and undernourished cancer patients to a normal control group, Newman *et al.*[93] found no difference in muscle protein synthesis and break-

down. Our group Dworzak et al.[94] found a significant decrease in synthesis in patients versus control, whereas breakdown was similar in the two groups; the decrease accounted for the negative net balance in patients and the apparent equilibrium in controls.

These data are in agreement with the analysis of Lundholm et al.,[95] who reported a decreased incorporation of 10C leucine into the skeletal muscle protein and an increase in catabolism. Emery et al.[83] have also reported a significantly decreased synthesis of skeletal muscle protein, as demonstrated by the 13C leucine enrichment in the quadriceps in cancer compared to normal controls. In contrast, Shaw et al.[91] have reported an increase in the muscle fractional protein synthesis rate. However, neither of these authors measured breakdown.

Protein metabolism in the liver

Studies in radio-labelled leucine have shown that while in normal subjects 53% of protein synthesis derives from muscle, it accounts for only 8% in malnourished cancer patients.

Synthesis of structural liver proteins is normal, and that of the acute phase is increased.[96] As far as albumin is concerned, there is a correlation between hypoalbuminaemia and tumour bulk. Studies with labelled precursors have reported a reduction in albumin synthesis, which is partially corrected by increased protein intake, and an increase in the catabolised fraction. There is also an increase in transcapillary escape with a decrease in the intravascular and extravascular ratio. In rare cases, hypoalbuminaemia is also due to its sequestration in pathological compartments or loss to the outside (nephrosic syndromes, protein-losing enteropathy, aminoaciduria in acute leukemias).

Such findings could explain the frequent occurrence of hypoalbuminaemia even when degradation is normal and synthesis is increased, as reported in recent investigations.

Amino acid profile

Some authors have reported specific alterations of the plasma amino acid profile.[68,97,98] Cancer patients have plasma concentrations of amino acids that are low in valine and leucine and high in tryptophan. Weight-losing cancer patients maintain a normal concentration of branched-chain amino acids, in contrast to malnourished or starved subjects.

Tumour interference in the host protein metabolism

It has been suggested that the tumour acts as a 'one-way nitrogen trap', and that this may have an influence on body economy when the mass accounts for 20% of the body weight of the host. However, it has been found that experimental tumours containing less than 6% of total body nitrogen have a protein metabolism equal to 35% of all protein synthesis. In humans it has been demonstrated that, when the tumour is localised and resectable (e.g. colorectal cancer), there is no substantial impact on overall protein kinetics, while the measurement of the difference in arteriovenous concentrations of amino acids in tumour-bearing limbs versus normal extremities has shown that less than half of the output of amino acids is released in the circulation by the tumour-bearing limb.

Cytokines: mediators of cancer cachexia

Extensive investigation has failed to identify altered classic hormonal pathways as a cause of cancer cachexia. The most common alterations in hormone profiles include increased cortisol secretion and urinary excretion of adrenaline and non-adrenaline,[99] increased glucagon levels,[100] a decreased insulin/glucagon ratio and changes in thyroid hormones. These alterations can often be attributed to the associated anorexia and cannot be considered the cause of the changes in energy expenditure and body composition.

Recent studies have investigated the role of cytokines, which are produced by immunocytes as an endogenous immune response to the tumour. Cytokines are polypeptide signals produced by the host's cells in response to a growing tumour, which regulate many of the nutritional and metabolic disturbances that occur in the host with cancer. They lead to:

- Decreased appetite
- Stimulation of the basal metabolic rate
- Stimulation of glucose uptake
- Stimulation of the mobilisation of fat and protein stores
- Reduction in adipocyte lipoprotein lipase activity
- Enhanced muscle amino acid release
- Stimulation of hepatic amino acid transport activity.

Elevated concentrations of tissue and circulating cytokines have been found in cancer patients and enhanced hepatic cytokine gene expression has been found in tumour-bearing animals. These cytokines include tumour necrosis factor, interleukins 1, 2, 4 and 6 and interferons α, β and γ and have been recently reviewed by Tisdale[101] and by Toomey et al.[102] The effects of the administration of some cytokines to experimental animals are shown in Table 37.5.

TNF-α
Both animal and human studies show that administration of TNF-α causes an initial drop in body weight followed by the development of tachyphylaxis with repeated administration.

Acute administration of TNF-α causes effects similar to those seen in cancer cachexia,[103,104] including a 30% increase in the metabolic rate, as well as increased temperature, heart rate, epinephrin and ACTH levels. In these studies, these responses were blunted by ibuprofen despite the absence of changes in the plasma levels of TNF-α. The glycerol turnover increased by more than 80% and fatty acid turnover increased by more than 60%. There was also an increased whole-body protein turnover and increased total amino acid efflux.[105] However, in chronic administration the alterations were resolved despite continuous administration of TNF-α.[106] Moreover, in no phase I clinical investigation of TNF-α was cachexia a major side-effect; instead, fluid retention through damage of the vascular endothelium and increased capillary permeability were reported. Only hypertriglyceridaemia persisted despite the development of tachyphylaxis, but this seems to be unrelated to cachexia since, for instance, AIDS with hypertriglyceridaemia patients maintain their weight for prolonged periods of time.

Experimental studies suggest that the increase in serum triglycerides due to TNF-α administration is mainly due to hepatic synthesis and secretion of VLDL rather than from adipose tissue. Depletion of skeletal muscle would be due to the induction of oxidative stress and nitric oxide synthase and consequent decreased myosin creatinine phosphokinase expression and binding activity.

Studies aimed at detecting levels of TNF-α in the serum of cancer patients or at correlating it with cachexia have usually been unsuccessful. No TNF-α has been detected in serum samples of patients with solid tumour and weight loss of 8–40%[107] or in mixed patient populations.[108] Balkwill et al.[109] have been able to detect a 'TNF-like' activity in the serum of 50% of cancer patients, but there was no correlation with weight loss. In a population of paediatric cancer patients, however, TNF-α levels were often elevated in the serum.

It is possible that naturally occurring TNF-α inhibitors in the circulation may hide TNF-α pro-

Table 37.5 – Cytokine-mediated effects on protein, carbohydrate and lipid metabolism.

| Cytokine | Metabolism | | |
	Protein	Carbohydrate	Lipid
TNF	increased muscle proteolysis increased protein oxidation increased hepatic protein synthesis	increased glycogenolysis decreased glycogen synthesis increased gluconeogenesis increased glucose clearance increased lactate production	decreased lipogenesis
IL-1	increased hepatic protein synthesis	increased gluconeogenesis increased glucose clearance	increased lipolysis decreased LPL synthesis increased fatty acid synthesis
IL-6	increased hepatic protein synthesis		increased lipolysis increased fatty acid synthesis
IFN-γ			decreased lipogenesis increased lipolysis decreased LPL activity

LPL: lipoprotein lipase, TNF: tumour necrosis factor, IL: interleukin, IFN: interferon.

duction by the monocytes of the host. In fact, Moldawer et al.[110] found these inhibitors to be circulating freely in healthy volunteers and increased in individuals with ovarian cancer.

The inability to detect TNF-α in cachectic patients has led to the suggestion that it acts as a paracrine/autocrine mediator rather than as the circulating messenger in cachexia. Thompson et al.[111] did not find elevated TNF-α levels in cancer patients. Nevertheless, there was a twofold increase in the relative levels of mRNA for hormone-sensitive lipase in adipose tissue of cancer patients compared with controls. These findings suggest that TNF-α may not contribute to the development of cachexia in cancer but indicates a stimulation of lipolysis in adipose tissue.

AntiTNF-α antibodies have had minimal effects in tumour-bearing animals even when, in a human squamous cell carcinoma of the maxilla grown as a xenograft in nude mice, antiTNF-α antibodies partially reversed but did not completely normalise body weight.[112] Pentoxifylline has been reported to decrease TNF mRNA levels in cancer patients. However, it failed to show any benefit in a recent trial on cachectic patients with lung or gastrointestinal tumours.[113]

IL-1

Elevated IL-1 plasma levels are seldom found in cancer patients,[96,114] but antibodies against an IL-1 receptor mitigate cachectic symptoms in tumour-bearing mice to a similar degree as antiTNF-α antibodies.[115,116]

IL-6

Unlike TNF-α and IL-1, increased levels of IL-6 are measured in the serum of cancer patients. IL-6 is the main cytokine involved in the induction of acute phase proteins (APP) and fibrinogen synthesis, and elevated levels have been reported in 39% of patients with lung or colon cancer and an ongoing APP response.[96,117] However, since all of the patients had lost weight, it is difficult to determine whether IL-6 was elevated in cachectic patients alone.

The increase in circulating IL-6 is closely related to tumour burden and is thought to originate from tumour cells as well as from various tissues of the cancer-bearing host (e.g. liver, kidney, small intestine, etc.) and to be induced by the IL-1 production of tumour-infiltrating macrophages.

Interferon-γ

IFN-γ is known to have effects on fat metabolism similar to those of TNF-α, namely the inhibition of LPL and decreased protein synthesis; polyclonal antibodies in rat IFN-γ partly mitigate cancer-induced anorexia and weight loss. However, like TNF-α, increased serum IFN-γ levels have not been found in cachectic patients with cancer.

Effects on glucose metabolism

Studies evaluating the effects of cytokine administration on the circulating glucose concentration indicate that the plasma glucose level rises or falls depending on the dose of cytokine administered, the timing of the measurement and the specific cytokine given.

There are experimental data that indicate that TNF-α administration can induce a marked increase in whole-body glucose utilization even though glucose uptake does not increase equally in all organs or tissues.

Effects on fat metabolism

It is likely that the loss of fat stores in patients with cancer is due in part to the ability of TNF-α and IL-1 to mobilise fat stores. In the experimental setting TNF-α is able to reduce the adipocyte lipoprotein-lipase (LPL) activity and heparin-releasable LPL activity and to increase the serum triglyceride levels, which also depend on a stimulation of the hepatic lipid secretion. IL-6 is also able to reduce adipose tissue LPL activity and heparin-releasable LPL activity.

Effects on nitrogen metabolism

Warren et al.[105] have measured the acute response to TNF-α in healthy volunteers and found a rise in C-reactive protein, a decrease in serum zinc level and a doubling of forearm amino-acid efflux, which was primarily attributable to increases in glucogenic amino-acid alanine and glutamine, although this accelerated nitrogen release may have been due to the effects of starvation. These results were replicated in animals and with IL-1. It is unclear, however, which distal mediators in the cytokine cascade are the key players.

Interleukin-6 and glucocorticords have been shown to work in a coordinated fashion to stimulate hepatic amino-acid transport both in vivo and in vitro.

Recently Kern and Norton[118] speculated on the mechanisms underlying host cachexia and proposed that cytokines elaborated by activated immunocytes in response to the tumour have secondary effects which exhibit an acute-phase reaction, re-routing nutrients from the periphery to the liver. Over the long term, however, a vicious cycle is activated that results in anorexia and widespread abnormalities in carbohydrate, protein and lipid metabolism (Fig. 37.1).

Catabolic factors in cancer cachexia

In addition to cytokines, some studies have reported circulating human factors that act directly on skeletal muscle and adipose tissues in a hormone-like manner. The most important are the lipid-mobilising factors.

LMF (lipid mobilising factor)

LMF include the toxohormone-L isolated from the ascitic fluid of patients with hepatoma[119] and that isolated from culture media of the human A375 melanoma cell line.[120]

The level of LMF in the sera of cancer patients has been found to be proportional to the extent of weight loss and reduced in patients responding to chemotherapy.[121]

Following some preliminary *in vitro* investigations showing inhibition of the tumour LMF by the PUFA eicosopentaenoic, Wigmore *et al.*[122] treated cachectic patients suffering from pancreatic cancer with fish oil capsules containing 18% EPA and 12% docosahexaenoic acid. This supplement reversed the weight loss of 2.9 kg/month and led to a weight gain of 0.3 kg/month, which was associated with a temporary reduction of acute phase proteins and stabilisation of the REE. The mechanism involved may be the continuous stimulation of LMF on the cyclic adenosine monophosphate (cAMP) that results in the activation of protein kinase which phosphorylates an inactive form of triglyceride lipase, otherwise known as hormone-sensitive lipase.

PMF (Protein mobilising factor)

There is some evidence that PMF plays a role in human cancer cachexia. Belizario *et al.*[123] found the presence of colpains, a group of cytosolic, calcium-dependent proteases able to induce proteolysis when incubated with rat diaphragm, in the serum of cachectic patients.

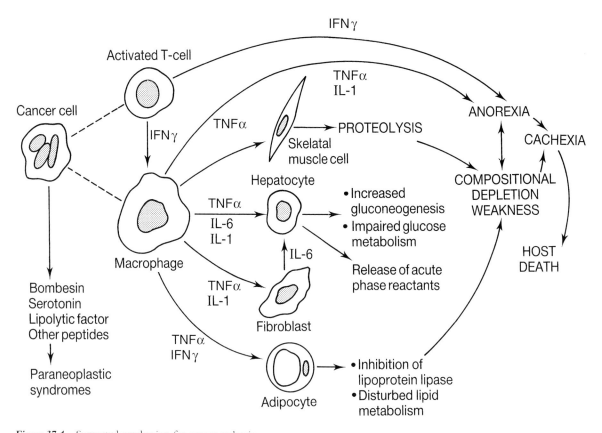

Figure 37.1 – Suggested mechanism for cancer cachexia.

Todorov *et al.*[124] recently succeeded in isolating the 24 k proteoglycan from the urine of cancer cachectic patients, regardless of the tumour type. This factor was able to accelerate the breakdown of skeletal muscle *in vitro* and *in vivo* and to produce weight loss *in vivo* by a process that did not involve anorexia.

Iatrogenic malnutrition

Hypophagia

Anorexia and hypophagia may involve a psychological component which is related to the communication of the diagnosis or of therapeutic decisions such as the need for hospitalisation or disabling therapies. In paediatric patients in particular, conditioning mechanisms can lead to anorexia or food aversion. Nutrition changes resulting from iatrogenic lesions of the alimentary tract are also important. Table 37.6 lists the nutrition changes related to the radical resection of organs of the digestive tract.

Table 37.6 – Nutrition consequences of radical resection of alimentary tract organs.

Organ	Consequences
Tongue or pharynx	Need for nutrition by tube (dysphagia)
Thoracic oesophagus	Gastric stasis (due to vagotomy) Malabsorption of fats (due to vagotomy)
Stomach	Dumping syndrome, anaemia, malabsorption of fats, iron, calcium and vitamins
Duodenum	Biliary-pancreatic deficiency
Jejunum (up to 120 cm)	Reduced absorption of glucose, fats, protein, folic acid, vitamin B_{12}, etc.
Ileum (60 cm) or ileocaecal valve	Malabsorption of vitamin B_{12}, biliary salts and fats
Small intestine (75%)	Malabsorption of fats, glucose, protein, folic acid, vitamin B_{12}, etc., diarrhoea
Jejunum and ileum	Complete malabsorption
Colon (subtotal or total resection)	Water and electrolyte loss
Pancreas	Malabsorption and diabetes
Liver	Transient hypoalbuminaemia

Without going into detail, it may be noted that malnutrition is only rarely related to reduced caloric and protein intake as a result of certain procedures (interference in chewing and swallowing due to glossectomy, dysphagia, total gastrectomy, etc. due to supraglottic laryngectomy). Instead, it is usually due to malabsorption.

Nutrition complications associated with radiotherapy are frequent (Table 37.7). It has been demonstrated that approximately 90% of patients submitted to intensive treatment in the head and neck region, the abdomen or the pelvis lose weight unless nutrition support is provided. More than 10% of patients lose over 10% of their usual weight when radiotherapy is continued for a period of 6–8 weeks. The pathophysiology of malnutrition from radiotherapy is twofold:

- Direct hypophagia in patients receiving radiotherapy to regions of the head and neck and chest
- Hypophagia associated with malabsorption in patients receiving radiotherapy to the abdomen.

The minimum tolerated dose for other regions (i.e., the dose that may cause severe complications within 5 years of completion of radiotherapy using the standard high energy therapeutic modality fractioned into 10 Gy a week, with 5 sessions a week) varies from 35 to 50 Gy, depending on the organs and tissue of the region (Table 37.8).

Table 37.7 – Nutrition complications associated with radiotherapy.

Region irradiated	Early effects (days)	Late effects (weeks/months/year)
Head and neck	Odynophagia Xerostomia Mucositis Anorexia Dysosmia Hypogeusia	Ulceration Xerostomia Dental caries Osteoradionecrosis Trismus Hypogeusia
Thorax	Dysphagia	Fibrosis Stenosis Fistula
Abdomen and pelvis	Anorexia Nausea Vomiting Diarrhoea Acute enteritis Acute colitis	Ulceration Malabsorption Diarrhoea Chronic enteritis Chronic colitis –

Table 37.8 – Radiation tolerance of the gastrointestinal tract.

Organ	TD 5/5 (rads)	TD 50/5 (rads)
Stomach	4500	5000
Small intestine	4500	6000
Colon	4500	6500
Rectum	5500	8000

TD 5/5 = total dose of radiation which will give rise to a 5% increase in significant complications in 5 years.
TD 50/5 = total dose of radiation which will give rise to a 50% incidence of significant complications in 5 years.

Head and neck irradiation interferes with nutrition because it causes a rapid exponential loss in the sense of taste. After 3-4 weeks, patients begin to suffer from an affected taste sensation due to lesion of the microvilli of the gustatory cells or their surfaces. This condition returns to normal 2-4 months after the end of treatment. Another change caused by head and neck irradiation is the decrease in salivation that occurs in the first 3-4 days of therapy, causing nausea and dysphagia and facilitating the onset of caries. Erythema, mucositis and oropharyngeal ulceration with odynophagia (which may be very pronounced) may develop during the second or third week. Radiotherapy to the chest may lead to dysphagia when the field of irradiation includes the esophagus; it occurs with fractioned doses of approximately 30 Gy over 3 weeks and may persist for several weeks after completion of therapy. Radiotherapy to the abdomen and pelvis may cause two different types of nutritional disturbances: a) those related to decreased food intake due to anorexia, nausea and vomiting, and b) those due to chronic x-ray enteropathy.

Negative side-effects from chemotherapy occur in several forms (Table 37.9): anorexia due to changes in the sense of taste with perception of a metallic tinge, dysphagia due to ulceration of the mucosa of the lip, tongue, oropharyngea cavity and oesophagus, decrease in food intake due to nausea and vomiting, as

Table 37.9 – Chemotherapeutic drugs commonly associated with severe nausea and vomiting.

Drug	Severity and duration
Nitrogen mustard (mustine hydrochloride; mechlorethamine hydrochloride *USP*)	Occurs in virtually all patients
	May be severe, but usually subsides within 24 hours
Chloroethyl nitrosoureas	Variable, but may be severe
Streptozotocin (streptozocin)	Occurs in nearly all patients
	Tolerance improves with each successive dose given on a 5-day schedule
Cis-platinum (cisplatin)	May be very severe
	Tolerance improves with intravenous hydration and continuous 5-day infusion
	Nausea may persist for several days
Imidazole carboxamide (DTIC; dacarbazine)	Occurs in virtually all patients
	Tolerance improves with each successive dose given on a 5-day schedule
Chemotherapeutic drugs commonly associated with mucositis	
Methotrexate	May be quite severe with prolonged infusions or if renal function is compromised
	Severity is enhanced by irradiation
	May be prevented with administration of adequate citrovorum rescue factor (folinic acid; leucovorin)
5-Fluorouracil (fluorouracil *USP*)	Severity increases with higher doses, frequency of cycles, and arterial infusions
Actinomycin D (dactinomycin *USP*)	Very common; may prevent oral alimentation
	Severity enhanced by irradiation
Adriamycin (doxorubicin)	May be severe and ulcerative
	Increased in presence of liver disease
	Severity enhanced by irradiation
Bleomycin	May be severe and ulcerative
Vinblastine	Frequently ulcerative

well as constipation or adynamic ileus. The most toxic treatment combination is vinblastine, bleomycin and cisplatinum (PVB), used for testicular cancer.

The combination of chemo- and radiotherapy produces cytotoxicity as a result of their simple additive effect and as a result of synergism (the final response is greater than the sum of the effects of the single modalities as a result of the use of sensitising drugs). Anti-tumour antibiotics (adriamycin, actinomycin D, bleomycin) are generally more toxic when administered to patients undergoing radiotherapy. The incidence and severity of oesophagitis from irradiation increase with the use of actinomycin D, vinblastine, hydroxyurea, procarbazine and the combination of cyclophosphamide, vincristine and actinomycin D. Adriamycin and daunomycin are sensitising agents which, when combined with radiotherapy, may cause oesophageal stenosis. Fluorouracil, actinomycin D and adriamycin may enhance damage from irradiation in other regions of the digestive tract. Actinomycin D and adriamycin are responsible for the so-called 'recall reaction', in which there is a reactivation of the latent effects of irradiation during medical therapy. In this case, severe irritation of the gastrointestinal mucosa may recur periodically.

Malabsorption

The malabsorption that occurs in cancer patients may be iatrogenic in origin, or directly related to disease. Recently it has been reported that patients with advanced breast cancer exhibit a markedly reduced capacity for active and facilitated absorption of some substrates.[125] However, it should be noted that intestinal enzyme deficiency and significant biochemical changes in the intestinal mucosa (with consequent malabsorption of protein) appear very early under conditions of fasting and hypoalbuminaemia, even in the absence of morphological changes. For this reason, it is difficult to determine whether there is a true 'neoplastic enteropathy', or if malabsorption is attributable to simple malnutrition and to what degree.

As far as postoperative malabsorption is concerned (Table 37.6), pancreatectomy may cause digestive enzyme deficiency with loss through the stool of fats and proteins as well as a considerable quantity of vitamins and minerals.

Radiotherapy to the small and large intestine may cause immediate and late damage, since the epithelium of the small intestine is second only to bone marrow in radiosensibility. Damage from irradiation, which appears in 70–80% of patients who receive abdominopelvic radiotherapy, is clinically expressed as malabsorption of glucose, fat, electrolytes and, in part, proteins (due to peptidase deficiency). Morphological lesions consistent with flattening of the villi and reduction in mitosis have been demonstrated in asymptomatic patients after a dose of 20 Gy over 3 weeks or 33 Gy over 4 weeks. Spontaneous recovery usually occurs within 2 weeks of completion of radiotherapy. One-third of patients who have had acute enteritis subsequently develop late enteritis.

Treatment with growth-inhibiting compounds (thioguanine, methotrexate, fluorouracil, vinca alkaloids, hydroxyurea, daunomycin and alkylating agents) may also cause malabsorption. Folic acid antagonists may cause changes in the intestinal mucosa which are similar to those of sprue, with a reduction in epithelial cell mitosis and absorption of xylose and other nutrients. The administration of fluorouracil leads to a dipeptidase deficiency, and a single intravenous administration of methotrexate (2–5 mg/kg) is followed by inhibition of cell mitosis of the jejunal mucosa as well as other cellular changes.

Malabsorption which is directly related to the tumour may be present in a series of circumstances:

- When the pancreas is involved and there is obstruction of the biliary-pancreatic ducts

- When there are lesions in the small intestine from leukaemic foci or lymphoma or solid tumours that may directly infiltrate the wall, obstruct lymphatic flow or affect the mucosa and villi

- When protein-losing syndromes are present in patients with lymphoma or gastric carcinoma

- When the digestive tract is the target organ of powerful pharmacological agents secreted by certain tumours (e.g. apudomas), such as trophic hormones, steroids, hormonal polypeptides with low molecular weight, quinines and prostaglandins

- When alterations in the villi and their function are observed in patients with tumours whose origin is extragastrointestinal.

Impact on prognosis

The concept that malnutrition is associated with a poor outcome in cancer patients has been amply documented in the literature.

There is a relationship between weight loss and poor quality of life,[15] and high morbidity and mortality rates have been demonstrated in malnourished cancer patients in both medical and surgical series.[31,32,126–128] Malnourished or weight-losing patients with breast cancer[129,130] or testis or Hodgkin's disease[131] have a poorer response to chemotherapy.

Cachexia is the principal cause of death in one out of 20 to one out of 4 cancer patients.[132–135]

In studies involving the paediatric population,[34] nutrition status has been correlated with survival time in lymphoma (and histiocytosis) and solid tumours, the greatest impact being most evident in patients with limited tumour spread. The effect of nutrition status on the response to chemotherapy is especially evident in patients with solid tumours, both children and adults; it has been reported that nutrition status is likely to have an impact on response when the response rate to chemotherapy is in the 40–80% range.

Rationale for nutrition support

The rationale for using artificial nutrition (TPN or EN) in cancer patients is primarily based on the assumption that although the final outcome of cancer patients mainly reflects the prognosis of the primary tumour, concomitant malnutrition can affect survival by increasing the complications of the oncological therapy, reducing tolerance to these treatments and, in some cases, decreasing both the length and the quality of survival. This approach tends to correlate cancer cachexia with undernutrition, a concept which is partially true, since, as we have already seen, reduced intake only partially accounts for the onset and progression of cachexia.

Effects of nutrition support on nutrition status

This is a pivotal aspect of nutrition support: in fact, since hypophagia 'alone' does not account for the onset and progression of cachexia, the effects of TPN and EN are expected to be more limited than in conditions of simple undernutrition; however, if TPN or EN were totally inefficient in reversing malnutrition or in preventing the progressive deterioration of the nutrition status, there would be no rationale for feeding malnourished cancer patients either in current clinical practice or in randomised trials.

The effects of TPN and EN on nutrition status have been reviewed in previous publications[136,137] and are summarised in Tables 37.10 and 37.11. The beneficial effects of TPN are more evident when compared in controlled studies to a standard oral diet (Table 37.12). It is worth noting that there is a nutritional benefit even when vigorous nutrition support is administered to patients undergoing cancer treatment (Table 37.13).

Special interest has focused on the effects of TPN and EN on body cell mass, the component of body compartment which contains the oxygen-exchanging,

Table 37.10 – Effects of TPN on the nutrition status of cancer patients.

Variable	Response
Body weight	always increases[14,15,138,139]
	usually increases[140,141]
Body fat	
Muscle mass	
Anthropometry	no change or increases[139,140,141]
urinary creatinine or	no change or decreases[139,142,143]
3-CH$_3$-histidine	
Lean body mass	
nitrogen balance	always positive[139,144,142–146]
total body nitrogen	no change or increases[55,145,146]
Whole-body potassium	increases or no change[143,144,146]
Serum protein	
total protein	no change[67,148]
albumin	usually no change[15,139,140–142,149–151]
transferrin	usually no change[139,141,142,149–151]
prealbumin	no change or increases[141,143,150–152]
retinol-binding protein	usually increases or no change[139,141,150–152]
cholinesterase and	no change[139,149]
ceruloplasmin	
immune humoral	
response	
IgA, C$_3$, C$_4$	no change[149,150]
IgG, IgM, IgA	no change or sometimes increases[149,150]
Non-specific cellular	
response	
neutrophils, total	
lymphocytes	
B, T lymphocytes	
helper T, suppressor	no change[128,149,150]
T, chemotaxis	
phagocitosis killing index	
natural killer	no change or increases[140,150]

Table 37.11 – Effects of EN on the nutrition status of cancer patients.

Variable	Response
Body weight	usually increases, sometimes no change[138,142–145,148,153–157]
Body fat	increases or no change[143,145,148,156,157]
Muscle mass	
anthropometry	no change, sometimes increases[148,155,156,157]
urinary creatinine or 3-CH$_3$-histidine	no change[142,143,157]
3-CH$_3$-histidine efflux from the leg	decreases[158]
Tyrosine, AA and BCAA efflux from the leg	no change[159]
Lean body mass	
nitrogen balance	usually positive or equilibrium[138,143,157,160]
total body nitrogen	no change[145]
Whole-body potassium	increase or no change[138,143,145]
Serum protein	
total protein	no change or increases[142,157]
albumin	usually no change, sometimes increases or decreases[143,148,155,156,158]
TIBC, CHE, TBPA	no change or increases[142,143,148,156,157]
ceruloplasmin	no change
immune humoral response	
IgG, IgA, IgM, CH$_{50}$	no change[160]
C$_3$-C$_4$, C$_3$PA	increases[148,160]
Non-specific cellular response	increases or no change[148,157,160]

TIBC = total iron-binding capacity.
CHE = cholinesterase.
TBPA = thyroxin-binding prealbumin.

Table 37.12 – Nutrition effects of TPN versus standard oral diet (OD).

Variable	TPN	OD
Weight	↑ or =	= or ↓
Nitrogen balance	positive	negative
Total body potassium	=	=
Urinary 3-methylhistidine	↓	=
Total protein	= or ↑	= or ↓
Albumin	= or ↓	= or ↓
Transferrin	↑ or =	= or ↓ ↑
CHE, RBP	↑	↓
TBPA	=	=
Ceruloplasmin, Fibrinogen, IgA	=	=
IgG, IgM, C$_3$A	↑	=

CHE = cholinesterase.
RBP = retinol-binding protein.
TBPA = thyroxin-binding prealbumin.

Table 37.13 – Effects of TPN and EN in cancer patients receiving chemotherapy or radiotherapy.

Variable	Type of nutrition	Response
Body weight	TPN	increases or no change
	EN	increases or no change
Body fat	TPN	increases
Muscular mass	TPN	increases
Lean body mass		
nitrogen balance	TPN	positive
total body nitrogen	TPN	no change
Serum protein		
total protein		
albumin		
transferrin	TPN	no change
retinol-binding protein		
Immune humoral response		
IgA, IgM	TPN	increases

potassium-rich, glucose-oxidising, work-performing tissue, and on the protein component of the body which represents the 'functional compartment' *par excellence*. Studies evaluating whole-body potassium (WBK) have generally had better results than those evaluating total body nitrogen (TBN). There are probably several explanations for the discrepancy between the response of WBK and that of TBN, aside from the intrinsic error of the two techniques, since neutron activation measures all protein nitrogen (cellular protein + extracellular collagen) equally without differentiating the site or the metabolic activity of the nitrogen measured. In fact, the intracellular potassium concentration is also influenced by the state of cellular hydration, by glycogen stores, and by the level of insulin and catecholamines; and its depletion may be independent of the loss of body protein.[161] In addition, the K/N ratio changes in different tissues of the body (3 mol of K/Kg of N in muscle, to about 1.3 mol/Kg in the rest of the lean body mass, to 1 mol/Kg in adipose tissue). The low nitrogen accretion with TPN or EN should come as no surprise. Studies on body composition during weight recovery[162] suggest that the initial percentage of body fat is the most important determinant variable in energy partitioning: the higher it is, the lower the proportion of energy mobilised as protein will be, and thus the greater the propensity the body has to mobilise fat during semi-starvation and to deposit it subsequently during refeeding.[163-166] Consequently, different results may simply reflect different types of tissue depletion and renewal in response to the nutrition support administered.

A number of studies have examined specific protein kinetic response to TPN in malnourished cancer patients. Whole-body protein turnover has been shown to increase with TPN,[71,75,138,142] but whole-body protein synthesis has been reported both to increase[91,167,168] and to decrease.[75] Whole-body protein catabolism has been reported to decrease in cancer patients on TPN.[75,167] Few studies have investigated

the two components of protein kinetics, namely the muscle compartment and the extra-muscle compartment. Shaw et al.[91] have reported an increase in whole-body protein synthesis and in the fractional synthetic rate of protein in muscle, with no change in whole-body protein catabolism.

In our experience in severely malnourished patients with gastric cancer,[94] whole-body protein synthesis and catabolism did not significantly change from 'before' to 'during' TPN, even while the net balance moved from negative to positive. In contrast, the skeletal muscle protein synthesis and the protein synthesis rate significantly increased, converting the net balance to a positive value. Generally it has been shown that TPN does not increase the serum level of proteins, albumin,[144,169] transferrin, cholinesterase or ceruloplasmin.

As regards TPN and immunological response, Monson et al.[170] have reported an increase of lymphocyte blastogenesis and production of the helper T-lymphocyte lymphokine Interleukin-2 after 7 days of a TPN regimen, but also a significant impairment of basal natural killer and Interleukin-2 activated natural killer activity. In contrast,[171] it has been recently reported that a 10-day course of TPN was able to restore to normal a depressed basal or interleukin- or

Table 37.14 – Response to TPN and EN in cancer versus non-cancer patients.

Variable	TPN		EN	
	Cancer	Non-cancer	Cancer	Non-cancer
Weight	↑	↑↑	↑	↑ or ↑↑
Arm circumference				
Triceps skinfold	↑	↑	= or ↑	↑
Arm muscle area	↑	↑↑	↑	↑
Creatinine–height index	↑	↑↑	↑	↑
N balance	+	+	+	+
Total-body K	–	–	↑	↑
Tyrosine balance	–	–	=	+
Albumin	↑	↑↑	↑	↑
Prealbumin	=	=	=	=
Retinol-binding protein	=	=	–	–
Balance of:				
Na	+	+	–	+
K	+	+	–	+
Cl	+	+	–	+
Mg	+	++	–	+
P	+	+	+	+
Ca	=	=	+	+

interferon-stimulated natural killer activity in cachectic cancer patients.[176]

The available data show that TPN and EN are usually able to prevent further deterioration of the nutritional state and may sometimes improve some metabolic indices. These results are probably dependent on the length of the nutrition support, the biological aggressiveness of the tumour and the efficacy of the available cancer therapy.

It must be emphasised that even while the nutritional benefit often seems to be limited to maintaining a 'status quo', it does so in patients who would be condemned to a progressive chronic 'autocannibalism' without a nutrition support. However, the nutritional response of cancer patients is always more sluggish and limited than that of undernourished non-cancer patients (Table 37.14).

Jeevanandam et al.[75] have shown that a 10-day course of TPN including 29 non-protein kcal/kg/day + 1.6 g amino acid/kg/day significantly decreased protein breakdown (by 50% and 59%) and protein synthesis (by 21% and 33%) in cancer and non-cancer patients, respectively, while it increased protein turnover (by 15%) in cancer patients only. The utilization efficiency of infused amino acid for synthesis of body protein was 39% in both cancer and non-cancer patients.

Table 37.14 reports data comparing TPN and EN[142,143,145,153] and Tables 37.15, 37.16 summarise the effects of TPN and EN on protein turnover. It is noteworthy that both techniques are able to improve some nutrition indices, such as body weight, fat mass, nitrogen balance and whole-body potassium. Thyroxin-binding prealbumin and retinol-binding protein levels increase only with TPN, while some immune response indices (complement factors and lymphocyte number) improve only with EN. Total body nitrogen shows a small gain only with TPN. Dresler et al.[172] have demonstrated that only 32% of the parenterally-infused nutrient was utilised for protein synthesis, as compared with 61% of the oral intake. The results of three randomised studies[138,142,153] comparing TPN and EN were partially conflicting, but only TPN showed some significant advantages with regard to weight gain, nitrogen balance, maintenance of serum albumin levels, and some mineral balances (K, Mg, P, Na, and Cl). However, differences were marginal, and the slight advantage of TPN does not support its being used indiscriminately in mal-

Table 37.15 – Effects of TPN and EN on nutrition variables.

Variable	Response	
	TPN	EN
Weight	↑	↑
Body fat	↑	↑
Muscle mass (★)	=	=
Lean body mass		
N balance	+	+
total body K	↑	↑ (=)
total body N	= ↑	= ?
Serum proteins		
total protein	=	=
albumin	=	= ↓
TIBC, CHE	=	= ↑
Ceruloplasmin	=	=
TBPA	↑ or =	= or ↑
RBP	↑	–
Protein flux,	↑ or =	=
synthesis, catabolism	=	=
Immune humoral response		
IgG, IgA, IgM	=	↑
C_3, C_4	=	↑
C_3PA	–	↑
CH_{50}	=	–
Immune cellular response		
neutrophils	=	–
lymphocytes		
(total/subpopulations)	=	↑ or =
chemotaxis/phagocytosis	=	–

(★): 3-methylhistidine, amino acid efflux, anthropometry, creatinine–height index.
TIBC = total iron-binding capacity.
CHE = cholinesterase.
TBPA = thyroxin-binding prealbumin.
RBP = retinol-binding protein.

nourished cancer patients with a working gastro-intestinal tract.

Effects of nutrition support on clinical outcome

Effects in cancer patients submitted to surgery

The rationale for perioperatively treating malnourished cancer patients with TPN or EN is mainly based on the following assumptions:

- Malnourished cancer patients are at higher risk for postoperative complications (especially infections)

Table 37.16 – Effects of TPN and EN★ on daily protein turnover in cancer patients.

Author	Tumour	Regimen		Synthesis (g/kg)		Catabolism	
		kcal/kg	AA/kg	pre	post	pre	post
Burt[14]	Oesophagus	38	1.68	2.2	2.7	2.8	2.4
	Oesophagus	44	0.87	2.4	2.3	2.9	2.3
Dresler[177]	UGI	BEE.	C/N				
		1.2	200	2.0	1.8•	2.3	1.1•
Jeevanandam[78]	GI	29	1.6	2.1	1.3•	2.6	1.3•

UGI = upper gastrointestinal tumour. GI = gastrointestinal tumour. • = statistically significant pre *vs* post.
C/N = kcal/g nitrogen.

- Cancer malnutrition can be reversed with nutrition support and consequently the surgical risk can be reduced.

However, the value of the above statements is limited, since malnutrition is not the only (and also perhaps not the most important, except in extreme cases) cause of surgical complications. Cancer malnutrition can probably be controlled by TPN or EN but this is less easy. Moreover, it takes more time than in non-cancer patients, and the length of the preoperative hospital stay has been correlated with increased surgical infection rates. Finally, we do not know whether the parameters of nutrition assessment we use to define a malnourished patient (weight loss, low serum albumin, lymphocyte number, etc.) are the same ones which are pathogenetically involved in the defective defence of the host against the microorganisms, and consequently whether we should aim at normalising them with TPN or EN before operating on the patient. Furthermore, it is a common experience that the more severe the malnutrition, the more advanced the stage of the tumour,[29] so that the probability of performing an explorative surgery which annuls the benefit of artificial nutrition is magnified in severely malnourished patients. Is it possible to find a statistically significant advantage in terms of reduction of the complication rate in patients receiving TPN, while the apparent reduction in mortality is dubious.[173,174]

A recent review of 21 studies on preoperative artificial nutrition in cancer patients revealed that 16 were randomised clinical trials, but only six focused on malnourished patients with GI tract cancers.[175–180] Two of these were non-randomised studies involving patients with oesophageal carcinoma who had metabolic[175] and clinical benefits (reduction of complications).[178] The other four studies included a randomised study on patients with gastrointestinal carcinoma which showed a reduction in septic complications only in those patients who had a weight loss of >10%[180] and three[144,176,177] which showed no reduction in complications.

The discrepancy in the results obtained by these randomised studies involving parenteral nutrition (TPN) in the pre- and postoperative periods[176,177,180] may be related to the different lengths of preoperative feeding (11 days, 3 days and >5 days). For example, the lowest rate of septic complications occurred in the group that received preoperative parenteral nutrition for the longest period of time.

Recently, a prospective randomised study involving cirrhotic patients who were submitted to hepatic resections for hepatocarcinoma reported that preoperative nutrition support can reduce postoperative complications.[181]

A recent study[182] on 90 patients with gastrointestinal cancer and weight loss ±>10% showed that preoperative TPN (10 days, calorie regimen at RME × 1.5, kcal(kJ)/N=150(628)/1, CHO/fat ratio 70:30) is able to reduce both the overall complication rate and mortality at a statistically significant level.

Preoperative TPN *vs* EN

Two studies[153,183] have compared two ways of preoperatively administering random nutrition support to patients with cancer of the oesophagus or head/neck, demonstrating a marginal advantage for TPN as regards body weight[153] and nitrogen balance,[153,183] with no difference in morbidity and mortality.

Postoperative TPN *vs* EN

Woolfson and Smith[184] investigated the effect of TPN for 7 days after elective thoracoabdominal procedures or after total cystectomy in 122 randomised patients, but found no advantage in terms of morbidity, mortality or duration of hospital stay. However, they did report a reduction in the net nitrogen loss.

Similar results were reported by Daly et al.,[185] who randomised 20 patients to immediate postoperative jejunostomy feeding or standard 5% dextrose solution. However, the improved nitrogen balance was counterbalanced by a 36% gastrointestinal complication rate in the patients who were fed enterally.

In a short randomised study on patients submitted to gastrectomy for advanced cancer who were given TPN for 18 days postoperatively (compared with a group receiving oral intake), Yamada et al.[186] reported not only a benefit in terms of the nutrition-related variable counts (body weight, serum albumin, total lymphocyte), but also an improvement in the survival rate in non-curative resection and in the disease-free interval.

Other studies compared different modalities of nutrition support: standard TPN versus modified TPN (30 ml of water/kg/day, no sodium, 70% of non-protein calories as fat),[187] TPN versus EN,[188] parenteral versus enteral glucose,[189] and system versus intraportal nutrition[190] at equal energy and nitrogen intake.

No significant differences were reported between parenteral and enteral regimens, whereas some metabolic advantages were observed in patients who received nutrients intraportally rather than through a peripheral vein.

Effects on outcome in oncologic patients

To date, 13 randomised clinical trials in adults[17–21,23,191–197] with the exclusion of bone marrow transplantation,[198,199] and five in children[24,34,200–202] have explored the effects of TPN as an adjunct to chemotherapy on survival and remission.

The majority of these studies in adult patients have been critically reviewed in meta-analyses (Table 37.17).[178,179] Briefly, only one study in patients with limited-disease small cell lung cancer receiving TPN showed an increased number of complete remissions,[200] while three studies revealed decreased survival or shortened remission in subgroups receiving TPN.[125,191,193]

In the remaining studies, benefits with respect to survival or remission were either not demonstrated or not tested.

However, the results of these meta-analyses – which were the basis for a paper published by the American College of Physicians[203] on the indications for parenteral nutrition in cancer patients undergoing chemotherapy – have been severely criticised because of the many flaws contained in the trials.

The criticism mainly concerns two aspects, the first regarding the statistical and methodological aspects of the studies and the second regarding some practical issues in the selection of the patients and the administration of TPN. It is important to point out that although formal sample size calculations for performing meta-analyses do not exist, if this were a single trial, there would be only a 50% chance of detecting and labelling as statistically significant at the 0.05 level a benefit of 10–20% over a baseline of 85 and 50%, respectively (i.e. the expected advantage in 3-month

Table 37.17 – Results of two meta-analyses of randomised cancer clinical trials of patients given TPN during chemotherapy.

Outcome	Odds ratio (95% CI)		p value	
	Klein et al.[173]	McGeer et al.[174]	Klein et al.[173]	McGeer et al.[174]
Survival	–	0.74 (0.42–1.3)	0.30	0.20
		0.81 (0.62–1.0)	–	0.06
Response	0.61 (0.34–1.1)	0.68 (0.40–1.1)	0.08	0.12
Infection	3.9 (2.0–8.0)	4.1 (2.4–6.9)	0.0001	0.001

survival and in the response rate, respectively) due to the small number of enrolled patients (190 for each outcome, or 15–20 per arm and per study). Moreover, the quality of the various studies was generally poor, with a score of 0.53 in a scale ranging from 0 to 1.0 by McGeer and colleagues;[174] and only 46% of the studies met the quality criteria for reporting randomised trials.[173]

The most crucial point, however, was that since the rationale for using TPN was the poor tolerance and poor compliance of malnourished patients receiving chemotherapy, one would have expected only severely malnourished patients to be randomised for TPN or no TPN. Instead, in 20% of the patients nutrition status was not assessed at all; in 16% it was good; only half of the remaining patients were mal-nourished. Moreover, in some studies a 5% weight loss or serum albumin level less than 3.6 g/dl were sufficient to consider the patients suitable for random-isation. Patients with gastrointestinal cancer, a group at high risk for developing malnutrition during therapy, were involved in only one or two studies. The technical quality of the TPN regimen was also sometimes inadequate (1500 kcal (6276 kJ) + 0.2 g AA/kg only during the 8 hours of chemotherapy[130], or sometimes excessive (more than 50 kcal (209 kJ)/kg/day) and potentially toxic because of CO_2 retention, particularly in patients with cancer of the lung.[191,192,196]

These problems make it difficult to accept the point which the randomised clinical trials attempted to establish: that TPN does not play a beneficial role in malnourished cancer patients undergoing chemo-therapy.

There is a paucity of prospective, controlled investi-gation on oral/enteral feeding in oncology patients. Douglass et al.[204] compared a supplemental elemental diet to between-meal feeding in addition to the standard diet in 30 patients undergoing radiotherapy with or without adjuvant chemotherapy for a variety of locally advanced, non-resectable gastrointestinal tumours. There was a trend towards improved skin test responses in patients receiving the elemental nutrition. There were no differences in weight, total lymphocyte count or survival.

Daly et al.[155] investigated intensive nasogastric tube feeding versus optimal oral nutrition in patients with advanced head and neck cancer who were undergoing 8 weeks of radiation treatment. There

was less weight loss in the tube-fed group, and the median value for albumin had returned to normal in the tube-fed group by the end of therapy. However, no differences were found in response or survival rates; tube-fed patients had significantly longer radiation toxicity (3.3 + 1.9 weeks versus 1.8 + 0.8 weeks).

Effects on performance status and quality of life

Three trials have reported improved performance status in TPN groups, but documentation for the reported improvement was lacking in the reports.[24,191,205] In three trials[34,193,201] no difference in quality of life or performance status was found, while this issue was not examined in the others.

Effects of oncological therapy on iatrogenic toxicity

It is well-known that aggressive chemotherapy may decrease spontaneous oral intake because of the side-effects of the treatment.[206]

Seven trials[17,24,200,201,202,205,207,208] have reported some benefit with respect to chemotherapy or radiotherapy toxicity in patients receiving TPN. Such benefits included a decrease in the number of medications needed for symptom control, decreased radiation enteritis, minimising reduction in white blood count, decreased duration of chemotherapeutic-induced nausea and vomiting, improved compliance to chemotherapy and fewer treatment delays. In other studies, however, there was poorer tolerance to therapy in patients receiving TPN, manifested by severe stomatitis, prolonged hospitalisation, decreased haemoglobin and white cell count, and increased frequency of bowel movements.

More recently, DeCicco et al.[205] have shown that TPN is able to reduce chemotherapy-associated toxicity in malnourished subjects, and Cozzaglio et al.[210] have demonstrated that EN is able to prevent deterioration of the nutritional state in dysphagic malnourished patients with oesophageal cancer receiving chemo-therapy and radiation therapy (while the opposite occurred in non-dysphagic patients without EN support). In conclusion, there has been no uniform pattern or tolerance to chemotherapy or radiotherapy, but a possible benefit has been found in the majority of the studies.

Effects on tumour growth

It has been widely demonstrated in tumour-bearing animals that the intravenous administration of TPN and especially amino acids can lead to an increase in absolute tumour volume, weight, mitotic activity and number of metastases, even if the tumour weight/carcass weight ratio sometimes remains unchanged. This effect has been explained by the fact that some components of the diet are able to bring about a uniform reduction of the cell proliferation cycle or a recruitment of dormant cells from GO into the active phase of cell replication.

It must be pointed out that in these experimental studies, refeeding after a period of nutrition deprivation resulted in a measurable increase in tumour volume after only 24 hours[211] and an increase in the S-phase tumour cell population could be observed by flow cytometry[212] only 2 hours after the start of TPN, with gradual normalisation of tumour growth kinetics within 24–48 hours of initiating TPN. This short-term effect of TPN on tumour growth kinetics represents a biological response at the cellular level which is independent of the nutrition status of the host.

Results from animal studies cannot, however, be extrapolated directly to the clinical field, since animal tumours usually become very large, accounting for up to 20% of the carcass weight. Such a condition never occurs in man, since human tumour mass rarely exceeds 1–2% of the host's weight. Furthermore, these experimental tumours have doubling times of a few days and can kill the animal host in a few weeks from the time of their onset – conditions which are never found in clinical practice. Therefore, the administration of TPN

to these animals even for just one week means feeding them for a substantial part of the natural history of their tumour, which would correspond to a TPN regimen of several months or years in human cancer patients.

The literature on the modulation of tumour cell proliferation in humans by parenteral or enteral nutrition is scanty. Apart from anecdotal reports,[213-215] there are only a few published studies whose aim was to determine the impact of TPN (Table 37.18) or EN (Table 37.19) on tumour cell kinetics.[151,216-220] A study was undertaken of 19 patients with histologically-proven gastric cancer who were severely malnourished and randomised either to preoperative TPN or no TPN.[221] The nutrition regimen was: energy = 1.5 × Harris-Benedict equation, with glucose/lipid (LCT) ratio of 70/30 and kcal/N ratio of 150/1. Tumour cell replication was investigated through assessment of ^{3}H-thymidine incorporation (labelling index) on cell suspension obtained from endoscopic biopsy samples at the time of randomisation and subsequently on the operative specimen. Data are summarised in Table 37.20.

The preliminary findings from these studies are the following:

- Tumour growth increased in two of five GI cancer studies and in two of five head/neck cancer studies

- Tumour growth increased in one of five EN studies. This study[225] included a caloric regimen of 120–150% of the REE

- There was no increase in tumour growth when nutrition was hypocaloric (< 20 kcal/kg with TPN or < 1000 kcal with EN).

Table 37.18 – TPN and tumour growth in malnourished patients.

Author (year)	Ota[151]	Baron[216]	Westin[217]	Dionigi[218]	Frank[219]
No. patients	25	8	9	7	10
Tumour	GI	Head/Neck	Head/Neck	GI	Head/Neck
Duration (days)	11	9	5–7	18	7
Kcal/kg/day	40–60	59	RME × 1.5	48	?
AA/kg/day	2–3	1.9	1.5	2.3	?
Tumour growth	(1) ↑	(2) ↑	(3) =	(4) =	(4) ↑

(1): RBC polyamine.
(2): % hyperdiploid cells.
(3): % aneuploid cells.
(4): labelling index.
↑: tumour growth increase.
=: tumour growth unchanged.

Table 37.19 – Enteral nutrition and tumour growth in malnourished patients.

Author (year)	Baron[216]	Edstrom[220]		Dionigi[218]
No. patients	6	13	13	9
Tumour	Head/Neck	Head/Neck		GI
Duration (days)	8	6–8	6–8	–
Kcal/kg/day	43	RME × 1.2–1.5	1000 kcal	19
AA/kg/day	1.4	1	0.5	11
Tumour growth	(1) =	(2) ↑	(2) =	(3) =

(1): % hyperdiploid cells.
(2): % aneuploid cells.
(3): labelling index.
↑: tumour growth increase.
=: tumour growth unchanged.

Table 37.20 – Effects of TPN on labelling index of gastric cancer.

Variable	TPN (10)	Controls (9)
Age (years)	60 (± 16)	68 (± 7)
Weight loss (%)	15.2 (± 4.8)	15.1 (± 4)
Serum albumin (g/dl)	3.6 (± 0.4)	3.4 (± 0.3)
Serum transferrin (µg/dl)	295 (± 38)	256 (± 60)
Serum cholinesterase U/l	1834 (± 551)	1772 (± 476)
Total lymphocytes n/mm^3	1647 (± 414)	1654 (± 398)
Stage II/III/IV	1/3/6	1/4/4
L1–L2 (interval, days)	9	11
L1 → L2	10.0% (± 6.8) → 15.0% (± 7.1)	19.9% (± 10) → 14.0% (± 6.9)
p	0.03	N.S.

The overall impression is that none of these studies has provided a definitive conclusion. As regards our investigation, we observed a statistically significant increase in the labelling index from 10.0% (± 6.8) to 15% (± 7.1) in patients receiving TPN, whereas the control group maintained unchanged values: 19.9% (± 10)–14% (± 6.9). The intriguing fact is that the final values for both the TPN group and the control group were equal, with both groups belonging to the fast-proliferating tumour type. In fact, the median value of the labelling index distinguishing between slow-versus fast-proliferating tumours and good versus bad prognosis is about 9%, according to the literature[227] and to our unpublished series.

Studies on protein synthesis not only give conflicting results; they also respond to the question of tumour growth in an indirect manner, since they measure the tumour protein synthesis but ignore the protein breakdown.

In contrast, methods which evaluate the kinetics of the cancer cells with the use of marked precursors of nucleic acids which are incorporated in the DNA in the S phase are more persuasive, since the growth fraction is a determinant of tumour growth.

Table 37.21 clearly shows that whatever the variable considered – type of tumour: gastrointestinal[151,218] or head-neck,[216,217,220] or type of nutrition: TPN[151,216,217] or EN[216,220] – there are conflicting results. However, it is impressive that increased tumour growth was reported especially when the amount of calories[151,216] and of proteins[151] was excessive.

It has been speculated that if it was true that there is a relationship between nutrient availability and tumour growth, then it would be appropriate to observe the highest cancer cell proliferation rate in well-nourished patients. This hypothesis was tested statistically in 136 adult patients with non-Hodgkin's lymphoma by evaluating the correlation between some nutrition variables (albumin, cholinesterase, number of lymphocytes and body weight loss) with the labelling index. The results obtained (Table 37.22)[223] in this large population of patients do not support the theory that good nutrition status result in faster tumour growth, since the opposite statistical association was found.

Not only was there no evidence that good nutrition status stimulates tumour growth, but the opposite seemed to be a possibility. Therefore, any conclusion about the deleterious effect of artificial nutrition on tumour growth is still preliminary.

TPN-related complications

Seven studies[18,20,192,193,194,200,202,208] have demonstrated an increased complication rate in patients receiving TPN (catheter and noncatheter sepsis, other infections, febrile, episodes, venous thrombosis and fluid overload). Seven other trials did not demonstrate any difference in complications, while four others did not investigate complications.

Table 37.21 – Artificial nutrition and tumour growth in malnourished cancer patients.

	Ota[151]	Baron[216]	Edstrom[220]	Westin[217]	Dionigi[218]	Gavazzi[219]
No. of patients	25	8/6	13/13	9/7	9	8
Tumour	GI	Head/Neck	Head/Neck	Head/Neck	GI	GI
Nutrition	TPN	TPN/oral	EN/oral	TPN/TPN	Oral	TPN
Kcal/kg/day	40–60	59/43	RME × 1.2–1.5/1000 kcal	RME × 1.5/48	19	RME × 1.5
AA/Kg/day	2–3	1.9–1.4	1/0.5	1.5/2.3	1.1	1.5
Tumour growth	(1)↑	(2)↑/=	(3)↑/=	(4)=/(5)=	(5) =	(5) =

GI: gastrointestinal.
(1): RBC polyamine.
(2): % hyperdiploid cells.
(3): % aneuploid cells.
(4): % aneuploid cells, % proliferating cells and ornithine decarboxylase activity.
(5): labelling index.
↑: tumour growth increase.
=: tumour growth unchanged.

Table 37.22 – Association between labelling index and nutrition variables in 136 patients with non-Hodgkin's lymphoma: odds ratio and 95% confidence ratio.

Variable	95% lower limit	Odds ratio	95% upper limit
Albumin (g/dl)			
(3.54–3.99) *vs* (>4)	0.6	1.3	3
(0–3.53) *vs* (>4)	1.4	3.3★	7.9
Cholinesterase (mU/ml)			
(2140–2739) *vs* (>2740)	1.2	2.9★	6.9
(0–2139)	1.7	4★	9.4
Lymphocytes (no/mm3)			
(1480–2129) *vs* (>2130)	0.4	0.9	2
(0–1479) *vs* (>2130)	0.9	2	4.7
Body weight loss			
Yes *vs* No	1.1	2.3★	4.9

★ odds ratio significantly different from 1.0 at 5% level.

A recent analysis of the prospective trials of TPN and cancer evaluated the potential role played by intravenous lipids in contributing to infectious complications. It was found that the risk of infection in chemotherapy patients receiving TPN increased when intravenous fat emulsion was included in the therapy, increasing 2.3-fold when IV fat was used intermittently and 6.3-fold when IV fat was used daily. No increase in infectious complications was found when IV fat was not used. Although there is no clear explanation for this, it has been postulated that intravenous fat emulsions, which are high in omega-6 fatty acids, may result in impaired immune function.

Bone marrow transplantation

Despite the fact that TPN has been used extensively in cancer patients undergoing bone marrow transplantation, there have been few controlled studies investigating outcome factors other than nutrition status. Weisdorf et al.[199] reported that well-nourished bone marrow transplant recipients receiving prophylactic TPN prior to and during transplantation were found to have a significantly increased length of median and 2-year survival (21 vs. 7 months, and 50 vs. 35% for TPN group vs. control group, respectively). Increased disease-free survival and longer time to relapse were also found in patients receiving TPN. These beneficial results were independent of nutrition status.

A subsequent study in a similar but smaller population was unable to find any TPN benefit as compared to an aggressive oral/enteral programme involving closely supervised intake, encouragement, between-meal snacks, supplements and tube feeding when necessary.[198]

It would seem, therefore, that there is a benefit in patients in whom nutrition support is begun early, as opposed to patients without nutrition support. However, this advantage is lost if TPN is begun late and the control group receives adequate nutrition surveillance and counselling.

Recent randomised double-blind trials with glutamine-enriched TPN have shown that this regimen affects outcome favourably because it reduces the infection rate and the length of hospital stay.[224,225]

Home TPN and EN

There is some controversy as to the indications for artificial nutrition (TPN in particular) in cancer patients. The high cost of TPN, coupled with the limited life expectancy of these patients, has led some countries to consider cancer as a relative contra-indication for providing such support.

Despite this fact, cancer patients account for 33.4% of those entered in the OASIS Home Registry (the largest single group),[226] 17% of the European Registry (the second largest group),[227,228] and more than 50% of the Italian Registry of Home TPN (Balzola, personal communication).

As regards survival, 50% of cancer patients survived 6 months, and 12–13% survived 2 years.[226] A similar percentage of patients (13–18%) in the American and European registries were completely rehabilitated, and another 27% were partially socially rehabilitated.[227] The hospital readmission rate per year was 3.5. Longer survival was associated with treatable neoplasms such as lymphoma and leukaemia, as well as good performance status[226] at the beginning of TPN.

The recent experience of the Italian Society of Parenteral and Enteral Nutrition[229] has demonstrated a longer survival in patients with a Karnofsky performance status >50 at the start of TPN and a benefit in the nutrition status and quality of life in patients surviving longer than 3 months with home TPN.

Cancer patients, most of whom were affected by GI tract tumours, also account for the majority (40%) of patients receiving home EN in the American study.[226] Survival was limited, with an average of more than 4 months in an Italian experience.[230]

Nutrition regimen

There is no definite consensus on the optimum calorie and protein requirements of the cancer patient. The minimum daily regimen in the literature which improved lean body mass and visceral proteins has ranged from 35 to 55 kcal (146–230 kJ)/kg and from 1.2 to 2 g amino acids/kg for TPN and 35 kcal (146 kJ)/kg and 1.3 g amino acids/kg for EN. The enteral regimen able to improve some immune responses has included 42 kcal (176 kJ)/kg and 2.3 g amino acids/kg.

The calorie requirement of cancer patients has been evaluated in different ways. Using calorimetry, Merrick et al.[231] showed that an energy intake of 30 kcal(126 kJ)/kg (approximately 1.4 times the calculated RME) is required to provide a respiratory quotient of 1.0 in well-nourished cancer patients. However, in malnourished cancer patients, a TPN corresponding to 200% of the non-protein energy resting expenditure (49 kcal (205 kJ)/kg) and 2.0 g amino acids/kg was necessary to stimulate whole-body protein synthesis,[168] an almost identical regimen to the one reported by Bozzetti[232] as being able to promote weight gain in cancer patients. Recently Shaw[233] reported that a TPN regimen providing 40 kcal (167 kJ)/kg/day (50% glucose and 50% lipid) and protein (1.7 g/kg/day) virtually abolished the net protein catabolism. Current opinion holds that most malnourished cancer patients require a daily regimen of about 35–40 kcal/kg plus 2 g or more amino acid/kg.

The future

In conclusion, four different approaches are possible in order to meet the requirements of the host and to feed patients without stimulating tumour growth.

- The use of appetite stimulant substances or anti-cachectic drugs
- The modulation of nutrients
- Glutamine supplementation
- Metabolic manipulation.

Appetite stimulant substances and anticachectic drugs

Medroxyprogesterone acetate (MAP)

There is wide experience with MAP for treating hormone-sensitive breast and endometrial carcinomas. Since its introduction into clinical practice in 1983, it has been reported that MAP at high doses (>500 mg/day) has anabolic effects.[234] A double-blind, placebo-controlled trial further demonstrated that MAP at 100 mg orally three times a day increased appetite in cachectic patients.

Megestrol acetate

Megestrol acetate is available in 20 and 40 mg tablets and in suspension at a concentration of 40 mg/ml.

The precise weight gain mechanism of megestrol is unknown; however, it does increase appetite and non-fluid weight gain.[235] In addition, megestrol produces antigonadotrophic effects and could stimulate adipocyte differentiation.

The effects of megestrol administration and dose response have been investigated in several randomised, double-blind, placebo-controlled studies.[236–239] A dose of 240 mg/day was associated with an increase in appetite along with a moderate increase in weight.[238] A dose of 480 mg/day increased both appetite and subjective energy level.[236] At a dose of 800 mg, it was reported that patients also had less nausea and emesis due to chemotherapy, but 13% of them suffered from oedema.[237] Tchekmedyian et al.[239] studied patients with advanced hormone-insensitive malignant lesions using 1600 mg/day versus placebo, and reported weight gain, increased appetite and food intake and increased prealbumin levels.

Several randomised trials have evaluated different dosages of megestrol.[240,241] In particular, Loprinzi et al.[240] have demonstrated that 800 mg/day caused an improvement in appetite as compared with the other dosages. There was however a certain risk of thromboembolic events with the dosage; in addition, 26% of the male patients reported impotence. In a randomised study of patients with hormone refractory cancer Gebbia et al.[241] concluded that dosages >480 mg/day were probably of no value in the majority of patients, and suggested two weeks of therapy before altering the dosage to meet the needs of the patients.

The same benefits were observed in a paediatric population.[242] At a dose of 10 mg/kg/day there was a significant increase in appetite, calorie intake and performance status score, often requiring a decrease in the dosage. In contrast with a previous study,[235] these authors proved the weight gain consisted of functionally adipose tissue rather than fat-free mass.

Potential side-effects of megestrol acetate administration include impotence in sexually active males and vaginal spotting or bleeding in females. Individual reports of reversible suppression of the pituitary-adrenal axis, hepatic toxicity, diabetes, mellitus and withdrawal response have been published.

Cyproheptadine hydrochloride

Cyproheptadine is available as 4 mg tablets and syrup in a concentration of 2 mg/5 ml and has been proposed as a means of encouraging weight gain by serotonin antagonism. However, a randomised double-blind trial[243] in cancer patients with anorexia or cachexia failed to prevent weight loss compared with the placebo group. Patients receiving cyproheptadine had less nausea, less energy and more sedation and dizziness compared with placebo patients.

Dronabinol

The literature reporting on the use of cannibinoids in the treatment of cancer cachexia is scanty.[244,245] It would seem that some benefit in appetite and mood is obtained by an administration of 5 mg/day, with about two-thirds of patients reporting that their appetites are stimulated. There is increased calorie intake and weight gain with 2.5 mg three times daily one hour after meals, but neuropsychological effects are not uncommon, including nausea and slurred speech.

Branched-chain amino acids (BCAA)

The use of BCAA has been proposed recently based on the postulate that increased hypothalamic serotinergic activity could play a role in the development of anorexia.[37] BCAA might slow down the entry of the precursor of serotinin, tryptophan, into the brain by competing for the same transport system across the blood–brain barrier. Encouraging results have been reported in a pilot study where anorectic patients received oral supplementation of BCAA.[246]

Corticosteroids

The mechanism underlying the ability of corticosteroids to increase the appetite is unknown, but it may be related to the euphoria produced by these agents. The literature includes at least four randomised, double-blind, placebo-controlled trials with steroids.[247,250] Despite the fact that these agents were effective in stimulating patients' appetites, none of these studies documented a significant weight gain.

Moertel et al.[247] demonstrated that dexamethasone administered both 0.75 or 1.5 mg four times daily produced a significant increase in appetite after 4 weeks of therapy in patients with advanced gastro-intestinal cancer who were not being submitted to chemotherapy.

Bruera et al.[249] showed that 16 mg methylprednisolone taken orally twice daily increased appetite, food intake and performance status as well as reducing pain and analgesic consumption in terminal cancer patients. However, this effect was short-term, and all nutritional indices returned to baseline after 20 days.

Another study[250] was performed in terminal cancer patients using methylprednisolone at a dose of 125 mg IV daily for 56 days. This led to a significant increase in baseline appetite entry during the second week. Other benefits include decreased nausea, vomiting and anxiety and improved alertness along with a sense of well-being. The effect on appetite was, however, quite transient. Moreover, there was an increase in gastrointestinal and cardiovascular side-effects.

Yet another study[248] involving the oral administration of 5 mg prednisolone three times daily for 2 weeks followed by a dosage reduction in the third week resulted in improved appetite and a sense of well-being compared to the placebo group.

The practical conclusion that can be drawn from these studies is that the ability of steroids to stimulate the appetite is short-lived, and that the administration of these drugs may entail long-term complications such as cataract formation, weakness, delirium, diabetes, osteoporosis and immunosuppression.

Anabolic steroids

There is only one randomised clinical trial[251] evaluating the effect of nandrolone decanoate in lung cancer patients with weight loss and receiving chemotherapy. These patients were administered 200 mg of the drug by intramuscular injection every week for 4 weeks, but continued to lose weight.

Insulin

Administration of insulin has resulted in a decreased whole-body protein breakdown rate[84] and an appropriate response of muscle protein synthesis.[93]

Growth hormones (GH)

There is some concern regarding the use of growth hormones because of the possible stimulation of tumour growth, despite the fact that experimental data have not shown tumour progression.[252,253] One clinical study[254] reported an increase in whole-body protein synthesis greater than the stimulation of whole-body protein breakdown, with no change in muscle protein turnover.

Metabolic inhibitors and anticytokine therapy

Inhibitors of gluconeogenesis
The enzyme that catalyses the conversion of oxalo-acetate to phosphenolpyruvate is phosphoenolpyruvate-carboxykinase (PEPCK). Hydrazine sulphate is a non-competitive inhibitor of PEPCK which inhibits *in vitro* gluconeogenesis in animal systems. Gold proposed that it be used as a potential therapy for cancer cachexia[255] and some benefit in terms of subjective parameters has been reported in cancer populations.[256,257]

Subsequent controlled studies[251,258] have demonstrated an improved tolerance to glucose and weight stabilisation with the administration of hydrazine sulphate, while little benefit has been reported in clinical trials aimed at decreasing tumour size.[259–261] It would seem that, while this agent has a limited efficacy alone, it would be opportune to test it in association with modulated diets.

Pentoxifylline

The ability of pentoxifylline to decrease TNF messenger RNA levels has been tested in cancer patients with contrasting results. Pentoxifylline has been reported to decrease TNF secretion[235] and increase appetite and promote weight gain,[263] while a randomised clinical trial[113] failed to report any benefit deriving from its administration.

Pentoxifylline has also been tested in patients receiving radio-chemotherapy for bone marrow transplantation, but here too, there were no consistent results.[264,265]

Melatonin

Melatonin, the pineal hormone that regulates the circadian rhythm, has recently been investigated for the treatment of cancer cachexia.[266] The proposed explanation for its use in cancer cachexia is that cancer patients have disrupted circadian rhythms, which in turn stimulate the release of TNF. Patients receiving a daily 20 mg oral dose of melatonin in the evening for three months had lower TNF serum levels and less weight loss compared to the control group.

Other anticachectic agents

Recently Lundholm *et al.*[158] reported that simple therapy with anti-inflammatory agents may prolong survival in undernourished patients with metastatic solid tumours. The potential role of ω-3-fatty acid as a cytokine inhibitor for cancer cachexia has recently been explored in phase I or II studies[122,267] with promising results.

IGF-1 (also known as somatomedin-C) stimulates amino acid uptake and protein synthesis while inhibiting lipolysis. No human data in cancer cachexia are available so far.

The modulation of nutrients

Further formulations will surely investigate the effects of the incorporation of new substrates such as ω-3 fatty acids, MCT, nucleotides, arginine and glutamine in nutrition regimens which are of great interest. The safety and efficacy of these nutrients are being tested in many experimental conditions and in injured patients, and future trials will undoubtedly include patients with cancer as well. Present experience is more limited and mainly concerns the composition of the amino acid content and the calorie component of the diet.

Tayek *et al.*[268] have shown that a 50% BCAA-enriched TPN formula (energy at 1.3 x BEE) and 1.2 g protein/kg/day had a significantly positive effect as compared to 19% BCAA-enriched TPN formula with regard to the increase in whole-body protein synthesis, leucine balance and incorporation of 14C leucine into plasma albumin. It has also been suggested that the BCAA-enriched solution could be less efficient than standard solution at increasing tumour protein synthesis.

As regards the quality of the caloric source, few studies have compared two different TPN regimens, one based on glucose and amino acids and the other on glucose, fat and amino acids. Data are summarised in Table 37.23 and show either no difference or only a marginal advantage for glucose-based TPN.

Similarly, few authors have compared a total or 'near total' glucose regimen to a total or 'near total' fat regimen. Shaw and Wolfe[167] have found that the infusion of glucose (23 kcal/kg/day) or fat (31 kcal/kg/day) resulted in a significant suppression of the net protein catabolism (approximately 15%) in

Table 37.23 – Effects of glucose (G) and glucose lipid (GL) TPN on nutrition status.

Category	G	GL
Body weight	↑ usually or = ↑	↑ usually or =
Albumin	=	=
TBPA, RBP	↑ or =	=
Transferrin	↑ or =	↑ or =
Total protein, fibrinogen, IgA, C₄	=	=
IgG	↑	=
IgM, C₃A	↑	↑

TBPA = thyroxin-binding prealbumin.
RBP = retinol-binding protein.

patients with lower gastrointestinal cancer, but was ineffective in those with upper gastrointestinal cancer. Glucose infusion resulted in a suppression of endogenous glucose production (at least 55%), while lipid infusion was associated with a minor suppression (9%). Lipid infusion did not decrease the glucose production.

Only one study[60] has compared the metabolic effect of two enteral isonitrogenous (1.5 g protein/kg/day), isocaloric (4.4 kcal/kg/day) diets containing different qualities of energy, one 31% as fat and the other 70% as MCT plus arginine D-3-hydroxybutirate. There was no significant alteration in host N balance, whole-body protein synthesis, degradation, or turnover rates.

Glutamine supplementation

There is some debate regarding the role of glutamine-supplemented diets in the cancer patient, since the potential benefits in protecting the gut from the enterotoxic effects of chemotherapy and radiation therapy might be counteracted by the stimulation of tumour cell metabolism. Experimental work in tumour models has shown that glutamine-supplemented TPN is able to maintain higher intestinal levels of gluthathione,[269] to promote the jejunal villous height in rats treated with 5-fluorouracil,[270–272] and to decrease bacterial translocation[273] compared with standard TPN formulas. A glutamine-supplemented enteral diet given to tumour-bearing rats increased the small bowel mucosal content of DNA[274] and resulted in a significant reduction in the severity of methotrexate-induced enterocolitis, as reflected by improved morphometric parameters,[275] as well as in

the incidence of positive cultures in the spleen,[276] and in morbidity and mortality associated with chemotherapy.[277] A substantial body of experimental evidence indicates that glutamine is the major respiratory fuel cell in some experimental tumours,[278–280] e.g. in hepatomas[281,282] and fibro-sarcomas[282] where the rate of glutamine uptake was quantified, leading to the concept that the tumour behaves as a type of 'glutamine trap'.

In 1935, it was demonstrated that the proliferation of cultured HELA cells (malignant cervidal cells) is greatest when glutamine concentrations are at least 1mmol/l.[278] This *in vitro* requirement may reflect the continuous demand for glutamine in the absence of the normal *in vivo* supply (0.6-0.9 mmol/l). Failure to provide glutamine in the growth medium of cultured malignant cells retards cell division and usually results in cell death. In contrast, *in vivo* studies using tumour-bearing rats have shown that glutamine-supplemented enteral or parenteral nutrition did not apparently stimulate tumour growth[269,283] even though the ratio of euploid to diploid cells in the tumour mass increased by 20% in animals receiving glutamine intravenously.

However, no data is available on humans, and it is important to keep in mind that due to the discrepancy between tumour weight/host weight ratio and cell kinetics in experimental versus human tumours, it is quite difficult to extrapolate laboratory findings to the clinical setting.

Data on human cancer are scanty. Bode *et al.*[284] reported that human hepatoma cells consume glutamine at a rate five to ten times faster than do normal hepatocytes, and Brand *et al.*[285] have demonstrated that patients with leukaemia exhibit an extremely high rate of glutamine consumption. *In vivo* human data show a considerable range in the exchange rate of glutamine in gastrointestinal cancer,[286–288] with the most common finding being a slightly negative balance.

A double-blind randomised study in breast cancer patients receiving glutamine supplementation versus placebo during chemotherapy failed to demonstrate a different oncological response in the two groups.[289]

As regards the protective effect of glutamine against chemotherapy-induced mucosity, our results are in keeping with recent clinical reports on patients with gastrointestinal cancer receiving 5-fluorouracil and folinic acid as well as in patients receiving bone marrow transplants for haematological malignancies,[290-291] which show neither a reduction in the extent of oral mucosity nor any difference in stool frequency or consistency.

These data are also in keeping with a recent investigation by Earl et al.[292] on rats receiving 5-fluorouracil showing that intestinal absorptive activity was less damaged when animals were fed with elemental diets, regardless of whether they contained equienergetic amounts of glutamine or glycine. Moreover, there is evidence that rat intestinal mucosa permeability behaves similarly to that of humans.[293]

These findings disagree in part with a report by Conversano et al.,[294] which showed no reduction in the prevalence of diarrhoea but a decrease in both duration and severity with glutamine supplementation. This, however, was not a randomised study.

A possible explanation for the discrepancy between the experimental literature and clinical results is the fact that changes in circulating glutamine concentration occur when tumour size accounts for at least 10% of the body weight.[295-297] At this point there is a 20% drop in the muscle glutamine concentration, with an accelerated glutamine efflux from the hind quarter,[297] a drop in gut glutamine extraction,[295] and a consequent increase in bacterial translocation,[298,299] suggesting a defect in the gut mucosal barrier. Usually at this stage the animal begins to show visible signs of cachexia, and appears unwell. However, in clinical practice the majority of patients reported in the literature and receiving oral glutamine were not severely depleted, and tumour weight almost never accounted for as high a percentage of the host body weight in humans as it does in experimental tumours. It is therefore possible that antineoplastic chemotherapy intestinal toxicity occurs by way of a mechanism that is completely independent from that mediated by the glutamine intracellular concentration that occurs during nutrition depletion.

Metabolic manipulation

The hypothesis of feeding the host without stimulating tumour growth through the use of selective nutrition has been extensively investigated in animals, but clinical applications have been very few, and mainly based on diets which were selectively deficient in some amino acids. Experimental data are extremely controversial. Some studies have shown that polyunsaturated fatty acids may be capable of promoting tumour growth by directly stimulating mitosis.[300,301]

Others have suggested that tumours may not actually deplete host lipid stores to support their own growth,[302] since fat utilisation by the tumour is poor[303] due to the lack of key enzymes for FFA and ketone body degradation.[101] In human trials, dietary supplementation with omega-3-fatty acids has been shown to inhibit tumour genesis.[304]

There is some evidence however that the energy metabolism of in vivo sarcoma and carcinoma in humans relies predominantly on glucose, with fat-derived calories making no appreciable contribution.[62,142,287,288,305] In our own unit we tested a clinical randomised trial (unpublished data) to see whether two isonitrogenous (1.5 g AA/kg) regimens of 36 (glucose) kcal/kg versus 27 (lipid) + 9 (glucose) kcal/kg could affect the tumour's response to the continuous intra-arterial administration of adryamycin or adryamycin plus ifosphamide. However, preliminary data on the objective response rate and on the percentage of necrosis on the surgical specimen of these soft tissue sarcomas of the limbs showed no difference between the two groups (18 patients each).

The association of lipid TPN with hydrazine sulphate, a gluconeogenic blocking agent, aims at selectively starving the tumour by interrupting the cycle of tumour energy gain–host energy loss at the enzymatic level of phosphoenolpyruvate-carboxy-kinase. The inhibition of gluconeogenesis was originally proposed by Gold[255] and Ray and Hanson[306] and the metabolic efficacy of hydrazine sulphate has been tested in a randomised clinical trial[307] where patients, however, were given a free diet. We tested this regimen on a patient with encouraging results in tolerance and feasibility.[308]

The role of nutrition support in the treatment of the cancer patient is becoming clearer; however, the mechanisms of cachexia development and the means of preventing it will remain a priority in research for many years.

References

1. Edsall DL. Case of acute leukaemia. Am J Med Sc 1905; **130:** 589–600.

2. Musser JH, Edsall DL. Study of metabolism of leukemia under influence of x-ray. Tr Ass Am Phys 1905; **20:** 294–321; also: Univ. Pennsylvania M. Bull 1905–1906; **18:** 174–184.

3. Murphy JB, Means JH, Aub JC. Effect of roentgen ray and radium therapy on metabolism of patient with lymphatic leukemia. Arch Int Med 1917; **19:** 890–900.

4. Waddell WR, Grillo HC. Metabolic effect of fat emulsion. *Am J Clin Nutr* 1949; **7:** 43–50.

5. Bolker N. Nitrogen balance in malignant disease. *Am J Roentgen* 1953; **69:** 839–848.

6. Pareira MD, Conrad EJ, Hicks W, Elman R. Therapeutic nutrition and tube feeding. *JAMA* 1954; **156:** 810–820.

7. Pareira MD, Conrad EJ, Hicks W, Elman R. Clinical response and changes in nitrogen balance, body weight, plasma proteins, and hemoglobin following tube feeding in cancer cachexia. *Cancer* 1955; **8:** 803–808.

8. Terepka AR, Waterhouse C. Metabolic observations during the forced feeding of patients with cancer. *Am J Med* 1956; **20:** 225–230.

9. Watkin D, Steinfeld JL. Nutrient and energy metabolism in patients with and without cancer during hyperalimentation with fat administered intravenously. *Am J Clin Nutr* 1965; **16:** 182–212.

10. Schwartz GF, Green HL, Bendon ML, *et al*. Combined parenteral hyperalimentation and chemotherapy in the treatment of disseminated solid tumors. *Am J Surg* 1971; **121:** 169–173.

11. Roubenhoff R, Heymsfield SB, Kehayias JJ, Cannon JG, Rosenberg IH. Standardization of nomenclature of body composition in weight loss. *Am J Clin Nutr* 1997; **66:** 192–196.

12. Morrison SD. Control of food intake in cancer cachexia: a challenge and a tool. *Physiol Behav* 1976; **17:** 705–714.

13. Nixon DW, Heymsfield SB, Cohen A, *et al*. Protein-calorie undernutrition in hospitalized cancer patients. *Am J Med* 1980; **68:** 683–690.

14. Chute C, Greenberg R. Presenting conditions of 1539 population-based lung cancer patients by cell type and stage in New Hampshire and Vermont. *Cancer* 1985; **56:** 2107–2111.

15. DeWys WD, Begg C, Lavin PT, *et al*. Prognostic effect of weight loss prior to chemotherapy in cancer patients. *Am J Med* 1980; **69:** 491–497.

16. Shils ME. Principles of nutritional support. *Cancer* 1979; **43:** 2093–2102.

17. Issell BF, Valdivieso M, Zaren HA, *et al*. Protection against chemotherapy toxicity by IV hyperalimentation. *Cancer Treat Rep* 1978; **62:** 1139–1143.

18. Samuels ML, Selig DE, Ogden S, *et al*. IV hyper-alimentation and chemotherapy for stage III testicular cancer: a randomized study. *Cancer Treat Rep* 1981; **65:** 615–627.

19. Nixon DW, Moffit S, Lawson DH, *et al*. Total parenteral nutrition as an adjunct to chemotherapy of metastatic colorectal cancer. *Cancer Treat Rep* 1981; **65:** 121–128.

20. Popp MB, Fisher RI, Simon RM, Brennan MF. A prospective randomized study of adjuvant parenteral nutrition in the treatment of diffuse lymphoma: effect on drug tolerance. *Cancer Treat Rep* 1981; **65 (suppl 5):** 129–135.

21. Shamberger RC, Brennan MF, Goodgame JT Jr., *et al*. A prospective, randomized study of adjuvant parenteral nutrition in the treatment of sarcomas: results of metabolic and survival studies. *Surgery* 1984; **96:** 1–12.

22. Goodwin WJ, Torres J. The value of the prognostic nutritional index in the management of patients with advanced carcinoma of the head and neck. *Head Neck Surg* 1984; **6:** 932–938.

23. Clamon GH, Gardner L, Pee D, *et al*. The effect of intravenous hyperalimentation on the dietary intake of patients with small cell lung cancer: a randomized trial. *Cancer* 1985; **55:** 1572–1578.

24. Rickard KA, Logmani ES, Grosfeld JL, *et al*. Short- and long-term effectiveness of enteral and parenteral nutrition in reversing or preventing protein-energy malnutrition in advanced neuroblastoma: a prospective randomized study. *Cancer* 1985; **56:** 2881–2897.

25. Bashir Y, Graham TR, Torrance A, Gibson GJ, Corris PA. Nutritional state of patients with lung cancer undergoing thoracotomy. *Thorax* 1990; **45:** 183–190.

26. Larrea J, Vega S, Martinez T, *et al*. The nutritional status and immunological situation of cancer patients. *Nutricion Hospitalaria* 1992; **7:** 178–187.

27. Tan YS, Nambiar R, Yo SL. Prevalence of protein calorie malnutrition in general surgical patients. *Ann Acad Med* (Singapore) 1992; **21:** 334–341.

28. Bozzetti F, Pagnoni A, Del Vecchio M. Excessive caloric expenditure as a cause of malnutrition in patients with cancer. *Surg Gynecol Obstet* 1980; **150:** 229–234.

29. Cassell P, Robinson JO. Cancer of the stomach: a review of 854 patients. *Br J Surg* 1976; **63:** 603–607.

29a. Bozzetti F, Migliavacca S, Scotti A, *et al*. Impact of cancer, type, site, stage, and treatment on the nutritional status of patients. *Ann Surg* 1982; **196:** 170–179.

30. Belghiti J, Longonnet F, Bourstyn E, Feketé F. Surgical implications of malnutrition and immunodeficiency in patients with carcinoma of the oesophagus. *Br J Surg* 1983; **70:** 339–341.

31. Fein R, Kelsen DP, Geller N, *et al*. Adenocarcinoma of the esophagus and gastroesophageal function: prognostic factors and results of therapy. *Cancer* 1985; **56:** 2512–2518.

32. Meguid MM, Meguid V. Preoperative identification of the surgical patient in need of a postoperative supportive total parenteral nutrition. *Cancer* 1985; **55:** 258–262.

33. Gail MH, Eagan RT, Feld R, *et al.* Prognostic factors in patients with resected Stage I non-small cell lung cancer: a report from the lung cancer study group. *Cancer* 1984; **54:** 1802–1803.

34. Donaldson SS, Wesley MA, DeWys W, *et al.* A study of the nutritional status of pediatric cancer patients. *Am J Dis Child* 1981; **135:** 1107–1112.

35. Grosvenor M, Bulcavage L, Chlebowski RT. Symptoms potentially influencing weight loss in a cancer population. Correlations with primary site, nutritional status, and chemotherapy administration. *Cancer* 1989; **63:** 330–334.

36. Bozzetti F, Agradi E, Ravera E. Anorexia in cancer patients: prevalence and impact on the nutritional status. *Clin Nutr* 1989; **8:** 35–43.

37. Rossi Fanelli F, Cangiano C. Increased availability of tryptophan in brain as a common pathogenic mechanism for anorexia associated with different diseases. *Nutrition* 1991; **7:** 364–367.

38. DeWys WD and Walters K. Abnormalities of taste sensation in cancer patients. *Cancer* 1975; 36: 1888–1896.

39. Shivshanker K, Bennett RW, Jr., Haynie TP. Tumor associated gastroparesis: correction with metoclopramide. *Am J Surg* 1983; **145:** 221–225.

40. Bernstein IL, Bernstein ID. Learned food aversions and cancer anorexia. *Cancer Treat Rep* 1981; **65 (suppl. 5):** 43–47.

41. Brooks SL, Neville AM, Rothwell NH, *et al.* Sympathetic activation of brown adipose tissue thermogenesis in cachexia. *Bioscience Rep* 1981; **1:** 509–517.

42. McFie J, Burkinshaw L, Oxby C, *et al.* The effect of gastrointestinal malignancy on resting metabolic expenditure. *Br J Surg* 1982; **69:** 443–446.

43. Lindmark L, Bennegard K, Eden E, *et al.* Resting expenditure in malnourished patients with and without cancer. *Gastroenterol* 1984; **87:** 402–408.

44. Hyltander A, Drott C, Korner U, Sandstrom R, Lundholm K. Elevated energy expenditure in cancer patients with solid tumours. *Eur J Cancer* 1991; **27:** 9–15.

45. Wallersteiner U. A study on resting metabolic expenditure in cancer patients. 1914.

46. Minot GR and Means JH. The metabolism-pulse ratio in exophthalmic goitre and leukaemia. *Arch Inst Med* 1924; **32:** 576–580.

47. Silver S, Paroto P, Crohn EB. Hypermetabolic states without hyperthyroidism. *Arch Intern Med* 1950; **85:** 479–482.

48. Waterhouse CL, Fenninger LD, Keutmann EH. Nitrogen exchange and caloric expenditure in patients with malignant neoplasm. *Cancer* 1951; **4:** 500–514.

49. Warnold I, Lundholm K, Scherstén T. Energy balance and body composition in cancer patients. *Cancer Res* 1978; **38:** 1801–1807.

50. Burke M, Bryson EI, Kark AE. Dietary intakes, resting metabolic rates, and body composition in benign and malignant gastrointestinal disease. *Br Med J* 1980; **1:** 211–215.

51. Long CL. Energy expenditure during parenteral nutrition. *Ann Surg* 1982; **196(6):** 737–738.

52. Knox L, Crosby L, Feurer I, Hansell J, Mangan C, Mullen JL. Energy expenditure and gynecologic cancer (abstract). *Clin Res* 1980; **28:** 620A.

53. Dempsey DT, Feurer ID, Crosby LO, Knox LS, Buzby GP, Mullen JL. Energy expenditure in malnourished gastrointestinal cancer patients. *Cancer* 1984; **53:** 1265–1273.

54. Axelrod L, Halter JB, Cooper DS, *et al.* Hormone levels and fuel flow in patients with weight loss and lung cancer. Evidence for excessive metabolic expenditure and for an adaptive response mediated by a reduced level of 3,5,3′-triiodothyronine. *Metabolism* 1983; **32:** 924–937.

55. Shike M, Russell D, Detsky AS, Harrison JE, *et al.* Changes in body composition in patients with small-cell lung cancer. The effect of TPN as an adjunct to chemotherapy. *Ann Intern Med* 1984; **101:** 303–309.

56. Russell DM, Shike M, Marliss EB, *et al.* Effects of total parenteral nutrition and chemotherapy on the metabolic derangements in small cell lung cancer. *Cancer Res* 1984; **44:** 1706–1711.

57. Hansell DT, Davies JWL, Burns HJG. The effects on resting energy expenditure of different tumor types. *Cancer* 1986; **58:** 1739–1744.

57a. Hansell DT, Davies JWL, Shenkin A, Burns HJG. Body fuel oxidation in cancer patients and controls. *Clin Nutr* 1986; **15(suppl):** 62.

58. Shaw JHF, Humberstone DA, Wolfe RR. Energy and protein metabolism in sarcoma patients. *Ann Surg* 1988; **207:** 283–289.

59. Nixon DW, Kutner M, Heymsfield S, Foltz AT, Carty CH, Seitz S, *et al.* Resting energy expenditure in lung and colon cancer. *Metabolism* 1988; **37:** 1059–1064.

60. Fearon KCH, Borland W, Preston T, Tisdale MJ, Shenkin A, Calman KC. Cancer cachexia: influence of systemic ketosis on substrate levels and nitrogen metabolism. *Am J Clin Nutr* 1988; **47:** 42–48.

61. Merli M, Riggio O, Romiti M, Caschera A, Attili A, Santis AD, *et al*. Increased resting energy expenditure in patients with hepatocellular carcinoma. *Clin Nutr* 1990; **9(suppl):** 37.

62. Norton JA, Burt ME, Brennan MF. In vivo utilization of substrate by human sarcoma-bearing limbs. *Cancer* 1980; **45:** 2934–2939.

63. Falconer JS, Fearon KCH, Plester CE, *et al*. Cytokines, the acute-phase response and resting energy expenditure in cachectic patients with pancreatic cancer. *Ann Surg* 1994; **219:** 325–331.

64. Grafe E. Die Steigerung des Stoffwechsels bei chronische Leukamie und ihre Ursachen. *Deutsch Arch F Klin Med* 1911; **102:** 406–430.

65. Gunderson AH. The basal metabolism in myelogenous leukemia and its relationship to the blood findings. *Boston Med Surg J* 1921; **185:** 785–787.

66. Boothby WM, Sandiford I. Summary of the basal metabolism data on 8,614 subjects and special reference to the normal standards for the estimation of the basal metabolic rate. *J Biol Chem* 1922; **54:** 783–803.

67. Muller JM, Brenner U, Dienst C, Pichlmayr R. Preoperative parenteral feeding in patients with gastrointestinal carcinoma. *Lancet* 1982; **1:** 68–71.

68. Cascino A, Cangiano C, Ceci F, *et al*. Plasma amino acids in human cancer. Individual role of tumor, malnutrition and glucose tolerance. *Clin Nutr* 1988; **7:** 213–218.

69. Waterhouse C, Jeanpretre N, Keilson J. Gluconeogenesis from alanine in patients with progressive malignant disease. *Cancer Res* 1979; **39:** 1968–1972.

70. Holroyde CP, Gabuzda TG, Putnam RC, *et al*. Altered glucose metabolism in metastatic carcinoma. *Cancer Res* 1975; **35:** 3710–3714.

71. Burt ME, Brennan MF. Nutritional support of the patient with esophageal cancer. *Semin Oncol* 1984; **11:** 127–135.

72. Holroyde CP and Reichard GA. Carbohydrate metabolism in cancer cachexia. *Cancer Treat Rep* 1981; **65(5):** 61–65.

73. Holroyde CP, Skutches CL, Boden G, *et al*. Glucose metabolism in cachectic patients with colorectal cancer. *Cancer Res* 1984; **44:** 5910–5913.

74. Mosconi C, Agradi E, Gambetta A, Bozzetti F, Galli C. Decrease of polyunsaturated fatty acids and elevation of the oleic stearic acid ratio in plasma and red blood cell lipids of malnourished cancer patients. *J Parent Enter Nutr* 1989; **13:** 501–504.

75. Jeevanandam M, Legaspi A, Lowry SF, *et al*. Effect of total parenteral nutrition on whole body protein kinetics in cachetic patients with benign or malignant disease. *J Parent Enter Nutr* 1988; **12:** 229–236.

76. Waterhouse C, Nye WHR. Metabolic effects of infused triglycerides. *Metabolism* 1961; **10:** 403–414.

77. Shaw JHF, Wolfe RR. Glucose and urea kinetics in patients with early and advanced gastrointestinal cancer: the response to glucose infusion, parenteral feeding, and surgical resection. *Surgery* 1987; **101:** 181–191.

78. Muscaritoli M, Cangiano C, Cascino A, *et al*. Plasma clearance of exogenous lipids in patients with malignant disease. *Nutrition* 1990; **6:** 147–151.

79. Chapman HA, Jr., Hibb JB, Jr. Modulation of macrophage tumoricidal capability by components of normal serum: a central role for lipid. *Science* 1977; **197:** 282–285.

80. Shaw JHF, Wolfe RR. Fatty acid and glycerol kinetics in septic patients and in patients with gastrointestinal cancer. *Ann Surg* 1987; **205:** 368–376.

81. Mueller PS, Watkin DM. Plasma unesterified fatty acid concentrations in neoplastic disease. *J Lab Clin Med* 1961; **57:** 95–100.

82. Hays ET. Serum lipids in human cancer. *J Surg Res* 1969; **57:** 95–100.

83. Emery PW, Edwards RHT, Rennie MJ, Souhami RL, Halliday D. Protein synthesis in muscle measured in vivo in cachectic patients with cancer. *Br Med J* 1984; **289:** 584–586.

84. Heslin MJ, Newman E, Wolf RF, Pisters PWT, Brennan MF. Effect of systemic hyperinsulinemia in cancer patients. *Cancer Res* 1992; **52:** 3845–3850.

85. Waterhouse C, Mason J. Leucine metabolism in patients with malignant disease. *Cancer* 1981; **48:** 939–944.

86. Norton JA, Stein TP, Brennan MF. Whole body protein synthesis and turnover in normal man and malnourished patients with and without known cancer. *Ann Surg* 1981; **194:** 123–128.

87. Heber D, Chlebowski RT, Ishibashi DE, Herrold JN, Block JB. Abnormalities in glucose and protein metabolism in non-cachectic lung cancer patients. *Cancer Res* 1982; **42:** 4815–4819.

88. Edén E, Ekman L, Bennegård K, Lindmark L, Lundholm K. Whole-body tyrosine flux in relation to energy expenditure in weight-losing cancer patients. *Metabolism* 1984; **33:** 1020–1027.

89. Jeevanandam M, Horowitz GD, Lowry SF, Brennan MF. Cancer cachexia and protein metabolism. *Lancet* 1984; **1:** 1423–1426.

90. Melville S, McNurlan MA, Calder AG, Garlick PJ. Increased protein turnover despite normal energy metabolism and responses to feeding in patients with lung cancer. *Cancer Res* 1990; **50:** 1125–1131.

91. Shaw JHF, Humberstone DA, Douglas RG, Koea J. Encine kinetics in patients with benign disease, non-weight-losing cancer, and cancer cachexia: studies at the whole-body and tissue level and the response to nutritional support. *Surgery* 1991; **109**: 37–50.

92. O'Keefe SJD, Ogden J, Ramjee G, *et al.* Contribution of elevated protein turnover and anorexia to cachexia in patients with hepatocellular carcinoma. *Cancer Res* 1990; **50**: 1226–1230.

93. Newman E, Heslin MJ, Wolf RF, Pisters PWT, Brennan MF. The effect of insulin on glucose and protein metabolism in the forearm of cancer patients. *Surg Onol* 1992; **1**: 257–267.

94. Dworzak F, Ferrari P, Gavazzi C, Maiorana C, Bozetti F. Effects of cachexia due to cancer on whole body and skeletal muscle protein turnover. *Cancer* 1998; **82**: 42–48.

95. Lundholm K, Bylund AC, Holm J, Scherstén T. Skeletal muscle metabolism in patients with malignant tumour. *Eur J Cancer* 1976; **12**: 465–473.

96. Fearon KCH, McMillan DC, Preston T, *et al.* Elevated circulating interleukin-6 is associated with an acute phase response, but reduced fixed hepatic protein synthesis in patients with cancer. *Ann Surg* 1991; **213**: 26–31.

97. Meguid MM, Muscaritoli M, Beverly JL, *et al.* The early cancer anorexia paradigm: changes in plasma free tryptophan and feeding indexes. *J Parent Enter Nutr* 1992; **16(6)**: 56S–59S.

98. Kubota A, Meguid MM, Hitch DC. Amino acid profiles correlate diagnostically with organ site in three kinds of malignant tumors. *Cancer* 1992; **69**: 2343–2348.

99. Drott C, Svaninger G, Lundholm K. Increased urinary excretion of cortisol and catecholamines in mal-nourished cancer patients. *Ann Surg* 1988; **208**: 645–650.

100. Burt ME, Aoki TT, Gorschboth CM, Brennan MF. Peripheral tissue metabolism in cancer-bearing man. *Ann Surg* 1983; **198**: 685–691.

101. Tisdale MJ. Cancer cachexia: metabolic alterations and clinical manifestations. *Nutrition* 1997; **13**: 1–7.

102. Toomey D, Redmond HP, Bouchier-Hayes D. Mechanisms mediating cancer cachexia. *Cancer* 1995; **76**: 2418–2426.

103. Starnes HF, Jr., Warren RS, Jeevanandam M, *et al.* Tumor necrosis factor and the acute metabolic response to tissue injury in man. *J Clin Invest* 1988; **82**: 1321–1325.

104. Michie HR, Manogue KR, Spriggs DR, *et al.* Detection of circulating tumor necrosis factor after endotoxin administration. *N Engl J Med* 1988; **318**: 1481–1486.

105. Warren RS, Starnes HF, Jr., Gabrilove JL, Oettgen MF, Brennan MF. The acute metabolic effects of tumor necrosis factor administration in humans. *Arch Surg* 1987; **122**: 1396–1400.

106. Bartsch HH, Pfizenmaier K, Schroeer M, *et al.* Intralesional application of recombinant human tumor necrosis factor alpha induces local tumor regressions in patients with advanced malignancies. *Eur J Cancer Clin Oncol* 1989; **25**: 287–291.

107. Socher SH, Martinez D, Craig JB, *et al.* Tumor necrosis factor not detectable in patients with clinical cancer cachexia. *J Natl Cancer Inst* 1988; **80**: 595–598.

108. Selby P, Hobbs S, Viner C, *et al.* Tumor necrosis factor in man. Clinical and biological observations. *Br J Cancer* 1987; **56**: 803–808.

109. Balkwill F, Burke F, Talbot D, *et al.* Evidence for tumour necrosis factor/cachectin production in cancer. *Lancet* 1987; **ii**: 1229–1232.

110. Moldawer L, Rogy M, Lowry S. The role of cytokines in cancer cachexia. *J Parent Enter Nutr* 1992; **16**: 43S–49S.

111. Thompson MP, Cooper ST, Parry BR, *et al.* Increased expression of the mRNA for hormone-sensitive lipase in adipose tissue of cancer patients. *Biochim Biophys Acta* 1993; **1180**: 236–242.

112. Yoneda T, Alsira MA, Chavez JB, *et al.* Evidence that tumor necrosis factor plays a pathogenetic role in the paraneoplastic syndrome of cachexia, hypercalcemia and leukocytosis in a human tumor in nude mice. *J Clin Invest* 1991; **87**: 977–985.

113. Goldberg RM, Loprinzi CL, Mailliard JA, *et al.* Pentoxifylline for treatment of cancer treatment of cancer cachexia and cachexia? A randomized, double-blind, placebo-controlled trial. *J Clin Oncol* 1995; **13**: 2856–2859.

114. Nakazaki H. Preoperative and postoperative cytokines in patients with cancer. *Cancer* 1992; **70**: 709–713.

115. Gelin J, Moldawer LL, Lonnroth C, Sherry B, Chizzonite R, Lundholm K. Role of endogenous tumor necrosis factor alpha and interleukin 1 for experimental tumor growth and the development of cancer cachexia. *Cancer Res* 1991; **51**: 415–421.

116. Strassmann G, Masui Y, Chizzonite R, Fong M. Mechanism of experimental cancer cachexia. Local involvement of IL-1 in colon-26 tumor. *J Immunol* 1993; **150**: 2341–2345.

117. Yamegewa H, Sone S, Takahashi Y, *et al.* Serum levels of interleukin 6 in patients with lung cancer. *Br J Cancer* 1995; **71**: 1095–1098.

118. Kern KA, Norton JA. Cancer cachexia. *J Parent Enter Nutr* 1988; **12**: 286–295.

119. Masuno H, Yoshimura H, Ogawa N, et al. Isolation of a lipolytic factor (toxohormone-L) from ascites fluid of patients with hepatoma and its effect of feeding behaviour. Eur J Cancer Clin Oncol 1984; **20:** 1177–1185.

120. Taylor DD, Gercel-Taylor C, Jenis LG, et al. Identification of a human tumor-derived lipolysis-promoting factor. Cancer Res 1992; **82:** 829–834.

121. Beck SA, Groundwater P, Barton C, et al. Alterations in serum lipolytic activity of cancer patients with response to therapy. Br J Cancer 1990; **62:** 822–825.

122. Wigmore SJ, Ross JA, Falconer JS, et al. The effect of polyunsaturated fatty acids on the progress of cachexia in patients with pancreatic cancer. Nutrition 1996; **12(1 suppl):** S27–S30.

123. Belizario J, Katz M, Chenker E, Raw I. Bioactivity of skeletal muscle proteolysis inducing factors in the plasma proteins from cancer patients with weight loss. Br J Cancer 1993; **63:** 705 –710.

124. Todorov P, Cariuk P, McDevitt T, et al. Characterization of a cancer cachectic factor. Nature 1996; **379:** 739–742.

125. Parrilli G, Iaffaioli V, Martorano M, et al. L'assorbimento intestinale in pazienti con neoplasia mammaria. Riv Ital Nutr Parent Enter 1989; **7:** 21–27.

126. Smale BF, Mullen JL, Buzby GP, et al. The efficacy of nutritional assessment and support in cancer surgery. Cancer 1981; **47:** 2375–2381.

127. Harvey KB, Moldawer LL, Bistrian BR, et al. Biological measures for the formulation of a hospital prognostic index. Am J Clin Nutr 1981; **34:** 2013–2022.

128. Bozzetti F, Migliavacca S, Gallus G, et al. Nutritional markers as prognostic indicators of postoperative sepsis in cancer patients. J Parent Enter Nutr 1985; **9:** 464–470.

129. Swenerton KD, Legha SS, Smith T, et al. Prognostic factors in metastatic breast cancer treated with combination chemotherapy. Cancer Res 1979; **39:** 1552–1562.

130. DeWys WD, Begg C, Band P, et al. The impact of malnutrition on treatment results in breast cancer. Cancer Treat Rep 1981; **65:** 87–91.

131. Bonadonna G, Valagussa P, Santoro A. Alternating noncross-resistant combination chemotherapy or MOPP in stage IV Hodgkin's disease: a report of 8-year results. Ann Int Med 1986; **104:** 739–746.

132. Waren S. The immediate cause of death in cancer. Am J Med Sci 1932; **184:** 610–615.

133. Klastersky J, Daneau D, Verhest A. Causes of death in patients with cancer. Eur J Cancer 1972; **8:** 149–154.

134. Inagaki J, Rodriguez V, Bodey GP. Causes of death in cancer patients. Cancer 1974; **33:** 568–573.

135. Ambrus JL, Ambrus CM, Mink IB. Causes of death in cancer patients. J Med 1975; **6:** 61–64.

136. Bozzetti F. Effects of artificial nutrition on the nutritional status of cancer patients. J Parent Enter Nutr 1989; **13:** 406–420.

137. Bozzetti F. Nutritional support in adult cancer patients. Clin Nutr 1992; **11:** 167–179.

138. Burt ME, Gorschboth CM, Brennan MF. A controlled, prospective, randomized trial comparing the metabolic effects of enteral and parenteral nutrition in the cancer patient. Cancer 1982; **49:** 1092–1105.

139. Bozzetti F, Ammatuna M, Migliavacca S, et al. Total parenteral nutrition prevents further nutritional deterioration in patients with cancer cachexia. Ann Surg 1987; **205:** 138–143.

140. Evans WK, Makuch R, Clamon GH. Limited impact of total parenteral nutrition on nutritional status during treatment for small cell lung cancer. Cancer Res 1985; **45:** 3347–3353.

141. Ota DM, Frasier P, Guevara J, Foulkes M. Plasma protein as indices of response to nutritional therapy in cancer patients. J Surg Oncol 1985; **29:** 160–165.

142. Burt ME, Stein TP, Brennan MF. A controlled, randomized trial evaluating the effects of enteral and parenteral nutrition on protein metabolism in cancer-bearing man. J Surg Res 1983; **34:** 303–314.

143. Bennegard K, Eden E, Ekman L, Scherstén T, Lundholm K. Metabolic response of whole body and peripheral tissues to enteral nutrition in weight-losing cancer patients. Gastroenterology 1983; **85:** 92–99.

144. Fan ST, Law WY, Wong KK, Chan WP. Preoperative parenteral nutrition in patients with oesophageal cancer: a prospective, clinical trial. Clin Nutr 1989; **8:** 23–27.

145. James H, Fabricius P, Chettle D, Dykes P. Whole body nitrogen and potassium measured by neutron activation analysis and whole body counting in malnourished cancer patients. Riv Ital Nutr Parent Enter 1985; **3:** 93–104.

146. Moghissi K, Hornshaw J, Teasdale PR, Dawes EA. Parenteral nutrition in carcinoma of the oesophagus treated by surgery: nitrogen balance and clinical studies. Br J Surg 1977; **64:** 125–128.

147. Cohn SH, Vartsky D, Vaswani AN, et al. Changes in body composition of cancer patients following combined nutritional support. Nutr Cancer 1982; **4:** 107–119.

148. Braga M, Cristallo M, Spiegel P, Staudacher C, et al. Valutazione dello stato nutrizionale e alimentazione enterale nel paziente portatore di neoplasia del tubo digerente. Riv Ital Nutr Parent Ent 1983; **2:** 30–40.

149. Rasmussen A, Segel E, Trier E, Aagaard M, Hessov I. The effect of preoperative nutrition on the immune system. *Clin Nutr* 1985; **4:** 175–178.

150. Ota DM, Jessup JM, Babcock GF, *et al.* Immune function during intravenous administration of a soybean oil emulsion. *J Parent Enter Nutr* 1985; **9:** 23–27.

151. Ota DM, Nishioka K, Foulkes M, Grossie VB. Nutritional parameters affecting erythroctye polyamine levels in cancer patients. *J Clin Oncol* 1984; **2:** 1157–1164.

152. Ota DM, Nishioka K, Grossie B, Dixon D. Erytrocyte polyamine levels during intravenous feeding of patients with colorectal carcinoma. *Eur J Cancer Clin Oncol* 1986; **7:** 837–842.

153. Lim STK, Choa RG, Lam KH, Wong J, Ong GB. Total parenteral nutrition versus gastrostomy in the perioperative preparation of patients with carcinoma of the oesophagus. *Br J Surg* 1981; **68:** 69–72.

154. Balzola F, Palmo A, Protta F, Avagnina S, *et al.* La terapia nutrizionale in pazienti portatori di neoplasia del capo colla in trattamento radiante. Parte prima: dati antropometrici. *Riv Ital Nutr Parent Ent* 1984; **3:** 30–54.

155. Daly JM, Hearne B, Dunaj J, *et al.* Nutritional rehabilitation in patients with advanced head and neck cancer receiving radiation therapy. *Am J Surg* 1984; **148:** 514–520.

156. Cristallo M, Braga M, Villa E, Baccari P, Di Carlo V. Nutrizione enterale palliativa nel trattamento della malnutrizione del paziente neoplastico. *Riv Ital Nutr Parent Enter* 1984; **3:** 19–30.

157. Ravera E, Radaelli G, Migliavacca S, Bozzetti F. Effetti della nutrizione enterale sullo stato nutrizionale dei pazienti con cachessia neoplastica. *Riv Ital Nutr Parent Ent* 1986; **4:** 43–50.

158. Lundholm K, Gelin J, Hyltander A, *et al.* Anti-inflammatory treatment may prolong survival in undernourished patients with metastatic solid tumors. *Cancer Res* 1994; **S4(21):** 5602–5606.

159. Bennegard K, Lindmark L, Eden E, *et al.* Flux of amino acids across the leg in weight-losing cancer patients. *Cancer Res* 1984; **44:** 386–393.

160. Haffejee AA, Angorn IB. Nutritional status and non-specific cellular and humoral immune-response in oesophageal carcinoma. *Ann Surg* 1979; **189:** 457–479.

161. Almond DY, King RF, Burkinshaw L, Laughland A, McMahon MJ. Potassium depletion in surgical patients: intracellular cation deficiency is independent of loss of body protein. *Clin Nutr* 1987; **6:** 45–50.

162. Dulloo AG. Regulation of body composition during weight recovery: integrating the control of energy partitioning and thermogenesis. *Clin Nutr* 1997; **16:** 25–35.

163. Forbes GB. Lean body mass–body fat interrelationships in humans. *Nutr Rev* 1987; **45:** 225–231.

164. Henry CJK, Rivers JPW, Payne PR. Protein and energy metabolism in starvation reconsidered. *Eur J Clin Nutr* 1988; **42:** 543–549.

165. Elia M. Effect of starvation and very low calorie diets on protein-energy interrelationships in lean and obese subjects. In: Scrimshaw NS, Schurch B (eds) Protein-Energy Interactions, IDECG, Lausanne, Switzerland, 1991, pp. 249–284.

166. Prentice AM, Goldberg GR, Jebb SA, Black AE, Murgatroyd PR. Physiological responses to slimming. *Proc Nutr Soc* 1991; **50:** 441–458.

167. Shaw JHF, Wolfe RR. Whole-body protein kinetics in patients with early and advanced gastrointestinal cancer: the response to glucose infusion and total parenteral nutrition. *Surgery* 1988; **103:** 148–155.

168. Hyltander A, Warnold I, Eden E, Lundholm K. Effect on whole-body protein synthesis after institution of intravenous nutrition in cancer and non-cancer patients who lose weight. *Eur J Cancer* 1991; **27:** 16–21.

169. Gray G, Meguid M. Can total parenteral nutrition reverse hypoalbuminemia in oncology patients? *Clin Nutr* 1990; **6:** 225–228.

170. Monson JRT, Ramsden CW, MacFie J, Brennan TG, Guillou PJ. Immunorestorative effect of lipid emulsions during total parenteral nutrition. *Br J Surg* 1986; **73:** 843–846.

171. Bozzetti F, Cozzaglio L, Villa ML, Ferrario E, Trabattoni D. Restorative effect of total parenteral nutrition on natural killer cell activity in malnourished cancer patients. *Eur J Cancer* 1995; **12:** 2023–2027.

172. Dresler CM, Jeevanandam M, Brennan MF. Metabolic efficacy of enteral feeding in malnourished cancer and noncancer patients. *Metabolism* 1987; **36:** 82–88.

173. Klein S, Simes J, Blackburn GL. Total parenteral nutrition and cancer clinical trials. *Cancer* 1986; **58:** 1378–1386.

174. McGeer AJ, Detsky AS, O'Rourke K. Parenteral nutrition in cancer patients undergoing chemotherapy: a meta-analysis. *Nutrition* 1990; **6:** 233–240.

175. Haffejee AA, Angorn IB. Oral alimentation following intubation for esophageal cancer. *Ann Surg* 1977; **186:** 165–170.

176. Holter AR, Fisher JE. The effects of perioperative hyperalimentation on complications in patients with carcinoma and weight loss. *J Surg Res* 1977; **23:** 31–34.

177. Thompson BR, Julian TB, Stremple JF. Perioperative parenteral nutrition in parents with gastrointestinal cancer. *J Surg Res* 1981; **30:** 497–500.

291. Jebb SA, Marcus R, Elia M. A pilot study of oral glutamine supplementation in patients receiving bone marrow transplants. *Clin Nutr* 1995; **14:** 162–165.

292. Earl S, Wood D, Gardner MLG. The effects of elemental diets and glutamine supplementation on intestinal absorptive function. *Clin Nutr* 1995; **14:** 134 (abstract).

293. Van der Hulst RRW, Van Kneel BK, von Meyenfeldt MF, *et al.* Glutamine and preservation of gut integrity. *Lancet* 1993; **34:** 1363–1365.

294. Conversano L, Muscaritoli M, Petti MC, *et al.* Effects of oral glutamine on high-dose chemotherapy (HDCT)-induced gastrointestinal toxicity in acute leukaemia patients: a pilot study. *Clin Nutr* 1995; **14:** 6 (abstract).

295. Souba WW, Strebel FR, Bull JM, *et al.* Interorgan metabolism in the tumour-bearing rat. *J Surg Res* 1988; **44:** 720–726.

296. Chen MK, Sallourm RM, Austgen TR, *et al.* Tumor regulation of hepatic glutamine metabolism. *J Parent Enter Nutr* 1991; **15:** 159–164.

297. Chen MK, Espat NJ, Bland KI, *et al.* Influence of progressive tumor growth on glutamine metabolism in skeletal muscle and kidney. *Ann Surg* 1993; **217:** 655–667.

298. Penn RL, Maca RD, Berg RD. Increased translocation of bacteria from the gastrointestinal tracts of tumour-bearing mice. *Infect Immun* 1985; **47:** 793–798.

299. Souba WW, Klimberg VS, Salloum RM, *et al.* Tumor modulation of intestinal glutaminase activity. *FASEB J* 1990; **4:** A1042 (abstract).

300. Tsai M, Yu C, Wei F, Stacey D. The effect of GTPase activating protein upon Ras is inhibited by mitogenically responsive lipids. *Science* 1988; **243:** 522–525.

301. Imagawa W, Bandyopadhyay G, Wallace D, Nandi S. Phospholipids containing polyunsaturated acyl groups are mitogenic for normal mouse mammary epithelial cells in serum free primary cell culture. *Proc Natl Acad Sci USA* 1989; **86:** 4122–4126.

302. Ookhtens M, Kannan R, Lyon I, Baker N. Liver and adipose tissue contributions to newly formed fatty acids in an ascites tumor. *Am J Physiol* 1984; **247:** R146–153.

303. Cederbaum AI, Rubin E. Fatty acid oxidation, substrate shuttles, and activity of the citric acid cycle in hepatocellular carcinomas of varying differentiation. *Cancer Res* 1976; **36:** 2980–2987.

304. Anti M, Marra G, Armelao F, *et al.* Effect of omega-3 fatty acids on rectal mucosal cell proliferation in subjects at risk for colon cancer. *Gastroenterology* 1992; **103:** 883–891.

305. Holm E, Hagmüller E, Staedt U, *et al.* Substrate balances across colonic carcinomas in humans. *Cancer Res* 1995; **55:** 1373–1378.

306. Ray PD, Hanson RL. Inhibition of gluconeogenesis by hydrazine. *Fed Proc* 1969; **28:** 411 (abstract).

307. Tayek JA, Heber D, Chlebowski RT. Effect of hydrazine sulphate on whole-body protein breakdown measured by 14C-lysine metabolism in lung cancer patients. *Lancet* 1987; **2:** 241–243.

308. Bozzetti F, Cozzaglio L, Gavazzi C, *et al.* Total nutritional manipulation in humans: report of a cancer patient. *Clin Nutr* 1996; **15:** 207–209.

38

Nutrition support in the elderly

DG Smithard, G Blandford and GK Grimble

Introduction

The concept of what is 'elderly' is fraught with difficulty. For insurance purposes, actuaries set the threshold of becoming 'old' at 60–65 years, which is typically marked by retirement. The arbitrary decision by the German Chancellor, Prince Otto von Bismarck, in the 19th century set retirement at 70 years (later 65 years) as part of a group of social security reforms which included health and accident insurance and old-age pensions. The distinction is artificial, however, and nowadays many people more than 65 years of age feel affronted to be called elderly. Indeed, it is salutary to consider that two of the most out-standing European leaders of the 20th century (Winston Churchill and Konrad Adenauer), who took office at very trying moments, did so at the ages of 65 and 73, respectively.

The trend of increasing longevity means that some people will spend as many years in retirement as they have done in paid work. This 'third age' has been artificially divided into three periods or phases, the young-old (65–75), the middle-old (76–85) and the old-old (more than 85). The burden of disability typically increases with age, and it is the oldest-old who have the greatest levels of dependency.

Between 1960 and 1994, the population of the United States increased by 45% but those over the age of 65 years of age increased by 100%, whilst the old-old (>85 years) increased by 274% to a total of three million. On this basis the elderly represent the fastest growing cohort, such that it is projected that, by 2041, two-thirds of the population will be older than 60 years and 36.5% will be older than 70 years.[1,2] Within these age groups there is a predominance of women, particularly in the oldest age groups. This phenomenon is often associated with poverty, loneliness and isolation.

Ageing

Growing older is not a disease process, nor are elderly people just 'old' young people. Increasing age brings physiological changes that affect homeostasis. For instance, renal glomerular filtration and hepatic blood flow both decrease with age even though there may be no diminution of function (Baltimore longitudinal study). However, the reduction in reserve capacity may mean that the body is less able to handle nutrient loads, or toxins or insults and stressors such as injury and infection, respectively.[3]

In addition, ageing is associated with a change in body composition. A general reduction occurs in lean body mass (in excess of that predicted by reduced dietary intake alone),[4] in total body water, cell mass and bone mineral density.[5] In contrast, central adiposity increases although this is not universally accepted.[6] Finally, in the very old, body fat and lean mass are lost in concert, perhaps mediated via a leptin mechanism.[7]

Loss of muscle during ageing has serious consequences and is associated with increased mortality and morbidity within the 2–3-day time-frame after illness or stress which results also in a reduced caloric intake.[8] The scale of muscle loss (sarcopenia) ranges from 15% of muscle strength (50–60 years) to 30% between 70 and 80 years although it is not inevitable and can be reversed by exercise programmes.[9,10]

Ageing itself, social isolation and the impact of chronic diseases and disabilities often impair both the ability to acquire and prepare food and the desire to eat. This can arise from age-related changes in taste and smell: a reduction in the number of taste buds/papillae in the tongue leads to a relative preponderance of bitter and sweet receptors. Older people tend to prefer salty to sweet food, and in many instances food which they had previously enjoyed can taste bland. All of these factors mean that careful attention has to be paid to nutrition require-ments in elderly people.

Energy requirements

Several prevalence studies have shown that, between the ages of 20 and 80 years, energy intake declines linearly to approximately 2000 kcal/day or less.[11,12] This is associated with a tendency to eat a diet containing relatively less fat than carbohydrate,[6,13] but this does not necessarily lead to malnutrition. This change is driven partly by a reduction in basal metabolic rate and partly by a dysregulation of appetite.[14,15] The ability to regulate energy intake appears to be reduced. This affects weight regulation in that the ability to return to the previous body weight after a period of weight gain (or loss) is markedly impaired.[6]

This loss of fine tuning of the appetite–energy balance loop has one benefit. When food supple-ments (e.g. drinks, snacks) are provided in order to boost energy intake[16,17] then it has been found that, if they are given 90 minutes before a main meal, there is no diminution of energy intake from that meal. The net result is an increase in daily energy intake. Older people have a greater degree of satiation with food; however the mechanism is not food-specific, unlike in younger patients,[18] but may predominantly be controlled by feedback from stomach stretch receptors combined with an age-related delay in gastric emptying.[19]

Energy expenditure is best represented by two measures: basal metabolic rate (BMR) and total energy expenditure (TEE). BMR can reasonably be calculated from FAO/WHO estimates,[20] but the issue has recently been re-examined. Indirect calorimetry on 40 healthy aged men and women suggested that present predictive equations underestimate BMR by about 6%.[21] The equation which best fits this data is:

$$\text{TEE (kcal)} = 1641 + [10.7 \times \text{weight (kg)}] - [9.0 \times \text{age (years)}] - 203 \times \text{sex (1 = male, 2 = female)}$$

More recently, the combination of the double-labelled water technique and portable indirect calorimetry in healthy, free-living aged people[22] has shown that BMR calculated from Schofield's equations[23] was most accurate whilst TEE could be predicted best from the equations developed by Fredrix and colleagues.[21]

In hospitalised older people, however, the effects of stress further increase energy requirements.[24] As a rule of thumb, energy expenditure can be calculated in this group using a formula based both on the level of clinical stress (i.e. severity of illness) and on the level of physical activity, which is generally assumed to be 400–600 kcal/day for hospital patients:

Low stress – 20 kcal/kg/day

Moderate stress – 25–35 kcal/kg/day

Severe stress – 35 kcal/kg/day

Whilst this method may overestimate needs, its simplicity and economy recommend it. Physical activity may use up to 35% of energy expenditure,[25] and with increasing age the efficiency of energy use declines; this may contribute to the slowing of pace of tasks that is often observed.[26] Thus a healthy woman of 70 years of age will expend 20% more energy than a younger woman walking at the same standard speed. Maintaining an active lifestyle is associated with better health and lower morbidity and mortality.[27]

Nutritional needs of the elderly

There have been several recent reviews of the nutritional needs of the elderly.[6,15,28–32] The accepted measure for daily nutrient intake in the USA and the UK is still the recommended dietary allowance (RDA) (Food and Nutrition Board, National Research Council 1989) but, unfortunately, 'elderly' is defined as anyone over the age of 50 years. More recently, dietary reference intakes (DRI) have been published and provide values up to the age of 70 years.

Protein

It is not clear whether protein requirements are increased or decreased in elderly patients. It is estimated that 10–25% of American women over the age of 75 years eat less than 30 g of protein per day.[33] Certainly, the presence of sarcopenia would suggest a lower skeletal muscle mass and thus reduced protein synthesis and amino acid requirements. This is a controversial topic since it depends on experimental data which suffer from the limitations of nitrogen balance and protein turnover methods discussed by Rennie and colleagues in Chapter 2. In brief, the earliest ^{15}N turnover studies suggested that protein synthesis decreases with age,[34] and this view has been reinforced by more recent studies which suggest that metabolic demand for the tracer amino acid (^{13}C-leucine) is lower in elderly subjects (68–91 years) than in younger controls.[35] In contrast, Young and colleagues have consistently argued that tracer-labelling and nitrogen balance studies support a mean protein requirement somewhat higher than the 0.60 g/kg/d recommended by the 1985 Joint FAO/WHO/UNU Expert Consultation. They suggest that a safer protein intake would be in the range 1.0–1.25 g/kg/d.[36,37] The key to this argument is whether one considers it possible to manipulate protein supplementation in such a way that the inevitable muscle loss that occurs with ageing can be reversed or at least halted.[38] It is intriguing that protein pulse-feeding (i.e. 80% of protein intake at midday) led to improved protein retention in elderly women[39] but not in young women.[40] There is clearly scope for specific interventions in the frail elderly in whom there has been loss of skeletal muscle with its consequent reduction in mobility and increase in dependency.[41]

Carbohydrates and fibre

It is recommended that 55–60% of total calories should consist of carbohydrate, predominantly complex carbohydrates,[42] with a concomitant reduction in simple sugars.[43] A modest increase in dietary fibre may improve glucose tolerance, which is beneficial as insulin resistance may develop with increasing age. It may also lower serum lipids, reduce constipation and the possible formation or complications of colonic diverticuli, and reduce the incidence of colonic cancer.[44] Fresh fruits and vegetables, a good source of fibre, reduce the relative risk of stroke and cardio-vascular disease.[45] Foods that are high in fibre may be difficult to chew or digest and may be relatively expensive. Cereals, though easy to eat and relatively inexpensive, generally have a low fibre content. The addition of fibre (bran) to food reduces the nutritional density of the total diet,[46] so that, whenever high-fibre foods are recommended, the target of 20–35 g fibre/day should also include attempts to increase the energy density of the diet. It is often useful to instruct patients to eat fruits and vegetables that 'crunch'; how-ever, it should be recognised that phytate present in some fibre sources (cereals, legumes, and vegetables) may impair calcium, zinc and iron absorption.

Fat

Fat deficiency is rarely encountered because the western diet is often overloaded with fat; indeed, it estimated that the American diet comprises 40% fat. Essential fatty acid deficiency can be observed in patients who receive long-term tube-feeding with diets that are either low in fat (e.g. elemental diets, see Ch. 18) or in which the essential fatty acid content is low but there is a high proportion of medium chain triglycerides.

In contrast, obesity is often associated with diseases that improve with weight reduction (e.g. hypertension, diabetes, and arthritis of weight-bearing joints). In an effort to improve health (heart disease, hypertension, cholesterol levels, diabetes) an attempt has been made to reduce the fat content of the diet to 30%. This may often make food relatively unpalatable and, since the diet of many elderly people living in reduced circum-stances may be marginal at best,[9] further nutrient reductions may be ill advised . Dietary weight reduc-tion is usually unsuccessful and the benefits are hard to measure. Increased physical activity and education are, therefore, generally better than dieting to manage obe-sity complicated by hypertension and diabetes.[47]

Vitamins

Much of what is known about vitamin deficiency in the elderly in Europe has been obtained from the SENECA project, which investigated the nutrition status of the healthy, free-living elderly population in 18 communities across Europe.[48] Despite the cultural and gastronomic diversity of Europe, folate and retinol status was found to be adequate, and prevalence of vitamin B_{12} and vitamin E deficiency was low, whereas vitamin B_6 deficiency was widespread.[49] The trend between 1988/89 and 1993 was for vitamin E, folate and vitamin B_6 status to improve but vitamin B_{12} status worsened (deficiency increased from 2.7% to 7.3%), primarily amongst women.[50] Deficiency, or at least marginal vitamin status of a different pattern, has also been observed in healthy elderly kibbutzniks in Israel,[51] in health-conscious elderly Parisians,[52] in rural Italians,[53] and in the citizens of Framingham.[54] If institutionalised elderly people are considered, the situation is more serious, since Dutch and British studies found that 73% of subjects had deficient 25-hydroxyvitamin D status, 28% were folate deficient and 28–56% had biochemical vitamin B_6 deficiency.[55,56] A similar Australian study[57] considered weighed dietary records and found that the overwhelming majority of long-stay subjects had intakes of macronutrients, vitamins (A, B_6, D, E), folate, magnesium and zinc which were less than 70% of the recommended daily allowance (RDA). Hospitalisation of the elderly is associated with a further reduction in vitamin status (especially in patients with infection), particularly in relation to antioxidant defences.[58,59] The theoretical basis of these observations is described in detail in Chapters 5 and 11. As will be discussed later, the relationship between neurocognitive disorders in elderly patients and vitamin deficiency (especially of the B group) has been known for many years,[60] even though its aetiology is still unclear.[61]

The progressive and selective reduction in vitamin status during ageing, especially in the face of illness, arises from several causes. Reduced macronutrient intake is probably the most common global reason[57] and is exacerbated by a poor-quality diet. Specific vitamin deficiencies may arise for clinical reasons. Although atrophic gastritis is more common in elderly subjects and is thought to be the main reason for loss of intrinsic factor release and subse-quent B_{12} malabsorption, it arises from several causes (bacterial overgrowth, *H. pylori* infection and impaired acid secretion).[62] Malignancy is a common cause of folate deficiency, as is associated chemotherapy. Impaired renal function is related to poor vitamin D and calcium status. Alcohol abuse is closely related to osteoporosis in men,[63] to vitamin B_1 deficiency (a major cause of neurocognitive dysfunction – Wernicke's encephalopathy) and, more rarely, to nicotinamide deficiency,[64] in addition to vitamin A,[65] riboflavin and B_6 deficiency. Alcohol abuse also depresses folate status and increases plasma homocysteine concentration,[66] an independent risk factor for stroke and cardiovascular disease. In the context of nutritional treatment of the elderly, in healthy individuals the combined likelihood of alcohol abuse and 'heavy drinking' is 1 in 7,[67] whereas in cognitively impaired elderly institutionalised patients approximately 1 in 4 have alcohol-related dementia compared to 1 in 3 with Alzheimer's disease.[68]

In the United States, where megadoses of vitamins are often taken, hypervitaminosis is rarely diagnosed. The most common form, hypervitaminosis A, arises insidiously from excess intake of fish-oil capsules (with hypervitaminosis D), from use of topical retinoic acid to prevent photo-ageing of the skin, and from excessive dietary intake of liver.

Minerals (Table 38.1)

Few data are available to help formulate requirements for minerals in the elderly, and dietary recom-

Table 38.1 – Mineral deficiency, causes and effects

Mineral	Cause of deficiency	Effects of deficiency
Sodium	Diuretics Fluid overload Inappropriate ADH Sweat	Hypotension Reduced skin turgor Fits
Potassium	Diuretics Steroids B_{12} replacement Diarrhoea Villous adenoma Adrenal or renal disease	Hypertension Lethargy Weakness Arrhythmias
Calcium	Vitamin D_3 deficiency Low albumin Renal disease Bisphosphonates Hypoparathyroidism Some malignancies	Tetany Osteomalacia
Zinc	Protein deficiency Diuretics Urinary loss	Impaired immune function and wound healing Impaired night vision ?Macular degeneration ?Loss of taste
Magnesium	Diuretics	Angina Stroke
Iron	Blood loss Atrophic gastritis Post gastrectomy Inflammatory bowel disease ?Vitamin C deficiency	Anaemia
Selenium	?	Ageing, reduced defence against free radicals, poor enzymatic function
Other trace elements, copper, iodine	Diet Amiodarone	Hypothyroidism

mendations must therefore remain tentative.[69] In view of the well-understood relationship between calcium intake and osteoporosis, this subject has been carefully reviewed and it is thought that the RDA is too high. In contrast, the recommendations for magnesium and chromium are probably too low. Use of diuretics can result in excessive losses of magnesium, sodium and potassium.

Reasons for poor dietary intakes

A healthy diet contributes to the health, well-being and survival of the older person.[6,70] With increasing age, however, the risk of poor nutrition status is increased, often secondary to a poor diet. Those aged over 79 years are most likely to be undernourished; of those admitted to hospital, up to 30% will have a degree of malnutrition.[71]

There are many reasons why some older people are unable to meet their physiological needs (Table 38.2) and there are often several factors (medical, social, psychological and economic) which should be considered.

Table 38.2 – Percentages of older people unable to meet their own needs

Factor	Age group	Prevalence (%)
Assistance with feeding	65–84	2
	>85	7
Food preparation	65–69	3.5
	75–84	16
	>85	26.1
Difficulty shopping	65–69	1.9
	75–84	29
	>85	37
Not shopping	65–74	11
	>75	30
Not cooking	65–74	6
	>75	12
Unable to climb stairs	>85	50
Help with finances	75–84	12

adapted from [6]

Altered appetite

Taste perception is altered during ageing and this has consequences for appetite, especially in the very old.[72] One study has noted that impaired olfactory functioning (i.e. preference for sour/sweet and pungent foods and high-fat foods) in free-living elderly people was strongly related to nutritional risk (e.g. waist:hip ratios).[73]

Inadequate chewing

Eating will be impaired by local oral pathology such as pain from gingivitis, fractured and decayed teeth, loss of dentition, and impaired salivation or other conditions such as candidiasis or cancer.[74,75] In addition, a high percentage (74%) of older people are edentulous following a lifetime of dental neglect;[76,77] ill-fitting dentures cause pain and may result in social embarrassment, sitophobia and isolation. Two studies have characterised the way in which food intake differs between elderly subjects with adequate natural dentition or inadequate natural dentition, with or without dentures. As expected, ease of eating and ultimately dietary intake were determined by the number of functional units (i.e. opposable teeth), not the number of teeth. The Italian study suggested that dentures were a fully effective replacement for natural teeth,[78] whereas an American study suggested otherwise.[79]

Impaired swallowing

The 'normal swallow' that occurs in more than 80% of young individuals is a symmetrical and synchronised act[80] which may be present in only 16% of those over the age of 70 who otherwise have no evidence of dysphagia.[81] Healthy ageing itself is not associated with swallowing difficulties.[82] Rather, with age, nerve conduction velocity slows, tongue muscle strength reduces and there is reduced compliance in the pharyngo-oesophageal segment of the pharynx[83] which results in variability in the swallowing process.[81,84,85] Swallowing problems are caused by concomitant disease rather than ageing *per se*[86,87] and may affect 16% of those over 87 years of age,[88] 10% of the acutely hospitalised elderly[29] and 30–60% of nursing and residential home residents.[89,90] The greater the level of dependence, the greater the prevalence of dysphagia. Oropharyngeal dysphagia may often be mild and its detection requires good observation of the way patients eat; it may require further investigation. Oral incontinence (dribbling, spillage of food from the mouth) is embarrassing and may lead the older person to decide not to eat in social situations where food is available, because of anxiety.

Social factors (Table 38.3)

Co-morbidity and dependency increase with age and approximately half of the retirement years will be spent with disability. In addition, loneliness, isolation (bereavement, loss of friends) and poverty all take their toll. Mobility may be reduced because of arthritis, and lack of personal and public transport (especially in rural areas) may reduce access to foodstuffs forming a balanced diet. Illness may also impair the person's ability to cook. The housebound and those on a low income often eat diets that are low in meat, fish, eggs and green vegetables. Those on low incomes need to spend a higher proportion of their income on food, but there is often competition from heating, lighting and medical bills. Many of these issues are admirably reviewed by Köhler and colleagues.[91] Feinberg et al.[92] suggest that social isolation and reduced oral intake may lead to disuse deconditioning and an increased risk of aspiration, though they offer no evidence to support this. Attendance at luncheon clubs or day centres increasing socialisation, or, in the case of institutions, more pleasant surroundings, results in an increased intake of energy and protein during meal-times.[93,94]

The need for nutrition support

Body composition changes with age: an initial increase in adiposity (middle-aged spread) is followed by a loss of adiposity in later years (old-old). Both have implications for prognosis. Whilst the risks of obesity are well known, the reverse of the coin is less well described (Table 38.4). Significant weight loss with age often precedes significant disease.[95,96]

Table 38.3 – Reasons why older people are unable to meet their nutritional needs

Social
- Isolation
- Poverty
- Lack of facilities
- Elder abuse (physical, financial)
- Institutionalisation
- Lack of access to shops
- No transport

Medical
- Special diets (low-salt, low-cholesterol)
- Endocrine disorders (diabetes, hyperparathyroidism, hyperthyroidism)
- Malabsorption
- Medication
- Malignancy
- Immobility (stroke, arthritis, amputation)
- Infection
- Loss of taste or of desire to eat
- Dysphagia (oral, candidiasis)
- Dry mouth (drugs, Sjögren's)
- Edentulous
- Vitamin/iron deficiency
- Malignancy
- Ulceration (oesophageal, gastric, duodenal)
- Presbyoesophagus

Psychiatric/psychological
- Depression
- Late-life paranoia
- Food avoidance
- Recurrence of anorexia nervosa
- Cognitive loss
- Alcohol or drug abuse

Table 38.4 – Effects and consequences of undernutrition

Effects
- Weight loss
- Reduced cell-mediated immunity
- Osteopenia
- Sarcopenia
- Altered drug metabolism
- Reduced response to antibiotics and vaccines

Consequences
- Anaemia
- Infection
- Falls
- Immobility
- Confusion
- Depression
- Decubitus ulcers
- Poor response to surgery
- Poor wound healing
- Respiratory problems
- Death

Anorexia of ageing

Anorexia of ageing has been called the idiopathic pathological state, or senile anorexia, and occurs in response to a reduction in metabolism and physical inactivity.[6] Anorexia of ageing has also been defined as age-enhanced dysfunction of the physiological regulation of appetite.[14] Its main nutritional characteristics are weight loss, low serum albumin and low cholesterol. There may be an associated increase in cytokines (IL-6 and TNF) and a reduction in cortical neuropeptide Y and hypothalamic noradrenaline.[96] The condition is characterised by thin, deconditioned people with poor balance[3] whose failure to thrive may be irreversible. Part of the syndrome arises from undernutrition itself.

Undernutrition in hospitalised patients

In 1974, Butterworth declared that malnutrition was the skeleton in the acute hospital closet.[97] This skeleton is still to be found in other health care settings and in the community at large. In the United States, malnutrition is estimated to affect 10–25% of the elderly in the community, 30–61% of hospital patients, and 17–85% of nursing home residents.[33,98–102] These numbers are highest for those aged over 80. McWhirter and Pennington[103] noted that 40% of 500 admissions to hospital in the UK were undernourished (BMI <20); in this group, by the time of discharge, there had been a mean loss in weight of 5.4%. Only 96 cases had any nutrition assessment, and only 10 had contact with a dietitian.

Protein–energy malnutrition (i.e. loss of more than 10% of body weight in less than 6 months, low BMI, serum albumin (<35 g/l) and low cholesterol (<130 g/dl) is present in 15% of those living independently in the community, 5–12% of the housebound, 20–65% of those in hospital, and 5–85% of those in institutional care. Incalzi[104] noted that nutrition depletion occurred in 27% of those admitted to an acute setting. In this group, the stress of illness or surgery will lead to increased energy expenditure and decreased energy intake (see Ch. 3).

Undernutrition in free-living elderly people

Depression, debility and a sedentary lifestyle result in reduced active metabolic mass and contribute to protein loss (see Ch. 3). Many older people take less exercise because of social isolation and the presence of concurrent disabilities such as osteoarthritis. This lack of activity results in a loss of muscle tone and mass and a consequent vicious circle.[105] Consequently, nutrition support in the elderly requires a parallel and appropriate exercise programme, and the appropriate management of any psychiatric/cognitive problems.

A more individualised approach to the management of energy and protein requirements is needed.[30] If this recommendation is followed, the diet should reflect the need for both increased energy expenditure and extra protein for muscle building. Unfortunately, high-quality protein is often expensive, as is attendance at the gym, and both are often beyond the means of the socially and economically compromised elderly.

Effects of undernutrition

A 50% mortality rate has been noted in those who are poorly nourished, compared to 16% in the adequately nourished.[106] Low serum albumin is associated with an increase in mortality, ranging from 1.7% with a level of 35 g/l to 62% with a level less than 20 g/l. Abnormal lymphocyte levels are associated with a 4-fold increase in mortality, an abnormal albumin six times and both an 8-fold increase in morbidity and a 9-fold increase in mortality. A cholesterol level of less than 4.0 mmol is associated with increased mortality.

Water

Total body water declines with age, from 60% in young adults to 50% at the age of 80 years, being more marked in women. Philips et al.[107] in a landmark paper stated that there was a decline in thirst with age, possibly because of changes in endocrine and renal function.

Dehydration in the elderly is a common and very serious problem constituting a potential threat to life and often requiring hospitalisation. A small shift in fluid balance and increase in osmolality[108] may have severe consequences, exacerbated by the presence of co-morbid conditions. Dehydration is difficult to diagnose, may occur very rapidly, and causes fever, leucocytosis, marked postural hypotension, constipation, nausea and vomiting, decreased urine output, and delirium or death.

The commonest causes are urinary and respiratory infections, low fluid intake, diuretic use, diabetes mellitus, hypercalcaemia and reduced concentrating ability of the renal tubules.[109] In the hospital setting, dehydration may occur if a person is sitting by a window on a hot day, with no ready supply of fluid.

The healthy elderly should be encouraged to drink about 30 ml/kg/d. Unfortunately, however, they are often reluctant to drink adequate amounts of liquids, often due to concomitant incontinence or nocturia. In most care settings the nursing staff and/or family should be encouraged to use specific fluid intake goals (e.g. 2 l/d) rather than being given the meaningless instruction to 'push fluids'.

Nutrition assessment

This subject has been dealt with in detail in Chapter 9 and only aspects peculiar to ageing will be considered here.

Nutrition assessment is multifaceted and constitutes part of a comprehensive geriatric assessment[110] involving many members of the multidisciplinary team (recall, dietitian, swallowing, speech and language therapist; doctor, medical aspects (Table 38.5); nursing, mattress assessment).[111,112] There may be a need to discuss the case with the family and the patient's general practitioner (family physician). The older

Table 38.5 – Assessment of nutrition status

		Factors to look for:
History	Eating difficulties Weight loss Bowel habit Chronic disease Smoking Alcohol Living alone Ability to shop Ask GP, relatives, carers	Look for presence of cardiac disease, obstructive lung disease, rheumatoid arthritis Neurological disease (Parkinson's disease, motor neurone disease, stroke, dementia)
Examination	Physical size Obesity, body fat Thin Tremor Strength Skin turgor Dry mouth, state and/or presence of teeth Mucosae, nails Weight Neurological assessment including swallowing Demispan/Body Mass Index	Look for evidence of body fat, skin turgor Any clinical evidence of anaemia, recent or sudden weight loss Compare with photographs, fitting of clothes Check for presence of dysphagia, may require referral to speech and language therapist Body Mass Index and weight may be inaccurate
Investigation	Full blood count Vitamins B$_{12}$ and folic acid Urea, creatinine Electrolytes Glucose Thyroid function tests Liver function tests (albumin) Cholesterol Chest radiograph (Consider barium meal, enema, endoscopy, ultrasound of abdomen)	Haemoglobin, mean cell volume, haematocrit Leucocytes and lymphocytes

person and his or her carers often have great difficulty in recognising and acknowledging the presence and consequences of undernutrition or 'failure to thrive'. A low threshold to diagnosis is essential: often, by the time the overt clinical picture has been recognised, the underlying causes are not reversible.

Many tools are available for the assessment of nutrition status.[113] The Mini-Nutritional Assessment (MNA)[114] has been validated for all settings, from the community to the nursing home, and is currently in widespread use in continental Europe. Adding the MNA to the interdisciplinary assessment facilitates early diagnosis and identification of reversible causes of undernutrition. Repeated assessments permit the monitoring of therapeutic interventions. A recent study[115] suggested that observation of a person eating was more sensitive than the Residents Assessment Instrument in detecting undernutrition.

Early and repeated nutritional screenings to identify those at risk or those with early malnutrition, with appropriate supplemental diets to correct nutritional deficits, would appear to be an appropriate public health measure. Unfortunately, even when malnutrition is accurately diagnosed, appropriate non-nutritional therapeutic interventions (e.g. personal assistance with feeding, transportation) may be unavailable or unaffordable, and nutritional support may also be too expensive. No satisfactory cost–benefit study has confirmed a consistent and beneficial outcome for widespread use of nutrition supplements in malnourished elderly persons.[28,116] Without this, and with the current fiscal restraint being imposed on national health care systems worldwide, preventative nutrition support for the elderly would appear to have little chance of being adequately financed. Only education and appropriate, longitudinal clinical research can offer opportunities to resolve this dilemma.

Dementia and nutrition support

Dementia (of Alzheimer's type or vascular dementia) results in global cognitive and physical functional decline, with increasing dependence on others for all activities of daily living, and particularly in later stages the provision of nutrition and hydration.

Nutrition status often becomes compromised due to forgetting to eat, being distracted while eating, non-

oral agnosia/dyspraxia (inability to feed), the exhibition of behaviour that is sometimes inaccurately called 'refusal to eat' or 'dysphagia' (evidence of oropharyngeal dysphagia). 'Refusal to eat' usually derives from the display of physically resistive or aversive feeding behaviours (AFB), most likely caused by protective reflexes when a spoon is thrust towards the face or the hands are held away from the mouth.[117]

Once oral dysphagia appears and is persistent, the question arises whether or not to provide nutrition support for the impending dehydration and malnutrition.[118] There are no data to support the notion that the provision of adequate nutrition will either restore normal eating and brain function or arrest disease progression. Careful consideration must therefore be given to whether nutrition support is an appropriate goal of care. This is discussed later.

Stroke and nutrition support

A hypercatabolic state often ensues after an acute stroke,[119,120] with deterioration in the nutrition status being most marked in the first week.[120a]

In the presence of dysphagia, nutrition is often ignored for several weeks, managed only by a dextrose infusion, despite the desire for rehabilitation to continue. If the various techniques used by the speech and language therapist, with or without equipment provided by the occupational therapist and dietitian (special cups and cutlery) do not enable the patient to swallow safely or to independently meet nutritional demands, then provision of calories needs to be considered. This may be by the provision of sip-feeds[121] or the use of enteral feeding to provide part or all of the nutritional needs of the patient. Patients who do not take nutrition, either independently or via means of support, tend to die of protein–energy malnutrition within 60–70 days.[122] In those with persistent dysphagia following stroke, the use of enteral feeding would appear to be morally and ethically justifiable but at this time lacks a significant evidence base.

Management of undernutrition

Accurate, reproducible clinical and laboratory assessment of malnutrition in the elderly remains elusive.[123]

Moreover, while it may be reasonable, humane, ethical, moral and legal to attempt to correct malnutrition in the elderly, evidence is increasing that nutritional supplementation improves anthropometric indices but may not affect outcome. Results have been more encouraging where there has been a concomitant disease state.[124,125] The causes for these disappointing results are directly related to the heterogeneity of the problems that impair eating in the elderly population.

General

When the causes of undernutrition have been identified by a multidimensional geriatric assessment, an interdisciplinary approach is essential to coordinate and integrate the patient's medical treatment with his or her nutritional needs and other goals of care. It is important for all care providers to recognise that the financial and functional assistance necessary to obtain, prepare, and eat food is as important as providing the appropriate constituents in the diet, the treatment of oral pathology and co-morbidities (e.g. diabetes) and review of all medication.

Environment

In many cases very simple approaches to the management of nutrition are all that are required. The provision of pleasant surroundings within a nursing home setting often results in an increase in food intake. Some older people do not prepare food because of the tedium of cooking for one, particularly when they used to cook for two, and the provision of company, such as at a luncheon club or Age Concern, may provide the stimulus to eat again.

It may also be helpful to provide carers to help people eat, if there are difficulties transferring food from the plate to the mouth. For those with mild oropharyngeal dysphagia, modified foods, the provision of water at the table and the time to eat are all important components in the process.

It has been clearly shown that an aggressively promoted exercise and rehabilitation programme is essential to increasing calorie intake.[126] Many elderly patients are either very reluctant or simply unable to increase their physical activity.

Dietary modification

It is important to pay attention to the presentation of food, particularly if it is thickened or pureed.

Thickened drinks do not taste pleasant, and pureed food is often presented as an amorphous mass, like something from a jar of baby food. Presentation of pureed food to look like real food can often recreate interest.

Many therapeutic diets for common co-morbid conditions (e.g. low-salt, low-fat, low-carbohydrate diets) significantly reduce the palatability of meals. The problems they address may often be managed with alternate therapies permitting the use of favourite foods and thus improving nutrition intake. General strategies include frequent small meals (for those who are easily fatigued), favourite foods and oral nutritional supplements (snacks or proprietary liquids).

In those patients for whom swallowing is difficult, strategies to aid swallowing[86] and modified diets may be useful (e.g. thickeners, chopping, pureeing, attention to flavour and temperature, etc.). Appropriate seating and support of the head while swallowing help to improve the safety of the swallow.

Sip-feeds

The use of sip-feeds is controversial because evidence for efficacy depends on the disease group in which their use has been studied. In stroke patients there has been a suggestion of benefit;[121,127] this has also been the case in malnourished patients with cognitive disorders. The strongest evidence for benefit has been found in patients with fractured neck of femur;[128] however a recent study by Espaulella et al.[129] has questioned these findings on the grounds that whilst complication rates were decreased there was no improvement in functional recovery or fracture-related mortality. The general use of sip-feeds in the healthy elderly is not evidence based[6] but there is evidence for the provision of nutrients for the frail older person and those in hospital.[121] A systematic review by Potter and colleagues suggests that sip-feeds may help to improve the nutritional markers of the frail older person, but may not improve outcome.[127] This issue is discussed in more detail in Chapter 41.

Enteral feeding

In those with more severe problems and those who can not take food orally, enteral provision of nutrition needs to be considered. The routes available for feeding include a nasogastric tube, gastrostomy (commonly a percutaneous endoscopic gastrostomy – PEG) and the now discontinued technique of rectal infusion.[130] There has been an increasing use of fine-bore nasogastric tubes and gastrostomy feeding.[131] Techniques for this are described in Chapter 17.

When using either a nasogastric tube (NGT) or PEG, the aim is to provide nutrition, not to prevent aspiration. Nasogastric tubes if anything may increase the risk of aspiration by slowing pharyngeal transit, by premature triggering of the swallow[132] and by reducing the competence of the oesophagogastric sphincter and increasing pharyngeal secretions. There is ample evidence that the risk of aspiration of oropharyngeal secretions and even feeds persists or increases with gastrostomy feeding.[133,134]

Those patients who have had a PEG inserted are often the most vulnerable or have had the most profound strokes, and it is not surprising that 67% of stroke patients die within 3 months of the gastrostomy being inserted. Infection around the gastrostomy site is common; recent work has suggested that prophylactic antibiotics may reduce this.[135] Gastrostomy feeding may be associated with reflux of feed and delayed gastric emptying. Prokinetic drugs have been used successfully to treat this, as have proton pump inhibitors. An alternative is to ensure that the feeding tube is placed into the jejunum.[136,137] Rimmer et al.[138] suggest that the complication rate is lower if the PEG has been inserted by a team orientated towards the older adult.

PEG vs NGT

Many patients find the nasogastric tube physically and psychologically uncomfortable. This may result in treatment failures.[139–141] It has been generally considered that a PEG is preferred over a nasogastric tube on the grounds of body image, however this is not true for all. There are many psychological and social implications, not only for the patient with a PEG but also for the carer.

How long should a nasogastric tube be persevered with? It should remain *in situ*, if possible, until either the swallow has improved sufficiently to enable the patient to meet his or her own nutrition requirements; if the tube has been removed by the patient on numerous occasions and it is considered that this is not a statement of intent then a PEG should be considered. In the case of a patient with stroke, the swallow needs to be continually assessed between day 7 and day 14. If it is improving, then oral feeding should be instituted; if not, then a PEG should be considered. Evidence has been presented[142] that those

later provided with PEG feeding tend to be older and to fare worse.

The majority of those patients in whom a PEG has been sited are heavily dependent and may be terminally ill. All patients discharged from hospital with a PEG require follow-up to review their physical needs and, if appropriate, to reassess the ability to swallow.[143,144] PEGs need replacing, and advice is often required on how to clear blocked tubes.

Parenteral nutrition

Parenteral nutrition should rarely be used unless the gastrointestinal tract is compromised. It does have a role when there is a delay in having a PEG placed and the patient will not allow a nasogastric tube to stay in place.

Ethical dilemmas

The medical profession and other care providers need to be persuaded that persistent failure to eat is a terminal event in irreversible progressive brain failure, and is equivalent to other organ system failures that result in death. Although life can be physiologically sustained with artificial nutrition and hydration, there is no evidence that quality of life is improved (on balance it is usually made worse by artificial feeding) and no improvement in the primary pathology can be expected.

At present, in the United Kingdom, there is much debate about the provision of nutrition to patients with brain injury. A balance needs to be struck between the prevention of death and the postponement of the inevitable. In many situations the decisions are simple. In some situations, however, the patient is neither dying nor rapidly improving. When the cognitive dysfunction is not the result of vitamin deficiency, it is these patients who present us with ethical and moral dilemmas. What should one do? Should enteral nutrition be used as a curative tool, could it not also be a palliative tool?

It is important that the patient's loved ones are aware that withholding or withdrawing tube feeding in terminal patients does not mean no treatment. All patients should be offered whatever care is necessary to relieve pain and suffering. It should also be made clear that dying from dehydration is a peaceful and pain-free death, that death is not optional, and that what we perceive as life may have been considered intolerable and undignified suffering by the patient. In the United States, where pro-life forces are extremely active, laws now exist to ensure that previously stated patient preferences regarding all medical and life-sustaining treatments are honoured.

One point, however, is clear cut: doing nothing will result in the death of the individual, but providing nutrition may not be of benefit. It is in this situation that the cost–benefit (burden) ratio for the patient needs to be considered. Lennard-Jones[145] suggested that enteral nutrition is a treatment that can be switched on and off. This view is supported by the British Medical Association[146] and the Nursing Board of Control.[128] However, how can the success of enteral nutrition be assessed over a short period of time? What would be assessed/measured? How can quality of life be assessed?

The provision of enteral nutrition requires consent, but often this is assumed to have been given for the passing of a NGT, unless it is refused. What might refusal of a NGT mean? What statement is being made by the patient who persistently removes the NGT? The insertion of a PEG requires formal consent. How can we ensure that *informed* consent has been obtained, especially in the dysphasic or cognitively impaired patient? What is the best interest of the patient? What is quality of life, and whose quality of life is being considered? What about autonomy?

Finally, we must consider whom we are treating: the patient, the family or ourselves. Whatever decisions are made must be for the good of the patient; often, however, they are made for the good of the relatives or clinical staff and this may not be justifiable. Whatever decision is made, it must be done after con-sultation with the relatives and the multidisciplinary team and after everyone is made aware that any decision not to feed will lead to death.

The future

There is still a great deal to be learned with respect to the management of nutritional care. The authors would suggest that the following areas require high-quality investigation:

- Many carers are not aware of ways in which they can assess the nutritional needs of an older person. In the hospital and institutional setting, nutrition is

often forgotten, and in the United Kingdom dietetic support is limited.

- The use of afternoon snacks needs to be explored more systematically.

- The effect of sip-feeds on outcome for the frail older person needs to be explored in greater depth to understand its effect on outcome (length of stay, Barthel score, Modified Rankin Index mortality).

- The use of supplemental and/or enteral feeding in various disease-specific areas needs further exploration (FOOD Trial).[147] Does the provision of extra calories improve outcome?

- What are the physiological and biochemical changes that occur after the withdrawal of nutrition and/or fluids? Does someone feel thirst when fluids are withdrawn but the mouth is kept wet?

References

1. Grundy E. Ageing, ill health and disability. In: Tallis RC (ed) *Increasing longevity*. Royal College of Physicians, London, 1998.

2. Warnes MA. Population ageing over the next few decades. In: Tallis RC (ed) *Increasing longevity*. Royal College of Physicians, London, 1998.

3. Horan MA. Advances in understanding the concept of biological ageing. In: Tallis RC (ed) *Increasing longevity*. Royal College of Physicians, London, 1998.

4. Ruiz-Torres A, Gimeno A, Munoz FJ, Vincent D. Are anthropometric changes in healthy adults caused by modifications in dietary habits or by ageing? *Gerontology* 1995; **41:** 243–251.

5. Yearick ES. Nutritional status of the elderly: Anthropometric and clinical findings. *J Gerontol* 1978; **33(5):** 657–662.

6. Morley JE. Anorexia of aging: physiologic and patho-logic. *Am J Clin Nutr* 1997; **66:** 760–773.

7. Mizuno TM, Ross A, Mobbs CV. Age-related changes in leptin: consequences and mechanisms. *Rev Clin Gerontol* 2000; **10:** 99–108.

8. Schlenker ED. Nutrition in Ageing. St Louis: Mosby 1993; pp 105–34.

9. Evans WJ, Cyr-Campbell D. Nutrition, exercise, and healthy aging. *J Am Diet Assoc* 1997; **97(6):** 632–638.

10. Fielding RA. Effects of exercise training in the elderly: impact of progressive-resistance training on skeletal muscle and whole-body protein metabolism. *Proc Nutr Soc* 1995; **54(3):** 665–675.

11. McGandy RB, Barrows CH, Spanias A. Nutrient intakes and energy expenditure in men of different ages. *J Gerontol* 1966; **21:** 581–587.

12. NHANES 3rd National Health and Nutrition Examination Survey, phase III 1988–91. Daily dietary fat and total food energy intakes. *MMWR Morb Mortal Weekly Rep* 1994; **43:** 116–125.

13. Wurtman JJ, Lieberman H, Tsay R. Calorie and nutrient intakes of elderly young subjects measured under identical conditions. *J Gerontol* 1988; **43:** B174–180.

14. Sinclair AJ. Anorexia of aging as a risk factor for weight loss in older humans. *Rev Clin Gerontol* 2000; **10:** 97–98.

15. Gariballa SE, Sinclair AJ. Assessment and treatment of nutritional status in stroke patients. *Postgrad Med J* 1998; **74:** 395–399.

16. Gall MJ, Grimble GK, Reeve NJ, Thomas SJ. The effect of providing fortified meals and between meal snacks on energy and protein intake of hospital patients. *Clin Nutr* 1998; **17(6):** 259–264.

17. Olin AÖ, Österberg P, Hadell K, Armyr I, Jerstrom S, Ljungqvist O. Energy-enriched hospital food to improve energy intake in elderly patients. *J Parent Enteral Nutr* 1996; **20:** 93–97.

18. Blundell JE, Stubbs RJ. High and low carbohydrate and fat intakes: limits imposed by appetite and palatability and their implications for energy balance. *Eur J Clin Nutr* 1999; **53 Suppl 1:** S148–S165.

19. Wegener M, Borsch G, Schaffstein J, Luth I, Rickels R, Ricken D. Effect of ageing on the gastro-intestinal transit of a lactulose-supplemented mixed solid-liquid meal in humans. *Digestion* 1988; **39:** 40–46.

20. WHO/FAO/UNU Report. *Energy and protein requirements.* WHO, Geneva, Technical Report Series 724, 1985.

21. Fredrix EW, Soeters PB, Deerenberg IM, Kester AD, von Meyenfeldt MF, Saris WH. Resting and sleeping energy expenditure in the elderly. *Eur J Clin Nutr* 1990; **44(10):** 741–747.

22. Fuller NJ, Sawyer MB, Coward WA, Paxton P, Elia M. Components of total energy expenditure in free-living elderly men (over 75 years of age): measurement, predictability and relationship to quality-of-life indices. *Br J Nutr* 1996; **75:** 161–173.

23. Schofield WN. Predicting basal metabolic rate, new standards and review of previous work. *Hum Nutr Clin Nutr* 1985; **39 Suppl 1:** 5–41.

24. Klipstein-Grobusch K, Reilly JJ, Potter J, Edwards CA, Roberts MA. Energy intake and expenditure in elderly patients admitted to hospital with acute illness. *Br J Nutr* 1995; **73(2):** 323–334.

25. Elia M. Energy expenditure in the whole body. In: Kinney JM, Tucker HN (eds) *Energy metabolism: Tissue determinants and cellular corollaries.* Raven Press, New York, 1992: 19–59.

26. Bassey EJ, Terry AM. The oxygen cost of walking in the elderly. *J Physiol* 1986; **42:** 373.

27. Bassey EJ. The benefits of exercise for the health of older people. *Rev Clin Gerontol* 2000; **10:** 17–31.

28. Thomas N. Nutrition in practice: nutrition in the elderly. *Nursing Times* 1998; **94(8): suppl** 1–6.

29. Hudson HM, Daubert CR, Mills RH. The interdependency of protein–energy malnutrition, aging, and dysphagia. *Dysphagia* 2000; **15(1):** 31–38.

30. Sullivan D, Lipschitz D. Evaluating and treating nutritional problems in older patients. *Clin Geriatr Med* 1997; **13(4):** 753–768.

31. Chernoff R. Baby boomers come of age: nutrition in the 21st century. *J Am Diet Assoc* 1995; **95(6):** 650–54.

32. Lehman AB. Nutrition and health: what is new? *Rev Clin Nutr* 1996; **6:** 147–168.

33. Mowe M, Bohmer T, Kindt E. Reduced nutritional status in an elderly population (>70) is probably before disease and possibly contributes to the development of disease. *Am J Clin Nutr* 1994; **33:** 3–15.

34. Golden MHN, Waterlow JC. Total protein synthesis in elderly people: a comparison of results with ^{15}N-glycine and ^{14}C-leucine. *Clin Sci Mol Med* 1977; **53:** 277–288.

35. Fereday A, Gibson NR, Cox M, Pacy PJ, Millward DJ. Protein requirements and ageing: metabolic demand and efficiency of utilization. *Br J Nutr* 1997; **77(5):** 685–702.

36. Campbell WW, Crim MC, Dallal GE, Young VR, Evans WJ. Increased protein requirements in elderly people: new data and retrospective reassessments. *Am J Clin Nutr* 1994; **60(4):** 501–509.

37. Gersovitz M, Motil K, Munro HN, Scrimshaw NS, Young VR. Human protein requirements: assessment of the adequacy of the current Recommended Dietary Allowance for dietary protein in elderly men and women. *Am J Clin Nutr* 1982; **35(1):** 6–14.

38. Short KR, Nair KS. The effect of age on protein metabolism. *Curr Opin Clin Nutr Metab Care* 2000; **3(1):** 39–44.

39. Arnal MA, Mosoni L, Boirie Y, *et al.* Protein pulse feeding improves protein retention in elderly women. *Am J Clin Nutr* 1999; **69(6):** 1202–1208.

40. Arnal MA, Mosoni L, Boirie Y, *et al.* Protein feeding pattern does not affect protein retention in young women. *J Nutr* 2000; **130(7):** 1700–1704.

41. Millward DJ. Optimal intakes of protein in the human diet. *Proc Nutr Soc* 1999; **58(2):** 403–413.

42. Macdonald IA. Carbohydrate as a nutrient in adults: range of acceptable intakes. *Eur J Clin Nutr* 1999; **53 Suppl 1:** S101–S106.

43. Sheiham A. Why free sugars consumption should be below 15 kg per person per year in industrialised countries: the dental evidence. *Br Dent J* 1991; **171(2):** 63–65.

44. O'Keefe SJ. Nutrition and gastrointestinal disease. *Scand J Gastroenterol (Suppl)* 1996; **220:** 52–59.

45. Gariballa SE. Nutritional factors in stroke. *Br J Nutr* 2000; **84(1):** 5–17.

46. Hermann JR, Hanson CF, Kopel BH. Fiber intake of older adults: Benefits not yet proved. *J Nutr Elderly* 1992 **11:** 21–32.

47. Marks DL, Cone RD. Central melanocortins and the regulation of weight during acute and chronic disease. *Recent Prog Horm Res* 2001; **56:** 359–375.

48. 't Hof MA, Hautvast JG, Schroll M, Vlachonikolis IG. Design, methods and participation. Euronut SENECA investigators. *Eur J Clin Nutr* 1991; **45 Suppl 3:** 5–22.

49. Haller J, Weggemans RM, Lammi-Keefe CJ, Ferry M. Changes in the vitamin status of elderly Europeans: plasma vitamins A, E, B-6, B-12, folic acid and carotenoids. Investigators. *Eur J Clin Nutr* 1996; **50 Suppl 2:** S32–S46.

50. Haller J, Lowik MR, Ferry M, Ferro-Luzzi A. Nutritional status: blood vitamins A, E, B6, B12, folic acid and carotene. Euronut SENECA investigators. *Eur J Clin Nutr* 1991; **45 Suppl 3:** 63–82.

51. Havivi E, Levin N, Reshef A. Nutritional status in elderly population in kibbutzim. *Int J Vitam Nutr Res* 1985; **55(3):** 351–355.

52. Cals MJ, Bories PN, Devanlay M, *et al.* Extensive laboratory assessment of nutritional status in fit, health-conscious, elderly people living in the Paris area. Research Group on Aging. *J Am Coll Nutr* 1994; **13(6):** 646–657.

53. Alberti-Fidanza A, Coli R, Genipi L, *et al.* Vitamin and mineral nutritional status and other biochemical data assessed in groups of men from Crevalcore and Montegiorgio (Italy). *Int J Vitam Nutr Res* 1995; **65(3):** 193–198.

54. Selhub J, Jacques PF, Wilson PW, Rush D, Rosenberg IH. Vitamin status and intake as primary determinants of homocysteinemia in an elderly population. *JAMA* 1993; **270(22):** 2693–2698.

55. Lowik MR, van den BH, Schrijver J, Odink J, Wedel M, van Houten P. Marginal nutritional status among institutionalized elderly women as compared to those living more independently (Dutch Nutrition Surveillance System). *J Am Coll Nutr* 1992; **11(6):** 673–681.

56. Smith JL, Wickiser AA, Korth LL, Grandjean AC, Schaefer AE. Nutritional status of an institutionalized aged population. *J Am Coll Nutr* 1984; **3(1):** 13–25.

57. Lipski PS, Torrance A, Kelly PJ, James OF. A study of nutritional deficits of long-stay geriatric patients. *Age Ageing* 1993; **22(4):** 244–255.

58. Pfitzenmeyer P, Guilland JC, d'Athis P. Vitamin B6 and vitamin C status in elderly patients with infections during hospitalization. *Ann Nutr Metab* 1997; **41(6):** 344–352.

59. Schmuck A, Roussel AM, Arnaud J, Ducros V, Favier A, Franco A. Analyzed dietary intakes, plasma concentrations of zinc, copper, and selenium, and related antioxidant enzyme activities in hospitalized elderly women. *J Am Coll Nutr* 1996; **15(5):** 462–468.

60. Wallace JI, Schwartz RS, LaCroix AZ, Uhlmann RF, Pearlman RA. Involuntary weight loss in older outpatients: incidence and clinical significance. *J Am Geriatr Soc* 1995; **43:** 329–337.

61. Selhub J, Bagley LC, Miller J, Rosenberg IH. B vitamins, homocysteine, and neurocognitive function in the elderly. *Am J Clin Nutr* 2000; **71(2):** 614S–620S.

62. Carmel R, Aurangzeb I, Qian D. Associations of food-cobalamin malabsorption with ethnic origin, age, Helicobacter pylori infection, and serum markers of gastritis. *Am J Gastroenterol* 2001; **96(1):** 63–70.

63. Vanderschueren D, Boonen S, Bouillon R. Osteoporosis and osteoporotic fractures in men: a clinical perspective. *Baillieres Best Pract Res Clin Endocrinol Metab* 2000; **14(2):** 299–315.

64. Cook CC, Hallwood PM, Thomson AD. B Vitamin deficiency and neuropsychiatric syndromes in alcohol misuse. *Alcohol Alcohol* 1998; **33(4):** 317–336.

65. Lieber CS. Biochemical factors in alcoholic liver disease. *Semin Liver Dis* 1993; **13(2):** 136–153.

66. Cravo ML, Gloria LM, Selhub J, *et al.* Hyperhomocysteinemia in chronic alcoholism: correlation with folate, vitamin B-12, and vitamin B-6 status. *Am J Clin Nutr* 1996; **63(2):** 220–224.

67. Adams WL, Cox NS. Epidemiology of problem drinking among elderly people. *Int J Addict* 1995; **30(13–14):** 1693–1716.

68. Carlen PL, McAndrews MP, Weiss RT, *et al.* Alcohol-related dementia in the institutionalized elderly. *Alcohol Clin Exp Res* 1994; **18(6):** 1330–1334.

69. Wood RJ, Suter PM, Russell RM. Mineral requirements of elderly people. *Am J Clin Nutr* 1995; **62(3):** 493–505.

70. Department of Health. Nutrition in the Elderly. Report on Health and Social Subjects No. 43 1992 HMSO.

71. Larsson J, Unosson M, Ek A-C, Nilsson L, Thorslund S, Bjurulf P. Effect of dietary supplement on nutritional status and clinical outcome in 501 geriatric patients – a randomised study. *Clin Nutr* 1990; **9:** 179–184.

72. Hetherington MM. Taste and appetite regulation in the elderly. *Proc Nutr Soc* 1998; **57(4):** 625–631.

73. Duffy VB, Backstrand JR, Ferris AM. Olfactory dysfunction and related nutritional risk in free-living, elderly women. *J Am Diet Assoc* 1995; **95(8):** 879–884.

74. MacEntee MI, Stolar E, Glick N. Influence of age and gender on oral health and related behaviour in independent elderly population. *Community Dent Oral Epidemiol* 1993; **21:** 234.

75. Ship JA, Duffy V, Jones JA, Langmore S. Geriatric oral health and its impact on eating. *J Am Geriatr Soc* 1996; **44:** 456–464.

76. Todd JE, Walker AM. Adult dental health, England and Wales, 1968–1978, Volume 1. HMSO, London, 1980.

77. Fiske J, Watson RM. The benefit of dental care to the elderly population assessed using sociodental measure of oral handicap. *Br Dent J* 1990; **168:** 513–516.

78. Appollonio I, Carabellese C, Frattola A, Trabucchi M. Influence of dental status on dietary intake and survival in community-dwelling elderly subjects. *Age Ageing* 1997; **26(6):** 445–456.

79. Hildebrandt GH, Dominguez BL, Schork MA, Loesche WJ. Functional units, chewing, swallowing, and food avoidance among the elderly. *J Prosthet Dent* 1997; **77(6):** 588–595.

80. Ekberg O, Nylander G. Cineradiography of the pharyngeal stage of deglutition in 150 individuals without dysphagia. *Br J Radiol* 1982; **55:** 253–257.

81. Ekberg O, Feinberg MJ. Altered swallowing function in elderly patients without dysphagia: radiologic findings in 56 cases. *AJR Am J Roentgenol* 1991; **156(6):** 1181–1184.

82. Blonsky ER, Logemann JA, Boshes B, Fisher HB. Comparison of speech and swallowing function in patients with tremor disorders and in normal geriatric patients: A cinefluorographic study. *J Gerontol* 1975; **30(3):** 299–303.

83. Tracy JF, Logemann JA, Kahrilas PJ, Jacob P, Kobara M, Krugler C. Preliminary observations on the effects of age on oropharyngeal deglutition. *Dysphagia* 1989; **4:** 90–94.

84. Robbins JA, Levine R, Maser A, Rosenbek JC, Kempster GB. Swallowing after unilateral stroke of the cerebral cortex. *Arch Phys Med Rehabil* 1993; **74:** 1295–1299.

85. Light KE, Spirduso WW. Effects of adult aging on the movement complexity factor of response programming. *J Gerontol* 1990; **45(3):** 107–109.

86. Logemann JA. *Evaluation and treatment of swallowing disorders*. College-Hill Press, San Diego, 1983.

87. Elliot JL. Swallowing disorders in the elderly: A guide to diagnosis and treatment. *Geriatrics* 1988; **43(1):** 95–113.

88. Bloem BR, Lagaay AM, van Beek W, Haan J, Roos RA, Wintzen AR. Prevalence of subjective dysphagia in community residents aged over 87. *BMJ* 1990; **300(6726):** 721–722.

89. Smithard DG. Swallowing and eating difficulties in institutionalised patients. *Clin Rehab* 1996; **2:** 153–4.

90. Mendez L, Friedman LS, Castell DO. Swallowing disorders in the elderly. *Clin Geriatr Med* 1991; **7:** 215–230.

91. Köhler BM, Feichtinger E, Barlösius E, Dowler E (eds) *Poverty and food in welfare societies*. Edition Sigma, Reiner Bohn Verlag, Berlin, 1997.

92. Feinberg MJ, Knebl J, Tully J, Segall L. Aspiration and the elderly. *Dysphagia* 1990; **5:** 61–71.

93. De Castro JM, Brewer EM, Elmore DK, Orazco S. Social facilitation of the spontaneous meal size of humans occurs regardless of time, place, alcohol or snacks. *Appetite* 1990; **15:** 89–101.

94. Isaksson B. How to avoid malnutrition during hospitalization? *Hum Nutr Appl Nutr* 1982; **36A:** 367–370.

95. Morley JE. Anorexia in older persons: epidemiology and optimal treatment. *Drugs Aging* 1996; **8(2):** 134–155.

96. Morley JE, Thomas DR. Anorexia and aging: pathophysiology. *Nutrition* 1999; **15(6):** 499–503.

97. Butterworth CE Jr. Malnutrition in hospital. *JAMA* 1974; **230:** 879.

98. Morley JE, Silver AJ. Nutritional issues in nursing home care. *Ann Intern Med* 1995; **123(11):** 850–859.

99. Verdery RB. Failure to thrive in the elderly. *Clin Geriat Med* 1995; **11:** 653–659.

100. Wallace JI, Schwartz RS, LaCroix AZ, Uhlmann RF, Pearlman RA. Involuntary weight loss in older outpatients: incidence and clinical significance. *J Am Geriatr Soc* 1995; **43:** 329–337.

101. Sullivan PH, Walls RC. Impact of nutritional status on morbidity in a population of geriatric rehabilitation patients. *J Am Geriatr Soc* 1994; **42:** 471–477.

102. Sullivan DH. Impact of nutritional status on health outcomes of nursing home residents. *J Am Geriatr Soc* 1995; **43(2):** 195–196.

103. McWhirter JP, Pennington CR. Incidence and recognition of malnutrition in hospital. *BMJ* 1994; **308:** 945–948.

104. Incalzi RA, Gemma A, Capparella O, *et al.* Energy intake and in-hospital starvation. A clinically relevant relationship. *Arch Intern Med* 1996; **156:** 425–429.

105. Gariballa SE, Sinclair AJ. Diagnosing undernutrition in elderly people. *Rev Clin Gerontol* 1997; **7:** 367–371.

106. Friedman PJ, Campbell AJ, Caradoc-Davies TH. Prospective trial of a new diagnostic criteria for severe wasting malnutrition in the elderly. *Age Ageing* 1985; **14:** 149–154.

107. Philips PA, Rolls BJ, Ledingham JGG, *et al.* Reduced thirst after water deprivation in health elderly men. *N Engl J Med* 1984; **311:** 753–759.

108. O'Neill PA, Faragher EB, Davies I *et al.* Reduced survival with increasing plasma osmolality in elderly continuing care patients. *Age and Ageing* 1990; **19:** 68–71.

109. de Castro JM, Brewer EM, Elmore DK, Orazco S. Social facilitation of the spontaneous mealsize of humans occurs regardless of the time, place, alcohol or snacks. *Appetite* 1990; **15:** 89–101.

110. Rubenstein LZ, Rubenstein LV. Multidimensional assessment of elderly patients. *Adv Int Med* 1991; **36:** 81–108.

111. American Dietetic Association Reports 1996.

112. Blandford G. "Gerontoscopy: An investigative Procedure in the Care of the Elderly" *Clinical Therapeutics* 1987; **10:** 9–17.

113. Barrocas A, Belcher D, Champagne C, Jastram C. Nutrition assessment: practical approaches. *Clin Geriatr Med* 1995; **11(4):** 675–713.

114. Guigoz Y, Vellas B, Garry PJ. Assessing the nutritional status of the elderly: The Mini Nutritional Assessment as part of the geriatric evaluation. *Nutr Rev* 1996; **54(1 Pt 2):** S59–65.

115. Beck AM, Ovensen L, Schroll M. Validation of the resident assessment instrument triggers in the detection of under-nutrition. *Age Ageing* 2001; **30:** 161–165.

116. Sullivan DH. The role of nutrition in increased morbidity and mortality. *Clin Geriatr Med* 1995; **11:** 661–674.

117. Blandford G, Watkins LB, Mulvihill MN, Taylor B. Assessing abnormal feeding behavior in dementia: a taxonomy and initial findings. In Research and Practice in Alzheimer's Disease: "Weight loss and eating behavior in Alzheimer's Disease. Eds. Vellas B, Riviere A, Fitten J. 1998 Serdi, Paris and Springer Publishing. Pp 49–65.

118. Volicer L, Volicer BJ, Hurley AC. Is hospice care appropriate for Alzheimer patients? *Caring* 1993; **12(11):** 50–55.

119. Touho H, Karasawa J, Shishido H, Morisako T, Yamada K, Shibamoto K. Hypermetabolism in the acute stage of hemorrhagic cerebrovascular disease. *J Neurosurg* 1990; **72:** 710–714.

120. Dávalos A, Ricart W, Gonzalez-Huix F, Soler S, Marrugat J, Molins A, Suñer R, Genís D. Effect of malnutrition after acute stroke on clinical outcome. *Stroke* 1996; **27:** 1082–1032.

120a. Smithard DG, O'Neill PA, Park C *et al.* Complications and outcome following acute stroke: does dysphagia matter? *Stroke* 1990; **27:** 1200-04

121. Gariballa SE, Parker SG, Taub N, Castleden CM. A randomized, controlled, single-blind trial of nutritional supplementation after acute stroke. *J Parenter Enteral Nutr* 1998; **22:** 315–319.

122. Macfie J. Ethics and nutritional support. *Supplement to Nutrition* 1995; **11(2):** 213–216.

123. Reuben DB, Greendale GA, Harrison GG. Nutrition screening in older persons. *J Am Geriatr Soc* 1995; **43:** 415-425.

124. Potter JN, Langhorne P. Nutritional supplementation in the elderly: a statistical overview. *Age and Ageing* 1996; **25 (S1):** 42.

125. Woo J, Ho SC, Mak YT, Law LK, Cheung A. Nutritional status of elderly patients during recovery from chest infection and the role of nutritional supplementation assessed by a prospective randomised single-blind trial. *Age Ageing* 1994; **23:** 40–48.

126. Fiatarone MA, O'Neill EF, Ryan ND. Exercise training and nutritional supplements for physical frailty in very elderly people. *N Engl J Med* 1994; **3330:** 1769–1775.

127. Potter J, Langhorne P, Roberts M. Routine protein energy supplementation in adults: systematic review. *BMJ* 1998; **317:** 495–501.

128. Delmi M, Rapin CH, Bengoa JM. Dietary supplementation in elderly patients with fractured neck of femur. *Lancet* 1990; **I:** 1013–1016.

129. Espaulella J, Guyer H, Diaz-Escriu F, Mellado-Navas JA, Castells M, Pladevall M. Nutritional supplementation of elderly hip fracture patients. A randomized, double-blind, placebo-controlled trial. *Age Ageing* 2000; **29(5):** 425–431.

130. Bastin HC. A treatise on aphasia and other speech defects. HK Lewis, London, 1898.

131. O'Mahony D, McIntyre AS. Artificial feeding for elderly patients after stroke. *Age Ageing* 1995; **24:** 533–535.

132. Huggins PS, Tuomi SK, Young C. Effects of nasogastric tubes on the young, normal swallowing mechanism. *Dysphagia* 1999; **14:** 157–161.

133. Hassett JM, Sunby C, Flint MW. No elimination of aspiration pneumonia in neurologically disabled patients with feeding gastrostomy. *Surg Gyn Obstet* 1988; **167:** 383–388.

134. Short TP, Patel NR, Thomas E. Prevalence of gastro-esophageal reflux in patients who develop pneumonia following percutaneous endoscopic gastrostomy: a 24-hour pH monitoring study. *Dysphagia* 1996; **11:** 87–89.

135. Preclik G, Grune S, Leser HG, Lebherz J, Heldwein W, Machka K, Holstege A, Kern WV. Prospective, randomised, double blind trial of prophylaxis with single dose of co-amoxiclav before percutaneous endoscopic gastrostomy. *BMJ* 1999; **319:** 881–884.

136. Wijdicks EFM, McMahon MM. Percutaneous endoscopic gastrostomy after acute stroke: complications and outcome. *Cerebrovasc Dis* 1999; **9:** 109–111.

137. Rosser JC, Rodas EB, Blancaflor J, Prosst RL, Rosser LE, Salem RR. A simpler technique for laparoscopic jejunostomy and gastrostomy tube placement. *Am J Surg* 1999; **177:** 61–65.

138. Rimmer E, Berner YN, Gindin J, Barr DD, Levy S. Low complication rate after percutaneous endoscopic gastrostomy by a geriatrics orientated team. *J Am Geriatr Soc* 1999; **47:** 765–766.

139. Park RHR, Allison MC, Spence E, Morris AJ, Danesh BJZ, Russell RI, Mills PR. Randomised comparison of percutaneous endoscopic gastrostomy and naso-gastric tube feeding in patients with persisting neurological dysphagia. *BMJ* 1992; **304:** 1406–1409.

140. Wicks C, Gimson A, Valavianos P, *et al.* Assessment of the percutaneous endoscopic gastrostomy feeding tube as part of an integrated approach to enteral feeding. *Gut* 1992; **33:** 613–616.

141. Norton B, Homer-Ward M, Donnely MT, Long RG, Holms GKT. A randomised prospective comparison of percutaneous endoscopic gastrostomy and nasogastric tube feeding after dysphagic stroke. *BM J* 1996; **312:** 13–16.

142. Nyswonger GD, Helmechen RH. Early enteral nutrition and length of stay in stroke patients. *J Neurosci Nursing* 1992; **24:** 220–223.

143. Raha SK, Woodhouse KW. Who should have a PEG? *Age and Ageing* 1993; **22:** 313–315.

144. Klor BM, Milianti FJ. Rehabilitation of neurogenic dysphagia with percutaneous endoscopic gastrostomy. *Dysphagia* 1999; **14:** 162–164.

145. Lennard-Jones JE. Giving or withholding fluid and nutrients: ethical and legal aspects. *J R Coll Physicians* 1999; **33:** 39–45.

146. British Medical Association. *Withholding and withdrawing life-prolonging medical treatment.* BMJ Books, London, 1998.

147. Dennis M on behalf of the International Stroke Trials Collaboration – FOOD. FOOD (Feed or ordinary diet): A "Family" of 3 randomised trials evaluating feeding policies for patients admitted to hospital with a recent stroke. *Cerebrovascular Diseases* 1999; **9(S1):** 107.

39

Management of patients with a short bowel

Jeremy Nightingale and John Lennard-Jones

Historical background

In 1912, Flint reviewed 55 adults who had lost more than 200 cm of small intestine mainly due to strangulated hernias or abdominal tumours.[1] Terms such as 'massive' small-bowel resection were used in subsequent reports and reference was made to the proportion of small bowel length removed.[2] It is now recognised that it is not the length removed, nor the proportion, but rather the length and type of small bowel remaining which are the important determinants of outcome.[3] In the 1960s Booth and his colleagues studied a series of patients who had undergone a small bowel resection in all of whom the residual gut was anastomosed to colon. From this work, supplemented by experimental studies, they were able to define the site of absorption of major nutrients and vitamins, particularly the localized absorption of vitamin B_{12} from the distal ileum.[4]

While most early reports were of patients with a retained colon it is becoming increasingly common to see patients in whom the ileum and colon have been removed and who thus have a jejunostomy.[5]

In 1981 Fleming and Remington proposed that intestinal failure occurred when there was a 'reduction in functioning gut mass below the minimal amount necessary for adequate digestion and absorption of nutrients'.[6] In order to identify easily patients with intestinal failure, we propose that intestinal failure occurs when there is reduced intestinal absorption so nutrient and/or fluid supplements are needed to maintain health. These supplements may be given by the oral, enteral or parenteral routes. Intestinal failure can be acute or chronic. Acute intestinal failure is reversible and usually due to perioperative problems (e.g. fistulae/sepsis) or to chemotherapy or irradiation. Chronic intestinal failure most commonly arises from an intestinal resection that leaves behind a short small bowel, but is occasionally due to gut dysmotility (e.g. scleroderma or visceral myopathy or neuropathy) or inflammation (e.g. extensive small bowel Crohn's disease or long-term irradiation damage).

Anatomical and physiological considerations

Small intestinal length

The normal human small intestinal length, measured at autopsy or at surgery from the duodeno-jejunal flexure to the ileocaecal valve varies from about 275 to 850 cm (Table 39.1)[7-12] and tends to be shorter in

Table 39.1 – Measured lengths of adult small intestine.

Author	Date	Number	Small intestinal length	
			mean	range (cm)
Autopsy★				
Bryant[5]	1924	160	620	300–850
Underhill[6]	1955	100	620	340–790
Radiological				
intubation				
Hirsch *et al*[7]	1956	10	260	210–320
small bowel enema				
Fanucci *et al*[8]	1988	158	290	160–430
Surgery				
Backman and Hallberg[9]	1974	42	660	400–850
Slater and Aufses†[10]	1991	38	500	300–780

★ Autopsy measurements from pylorus, all others from duodeno-jejunal flexure (duodenum is about 25 cm in length).
† 21 of these patients had small bowel and 4 others colonic Crohn's disease but their small intestinal lengths were not different from 13 patients without Crohn's disease.
From the autopsy and surgical studies the small bowel length from the duodeno-jejunal flexure varies from 275 to 850 cm. It is important to refer to the length of bowel remaining rather than the length resected.

women. Radiological measurements give shorter measurements partly as the bowel telescopes around an intubation tube and on a barium film is only seen in two dimensions. Congenital cases of a short bowel have been reported[13] and many patients with a short bowel do indeed start with a short intestinal length before they have undergone any resections.[14] Due to this wide variation in normal small intestinal length, it is more important, after an intestinal resection, to refer to the length of bowel remaining rather than to the length resected. A resection of 300 cm of intestine might remove all the small gut from one patient and leave another with a length that is average in the general population.

If small bowel length has not been measured at surgery, it may be measured with moderate accuracy from a barium follow-through film providing the remaining small-bowel length is less than 200 cm.[15]

Volume of gastrointestinal secretions

The normal gastrointestinal secretions are usually made up of 0.5 l saliva, 2 l gastric acid, 1.5 l pancreatico-biliary secretions, which are added to a volume of 2 l food and drink. Thus each day about 6 l of chyme pass the duodeno-jejunal flexure and this is mostly reabsorbed before the colon is reached. Studies using non-absorbed markers in healthy subjects have shown that food or drink is diluted between two and three times by secretions when it passes through the distal duodenum. On entering the jejunum, water and sodium are absorbed but dilution of the original meal is still detectable up to 100 cm or more distal to the duodeno-jejunal flexure.[16,17] Thus if a patient has a stoma situated in the upper 100 cm of jejunum, the volume which emerges from the stoma is likely to be greater than the volume taken by mouth and so such a patient will be in negative fluid and sodium balance after any food or drink.[18] The sodium concentration at the duodeno-jejunal flexure is about 90 mmol/l and this gradually increases to about 140 mmol/l in the terminal ileum.[17]

Gastrointestinal motility

In health, there are neuro-endocrine mechanisms by which gastric emptying and the rate of small intestinal passage are delayed by unabsorbed nutrients, particularly fat, entering the distal ileum or colon.[19,20] These 'ileal and colonic brakes' are lost if the distal ileum and/or colon are removed. Thus patients with a jejunostomy have rapid liquid gastric emptying[20]

associated with low plasma peptide YY levels.[21] Patients with a retained colon have a normal overall rate of liquid and solid gastric emptying[20] associated with high plasma peptide YY levels.[21]

Jejunal, ileal and colonic absorption

Water and electrolytes

The jejunal mucosa is more permeable than the ileum to water, sodium and chloride. In two studies, water movements in response to an osmotic gradient were nine times[22] and sodium fluxes twice,[23] as great in the jejunum compared with the ileum. Sodium absorption in the jejunum can take place against only a small concentration gradient, it is dependent on water movement, and it is coupled to absorption of glucose and some amino acids.[24] Movement of sodium into the lumen occurs if the luminal sodium concentration is low. Perfusion experiments show that absorption from the perfusate occurs if its sodium concentration is 90 mmol/l or more, while secretion of sodium into the lumen occurs if its concentration is less. Several studies have shown that maximal jejunal absorption of sodium from a perfused solution occurs at a concentration around 120 mmol/l[25–27] (Fig. 39.1).

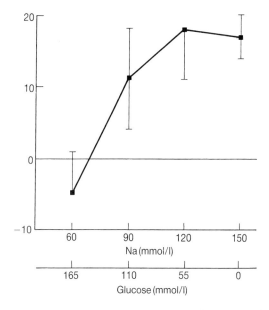

Figure 39.1 – Results of an experiment in which patients with a high jejunostomy drank on different days 500 ml of four different isotonic test solutions with varying ratios of sodium to glucose. Loss of sodium occurred with a solution containing 60 mmol/l of sodium but absorption with higher concentrations. Drawn from data in Rodrigues et al.[27]

In contrast, the ileum can absorb sodium against a concentration gradient and movement of sodium is not coupled with glucose or other nutrients. The colon avidly absorbs sodium against high concentration gradients and, whereas jejunal and ileal effluent contains sodium at a concentration of about 90 and 140 mmol/l respectively, normal stool contains very little sodium.

Macronutrients

In health, intubation studies have shown that polysaccharides, proteins and fats are digested and absorbed within the upper 200 cm of the small intestine.[16] However, increasing amounts of fat reach more distal parts of the intestine as the dietary load increases, and thus steatorrhoea is likely with a normal or high-fat diet if the length of small intestine is reduced.[4] Fat digestion in the short bowel may be impaired by a low bile–salt concentration in the jejunum owing to failure of normal reabsorption of bile salts from the distal ileum. The fact that digestion and absorption of carbohydrate and protein normally occurs in the upper jejunum explains why an elemental or hydrolysed diet does not have an advantage over a polymeric diet in the treatment of most patients with a short gut [28] (Fig. 39.2).

Micronutrients

Most water-soluble vitamins are absorbed from the upper intestine and deficiencies are unlikely in patients with a short bowel who are eating normal food. The exception is vitamin B_{12} which is selectively absorbed from the distal 60 cm of ileum.[29]

Absorption of fat-soluble vitamins may be impaired if there is malabsorption of fat. Patients with a short bowel may therefore need supplements of vitamin A, D, E and K. In patients taking food with or without enteral supplements, iron deficiency may occur. Zinc deficiency is rare unless stool volumes are very large.

Anatomical types of short bowel

In clinical practice there are two types of patient with a short bowel (Fig. 39.3). Those who have had their ileum and some of their jejunum resected, usually leaving a jejuno-colic anastomosis, though sometimes the ileocaecal valve is preserved. Others have had their

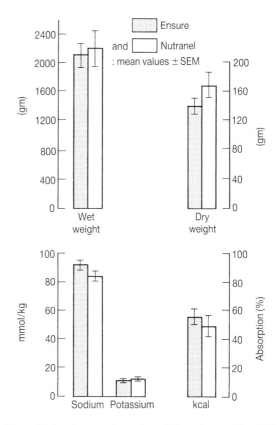

Figure 39.2 – An experiment in which patients with a high jejunostomy took on different days equivalent amounts of either a polymeric diet (Ensure, Abbott, Maidenhead, UK) or a hydrolysed diet (Nutranel, Nutricia Chemical, Wilts, UK). There was no significant difference in jejunal output of fluid, dry weight or monovalent cations, nor in percentage absorption of energy. From data of Dr P. B. Mcintyre, with permission.

colon, ileum and some of their jejunum resected and have a jejunostomy. Both patient types commonly result from bowel resections for Crohn's disease (Table 39.2). There are more women than men with a short bowel possibly because women start with a shorter length of small bowel.[7]

The presence or absence of a colon affects the small intestinal length at which nutrient and/or fluid supplements are needed.[5,18,30] In those with a retained colon long-term parenteral nutrient supplements are likely if less than 50 cm residual jejunum remains. Most patients with a jejunostomy will need parenteral nutrition if the jejunal length is less than 75 cm, parenteral saline if less than 100 cm, and oral sodium and water supplements if it is 100–200 cm.[5,18]

Jejunostomy   Jejuno-colic anastomosis

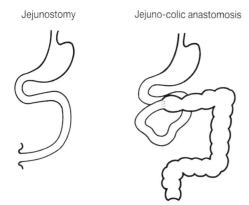

Figure 39.3 – The two common types of patient seen in clinical practice with a short bowel. Before 1970, most published reports described the consequences and treatment of a resection in which a small intestinal remnant was anastomosed to colon. During the last two decades, the proportion of patients with a high jejunostomy, having lost both the distal small intestine and colon, has increased. There are important physiological and clinical differences between patients with or without the colon.

Table 39.2 – Causes of a short bowel.[28]

	Jejunum-colon	Jejunostomy
Number	38 (26F)★	46 (31F)
Age	46 (7–70)	42 (16–68)
Crohn's disease	16	33
Ischaemia	6	2
Irradiation	5	3
Ulcerative colitis	–	5
Volvulus	5	–
Other	6	3

★ 7 have an ileocaecal valve and 31 a jejuno-colic anastomosis.

Patients who have had a predominantly jejunal resection are uncommon. However they are managed in the same way as patients with an ileal resection, but their long-term outlook is much better as the remaining ileum can absorb sodium against a concentration gradient and with time its absorption of nutrients and minerals will increase. Vitamin B_{12} injections may not be needed.

Presentation, problems and treatments (Table 39.3)

Problems and treatments common to all types of patient

Protein-energy malnutrition

Loss of muscle bulk leads to physical weakness and lack of stamina. Loss of body fat can result in a permanent feeling of coldness and a gaunt facial appearance. Dry wrinkled skin, dull hair and nails, and a stooped posture combine to give an impression of premature ageing. Many patients who are wasted dislike looking in a mirror and avoid company because of self-consciousness about their appearance. Mental effects of undernutrition include apathy, depression and irritability, effects which deprive the patient of their motivation for recovery.

Table 39.3 – Problems of a short bowel.[28]

	Jejunum-colon	Jejunostomy
Water, sodium and magnesium depletion	uncommon	common
Nutrient malabsorption	common★	common
Renal stones	25%	none
Gallstones	45%	45%
Adaptation	possibly	no evidence
Social problems	occasional	common

★ Bacterial fermentation of carbohydrate salvages some energy, but D(-)lactic acidosis can occur if the diet is high in mono and oligosaccharides.

All short-bowel patients who can be maintained on an oral diet need to consume more energy than normal subjects because as much as 50% of the energy from the diet may be malabsorbed. Most patients can achieve this by eating more high-energy food. Enteral sip-feeds may be given in addition to food, preferably taken between meals and at bedtime. By these means, a patient may increase energy intake by at least 1000 kcal/day. If enteral supplements during the day fail to achieve weight gain or maintain nutrition, a naso-gastric or gastrostomy tube may be inserted and a feed given at night so that the short residual length of intestine is used at a time when usually inactive. Once weight is regained, the daily energy requirement may decrease so that the nocturnal feed can be stopped and sip-feeds during the day become adequate.

Only if these measures fail and the patient continues to lose weight, or fails to regain lost weight, is parenteral nutrition given. Even then, parenteral supplements may be needed for only a limited period of weeks or months, and thereafter oral supplements may be adequate. In the long term, parenteral nutrition is always needed if a patient absorbs less than one-third of the oral energy intake[18] and in young people with a high energy requirement when absorption is 30–60% of normal.

Vitamin B_{12} deficiency

All patients who have had more than 60 cm of their terminal ileum removed need long-term vitamin B_{12} therapy with hydroxycobalamin 1 mg every three months.

Gallstones

Gallstones are common (45%) in both types of patient and are more common in men.[5] It was originally thought that gallstones in this circumstance were due to deposition of cholesterol because of a depleted bile-salt pool. However, the gallstones tend to contain calcium bilirubinate. Such stones probably result from gallbladder stasis which predisposes to biliary sludge formation and subsequently calcium bilirubinate stones which often appear calcified on abdominal radiographs.[31] Calcium bilirubinate crystals occur more commonly in men with biliary sludge than women.[32] Cholecystokinin injections have been used to prevent gallbladder stasis;[33] there may be a role for a prophylactic cholecystectomy.[34]

Social problems

Most long-term patients with a short bowel have a body mass index within the normal range and most are at full-time work or looking after the home and family unaided.[5] Both groups may have diarrhoea which causes problems, especially if housing conditions are poor. For those with a colon the diarrhoea is mal-odorous and bulky due to steatorrhoea. The effluent from a small-bowel stoma, unlike from a colostomy, is not offensive. However, the patient may be troubled by the large volume of fluid which emerges, some-times three or more litres during the 24 hours. The bag then has to be emptied frequently and, if it becomes overfull, the adhesive flange may separate from the skin with embarrassing leakage of fluid, and with the likelihood of skin soreness.

Short bowel patients with a preserved colon

Presentation

These patients have a short length of jejunum anasto-mosed either to the ileum just proximal to the ileo-caecal valve, or directly to the colon. They are often moderately well after their resection except for diarrhoea/steatorrhoea, but in the succeeding months may lose weight and become severely under-nourished.

Nutrient absorption

Most, if not all, of these patients are able either immediately, or after an interval of some months, to maintain satisfactory nutrition without troublesome diarrhoea while taking a normal diet. If the length of jejunum exceeds 200 cm, few problems arise and little treatment is needed. If the jejunal length is between 100 and 200 cm, patients can usually be maintained in good health with simple oral supplements. When the jejunal length is between 50 and 100 cm, some or all patients (if the residual jejunum is less than 30–50 cm), need long-term parenteral supplements[5,30] (Fig. 39.4).

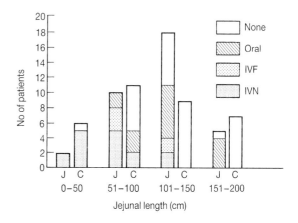

Figure 39.4 – Differences in the need for nutrition supplements in patients with a similar jejunal length ending either at a stoma (J) or anastomosed to colon (C) two years after operation. Patients without the colon usually needed oral supplements if the jejunal length was 100–200 cm and parenteral supplements of fluid and electrolytes (IVF), often with nutrients (IVN), when the length of intestine was less than 100 cm. Most patients with a colon needed parenteral supplements only if the jejunal length was less than 50 cm. Reproduced from Nightingale *et al.*[5]

In order to increase the energy absorption and reduce the risk of renal stones, patients with a retained colon need to be given information about their oral intake. They need a large total energy intake with a diet high in carbohydrate (polysaccharides), but not increased in fat, and low in oxalate.

Carbohydrate

Carbohydrate, unabsorbed by the small bowel, is fermented by colonic bacteria to short chain fatty acids which are absorbed, and so provide an important mechanism by which energy is salvaged.[35–39] As much as 1000 kcal (4.2 MJ) can be salvaged each day in these patients.[35] Experimentally this process can be prevented by giving metronidazole which also inhibits intestinal adaptation.[40] Thus a diet high in carbo-hydrate is beneficial, but in addition to being very bulky, such a diet (especially if rich in mono and oligosaccharides) can rarely cause D-lactic acidosis.[41] Lactic acid produced by man is the L(+) isomer but abnormal bacterial or fungal colonisation of the colon can result in a metabolic acidosis due to formation and absorption of the D(-) isomer which cannot be metabolised. It is more likely if thiamine deficiency coexists. D(-) lactic acidosis can cause a syndrome of ataxia, blurred vision, ophthalmoplegia and nystagmus. It is suspected when a patient is found to have a metabolic acidosis with a large anion gap. Treatment is with broad spectrum antibiotics (neomycin or vancomycin), thiamine and changing the diet to one high in polysaccharides but low in mono and oligosaccharides.[42]

Fat

The proportion of fat absorbed from different diets remains constant.[4,36] Unabsorbed long chain fatty acids in the colon may worsen diarrhoea by reducing water and sodium absorption[43] and increasing the colonic transit rate.[44] They are toxic to bacteria so reducing the amount of carbohydrate fermented.[45,46] They bind to calcium and magnesium[4] so increasing the stool losses, and they increase oxalate absorption. Theoretically, a low fat diet is indicated, especially in the early months after the resection, but in practice it is hard to implement. Fat yields twice as much energy as comparable weights of carbohydrate and it also makes food palatable. A balance has to be struck therefore between maintaining weight and strength, and worsening diarrhoea with pale bulky offensive stools. Medium chain triglycerides are an alternative source of energy and can be absorbed from the small and large bowel.[47]

Some patients may need supplements of fat-soluble vitamins by mouth. Essential fatty acids can be obtained by rubbing sunflower oil on the skin.[48]

Oxalate

Any patient who is chronically dehydrated and passes low volumes of concentrated urine is at risk of renal stone formation. Calcium oxalate renal stones occur in a quarter of patients with a retained colon.[5] After an ileal resection there is increased colonic absorption of dietary oxalate.[49] Several mechanisms may be responsible for the increased absorption and renal excretion of oxalate. Calcium and oxalate usually form an insoluble complex in the colon but if free fatty acids are present in the colon they preferentially bind the calcium to form soaps; thus the oxalate becomes soluble and is absorbed giving rise to hyperoxaluria.[50,51] Unabsorbed bile salts in the colon increase colonic permeability to oxalate.[52] Oxalate may be manufactured by organisms within the colon.

Calcium oxalate stones are prevented by giving a low oxalate diet, which avoids rhubarb, spinach, beetroot, peanuts and excessive amounts of tea.[53] In addition fat in the diet may be reduced.[51] Oral calcium supplements,[54] calcium-containing organic marine hydro-colloid[55] and cholestyramine (which binds bile salts)[56] may be given.

Water and mineral losses

The colon has a large capacity to absorb sodium and water; thus patients with a short bowel and a preserved colon are rarely in negative water and sodium balance and rarely need water or sodium supplements.[5,57] If sodium deficiency does develop, a glucose-saline drink can be given as for patients with a jejunostomy.

Fatty acids from digestion of dietary fat and from bacterial fermentation of malabsorbed carbohydrate combine with calcium and magnesium to increase faecal losses. A low-fat diet decreases these losses.[38] The need for magnesium supplements is less than in patients with a jejunostomy (about 40%)[5] and can be treated in the same way as for patients with a jejunostomy with magnesium oxide, vitamin D and reduced fat diet.

Diarrhoea

The oral intake determines the amount of stool passed. The diarrhoea, which may severely limit a patient's lifestyle, occasionally can be managed by reducing food intake, but this may increase the problems of undernutrition. Rarely a patient may need parenteral nutrition to offset a reduced food intake during management.

Diarrhoea may be treated with loperamide 2–8 mg given half an hour before food. Loperamide is usually given in preference to codeine phosphate as it is non-sedative and non-addictive, however occasionally both are needed. As the enterohepatic circulation, round which loperamide circulates, is disrupted, higher doses than usual may need to be given. Rarely bile salt malabsorption contributes to the diarrhoea and is helped by cholestyramine, which has the additional advantage of reducing oxalate absorption but may reduce fat absorption by further reducing the bile-salt pool. Occasionally a gastric antisecretory drug can be tried, but this is not usually effective in the long-term in this group of patients.

Adaptation

After a jejunal resection in animals, the remaining ileum gradually compensates for loss of surface area by increasing its absorptive capacity. Structural changes occur in the remaining bowel with elongation of villi, deeper crypts and there are more absorptive cells in a given length of villus. As a result of these structural changes and probably a slowing of gut transit time, an increase in the absorption of water, nutrients and minerals occurs. These changes are less apparent if the ileum has been resected and jejunum remains.

In humans, who eat a normal diet and who have jejunum anastomosed to a functioning colon, no major structural changes in the jejunum have been reported. Two reports of jejunal biopsies from 4 patients showed a greater number of cells lining each villus (epithelial hyperplasia),[58,59] but in contrast another study of 10 patients has shown the reverse, that is intestinal atrophy.[60] Functional adaptation with a small reduction in faecal weight in the 3 months following the small bowel resection does occur.[61] There is also increased jejunal absorption of water,[59] sodium,[60] glucose,[62] and calcium[63] with time. Intestinal calcium absorption may continue to increase for more than two years after a resection.[63]

Luminal nutrients are important in causing intestinal adaptation to occur; hence, it is important that patients should eat even though parenteral nutrition may be needed. If they do not eat, villous atrophy occurs.

Pancreatico-biliary secretions and some gastro-intestinal hormones (e.g. gastrin and glucagon-like peptide-2 (GLP-2) for structural changes and peptide YY to reduce gastrointestinal motility) may be important. The presence of nutrients in the colon may be important, as jejunal adaptation occurs in rats if the colon is perfused with nutrients.[64]

Short bowel patients with a jejunostomy

Presentation

The main problem experienced immediately after surgery by patients with a jejunostomy is of a high stomal output especially after food. Malabsorption of nutrients is important but does not cause such immediate problems. These patients are very dependent on treatment to compensate for the water and sodium losses. If they miss their treatment for one day they are likely to be unwell due to sodium and water depletion.

Water and mineral losses

Large stomal water, sodium and magnesium losses cause major problems.

The normal daily intestinal secretions (about 4 litres/day) cannot be reabsorbed in the short length of bowel remaining, and so are lost through the stoma. High gastrin levels could cause gastric acid hyper-secretion and thus contribute to the jejunostomy out-put.[21,65] However in man gastric acid hypersecretion has only been demonstrated in the immediate post-operative period in patients with a retained colon.[66] Rapid liquid gastric emptying may increase the stomal output[20] and may be due to low plasma peptide YY levels.[21]

Water and sodium losses

Jejunostomy patients can be divided into two groups depending upon the relative weight of oral intake and stomal output and corresponding sodium content (Fig. 39.5).

● 'Absorbers' usually have more than 100 cm residual jejunum and they absorb more water and sodium from their diet than they take by mouth, thus they can be managed without needing parenteral fluids. Their usual daily jejunostomy output is about 2 kg.

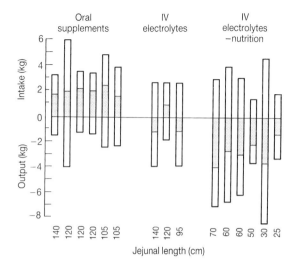

Figure 39.5 – Balance between total input and output (kg) in 15 patients with a short intestine ending in a jejunostomy. The patients are divided into three groups by their clinical need for nutrition support. Six patients maintained good nutrition status with oral supplements; three needed a parenteral supplement of water and electrolytes but maintained satisfactory nutrition status with food; and six patients needed parenteral electrolyte and nutrient supplements. The outcome correlated with residual jejunal length. Patients in negative balance needed parenteral supplements; most of those in positive balance could be maintained by oral supplements. Reproduced with permission of the publisher from *Hospital Update,* October 1991.

- 'Secretors' usually have less than 100 cm jejunum and they lose more water and sodium from their stoma than they take by mouth. These patients need long-term parenteral supplements[18] and these requirements change very little with time.[5] Their usual daily jejunostomy output may be 4–8 kg/24 hours.

Magnesium deficiency

Patients with a jejunostomy are often in precarious magnesium and calcium balance[28,67] though the balance does not correlate with residual jejunal length. Magnesium deficiency is common (70% of patients not receiving parenteral nutrition needed magnesium supplements)[5] and may cause fatigue, depression, irritability, muscle weakness, occasionally tetany and, if very severe, convulsions.[67]

Potassium deficiency

The effluent from a jejunostomy or ileostomy contains relatively little potassium (about 15 mmol/l), whereas the colon secretes potassium.[18,68] Potassium

problems are unusual and patients maintained on enteral nutrition rarely need a potassium intake greater than normal. Net loss through the stoma occurs only when less than 50 cm jejunum remains.[18] A low serum potassium level may be due to sodium depletion with secondary hyperaldosteronism and thus greater than normal urinary losses of potassium[68] or magnesium depletion.[69]

Treatment

Total loss of sodium increases in a linear relationship with volume (at a concentration of about 90 mmol/l) so that the clinician can predict with reasonable accuracy that an effluent volume of 3 litres contains 270 mmol of sodium (Fig. 39.6). There is an obligatory stomal loss which may be up to 2 litres/24 hours even if a patient fasts, but the output increases after food or drink.

Restrict oral fluids

Jejunal mucosa is 'leaky' and rapid sodium fluxes occur across it. If water or indeed any solution with a sodium concentration of less than 90 mmol/l is drunk there is a net efflux of sodium from the plasma into the bowel lumen[69] until a luminal sodium concentration of 90–100 mmol/l is reached; this fluid is then lost in the jejunostomy fluid. It is a common mistake for patients to be encouraged to drink oral hypotonic solutions to quench their thirst, as this literally washes sodium out of the body.[70,71]

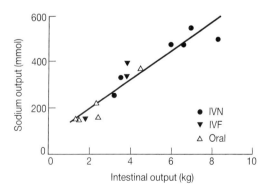

Figure 39.6 – Sodium output bears a linear relationship to daily intestinal output in patients with a jejunostomy. The concentration of sodium is about 90 mmol/l of output. The patients with a daily sodium loss greater than about 250 mmol usually need an intravenous supplement (IVF = intravenous fluid and electrolyte; IVN = intravenous nutrition). r = 0.96; p < 0.0001.

Treatment for a high output from a jejunostomy (or indeed an ileostomy or upper small bowel entero-cutaneous fistula) begins with the patient restricting the total amount of hypotonic fluid (water, tea, fruit juices, tea, coffee, alcohol or dilute salt solutions) to less than a litre daily. To make up the rest of the fluid requirement the patient is encouraged to drink a glucose–saline replacement solution as described.

If there is marked sodium and water depletion and thus severe thirst, it is often difficult to replace previous losses with an oral regimen. It is then best to give intra-venous normal saline (2–4 litres over 1–2 days) and maintain subsequent balance with oral supplements.

Take an oral glucose–saline solution

Patients with stomal losses of less than 1200 ml daily can usually maintain sodium balance by adding extra salt to the limit of palatability at the table and when cooking. When stoma losses are in the range 1200–2000 ml, or sometimes more, it is possible for a patient to maintain sodium balance by taking a glucose–saline solution or salt capsules.

As the sodium content of jejunostomy (or ileostomy) effluent is relatively constant at about 90 mmol/l and as there is coupled absorption of sodium and glucose in the jejunum, patients are advised to sip a glucose–saline solution with a sodium concentration of at least 90 mmol/l throughout the day.[72] The World Health Organization (WHO) cholera solution has a sodium concentration of 90 mmol/l[72] and is commonly used (without the potassium chloride).

Sodium chloride	60 mmol (3.5 g)
Sodium bicarbonate (or citrate)	30 mmol (2.5 g) (2.9 g)
Glucose	110 mmol (20 g)
Tap water	One litre

The concentration of sodium in this solution is much higher than many commercial preparations used to treat infective diarrhoea. Patients can prepare this solution at home using simple measuring scoops. There is no evidence that the sodium bicarbonate adds to the effectiveness of this solution[73] and it may be more palatable if sodium bicarbonate is replaced by sodium citrate. There is an advantage in using a more concentrated and simpler solution of:

Sodium chloride	120 mmol (7.0 g)
Glucose	44 mmol (8 g)
Tap water	One litre

Although taste perception changes in patients who are salt and water depleted they still may find this solution too salty to drink. A glucose-polymer may be sub-stituted for glucose to slightly increase the energy intake[74] and additionally to cause smaller changes in blood glucose in diabetic patients. The patient should be encouraged to sip a total of one litre or more of one of these solutions in small quantities at intervals throughout the day. The solution may be chilled or flavoured with fruit juice (provided that it is not diluted). Since it tastes like sweet dilute sea water and a large daily volume is needed, the patient needs to understand why it is necessary or else motivation and self-discipline will be lacking. Some patients cannot be maintained with an oral regimen and regular parenteral supplements are needed. Most such patients also need nutrition supplements but a few need only one or two litres of normal saline, sometimes with added magnesium sulphate (14 mmol) by regular infusion at home.

Sodium chloride capsules (500 mg each) are effective when taken in large amounts (14/24 hours), but can cause some patients to feel sick and even vomit.[74]

Drug therapy

If restricting oral fluids and giving a glucose-saline solution to drink are not adequate, drugs may be needed. As the intestinal output, especially in net 'secretors' rises after meals, it is important to give the drugs before food. Drugs used to reduce jejunostomy output act to reduce either intestinal motility or secretions.

Antisecretory drugs. Since food and drink are diluted by digestive juices, the volume of stomal effluent can be reduced in 'secretors' by drugs designed to reduce the output of fluid from the stomach, liver and pancreas. Drugs that reduce gastric acid secretion (e.g. the H_2 receptor antagonists[75] or proton pump inhibitors[76] or the somatostatin analogue octreotide[77–81]) are effective. Octreotide also reduces gastrointestinal motility and other exocrine secretions; however, it only reduces jejunostomy water and sodium losses in 'secretors' not 'absorbers'. 50 mg of octreotide can be injected subcutaneously before breakfast and supper, but the injection is painful and may further increase the risk of the patient developing gallstones. A proton pump inhibitor (omeprazole 40 mg daily) has the same effect as octreotide, so it seems likely that the effect of octreotide is mainly to reduce gastric secretion.[75,76] Ranitidine (300) mg before breakfast and supper is often as effective as omeprazole. While the reduction in stomal output with octreotide, proton pump inhibitors and the H_2 antagonists decreases the social disability of the jejunostomy effluent and reduces the volume of parenteral fluid needed each day, they do not obviate the need for parenteral therapy[80] (Fig. 39.7). Occasional patients use these preparations (particularly octreotide) before meals to diminish the social inconvenience of a profuse jejunostomy output after food.

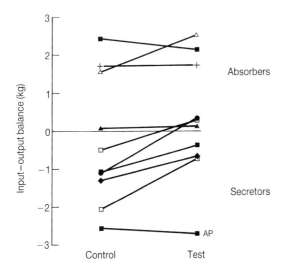

Figure 39.7 – Effect of oral omeprazole, 40 mg daily, on the stomal effluent of 10 patients with a high jejunostomy. The drug had no effect on the effluent of patients whose output was less than the oral intake. Omeprazole decreased the effluent in patients whose output was greater than the oral intake (patient AP probably did not absorb the drug and responded to intravenous cimetidine), but the patients remained in negative balance and thus continued to require an intravenous supplement.

Antidiarrhoeal drugs. Loperamide (often in high dose) and codeine phosphate mainly reduce intestinal motility and thus decrease water and sodium output from an ileostomy by about 20%.[82] These drugs also appear to be effective in some patients with a jejunostomy[78] though their efficacy in net 'secretors' is uncertain. A combination of both of these drugs, taken before food, together with a glucose-saline solution, has liberated at least one patient from dependence on parenteral electrolyte supplements.[83]

Magnesium supplements

Magnesium deficiency can often be corrected by oral supplements. Magnesium supplements may be given as gelatine capsules of 4 mmol magnesium oxide (160 mg of MgO) to a total of 12–24 mmol daily. This regimen increases magnesium absorption[67,84] and does not appear to increase stomal output. If this supplement does not bring the magnesium level into the normal range, oral 1-alpha hydroxy-cholecalciferol in a dose of 2–6 μg daily may be given.[67] Occasionally magnesium can be given as a subcutaneous injection of 4 mmol magnesium sulphate every 2 or more days or as a regular intravenous infusion of 12 or more mmol usually in a litre of saline.

Clinical assessment/monitoring

Patients with the shortest lengths of residual intestine are liable to sodium deficiency with corresponding loss of extracellular fluid volume, hypotension and pre-renal failure. During the initial stages of management, daily body weight and an accurate fluid balance (to include stomal effluent) are essential measurements. Acute sodium and water deficiencies are detected by a rapid fall in body weight, postural hypotension, low urine volume and, if it is severe, by a rising serum creatinine and urea. Chronic sodium deficiency is less easy to detect clinically, though a low urine volume is suggestive. A most useful guide to deficiency is measurement of sodium concentration in a random urine sample: lack of body sodium is suggested by a concentration of only 1–5 mmol/l. One aim is for a daily urine volume of at least 800 ml with a sodium concentration greater than 20 mmol/l. In addition to relatively normal haematological and biochemical measurements another aim is to have a plasma magnesium level greater than 0.6 mmol/l. These goals are not always attainable.

Nutrient absorption

Need for parenteral nutrition

If patients absorb less than 35% of their oral energy intake they are likely to need long-term parenteral nutrition with additional fluids; this tends to occur at a jejunal length of less than 75 cm. In the range 75–100 cm most patients at least need parenteral saline (sometimes with added magnesium) but manage to maintain nutrition status with an enteral regimen (Figs. 39.4 and 39.5). All patients wish to eat food so as to feel normal and to maintain their social relationships. The proportion of their energy requirements contributed by normal food varies from patient to patient. Patients who are 'absorbers' can usually maintain adequate nutrition on an enteral regimen but they will need to eat more than normal subjects. Most patients, who have less than 100 cm small bowel remaining and who are maintained on oral supplements, absorb only about 50–60% of their oral energy intake, so they need to consume twice as much energy as before the resection.[18]

Type of food

Patients with a jejunostomy absorb a constant proportion of the nitrogen, energy and fat from their diet.[28,36,84] Increasing fat in the diet raises fat excretion but does not increase stomal output, nor make the output offensive.[28,36,84] One study showed that increasing fat in the diet increased the loss of the divalent cations (Mg and Ca),[84] but this was not the case in another.[28] There is no advantage in giving a diet of small molecules (e.g. an elemental diet) which causes a feed to be hyperosmolar[28] and usually contains little sodium, so increasing the losses of water and sodium from the stoma. Little advantage comes from taking a diet in which water-soluble MCTs replace normal fat.[47] The fibre content of the diet plays a minor role in determining jejunal output.[27] So far, no unabsorbed carbohydrate has been found to improve the nutrient absorption by increasing the viscosity of a liquid supplement and, by decreasing the rate of gastric emptying.[82] Thus jejunostomy patients need a large total oral energy intake of a polymeric, iso-osmolar diet relatively high in fat with added salt. The limiting factor is the volume of the stomal output. This may become so high with a normal diet or with extra feeding that it is a major social disability and a cause of high sodium loss. If this is the case, parenteral feeding becomes necessary to improve quality of life by enabling oral intake to be reduced.

Adaptation

It has been shown[84] in patients with an 'ileostomy' following an ileal resection, that there was no decrease in ileostomy water, sodium and potassium losses for 11 days after the resection and up to 6 months later.[85] There is no structural change in distal duodenal mucosa in patients with an established jejunostomy.[86] Thus there is no evidence for any structural or functional adaptive changes occurring in the remaining jejunum of patients with a jejunostomy.

Outcome for patients with a short bowel

The outcome for adult patients with a short bowel with or without a colon is now good. Most (85%) achieved a normal body mass index and most (70%) were in full-time work or looking after their home and family unaided.[5] Although anaemia is common, most achieve normal liver and bone biochemical values. Five years after the resection parenteral nutrition is likely to be needed if a patient has a jejunostomy and less than 100 cm jejunum remaining, if they have a jejuno-colic anastomosis and less than 65 cm jejunum remaining or if they have a jejuno-ileal anastomosis leaving a remaining small bowel length of less than 30 cm.[87] The overall survival rate for patients on home parenteral nutrition for non-neoplastic reasons is 70% at 3 years.[88] Patients with a preserved colon have a higher survival rate than those with a jejunostomy.

The two-year survival for infants born after 1980 with a short bowel and usually a retained colon is good: 97% survival if more than 40 cm small bowel remains and 94% if less.[89] Thus with time a few of these patients may be seen in adult clinics; however most will have adapted and not need any nutrition support.

Surgery for short bowel and intestinal transplantation

Surgical techniques

Over the years several surgical treatments have been tried with the aim of slowing intestinal transit or increasing surface area for absorption. Reversal of a 10 cm segment of intestine can slow transit but may also cause functional obstruction.[90,91] Intestinal lengthening and tailoring has been used in children with a short gut due to congenital anomalies.[92] In this procedure the mucosal area is increased by dividing the intestinal lumen into two, utilising a vascular plane at the mesenteric border which permits splitting the blood supply to each side of the gut. The two narrowed intestinal tubes are then separated along their length and joined end-to-end, so creating a double length of intestine with reduced calibre. The narrowed segment of gut dilates with time to give a length of intestine twice as long as the original. In adults, procedures of this type are generally regarded as having too great a risk of damaging the already shortened gut.

Small bowel transplantation

Currently 40–47% of patients having a small bowel transplant will be alive 3 years later if tacrolimus is used for immunosuppression and 29–38% will have a functioning graft. Only 78% of those who survive with the transplant are able to stop parenteral nutrition.[93] Although there are problems with rejection, graft-versus-host disease and denervation of the transplanted segment, most deaths result from immunosuppression.[93] As patients on home parenteral nutrition have a relatively good quality of life[5] and as small bowel transplantation is a life endangering procedure, small intestinal transplantation cannot currently be recommended for most adult patients. In addition, many patients currently receiving home parenteral nutrition for intestinal failure are unlikely to be good candidates for transplantation owing to the complexity of the underlying disease and of previous surgery.[94] Crohn's disease may recur after a transplant.[95]

Future treatments

The increased number of patients with a short bowel, particularly of those with a high jejunostomy, is largely due to the greater incidence and prevalence of Crohn's disease. Development of an effective medical treatment for this condition would reduce the numbers of patients with a short bowel.

Once a major small-bowel resection has occurred, in addition to improved techniques with small bowel transplantation, other medical treatments may affect the outcome.

Dietary or drug therapy to improve absorption

Drugs, which delay gastric emptying or slow down small-gut transit, might improve absorption. Since these patients often need to eat more than normal, it is important that such drugs should not decrease appetite. Any measure, which improves sodium absorption by the small bowel, would be beneficial. Similarly, any dietary formulation, which improves

nutrient absorption by the upper gut, could be helpful. Peptide YY analogues may reduce gastric emptying and small bowel transit and thus reduce the output from a high jejunostomy.

Conjugated bile acid treatment

Since fat malabsorption occurs in patients with a short bowel, partly due to bile acid depletion, there is interest in giving cholylsarcosine, which is a synthetic bile acid that is resistant to bacterial deconjugation and dehydroxylation, and does not itself cause colonic secretion so does not usually cause diarrhoea. Four grams taken three times a day causes a variable improvement in fat and calcium absorption in patients with a short bowel with and without a retained functioning colon. It does occasionally cause nausea.[96,97]

Mucosal growth factors

Treatment, which leads to increased growth of the jejunal mucosa, may be effective. Therapy with growth hormone, glutamine and, fibre were initially encouraging[98] but a later study showed no benefit.[99] In addition there are concerns that long-term growth hormone therapy may increase the risk of colon cancer, as patients with acromegaly are more prone to colonic polyps and colon cancer.[100] Recombinant epidermal growth factor was used with some success to treat an infant with microvillous atrophy.[101] Polyamines are derived from ornithine through the action of ornithine decarboxylase and they induce epithelial hyperplasia. Any mechanism, which increases the synthesis or slows the removal of polyamines, could lead to cellular hyperplasia and improved absorption. Aminoguanidine inhibits diamine oxidase, which breaks down polyamines, and has been used successfully in animals.[102] GLP-2 is an enterocyte specific growth hormone that causes small and large bowel villus/crypt growth; it also increases small and large bowel length in mice. GLP-2 is found in low concentrations in the plasma of patients with a jejunostomy[103] and in high concentrations in those with a retained colon. Current research involves giving injections of GLP-2 to patients with a short bowel, particularly those with a jejunostomy, to study if it induces structural adaptation.

A novel, still experimental, way of improving absorption in those with a retained colon is to replace colonic mucosa with small intestinal mucosa.[104]

References

1. Flint JM. The effect of extensive resections of the small intestine. *Bull Johns Hopkins Hosp* 1912; **23:** 127–144.

2. Haymond HE. Massive resection of the small intestine: an analysis of 257 collected cases. *Surg Gynecol Obst* 1935; **61:** 693–705.

3. Krejs GJ. Intestinal resection. *Clin Gastroenterol* 1979; **8:** 373–386.

4. Booth CC. The metabolic effects of intestinal resection in man. *Postgrad Med J* 1961; **37:** 725–739.

5. Nightingale JMD, Lennard-Jones JE, Gertner DJ, Wood SR, Bartram CI. Colonic preservation reduces the need for parenteral therapy, increases the incidence of renal stones but does not change the high prevalence of gallstones in patients with a short bowel. *Gut* 1992; **33:** 1493–1497.

6. Fleming CR, Remington M. Intestinal failure. In: Hill GL (ed) *Nutrition and the Surgical Patient.* Churchill Livingstone, New York, 1981; pp. 219–235.

7. Bryant J. Observations upon the growth and length of the human intestine. *Am J Med Sci* 1924; **167:** 499–520.

8. Underhill BML. Intestinal length in man. *Br Med J* 1955; **2:** 1243–1246.

9. Backman L, Hallberg D. Small intestinal length. An intraoperative study in obesity. *Acta Chir Scand* 1974; **140:** 57–63.

10. Hirsch J, Ahrens EH, Blankenhorn DH. Measurement of the human intestinal length in vivo and some causes of variation. *Gastroenterology* 1956; **31:** 274–284.

11. Fanucci A, Cerro P, Fraracci L, Ietto F. Small bowel length measured by radiology. *Gastrointest Radiol* 1984; **9:** 349–351.

12. Slater G, Aufses Jr AH. Small bowel length in Crohn's disease. *Am J Gastroenterol* 1991; **86:** 1037–1040.

13. Wu T-J, Teng R-J, Chang M-H, Chen C-C. Congenital short bowel syndrome: report of a case treated with home central parenteral nutrition. *J Formosan Med Assoc* 1992; **91:** 470–472.

14. Nightingale JMD, Lennard-Jones JE. Patients with a short bowel due to Crohn's disease often start with a short normal bowel. *Eur J Gastroenterol Hepatol* 1995; **7:** 989–991.

15. Nightingale JMD, Bartram CI, Lennard-Jones JE. Length of residual small bowel after partial resection: Correlation between radiographic and surgical measurements. *Gastrointest Radiol* 1991; **16:** 305–306.

16. Borgström B, Dahlqvist A, Lundh G, Sjövall J. Studies of intestinal digestion and absorption in the human. *J Clin Invest* 1957; **36:** 1521–1536.

17. Fordtran JS, Locklear TW. Ionic constituents and osmolality of gastric and small intestinal fluids after eating. *Am J Dig Dis* 1966; **11:** 503–521.

18. Nightingale JMD, Lennard-Jones JE, Walker ER, Farthing MJG. Jejunal efflux in short bowel syndrome. *Lancet* 1990; **336:** 765–768.

19. Spiller RC, Trotman IF, Higgins BE *et al.* The ileal brake-inhibition of jejunal motility after ileal fat perfusion in man. *Gut* 1984; **25:** 365–374.

20. Nightingale JMD, Kamm MA, van der Sijp JRM *et al.* Disturbed gastric emptying in the short bowel syndrome. Evidence for a 'colonic brake'. *Gut* 1993; **34:** 1171–1176.

21. Nightingale JMD, Kamm MA, van der Sijp JRM, Walker ER, Ghatei MA, Bloom SR, Lennard-Jones JE. Gastrointestinal hormones in the short bowel syndrome. PYY may be the 'colonic brake' to gastric emptying. *Gut* 1996; **39:** 267–272.

22. Fordtran JS, Rector FC Jr, Ewton MF, Soter N, Kinney J. Permeability characteristics of the human small Intestine. *J Clin Invest* 1965; **44:** 1935–1944.

23. Davis GR, Santa Aria CA, Morawski SG, Fordtran JS. Permeability characteristics of human jejunum, ileum, proximal colon and distal colon: results of potential difference measurements and unidirectional fluxes. *Gastroenterology* 1982; **83:** 844–850.

24. Fordtran JS, Rector FC Jr, Carter NW. The mechanisms of sodium absorption in the human small intestine. *J Clin Invest* 1968; **47:** 884–900.

25. Spiller RC, Jones BJM, Silk DB. A. jejunal water and electrolyte absorption from two proprietary enteral feeds in man: importance of sodium content. *Gut* 1987; **28:** 681–687.

26. Sladen GE, Dawson AM. Inter-relationships between the absorptions of glucose, sodium and water by the normal human jejunum. *Clin Sci* 1969; **36:** 119–132.

27. Rodrigues CA, Lennard-Jones JE, Thompson DG, Farthing MJG. What is the ideal sodium concentration of oral rehydration solutions for short bowel patients? *Clin Sci* 1988; **74 (suppl 18):** 69p.

28. McIntyre PB, Fitchew M, Lennard-Jones JE. Patients with a jejunostomy do not need a special diet. *Gastroenterology* 1986; **91:** 25–33.

29. Thompson WG, Wrathell E. The relation between ileal resection and vitamin B_{12} absorption. *Can J Surg* 1977; **20:** 461–464.

30. Gouttebel MC, Saint-Aubert B, Astre C, Joyeux H. Total parenteral nutrition needs in different types of short bowel syndrome. *Dig Dis Sci* 1986; **31:** 718–723.

31. Heaton KW, Read AE. Gallstones in patients with disorders of the terminal ileum and disturbed bile-salt metabolism. *Br Med J* 1969; **3:** 494–496.

32. Lee SP, Nicholls JF, Park HZ. Biliary sludge as a cause of acute pancreatitis. *N Engl J Med* 1992; **326:** 589–593.

33. Doty JE, Pitt HA, Porter-Fink V, Denbesten L. Cholecystokinin prophylaxis of parenteral nutrition-induced gallbladder disease. *Ann Surg* 1985; **201:** 76–80.

34. Thompson JS. The role of prophylactic cholecyst-ectomy in the short bowel syndrome. *Arch Surg* 1996; **131:** 556–560.

35. Nordgaard I, Hansen BS, Mortensen PB. Importance of colonic support for energy absorption as small-bowel failure proceeds. *Am J Clin Nutr* 1996; **64:** 222–231.

36. Nordgaard I, Hansen BS, Mortensen PB. Colon as a digestive organ in patients with short bowel. *Lancet* 1994; **343:** 373–376.

37. Royall D, Wolever TMS, Jeejeebhoy KN. Evidence for colonic conservation of malabsorbed carbohydrate in short bowel syndrome. *Am J Gastroenterol* 1992; **87:** 751–756.

38. Messing B, Pigot F, Rongier M, Morin MC, Mdeindoum U, Rambaud JC. Intestinal absorption of free oral hyperalimentation in the very short bowel syndrome. *Gastroenterology* 1991; **100:** 1502–1508.

39. Briet F, Flourie B, Achour L, Maurel M, Rambaud J-C, Messing B. Bacterial adaptation in patients with short bowel and colon in continuity. *Gastroenterology* 1995; **109:** 1446–1453.

40. Aghdassi E, Plapler H, Kurian R, Raina N, Royall D, Jeejeebhoy K N, Cohen Z, Allard JP. Colonic fermentation and nutritional recovery in rats with massive small bowel resection. *Gastroenterology* 1994; **107:** 637–642.

41. Editorial. The colon, the rumen, and D-lactic acidosis. *Lancet* 1990; **336:** 599–600.

42. Mayne AJ, Handy DJ, Preece MA, George RH, Booth I. Dietary management of D-lactic acidosis in short bowel syndrome. *Arch Dis Child* 1990; **65:** 229–231.

43. Ammon HV, Phillips SF. Inhibition of colonic water and electrolyte absorption by fatty acids in man. *Gastroenterology* 1973; **65:** 744–749.

44. Spiller RC, Brown ML, Phillips SF. Decreased fluid tolerance, accelerated transit, and abnormal motility of the human colon induced by oleic acid. *Gastroenterology* 1986; **91:** 100–107.

45. Knapp HR, Melly MA. Bactericidal effects of poly-unsaturated fatty acids. *J Infect Dis* 1986; **154:** 84–94.

46. Thompson L, Edwards RE, Greenwood D, Spiller RC. Inhibitory effect of long chain fatty acids (LCFA's) on colonic bacteria. *Gut* 1990; **31:** A1167.

47. Jeppesen PB, Mortensen PB. Colonic digestion of medium-chain fat in patients with a short bowel. *Gastroenterology* 1997; **112:** A882.

48. Press M, Hartop PJ, Prottey C. Correction of essential fatty-acid deficiency in man by cutaneous application of sunflower-seed oil. *Lancet* 1974; **ii:** 597–599.

49. Dobbins JW, Binder HJ. Importance of the colon in enteric hyperoxaluria. *N Engl J Med* 1977; **296:** 298–301.

50. Earnest DL, Johnson G, Williams HE, Admirand WH. Hyperoxaluria in patients with ileal resection: an abnormality in dietary oxalate absorption. *Gastroenterology* 1974; **66:** 1114–1122.

51. Andersson H, Jagenburg R. Fat-reduced diet in the treatment of hyperoxaluria in patients with ileopathy. *Gut* 1974; **15:** 360–366.

52. Dobbins JW, Binder HJ. Effect of bile salts and fatty acids on the colonic absorption of oxalate. *Gastroenterology* 1976; **70:** 1096–1100.

53. Chadwick VS, Modha K, Dowling RH. Mechanism for hyperoxaluria in patients with ileal dysfunction. *N Engl J Med* 1973; **289:** 172–176.

54. Barilla DE, Notz C, Kennedy D, Pak CYC. Renal oxalate excretion following oral oxalate loads in patients with ileal disease and with renal and absorptive hypercalciurias. Effect of calcium and magnesium. *Am J Med* 1978; **64:** 579–585.

55. Lindsjo M, Ljunghall S, Fellstrom B, Wikstrom B, Danielson BF. Treatment of enteric hyperoxaluria with calcium-containing organic marine hydrocolloid. *Lancet* 1989; **ii:** 701–704.

56. Smith LH, Fromm H, Hofmann AF. Acquired hyper-oxaluria, nephrolithiasis and intestinal disease. *N Engl J Med* 1972; **286:** 1371–1375.

57. Ladefoged K, Olgaard K. Sodium homeostasis after small-bowel resection. *Scand J Gastroenterol* 1985; **20:** 361–369.

58. Porus RL. Epithelial hyperplasia following massive small bowel resection in man. *Gastroenterology* 1965; **48:** 753–759.

59. Weinstein LD, Shoemaker CP, Hersh T, Wright HK. Enhanced intestinal absorption after small bowel resection in man. *Arch Surg* 1969; **99:** 560–562.

60. De Francesco A, Malfi G, Delsedime L *et al.* Histological findings regarding jejunal mucosa in short bowel syndrome. *Transplant Proc* 1994; **26:** 1455–1456.

61. Cosnes J, Carbonnel F, Beaugerie L, Ollivier J-M, Parc R, Gendre J-P, Le Quintrec Y. Functional adaptation after extensive small bowel resection in humans. *Eur J Gastroenterol Hepatol* 1994; **6:** 197–202.

62. Dowling RH, Booth CC. Functional compensation after small bowel resection in man: Demonstration by direct measurement. *Lancet* 1966; **ii:** 146–147.

63. Gouttebel MC, Saint Aubert B, Colette C, Astre C, Monnier LH, Joyeux H. Intestinal adaptation in patients with short bowel syndrome. Measurement by calcium absorption. *Dig Dis Sci* 1989; **34:** 709–715.

64. Miazza BM. Hyperenteroglucagonaemia and small intestinal mucosal growth after colonic perfusion of glucose in rats. *Gut* 1985; **26:** 518–524.

65. Buxton B. Small bowel resection and gastric acid hypersecretion. *Gut* 1974; **15:** 229–238.

66. Windsor CWO, Fejfar J, Woodward DAK. Gastric secretion after massive small bowel resection. *Gut* 1969; **10:** 779–786.

67. Selby PL, Peacock M, Bambach CP. Hypomagnesaemia after small bowel resection: treatment with 1 alpha-hydroxylated vitamin D metabolites. *Br J Surg* 1984; **71:** 334–337.

68. Ladefoged K, Olgaard K. Fluid and electrolyte absorption and renin-angiotensin-aldosterone axis in patients with severe short-bowel syndrome. *Scand J Gastroenterol* 1979; **14:** 729–735.

69. Whang R, Whang DD, Ryan MP. Refactory potassium repletion. A consequence of magnesium deficiency. *Arch Intern Med* 1992; **152:** 40–45.

70. Newton CR, Gonvers JJ, McIntyre PB, Preston DM, Lennard-Jones JE. Effect of different drinks on fluid and electrolyte losses from a jejunostomy. *J Roy Soc Med* 1985; **78:** 27–34.

71. Griffin GE, Fagan EF, Hodgson HJ, Chadwick VS. Enteral therapy in the management of massive gut resection complicated by chronic fluid and electrolyte depletion. *Dig Dis Sci* 1982; **27:** 902–908.

72. Avery ME, Snyder JD. Oral therapy for acute diarrhoea. The underused simple solution. *N Engl J Med* 1990; **323:** 891–894.

73. Fordtran JS. Stimulation of active and passive sodium absorption by sugars in the human jejunum. *J Clin Invest* 1975; **55:** 728–737.

74. Nightingale JMD, Lennard-Jones JE, Walker ER, Farthing MJG. Oral salt supplements to compensate for jejunostomy losses: comparison of sodium chloride capsules, glucose electrolyte solution and glucose polymer electrolyte solution (Maxijul). *Gut* 1992; **33:** 759–761.

75. Jacobsen O, Ladefoged K, Stage JG, Jarnum S. Effects of cimetidine on jejunostomy effluents in patients with severe short bowel syndrome. *Scand J Gastroenterol* 1986; **21:** 824–828.

76. Nightingale JMD, Walker ER, Farthing MJG, Lennard-Jones JE. Effect of omeprazole on intestinal output in the short bowel syndrome. *Aliment Pharmacol Therap* 1991; **5:** 405–412.

77. Cooper JC, Williams NS, King RFGJ, Barker MCJ. Effects of a long acting somatostatin analogue in patients with severe ileostomy diarrhoea. *Br J Surg* 1986; **73:** 128–131.

78. Rodrigues CA, Lennard-Jones JE, Walker ER, Thompson DG, Farthing MJG. The effects of octreotide, soy polysaccharide, codeine and loperamide on nutrient, fluid and electrolyte absorption in the short bowel syndrome. *Aliment Pharmacol Therap* 1989; **3:** 159–169.

79. Ladefoged K, Christensen KC, Hegnhoj J, Jarnum S. Effect of a long acting somatostatin analogue SMS 201–995 on jejunostomy effluents in patients with severe short bowel syndrome. *Gut* 1989; **30:** 943–949.

80. Nightingale JMD, Walker ER, Burnham WR, Farthing MJG, Lennard-Jones JE. The short bowel syndrome. *Digestion* 1990; **45(suppl 1):** 77–83.

81. O'Keefe SJD, Peterson ME, Fleming CR. Octreotide as an adjunct to home parenteral nutrition in the management end-jejunostomy syndrome. *J Parent Enteral Nutr* 1994; **18:** 26–34.

82. Newton CR. Effect of codeine phosphate, Lomotil and Isogel on ileostomy function. *Gut* 1978; **19:** 377–383.

83. Nightingale JMD, Lennard-Jones JE, Walker ER. A patient with jejunostomy liberated from home intra-venous therapy after 14 years; contribution of balance studies. *Clin Nutr* 1992; **11:** 101–105.

84. Hill GL, Mair WSJ, Goligher JC. Impairment of 'ileostomy adaptation' in patients after ileal resection. *Gut* 1974; **15:** 982–987.

85. Ovesen L, Chu R, Howard L. The influence of dietary fat on jejunostomy output in patients with severe short bowel syndrome. *Am J Clin Nutr* 1983; **38:** 270–277.

86. O'Keefe SJD, Haymond MW, Bennet WM, Oswald B, Nelson DK, Shorter RG. Long-acting somatostatin analogue therapy and protein metabolism in patients with jejunostomies. *Gastroenterology* 1994; **107:** 379–388.

87. Messing B, Crenn P, Vahedi K, Panis Y, Matuchansky C. Short bowel as a model of intestinal failure. *Gut* 1997; **41 (suppl 3):** A14.

88. Messing B, Leman M, Landais P *et al*. Prognosis of patients with nonmalignant chronic intestinal failure receiving long-term home parenteral nutrition. *Gastroenterology* 1995; **108:** 1005–1010.

89. Goulet OJ, Revillon Y, Jan D *et al*. Neonatal short bowel syndrome. *J Paediatr* 1991; **119:** 18–23.

90. Thompson JS. Surgical considerations in the short bowel syndrome. *Surg Gynecol Obstet* 1993; **176:** 89–101.

91. Shanbhogue LKR, Molenaar JC. Short bowel syndrome: metabolic and surgical management. *Br J Surg* 1994; **81:** 486–499.

92. Bianchi A. Longitudinal intestinal lengthening and tailoring: results in 20 children. *J Roy Soc Med* 1997; **90:** 429–432.

93. Grant D. Current results of intestinal transplantation. *Lancet* 1996; **347:** 1801–1803.

94. Ingham Clark CL, Lear PA, Wood S, Lennard-Jones JE, Wood RFM. Potential candidates for small-bowel transplantation. *Br J Surg* 1992; **79:** 676–679.

95. Sustento-Reodica N, Ruiz P, Rogers A, Viciana AL, Conn HO, Tzakis AG. Recurrent Crohn's disease in transplanted bowel. *Lancet* 1997; **349:** 688–691.

96. Gruy-Kapral C, Little KH, Fortran JS, Meziere TL, Hagey LR, Hofmann AF. Conjugated bile acid replacement therapy for short-bowel syndrome. *Gastroenterology* 1999; **116:** 15–21.

97. Heydorn S, Jeppesen PB, Mortensen PB. Bile acid replacement therapy with cholylsarcosine for short-bowel syndrome. *Scand J Gastroenterol* 1999; **34:** 818–823.

98. Byrne TA, Persinger RL, Young LS, Ziegler TR, Gatzen C, Wilmore DW. A new treatment for patients with short-bowel syndrome. Growth hormone, glutamine, and a modified diet. *Ann Surg* 1995; 222.

99. Scolapio JS, Camilleri M, Fleming CR, Oenning LV, Burton DD, Sebo TJ, Batts KP, Kelly DG. Effect of growth hormone, glutamine, and diet on adaptation in short-bowel syndrome: a randomized, controlled study. *Gastroenterology* 1997; **113:** 1074–1081.

100. Delhougne B, Deneux C, Abs R, Chanson P, Fierens H, Laurent-Puig P, Duysburgh I, Stevenaert A, Tabarin A, Delwaide J *et al.* The prevalence of colonic polyps in acromegaly: a colonoscopic and pathological study in 103 patients. *J Clin Endocrinol Metab* 1995; **80:** 3223–3226.

101. Walker-Smith JA, Phillips AD, Walford N, Gregory H, Fitzgerlad JD, MacCullagh K, Wright NA. Intravenous epidermal growth factor/urogastrone increases small-intestinal cell proliferation in congenital microvillous atrophy. *Lancet* 1985; **88:** 1239–1240.

102. Rokkas T, Vaja S, Murphy GM, Dowling RH. Aminoguanidine blocks intestinal diamine oxidase (DAO) activity and enhances the intestinal adaptive response to resection in the rat. *Digestion* 1990; **46 (suppl 2):** 447–457.

103. Nightingale JMD. Short gut, short answer? *Gut* 1999; **45:** 478–479.

104. Campbell FC, Tait IS, Flint N, Evans GS. Transplantation of cultured small bowel enterocytes. *Gut* 1993; **34:** 1153–1155.

40

Nutrition support in pancreatitis

Stephen A McClave and David A Spain

Introduction and historical background

Throughout the recent history of the science of clinical nutrition, the central strategy of nutrition support for the patient with acute pancreatitis has focused on the single issue of reducing pancreatic exocrine secretion and placing the pancreas 'at rest' by the use of total parenteral nutrition (TPN). In the past 5 years, this focus has begun to change with evidence that routine use of TPN may not be beneficial to the patient.[1,2] A number of other issues also require the attention of the clinician, such as the overall stress response, maintenance of gut integrity and reduction in late complications of nosocomial infection and multiple organ failure.[3–5] This chapter reviews the historical events that helped determine the use of nutrition support for the patient with acute pancreatitis, discuss the pertinent issues related to the need for reduction of pancreatic stimulation while providing enteral nutrients, and discuss the practical application of enteral and parenteral nutritional alimentation in patients with this disease process.

A chronology of the key events over the second half of the 20th century helps to understand our current practice of nutrition support (Fig. 40.1). The decade of the 1960s saw leaders in the field of pancreatitis convene in 1963 to define pancreatitis and to differentiate acute and chronic disease.[6] In 1968, Dudrick reported the first case of human growth and development sustained by parenteral feeding, giving birth to the practice of TPN.[7] The concept of avoiding enteral nutrients to reduce stimulation of exocrine secretion and place the pancreas 'at rest' was crystallised in 1977 when Ranson warned that early advancement to an oral diet in a patient with acute pancreatitis was associated with increased risk of late complications, such as parapancreatic infection and abscess.[8] Numerous studies demonstrated that pancreatic enzyme secretion changed very little in response to parenteral substrates and helped forge the era of TPN throughout the 1970s and early 1980s.[9–16] In 1986, however, prospective randomised controlled trials (PRCTs) in trauma patients comparing TPN with enteral nutrition by tube (EN) were first reported, with results suggesting that EN was less costly and was associated with less nosocomial infection, multiple organ failure and shorter length of hospitalisation when compared to TPN.[4,17–21] In 1987, Sax set out to provide the definitive study substantiating the usefulness of TPN in the treatment of patients with acute pancreatitis.[1] Much to the surprise of these investigators, this study found that the patients with acute pancreatitis receiving early TPN had a significantly

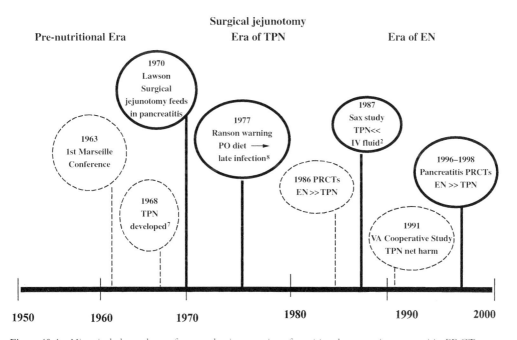

Figure 40.1 – Historical chronology of events shaping practice of nutritional support in pancreatitis. PRCT = prospective randomised controlled trials, PO = per os.

higher rate of catheter sepsis (10.5% vs 1.5%; $P < 0.003$) and a longer length of hospitalisation (16 vs 10 days; $P < 0.05$) than a similar group receiving only intravenous fluid resuscitation and analgesia.[1] This was the first study to indicate that routine use of TPN in acute pancreatitis might not be warranted. Shortly afterwards in 1991, the VA Cooperative Study which was undertaken to substantiate the benefit of TPN in the management of patients through the perioperative period, provided results which were opposite of what was expected.[2] A 4-fold increase in septic complications was seen in those patients receiving TPN, compared to a similar group receiving intravenous fluids alone without nutrition support. These results prompted the investigators to conclude that TPN caused net harm over the entire study population, and that preoperative TPN should be reserved only for those patients found to be severely malnourished.[2]

With these events in place, a general preference for EN over TPN began to develop. By the mid 1990s, PRCTs comparing early enteral with early parenteral feeding in acute pancreatitis were finally emerging. Results from these trials showed that jejunal feeds were tolerated as well as parenteral feeding.[22-26] Use of the enteral route incurred less expense, attenuated the acute phase response to a greater extent and reduced long-term complications associated with pancreatitis when compared to parenteral feeding.[22,24,25] The most surprising aspect of this chronology is the reference from Lawson reporting on his experience operating on pancreatitis from 1968 to 1970.[27] Just as TPN was being developed, Lawson emphasised for the first time the importance of placing jejunal tubes in the pancreatitis patient at the time of surgery for long-term enteral support postoperatively.[27] The science of clinical nutrition seems to have come full circle over the past 30 years back to where it started, with the emphasis shifting back to the enteral route of nutrition support for patients with acute pancreatitis.

Theoretical concepts and benefits of nutrition support

The focus of management of the patient with acute pancreatitis or an acute flare of chronic pancreatitis has been reduction of pancreatic secretion. The need for gut and pancreatic rest appeared to be universal and has been applied to all patients without regard to the severity of pancreatitis. However, this practice has never been proven to affect patient outcome. The only clear benefit of gut rest has been the relief of pain.[28] Slight increases in pain with early attempts at refeeding are usually well tolerated and may only lead to disease exacerbation in a small percentage of cases.[29] The entire concept of pancreatic rest has been poorly defined. Pancreatic secretory function may be assessed by volume, bicarbonate and enzyme output. The method and degree of stimulation varies for each. With the main concern being reduction of enzyme output and avoidance of autodigestion of the pancreas, then measures which produce an alkaline, watery, enzyme-poor secretion from the gland (reduced enzyme output with continued secretion of volume and bicarbonate) may successfully put the pancreas to rest.[30] The concept of pancreatic rest implies that pancreatic enzyme secretion has been reduced to a level at or below basal output. In practice, reducing secretion to a subclinical level (which may still be above basal levels) may be adequate enough to allow resolution of the disease process and overall clinical improvement.

Gut disuse has not been the only modality utilised to 'rest' the pancreas. A number of PRCTs have evaluated the clinical use of nasogastric suction, hormones (i.e. somatostatin, calcitonin, glucagon), or pharmacologic agents (i.e. cimetidine, anticholinergic agents) to reduce pancreatic stimulation.[31] None of them showed a significant effect of pancreatic rest by these methods on complications, length of hospitalisation, or mortality.[31] Furthermore, reducing pancreatic secretion at the time of acute inflammation may be a moot point; that there may be no secretion to suppress.[31]

A number of equally important clinical issues have emerged which compete with, and potentially contradict the concept of gut and pancreatic rest with TPN. The disease process of pancreatitis itself is notorious for generating a dramatic stress response indistinguishable from sepsis.[32] On admission, this stress response to the pancreatitis is associated with its own risk for early complications including organ failure and nosocomial infection. Prolonged placement of a patient nil by mouth with a hypercatabolic/hypermetabolic disease process such as acute pancreatitis, promotes deterioration of nutrition status which in turn may reduce systemic immunity and wound healing capabilities. Complications arising directly from use of TPN (i.e. catheter line sepsis) may occur due to the immunosuppressant effects of intravenous fat emulsions or the frequent occurrence of hyperglycaemia.[24] Loss of gut integrity from prolonged disuse may promote bacterial translocation and loss of gut-associated lymphoid tissue.[4] These late complications with further increases in organ failure, nosocomial infection and length of hospitalisation may result from iatrogenic factors related to patient management. Focusing solely on the issue of gut and pancreatic rest at the exclusion of these other equally important issues may lead to adverse effects on patient outcome. An increasing amount of data from the literature suggests that maintenance of gut integrity, attenuation of stress response and reduction in late complications of nosocomial infection and multiple organ failure are critically important in the disease process of pancreatitis.[24,25,33]

An adverse effect of TPN on intestinal morphology was recently reported in patients with chronic pancreatitis.[34] In this prospective, non-randomised study, ten patients with chronic pancreatitis anticipated to require surgery were placed on enteral feeding (n = 3) or TPN (n = 7), and compared to controls on enteral feeding without pancreatitis undergoing

surgery for other reasons. After receiving preoperative enteral or parenteral feeding for 1–12 weeks, a section of jejunum 15 cm below the ligament of Treitz was resected at the time of surgery and compared among the three groups. Results showed that the disease process of chronic pancreatitis itself was associated with a decrease in height of the small intestinal villi in pancreatitis patients on enteral feeding compared to the controls. However, further decreases in the height of the villi were seen in those pancreatitis patients receiving TPN (Fig. 40.2). Of concern were the morphologic changes associated with use of TPN, which included the formation of short, stubby villi with shallow crypts, broad leaf-like villi and even fusion of villi into indistinct ridges (Fig. 40.3). Prolonged use of TPN was associated with greater decreases in overall villous height. As seen in Figure 40.4, the frequency of villi below 500 μm increased from 22% in the control group, to 47% with 1 week of TPN, 64% with 2 weeks of TPN and up to 87% with 12 weeks of TPN.[34]

Data from animal and human studies suggest that loss of gut integrity with increased bacterial translocation

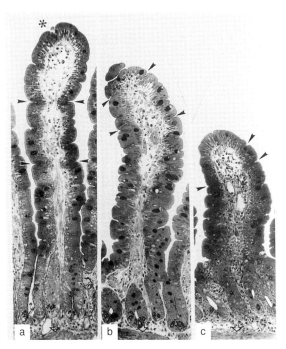

Figure 40.2 – Comparison of height of villi in non-pancreatitis patients receiving enteral nutrition (A), pancreatitis patients receiving enteral nutrition (B) and pancreatitis patients receiving TPN (C).[34]

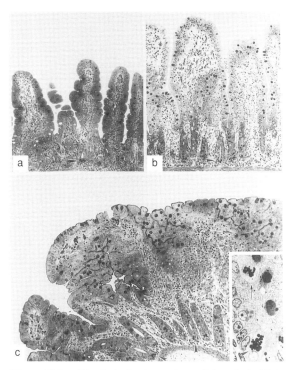

Figure 40.3 – Morphologic change in small intestinal villi in pancreatitis patients on TPN – from short stubby villi (A), to broad leaf-like villi (B), to fused ridge-like villi (C).[34]

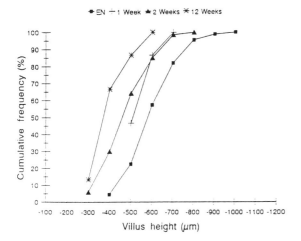

Figure 40.4 – Effect of duration of TPN therapy on small intestinal villous height.[34]

may contaminate the pancreas with intestinal organisms and lead to increases in nosocomial sepsis.[28,35–37] Potential mechanisms proposed in these studies include transportation of bacteria to areas of pancreatic necrosis by intestinal lymphatics, passage of bacteria into the portal vein with return to the pancreas via the common bile duct, or direct contamination of the pancreas through colonic microperforations. In an animal model, intestinal bacteria were shown to contaminate inflamed pancreatic tissue.[28] Gut decontamination with antibiotic therapy significantly reduced the rate of positive mesenteric lymph node cultures and overall mortality in response to pancreatitis.[36] In human studies, an association between intestinal bacteria and pancreatic infection was suggested by the fact that pancreatic phlegmons and infected fluid collections cultured positive for Gram-negative organisms in 60% of cases.[28,35,37] A recent study comparing enteral with parenteral feeding over 7 days[25] showed that serum IgM anticore endotoxin antibodies increased by 28.5% in the group receiving TPN, compared to a decrease of 1.1% in the group receiving enteral feeding ($P < 0.05$). Furthermore, total antioxidant capacity (measured by an enhancement chemiluminescence assay) fell by a median of 27.7% in the parenterally fed group, but increased by 32.6% in the enterally fed group ($P < 0.05$).[25] The IgM anti-endotoxin response in the TPN group suggested that loss of gut integrity may have led to significant systemic exposure to endotoxin, while the reduction in antioxidant capacity implied an increase in endotoxin-derived oxidant stress. In contrast, the enterally fed group showed no

IgM antibody response and actually improved their antioxidant capacity following 7 days of nutrition support, suggesting that maintenance of gut integrity by enteral feeding reduced exposure of the host to systemic bacterial endotoxin.[25]

Since the dramatic stress response induced by pancreatitis may promote early organ failure and nosocomial infection, efforts to attenuate this response may impact significantly on patient outcome. One example is the recent multicentre PRCT using a platelet activating factor antagonist in the treatment of patients with acute pancreatitis or an acute flare of chronic pancreatitis.[33] Patients given the antagonist within 48 h of the onset of pain showed a significant decrease in the incidence of multiple organ failure compared to placebo controls.[33] Similar studies in an animal model showed that blocking the activity of tumour necrosis factor (TNF) or interleukin 1 (IL-1) significantly reduced tissue damage and overall severity of pancreatitis.[38,39]

The route by which nutrition support is provided may further attenuate or provoke the stress response as well and thereby affect the patient's risk of developing late complications. In a recent PRCT of patients with acute pancreatitis,[24] we demonstrated that patients receiving TPN had a steady statistically significant rise in stress-induced hyperglycaemia over the first 6 days of infusion, an effect which was not seen in the group receiving EN. By the sixth day of hospitalisation, the mean serum glucose was 210 units in the TPN group compared to 151 units in the EN group ($P = 0.07$).[24] Serial mean Ranson criteria, Marshall multiorgan failure score, and APACHE III score suggested that the TPN group was slower to resolve the stress response associated with pancreatitis. However, only the mean Ranson criteria at day 6 for the TPN group was significantly higher than the EN group ($P = 0.002$).[24] In the recent Windsor study, C-reactive protein levels (a marker for the acute phase response) did not change significantly following 7 days of nutrition support in the TPN group, but decreased significantly in the EN group.[25] Also, no significant change in the mean APACHE II score in the TPN group was seen (9.5 to 8.0; $P = $ NS) over 7 days of nutrition support, while the mean score in the EN group decreased significantly (8.0 to 6.0; $P < 0.001$) over the same time interval.[25] The overall incidence of the systemic inflammatory response syndrome (SIRS) decreased significantly in the EN group from 69% of patients on admission to 12.5% after 7 days of nutrition support ($P < 0.05$).[25] There was no significant change in incidence of this syndrome (66.7% to 55.5% of patients) over the same time interval in the TPN group. Reductions in nosoconial infection, multiple organ failure and length of stay in the intensive care unit were seen in the EN group compared to the TPN group.[25] In a third PRCT in severe acute pancreatitis, Kalfarentzos showed that use of EN reduced overall complications (44% vs 75%; $P < 0.01$) and specifically, septic complications (28% vs 50%; $P < 0.01$) when compared respectively to use of TPN.[22] These three studies suggest that early EN may attenuate the stress response and improve patient outcome.

Several factors exist which determine the degree to which the pancreas is stimulated in response to nutrition support. The most significant of these factors is the level of the gastrointestinal tract into which enteral nutrients are infused (Fig. 40.5). Three distinct phases of pancreatic stimulation (cephalic, gastric and intestinal phases) correspond to the various levels in the gastrointestinal tract from which the stimulating factors originate.[40] Each phase has multiple components ranging from neurovagal or mechanical, to hormonal and chemical stimulants of pancreatic secretion. The higher the level at which nutrients are infused, the greater the number of factors that are brought into play, and the greater the degree of response from the pancreas that ensues. Conceivably, feeding low enough in the gastrointestinal tract (i.e.

jejunum) may invoke very few, if any, of these stimulating factors (Fig. 40.5). Alternatively, the few stimulatory factors which are invoked at this level may be offset by inhibitory factors, such that the end result is a negligible increase in pancreatic stimulation. Pancreatic inhibitory factors generated in the intestinal phase include luminal proteases and bile acids, rising pH and hormones such as somatostatin, pancreatic polypeptide, or peptide YY. In a dog model, infusion of nutrients into the stomach increased volume, bicarbonate and enzyme output from the pancreas, while duodenal infusion increased only volume output.[41] Only the jejunal infusion of enteral formula showed no significant increase in any of the three components of pancreatic secretion (in comparison to the infusion of saline).[41] While other studies looking at the change in specific enzyme levels in response to jejunal feeding supported[42] or refuted[43-45] the data from this study, the clinical effect of the level of ETF infusion on the patient's course of hospitalisation was demonstrated in our recent clinical trial.[24] Three patients who resolved their clinical symptoms and normalised their serum amylase levels over 5 days of jejunal feeding, developed an exacerbation of their disease process with recurrence of pain and hyper-amylasaemia when advanced to clear liquids by mouth. Two of these patients were placed back on jejunal feeds and their symptoms resolved with normalisation of amylase levels.[24] A fourth patient had

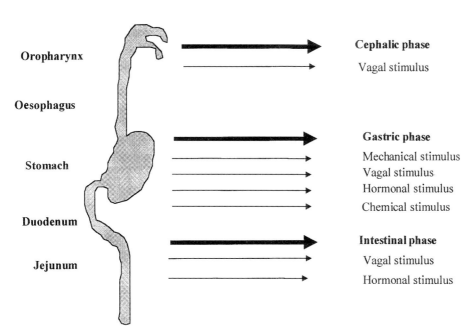

Figure 40.5 – Source of pancreatic secretory stimulants by level of the gastrointestinal tract.

a similar experience when the feeding tube was displaced from the jejunum back to the stomach.[24]

Irrespective of the level of the gastrointestinal tract from which they arise, a number of factors related to the quality and characteristics of food substances are involved which have a variable effect in stimulating the pancreas (Fig. 40.6). The sight and smell of food, acid produced in response to digestion and mechanical distention of the stomach from the volume of the meal are all potent stimulants of pancreatic secretion. A graded response to food components exists, such that fat has a greater stimulatory effect than protein and carbohydrate. Greater stimulation occurs in response to ingestion of long-chain compared to medium-chain fat, oligopeptides compared to intact protein or individual amino acids, and hyperosmolar compared to isosmolar formulas.[40,46] The greater the number of these factors that are invoked by a particular diet, the greater the degree of pancreatic stimulation. Thus, an odourless, isosmolar, nearly fat-free elemental diet with individual amino acids ingested by mouth might be well tolerated without pain in a patient who is otherwise intolerant of regular food.[46] A case series report of 17 patients with acute pancreatitis showed clinical improvement in symptoms and resolution of hyperamylasaemia when given an elemental diet by mouth or by nasogastric infusion.[46] Several patients showed an exacerbation of symptoms and an increase

in amylase when advanced to a full diet, all of which resolved when placed back on the elemental feeding.[46]

Therefore, a graded balance of management seems to exist, such that the greater the degree of disease severity, the fewer the number of stimulating factors that can be invoked and still result in clinical remission (Fig. 40.7). Factors determining the degree of disease severity are most likely related to the presence or absence of pancreatic necrosis on dynamic computerised tomography (CT) scan[47] (Fig. 40.7). A hierarchy exists in the type of factors which stimulate pancreatic secretion, with fat at one end of the scale with the greatest capacity to increase enzyme output, and intact protein and carbohydrate are at the opposite end. Generally, the level of the gastrointestinal tract at which nutrients are infused seems to have a greater clinical impact than the specific factors related to food substances in determining the degree of pancreatic stimulation. Oral feedings are at one end of the scale invoking the greatest stimulation of the pancreas, while jejunal feeds or parenteral feeding are at the opposite end of the scale invoking the least. Gastric infusion or oral ingestion of a low fat diet might be tolerated with a mild degree of pancreatitis, while greater degrees of disease severity may require infusion of a fat-free isosmolar elemental diet into the jejunum to resolve symptoms and allow the inflammatory response to abate.

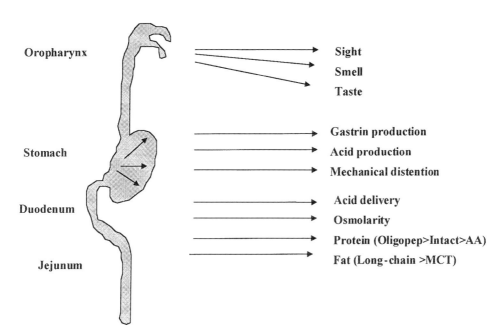

Figure 40.6 – Source of pancreatic secretory stimulants related to quality and characteristics of food substances.

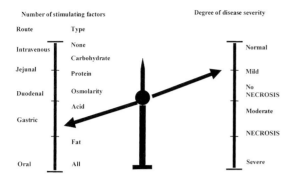

Figure 40.7 – Graded balance of nutritional management between degree of disease severity in pancreatitis and the number and characteristics of stimulatory factors involved.

Practical application including enteral and parenteral nutrition

One of the most difficult aspects in the clinical management of acute pancreatitis involves nutritional assessment and determination of when resumption of oral diet is appropriate. Clinicians must make several key determinations related to patient selection, timing and overall risk: which patients are likely to advance early to oral diet, when is a particular patient ready to advance to an oral diet and what deleterious effects may occur by advancing diet too early. Overshadowing these decisions is the long-held fear that poorly-timed advancement to oral intake may result in late complications of major parapancreatic infection and pancreatic abscess.[8] A recent prospective, non-randomised trial investigated several issues related to early advancement to oral diet in 116 consecutive patients with pancreatitis, and evaluated those factors which might predict the likelihood for relapse of symptoms once oral diet was resumed.[29] Physicians in this trial were allowed to decide when patients could advance to oral diet. Once advanced, patients were restricted to a uniform diet characterised by a slow increase in the number of total calories with an increasing percentage of fat over the first 5 days.[29] Results showed that 21.0% of these patients developed an exacerbation of symptoms when advanced to oral diet, but only 4.3% developed an actual exacerbation of their disease process. Of interest was the effect of relapse on patient outcome. Total length of hospitalisation was almost twice as long in those patients with relapse compared to those who showed no relapse (33.0 vs 18.0 days; $P < 0.002$). Length of hospital-

isation after the first attempt at oral diet was almost three times longer in the relapse group (18.0 days vs 7.0 days, $P < 0.002$) compared respectively to the group which showed no relapse.[29] Factors not associated with risk for relapse were maximum amylase and lipase levels, C-reactive protein, presence of fluid collection, pancreatic calcifications, dilation of the pancreatic ducts, or need for therapeutic procedures. However, duration of painful period was significantly longer in those patients who relapsed upon advancement to oral diet compared to those who did not (11.0 vs 6.0 days respectively; $P < 0.002$).[29] If the serum lipase drawn 1 day prior to oral diet was greater than three times normal, 39% of the patients developed relapse. In contrast, lipase levels less than or equal to three times normal were associated with a 16% chance of relapse ($P < 0.03$). Additionally, evidence of pancreatic necrosis on CT scan (Baltazar's score ≥ D) was associated with a 35% chance of relapse, whereas absence of necrosis (Baltazar's score < D) was associated with a 12% chance of relapse ($P < 0.002$).[29] Thus, the results of this study provide some criteria for determining the risk of the patient for advancement to oral diet. The clinical criteria include a long, painful period ≥ 6 days, serum lipase level greater than three times normal, or evidence of pancreatic necrosis on CT scan. The likelihood of relapse if one or more of these criteria are present is 35–39%, while the absence of the three criteria are associated with a relapse rate of only 12–16%.[29]

The determination of which patients will require early aggressive nutrition support involves differentiating patients with mild versus severe pancreatitis. Recent studies have begun to provide very specific information to allow the clinician to make this distinction (Fig. 40.8).[48–51] Patients with ≤ 2 Ranson criteria and an APACHE II score ≤ 9 have a mild degree of acute pancreatitis and are unlikely to have pancreatic necrosis.[49,50] These patients account for 80% of admissions for acute pancreatitis.[47,49] Their APACHE II score should decrease by at least 1 point during the first 48 h of admission. The overall likelihood of complications is only 7.7% and their mortality rate is near 0%.[48,51] These patients should advance to oral diet without incidence by the fifth day of hospitalisation.[1] These patients do not need aggressive nutrition support, but simple fluid resuscitation, analgesia and general supportive care. In contrast, patients with ≥ 3 Ranson criteria or an APACHE II score ≥ 10 have a severe degree of pancreatitis.[49,50] These patients make up 20% of hospital admissions for pancreatitis and

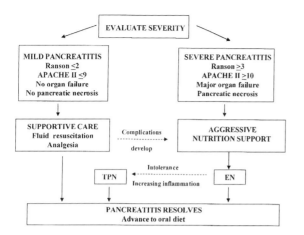

Figure 40.8 – Algorithm for nutritional hyperalimentation in pancreatitis.

usually have evidence of pancreatic necrosis on CT scan.[47,49] During the first 48 h of hospitalisation, the APACHE II score usually increases by a mean of 3 points.[48] Complications develop in 38% of these patients and the mortality rate is 20%.[51] These patients are unlikely to progress to oral diet within the first 5 days of hospitalisation.[1] They are candidates for aggressive nutrition support, hopefully by achievement of enteral access and early infusion of EN.

Greatest severity of pancreatitis does not preclude use of the enteral route of feeding, but it may affect the likelihood for overall tolerance. Early evidence would suggest that safety issues related to jejunal feeding and suppression of pancreatic secretion to subclinical levels should be no different in patients with more severe pancreatitis.[22,24,25] However, increasing degrees of intestinal ileus may reduce tolerance.[25]

A prospective non-randomized trial evaluated this issue of tolerance of enteral feeding in 102 consecutive patients with acute pancreatitis.[52] Unfortunately, no information was provided on degree of severity of pancreatitis. Patients who had an intestinal ileus lasting greater than 6 days had to be placed on TPN ($n = 11$). Patients who showed no ileus at 48 h were advanced to enteral feeding ($n = 83$), as were patients who had no ileus at 5 days ($n = 8$).[52] Tolerance of EN occurred in 92% of the patients in the early group and in only four out of eight (50%) patients in the late group.[52] Although ileus and tolerance were not well defined, these results suggest that any evidence for intestinal ileus at 48 h should alert the clinician to problems with tolerance when enteral feedings are begun. EN intolerance was common (31.2% of patients) in the

study by Windsor *et al*, which included a significant number of patients with severe pancreatitis.[25] However, most required only a temporary decrease in the volume of enteral feedings for a duration of 2–4 days.[25] Feeding was able to be continued at a lower rate during this time period as the signs of ileus resolved. Although patients on EN received significantly fewer non-protein calories, they had a lower complication rate and resolved their disease process more quickly than patients on TPN.[25]

The presence of complications from pancreatitis is not necessarily a contraindication to the use of enteral feeding. Several uncontrolled, mostly retrospective case series have described the use of enteral feeding in patients with complications arising from pancreatitis such as ascites, fistulae, or fluid collections.[46,53–57] In many of these cases, enteral feeding was given in the middle of their hospital course after most of the acute inflammation had subsided to some degree. Faced with prolonged hospitalisation due to the complication, efforts were made to use the enteral route. In some cases, patients clearly failed TPN or developed complications from intravenous access, while in other cases the clinicians made a legitimate effort to use EN earlier. Surprisingly, the enteral feedings were often given as an elemental formula by mouth or by nasogastric infusion. In most cases, complications resolved during several weeks of enteral nutrition. Only one patient in these case series developed a new pseudocyst (but was otherwise asymptomatic) while on EN.[46] Diarrhoea was the only complication arising infrequently from enteral feeding. When complications failed to resolve, patients went to surgery uneventfully. In one of the larger series involving 17 patients,[46] tolerance of elemental formulas ingested by mouth or given by nasogastric infusion was seen in five cases of pancreatic ascites, three cases of pleural effusion and four cases of acute fluid collections, many of whom had shown exacerbation of symptoms when placed on an oral diet.[46]

Surgical intervention to treat the complications of severe pancreatitis does not preclude use of enteral feeding and, in fact, provides an opportunity to secure enteral access.[27,58] Critically ill patients with severe haemorrhagic and infectious complications from pancreatitis in a recent case series were treated aggressively with jejunal feeding in the immediate postoperative period.[58] Although two of 11 patients died due to complications arising from placement of a needle jejunostomy, the nine patients who had successful tube placement tolerated their feedings well and showed no evidence of exacerbation of pancreatitis.[58] Two recent prospective studies, in which patients undergoing surgery for complications of acute pancreatitis were randomised postoperatively to either enteral feeding (through a surgical jejunostomy) or TPN, showed no significant differences in outcome or tolerance between the two routes of feeding.[23,26] Of interest was the fact that catheters placed in the pancreatic duct at the time of surgery showed no significant differences in pancreatic volume, bicarbonate, protein, amylase, or chymotrypsin output between the two routes of feeding.[23]

An algorithm for nutrition support in acute pancreatitis is provided in Figure 40.8. Upon initial examination, patients with acute pancreatitis or an acute flare of chronic pancreatitis should be evaluated for Ranson criteria, APACHE II score, evidence of organ failure and presence of necrosis on CT scan. Patients with ≤ 2 Ranson criteria or an APACHE II score ≤ 9 may be designated as having mild pancreatitis and, in the absence of pancreatic necrosis or organ failure, can be placed on fluid resuscitation, analgesia and supportive care.[49,50] Duration of pain < 6 days, absence of necrosis on CT scan and a decrease in lipase levels to less than three times normal may identify patients ready to progress to oral diet.[29] The presence of any of these three criteria may necessitate delay in advancement to oral diet for up to 5 days. Those patients with ≥ 3 Ranson criteria with an APACHE II score of ≥ 10, particularly if the APACHE II score increases during the first 48 h, may be identified as having severe pancreatitis and will require aggressive nutrition support.[49,50]

In those patients determined to require aggressive nutrition support, enteral access may be obtained by endoscopic or fluoroscopic placement of a nasoenteric tube at or below the ligament of Treitz (see Chapter 17). An elemental formula, which is nearly fat-free and has a high percentage of amino acids as the protein source, may be the optimal choice for this disease process. An acceptable alternative would be a semielemental small peptide formula. Any slight disadvantage these formulas have due to the oligopeptides and long-chain fat (which cause greater stimulation of pancreatic secretion than the elemental formulas) may be offset by greater absorption in an environment where the pancreas has been put to rest and enzymes are absent.[59,60]

Patients receiving enteral tube feeding should be monitored closely for evidence of tube migration.

Residual volumes, development of nausea, vomiting and diarrhoea, and risk of aspiration should be followed closely. Patients should receive adequate analgesia and aggressive fluid volume resuscitation. Care should be taken to identify any nutrient deficiencies and a vitamin/trace mineral solution should be added if the volume of enteral feeding does not provide adequate micronutrients.

Patients on EN who demonstrate clear-cut intolerance or have increasing pain with significant increases in amylase and lipase, should be considered for conversion to TPN. A central line should be placed and a mixed fuel regimen started. The majority of earlier studies which evaluated the effect of intravenous nutrients on pancreatic stimulation found that in the absence of hypertriglyceridaemia, the provision of fat, protein and carbohydrate by the parenteral route is well tolerated and should not lead to an exacerbation of the disease process.[61,62] The overall amount of fat should be kept at 15–30% of total calories. TPN should be slowly advanced to avoid problems with hyperglycaemia. Any hyperglycaemia that develops should be treated aggressively with insulin infusion. Serum triglyceride levels, glucose levels and electrolytes (i.e. calcium, magnesium and potassium) should all be monitored closely. Hypercalcaemia, which can cause exacerbation of pancreatitis by itself,[63] should obviously be avoided.

The future

It is difficult to predict how the nutritional management of pancreatitis will change in the new millennium. Certainly, clinicians will become more comfortable with aggressive use of the enteral route in patients with pancreatitis. New pharmacologic agents and treatments to attenuate the stress response, such as platelet activating factor antagonists or leukotriene inhibitors, may become available for widespread use. Increasing use of endoscopic and CT-guided percutaneous procedures may be utilised to manage complications arising from pancreatitis. Changes in the management of the patients with acute pancreatitis must focus on cost containment and reduction in overall mortality and length of hospitalisation.

The most important message for the clinician is that multiple concepts related to the nutritional management of the patient with acute pancreatitis are simultaneously important and require an equivalent degree of attention. The nutrition support regimen should be designed to reduce stimulation of the pancreas to subclinical levels, while simultaneously reducing the stress response, maintaining gut integrity and avoiding iatrogenic complications. While the competing issues of pancreatic rest and the benefits of early EN in critical illness are not completely resolved, the balance has shifted towards more aggressive use of EN. As with all patients with critical illness, the clinician must be aware of the full range of treatment options available and be flexible enough to individualise those methods specific to the patient needs.

References

1. Sax HC, Warner BW, Talamini MA et al. Early total parenteral nutrition in acute pancreatitis: lack of beneficial effects. Am J Surg 1987; 153(1): 117–124.

2. The Veterans Affairs Total Parenteral Nutrition Cooperative Study Group. Perioperative total parenteral nutrition in surgical patients. N Engl J Med 1991; 325: 525–532.

3. Moore EE, Moore FA. Immediate enteral nutrition following multisystem trauma: a decade perspective. J Am Coll Nutr 1991; 10: 633–648.

4. Zaloga GP, MacGregor DA. What to consider when choosing enteral or parenteral nutrition. J Crit Illness 1990; 5: 1180–1200.

5. Kudsk KA, Croce MA, Fabian TC et al. Enteral versus parenteral feeding: effects on septic morbidity after blunt and penetrating abdominal trauma. Ann Surg 1992; 215: 503–511.

6. Sarles H. Clinical classification. Bibl Gastroenterol 1965; 7: 7.

7. Dudrick SJ, Wilmore DW, Vars HM, Rhoads JE. Long-term total parenteral nutrition with growth, development, and positive nitrogen balance. Surgery 1968; 64: 134–142.

8. Ranson JHC, Spencer FC. Prevention, diagnosis and treatment of pancreatic abscess. Surgery 1977; 82: 99–106.

9. Klein E, Shnebaum S, Ben-Ari G et al. Effects of total parenteral nutrition on exocrine pancreatic secretion. Am J Gastroenterol 1983; 78: 31.

10. Buch A, Buch J, Carlsen A et al. Hyperlipidemia and pancreatitis. World J Surg 1980; 4: 307–314.

11. Silberman H, Dixon NP, Eisenberg D. The safety and efficacy of a lipid-based system of parenteral nutrition in acute pancreatitis. Am J Gastroenterol 1982; 77(7): 494.

12. Grant JP, James S, Grabowski V et al. Total parenteral nutrition in pancreatic disease. Ann Surg 1984; 200: 627.

13. Grundfest S, Steiger E, Selinkoff P et al. The effect of intravenous fat emulsions in patients with pancreatic fistula. JPEN 1980; 4(1): 27.

14. Bivins BA, Bell RM, Rapp RP et al. Pancreatic exocrine response to parenteral nutrition. JPEN 1984; 8: 34.

15. Edelman K, Valenzuela JE. Effect of intravenous lipid on human pancreatic secretion. Gastroenterology 1983; 85: 1063.

16. Variyam EP, Fuller RK, Brown FM et al. Effect of parenteral amino acid on human pancreatic exocrine secretion. Dig Dis Sci 1980; 30: 541.

17. Moore EE, Jones TN. Benefits of immediate jejunostomy feeding after major abdominal trauma: a prospective, randomized study. J Trauma 1986; 26: 874–880.

18. Moore FA, Moore EE, Jones TN et al. TEN versus TPN following major abdominal trauma: reduced septic morbidity. J Trauma 1989; 29: 916–922.

19. Adams S, Delinger EP, Wertz MJ et al. Enteral versus parenteral nutritional support following laparotomy for trauma: a randomized prospective trial. J Trauma 1986; 26: 882–890.

20. Young B, Ott L, Twyman D et al. The effect of nutritional support on outcome from severe head injury. J Neurosurg 1987; 67: 668–676.

21. Hadley MN, Grahm TW, Harrington T et al. Nutritional support and neurotrauma: a critical review of early nutrition in forty-five acute head injury patients. Neurosurgery 1986; 19: 367–373.

22. Kalfarentzos F, Kehagias J, Mead N et al. Enteral nutrition is superior to parenteral nutrition in severe acute pancreatitis: results of a randomized prospective trial. Br J Surg 1997; 84: 1665–1669.

23. Bodoky G, Harsanyi L, Pap A, Tihanyi T, Flautner L. Effect of enteral nutrition on exocrine pancreatic function. Am J Surg 1991; 161: 144–148.

24. McClave SA, Greene LM, Snider HL et al. Comparison of the safety of early enteral versus parenteral nutrition in mild acute pancreatitis. JPEN 1997; 21: 14–20.

25. Windsor ACJ, Kanwar S, Li AGK et al. Compared with parenteral nutrition, enteral feeding attenuates the acute phase response and improves disease severity in acute pancreatitis. Gut 1998; 42: 431–435.

26. Hernandez-Aranda JC, Gallo-Chico B, Ramirez-Barba EJ. Nutritional support in severe acute pancreatitis. Nutricion Hospitalaria 1996; 11: 160–166.

27. Lawson DW, Daggett WM, Civetta JM et al. Surgical treatment of acute necrotizing pancreatitis. Ann Surg 1970; 172: 605–615.

28. Helton WS. Intravenous nutrition in patients with acute pancreatitis. In: Rombeau JL (ed) *Clinical nutrition: Parenteral nutrition*. WB Saunders, Philadelphia, 1990; pp. 442–461.

29. Levy P, Heresbach D, Pariente EA *et al*. Frequency and risk factors of recurrent pain during refeeding in patients with acute pancreatitis: a multivariate multicentre prospective study of 116 patients. *Gut* 1997; **40:** 262–266.

30. Cassim MM, Allardyce DB. Pancreatic secretion in response to jejunal feeding of elemental diet. *Ann Surg* 1974; **180:** 228–231.

31. Koretz RL. Nutritional support in pancreatitis: feeding an organ that has eaten itself. *Semin Gastrointest Dis* 1993; **4:** 99–113.

32. DiCarlo V, Nespoli A, Chiesa R *et al*. Hemodynamic and metabolic impairment in acute pancreatitis. *World J Surg* 1981; **5:** 329–339.

33. Kingsworth AN, Galloway SW, Formela LJ. Randomized, double-blind phase II trial of Lexipafant, a platelet-activating factor antagonist, in human acute pancreatitis. *Br J Surg* 1995; **82:** 1414–1420.

34. Groos S, Hunefeld G, Luciano L. Parenteral versus enteral nutrition: morphological changes in human adult intestinal mucosa. *J Submic Cytol Pathol* 1996; **28:** 61–74.

35. Hancke E, Marlein G. Bacterial contamination of the pancreas with intestinal germs: a cause of acute suppurative pancreatitis. In: Berger HG (ed) *Acute pancreatitis*. Springer-Verlag, Berlin, 1987; pp. 87–89.

36. Lange JF, van Gool J, Tytgat GNJ. The protective effect of a reduction in intestinal flora on mortality of acute haemorrhagic pancreatitis in the rat. *Hepatogastroenterology* 1987; **34:** 28–30.

37. Russel JC, Welch JP, Clark DG. Colonic complications of acute pancreatitis and pancreatic abscess. *Am J Surg* 1983; **146:** 558–564.

38. Denham W, Fink G, Yang J *et al*. Small molecule inhibition of tumor necrosis factor gene processing during acute pancreatitis prevents cytokine cascade progression and attenuates pancreatitis severity. *Am Surg* 1997; **63:** 1045–1049.

39. Denham W, Yang J, Fink G *et al*. Gene targeting demonstrates additive detrimental effects of interleukin 1 and tumor necrosis factor during pancreatitis. *Gastroenterology* 1997; **113:** 1741–1746.

40. Corcoy R, Ma Sanchez J, Domingo P, Net A. Nutrition in the patient with severe acute pancreatitis. *Nutrition* 1988; **4:** 269–275.

41. Ragins H, Levenson SM, Singer R *et al*. Intrajejunal administration of an elemental diet at neutral pH avoids pancreatic stimulation. *Am J Surg* 1973; **126:** 606–614.

42. Keith RG. Effect of a low fat elemental diet on pancreatic secretion during pancreatitis. *Surg Gynecol Obstet* 1980; **151:** 337–343.

43. DiMagno EP, Vay LW, Summerskill HJ. Intraluminal and postabsorptive effects of amino acids on pancreatic enzyme secretion. *J Lab Clin Med* 1971; **82:** 241–248.

44. Vidon N, Hecketsweiler P, Butel J *et al*. Effect of continuous jejunal perfusion of elemental and complex nutritional solutions on pancreatic enzyme secretion in human subjects. *Gut* 1978; **19:** 194–198.

45. Ertan A, Brooks FF, Ostrow *et al*. Effect of jejunal amino acid perfusion and exogenous cholecystokinin on the exocrine pancreatic and biliary secretions in man. *Gastroenterology* 1971; **61:** 686.

46. Parekh D, Lawson HH, Segal I. The role of total enteral nutrition in pancreatic disease. *S Afr J Surg* 1993; **31:** 57–61.

47. Banks PA. Pancreatitis for the endoscopist-terminology, prediction of complications and management. ASGE Postgraduate Course, Digestive Disease Week, San Francisco, CA, 23–24 May 1996.

48. Agarwal N, Pitchumoni CS. Assessment of severity in acute pancreatitis. *Am J Gastroenterol* 1991; **86(10):** 1385–1391.

49. Corfield AP, Cooper MJ, Williamson RCN *et al*. Prediction of severity in acute pancreatitis: prospective comparison of three prognostic indices. *Lancet* 1985; **ii:** 403–407.

50. Larvin M, McMahon MJ. Apache-II score for assessment and monitoring of acute pancreatitis. *Lancet* 1989; **2:** 201–205.

51. Wilson C, Heath DI, Imrie CW. Prediction of outcome in acute pancreatitis: a comparative study of APACHE II, clinical assessment and multiple factor scoring system. *Br J Surg* 1990; **77:** 1260–1264.

52. Cravo M, Camilo ME, Marques A, Pinto Correia J. Early tube feeding in acute pancreatitis: A prospective study. *Clin Nutr* 1989; **8(suppl):** 14.

53. Voitk A, Brown RA, Echave V *et al*. Use of an elemental diet in the treatment of complicated pancreatitis. *Am J Surg* 1973; **125:** 223–227.

54. Bury KD, Stephens RV, Randall HT. Use of chemically defined, liquid elemental diet for nutritional management of fistulas of the alimentary tract. *Am J Surg* 1971; **121:** 174–183.

55. Nasrallah SM, Martin DM. Comparative effects of criticare HN and vivonex HN in the treatment of malnutrition due to pancreatic insufficiency. *Am J Clin Nutr* 1984; **39:** 251–254.

56. Cowley A, Dutta SK, Narang A *et al*. Evaluation of the efficacy of elemental diet therapy in patients with chronic alcoholic pancreatitis (Abstr). *Gastroenterology* 1983; **84:** 1130.

57. Simpson WG, Marsano L, Gates L. Enteral nutritional support in acute alcoholic pancreatitis. *J Am Coll Nutr* 1995; **14:** 663–665.

58. Kudsk KA, Campbell SM, O'Brien T, Fuller R. Postoperative jejunal feedings following complicated pancreatitis. *Nutr Clin Pract* 1990; **5:** 14–17.

59. Imondi AR, Stradley RP. Utilization of enzymatically hydrolyzed soybean protein and crystalline amino acid diets by rats with exocrine pancreatic insufficiency. *J Nutr* 1974; **104:** 793–801.

60. Milla PJ, Lilby A, Rassam UB, Harries JT. Small intestinal absorption of amino acids and a dipeptide in pancreatic insufficiency. *Gut* 1983; **24:** 818–824.

61. McClave SA, Snider HL, Owens N, Sexton LK. Clinical nutrition in pancreatitis. *Dig Dis Sci* 1997; **42:** 2035–2044.

62. Havala T, Shronts E, Cerra F. Nutritional support in acute pancreatitis. *Gastroenterol Clin N Am* 1989; **18(3):** 525–542.

63. Iszak EM, Shike M, Roulet M, Jeejeebuoy KN. Pancreatitis in association with hypercalcemia in patients receiving total parenteral nutrition. *Gastroenterology* 1980; **79:** 555–558.

41

The cost-effectiveness of nutrition support

Ceri J Green

Introduction

There is growing evidence to support the idea that individuals with disease-related malnutrition (DRM) are likely to have a poorer clinical outcome than well-nourished individuals, and that this is associated with increased hospital costs. Nutrition support techniques, such as oral supplements, enteral feeding via naso-enteric or percutaneous tube, and intravenous feeding via central or peripheral catheters are now widely available. These are employed in the belief that improving or preventing a deterioration of nutritional status will reduce the complications that are seen in poorly nourished patients. However, in this era of budgets and cost constraints, it is becoming increasingly important to demonstrate that employing these supportive therapies is not only clinically effective, but also cost-effective. This chapter addresses a number of the issues surrounding the question of whether nutrition support is cost-effective. Of relevance is the prevalence of DRM, its causes, its consequences in relation to clinical outcome, the costs associated with it, the clinical efficacy of nutritional intervention, and the costs associated with providing nutrition support relative to its effect on outcome. A number of these issues are also explored in more detail in other chapters.

The prevalence of disease-related malnutrition

Several studies published in the 1970s were the first indicators of a previously unrecognised problem in hospitals.[1–4] Since then, there have been many investigations into the prevalence of malnutrition in a wide variety of patient groups, varying in underlying disease state and age (see Table 41.1). Although the exact prevalence is unclear because of the lack of a universally accepted definition of malnutrition, it is apparent that this is a common phenomenon. Of the few studies that followed patients during the course of their hospitalisation, most have demonstrated that those who were malnourished on admission are at most risk for further deterioration during their hospital stay.[5–7] Relatively few studies have specifically set out to examine the prevalence of DRM outside the hospital setting, although poor nutritional status on admission may be regarded as an indicator that this problem is not confined to hospitals. Using anthropometric criteria, a prevalence of about 10% in patients

with malignant disease, non-malignant chronic disease and after discharge following surgery has been identified in the UK.[8–10] Variable incidences of malnutrition have been recorded at out-patient appointments in a number of patient groups.[11–13] Studies in institutionalised elderly in the USA using a variety of criteria suggest that between 10 and 85% of such residents may be undernourished.[14–15] Severely disabled individuals are also at risk, mainly because of motor dysfunction and feeding difficulties.[16] Even relatively independent tenants in sheltered accommodation may have deficiencies in their nutritional intakes and difficulties in preparing their own meals.[17] Taken together, this information demonstrates that DRM is not an insignificant problem.

Causes of disease-related malnutrition

The causes of DRM are summarised in Table 41.2. Often more than one factor is present. Financial and psychosocial factors may also play a role, including the effect of hospitalisation itself.

For many years it was assumed that the primary cause of DRM was increased energy expenditure (EE) and catabolism associated with metabolic stress. In fact, total EE (TEE) is not raised and is frequently lower than normal due to a decrease in physical activity level.[32] However, other consequences of the metabolic response to trauma, infection and inflammation are probably central in modifying the drive to eat, the assimilation of nutrients and the conservation of body composition.[33] Whether these factors may also influence absorption is not clear, but malabsorption may be an independent factor in patients with intestinal disease or as a result of surgical procedures.[34]

These factors alone are clearly not completely responsible for the development of DRM. In the sickest patients, with the lowest TEE, energy intake is even lower than energy requirements.[32] Inadequate intake *per se* has been documented in a variety of patient groups.[6,27,35–39] Furthermore, DRM may itself contribute to inadequate intake.[35] It is thus becoming evident that reduced food intake for a number of reasons is crucial in the development of DRM. These data underpin the belief that institution of nutrition support may be able to counteract the reduction in intake of normal foods and improve nutrition status.

Table 41.1 – Prevalence of disease-related malnutrition.

Investigator	Type of patients/n	Definition of malnutrition	Prevalence
Brookes[18]	Head and neck cancer/n=84	General nutrition score based on weight loss and arm muscle loss	39%
Bashir[19]	Bronchial carcinoma, preoperatively/n=39	BMI, TSF and subscapular skinfold < 25th centile	46%
		< 90% of ideal body weight	36%
		Creatinine height index < 80% of predicted	79%
		Serum albumin < 35 g/l	8%
		Serum transferrin < 2 g/l	67%
McWhirter and Pennington[5]	General surgical/n=100	BMI < 20 and TSF or MAMC < 15th centile (mild)	10%
		BMI < 18 and TSF or MAMC < 5th centile (moderate)	16%
		BMI < 16 and TSF or MAMC < 5th centile (severe)	1%
McWhirter and Pennington[5]	Orthopaedic surgery/n=100	BMI < 20 and TSF or MAMC < 15th centile (mild)	28%
		BMI < 18 and TSF or MAMC < 5th centile (moderate)	5%
		BMI < 16 and TSF or MAMC < 5th centile (severe)	6%
Lumbers et al[20]	Elderly orthopaedic surgery/n=60	Three or more criteria < 5th centile: serum albumin, haemoglobin, TSF, MAMC, body weight	41% (FNF) 4% (THR)
McWhirter and Pennington[5]	Respiratory medicine/n=100	BMI < 20 and TSF or MAMC < 15th centile (mild)	13%
		BMI < 18 and TSF or MAMC < 5th centile (moderate)	19%
		BMI < 16 and TSF or MAMC < 5th centile (severe)	13%
McWhirter and Pennington[5]	General medical/n=100	BMI < 20 and TSF or MAMC < 15th centile (mild)	11%
		BMI < 18 and TSF or MAMC < 5th centile (moderate)	27%
		BMI < 16 and TSF or MAMC < 5th centile (severe)	8%
Naber et al[21]	Non-surgical/n=155	Subjective Global Assessment	45%
		Nutritional Risk Index	57%
		Maastricht Index	62%
Larsson et al[22]	Elderly medical/n=501	Three or more criteria including weight index, TSF, MAMC, prealbumin, albumin, skin test	29%
Cederholm and Hellström[23]	Elderly medical/n=96	Weight index < 10th centile	35%
		TSF < 10th centile	32%
		Serum albumin < 10th centile	50%
		DCH < 10th centile	31%

Table 41.1 – (continued).

Investigator	Type of patients/n	Definition of malnutrition	Prevalence
Constans et al[24]	Elderly medical/n=324	Moderate: MAC < 10th centile or albumin < 35 g/l	30% (M) 41% (F)
		Severe: MAC < 10th centile and albumin < 35 g/l	16% (M) 21% (F)
McWhirter and Pennington[5]	Elderly medical/n=100	BMI < 20 and TSF or MAMC < 15th centile (mild) BMI < 18 and TSF or MAMC < 5th centile (moderate) BMI < 16 and TSF or MAMC < 5th centile (severe)	4% 20% 19%
Gariballa et al[7]	Acute stroke/n=201	BMI < 20 TSF < 25th centile MAC < 25th centile Serum albumin < 35 g/l	31% 49% 12% 19%
Carver and Dobson[35]	Elderly psychiatric/n=293	BMI 15.1–19.9 (underweight) BMI < 15.1 (emaciated)	27% 5%
Moy et al[26]	Hospitalised children/n=255	Stunted (SD score of –2 for height for age) Wasted (SD score of –2 for weight for height) Stunted and wasted At risk of stunting and/or wasting (SD score of between –1 and –2)	16% 14% 2% 20%
Smith et al[27]	Diagnosis of malignancy, children/n=100	Stunted (SD score of –2 for height for age) TSF (SD score of –2) Wasted (weight for height 80% of median) MAC (< 5th centile)	3% 23% 5% 20%
Cameron et al[28]	Congenital heart disease, children/n=160	Stunted (ratio of height: mean height for age < 0.94) Wasted (ratio of weight: mean weight for height < 0.89) Stunted and wasted	66% 33% 6%
Hendricks et al[29]	Hospitalised children/n=268	Stunted (height for age < 95% of median) Wasted (weight for height < 90% of median)	27% 25%
Hendrikse et al[30]	Hospitalised children aged 7 months to 16 years/n=226	Stunted (< 5th centile height for age) Wasted (< 80% weight for height) Underweight (< 5th centile weight for age)	15% 8% 16%

BMI: body mass index; TSF: triceps skinfold thickness; MAMC: mid-arm muscle circumference; MAC: mid-arm circumference; DCH: delayed cutaneous hypersensitivity; SD: standard deviation; M: male; F: female; FNF: fractured neck of femur; THR: total hip replacement.

Table 41.2 – Causes of disease-related malnutrition.

Category	Cause	Examples
Reduced food intake	Anorexia	Poor appetite, nausea or vomiting as a result of the disease process (e.g. malignancy or infection), treatment (e.g. chemotherapy) or depression
	Episodes of fasting	Prior to investigative procedures or operations, missed meals due to these procedures, or avoidance of food due to diarrhoea
	Pain on eating	Sore mouth (e.g. mucositis and candidiasis) due to the disease process (e.g. HIV infection) or treatment (e.g. chemotherapy), or partial gastrointestinal obstruction
	Swallowing difficulties	Dysphagia (e.g. due to upper gastrointestinal obstruction, cerebral palsy, stroke, motor neurone disease)
	Inability to eat independently	Physical handicap, arthritis, dementia
	Respiratory problems	Pulmonary disease
Malabsorption	Impaired digestion	Pancreatic insufficiency, enzyme deficiencies, intestinal pH alteration (e.g. cystic fibrosis)
	Impaired absorption	Intestinal resection (e.g. short bowel syndrome), mucosal damage (e.g. inflammatory bowel disease)
	Excess losses from the gut	High output fistulae, protein-losing enteropathy, short bowel syndrome
Modified metabolism	Metabolic response to disease resulting in changes in nutrient mobilisation and utilisation	Malignancy, trauma, chronic sepsis, multiple organ failure, advanced HIV infection
	Metabolic consequences of impaired organ function	Renal disease, liver disease, pulmonary disease

Reproduced with permission from Green.[31]

The influence of disease-related malnutrition on clinical outcome

Poor nutrition status is associated with impairments in growth and development,[26,27,30] functional capacity,[13,40–44] gut structure and function,[45] immune function,[46–49] wound healing[50,51] and resistance to development of pressure ulcers.[52,53] These consequences are important because they will impact on the incidence of complications and clinical outcome (i.e. morbidity and mortality), in turn having major implications for length of stay (LOS), convalescence and thus costs. Numerous publications have demonstrated associations between preoperative weight loss and increased morbidity and/or mortality after a variety of surgical procedures.[19,20,35,38,50,54–58] Similar findings have also been found in non-surgical patients.[7,21,59,60] Many of these studies and others[61] have also shown associations between the presence or risk of malnutrition and LOS. Although LOS can be influenced by many non-nutritional factors and is thus often regarded as an unsuitable outcome parameter, it is attractive because it captures the possible combined effects of poor wound healing, infections and impaired functional status, and an estimate of cost can be attached to it.[62]

The financial implications of disease-related malnutrition

Relatively few studies have examined the impact of poor clinical outcome and increased LOS on hospital costs, but of those that have, significant effects on costs have been calculated. These are summarised in Table 41.3.

The costs of DRM in the community have not yet been clearly identified, although patients who are malnourished utilise more community resources (e.g. require more contact with general practitioners and more prescriptions) and require 25% more hospital admissions than patients who are well-nourished.[67] If DRM does impact directly on costs in hospitals, then it could be argued that patients who are malnourished in the community (i.e. on admission to hospital) will contribute to increased hospital costs.

A number of broad estimates have been made of the financial impact of DRM, and by inference the amount of money that could be saved if appropriate nutrition support was instituted. In the US, Meguid[68] estimated that increased LOS in malnourished patients at a cost of $5000 per patient amounted to annual costs of $18 billion. Using more complicated techniques in 20 specific diagnosis related groups in the US Medicare system, the Nutrition Screening Initiative calculated a reduction in spending of $156 million in 1994 if appropriate nutrition support resulting in reduced LOS was applied. Over the 1996–2002 period, this would amount to cumulative savings of $1.3 billion.[69] Tucker & Miguel[61] calculated potential annual savings of over $1 million per average institution if patient stay in hospital could be reduced by nutrition support. Similarly, in the UK in 1992, calculations showed that nutrition support could result in annual savings of £266 million in the National Health Service (NHS) if hospital stay was reduced by 5 days in 10% of in-patients.[70]

It is over-simplistic, however, to deduce from these studies that provision of nutrition support will improve outcome and reduce hospital costs, as demonstration of a causal association between DRM and complications, LOS and thus costs was not sought in these studies. Indeed, some argue that DRM is simply a secondary phenomenon of disease and not an important cause of morbidity in itself.[71] Despite their limitations,[72] prospective, randomised controlled studies in patients with or at risk of DRM are necessary to determine whether nutritional intervention can positively influence clinical outcome, and ideally clusters of similar studies should be subjected to systematic review to distill the most important findings.

The clinical benefits of nutritional intervention

Greater choice and flexibility of food provision by hospital catering services could improve intake in some patient groups,[73] although ironically the costs of providing such a service may be even higher than for enteral nutrition (EN) or parenteral nutrition (PN). Food fortification (i.e. supplementation of normal foods with additional energy and/or protein) can also increase energy and/or protein intakes.[74] Despite these options, however, there are many patients who are simply unable to consume a sufficient, if any, oral diet to meet their nutritional requirements. For these

Table 41.3 – Costs associated with disease-related malnutrition.

Investigators	Study design	Types of patients/n	Classification of malnutrition	Outcome in malnourished versus well-nourished	Cost differences in malnourished versus well-nourished
Christensen[63]	Prospective	Small town community hospital/n=500 of which 22% malnourished	Serum albumin < 35 g/l or total lymphocyte count < 1500/mm3	• average LOS twice as long (10.8 days *vs* 5.4 days)	• 75% more costly • mean difference in charges was $1296 ($3017 *vs* $1721)
Reilly *et al*[64]	Retrospective	Acute care medical and surgical patients/n=771; 59% of medical and 48% of surgical patients at risk of malnutrition	At risk: serum albumin < 35 g/l, total lymphocytes < 1500/mm3, ht/wt < 80% of the 1979 Metropolitan Weight Table values, description by doctor or nurse as malnourished, or unintentional weight loss of 4.5 kg or 15% UBW in 3 months prior to admission	• 2.6 times more likely to have a minor complication (p < 0.001) • 3.4 times more likely to have a major complication (p < 0.001) • 3.8 times more likely to die (p < 0.001) • longer LOS (range 1.1–12.8 excess days)	• ↑ mean costs per patients of $1738 (p < 0.0001), and $2996 if complications occurred (p < 0.01) • ↑ mean charges per patient of $3557 (p < 0.0001), and $6157 if complications occurred (p < 0.01)
Robinson *et al*[65]	Prospective	Medical admissions/ n=100 of which 40% malnourished	Weight loss > 10% or global assessment (anthropometric and laboratory parameters)	• 45% hospitalised longer than allowed under diagnosis related group, compared with 30% for well-nourished group and 37% in borderline group • average LOS 15.6 days *vs* 10 days in other 2 groups (p < 0.01)	• ↑ actual hospital charges of $16691 in malnourished and $14118 in borderline groups compared with $7692 in normally nourished (p < 0.01)
Chima *et al*[66]	Prospective	General medicine/ n=173 of which 32% at risk of malnutrition	At risk: weight for height < 75% ideal body weight, admission serum albumin < 30 g/l, or > 10% unintentional weight loss 1 month before admission	• ↑ mean LOS: 6 days (4–8)★ *vs* 4 days (3–7)★ (p < 0.01) • less likely to be discharged home with self-care (41% *vs* 66%) (p < 0.05) • more likely to use home health care service (31% *vs* 12%) (p < 0.001)	• ↑ mean hospitalisation cost/patient ($6196 *vs* $4563) (p < 0.02)

★ 25th and 75th percentile; LOS: length of stay; UBW: usual body weight; IBW: ideal body weight; ↑: increased.

patients, oral supplements (sip feeds), supplementary nasogastric feeding, total EN or PN are indicated.

Some of the evidence of the benefits of providing different types of nutrition support is presented in the following sections.

Oral supplements and sip feeds

Oral supplements, consumed in addition to normal foods, can increase intake of protein and energy and maintain or improve parameters of nutrition status, recently demonstrated by systematic review.[75] Some studies also reported improvements in immune and muscle function,[42,76,77] although not all have done so.[78,79] Many studies with oral supplements have documented clinical benefits; some of these are summarised in Table 41.4.

Supplementary enteral tube feeding

Many patients may be able to partially meet their requirements *via* the oral route with normal diet and supplements, but may require supplementary EN to achieve target intake. Nocturnal EN is of particular value for patients who are at home, with the advantage that ambulatory patients are not confined to a feeding pump during the day. Improvements in a variety of nutrition parameters have been shown with nocturnal EN in malnourished patients with a variety of underlying causes.[83,84] The clinical value of this approach has been demonstrated in elderly malnourished women with fractured neck of femur.[54]

Complete enteral nutrition

In patients in whom failure to eat is likely to be prolonged, total EN may be required over weeks, months or even years. In these cases, nutrition support may be life-saving, similar in principle to renal replacement therapy for end-stage renal failure or artificial ventilation for respiratory failure. Ethical issues aside,[85] the goal is generally to prolong life and/or improve quality of life (QOL), and in children to maintain or improve growth.[86,87] In many cases, patients who require long-term feeding will receive it outside the hospital setting, i.e. at home or in long-stay institutions. Nutrition support at home has social and emotional benefits allowing a more normal integration into family life.[88]

Gastrostomy feeding is becoming the preferred method of gut access for long-term EN.[88,89] However, the median survival time following percutaneous endoscopic gastrostomy (PEG) may be limited[90,91] and complications associated with the procedure, although usually minor,[89,92] may sometimes be more problematic.[90] Although experience and involvement of a specialist nutrition team may play a role in improving outcome,[92] there is a need to improve the decision-making process for PEG placement.[91] These points may all have influence on the cost-effectiveness of nutrition support.

In some cases, an inability to eat may occur for a relatively short period (e.g. 2–10 days). This constitutes a grey area in terms of the need to provide nutrition support during this period and, if it is given, the preferred route of feeding, composition of formulation and timing of intervention. Some believe that the majority of patients can withstand a lack of nutrition for periods of up to seven days if they are not severely malnourished,[93] common practice in the UK following surgery. However, there is a growing feeling that periods of inadequate oral intake may be detrimental to outcome. Audits have revealed possible links between period of time of starvation prior to institution of EN and mortality,[94] and between delay in attempting aggressive EN and major complications and LOS.[35,61] In addition, rapid deficits in muscle function and wound healing have been documented to occur with reduced food intake well before changes in nutrition status as assessed by anthropometry become apparent.[95–98] In turn, deficits are quickly rectified by a return to normal food intake.[96,98]

The majority of short-term intervention studies have been performed in the perioperative period. Several have documented trends in decreased infections, improved wound healing and/or improved nitrogen retention with early EN compared with delayed feeding.[98–101] Beier-Holgersen & Boesby[102] showed convincingly that institution of EN within 4 hours of major abdominal surgery can result in a significant reduction in complications, even in the apparently well-nourished or only mildly malnourished. Two recent reports, however, make it difficult to suggest that early postoperative EN should be routinely prescribed,[103,104] and indicate that further research is required to determine which types of patients may benefit and which may not.

Another controversial area is the use of the enteral route in patients in whom it was previously thought that EN would not be tolerated, such as the critically ill.[105] Nutrition support in critically ill patients is

Table 41.4 – Prospective, randomised, controlled oral supplement studies that have recorded complications and LOS.

Authors	Patients	Intervention/n	Average no. days of nutrition support (n)	Complication rate (n)	Mean LOS (days)
Flynn and Leighrty[80]	Malnourished head and neck cancer	• Oral supplement (preoperative) + ward diet (n=19) • Ward diet (n=17)	18*	• 6 • 10	• 18 • 21
Delmi *et al*[81]	Elderly with fractured neck of femur	• Oral supplement + ward diet (n=27) • Ward diet (n=32)	32	• 4 • 14 (p=0.07)	• 24 • 40 (p < 0.02)
Rana *et al*[82]	Moderate/major gastrointestinal surgery	• Oral supplement + ward diet (n=20) • Ward diet (n=20)	7	• 3 • 10 (p < 0.02)	• 12.6 (SD1.1) • 15.9 (SD 1.9) (NS)
Keele *et al*[38]	Moderate/major gastrointestinal surgery	• Oral supplement + ward diet (n=43) • Ward diet (n=43)	5.5	• 5 (4 patients) • 14 (12 patients) (p < 0.05)	• 10.8 (CI 1.2) • 13.2 (CI 2.6) (NS)

Supplements given postoperatively unless otherwise stated; LOS: length of stay; SD = standard deviation; CI = 95% confidence interval; NS: not significant;
* Assumed based on LOS data.
Adapted with permission from Green.[169]

Table 41.5 – Difficulties encountered in assessing cost–effectiveness and cost–utility.

Assessment of costs	Assessment of outcome	Clinical study as environment for health economics assessment
True costs (charges)	Design of study	External validity
Discounting (inflation)	Choice of placebo	Publication bias
Inclusion of all costs	Choice of endpoints	Power usually set for clinical benefits not costs
Costs of surrounding services	Assessment of QOL	
Intangible costs	Period of follow-up	
Opportunity costs		
Cost shifting between sectors		
Comparison between institutions and countries		

Assessment of costs

It is difficult to assess the true cost of interventions, e.g. nutrition formulas. There may be large differences between the price paid by the hospital and the price charged to patients/insurance companies,[129] which may also be the case in the NHS as well as in the US.[126] Actual charges are thus probably of most relevance, but there may be large differences between institutions and certainly between countries. Difficulties arise over time when allowances for inflation (discounting) must be made. Costs of surrounding services may also have a large impact on the costs of a particular intervention and should be taken into account, but can be difficult to assess, as can indirect costs, such as those incurred by the family as a result of a patient's illness. The complications and negative effects of feeding, e.g. discomfort, immobility, psychological aspects, lost time from activities due to feeding or complications should also be considered.[129] These are intangible costs (i.e. items of unknown value). It is difficult to assess opportunity cost, defined in terms of the next best opportunity foregone (includes direct cost of treatment, knock-on costs of treatments averted or postponed, and time spent off work).[130] Finally, since health economics has its foundations in welfare economics (i.e. attempts to examine the welfare of the whole of society rather than just individuals), there is a need to acknowledge that funding within the hospital cannot be seen in isolation and cost shifting between sectors must also be considered. Furthermore, there is a danger in attributing savings based on average costs; actual savings are in fact a fraction of estimated costs due to overhead, running costs and possible increased patient turnover as a result of improved care. In practice, it is obviously impractical to include assessment of all costs. Pragmatically, some costs can be excluded if they are expected to make little impact on overall results (prioritisation),[131] and it is not inappropriate to consider only those costs that are of most relevance to the target audience.[132] Whichever approach is chosen, it is always important that the perspective of the study is explicitly defined.[126,131,133]

Assessment of outcome

Intangible benefits such as improved nutrition status, function and QOL are considered to have a relatively minor contribution to overall economic benefits compared with measurable reduction in morbidity and/or mortality.[129] However, interest is growing in the evaluation of QOL and this is essential in calculations of QALYs; but there is not yet clear consensus on how QOL should be measured. Quality of life assessment aims to measure general well-being based on objective and subjective changes in physical, functional, mental and social health.[134,135] Numerous scales exist, such as the EuroQOL, SF-36, Nottingham Health Profile, Quality of Well-Being Scale and WISP (well-being in surgical patients), but all seem to have inherent problems. Many are several pages long, they may not be validated in more than one target group or may be too generic, they may not be relevant to all individuals, they may not be valid in other languages, they may not be single index measures, and/or they may be influenced by the mode of administration. The best mode of assessment of QOL in children and adolescents is even less clear. In clinical practice, the simpler, shorter and less ambiguous the questionnaire the better, as patients will not all be willing or able to co-operate with more complex surveys. The time scale to collect QOL, morbidity and mortality data is relevant, i.e. patients must be followed up long enough to measure outcomes of interest but it must be a practical period of time so that results are available within a reasonable period.[126] Benefits must be real, not theoretical.[129] Surrogate markers may be used to infer final outcomes of interest,[126] but are only of real value if separate studies have demonstrated relationships with outcome. The selection of an appropriate control is also relevant in determining outcome benefits.[136] Ideally all possibilities should be compared (new intervention versus gold standard versus current practice versus no intervention), although ethical issues and patient availability will play a role in determining the most appropriate approach.

Appropriateness of a clinical study as a setting for economic analyses

Until recently, prospective economic analyses have rarely been included in clinical studies in the health care setting. Although the numbers of trials that include health economics are increasing, there is some controversy over whether a clinical trial is an appropriate environment for assessment of cost-effectiveness or utility. Some argue that this should be standard practice,[137] whilst others caution against it, mainly due to the suggestion that the study environment is atypical and results may not be readily generalised to the population as a whole.[128,133] In prospective clinical studies that include cost assessment, power calculations are generally based on the clinical endpoints rather than on the cost endpoint which may limit the interpretation of cost data.[130] However, alternative methods of economic assessment, such as modelling and simulations (e.g. decision analyses) have also been criticised due to openness to bias (e.g. publication bias: negative studies may not be reported).[130] For these reasons, it has been suggested that health economic assessments are more appropriate in settings that most closely resemble real life.[138] Furthermore, there is little to be gained from recording extremely detailed cost information or attempting to calculate QALYs; rather, data on individual dimensions should be reported separately.[128] Such a simplified approach would certainly be advantageous in the field of clinical nutrition. Nutrition support studies are usually more pragmatic than those for pharmaceuticals (due to lack of strict guidelines for their conduct and lower funding) and calculation of QALYs may be of little value outside the area of long-term feeding where nutrition support is used as a life-saving therapy. Simple standardised evaluation systems have been proposed for general use in health care.[130,133] For the purposes of assessing cost-effectiveness of nutrition support, such a simplified approach which aims to determine satisfactory rather than optimum solutions and facilitates choices for individual patients[133] would be welcomed by nutrition support practitioners.

Evidence of the cost-effectiveness of nutrition support

Most of the studies that have documented associations between malnutrition and poor clinical outcome, and thus increased hospital costs, have called for early, aggressive nutrition support as a means of reducing expenditure. In contrast, Reynolds et al[139] calculated the potential annual financial consequences of meeting guidelines for giving oral supplements and EN. They showed that despite the crude nature of the calculations, implementation could lead to large increases in expenditure on dietetic referrals and nutrition products. Thus, despite the limitations, the question of whether or not nutritional intervention can save money can best be answered by inclusion of economic analyses in well-designed nutritional intervention studies. Unfortunately, data are scarce in this respect. Examples of different approaches to assessing the cost-effectiveness of nutrition support are given in Table 41.6. Many of these are studies in which two forms of feeding are compared. A few economic

analyses performed in the 1980s[129,159,160] focused on studies of preoperative total PN compared with no PN and used models that estimated rather than measured PN costs and presumed PN-associated reductions in complications.[161] Results suggested that patient selection is important in ensuring cost-effective nutrition support, but the quality of the clinical and cost data has been criticised,[161] and the studies are difficult to interpret. One prospective cost-effectiveness analysis of perioperative PN versus no PN has been performed.[155] In this cohort of patients, there was no decrease in costs for any subgroup of patients, including the most malnourished who had a reduction in rate of complications, although incremental costs were lowest for high-risk patients. However, PN is the most costly method of nutrition support and therefore the most difficult for which to demonstrate cost-effectiveness,[162] although the cost differential with EN may be decreasing as the peripheral route offers a cheaper approach than central PN[149] and gut access techniques and enteral formulations become more sophisticated.[163]

There is even less data on the cost-effectiveness of EN or oral supplements, although more recent studies are now attempting to include a cost component. Beier-Holgersen & Boesby[102] showed that early postoperative EN was associated with a non-significant reduction in median costs compared with watery placebo (43.270 vs 58.385 Danish Kroner) although the exact method of calculating costs was not described. Retrospective cost analyses using a variety of assumptions applied to several studies of supplemental and sip feeds demonstrated that cost savings are probably possible compared with no feeding.[71,164,165] In order to attempt to achieve a comparable overview of the possible costs and savings that might be expected from providing oral supplements or tube feeding compared with not feeding on a per patient basis, a number of intervention studies, including those mentioned above, have been reviewed and are summarised in Tables 41.4 and 41.7. Using some simple assumptions, with one exception, potential cost savings of at least £81 per patient can be calculated for surgical patients (Table 41.8): £150/day for additional hospital stay; complications cost a mean of £80 per complication to treat; supplements cost on average £3.00/patient/day assuming a patient consumes 400 ml of a 1.5 kcal/ml product, EN costs on average £14/patient/day assuming an intake of 2000 kcal of a standard or energy-dense product plus use of a giving set.[165,167] Potential cost savings for elderly females with fractured neck of femur could be several times higher

Table 41.6 – Examples of different types of cost–effectiveness studies in the nutrition support literature.

Type of analysis	Study example	Reference
Cost identification/minimisation	Retrospective cost analysis of nutritional solutions and annual cost of hospitalisation in patients receiving home nutritional support	Reddy and Malone[140]
	Prospective cost analysis of long-term feeding by PEG	Sartori et al[141]
	Investigation of the reduction in costs associated with using the most appropriate method of nutrition support according to dietetic and/or nutrition support team input	Roberts and Levine[142]
		Hassell et al[143]
		Johansson et al[144]
		Schwartz[145]
		Moffitt et al[146]
		Silkroski et al[147]
		Trujillo et al[148]
	Prospective investigation of the costs associated with central versus peripheral PN	May et al[149]
	Prospective comparison of costs of PN versus oral semi-elemental diet in AIDS	Kotler et al[150]
	Retrospective cost–comparison of radiological, surgical and endoscopic gastro/jejunostomy	Barkmeier et al[151]
Retrospective comparison of costs to treat complications	Retrospective comparison of costs of treating complications in upper gastrointestinal surgery patients receiving specialised or standard EN	Senkal et al[152]
Retrospective comparison of total hospital costs	Retrospective cost–comparison of total hospital costs associated with PEG versus open gastrostomy in head injured patients	Harbrecht et al[153]
	Investigation of the costs associated with early EN versus early PN in trauma patients	Trice et al[154]
Prospective cost–effectiveness study	Does perioperative PN reduce medical care costs?	Eisenberg et al[155]
	Glutamine-enriched EN versus control formula in very low birth weight infants	Dallas et al[156]
	Do feeding assistants improve intake and clinical outcome, and is this cost-effective?	Hickson et al[157]
	Costs of glutamine-enriched EN versus control formula in ICU patients based on cost/Therapeutic Intervention Scoring (TISS) point	Jones et al[113]
	Long-term outcome and cost-effectiveness of PN for acute gastrointestinal failure	Shields et al[119]
Cost-utility analysis	Cost-utility analysis of home parenteral nutrition	Richards and Irving[158]
Decision analysis	Calculation of cost-effectiveness ratios for preoperative PN in major GI surgery	Detsky and Jeejeebhoy[159]
		Twomey and Patching[29]
		Jendteg et al[160]
	Calculation of cost-effectiveness ratios for use of steroids and elemental diet in steroid-refractory Crohn's disease, and lactulose and peripheral BCAAs in hepatic encephalopathy	Ofman and Koretz[71]

Table 41.7 – A selection of prospective, randomised, controlled EN studies that have recorded LOS.

Authors	Patients	Intervention	Average no. days of nutrition support (n)★	Complication rate (n)	Mean LOS (days)
Bastow et al[54]	Very thin elderly with fractured neck of femur	• Overnight tube feeding + ward diet (n=25) • Ward diet (n=23)	28	Not recorded	• median 29 • median 38 (p < 0.05)
Shukla et al[106]	Malnourished surgical patients	• Preoperative tube feeding (n=67) • No tube feeding (n=43)	10	• 7 • 16 (p < 0.05)	• 10 • 13
Beier-Holgersen and Boesby[102]	Major (predominantly lower) gastrointestinal surgery	• Early postoperative feeding (n=30) • Placebo (n=30)	5	• 8 • 19 (p < 0.01)	• median 8 • median 11.5 (p=0.08)
Heslin et al[103]	Major upper gastrointestinal surgery	• Early postoperative feeding (n=81) • Standard care (n=83)	7 (approx.)	• 34 • 24 (p=0.08)	• median 11 • median 10 (p=0.55)
Watters et al[104]	Major upper gastrointestinal surgery	• Early postoperative feeding (n=13) • Standard care (n=15)	6	• 1 (anastamatic leak) • 4 (anastamatic leak) (NS)	• 17 (SD 9) • 16 (SD 7) (NS)

LOS: length of stay; SD: standard deviation; NS: not significant; ★ Assumed based on LOS data if not stated.
Adapted with permission from Green.[169]

Table 41.8 – Additional mean costs per patient accrued with and without use of nutrition support (based on data in Tables 41.4 and 41.7).

Author	Group	Mean cost per patient of additional LOS (£)	Mean cost per patient of treating complications (£)	Mean cost per patient for nutrition support (£)	Mean total cost per patient (£)	Mean total saving per patient as a result of nutrition support (£)
Flynn and Leightty[80]	Treatment	0	25	54	79	418
	Control	450	47	0	497	
Delmi et al[81]	Treatment	0	12	96	108	2327
	Control	2400	35	0	2435	
Rana et al[82]	Treatment	0	12	21	33	502
	Control	495	40	0	535	
Keele et al[58]	Treatment	0	9	17	26	360
	Control	360	26	0	386	
Bastow et al[54]	Treatment	0	–	406	406	944
	Control	1350	–	0	1350	
Shukla et al[166]	Treatment	0	8	140	148	332
	Control	450	30	0	480	
Beier-Holgersen and Boesby[102]	Treatment	0	21	70	91	485
	Control	525	51	0	576	
Heslin et al[103]	Treatment	150	34	98	282	−259
	Control	0	23	0	23	
Watters et al[104]	Treatment	0	6	84	90	81
	Control	150	21	0	171	

LOS: length of stay. Assumptions: Hospital (hotel) costs: £150/day; treatment costs: £80/complication; enteral feeding: £14/day; oral supplements: £3/day.
Adapted with permission from Green.[169]

than the figure given above. Although these assumptions and method of calculation can be criticised, the data strongly suggest that when nutrition support (EN and oral supplements) is clinically effective, it is also cost-effective.

For patients who require long-term complete nutrition support, there is good evidence to suggest that treatment in the community is substantially more cost-effective (about 65% for home PN) than hospital care.[88,158,168] Money can thus be saved by keeping patients out of hospital. Furthermore, it does not seem unreasonable to suggest that if treatment of malnutrition in the community leads to reduced need for GP visits, less hospitalisation, and shorter periods of hospitalisation,[67] as well as contributing to clinical improvements, then it can be regarded as cost-effective. More work is needed to try to substantiate this concept.

Part of the future challenge of determining the cost-effectiveness of nutrition support will depend on identifying those patients most likely to benefit, and the cheapest route and formulation to achieve a positive outcome. Proving the cost-effectiveness of nutrition support is difficult, but saving money by avoiding the use of inappropriate nutrition support and the complications associated with it is less so (see Table 41.6 for references). Nutrition support teams appear to be of key importance in this respect.[119,142,154]

Conclusion

Malnutrition is prevalent in a large number of disease states, and poor intake is central in its development. Disease-related malnutrition is associated with poor clinical outcome and many, though not all, studies have shown clinical benefits of nutrition support, even when frank malnutrition is not present. This suggests that inadequate oral intake may also be a risk factor for poor clinical outcome. In some cases, the severity of the trauma or disease may overwhelm the capacity of nutrition support to have measurable benefit. Thus, in future indices of depletion may not be the key to selecting patients who will benefit most from nutrition support. The extent of inadequate oral intake and the severity of the trauma that a patient has undergone may be at least as crucial in this decision-making process.

There are growing calls to demonstrate the cost-effectiveness of nutrition support. This term is often poorly defined, and is frequently used to indicate that EN is cheaper than PN. Indeed, cost-containment is

an important issue and nutrition teams in particular may prevent inappropriate use of nutrition support and avoid unnecessary complications. Targeting interventions more specifically to those patients most likely to benefit will be a continuing challenge. Retrospective studies and calculations based on rough estimates of cost involved in feeding and preventing complications strongly suggest that appropriate nutrition support compared with no or inappropriate measures is not associated with increased expenditure and may even reduce costs per patient. However, true cost-effectiveness is difficult to measure, in view of the problems in assessing real costs, clinical outcomes and applying those figures obtained from clinical studies to routine practice. Few studies have thus far attempted this, but several prospective studies are in progress, in collaboration with health economists and using pragmatic assessments, to seek to fill this gap. Furthermore, new insights into metabolism and requirements may result in the development of more specific nutrition formulations which may have additional effects over and above those expected from standard ones. Cost versus outcome studies will be of even more relevance in this case. Thus there is a strong need for some simple guidelines for assessing cost-effectiveness that can be readily incorporated into future clinical study protocols.

Acknowledgement

This article was written whilst the author was employed at Numico Research, The Netherlands.

References

1. Butterworth CE. The skeleton in the hospital closet. *Nutr Today* 1974; March/April: 4–8.

2. Bistrian BR, Blackburn GL, Hallowell E, Heddle R. Protein status of general surgical patients. *J Am Med Assoc* 1974; **230:** 858–860.

3. Bistrian BR, Blackburn GL, Vitale J, Cochran D, Naylor J. Prevalence of malnutrition in general medical patients. *J Am Med Assoc* 1976; **235:** 1567–1570.

4. Hill GL, Blackett RL, Pickford I *et al.* Malnutrition in surgical patients. *Lancet* 1977; **I:** 689–692.

5. McWhirter JP, Pennington CR. Incidence and recognition of malnutrition in hospital. *Br Med J* 1994; **308:** 945–948.

6. Fenton J, Eves A, Kipps M, O'Donnell CC. Menu changes and their effects on the nutritional content of menus and nutritional status of elderly, hospitalised, mental health patients. *J Hum Nutr Diet* 1995; **8:** 395–409.

7. Gariballa SE, Parker SG, Taub N, Castleden M. Nutritional status of hospitalized acute stroke patients. *Br J Nutr* 1998; **79:** 481–487.

8. Edington J, Kon P, Martyn CN. Prevalence of malnutrition in patients in general practice. *Clin Nutr* 1996; **15:** 60–63.

9. Edington J, Kon P, Martyn CN. Prevalence of malnutrition after major surgery. *J Hum Nutr Diet* 1997; **10:** 111–116.

10. Edington J. Patients at risk of malnutrition. *Proc Nutr Soc* 1997; **56:** 267A.

11. Young GA, Kopple JD, Lindholm B *et al.* Nutritional assessment of continuous ambulatory peritoneal dialysis patients: an international study. *Am J Kidney Dis* 1991; **XVII:** 462–471.

12. Thulavath PJ, Triger DR. Evaluation of nutritional status by using anthropometry in adults with alcoholic and nonalcoholic liver disease. *Am J Clin Nutr* 1994; **60:** 269–273.

13. Bell SC, Bowerman AR, Davies CA, Campbell IA, Shale DJ, Elborn JS. Nutrition in adults with cystic fibrosis. *Clin Nutr* 1998; **17:** 211–215.

14. Rudman D, Feller AG. Protein-calorie undernutrition in the nursing home. *J Am Geriatr Soc* 1989; **37:** 173–183.

15. Kerstetter JE, Holhausen BA, Fitz PA. Malnutrition in the institutionalized older adult. *J Am Diet Assoc* 1992; **92:** 1109–1116.

16. Sullivan PB, Rosenbloom L. *Feeding the disabled child.* MacKeith Press, London, 1996.

17. Caughey P, Seaman C, Parry D, Farquar D, McNennan WJ. Nutrition of old people in sheltered housing. *J Hum Nutr Diet* 1994; **7:** 263–268.

18. Brookes GB. Nutritional status in head and neck cancer: observations and implications. *Clin Otolaryngol* 1982; **8:** 211–220.

19. Bashir Y, Graham TR, Torrance A, Gibson GJ, Corris PA. Nutritional state of patients with lung cancer undergoing thoracotomy. *Thorax* 1990; **45:** 183–186.

20. Lumbers M, Driver LT, Howland RJ, Older MWJ, Williams CM. Nutritional status and clinical outcome in elderly female surgical orthopaedic patients. *Clin Nutr* 1996; **15:** 101–107.

21. Naber THJ, Schermer T, de Bree A *et al.* Prevalence of malnutrition in nonsurgical hospitalized patients and its associations with disease complications. *Am J Clin Nutr* 1997; **66:** 1232–1239.

22. Larsson J, Unosson M, Ek A-C, Nilsson L, Thorslund S, Bjurulf P. Effect of dietary supplement on nutritional status and clinical outcome in 501 geriatric patients – a randomised study. *Clin Nutr* 1990; **9:** 179–184.

23. Cederholm T, Hellström K. Nutritional status in recently hospitalized and free-living elderly subjects. *Gerontology* 1992; **38:** 105–110.

24. Constans T, Bacq Y, Bréchot J-F, Guilmot J-L, Choutet P, Lamisse F. Protein-energy malnutrition in elderly medical patients. *J Am Geriatr Soc* 1992; **40:** 263–268.

25. Carver AD, Dobson AM. Effects of dietary supplementation of elderly demented hospital residents. *J Hum Nutr Diet* 1995; **8:** 389–394.

26. Moy RJD, Smallman S, Booth IW. Malnutrition in a UK children's hospital. *J Hum Nutr Diet* 1990; **3:** 93–100.

27. Smith DE, Stevens MCG, Booth IW. Malnutrition at diagnosis of malignancy in childhood: common but mostly missed. *Eur J Pediatr* 1991; **150:** 318–322.

28. Cameron JW, Rosenthal A, Olson AD. Malnutrition in hospitalized children with congenital heart disease. *Arch Pediatr Adolesc Med* 1995; **149:** 1098–1102.

29. Hendricks KM, Duggan C, Gallagher L *et al.* Malnutrition in hospitalized pediatric patients. *Arch Pediatr Adolesc Med* 1995; **149:** 1118–1122.

30. Hendrikse WH, Reilly JJ, Weaver LT. Malnutrition in a children's hospital. *Clin Nutr* 1997; **16:** 13–18.

31. Green CJ. Existence, causes and consequences of disease-related malnutrition in the hospital and the community, and clinical and financial benefits of nutritional intervention. *Clin Nutr* 1999; **18 (Suppl 2):** 3–28.

32. Jebb SA. Energy metabolism in cancer and human immunodeficiency virus infection. *Proc Nutr Soc* 1997; **56:** 763–775.

33. Chang HR, Bistrian B. The role of cytokines in the catabolic consequences of infection and injury. *J Parenter Enteral Nutr* 1998; **22:** 156–166.

34. Grant JP, Chapman G, Russell MK. Malabsorption associated with surgical procedures and its treatment. *Nutr Clin Prac* 1996; **11:** 43–52.

35. Meguid MM, Campos ACL, Meguid V, Debonis D, Terz JJ. IONIP, a criterion of surgical outcome and patient selection for perioperative nutritional support. *Brit J Clin Prac* 1988; **42 (Suppl 63):** 8–14.

36. Holmes S, Dickerson JWT. Food intake and quality of life in cancer patients. *J Nutr Med* 1991; **2:** 359–368.

37. Klipstein-Grobusch K, Reilly JJ, Potter J, Edwards CA, Roberts MA. Energy intake and expenditure in elderly patients admitted to hospital with acute illness. *Br J Nutr* 1995; **73:** 323–334.

38. Keele AM, Bray MJ, Emery PW, Silk DBA. Two phase randomised controlled clinical trial of postoperative oral dietary supplements in surgical patients. *Gut* 1997; **40:** 393–399.

39. Gariballa SE, Parker SG, Taub N, Castlden CM. A randomized, controlled, single-blind trial of nutritional supplementation after acute stroke. *J Parenter Enteral Nutr* 1998; **22**: 315–319.

40. Heymsfield SB, Bethel RA, Ansley JD, Gibbs DM, Felner JM, Nutter DO. Cardiac abnormalities in cachectic patients before and during nutritional repletion. *Am Heart J* 1978; **95**: 584–594.

41. Arora NS, Rochester DF. Respiratory muscle strength and maximal voluntary ventilation in undernourished patients. *Am Rev Respir Dis* 1982; **126**: 5–8.

42. Efthimiou J, Fleming J, Gomes C, Spiro SG. Effect of supplementary oral nutrition in poorly nourished patients with chronic obstructive pulmonary disease. *Am Rev Respir Dis* 1988; **137**: 1075–1082.

43. Windsor JA, Hill GL. Grip strength: a measure of the proportion of protein loss in surgical patients. *Br J Surg* 1988; **75**: 880–882.

44. Cederholm T, Jägrén C, Hellström K. Nutritional status and performance capacity in internal medical patients. *Clin Nutr* 1993; **12**: 8–14.

45. Lara TM, Jacobs DO. Effect of critical illness and nutritional support on mucosal mass and function. *Clin Nutr* 1998; **17**: 99–105.

46. Ek A-C, Larsson J, von Schenck H, Thorslund S, Unosson M, Bjurulf P. The correlation between anergy, malnutrition and clinical outcome in an elderly hospital population. *Clin Nutr* 1990; **9**: 185–189.

47. Chandra RK. Nutrition and the immune system. *Proc Nutr Soc* 1993; **52**: 77–84.

48. Welsh FKS, Farmery SM, Ramsden C, Guillou PJ, Reynolds JV. Reversible impairment in monocyte major histocompatability complex class II expression in malnourished surgical patients. *J Parenter Enteral Nutr* 1996; **20**: 344–348.

49. Van Bokhorst-de van der Schueren MAE, von Blomberg-van der Flier BME, Riezebos RK *et al.* Differences in immune status between well-nourished and malnourished head and neck cancer patients. *Clin Nutr* 1998; **17**: 107–111.

50. Haydock DA, Hill GL. Impaired wound healing in surgical patients with varying degrees of malnutrition. *J Parenter Enteral Nutr* 1986; **10**: 550–554.

51. Pedersen NW, Pedersen D. Nutrition as a prognostic indicator in amputations. *Acta Orthop Scand* 1992; **63**: 675–678.

52. Breslow R. Nutritional status and dietary intake of patients with pressure ulcers: review of research literature 1943 to 1989. *Decubitus* 1991; **4**: 16–21.

53. Trujillo EB. Effects of nutritional status on wound healing. *J Vasc Nurs* 1993; **11**: 12–18.

54. Bastow MD, Rawlings J, Allison SP. Benefits of supplementary tube feeding after fractured neck of femur: a randomised controlled trial. *Br Med J* 1983; **287**: 1589–1592.

55. Warnold I, Lundholm K. Clinical significance of pre-operative nutritional status in 215 noncancer patients. *Ann Surg* 1984; **201**: 299–305.

56. Windsor JA, Hill GL. Weight loss with physiological impairment. A basic indicator of surgical risk. *Ann Surg* 1988; **205**: 290–296.

57. Von Meyenfeldt MF, Meijerink WJHJ, Rouflart MMJ, Builmaassen MTHJ, Soeters PB. Perioperative nutritional support: a randomised clinical trial. *Clin Nutr* 1992; **11**: 180–186.

58. Van Bokhorst-de van der Schueren MAE, van Leeuwen PAM, Sauerwein HP, Kuik DJ, Snow GB, Quak JJ. Assessment of malnutrition parameters in head and neck cancer and their relation to postoperative complications. *Head Neck* 1997; **19**: 419–425.

59. Anker SD, Ponikowski P, Varney S *et al.* Wasting as independent risk factor for mortality in chronic heart failure. *Lancet* 1997; **349**: 1050–1053.

60. Galanos AN, Pieper CF, Kussin PS *et al.* Relationship of body mass index to subsequent mortality among seriously ill hospitalized patients. *Crit Care Med* 1997; **25**: 1962–1968.

61. Tucker HN, Miguel SG. Cost containment through nutrition intervention. *Nutr Rev* 1996; **54**: 111–121.

62. Booth K, Morgan S. Financial issues for clinical nutrition in NHS hospitals. Nutricia Clinical Care, 1995, Trowbridge; Pharmacia, Milton Keynes. (Available from Christine Russell, Nutricia Clinical Care, Trowbridge, or Cathy Craig, Burson Marsteller, 24–28 Bloomsbury Way, London WC1 2PX.)

63. Christensen KS. Hospitalwide screening increases revenue under prospective payment system. *JADA* 1986; **86**: 1234–1235.

64. Reilly JJ, Hull SF, Albert N, Waller A, Bringardener S. Economic impact of malnutrition: a model system for hospitalised patients. *J Parenter Enteral Nutr* 1988; **12**: 371–376.

65. Robinson G, Goldstein M, Levine GM. Impact of nutritional status on DRG length of stay. *J Parenter Enteral Nutr* 1987; **11**: 49–51.

66. Chima CS, Barco K, Dewitt MLA, Maeda M, Teran JC, Mullen KD. Relationship of nutritional status to length of stay, hospital costs, and discharge status of patients hospitalized in the medicine service. *J Am Diet Assoc* 1997; 975–978.

67. Martyn CN, Winter PD, Coles SJ, Edington J. Effect of nutritional status on use of health care resources by patients with chronic disease living in the community. *Clin Nutr* 1998; **17**: 119–123.

68. Meguid MM. An open letter to Hillary Rodham Clinton. *Nutrition* 1993; **9:** ix–xi.

69. Nutrition Screening Initiative. The clinical and cost-effectiveness of medical nutrition therapy: evidence and estimates of potential Medicare savings from the use of selected nutrition intervention. Prepared by Barents Group, LLC of KPMG Peat Marwick LLP for the Nutrition Screening Initiative, 1010 Wisconsin Ave, NW, Suite 800, Washington DC 20036, 1996.

70. Lennard-Jones JE (ed) A positive approach to nutrition as treatment. King's Fund Centre, London; 1992 (available from the King's Fund Centre, 126 Albert St., London NW1 7NF).

71. Ofman J, Koretz RL. Clinical economics review: nutritional support. *Aliment Pharmacol Ther* 1997; **11:** 453–471.

72. Wolfe BM, Mathiesen KA. Clinical practice guidelines: can they be based on randomized clinical trials? *J Parenter Enteral Nutr* 1997; **21:** 1–6.

73. Levine JA, Morgan MY. Weighed dietary intakes in patients with chronic liver disease. *Nutrition* 1996; **12:** 430–435.

74. Olin AO, Osterberg B, Hadell K, Armyr I, Jerström S, Ljungqvist O. Energy enriched hospital food to improve energy intake in elderly patients. *J Parenter Enteral Nutr* 1996; **20:** 93–97.

75. Potter J, Langhorne P, Roberts M. Routine protein energy supplementation in adults: systematic review. *Br Med J* 1998; **317:** 495–501.

76. Shepherd RW, Holt TL, Cleghorn G, Ward LC, Isles A, Francis P. Short-term nutritional supplementation during management of pulmonary exacerbations in cystic fibrosis: a controlled study, including effects of protein turnover. *Am J Clin Nutr* 1988; **48:** 235–239.

77. Fuenzalida CE, Petty TL, Jones ML *et al.* The immune response to short-term nutritional intervention in advanced chronic obstructive pulmonary disease. *Am Rev Respir Dis* 1990; **142:** 49–56.

78. Williams CM, Driver LT, Older J, Dickerson JWT. A controlled trial of sip-feed supplements in elderly orthopaedic patients. *Eur J Clin Nutr* 1989; **43:** 267–274.

79. Otte KE, Ahlburg P, D'Amore F, Stellfeld M. Nutritional repletion in malnourished patients with emphysema. *J Parenter Enteral Nutr* 1989; **13:** 152–156.

80. Flynn MB, Leightty FF. Preoperative outpatient nutritional support of patients with squamous cancer of the upper aerodigestive tract. *Am J Surg* 1987; **154:** 359–362.

81. Delmi M, Rapin C-H, Bengoa J-M, Delmas PD, Vasey H, Bonjour J-P. Dietary supplementation in elderly patients with fractured neck of the femur. *Lancet* 1990; **335:** 1013–1016.

82. Rana SK, Bray J, Menzies-Gow N *et al.* Short term benefits of post-operative oral dietary supplements in surgical patients. *Clin Nutr* 1992; **11:** 337–344.

83. Smith DL, Clarke JM, Stableforth PG. A nocturnal nasogastric feeding programme in cystic fibrosis adults. *J Hum Nutr Diet* 1994; **7:** 257–262.

84. McWhirter JP, Pennington CR. A comparison between oral and nasogastric nutritional supplements in malnourished patients. *Nutrition* 1996; **12:** 502–506.

85. Lennard-Jones JE (ed) Ethical and legal aspect of clinical hydration and nutritional support. King's Fund Centre, London; 1998 (available from the King's Fund Centre, 126 Albert St., London NW1 7NF).

86. Papadopoulou A, Holden CE, Paul L, Sexton E, Booth IW. The nutritional response to home enteral nutrition in childhood. *Acta Paediatr* 1995; **84:** 528–531.

87. Jamieson CP, Norton B, Day T, Lakeman M, Powell-Tuck J. The quantitative effect of nutrition support on quality of life in outpatients. *Clin Nutr* 1997; **16:** 25–28.

88. McCarey DW, Buchanan E, Gregory M, Clark BJ, Weaver LT. Home enteral feeding of children in the West of Scotland. *Scott Med J* 1996; **41:** 147–149.

89. Park RHR, Allison MC, Lang J *et al.* Randomised comparison of percutaneous endoscopic gastrostomy and nasogastric tube feeding in patients with persisting neurological dysphagia. *Br Med J* 1992; **304:** 1406–1409.

90. Wanklyn P, Cox N, Belfield P. Outcome in patients who require a gastrostomy after stroke. *Age Ageing* 1995; **24:** 510–514.

91. Rabeneck L, McCullough LB, Wray NP. Ethically justified, clinically comprehensive guidelines for percutaneous endoscopic gastrostomy tube placement. *Lancet* 1997; **349:** 496–498.

92. Hull MA, Rawlings J, Murray FE *et al.* Audit of outcome of long-term enteral nutrition by percutaneous endoscopic gastrostomy. *Lancet* 1993; **341:** 869–872.

93. FFSPEN. French Speaking Society for Parenteral and Enteral Nutrition. Perioperative artificial nutrition in elective adult surgery. *Clin Nutr* 1996; **15:** 223–229.

94. Taylor SJ. Audit of nasogastric feeding practice at two acute hospitals: is early enteral feeding associated with reduced mortality and hospital stay? *J Hum Nutr Diet* 1993; **6:** 477–489.

95. Brough W, Horne G, Blount A, Irving MH, Jeejeebhoy KN. Effects of nutrient intake, surgery, sepsis, and long term administration of steroids on muscle function. *Br Med J* 1986; **293:** 983–988.

96. Jeejeebhoy KN. Bulk or bounce – the object of nutritional support. *J Parenter Enteral Nutr* 1988; **12:** 539–549.

97. Windsor JA, Knight GS, Hill GL. Wound healing response in surgical patients: recent food intake is more important than nutritional status. *Br J Surg* 1988; **75**: 135–137.

98. Schroeder D, Gillanders L, Mahr K, Hill GL. Effects of immediate postoperative enteral nutrition on body composition, muscle function and wound healing. *J Parenter Enteral Nutr* 1991; **15**: 376–383.

99. Chiarelli A, Enzi G, Casadei A, Baggio B, Valerio A, Mazzoleni F. Very early nutrition supplementation in burned patients. *Am J Clin Nutr* 1990; **51**: 1035–1039.

100. Hasse JM, Blue LS, Liepa GU *et al*. Early enteral nutrition support in patients undergoing liver transplantation. *J Parenter Enteral Nutr* 1995; **19**: 437–443.

101. Carr CS, Ling KDE, Boulos P, Singer M. Randomised trial of safety and efficacy of immediate postoperative enteral feeding in patients undergoing gastrointestinal resection. *Br Med J* 1996; **312**: 869–871.

102. Beier-Holgersen R, Boesby S. Influence of postoperative enteral nutrition on postsurgical infections. *Gut* 1996; **39**: 833–835.

103. Heslin MJ, Latkany L, Leung D *et al*. A prospective, randomized trial of early enteral feeding after resection of upper GI malignancy. *Ann Surg* 1997; **226**: 567–580.

104. Watters JM, Kirkpatrick SM, Norris SB, Shamji FM, Wells GA. Immediate postoperative enteral feeding results in impaired respiratory mechanics and decreased mobility. *Ann Surg* 1997; **226**: 369–380.

105. Heyland DK. Nutritional support in the critically ill patients. A critical review of the evidence. *Crit Care Clin* 1998; **14**: 423–440.

106. Kudsk KA, Croce MA, Fabian TC *et al*. Enteral versus parenteral feeding. Effects on septic morbidity after blunt and penetrating abdominal trauma. *Ann Surg* 1992; **215**: 503–513.

107. Moore FA, Feliciano DV, Andrassy RJ *et al*. Early enteral feeding, compared with parenteral, reduces postoperative septic complications. The results of a meta-analysis. *Ann Surg* 1992; **216**: 172–183.

108. Bower RH, Cerra FB, Bershadsky B, Licari JJ, Hoyt DB, Jensen GL. Early enteral administration of a formula Impact supplemented with arginine, nucleotides, and fish oil in intensive care unit patients: results of a multicenter, prospective, randomized, clinical trial. *Crit Care Med* 1995; **23**: 436–449.

109. Kudsk KA, Minard G, Croce MA, Brown RO, Lowrey TS, Prichard FE. A randomized trial of isonitrogenous enteral diets after severe trauma. An immune-enhancing diet reduces septic complications. *Ann Surg* 1996; **224**: 531–543.

110. Griffiths RD, Jones C, Palmer TEA. Six-month outcome of critically ill patients given glutamine-supplemented parenteral nutrition. *Nutrition* 1997; **13**: 295–302.

111. Houdijk APJ, Rijnsburger ER, Jansen J *et al*. Randomised trial of glutamine-enriched enteral nutrition on infectious morbidity in patients with multiple trauma. *Lancet* 1998; **352**: 772–776.

112. Preiser J-C, Berre J, van Gossum A, Vincent J-L, Carpentier YA. Effects of enteral feeding supplementation with arginine and vitamins A, C and E in critically ill patients. *J Parenter Enteral Nutr* 1998; **22**: S4.

113. Jones C, Palmer TEA, Griffiths RD. Randomized clinical outcome study of critically ill patients given glutamine-supplemented enteral nutrition. *Nutrition* 1999; **15**: 108–115.

114. Fleming CR, Remington M. Intestinal failure. In: Hill GL (ed) *Nutrition and the surgical patient*. Churchill Livingstone, Edinburgh, 1981; pp. 219–235.

115. Haydock DA, Hill GL. Improved wound healing response in surgical patients receiving intravenous nutrition. *Br J Surg* 1987; **74**: 320–323.

116. Sacks GS, Brown RO, Teague D, Dickerson RN, Tolley EA, Kudsk KA. Early nutrition support modifies immune function in patients sustaining severe head injury. *J Parenter Enteral Nutr* 1995; **19**: 387–392.

117. Christie PM, Hill GL. Effect of intravenous nutrition on nutrition and function in acute attacks of inflammatory bowel disease. *Gastroenterology* 1990; **99**: 730–736.

118. Puntis JWL. Home parenteral nutrition. *Arch Dis Child* 1995; **72**: 186–190.

119. Shields PL, Field J, Rawlings J, Kendall J, Allison SP. Long-term outcome and cost-effectiveness of parenteral nutrition for acute gastrointestinal failure. *Clin Nutr* 1996; **15**: 4–68.

120. O'Hanrahan T, Irving MH. The role of home parenteral nutrition in the management of intestinal failure – report of 400 cases. *Clin Nutr* 1992; **11**: 331–336.

121. Johnston DA, Pennington CR. Home parenteral nutrition in Tayside 1980–1992. *Scott Med J* 1993; **38**: 110–111.

122. Carlson GL, Maguire G, Williams N, Bradley A, Shaffer JL, Irving MH. Quality of life on home parenteral nutrition: a single centre study of 37 patients. *Clin Nutr* 1995; **14**: 219–228.

123. Heys SD, Walker LG, Eremin O. The value of perioperative nutrition in the sick patient. *Proc Nutr Soc* 1997; **56**: 443–457.

124. Glade MJ. Workshop on cost-effectiveness in medicine. *Nutrition* 1997; **13:** 595–597.

125. Mirtallo JM. Cost-effectiveness of nutrition therapy. In: Torosian MH (ed) *Nutrition for the hospitalized patient.* Marcel Dekker, New York, 1995; pp. 653–667.

126. Kernick DP. Economic evaluation in health: a thumbnail sketch. *Br Med J* 1998; **316:** 1663–1665.

127. Rice DP. Cost-of-illness studies: fact or fiction? *Lancet* 1994; **344:** 1519–1520.

128. Fayers PM, Hand DJ. Generalisation from phase III clinical trials: survival, quality of life, and health economics. *Lancet* 1997; **350:** 1025–1027.

129. Twomey PL, Patching SC. Cost-effectiveness of nutritional support. *J Parenter Enteral Nutr* 1985; **9:** 3–10.

130. Raftery J. Economic evaluation: an introduction. *Br Med J* 1998; **316:** 1013–1014.

131. Byford S, Raftery J. Perspectives in economic evaluation. *Br Med J* 1998; **316:** 1529.

132. Roehrig CS, Lee JA. Cost analysis in nutrition-intervention outcome studies. *Nutrition* 1996; **12:** 558–559.

133. Kernick DP. Has health economics lost its way? *Br Med J* 1998; **317:** 197–199.

134. Testa MA, Simonson DC. Assessment of quality-of-life outcomes. *N Engl J Med* 1996; **334:** 835–840.

135. Muldoon MF, Barger SD, Flory JD, Manuck SB. What are quality of life measurements measuring? *Br Med J* 1998; **316:** 542–545.

136. Tramèr MR, Reynolds DJM, Moore RA, McQuay HJ. When placebo controlled trials are essential and equivalence trials are inadequate. *Br Med J* 1998; **317:** 875–880.

137. Jefferson T. Commentary: Concurrent economic evaluations are rare but should be standard practice. *Br Med J* 1998; **317:** 915–916.

138. Thompson S, Barber J. From efficacy to cost-effectiveness (letter). *Lancet* 1997; **350:** 1781–1782.

139. Reynolds N, Baxter JP, Pennington CR. The implementation of guidelines: another drain on the NHS purse? *Proc Nutr Soc* 1998; **57:** 107A.

140. Reddy P, Malone M. Cost and outcome analysis of home parenteral and enteral nutrition. *J Parenter Enteral Nutr* 1998; **22:** 302–310.

141. Sartori S, Trevisani L, Tassinari D, Gilli G, Nilesen I, Maestri A. Cost analysis of long-term feeding by percutaneous endoscopic gastrostomy in cancer patients in an Italian health district. *Support Care Cancer* 1996; **4:** 21–26.

142. Roberts MF, Levine GM. Nutrition support team recommendations can reduce hospital costs. *Nutr Clin Prac* 1992; **7:** 227–230.

143. Hassell JT, Games AD, Shaffer B, Harkins LE. Nutrition support team management of enteral fed patients in a community hospital is beneficial. *JADA* 1994; **94:** 993–998.

144. Johansson C, Backman L, Jakobsson J. Is enteral nutrition optimally used in hospitalized patients? A study of the practice of nutrition in a Swedish hospital. *Clin Nutr* 1996; **15:** 171–174.

145. Schwartz DB. Enhanced enteral and parenteral nutrition practice and outcomes in an intensive care unit with a hospital-wide performance improvement process. *J Am Diet Assoc* 1996; **96:** 484–489.

146. Moffitt SK, Gohman Sm, Sass KM, Faucher KL. Clinical and laboratory evaluation of a closed enteral feeding system under cyclic feeding conditions: a microbial and cost evaluation. *Nutrition* 1997; **13:** 622–628.

147. Silkroski M, Allen F, Storm H. Tube feeding audit reveals hidden costs and risks of current practice. *Nutr Clin Prac* 1998; **13:** 283–290.

148. Trujillo EB, Young LS, Chertow GM *et al.* Metabolic and monetary costs of avoidable parenteral nutrition use. *JPEN* 1999; **23:** 109–113.

149. May J, Sedman P, Mitchell C, MacFie J. Peripheral and central parenteral nutrition: a cost-comparison analysis. *Health Trends* 1993; **25:** 129–132.

150. Kotler DP, Fogleman L, Tierney AR. Comparison of total parenteral nutrition and an oral semielemental diet on body composition, physical function, and nutrition-related costs in patients with malabsorption due to acquired immunodeficiency syndrome. *JPEN* 1998; **22:** 120–126.

151. Barkmeier JM, Trerotola SO, Wiebke EA *et al.* Percutaneous radiologic, surgical endoscopic, and percutaneous endoscopic gastrostomy/gastro-jejenustomy: comparative study and cost analysis. *Cardiovasc Intervent Radiol* 1998; **21:** 324–328.

152. Senkal M, Mumme A, Eickhoff U, Geier B, Spaeth G, Wulfert D. Early postoperative enteral immuno-nutrition: clinical outcome and cost-comparison analysis in surgical patients. *Crit Care Med* 1997; **25:** 1489–1496.

153. Harbrecht BG, Moraca RJ, Saul M, Courcoulas AP. Percutaneous endoscopic gastrostomy reduces total hospital costs in head-injured patients. *Am J Surg* 1998; **176:** 311–314.

154. Trice S, Melnik G, Page CP. Complications and costs of early postoperative parenteral versus enteral nutrition in trauma patients. *Nutr Clin Prac* 1997; **12:** 114–119.

155. Eisenberg JM, Glick HA, Buzby GP, Kinosian B, Williford WO. Does perioperative total parenteral nutrition reduce medical care costs? *J Parenter Enteral Nutr* 1993; **17**: 201–209.

156. Dallas MJ, Bowling D, Roig JC, Auestad N, Neu J. Enteral glutamine supplementation for very low birth weight infants decreases hospital costs. *JPEN* 1998; **22**: 352–356.

157. Hickson M, Nicholl C, Bulpitt C, Fry M, Frost G, Davies L. The design of the feeding support trial – does intensive feeding support improved nutritional status and outcome in acutely ill older in-patients? *J Hum Nutr Dietet* 1999; **12**: 53–59.

158. Richards DM, Irving MH. Cost-utility analysis of home parenteral nutrition. *Br J Surg* 1996; **83**: 1226–1229.

159. Detsky AS, Jeejeebhoy KN. Cost-effectiveness of pre-operative parenteral nutrition in patients undergoing major gastrointestinal surgery. *J Parenter Enteral Nutr* 1984; **8**: 632–637.

160. Jendteg S, Larsson J, Lindgren B. Clinical and economic aspects on nutritional supply. *Clin Nutr* 1987; **6**: 185–190.

161. Lipman TO. The cost of total parenteral nutrition: Is the price right? *J Parenter Enteral Nutr* 1993; **17**: 199–200.

162. McCamish MA. Malnutrition and nutrition support interventions: costs, benefits and outcomes. *Nutrition* 1993; **9**: 556–557.

163. Lipman TO. Grains or veins: is enteral nutrition really better than parenteral nutrition? A look at the evidence. *J Parenter Enteral Nutr* 1998; **22**: 167–182.

164. Allison SP. Nutritional support: efficacy versus cost. *Nutrition Int* 1987; **3**: 19–24.

165. Silk DBA (ed) Organisation of nutritional support in hospitals. BAPEN, Maidenhead; 1994 (available from BAPEN, PO BOX 922, Maidenhead, Berks SL6 4SH).

166. Shukla HS, Rao RR, Banu N, Gupta RM, Yadav RC. Enteral hyperalimentation in malnourished surgical patients. *Indian J Med Res* 1984; **80**: 339–346.

167. MIMS. Monthly index of medical specialities. Haymarket Medical, London, 1997; May: 200–203.

168. Cade A, Puntis J. Economics of home parenteral nutrition. *Pharmacoeconomics* 1997; **12**: 327–338.

169. Green CJ. The role of peri-operative feeding. *S Afr Med J* 1998; **88**: 92–98.

42

The role of enteral and parenteral nutrition: enteral vs parenteral?

Simon M Gabe

There is no simple answer to the question of whether enteral or parenteral nutrition is the best form of nutrition support. It is important to understand that the purpose of nutrition is to support the appropriate nutrients necessary for cellular function. The challenge is to be able to supply the relevant nutrients to each organ in different clinical conditions in order that each organ may function optimally. In trying to achieve this goal it is necessary to disassociate our preconceptions and dogma from scientific evidence. The phrase 'if the gut works, use it' is commonly used – and for good reason. However, this belief is often based on the judgements about hazards and costs of parenteral relative to enteral nutrition. Cost seems to be the most important factor in selecting enteral over a parenteral route, with science taking second place. However, in recent years the composition, formulation and delivery of parenteral nutrition have changed substantially and it is essential to explore the question in further detail. This chapter compares the effects of enteral and parenteral nutrition on intestinal physiology, morphology, barrier function, patient morbidity and mortality.

Intestinal physiology

The obvious difference between enteral and parenteral nutrition is that enteral nutrition provides nutrients within the intestinal lumen and the instinctive feeling is that this must be more physiologically normal than parenteral nutrition. In many respects this is true but the intestinal mucosa is a dynamic structure which can adapt to its environment. The enzymes and transport processes on the mucosal surface are inducible and thus the absence of enteral nutrition will result in a down-regulation of these processes. Examples include the brush-border disaccharidases which decrease in healthy volunteers on total parenteral nutrition (TPN), returning to normal after reinstating an oral diet.[1,2] Factors that regulate intestinal adaptation are largely unknown but the current understanding is that multiple regulatory elements act in combination to control gene transcription patterns.[3] Homeodomain transcription factors are involved in establishing gradients of differentiation during development and in maintaining the gene patterns through continued expression in adult tissues. These transcription factors appear to be responsible for the intestinal phenotype expressed at any point in time and are therefore involved in the adaptive process.[4] These data suggest that the intestine adapts to change and it is not necessarily unphysiological to withhold enteral nutrition. The evolutionary advantage of this process is to be

able to induce the necessary enzymes for the ingested diet, which may vary considerably around the world. Unnecessary enzyme and transport systems may not be synthesised, improving digestive efficiency. It would be ridiculous to suggest that humans evolved to be able to tolerate TPN, but the same adaptive processes apply.

Another perspective is that artificial enteral nutrition is as unphysiological as parenteral nutrition. Normal human life is associated with episodic periods of high nutrient intake followed by periods of no nutrient intake. This results in the feed/fast cycle which may be necessary to achieve optimal metabolic efficiency. The continuous administration of nutrients by tube feeding will disturb this process and may contribute to insulin resistance. Furthermore, enteral tube feeding misses the cephalic and oral phases of digestion and parenteral nutrition misses first pass metabolism. Taking these factors into account, artificial enteral tube feeding appears to be as unphysiological as parenteral nutrition.

A final argument relates to the question as to the nutrient source for mucosal enterocytes. It can be suggested that when feeding parenterally, the body is fed but the intestine is starved. It has been suggested that glucose is taken up from the arterial blood and used for intestinal metabolism and lactate production, while luminal glucose is absorbed mainly unaltered and transferred to the portal blood.[5] Amino acid uptake may be different, however, as it has been demonstrated that both luminal and vascular amino acids contribute to protein synthesis within the intestine during feeding.[6] Teleologically it appears reasonable to conclude that the energy supply to enterocytes comes from a reliable source, while amino acids can be obtained from a less reliable source.

Overall, artificial enteral nutrition is less physiological than normal oral feeding. It may offer some advantages over parenteral feeding. These advantages are minimal and may not be clinically relevant. This is examined further below.

Intestinal morphology

Studies in rats demonstrate that both starvation and parenteral nutrition will result in intestinal atrophy with a decreased intestinal mass, protein and DNA content.[1] These alterations are paralleled by a functional impairment of the intestinal mucosa[1] and immunological impairment.[7] However, there appear to be significant species differences in this adaptive process, as studies in mice suggest that parenteral nutrition results in a functional decrease in disaccharidase activity without atrophy.[8] The mouse model may represent humans more closely than in rats. In humans, the evidence suggesting that TPN results in mucosal atrophy is conflicting. It has been demonstrated that TPN is associated with a decreased mucosal thickness and an increased intestinal permeability in healthy volunteers.[2] A further study examined duodenal biopsies from seven patients on TPN for 21 days.[9] There was no alteration in mucosal architecture as assessed by light microscopy, but electron microscopy demonstrated a decrease in the microvillus height and functional studies showed a decrease in functional (disaccharidase) activity. One week of preoperative parenteral nutrition results in a decreased transport enzyme activity.[10] Placed into the context that it is now better understood that the brush-border enzyme activity and transport mechanisms are induced by the presence of luminal nutrition, these studies simply suggest that it is the absence of luminal nutrition that leads to down-regulation of the intestinal mucosa rather than changes occurring as a result as a detrimental effect of TPN. This would seem to be a sensible perspective, but the picture is not so clear when assessing the literature further.

Some studies have not demonstrated that TPN alters the intestinal mucosal architecture.[11,12] Moreover, there are studies which demonstrate that artificial enteral formulations are associated with similar structural changes to the intestinal mucosa as has been attributed to TPN. Cummings demonstrated that an artificial feed (Isocal (Abbott, Maidenhead, UK) or Jevity (Abbott, Maidenhead, UK)) did not reverse the mucosal atrophy and functional (maltase) activity noted in patients with gastrostomies after 3 months of enteral feeding.[13] Hoensch showed that healthy volunteers taking three different types of artificial feed (whole protein, oligopeptide and amino acid) had a significant decrease in jejunal villous height and mucosal functional ability.[14] It could therefore be argued that these artificial enteral feeds must be missing a vital ingredient required for optimal mucosal growth. This is part of the rationale for using feeds with additional novel substrates such as glutamine, alanine and nucleosides. The studies in the literature that compare the physiological effects of enteral and parenteral feeding are presented in Table 40.1 (standard feeds) and Table 40.2 (augmented feeds). It can be seen that it is very difficult to compare results directly due to the diversity of the type of feeds, duration of feeding, quantity given as well as the different patient populations.

Perhaps the literature does not help us answer the question as to whether enteral nutrition is better than parenteral nutrition in maintaining the intestinal mucosal morphology. Most comparative studies look at nitrogen balance, outcomes and complications (see Tables 42.1 and 42.2). The few studies that aim to assess intestinal mucosal architecture differ substantially in the patients assessed and in the type of feed used. Two randomised studies comparing TPN with jejunal Osmolite (Abbott, Maidenhead, UK) found no difference in intestinal permeability in postoperative patients undergoing cancer surgery and elective liver transplantation.[15,16] Hadfield and colleagues studied intensive care patients by comparing TPN with a glutamine-enriched enteral feed (Alitraq, Ross Laboratories, UK).[17] They demonstrated that intestinal permeability was significantly lower in the enterally fed group on the ninth intensive care unit (ICU) day. Most patients had undergone cardiopulmonary bypass surgery and the severity of illness of these patients (APACHE II score) similar to the transplanted patients studied by Wicks. In both of these studies patients underwent a single insult and recovered on the ICU. The differing results highlight the uncertainty of the effect of TPN on the intestinal mucosal architecture, especially when other diseases coexist.

Thus overall there is insufficient evidence to suggest that artificial enteral nutrition offers significant benefits to the intestinal mucosa over parenteral nutrition. However, it would be reasonable to suggest that the absence of luminal nutrition results in a down-regulation of intestinal mucosal function.

Intestinal barrier function

Microbes are present throughout the gastrointestinal tract, from mouth to anus. The pharyngeal flora consists of aerobes, anaerobes and yeast species. With the exception of *Helicobacter pylori*, the stomach is sterile but the small bowel has a microfloral population of 10^3–10^4 per ml. This increases to 10^6–10^7 in the terminal ileum and further in the colon to 10^9–10^{11} per ml.[18]

The recognition of bacterial migration across the gastrointestinal epithelium dates back to the 19th century.[19] In 1979, Berg & Garlington defined bacterial translocation as the passage of viable bacteria through the epithelial mucosa into the lamina propria,

Table 42.1 – Non-outcome studies of enteral versus parenteral standard feeds.

Author, date	Patient group	Feed used	Feed duration	Amount per day	N balance	Serum proteins	Metabolic markers	Immune markers	Intestinal mucosa
Hindmarsh, 1973[85]	Surgery (GI)	7 EN[a], 8 TPN	3 days (weaned onto oral diet by day 7)	EN: 2015 kcal, 10.9 g N; TPN: 2130 kcal, 12.7 g N	EN: less −ve	–	–	–	–
Rowlands, 1977[86]	Surgery (GI)	7 EN[a], 25 TPN (+EN?), 14 IV fluids	8 days	EN: 2750 kcal, 12.7 g N; TPN: 0.23 g N/kg, 12–51 kcal/kg	No difference (EN vs TPN)	–	–	–	–
McArdle, 1981[87]	Recent weight loss	24 EN/TPN	10 days	EN: Aminosyn (Abbott, Maidenhead, UK) 7% and polycose 50%; TPN: 3600–6000 kcal, Aminosyn (Abbott, Maidenhead, UK) 7% for N	No difference	–	TPN: ↓FFA ↑insulin	–	–
Bennegard, 1984[88]	Healthy men	5 EN, 5 TPN cross-over (TPN to EN)	14 days	9.23 g N in 12 h	No difference	–	TPN: ↑glucagon	–	–
Adams, 1986[b][89]	Surgery (GI)	23 EN jejunal Traumacal (Mead Johnson, UK), 22 TPN	14 days	Initially REE × 1.68 Later REE × 2 (TPN) and REE × 2.4 (EN)	No difference	No difference	–	No difference	–
Fletcher, 1986[90]	Surgery (GI, vascular)	9 EN jejunal Criticare (Mead Johnson, UK), 16 TPN, 9 IV fluids	5 days	EN: 1014 kcal, 5.9 g N; TPN: 1010 kcal, 6.8 g N; IV: 300 kcal	No difference (EN vs TPN)	–	–	–	–
Young, 1987[26]	Head injury	96 EN/TPN (Traumacal (Mead Johnson, UK)/Vital (Ross laboratories, UK)/Ensure plus) (Abbott, Maidenhead, UK)	18 days	According to requirements (EN received less for the 1st 12 days)	TPN: ↑protein intake	–	–	–	–
Kudsk, 1994[91]	Surgery (GI) & trauma	34 EN jejunal Vital H/N, 34 TPN	10 days	According to requirements	–	EN ↑prealbumin & transferrin, ↓CRP	–	–	–
Wicks, 1994[16]	Surgery (OLT)	14 EN NJ Osmolite (Abbott, Maidenhead, UK), 1) TPN	10 days	According to requirements	–	–	–	–	No difference in int. permeability or CHO absorption
Suchner, 1996[44]	Surgery (neuro)	17 EN NG Osmolite (Abbott, Maidenhead, UK), 17 TPN	12 days	Increased slowly to requirements over 3–5 days	–	EN: ↑transferrin prealbumin, RBP	EN: ↑REE	EN: ↑lymphocyte count	TPN: ↓int A & D-xylose absorption
Reynolds, 1997[5]	Surgery (GI)	33 EN jejunal Osmolite (Abbott, Maidenhead, UK), 34 TPN	7 days	EN: 1680 kcal, 12.8 g N; TPN: 1800 kcal, 9.49 g N	No difference	No difference	–	–	No difference in permeability by day 7
Georgannos, 1997[g]	Malnourished patients	15 EN (semi-elemental), 15 TPN	10 days	2900 kcal, 14.5 g N both groups	No difference	No difference	TPN: ↑insulin	No difference	–

[a] Enteral feed formula used previously described by Hindmarsh. [b] Poor study with many cross-over patients and differing feeds and amounts given. IV = intravenous, EN = enteral nutrition, TPN = total parenteral nutrition, GI = gastrointestinal, FFA = free fatty acids, CRP = C-reactive protein, RBP = retinol-binding protein.

Table 42.2 – Non-outcome studies of augmented enteral versus parenteral feeds

Author, date	Patient group	Feed used	Feed duration	Amount	N_2 balance	Serum proteins	Metabolic markers	Immune markers	Intestinal mucosa
Burt, 1982, 1983a [103,104]	Cancer (oesophageal)	4 oral (ad libitum) / 6 TPN / 3 EN Vivonex (Norwich Eaton Pharmaceuticals) / 5 TPN	14 days	Isocaloric (except oral group) but not isonitrogenous	TPN: ↑N_2 balance, ↑weight, ↓muscle catabolism	—	No difference		—
Bower, 1986 [70]	Surgery (GI)	10 EN jejunal Vivonex (Norwich Eaton Pharmaceuticals) / 10 TPN	7 days	960–3000 kcal each group	No difference	EN ↓albumin			—
O'Keefe, 1987 [75]	Alcoholic encephalopathy	4 EN (semi elemental with BCAA) / 4 TPN BCAA enriched	7 days	Isocaloric but not isonitrogenous	No difference		No difference		—
Peterson, 1988 [76]	Surgery (GI) & trauma	18 EN Vivonex (Norwich Eaton Pharmaceuticals) / 18 TPN	10 days	According to requirements	No difference	EN: ↑alb, RBP TPN: ↑α1AT, orosomucoid			—
Borzotta, 1994 [6]	Head injury	27 EN jejunal Vivonex / 21 TPN	12 days	According to requirements	No difference	No difference	No difference		—
Hadfield, 1995 [27]	ICU (mainly post CPB)	12 EN Alitraq (Ross laboratories) / 12 TPN	9 days	According to requirements					TPN: Permeability ↑day 9, abs no difference
Pearlstone, 1995 [98]	Malnourished cancer (oesophageal)	6 EN jejunal Vivonex (Norwich Eaton Pharmaceuticals) / 5 TPN	14 days isonitrogenous	Isocaloric but not amino acid levels	TPN: improved	—	—		—
Braga, 1996 [5]	Surgery (GI)	20 EN (impact) (Novartis, UK) / 20 TPN / 20 EN (standard)	8 days	According to requirements	No difference	↑pre-albumin & RBP with Impact		Improved with Impact	
Fish, 1997 [?]	Surgery (GI)	7 EN Vivonex (Norwich Eaton Pharmaceuticals) / 10 TPN	5 days	According to requirements	No difference		No difference		—
Gianotti, 1997 [?]	Surgery (GI)	87 EN jejunal / 87 EN Impact / 86 TPN	7 days	25 kcal/kg/day		No difference	Significant improvement with Impact	Better with Impact	—
Shirabe, 1997 [72]	Surgery (hepatic)	13 EN BCAA / 13 TPN BCAA	7 days	EN 23.5 kcal/kg/day TPN 26 kcal/kg/day		No difference	No difference	Improved more with EN than TPN	—
Kotler, 1998 [?]	AIDS	11 EN (Alitraq, Ross laboratories) / 12 TPN	4–12 weeks	According to requirements but more calories in TPN group		No difference		No difference	—

a Same study split into two papers. EN = enteral nutrition, TPN = total parenteral nutrition, GI = gastrointestinal, α1AT = α anti trypsin, BCCA – branched-chain amino acids mesenteric lymph nodes and then possibly to other tissues.[20] In 1990, Alexander et al further suggested that this concept should be refined to include the translocation of microbes and all microbial products.[21]

However, not only is there disagreement as to the relevance of bacterial translocation to patient morbidity but also whether bacterial translocation actually occurs in humans. This is important to view the different levels of evidence to assess whether bacterial translocation occurs.

Animal studies

In animals, it appears that a variety of insults affect the intestinal barrier stimulating bacterial translocation including trauma, burns, endotoxaemia, shock, obstructive jaundice, intestinal obstruction, chemotherapy and radiotherapy. The methods that have been used to assess bacterial translocation include mesenteric lymph node culture, electron microscopy and detection of bacterial breakdown products. From this it can be inferred that almost any type of acute insult may alter the intestinal barrier function and permit the translocation of bacteria. It should be noted that starvation or protein malnutrition do not promote bacterial translocation themselves, but together with a systemic insult protein malnutrition will exacerbate the morbidity and mortality by promoting bacterial translocation.[22,23]

A number of animal studies have demonstrated that parenteral nutrition promotes bacterial translocation.[24-29] Kueppers et al evaluated the hypothesis that gut stasis, induced by morphine, would lead to enhanced bacterial translocation in parenterally fed rats.[25] Fifty per cent of rats on TPN developed infected mesenteric lymph nodes, but only one of these had > 100 colony-forming units (cfu) per node and distant organ cultures were all negative. With the addition of morphine, 100% of mesenteric lymph nodes were infected with > 100 cfu per node and 14 out of 15 animals manifested evidence of bacterial translocation at distant sites. Conversely, bacterial translocation associated with TPN may be inhibited by the concomitant administration of enteral fibre or 20% of the total calorie intake being given enterally.[24,27] These studies suggest that bacterial translocation occurs in rodents, especially in association with intestinal stasis and that the luminal contents may alter this process.

The relationship between parenteral nutrition–induced gut atrophy and bacterial translocation has been addressed and discussed above. In humans there is conflicting evidence that parenteral nutrition causes mucosal atrophy. However, it appears that the bacterial translocation that occurs in association with TPN is independent of the presence of mucosal atrophy. Illig et al demonstrated that bacterial translocation was not increased in animals with intestinal atrophy induced by TPN compared to control groups.[30] While intestinal permeability to lactulose correlated with intestinal atrophy, both of these variables were independent of bacterial translocation. Helton and Garcia demonstrated that oral prostaglandin E_2 attenuated the mucosal atrophy associated with parenteral feeding but did not prevent bacterial translocation.[26] These data suggest that the mechanism of bacterial translocation does not necessarily require an altered or damaged mucosa but may occur through morphologically intact enterocytes.

Human studies

The data supporting the existence of bacterial translocation in humans are less extensive and come from both direct and indirect studies. The direct studies assess bacterial translocation from mesenteric lymph node cultures in patients undergoing laparotomy. Deitch et al[31] studied 42 patients undergoing laparotomy for intestinal obstruction and demonstrated that mesenteric lymph node cultures were positive in 59% of patients, compared to 4% in patients operated on for other reasons. Sedman et al[32] examined 267 consecutive surgical patients for translocation by obtaining an ileal serosal biopsy and an ileal mesenteric node biopsy for cultures at the start of surgery. Translocation occurred in 10.3% of patients overall, but in only 5% when distal intestinal obstruction and inflammatory bowel disease were excluded. There was no correlation between translocation and nutrition status, preoperative TPN or intestinal villous height. Postoperative septic complications were twice as frequent (28% vs 11.5%) in those patients with evidence of bacterial translocation, but the organisms causing infection were rarely those that had translocated. The same group has recently published the largest study on bacterial translocation in humans to date.[33] They cultured mesenteric lymph nodes, serosal scrapings and peripheral blood in 448 surgical patients undergoing laparotomy. Bacterial translocation was identified in 15.4% of patients. Both enteric bacteria and non-enteric bacteria were isolated and the most common organism identified was *Escherichia coli* (54%). Postoperative septic complications developed in 23% of patients and enteric organisms were responsible in 74% of cases. Forty-one per cent of patients who had evidence of bacterial translocation developed sepsis compared with 14% in whom no organisms were cultured ($P < 0.001$). Brooks et al studied 114 patients undergoing abdominal surgery for varied reasons and found that mesenteric lymph node or serosal cultures were positive in 16% of cases.[34] Postoperative septic complications occurred in 28% of patients with translocation and in 14% of patients without translocation, but the difference did not reach statistical significance. It is worthy of note that blood cultures were positive in only four out of 18 patients with translocation and in only two of these patients the organisms cultured from both blood and tissue were identical. This study illustrates the ineffectiveness of performing blood cultures to assess bacterial translocation. Reed et al[35] examined the mesenteric lymph nodes in 16 patients operated for abdominal trauma. Nodes showed evidence of bacterial translocation in 13 patients by electron microscopy and nodal culture was positive in only four of the 13. Bacterial translocation did not correlate with the severity of injury, infection or the degree of haemorrhagic shock. A notable study by Braithwaite et al demonstrated that bacterial breakdown products can be detected in all mesenteric lymph node macrophages of patients undergoing laparotomy without intestinal perforation.[36] In this study lymph node cultures were positive on only one occasion and portal blood culture was positive on only three occasions. This suggests that translocation of bacteria occurs much more frequently than is detected by culturing and that this translocation is usually controlled by the mesenteric nodes and that in surgical patients, bacterial translocation is a real phenomenon and is associated with an increased prevalence of postoperative sepsis.

The indirect evidence that is often also used to promote the existence of bacterial translocation is much less convincing. This relates to studies assessing intestinal permeability and selective gut decontamination. A number of studies have demonstrated that the permeability of the intestinal mucosa to small molecules increases in the same situations where bacterial translocation may occur, e.g. burns,[37–39] trauma,[40–42] cardiothoracic bypass[43,44] and critical illness.[45,46] However, the mechanisms relating to an altered intestinal permeability and bacterial translocation are likely to be unrelated. One study of surgical patients assessed intestinal permeability, villus atrophy and bacterial translocation in 43 patients undergoing laparotomy.[47] Significant differences were

apparent in the incidence of bacterial translocation in patients with normal permeability (23%) compared with patients with increased permeability (19%). Similarly, no correlation was seen between the incidence of bacterial translocation and the index of villus atrophy. These data agree with the animal data that bacterial translocation is unrelated to an altered intestinal permeability or the development of intestinal mucosal atrophy.

Another avenue of indirect reasoning for the existence of bacterial translocation in humans derives from studies on selective gut decontamination in intensive care unit patients. It is suggested that many nosocomial infections in critically ill patients may come from either aspiration of colonised organisms from the oropharynx or stomach, or from bacterial translocation of intestinal organisms.[48,49] Fiddian-Green & Baker demonstrated that the best predictor for the development of nosocomial pneumonia in the critically ill was the development of gut mucosal injury.[50] The indices used to detect gastrointestinal mucosal injury were better predictors of nosocomial pneumonia than any of the factors known to predispose to the aspiration of contaminated nasopharyngeal secretions (the administration of antacids and/or cimetidine, gastric juice pH > 4 and requiring mechanical ventilation). However, a recent large prospective controlled trial of selective gut decontamination demonstrated that decontamination reduced intestinal bacterial colonisation but not the incidence of pneumonia, sepsis, multiple organ failure or death.[51]

Thus from the animal data, bacterial translocation seems to occur to a minor extent in normal animals and is significantly increased after a number of physical insults. Starvation and protein malnutrition do not lead directly to bacterial translocation but may potentiate translocation due to other causes. Enteral fibre and minimal enteral nutrition appear to decrease translocation in the animal model. In humans the direct evidence is more convincing than the indirect evidence for the existence of bacterial translocation, but there is little information on the effect of different types of nutrition on bacterial translocation. It is often suggested that bacterial translocation is more likely to occur when there is mucosal atrophy or an increased permeability, however, both animal and human data suggest that intestinal mucosal atrophy and intestinal permeability are unrelated to bacterial translocation. Some TPN regimens may be associated with the development of intestinal mucosal atrophy but this does not necessarily imply that bacterial translocation is more likely to occur as a result.

Morbidity and mortality

Animal studies suggest that there is a survival benefit of enteral over parenteral feeding in well nourished and malnourished rodents subjected to different insults. Kudsk and colleagues randomised rats to receive dextrose-amino acids solutions via the enteral or parenteral route.[52,53] Peritonitis was induced after 12–14 days of feeding and survival was significantly higher in the enteral groups (malnourished and well-nourished). Petersen and co-workers also studied normal and protein-depleted rats and demonstrated that survival following peritonitis and subsequent enteral or parenteral refeeding was significantly worse in the parenteral group than in the enterally fed group (0–5% vs 53% respectively).[54] Zaloga et al evaluated survival in rats following haemorrhagic hypotension fed via the parenteral and enteral routes.[55] The 24-h mortality was significantly increased in animals receiving TPN (63%) compared to peptide-based enteral diets (0%). The same group also demonstrated that following high-dose methotrexate the mortality is greater in parenterally than enterally fed rats.[56]

Many prospective randomised controlled trials of enteral and parenteral nutrition have been performed in humans and these are considered below.

Trauma

Randomised controlled trials in trauma patients suggest that there may be some benefit of enteral over parenteral feeding with regard to infectious complications, although there is little consistency in the type of enteral feed used. Moore et al studied 59 postoperative patients with abdominal trauma, comparing jejunal Vivonex (Norwich Eaton Pharmaceuticals) with TPN.[57] This group demonstrated a significant benefit of enteral feeding on the development of major infections but this benefit was not significant for the total number of infected patients in either group (five enteral vs 11 parenteral). There was no significant difference in non-infectious complications. Mortality was not noted in either of these studies. Subsequently Moore et al published a meta-analysis using combined data from two published trials as well as data from six unpublished studies.[58] The fact that previously unpublished data was included in the analysis undermines the validity of this meta-analysis where 118 postoperative patients receiving jejunal Vivonex were compared with 112 postoperative patients receiving TPN. The case-mix of the patients included both trauma and non-trauma patients. Overall, there were fewer septic complications in the enteral group and subgroup analysis demonstrated that this benefit was only seen in trauma patients. There were no differences in the non-infectious complications, mortality, length of stay or cost. Kudsk et al compared jejunal Vital HN (Ross Laboratories) to TPN in patients with abdominal trauma.[59] The enterally fed group had significantly fewer infections per patient as well as significantly fewer infections per infected patient. Mortality and wound healing were not studied.

Two randomised controlled trials have not shown any benefit of enteral feeding in this patient population. Adams et al randomised 46 patients to receive either a jejunal feed (Isocal or Traumacal, Mead Johnson, UK) or TPN after surgery for trauma (mostly abdominal trauma but some orthopaedic and head injuries were included).[60] There was no difference in nutritional outcome or morbidity (nutrition-related complications, infectious complications, non-infectious complications and wound healing). Dunham et al studied jejunal Traumacal, TPN and the provision of both enteral and parenteral feeding in three small patient groups.[61] Jejunal tubes were endoscopically placed and, in ventilated patients, endoscopic jejunal feeding tube placement had a 36% failure rate. There were no differences in mortality between the different groups. Intolerance to jejunal feeding had 100% mortality, demonstrating the importance of nutrition as a whole in this patient group.

One important question relates to the parenteral nutrition given to the patients in the studies where a benefit was observed in enteral feeding. In general these were balanced feeds with no hyperalimentation, although the study by Moore et al provided 84% of calories from carbohydrate.[57]

Head injury

Following a head injury there is no evidence that enteral is more beneficial than parenteral nutrition, in fact there is more evidence to suggest that parenteral feeding is better. These studies are, however, complicated by the problem of severe gastric atony which results in a major difficulty in providing an equal calorie and nitrogen intake in both groups under study. The observed differences may simply be related to differences in nutrient intake.

Rapp and colleagues compared parenteral with standard enteral nutrition after head injury in 38 patients.[62] Parenterally fed patients had a more positive nitrogen balance, a higher serum albumin and total lymphocyte count and an improved outcome at both 18 days and 1 year. A follow on study on 51 patients again demonstrated increased calorie intake and nitrogen balance in the TPN group. Patient outcome was improved at 18 days and 3 months but there was no difference at 6 months and 1 year.[63] A study by Suchner and investigators demonstrated an improved Glasgow Coma Score in patients on TPN after the first week, compared to enterally fed patients.[64] Two other studies have not shown any difference in the feeding route.[65,66]

Elective surgery

Preoperative nutrition support

Two randomised controlled trials have not shown any benefit of enteral feeding. Lim et al randomised 24 patients to receive TPN or gastrostomy feeding with a blended diet for 3–4 weeks.[67] The TPN group attained earlier positive nitrogen balance and more weight gain. Two episodes of catheter sepsis and one subclavian thrombosis occurred in the TPN group. There were no differences in postoperative wound infections, non-infective complications or mortality, although the study size is too small to show any differences between the groups for these variables. Von Meyenfeldt et al studied at least 10 days of pre-operative nutrition support.[68] They demonstrated no differences between enteral or parenteral nutrition with respect to septic complications, non-septic complications, nutrition support-related complications, length of stay or mortality.

Postoperative care

Two small studies from the same group looked at the effect of enteral versus parenteral nutrition after abdominal surgery.[69,70] Muggia-Sallam et al showed that both enteral and parenteral nutrition maintained a positive nitrogen balance and maintained the serum albumin and other synthesised proteins, but outcome was not recorded. The study by Bower et al demonstrated that although the serum albumin fell significantly more in the TPN group, there was no difference in wound healing and they concluded that the two routes were therapeutically equal. Larger studies have also been performed following abdominal surgery. Baigrie et al studied 97 oesophagogastrectomy patients,

randomised to receive either jejunal Osmolite (Abbott, UK) or TPN.[71] Mortality was not significantly different between the groups but the TPN group had more life-threatening complications than the enteral group (15 vs nine). Reynolds et al looked at the effects of jejunal Osmolite and TPN in postoperative patients with gastrointestinal cancer.[15] There were no differences in infectious complications, non-infectious complications, nutrition support-related complications or mortality. Following liver transplantation, there are no differences in nutritional outcome, nutrition support-related complications, infectious morbidity, non-infectious complications or mortality.[16] Following hepatic resection for liver cancer, no difference in mortality between a branched-chain amino acid-enriched enteral and parenteral feed has been demonstrated.[72] Following head and neck surgery, two randomised controlled trials have been performed comparing enteral with parenteral feeding. The first achieved a better nitrogen balance in the TPN group, but there were no significant differences in infective complications, nutrition support complications or mortality. The second did not find any differences in nutritional outcome or wound infections.[73,74]

Studies using augmented enteral feeds have found some benefit in morbidity postoperatively. The effect of a feed enriched with arginine, RNA and ω–3-fatty acids (Impact, Novartis, UK) was compared with a standard (unspecified) feed and TPN.[75] No differences were seen between the standard feed and TPN with respect to nutritional proteins, infections or mortality. The augmented feed affected markers of the inflammatory response and immune system but did not affect infection rates, although infections were less severe in the augmented group. A follow-up study by the same group on 166 patients with the same study design demonstrated a benefit of Impact over standard enteral nutrition and parenteral nutrition in patients undergoing major abdominal surgery. Further benefits were seen in previously malnourished patients.[76]

Thus in postoperative care there do not appear to be any consistent differences in outcome parameters when comparing a standard enteral or parenteral feed, but augmented feed may be promising in this area.

Critical illness

The crucial question to be adhered in the critically ill patient is not whether enteral or parenteral nutrition should be used, but whether there is any evidence that any nutrition is beneficial to this patient group. A systematic review by Heyland in 1998 revealed 27 prospective randomised controlled trials assessing supplemental parenteral nutrition in the critically ill.[77] Unfortunately this meta-analysis included studies comparing enteral with supplemental TPN versus enteral feeding as well as TPN versus no feeding. Amalgamating all this data demonstrated no effect of TPN on mortality. However, there seemed to be a trend toward a favourable effect on major complications. TPN seemed to reduce the complication rates in malnourished patients and lipid-free TPN was associated with a further reduction in complication rates. However, the trials analysed did have significant heterogeneity. When only the studies with higher quality scores were assessed, there was a trend for mortality and morbidity to be higher in TPN patients. TPN reduction in mortality was only seen in the lower quality trials. Similarly the beneficial effect on morbidity was restricted to the trials published before 1989. In the later trials, the morbidity tended to be higher in the TPN patients. Finally, in trials in non-surgical patients, mortality was significantly worse in TPN recipients, although most of these data are biased by a study in burn patients in which the patients received more calories than were needed.

A study not included in the meta-analysis by Heyland assessed surgical patients on the ICU given TPN or a standard enteral feed. No differences were found in the incidence of multiple organ failure, sepsis or mortality rate between the two groups. The type of formula given had an effect on the nutritional outcome. A formula with a non-protein calorie/nitrogen ratio of 100:1 was associated with more nitrogen retention, higher levels of visceral proteins and better gut tolerance. As expected, however, there was an increased incidence of diarrhoea in the enterally fed group.[78]

These studies have been comparing standard parenteral and enteral nutrition. Another area of interest relates to the provision of augmented feeds to modulate the inflammatory response in some way for the critically ill patient. It is suggested that the inflammatory response is responsible for the sepsis syndrome and multiple organ failure in these patients. Griffiths et al performed a double blind study on 84 critically ill patients in a single centre.[79] They compared a glutamine-containing TPN with an isonitrogenous, isocaloric equivalent and demonstrated significantly improved survival at 6 months in those receiving parenteral glutamine. Heys et al recently assessed the effects of augmented enteral feeds over standard enteral feeds in critically illness.[80] They demonstrated

that the use of a specialised enteral diet (with combinations of glutamine, arginine, ribonucleic acid and n-3 fatty acids) was associated with a reduction in infectious mortality (odds ratio 0.47). The overall odds ratio for mortality was 1.77 and the investigators state that the use of supplemented nutrition support was not associated with a significant decrease in the risk of death. Eight of the trials reported data regarding duration of hospitalisation and, when aggregated, the specialised nutrition recipients had a reduction in overall length of stay 2.5 days.

Overall, nutrition in the critically ill patient remains an open question and further good studies are warranted in this difficult area. We still need to ask whether there is a definite benefit from any nutrition.

Other conditions

Other studies cover acute pancreatitis, inflammatory bowel disease and bone marrow transplantation. Recent studies in acute pancreatitis favour post-pyloric enteral feeding.[81,82] With regard to inflammatory bowel disease, enteral and parenteral feeding appears equally efficacious.[83,84]

In conclusion, it would appear that it cannot be generally stated that enteral is the best form of nutrition support as it clearly depends upon the patient's diagnosis and situation. Differences are seen between animal and clinical studies and good randomised controlled trials are still required in this area. It is still reasonable to question whether any form of nutrition is appropriate in the early stages of critical illness. In some situations TPN may have some benefit over enteral nutrition, possibly as a result of reliable delivery of nutrients. Where there is insufficient evidence that parenteral nutrition is better, it is reasonable to choose enteral feeding because of cost but it should be borne in mind that tube feeding has recognised complications. Nevertheless significant advances have been made in the understanding and formulation of both enteral and parenteral nutrition over recent years and this field is constantly changing. This area is becoming more complicated with the development of immunonutrition and the use of minimal enteral feeding while using TPN.

References

1. Levine GM, Deren JJ, Steiger E, Zinno R. Role of oral intake in maintenance of gut mass and disaccharide activity. *Gastroenterology* 1974; **67**: 975–982.

2. Buchman AL, Moukarzel AA, Bhuta S *et al*. Parenteral nutrition is associated with intestinal morphologic and functional changes in humans. *J Parenter Enteral Nutr* 1995; **19**: 453–460.

3. Shaw-Smith CJ, Waters JR. Regional expression of intestinal genes for nutrient absorption. *Gut* 1997; **40**: 5–8.

4. Soubeyran P, Andre F, Lissitzky J-C *et al*. Cdx1 promotes differentiation in a rat intestinal epithelial cell line. *Gastroenterology* 1999; **117**: 1326–1338.

5. Fernandez-Lopez JA, Casado J, Argiles JM, Alemany M. Intestinal handling of a glucose gavage by the rat. *Mol Cell Biochem* 1992; **113**: 43–53.

6. Bouteloup-Demange C, Boirie Y, Dechelotte P, Gachon P, Beaufrere B. Gut mucosal protein synthesis in fed and fasted humans. *Am J Physiol* 1998; **274**: E541–E546.

7. Li J, Kudsk KA, Gocinski B, Dent D, Glezer J, Langkamp Henken B. Effects of parenteral and enteral nutrition on gut-associated lymphoid tissue. *J Trauma* 1995; **39**: 44–51.

8. Sitren HS, Bryant M, Ellis LM. Species differences in TPN-induced intestinal villus atrophy. *J Parenter Enteral Nutr* 1992; **16**: 30S.

9. Guedon C, Schmitz J, Lerebours E *et al*. Decreased brush border hydrolase activities without gross morphologic changes in human intestinal mucosa after prolonged total parenteral nutrition of adults. *Gastroenterology* 1986; **90**: 373–378.

10. Inoue Y, Espat NJ, Frohnapple DJ, Epstein H, Copeland EM, Souba WW. Effect of total parenteral nutrition on amino acid and glucose transport by the human small intestine. *Ann Surg* 1993; **217**: 604–612.

11. Rossi TM, Lee PC, Young C, Tjota A. Small intestinal mucosa changes, including epithelial cell proliferative activity, of children receiving total parenteral nutrition (TPN). *Dig Dis Sci* 1993; **38**: 1608–1613.

12. Sedman PC, MacFie J, Palmer MD, Mitchell CJ, Sagar PM. Preoperative total parenteral nutrition is not associated with mucosal atrophy or bacterial translocation in humans. *Br J Surg* 1995; **82**: 1663–1667.

13. Cummins A, Chu G, Faust L *et al*. Malabsorption and villous atrophy in patients receiving enteral feeding. *J Parenter Enteral Nutr* 1995; **19**: 193–198.

14. Hoensch HP, Steinhardt HJ, Weiss G, Haug D, Maier A, Malchow H. Effects of semisynthetic diets on xeno-biotic metabolizing enzyme activity and morphology of small intestinal mucosa in humans. *Gastroenterology* 1994; **86**: 1519–1530.

15. Reynolds JV, Kanwar S, Welsh FK *et al*. Does the route of feeding modify gut barrier function and clinical outcome in patients after major upper gastro-intestinal surgery? *J Parenter Enteral Nutr* 1997; **21**: 196–201.

16. Wicks C, Somasundaram S, Bjarnason I *et al*. Comparison of enteral feeding and total parenteral nutrition after liver transplantation. *Lancet* 1994; **344**: 837–840.

17. Hadfield RJ, Sinclair DG, Houldsworth PE, Evans TW. Effects of enteral and parenteral nutrition on gut mucosal permeability in the critically ill. *Am J Respir Crit Care Med* 1995; **152**: 1545–1548.

18. Lipman TO. Bacterial translocation and enteral nutrition in humans: an outsider looks in [Review]. *J Parenter Enteral Nutr* 1995; **19**: 156–165.

19. Fraenkel A. Ueber peritoneale infektion. *Wein Klin Wochenschr* 1895; **4**: 265–85.

20. Berg RD, Garlington AW. Translocation of certain indigenous bacteria from the gastrointestinal tract to the mesenteric lymph nodes and other organs in a gnotobiotic mouse model. *Infect Immunol* 1979; **23**: 403–411.

21. Alexander JW, Boyce ST, Babcock GF *et al*. The process of microbial translocation. *Ann Surg* 1990; **212**: 496–510.

22. Deitch EA, Berg R. Endotoxin but not malnutrition promotes bacterial translocation of the gut flora in burned mice. *J Trauma* 1987; **27**: 161–166.

23. Deitch EA, Winterton J, Li M, Berg R. The gut as a portal of entry for bacteremia. Role of protein mal-nutrition. *Ann Surg* 1987; **205**: 681–692.

24. Shou J, Lappin J, Minnard EA, Daly JM. Total parenteral nutrition, bacterial translocation, and host immune function. *Am J Surg* 1994; **167**: 145–150.

25. Kueppers PM, Miller TA, Chen CY, Smith GS, Rodriguez LF, Moody FG. Effect of total parenteral nutrition plus morphine on bacterial translocation in rats. *Ann Surg* 1993; **217**: 286–292.

26. Helton WS, Garcia R. Oral prostaglandin E$_2$ prevents gut atrophy during intravenous feeding but not bacterial translocation. *Arch Surg* 1993; **128**: 178–183.

27. Spaeth G, Berg RD, Specian RD, Deitch EA. Food without fiber promotes bacterial translocation from the gut. *Surgery* 1990; **108**: 240–246.

28. Alverdy JC, Aoys E, Moss GS. Total parenteral nutrition promotes bacterial translocation from the gut. *Surgery* 1988; **104**: 185–190.

29. Spaeth G, Gottwald T, Haas W, Holmer M. Glutamine peptide does not improve gut barrier function and mucosal immunity in total parenteral nutrition. *J Parenter Enteral Nutr* 1993; **17**: 317–323.

30. Illig KA, Ryan CK, Hardy DJ, Rhodes J, Locke W, Sax HC. Total parenteral nutrition-induced changes in gut mucosal function: atrophy alone is not the issue. *Surgery* 1992; **112:** 631–637.

31. Deitch EA. Simple intestinal obstruction causes bacterial translocation in man. *Arch Surg* 1989; **124:** 699–701.

32. Sedman PC, MacFie J, Sagar P *et al.* The prevalence of gut translocation in humans. *Gastroenterology* 1994; **107:** 643–649.

33. O'Boyle CJ, MacFie J, Mitchell CJ, Johnstone D, Sagar PM, Sedman PC. Microbiology of bacterial translocation in humans. *Gut* 1998; **42:** 29–35.

34. Brooks SG, May J, Sedman P *et al.* Translocation of enteric bacteria in humans. *Br J Surg* 1993; **80:** 901–902.

35. Reed LL, Martin M, Manglano R, Newson B, Kocka F, Barrett J. Bacterial translocation following abdominal trauma in humans. *Circ Shock* 1994; **42:** 1–6.

36. Brathwaite CE, Ross SE, Nagele R, Mure AJ, O'Malley KF, Garcia-Perez FA. Bacterial translocation occurs in humans after traumatic injury: evidence using immunofluorescence. *J Trauma* 1993; **34:** 586–590.

37. Ziegler TR, Smith RJ, O'Dwyer ST, Demling RH, Wilmore DW. Increased intestinal permeability associated with infection in burn patients. *Arch Surg* 1988; **123:** 1313–1319.

38. Shippee RL, Johnson AA, Cioffi WG, Lasko J, LeVoyer TE, Jordan BS. Simultaneous determination of lactulose and mannitol in urine of burn patients by gas-liquid chromatography. *Clin Chem* 1992; **38:** 343–345.

39. LeVoyer T, Cioffi WG Jr, Pratt L *et al.* Alterations in intestinal permeability after thermal injury. *Arch Surg* 1992; **127:** 26–29.

40. Roumen RM, Hendriks T, Wevers RA, Goris JA. Intestinal permeability after severe trauma and hemorrhagic shock is increased without relation to septic complications. *Arch Surg* 1993; **128:** 453–457.

41. Pape HC, Dwenger A, Regel G *et al.* Increased gut permeability after multiple trauma. *Br J Surg* 1994; **81:** 850–852.

42. Langkamp-Henken B, Donovan TB, Pate LM, Maull CD, Kudsk KA. Increased intestinal permeability following blunt and penetrating trauma. *Crit Care Med* 1995; **23:** 660–664.

43. Ohri SK, Somasundaram S, Koak Y *et al.* The effect of intestinal hypoperfusion on intestinal absorption and permeability during cardiopulmonary bypass. *Gastroenterology* 1994; **106:** 318–323.

44. Riddington DW, Venkatesh B, Boivin CM *et al.* Intestinal permeability, gastric intramucosal pH, and systemic endotoxemia in patients undergoing cardiopulmonary bypass. *JAMA* 1996; **275:** 1007–1012.

45. Harris CE, Griffiths RD, Freestone N, Billington D, Atherton ST, Macmillan RR. Intestinal permeability in the critically ill. *Intensive Care Med* 1992; **18:** 38–41.

46. Tremel H, Kienle B, Sacha Weilemann L, Stehle P, Furst P. Gluamine dipeptide-supplemented parenteral nutrition maintains intestinal function in the critically ill. *Gastroenterology* 1994; **107:** 1595–1601.

47. O'Boyle CJ, MacFie J, Dave K, Sagar PS, Poon P, Mitchell CJ. Alterations in intestinal barrier function do not predispose to translocation of enteric bacteria in gastroenterologic patients. *Nutrition* 1998; **14:** 358–362.

48. Kerver AJ, Rommes JH, Mevissen-Verhage EA *et al.* Prevention of colonization and infection in critically ill patients: a prospective randomized study. *Crit Care Med* 1988; **16:** 1087–1093.

49. Cerra FB, Maddaus MA, Dunn DL *et al.* Selective gut decontamination reduces nosocomial infections and length of stay but not mortality or organ failure in surgical intensive care unit patients. *Arch Surg* 1992; **127:** 163–167.

50. Fiddian-Green RG, Baker S. Nosocomial pneumonia in the critically ill: product of aspiration or translocation? *Crit Care Med* 1991; **19:** 763–769.

51. Lingnau W, Berger J, Javorsky F, Lejeune P, Mutz N, Benzer H. Selective intestinal decontamination in multiple trauma patients: prospective, controlled trial [see comments]. *J Trauma* 1997; **42:** 687–694.

52. Kudsk KA, Stone JM, Carpenter G, Sheldon GF. Enteral and parenteral feeding influences mortality after hemoglobin–E. coli peritonitis in normal rats. *J Trauma* 1983; **23:** 605–609.

53. Kudsk KA, Carpenter G, Petersen S, Sheldon GF. Effect of enteral and parenteral feeding in malnourished rats with E. coli–hemoglobin adjuvant peritonitis. *J Surg Res* 1981; **31:** 105–110.

54. Petersen SR, Kudsk KA, Carpenter G, Sheldon GE. Malnutrition and immunocompetence: increased mortality following an infectious challenge during hyperalimentation. *J Trauma* 1981; **21:** 528–533.

55. Zaloga GP, Knowles R, Black KW, Prielipp R. Total parenteral nutrition increases mortality after hemorrhage [see comments]. *Crit Care Med* 1991; **19:** 54–59.

56. Zaloga GP, Roberts P, Black KW, Prielipp R. Gut bacterial translocation/dissemination explains the increased mortality produced by parenteral nutrition following methotrexate. *Circ Shock* 1993; **39:** 263–268.

57. Moore FA, Moore EE, Jones TN, McCroskey BL, Petersen VM. TEN versus TPN following major abdominal trauma-reduced septic morbidity. *J Trauma* 1989; **29**: 916–923.

58. Moore FA, Feliciano DV, Andrassy RJ *et al*. Early enteral feeding, compared with parenteral, reduces postoperative septic complications. The results of a meta-analysis. *Ann Surg* 1992; **216**: 172–183.

59. Kudsk KA, Croce MA, Fabian TC *et al*. Enteral versus parenteral feeding. Effects on septic morbidity after blunt and penetrating abdominal trauma. *Ann Surg* 1992; **215**: 503–513.

60. Adams S, Dellinger EP, Wertz MJ, Orekovich MR, Simmonowicz D, Johansen K. Enteral versus parenteral nutritional support following laparotomy for trauma: a randomised prospective trial. *J Trauma* 1986; **26**: 882–890.

61. Dunham CM, Frankenfield MS, Belzberg H, Wiles C, Cushing B, Grant Z. Gut failure: predictor of or contributor to mortality in mechanically ventilated blunt trauma patients? *J Trauma* 1994; **37**: 30–34.

62. Rapp RP, Young B, Twyman D *et al*. The favorable effect of early parenteral feeding on survival in head-injured patients. *J Neurosurg* 1983; **58**: 906–912.

63. Young B, Ott L, Twyman D *et al*. The effect of nutritional support on outcome from severe head injury. *J Neurosurg* 1987; **67**: 668–676.

64. Suchner U, Senftleben U, Eckart T *et al*. Enteral versus parenteral nutrition: effects on gastrointestinal function and metabolism. *Nutrition* 1996; **12**: 13–22.

65. Hadley MN, Grahm TW, Harrington T, Schiller WR, McDermott MK, Posillico DB. Nutritional support and neurotrauma: a critical review of early nutrition in forty-five acute head injury patients. *Neurosurgery* 1986; **19**: 367–373.

66. Borzotta AP, Pennings J, Papasadero B, Paxton J, Mardesic S, Borzotta R. Enteral versus parenteral nutrition after severe closed head injury. *J Trauma* 1994; **37**: 459–468.

67. Lim ST, Choa RG, Lam KH, Wong J, Ong GB. Total parenteral nutrition versus gastrostomy in the pre-operative preparation of patients with carcinoma of the oesophagus. *Br J Surg* 1981; **68**: 69–72.

68. von Meyenfeldt MF, Meijerink WJHJ, Rouflart MMJ, Buil-Massen MTHJ, Soeters PB. Perioperative nutritional support: a randomised clinical trial. *Clin Nutr* 1992; **11**: 180–186.

69. Muggia-Sullam M, Bower RH, Murphy RF, Joffe SN, Fischer JE. Postoperative enteral versus parenteral nutritional support in gastrointestinal surgery. A matched prospective study. *Am J Surg* 1985; **149**: 106–112.

70. Bower RH, Talamini MA, Sax HC, Hamilton F, Fischer JE. Postoperative enteral vs parenteral nutrition. A randomized controlled trial. *Arch Surg* 1986; **121**: 1040–1045.

71. Baigrie RJ, Devitt PG, Watkin DS. Enteral versus parenteral nutrition after oesophagogastric surgery: a prospective randomized comparison. *Aust NZ J Surg* 1996; **66**: 668–670.

72. Shirabe K, Matsumata T, Shimada M *et al*. A comparison of parenteral hyperalimentation and early enteral feeding regarding systemic immunity after major hepatic resection: the results of a randomized prospective study. *Hepato-Gastroenterology* 1997; **44**: 205–209.

73. Sako K, Lore JM, Kaufman S, Razack MS, Bakamjian V, Reese P. Parenteral hyperalimentation in surgical patients with head and neck cancer: a randomized study. *J Surg Oncol* 1991; **16**: 391–402.

74. Iovinelli G, Marsili I, Varrassi G. Nutrition support after total laryngectomy. *J Parenter Enteral Nutr* 1993; **17**: 445–448.

75. Braga M, Vignali A, Gianotti L, Cestari A, Profili M, Carlo VD. Immune and nutritional effects of early enteral nutrition after major abdominal operations. *Euro J Surg* 1996; **162**: 105-112.

76. Braga M, Gianotti L, Vignali A, Cestari A, Bisagni P, Di Carlo V. Artificial nutrition after major abdominal surgery: impact of route of administration and composition of the diet [see comments]. *Crit Care Med* 1998; **26**: 24–30.

77. Heyland DK, MacDonald S, Keefe L, Drover JW. Total parenteral nutrition in the critically ill patient: a meta-analysis. *JAMA* 1998; **280**: 2013–2019.

78. Cerra FB, McPherson JP, Konstantinides FN, Konstantinides KM, Teasley KM. Enteral nutrition does not prevent multiple organ failure syndrome (MOFS) after sepsis. *Surgery* 1988; **104**: 727–733.

79. Griffiths RD, Jones C, Palmer TE. Six-month outcome of critically ill patients given glutamine-supplemented parenteral nutrition [see comments]. *Nutrition* 1997; **13**: 295–302.

80. Heys SD, Walker LG, Smith I, Eremin O. Enteral nutritional supplementation with key nutrients in patients with critical illness and cancer: a meta-analysis of randomized controlled clinical trials. *Ann Surg* 1999; **229**: 467–77.

81. Windsor AC, Kanwar S, Li AG *et al*. Compared with parenteral nutrition, enteral feeding attenuates the acute phase response and improves disease severity in acute pancreatitis [see comments]. *Gut* 1998; **42**: 431–435.

82. McClave SA, Snider H, Owens N, Sexton LK. Clinical nutrition in pancreatitis [Review]. *Dig Dis Sci* 1997; **42:** 2035–2044.

83. Greenberg GR, Fleming CR, Jeejeebhoy KN, Rosenberg IH, Sales D, Tremaine WJ. Controlled trial of bowel rest and nutritional support in the management of Crohn's disease. *Gut* 1988; **29:** 1309–1315.

84. Gonzalez-Huix F, Fernandez-Banares F, Esteve-Comas M *et al.* Enteral versus parenteral nutrition as adjunct therapy in acute ulcerative colitis. *Am J Gastroenterol* 1993; **88:** 227–232.

85. Hindmarsh JT, Clark RG. The effects of intravenous and intraduodenal feeding on nitrogen balance after surgery. *Br J Surg* 1973; **60:** 589–594.

86. Rowlands BJ, Giddings AE, Johnston AO, Hindmarsh JT, Clark RG. Nitrogen-sparing effect of different feeding regimes in patients after operation. *Br J Anaesth* 1977; **49:** 781–787.

87. McArdle AH, Palmason C, Morency I, Brown RA. A rationale for enteral feeding as the preferable route for hyperalimentation. *Surgery* 1981; **90:** 616–623.

88. Bennegard K, Lindmark L, Wickstrom I, Schersten T, Lundholm K. A comparative study of the efficiency of intragastric and parenteral nutrition in man. *Am J Clin Nut* 1984; **40:** 752–757.

89. Fletcher JP, Little JM. A comparison of parenteral nutrition and early postoperative enteral feeding on the nitrogen balance after major surgery. *Surgery* 1986; **100:** 21–24.

90. Young B, Ott L, Twyman D *et al.* The effect of nutritional support on outcome from severe head injury. *J Neurosurg* 1987; **67:** 668–676.

91. Kudsk KA, Minard G, Wojtysiak SL, Croce M, Fabian T, Brown RO. Visceral protein response to enteral versus parenteral nutrition and sepsis in patients with trauma. *Surgery* 1994; **116:** 516–523.

92. Georgiannos SN, Renaut AJ, Goode AW. Short-term restorative nutrition in malnourished patients: pro's and con's of intravenous and enteral alimentation using compositionally matched nutrients. *Int Surg* 1997; **82:** 301–306.

93. Burt ME, Gorschboth CM, Brennan MF. A controlled, prospective, randomized trial evaluating the metabolic effects of enteral and parenteral nutrition in the cancer patient. *Cancer* 1982; **49:** 1092–1105.

94. Burt ME, Stein TP, Brennan MF. A controlled, randomized trial evaluating the effects of enteral and parenteral nutrition on protein metabolism in cancer-bearing man. *J Surg Res* 1983; **34:** 303–314.

95. O'Keefe SJ, Ogden J, Dicker J. Enteral and parenteral branched chain amino acid-supplemented nutritional support in patients with encephalopathy due to alcoholic liver disease. *J Parenter Enteral Nutr* 1987; **11:** 447–453.

96. Peterson VM, Moore EE, Jones TN *et al.* Total enteral nutrition versus total parenteral nutrition after major torso injury: attenuation of hepatic protein reprioritization. *Surgery* 1988; **104:** 199–207.

97. Hadfield RJ, Sinclair DG, Houldsworth PE, Evans TW. Effects of enteral and parenteral nutrition on gut mucosal permeability in the critically ill. *Am J Respir Crit Care Med* 1995; **152:** 1–8.

98. Pearlstone DB, Lee JI, Alexander RH, Chang TH, Brennan MF, Burt M. Effect of enteral and parenteral nutrition on amino acid levels in cancer patients. *J Parenter Enteral Nutr* 1995; **19:** 204–208.

99. Fish J, Sporay G, Beyer K *et al.* A prospective randomized study of glutamine-enriched parenteral compared with enteral feeding in postoperative patients. *Am J Clin Nutr* 1997; **65:** 977–983.

100. Gianotti L, Braga M, Vignali A *et al.* Effect of route of delivery and formulation of postoperative nutritional support in patients undergoing major operations for malignant neoplasms. *Arch Surg* 1997; **132:** 1222–1229.

101. Kotler DP, Fogleman L, Tierney AR. Comparison of total parenteral nutrition and an oral, semielemental diet on body composition, physical function, and nutrition-related costs in patients with malabsorption due to acquired immunodeficiency syndrome. *J Parenter Enteral Nutr* 1998; **22:** 120–126.

Index

Note: page numbers in bold refer to tables

abdominal distension
  EN-related 339
    incidence rates 337
  enteral feeding contraindication
      296
abetalipoproteinaemia, predigested
    elemental diet 311
abscesses, intra-abdominal wall, PEG
    complications 290
acetoacetate (AcAc)
  hepatic synthesis 83
  and 3-hydroxybutyrate (beta-
    OHB) **11–13**
acetylcoenzyme A (CoA)
  AcCoA/CoA ratio 3, 10
  hepatic synthesis 84
acridine orange leucocyte cytospin
    test, catheter-related sepsis
    diagnosis 387
acrodermatitis enteropathica, zinc
    deficiency 140
actinomycin D
  chemotherapy combination 653
  mucositis 652
  recall reaction 653
acute phase proteins
  C-reactive protein 18–19
  in injury and sepsis, positive and
    negative phase **18**, 19–20
  serum albumin, zinc and iron **206**
  smoking 101
adipose tissue
  brown/white, MR **66**
  elderly people 688
adrenaline
  infusion, overnight fasted vs 48 h
    starvation **67**
  injury and sepsis 71–2
  thermogenesis 67–8
adriamycin
  mucositis 652
  radiotherapy combination 653
  recall reaction 653
aerobic/anaerobic metabolism 68–9

ageing
  muscle protein turnover 48–9
  physiological changes 683
  population trends 683
  vitamin B12 deficiency 109
  see also elderly patients
AIDS see HIV infection and AIDS
airway abnormalities, FBT placement
    285
airway obstruction, feeding tubes 336
alanine 17–18
  metabolism, inhibition by xylitol
    423–4
albumin
  changes, acute phase response
    18–19, **206**
  hepatic synthesis 85
  hypoalbuminaemia, enteral feeding
    intolerance 338
  as marker of ECW changes 173
  monitoring, EN 296
  negative acute phase response
    19–20
  protein–energy malnutrition 222
  in starvation, short term **20**
  and visceral proteins, assessment
    169–70
alcohol, catheter occlusion clearance
    388
alcohol misuse
  fatty acids 86
  hypoglycaemia 86
  lipase inhibition 87
  lipid metabolism 86–7
  malnutrition 86
  megaloblastic anaemia 87
  thiamine deficiency 109
  vitamin deficiencies 686
  see also hepatic disease
algorithms, hyperalimentation,
    pancreatitis **728**
alkalosis, hepatic encephalopathy 89
allergic disease, and n-6 PUFAs
    99–100

alpha-2-macroglobulin, and protein
    101–2
^{13}C-alpha-ketoisocaproate labelling,
    protein turnover
    measurement 44–5
aluminium 474
  HPN solutions 493
amino acids
  analysis 29–31
    intracellular measurements 30
    intramuscular measurements 31
    radioactive and stable-isotope
      tracers 29–30
    snapshots of metabolism 30–1
  arteriovenous (A-V) differences 32
  branched chain (BCAA) 83, 517
    cancer therapy 666
    hepatic encephalopathy enteral
      diets 89, 320–1
    hepatic regeneration 90
    plasma concentrations, hepatic
      disease 88
  cancer cachexia 647
  in catabolic response to injury
    17–18
  catabolism 43, 84–5
  conditionally essential 41
    protein turnover modification
      46
  cytokine biology 101–2
  depletion, injury and sepsis 516–17
  determination of body composition
    28–9
  dispensable/non-dispensable,
    classification 40–1
  essential, requirements **183**
  feeding effects 28
  formula for infants 356
  free pool
    composition 38
    membrane transport 37–9
    protein balance 39
    size regulation 39
  gluconeogenesis 83

amino acids – *continued*
  homeostasis, glutamine 408, 416
  hormonal stimulation 85
  hypercalcaemia, PN 453–4
  imbalance, anorexia 643
  immune function 139–41
  infants, blood composition 472
  intermediary metabolism 84–5
    abnormalities 88–9
    Krebs cycle activity 41
    protein turnover relationship
      39–41
    schema 40
    urea excretion 84
  limbs, splanchnic bed and blood
    exchange 32
  muscle fluxes, feeding/starvation
    effects 32–3
  N-acetylated 417–18
  as oral supplements, palatability
    272
  precursor labelling 35–7
    flooding dose method 36–7
  recommended intakes 42–3
  source, lipid emulsion stability
    438
  'tertiary amino acid transport' 39
  tissue-specific metabolism 42–3
  tracers
    dilution technique 33–4
    flooding dose method 36–7
    GC–MS assessment 35
    protein incorporation 34–5
      constant infusion method 34,
      44
    protein turnover information
      32–3
    tracer/tracee free pool
      relationship 36
  transporter proteins
    characteristics 38
    identification and isolation 38
  transporter systems, regulatory role
    39
  venous pattern 43
  venous transport 39
  see also named amino acids; proteins
aminoacyl-tRNA labelling 34–5
ammoniagenesis, glutamine substrate
  322
anabolic agents, amino acid transport
  defect reversal 158
anabolic steroids, protein turnover
  effects 48
anaemia *see* megaloblastic anaemia
anaerobic metabolism 68–9
anorectic peptides, food intake,
  appetite control 236

anorexia 102, 236–7
  of ageing 689
  amino acid imbalance 643
  cancer cachexia 642–3, 651–3
  cytokines 102, 228
  learned food aversion 643, 651
anthropometry, paediatric nutrition
  assessment 221–2
antibiotics
  catheter infections 476
  coated catheters 383
  diarrhoea association 124
  intrahepatic cholestasis 491
  prophylactic, PEG 290, 693
anticachectics 665–7
anticoagulants, CVT 490
antidiarrhoeal drugs 338, 712
antioxidants
  catabolic patients 159
  examples 100
  modulation of cytokines 100–1
antiretroviral agents
  dietary recommendations **627**
  HIV infection 619
antisecretory drugs, jejunostomy
  711–12
apoptosis, taurine modulation 407
appetite control 225–39
  body weight stability 228–9
  and disease, immune response 95
  dysregulation, elderly people
    683–4, 687
  hypothalamic control of energy
    balance **227**, 232–3
  leptin 230 2
  long-term regulation of body
    weight 229–32
    lipostat theory 230
    ob protein and *ob* receptor in
      mice 230
  peptides and neurotransmitters
    increasing food intake
    233–4
    galanin 234
    melanin-concentrating hormone
      234
    neuropeptide Y 233–4
    other peptides 234
  peptides and neurotransmitters
    reducing food intake 233–4
    corticotrophin-releasing factor
      235
    melanocyte-stimulating
      hormone 235
    other anorectic peptides 236
    serotonin 235
  short-term regulation 236
  see also anorexia

arginine 599
  immune response modulation 322
  insulin stimulation 125
  intestine utilisation 125
  lysine deprivation 406
  properties 139
  protein nutrition substrate 405–6
  surgical patients 611
  tumour protein synthesis increase
    46
  uptake in cystinuria 114
arteriovenous catheterization, burn
  injury 17
ascites
  complications of liver disease 506
  FPG 291
ascorbic acid *see* vitamin C
aspiration, enteral nutrition risks
  338–9, 373–4, 547
  and neurologic deficit 338
  prophylaxis 339
  recumbency 286
aspiration pneumonia 295, 338
assessment of nutrition 165–76
  aims 167–8
  elderly people 690–1
  history 167
  methods 168–73
    albumin and visceral proteins
      169–70
    body fat 169
    body water compartment
      volume 171–3
    hand grip strength **170**
    muscle protein 170–1
    prognostic indices 173–4
    whole-body 168–9
  proposal for parameters **174**
ATP, short term starvation 3
atrophic gastritis, elderly people 685–6
audit *see* hospital audit
aversive feeding behaviours (AFB),
  elderly people 691
azotaemia 453

bacterial translocation
  GI epithelium
    animal studies 765
    human studies 765–7
  multi-organ failure 610
  post-operative sepsis 766
basal metabolic rate (BMR) 3, **9–10**
  elderly people 684
  injury and sepsis 13–15
  and RMR 260
  see also resting energy expenditure
    (REE); total available
    energy (TEE)

beta blockers 72
bicarbonate–urea method,
          measurement of MR 65,
          65
bile, and vitamin absorption 85
bile acids
    cholesterol 84
    synthetic 714
biliary dysfunction, HPN 491–3
biliary obstruction, predigested
          elemental diet 311
biliary sludge and stones, HPN
          related 491–2
bioelectric impedance analysis (BIA)
          172, 505
biotin, RDA/effects 202–3
bleomycin
    mucositis 652
    radiotherapy combination 653
blood culture, catheter-related sepsis
          diagnosis 387
BMI *see* body mass index
body cell mass, cancer patients, TPN
          and EN effects 654–5
body composition
    determination 28–9
    DEXA 505
    fuel availability and survival time,
          lean vs obese **6**
    pre/post resuscitation, PEM **594**
body fat
    assessment 169
    BMR, protein oxidation,
          prolonged starvation **9**
    brown/white adipose tissue **66**
    metabolism, TNF-alpha and IL-1
          649
    oxidation/turnover
        activity and energy cost, burn
          injury **16**, 72
        modulation of cytokines 98–100
        oxygen consumption and RQ
          68
        sepsis, low and high REE, with
          i.v. glucose **74**
        synthesis 69
        standardizations of MR
          measurements and values,
          predictive equations, resting
          MR, same height, different
          BMI **66**
    see also lipids
body impedance analysis (BIA) 172,
          505
body mass index (BMI)
    ageing 683
    BMR, protein oxidation,
          prolonged starvation **9**

fat free mass (FFM), and MR 65
influence of disease, REE 181
metabolism/metabolic rate,
          predictive equations **66**
nutrition category definition 151
standardizations of MR
          measurements, resting MR
          66
body surface area (BSA), nomogram
          580
body water compartment volume
    albumin as marker of ECW
          changes 173
    assessment 171–3
    body impedance analysis 172
    clinical examination 172
    dilution techniques 172
    extracellular water volume 171
body weight stability 228–9
    AIDS 228
    cancer 229
    chronic inflammatory conditons
          228
    gain/loss prognosis 169
    leptin 229–32
    long-term 229–32
    see also anorexia; appetite control;
          obesity
bombesin, appetite control 236
bone disease
    HPN related 492–3
    inappropriate nutrients in PN
          454–5
    osteomalacia, vitamin D-induced,
          HPN related 87, 492
    osteoporosis
        calcium intake 687
        chronic hepatic disease 87
        HPN related 492–3
    vitamin D deficiency 87
bone marrow transplantation, TPN
          664
bowel transplantation, short bowel
          714
brain, MR **66**
brain injury, nutritional support,
          ethical dilemmas 693–4
breast feeding 42, 220
    HIV infection 633
breast milk 354
British Artificial Nutrition Survey
          369–71
brush border *see* enterocyte brush
          border
burn injury 575–89
    amino acids, catabolic response
          17–18
    anabolic agents 588

EN 149, 585–6
    commercial enteral feedings **587**
energy goals **578**, 580–1
    metabolic energy expenditure
          (MEE) of adults **582**
    metabolism/metabolic rate
          71–3
    nomogram, body surface area
          (BSA) **580**
    predictions of energy needs,
          BSAB **581**
fat turnover **16**, 72
fluid requirements and resuscitation
          577–80
glucose oxidation **16**, 72
hyperglycaemia 17
nitrogen metabolism **16**
nutritional immunomodulation
          586–8
protein goals **578**, 581–2
protein turnover **16**, 72
TPN 582–5
    adolescents and adults 585
    crystalloid central PN (CPN)
          solutions **584**
    infants/young children 585
    infusion rates and remaining
          energy deficit **583**
    see also injury and sepsis, metabolic
          response
button devices, gastrostomies and
          jejunostomies 293, 358
butyrate, colonic epithelium trophic
          effects 315–16

^{13}C-alpha-ketoisocaproate labelling,
          protein turnover
          measurement 44–5
cadmium, excess 141
calcium
    age and RDA 219
    deficiency 140, 453–4
    as glycerophosphate 473
    and osteoporosis 687
    sources, paediatric PN 473
calcium phosphate, PN mixture
          precipitation 439–40
Calman modular training 251
calorimetry, measurement of energy
          expenditure, direct and
          indirect 181
cAMP *see* cyclic adenosine
          monophosphate
cancer, *see also* tumour cells
cancer, nutrition support 156–7,
          639–80
    aetiology and pathogenesis of
          cancer cachexia 642–50

cancer, nutrition support – *continued*
  appetite stimulant substances and
      anticachectic drugs 665–7
  arginine adjunctive therapy 125
  cancer vs non-cancer patients 656
  catabolic factors 650–1
  chemotherapy and radiotherapy
      655
  children, nutrition status 642, 654
  clinical outcome 657–63
  defective starvation adaptation 644
  definition 641
  future developments 665–7
  glucose uptake increase 645–6
  glutamine supplementation 668–9
  historical background 641
  hypophagia and anorexia theory
      642–3
  iatrogenic malnutrition 651–3
      prognostic impact 653–4
  immune dysfunction 142–3
  lactic acid increase 645
  malnutrition, incidence rates 642
  mechanisms 649–50
  metabolic abnormalities 643–50
  metabolic competition theory 642
  metabolic manipulation 669
  mortality rates 654
  nutrient modulation 667–8
  nutrition regimen 664–5
  nutrition status effects 654–7
  omega-3: omega-6 fatty acids
      158–9
  oral supplements 275–6
  paediatrics 353
  prevalence of cachexia 641–2
  protein turnover 658
  quality of life and performance
      status 660
  surgical intervention 657–9
  TPN 661–2
      complications 663–6
      vs EN, pre- and postoperative
          658–9
      home TPN and EN 664
      outcome effects 659–60
      vs standard oral diet 655
  tumour growth 661–3
  weight loss and tumour type
      relationship 641–2
Candida, catheter-related infections
      386
Candida albicans, PEG tube
      colonisation 290
carbohydrates
  assimilation 126
      predigested elemental diets 318
      rate-limiting steps 118–19

digestion and absorption 117–22,
      126
  EN 120
  enterocyte brush border 118
  monosaccharide transport
      119–20
and fibre, elderly population
      requirements 685
homeostasis 83
hydrolysis, luminal and brush
      border alpha-glucosidases
      118–19
metabolism
  abnormalities 86
  cancer cachexia 645–6
  cytokine mediation 647–8
  hepatic 83–4
  oxygen consumption and RQ
      68
  total kJ in storage 69
paediatric requirements 217, 469
in respiratory failure 545
sources, paediatric PN 469
cardiac arrhythmias, risk reduction, n-
      3 long-chain fatty acids 422
cardiac function
  nutrition depletion effects 607
  protein turnover effects 46
cardiac MR **66**
cardiomyopathy
  congenital heart disease (CHD),
      indications for paediatric
      EN 353–4
  selenium depletion 156
  selenium-related, HPN 490
cardiopulmonary disease, enteral diets
      307
L-carnitine 472
  deficiency 597
casein
  feeding tube blockage 112
  tube obstruction association 336
cat, prolonged starvation, percentage
      loss of organs **5**
catabolic factors
  antioxidants 159
  cancer cachexia 650–1
      LMF 650
      PMF 650–1
catecholamines
  and cytokines 97
  protein turnover effects 48
catheters
  care 395–6
  catheter-related sepsis 386–7
      central vein thrombosis (CVT)
          490
      HPN 489–90

line or hub fracture 490
  tunnel swelling 490
central venous 382–5, 474–5
  complications
      mechanical 476
      paediatric PN 475–6
  cyclical infusions 393–5
  exit sites 395–6
  historical notes 381–2
  implantable devices 384
  infections 243, 386–7, 476
  insertion 395–6
      complications 386
      support team roles 244
      technique 385–6
  jejunostomy
      cuffed-tube (CTJ) 293
      needle catheter (NCJ) 292–3
  material 382–3, 395
  occlusion 387–8
  peripherally inserted central
      catheters (PICCs) 384–5
  PVT risks 391–2
  safer IV feeding 243–4
  single lumen vs multi-lumen 384
  tunnelling 385
  ultrafine, PPN 393–5
cellular hydration, glutamine effects
      413
central vein thrombosis (CVT),
      catheter-related sepsis 490
cerebral palsy, indications for EN
      351–2
cerebrospinal fluid, leptin 232
cerebrovascular disease
  enteral tube feeding 159
  stroke
      gastric atony 309
      nutritional support 691–2
chemical pathologist/biochemist,
      team role 246
chemotherapy
  cancer, glutamine supplementation
      412
  and radiotherapy combination,
      cytotoxicity 653
  side effects 652–3
  TPN, and EN 655, 659–60
chenodeoxycholic acid 477
chinidin, diarrhoea association 338
cholecystokinin (CCK) 159, 236,
      477
cholecystokinin–octapeptide therapy,
      HPN related biliary sludge
      and stone 491–2
cholestasis
  intrahepatic, HPN related 491
  lipoprotein X 87

paediatric PN 477–8
taurine-enriched HPN 491
cholesterol 99
bile acid synthesis 84
hepatic synthesis 84
n-6 PUFAs 99–100
cholestyramine, and vitamin D
deficiency 87
cholic acid 477
cholylsarcosine 714
chromium
age and RDA 219
deficiency 450
RDA/effects 204–5
chronic pulmonary disease see
respiratory disease
chylomicrons, lipid transport 123
cimetidine, PN formulation 440–1
cisapride, gastric emptying 287
clinician, team role 246
Clostridium difficile,
pseudomembranous colitis
338
CO₂, protein turnover measurement
32
co-carboxylase, degradation,
bisulphite 440
coagulation system
hepatic disease 88–9
protein synthesis 85
vitamin K deficiency 87–8, 89
coagulopathy 448
codeine phosphate, diarrhoea
treatment 338
coeliac disease, dietary LCT and
MCT 127
colitis, fish oil preparations 420
colon
preserved, short bowel 707–9
radiotherapy effects 653
colonic absorption, short bowel 705,
705
colonic anastomosis, fibre and SCFA
effects 316
commercial drinks/liquid
supplements, energy and
protein content **271**
computer-assisted TPN, Fresenius
Kabi nutrition programme,
paediatric PN **470**
congenital heart disease (CHD),
indications for paediatric
EN 353–4
constipation
EN-related, incidence rates 337,
338
fibre and EN 314, 337, 338
hepatic encephalopathy 89

continuous arteriovenous
haemofiltration, intra-
dialytic PN 532
copper
age and RDA 219
deficiency 140, 449
incidence rates 341
RDA/effects 204–5
supplement 474
Cori cycle 76
energy expenditure increase 645
corticosteroids
adrenal, amino acid stimulation 85
cancer therapy 666
protein turnover effects 47
corticotrophin-releasing factor, food
intake, appetite control 235
Corynebacterium, tunnelled catheter
infections 386
cost-effectiveness of treatment
733–51
audit see hospital audit
causes of disease-related
malnutrition 735, **738**
clinical benefits 739, 741–3
complete EN 741, 743
oral supplements, sip feeds 741,
742
PN 743
supplementary enteral tube
feeding 741
health economics 744–7
additional mean costs per patient
with/without nutrition
support **750**
application difficulties 744–7
assessment, costs/outcome 746
cost–benefit 744
cost–effectiveness 744, 748
cost–identification
(assessment/comparison or
minimisation) 744, **748**
cost–utility analysis 744, **745,**
748
decision analysis 744, **748**
economic analysis,
appropriateness of clinical
study 746–7
malnutrition 739, **740**
marginal analysis 744
prevalence of disease-related
malnutrition 735, **735–7**
sensitivity analysis 744
terminology 744
length of stay **748, 749**
support team roles 251
CPN see parenteral nutrition, central
venous route

critical illness see intensive care
Crohn's disease 555–66
fish oil preparations 420
HPN 488
indications for paediatric EN 351
nutritional management 564
PEG placement 290
vitamin K deficiency 493
CTJ see jejunostomy, cuffed-tube
cyclic adenosine monophosphate
(cAMP), LMF continuous
stimulation 650
cyclophosphamide, vincristine and
actinomycin D 653
cyproheptadine hydrochloride, cancer
therapy 665–6
cysteine 407–8
acetylcysteine, renal clearance
417–18
cysteine peptide
synthesis 408
taurine and glutathione
formation 417
cysteinyl–leukotriene (Cys–LT)
metabolism, glutamine
dipeptide influence 412
cystic fibrosis
dietary LCT and MCT 127
enteral diet 311
indications for paediatric EN
352–3
PEG placement 290
cystinuria, arginine uptake 114
cytokines 93–104
and amino acids 101–2
anorexia 102
anticytokines, cancer therapy 667
beneficial effects upon host 95
cancer cachexia mediation 647–8
chronic diseases 96
glucose metabolism 649
HIV replication **101**
in hyperalimentation 103
modulatory influences
amount/route of nutrient
delivery 102–3
effects on metabolism 97–8
fats 98–100
oxidants, and antioxidant status
100–1
pathological effects 95–6
protein/amino acids intake
101–2
and polyunsaturated fatty acids
(PUFA) 98–9
pro-inflammatory
actions upon immune system
and metabolism **95**

cytokines – *continued*
    pro-inflammatory – *continued*
        anorexia 102–3
        control by innate systems **96**
        endogenous modulators 97–8
        glutamine effects 412
        and HIV replication **101**
        pathological effects in diseases
            and conditions **96**
        protein metabolism 101–2, 647–8
        protein turnover effects 48
        and tissue wasting 155
        and unsaturated fatty acids,
            infection/trauma/inflam-
            matory disease **99**
        and viruses 96

daunomycin
    malabsorption 653
    oesophageal stenosis 653
deglutition disorders 159–60, 351
    diet regurgitation and aspiration
        risks 286
    gastric atony 309
dehydration
    elderly people 689–90
    hyperosmolar 451
dementia, PEG contraindication 290
Denmark, hospital food, two
    recommended diets **269**,
    270
Depage–Janeway gastrostomy 291
deuterium, doubly-labelled water
    method, measurement of
    MR **64**
dextrins
    alpha-limit, hydrolysis 117–18
    maltodextrins
        EN 120
        predigested elemental diets 318
diabetes mellitus
    with neuropathy
        diet regurgitation and aspiration
            risks 286
        FBT placement, prokinetic
            drugs 287
        gastric atony 309
dialysis
    peritoneal, FPG 291
    PN in 532
diarrhoea
    antidiarrhoeal drugs 338, 712
    chinidin 338
    EN-related 310, 337–8
        fibre supplements 315
        incidence rates 337
        non-infectious 124–5
    fibre and enteral nutrition 315

fluid balance maintenance 338
intermittent enteral feeding 295
lactose-induced, nucleotide
    supplementation 126
short bowel/syndrome 708–9
stool culture 338
stool output quantification 337
symptomatic therapy 338
water malabsorption 124–5
diet technicians, ward staffing,
    hospital 262
dietician, team role 245
digestion, humans, small intestine/
    caecum digesters 110
digoxin, diarrhoea association 338
dilution techniques, body water
    compartment volume
    assessment 172
DNA, cDNA, amino acid transporter
    114
dog, prolonged starvation, percentage
    loss of organs **5**
doubly-labelled water method,
    measurement of MR,
    isotope disappearance
    curves **64**
Douglas bag 63–4
drinks/liquid supplements, energy
    and protein content **271**
dronabinol, cancer therapy 666
drug abusers, intravenous, catheter-
    related sepsis risks 489
drug interactions, EN 340
drug therapy
    CNS, hepatic encephalopathy
        association 89
    diarrhoea related 338
    feeding tube administration, tube
        blockage 112
    jejunostomy 711–12
    PN formulation 440–1
duodenostomy, PED 291–2
dysgeusia, hypophagia association
    643
dysomia, food aversion 643
dysphagia, elderly people 687–8

eating
    disorders, enteral tube feeding
        159–60
    gastrocolonic response 310
    inadequate chewing 687
    oral incontinence 687–8
    see also oral diet
economics *see* cost-effectiveness of
    treatment
education and training, hospital food
    as treatment 262

eicosanoids
    cyclooxygenase pathway 542
        (prostaglandin, leukotriene and
        thromboxane), synthesis in
        IBD **564**
eicosapentaenoic acid (EPA),
    endotoxin stimulation 420
elderly patients 681–99
    adiposity 688
    aversive feeding behaviours (AFB)
        691
    dehydration 689–90
    dementia 691
    diet regurgitation and aspiration
        risks 286
    dietary intakes 687–8
        social factors 688
    dietary modifications 692
    dysphagia 687–8
    energy requirements 684
    ethical dilemmas 693–4
    exercise 689, 692
    malnutrition
        management 691–3
            dietary modification 692
            enteral feeding 692–3
            environment 692
            sip-feeds 692
    Mini-Nutritional Assessment
        (MNA) 691
    nutritional needs 684–7
        carbohydrates and fibre 685
        energy 683–4
        fat 685
        minerals 686–7
        protein 684
        vitamins 685–6
    nutritional status, assessment
        690–1
    nutritional support, future
        developments 694
    oral supplements 274–5
    orthopaedic department 274
    physiological needs 687
    third age, classification 683
    undernutrition as inpatients
        actual consumption 257–9
        recommendations 263–4, 277
    water requirements 689–90
electrolytes
    absorption 123–4
    concentrates, diarrhoea association
        338
    disturbances, EN 340
    lipid emulsion stability 438–9
        Davis equation 439
elemental diets, predigested 305–7,
    311, 317–19

emphysema
 enteral diets 319–20
 and MR 73
 subcutaneous, PEG complication
  290
EN *see* enteral nutrition
encephalopathy
 hepatic *see* liver disease
 Wernicke's
  alcoholic cirrhosis 87
  thiamine deficiency 156, 686
endoluminal brush, catheter-related
  sepsis 387
endoplasmic reticulum, lipid re-
  esterification 123
endoscopy
 duodenostomy/jejunostomy, EN
  292
 FBT placement 287
 gastrostomy 288–91
endothelial damage, PVT 390–1
endotracheal tube, cuffed, FBT risks
  285
energy expenditure 179–83
 direct and indirect calorimetry 181
 estimation 518–19
 measurements 180–1
 see also metabolism/metabolic rate;
  resting energy expenditure
  (REE); total available
  energy (TEE)
energy requirements 259–61, 307–8
 calorimetry measurement 308
 cancer cachexia 643–5, 665
  biochemical aberrations 645
  NEFA oxidation 645
  resting (REE) 643–4
 chronic fasting, oxygen
  consumption decrease
  644–5
 Cori cycle association 645
 elderly patients 683–4
 Harris & Benedict equation 179,
  260, 308
 macronutrients 177–91
 paediatric 216–17, 469
 recommendations 308
 in respiratory failure 544–5
 resting (REE), hormone-sensitive
  lipase 650
enteral nutrition 303–32
 audit, Oldchurch nutrition team
  249
 cancer patients, nutrition status 655
 carbohydrate absorption 120
 carbohydrate source 117
 clinical factors 305, 307–8
  gastrointestinal function 308–9

inflammatory bowel disease
  561–6
 pancreatitis 727–9
 surgical patients 610
 complications 333–46
  aspiration of food 338–9, 373–4,
   547
  contamination and infectious
   complications 293–4
  drug interactions 340
  infective 340
  management and prevention
   341–2
  metabolic 339–40
  monitoring guidelines (BAPEN)
   340–1
 disease-specific 307, 319–21
 elderly patients 692–3
  PEG vs NGT 693
 EN vs parenteral 759–73
  morbidity and mortality 767–9
  non-outcome studies 763–4
 fibre, and bowel function effects
  314–17
 formulations 306, 311–14
  maltodextrins 120
  modular 307
  specialised 307, 321–2
  sucrose 120–2
 paediatric requirements 213–24,
  349
 patient assessment 283, 305
 strategy development 311–12
 supplementary enteral tube feeding, cost-effectiveness 741
 variable effects 657
 see also enteral tube feeding; home
  enteral tube feeding;
  nasoenteral tubes; paediatric
  enteral nutrition
enteral tube feeding
 administration techniques
  closed system 294
  commercial feeds 294–5
  contamination and infectious
   complications 293–4
  continuous vs bolus 295
  HACCP 295
  starter regimens 295
 commencement 295–6
 complications 335–7
 continuous, diarrhoea association
  124
 historical considerations 283
 hospitalised patients 158, 159–60
 long-term 288–93
 minimal, post-abdominal surgery
  159

monitoring 296
 patient consent 283
 short-term 284–8
 see also enteral nutrition;
  nasoenteral tubes
Enterococcus, tunnelled catheter
  infections 386
enterocyte brush border
 carbohydrate absorption 118
 disaccharidases, decrease, TPN 761
 enterokinase binding 111
 fatty acid translocation 122–3
enterokinase, expression 111
enzymes, protein absorption 110–12
epithelial cells *see* gastrointestinal
  epithelium
ethane production, free radicals 100
ethanol, oxygen consumption and
  RQ **68**
eukaryotic initiation factors (eIFs),
  protein turnover 43
European countries, home enteral
  tube feeding, national
  register **376**
extracellular water volume (ECW),
  assessment 171

facial injuries, FBT risks 285
fasciitis, necrotising, PEG
  complications 290
fasting *see* starvation, short term
fat, body *see* body fat
fat free mass (FFM), and MR 65
fats, dietary *see* lipids
fatty acids
 alcohol misuse 86
 blood glucose and ketone bodies,
  prolonged starvation **13**
 enterocyte membrane translocation
  122–3
 essential, deficiency (EFAD), PN
  449
 free fatty acids (FFA), hepatic
  synthesis 84
 immune modulators 529
 monounsaturated (MUFA),
  Mediterranean diet 419
 non-esterified (NEFA) 13
  and disease **187**
  oxidation, energy expenditure
   645
 polyunsaturated (PUFA)
  in infection, and cytokines **99**
  long chain (LCP), premature
   infants 221
  n-3 403, 420–2
   cyclo-oxygenase pathway
    inhibition 420

fatty acids – *continued*
  polyunsaturated (PUFA) – *continued*
    n-3 – *continued*
      IBD 565
      immunoregulatory process effects 420
      and n-6 98, **99**, 140, 313
      surgical patients 597, 611
    omega-3: omega-6 ratio 158–9
    omega-3, fish oil emulsion 420–1
    omega-3 immune response modulation 322
    oxidative damage 197–8
    paediatric requirements 221
    prostaglandin metabolism 545–6
    response to cytokines 98–9
    synthesis **563**
  short-chain (SCFA)
    colonic epithelium trophic effects 315–16
    in IBD 565–6
    luminal microflora 112
    postoperative effects, experimental 316–17
    water and electrolyte absorption 124
  triglyceride–fatty acid metabolism activity and energy cost, burn injury **16**
  critical illness 74
  see also triglycerides
FBT *see* nasoenteral tubes, fine-bore
feeding care assistants, ward staffing 262
femur fractures 692
fetal and neonatal malnutrition, effects on adult health 220
fever, and cytokines 103
fibre and enteral nutrition 314–17
  bowel function effects 314–15
    constipation 314
    diarrhoea 315
  elderly requirements 685, 692
  epithelial cell proliferation
    experimental studies 315–16
    SCFA postoperative effects 316
  fibre concentration 317
  fibre source 317
  gut barrier function 317
  predigested elemental diets 319
fibre supplements
  particle size 314–15, 317
  sources 315
fibrinogen, acute phase proteins 19
fish oil
  anti-inflammatory effects 420–1
  circulating TNF-alpha reduction 421

fatty acid oxidation 421
preparations 420
see also fatty acids, polyunsaturated
fluid requirements
  burn injury 577–80
  composition of fluid loss 469
  Parkland formula 579
fluid retention, excessive glucose in PN 452
fluoride, RDA/effects 206–7
fluoroscopically guided percutaneous gastrostomy (FPG) 291
fluoroscopy, FBT placement 287
5-fluorouracil
  malabsorption 653
  mucositis 652
  radiotherapy combination 653
folic acid
  antagonists, malabsorption 653
  deficiency
    HIV infection 631
    malignancy 685–6
    megaloblastic anaemia 156
  IBD 558, 559
  and immune function 141
  RDA/effects 202–3
food *see* hospital food; oral diet; *specific nutrients*
food supplements *see* oral supplements
free radicals
  antioxidants, in cytokines 100–1
  ethane and pentane production 100
  ROS 197
  scavenging mechanisms 198
Fresenius Kabi nutrition programme, paediatric PN **470**
fructose 423
  uptake mediation, GLUT5 transporter 319

galanin, appetite control 234
gall bladder dysfunction, HPN related 491–2
gas chromatography–mass spectrometry (GC–MS), plasma and precursor pool labelling 35
gas exchange
  energy expenditure by direct and indirect calorimetry 181
  measurement of MR 63–4
gastric atony
  patient groups and associated diseases 309
  stasis, jejunal feeding 155
gastric cancer, labelling index, TPN effects 662

gastric emptying, postoperative delay 272
gastritis, atrophic, elderly patients 685–6
gastrocolonic response, eating 310
gastrointestinal bleeding
  EN contraindication 339
  hepatic encephalopathy 89
gastrointestinal epithelium
  bacterial translocation 762–5
    animal studies 765
    human studies 765–7
  permeability 123–4
  proliferation with fibre supplements 315–17
gastrointestinal function
  barrier function 317
  iatrogenic lesions, nutrition changes 649
  motility 309–11
    diet regurgitation and aspiration risks 286
    enteral diets 308–11, 337–9
    fasting state 309
    PN 155
    see also motility disorders
  nutrient deficiencies 155
  preoperative PN 156–7
  protein turnover effects 46
  radiotherapy tolerance 651–2
gastrointestinal secretions, volumes 704
gastrointestinal surgery, enteral feeding contraindication 296
gastrojejunal tubes, advantages/disadvantages 357
gastrostomy
  button devices 293, 358
  EN 288–92
  endoscopic 288–91
  laparoscopic 291–2
  PEG and FPG 288–91
  temporary, child 356–7
gastrostomy tubes
  HETF 371
  specifications **358**
GLP-2 714
glucagon
  carbohydrate homeostasis 84
  injury and sepsis 71–2
  protein turnover effects 47
glucocorticoids
  and cytokines 97, 98
  nitrogen metabolism 649
gluconeogenesis
  alcohol inhibitory effect 86
  amino acids 83–4

cancer 645
  inhibition, cancer therapy 667
  post injury 17–18
  starvation 70
glucose 422–3
  disposal, oxidation and storage, and
    insulin **185**
  EN monitoring 296
  hepatic 83
  homeostasis abnormalities 86
  lipid emulsion stability 438
  metabolic stress 423
  metabolism
    cytokine administration 649
    TNF-alpha 649
  oxidation
    during infusion **186**
    injured/burned subjects **16**, 72
    oxygen consumption and RQ
      68
    sepsis, low and high REE, with
      i.v. glucose **74**
  requirements in disease/health
    185–6, 422
  starch hydrolysis 118
  tolerance, and dietary fibre 685
  TPN regimens
    cancer therapy 667–8
    excessive administration 450–2
  see also monosaccharides
glucose–alanine shuttle 83
glucose–'lactate'
  activity and energy cost, burn
    injury **16**
  fructose-6P–fructose-1-6P **16**
  glucose–glucose-6P **16**
glutamate, cysteine uptake inhibition
  407
glutamine 18, 598–9
  acetylglutamine, renal clearance
    417–18
  cancer therapy 668–9
  concentrations in muscle **595**
  cysteine administration 408–9
  functions 322
  glutamine dipeptides
    animal studies 409–10
    arginine interaction 410
    glutathione preservation 410
    heat shock protein 70 expression
      and RNA transcription 410
    human studies
      clinical studies 411–16
      healthy volunteers 410–11
    immunostimulatory role 413
    intra/extracellular glutamine
      pools 410, 412, 416
    mechanism of action 416

  muscle protein balance 409
  nitrogen retention 411
  patient group benefits 416
  TPN effects 414–15
  injury and sepsis 516–17
  intestinal metabolism 126–7
  lymphocytes and macrophages
    139
  nitrogen loss amelioration 46
  PN solutions 159
  predigested elemental diets 318
  properties 610–11
  supplementation 322
  survival improvement 413
  TPN 517, 519, 610–11
  transporter system 38–9
glutathione 101–2
  glutamine preservation 410, 416
glyceryl trinitrate patches, PVT risk
  reduction 392, 395
[15]N-glycine ammonia, protein
  turnover measurement 32
glycogen
  metabolism, amino acid regulatory
    role 39
  pool, starvation 9–10
  storage and synthesis costs 69, 70–1
  synthesis, fructose 423
glycogenolysis 83–4
  insulin suppression 86
glycolysis, anaerobic, cancer tissue
  646
gold, excess 141
Golgi apparatus, triglyceride transfer
  123
Groshong catheter, HPN 383–4
growth, glutamine enhancement 414
growth factors, hepatic 90
growth hormone 599
  administration
    mortality risk 47–8
    nitrogen loss amelioration 48
  cancer therapy 666–7
  liver 90
  plasma, insulin resistance 86
  protein turnover effects 47–8
  secretion, insulin stimulation 125
guanethidine, diarrhoea association
  338

HACCP *see* Hazard Analysis Critical
  Control Point
haemodialysis, PN 532
haemorrhage, feeding tube insertion
  337
hand grip strength 170–1, **170**
Harris & Benedict equations
  energy requirements 308

REE 179
RMR 260
Havering Hospitals Trust, Oldchurch
  nutrition team 247–50
Hazard Analysis Critical Control
  Point (HACCP), EN
  administration 295
head injury, EN vs PN 767–8
health economics *see* cost-
  effectiveness of treatment
heart *see* cardiac
heat shock protein (HSP) 70,
  induction, glutamine 410
height
  children, malnutrition recognition
    151–2
  velocity, and height attained, boys
    and girls **215**
heparin
  catheter occlusion risk reduction
    388
  cyclical CPN, catheter care 396
  lipase and enterocytic brush border
    binding 122
  PN formulations 441
  PVT risk reduction 392
hepatic *see* liver
hepatobiliary dysfunction, HPN,
  associated factors 491
hepatocellular carcinoma, protein
  turnover rate increase 646
hepatocytes, replication 89
Hickman catheter, HPN 383
histidine, protein nutrition substrate
  405
HIV infection and AIDS 617–38
  background and history 619–20
  in developing countries 620
  drugs 627, 629
    anabolic drugs 629
    antiretroviral treatment
      (HAART) 619–20
    appetite stimulants 629
    pancreatic enzymes 629
  future perspectives 633
  mother-to-child transmission 626
  nutrition support 624–6
    asymptomatic HIV infection
      626–7
    dietary supplementation 627–8
    EN and PN 628–9
    energy and macronutrients
      624–5
    food hygiene 627
    guidelines 626
    micronutrients 625–6, 629
    side-effect management 627
    specialised diets 628

HIV infection and AIDS – *continued*
  nutrition support – *continued*
    vitamin A status and risk of
        mother-to-child
        transmission **626**
  paediatric HIV infection 629–33
    assessment and management of
        weight loss **630**
    breast feeding 633
    gastrointestinal investigation and
        management of diet **631**
    nutrition support scheme **632**
  pathophysiology of weight loss
      620–4
    body composition and protein
        synthesis 624
    body weight stability 228
    energy balance 622–3
    fat metabolism 623–4
    gastrointestinal infections 621–2
    HAART and energy metabolism
        623
    jejunal biopsy, villous atrophy
        and crypt hyperplasia **621**
    lipid abnormalities 620
    REE, TEE and energy intake
        73, **622**, **623**
  sulphydryl compounds 408
HIV replication
  cytokines, modulation of
      inflammatory response **101**
  nuclear factor (NF) kappa-beta 96
home enteral tube feeding 367–78
  age of patients 370, **370**
  benefits to patients 371
  complications 360
  ethical considerations 376
  European countries 376
  feeding routes 371–2
  feeds and administration methods
      372–3
    portable EN pump **372**
    portable feeding system (back
        pack) **373**
  follow-up and monitoring 375
  future care 376–7
  incidence and growth 369
  indications 369–70
    associated disorders **370**
    reasons for starting HETF **370**
  outcome and quality of life 375–6
  paediatric 357–61
  patient selection 370–1
  problems and complications 373–4
    aspiration of food 373–4
    feeding tubes 373
    funding issues 374
    nutrient deficiencies 374

returning patient to community
    374–5
home parenteral nutrition 485–98
  asepsis 489
  bone disorders 492–3
  catheter choice 383
  complications 489–93, 494
    catheter-related sepsis 489–90
    hepatobiliary 491–3
    of prescription 490
  controversial areas 493–5
    teams, specialist centres and
        small units 493–4
  cost-effectiveness 495
  epidemiology and indications
      487–8
  equipment
    all-in-one bags 490
    pumps 489
  historical aspects 487
  lipid energy supply 490
  mortality rates 494–5
  'paradox of rickets' 492
  PINNT 489
  practical considerations 488–9
  prescribing 490
  prevalence 487
  quality of life issues 494–5
  route of administration 489
  taurine-enriched, intrahepatic
      cholestasis therapy 491
hospital audit 247–50
  data assessment
    educational programme 248
    infection of feeding lines 248
    intake 248
    malnutrition 248
    total work load 248
  hospital food service 263
  results 248–50
    assessment, nutrient intake 249
    IV feeding by Oldchurch
        nutrition team **249**, **250**
    malnutrition, before/after
        education programme
        248–9
    monitoring of IV enteral and
        oral feeding 249–50
hospital food 255–65, 269–70
  audit, food chain management/
      finance 263
  Denmark, recommended diets **269**,
      270
  distribution and serving systems
      261–2
    central service trays/pates 261
    ward-based bulk service/
        kitchens 261

food chain management and
    finance
  audit 263
  control **263**, **264**
  production 261
food composition
  energy density 270
  satiety and intake 270
  history of provision 243
  low food consumption and high
      wastage 258–9
    catering/management 258,
        259
    environment 259
    medication 259
    menus, quality and quantity
        258–9, 262
    missed meals 258
    staffing and serving 259
    timing 259, 263
  nature of food, relevance to energy
      intake **270**
  patient requirements 259–61
  recommendations 263–4
  studies of healthy volunteers 270
  timing of meals/snacks/beverages
      259, 263
  undernutrition in inpatients
      149–64
    immune dysfunction 142
    recommendations 277
  ward staffing
    diet technicians 262
    education and training 262
    feeding care assistants 262
    volunteers, help with feeding
        262
    ward hostesses 262
hospital nutrition team 247
  support and liaison 248
hospitalised patients
  enteral tube feeding 159–60
  malnutrition 149–64
    screening 153
  nutrition support benefits/
      management 156–60
  oral supplements 159
  see also hospital food; surgical
      patients
hub fracture, catheter-related sepsis
    490
hydration, in respiratory failure
    547
hydrazine sulphate, cancer therapy
    667
hydrocortisone
  instability, PN formulations 441
  PVT risk reduction 392

hydropathy plots, Kyte–Doolittle, transport protein identification 114–15
beta-hydroxy–methylglutaryl CoA (HMG–CoA), hepatic synthesis 84
beta-hydroxybutyrate
and acetoacetate (AcAc) **11–13**
hepatic synthesis 83
starvation 10–13
hydroxyurea
malabsorption 653
radiotherapy combination 653
hyperalimentation 74
acute metabolic complications in PN 450–4
algorithm, practical application, pancreatitis **728**
and cytokines 103
HPN related 491
hyperammonaemia
arginine 405
arginine deficiency 125
hypercalcaemia 140
amino acids in PN 453–4
hypercapnia, excessive glucose administration in PN 451
hyperchloraemic acidosis 448
hypercholesterolaemia, lipid emulsions in PN 453
hyperglucagonaemia, insulin resistance 86
hyperglycaemia
burn injury 17
defined 448
diabetes of injury 20
excessive glucose administration in PN 450–1
incidence rates 341
hyperinsulinaemia, cirrhosis 86
hyperkalaemia
incidence rates 341
renal failure 530
hyperlipidaemia
cancer 646
TPN 453
hypernatraemia, incidence rates 341
hyperosmolar dehydration 451
hyperosmolar hyperglycaemic non-ketosis, defined 448, 451
hyperphagia, intestinal adaptation 110
hyperphosphataemia, renal failure 530
hypertriglyceridaemia
defined 448
lipid emulsions in PN 453
PN, metabolic complications 453
hyperuricaemia, fructose administration rate 423

hypoalbuminaemia
assessment of nutrition 169–70
cancer 647
enteral feeding intolerance 338
hepatic disease 88
negative acute phase response 19–20
hypocalcaemia
PN 448–9
renal failure 530
hypoglycaemia
cirrhosis 86
defined 448
incidence rates 341
PN 447–8
hypokalaemia 710
incidence rates 341
hypomagnesaemia 140, 493, 648
incidence rates 341
jejunostomy 710
renal failure 530
hyponatraemia, incidence rates 341
hypophagia, cancer cachexia 642–3, 651–3
hypophosphataemia
incidence rates 341
PN 448
renal failure 530
respiratory failure 544
hypothalamus, control of food intake and energy balance **227**, 232–3
hypothermia, malnutrition association 156
hypothyroidism
diet regurgitation and aspiration risks 286
gastric atony 309
hypozincaemia, incidence rates 341

iatrogenic malnutrition
hypophagia 651–3
malabsorption 653
IgM anti-endotoxin response, pancreatitis 724
ileal absorption, short bowel 705, **705**
imidazole carboxamide, side effects 652
immobility, tissue wasting 155
immune function 137–48
amino acids 139–41
calcium deficiency 140
clinical practice 142–8
cancer patients 142–3
immunosenescence 142
inflammatory bowel disease 143
nutritional supplements 142

protein–energy malnutrition 139, **139**
specific vitamin deficiency effects 141
TPN 143, 656–7
undernutrition 142
fish oil effects 420–1
glutamine requirement 42
immune-enhancing diets 322
immunosenescence 142
iron and zinc 140
lipids 140
malnutrition 155–6
nucleotides 139
trace elements 139–41
vitamins, water and fat-soluble 141
see also cytokines
immunomodulation
acute burns 586–8
arginine 405–6
fish oil emulsion 421
taurine 407
infant formulae 354
amino acid-based 356
infants
energy requirements 349
neonatal malnutrition, effects on adult health 220
neonates, PN formulation 441
preterm, glutamine TPN 414
very low birth-weight (VLBW), glutamine TPN 414
see also paediatric enteral nutrition
infections
bacterial translocation 765–7
complications, EN 340
respiratory 689–90
see also injury and sepsis
inflammatory bowel disease 553–73
administration technique and monitoring 564–5
background 555
Crohn's disease 564
eicosanoid (prostaglandin, leukotriene and thromboxane) synthesis **564**
EN 561–6
future trends 565–6
glutamine 566
management 563–5
micronutrients 566
n-3 fatty acids (marine oils) 565
short chain fatty acids (SCFA) 565–6
structured lipids 566
EN vs PN 769
immune dysfunction 143

inflammatory bowel disease – *continued*
  micronutrient deficiency 558–60
    minerals and trace elements
      559–60
    vitamins 558–9
  nutrition status 555–8
  protein–energy malnutrition
    (PEM) 555–8
    malabsorption 557–8
    nutrient intake 556
  PUFA synthesis **563**
  TPN 560–1
  ulcerative colitis 563–4
  weight loss 228
inflammatory diseases, sulphydryl
    compounds 408
inflammatory response 95, 99–101
  see also cytokines
inherited metabolic disease,
    indications for paediatric
    EN 351
injury and sepsis 13–24, 71–3,
    511–22
  abdominal, enteral feeding
    contraindication 296
  EN vs PN 767
  hepatic encephalopathy 89
  history 513
  intra-abdominal, gastric atony
    309
  intracellular amino acids 30
  metabolic response 13–24, 71–3
    acute phase proteins 18–20
    amino acids 17–18
    basal hypermetabolism in REE
      14, 72–3
    change in REE after elective
      surgery/injury **14–15**, 72
    clinical implications 20–1
    cytokines 101–2
    'ebb' and 'flow' phases 71–2
    energy metabolism 14–15, 72,
      517–18, **518**
    glucose–'lactate', activity and
      energy cost, burned
      subjects **16**
    hyperalimentation 74
    nitrogen metabolism 15–17,
      517–18, **518**
    triglyceride–fatty acid
      metabolism **16**
    variability in response 20
    see also metabolism/metabolic
      rate
  post-operative, bacterial
    translocation association
    766
  practical applications 515

recommendations for clinical
    practice 518–19
  energy requirements 518–19
  future perspectives 520
  protein requirements 519
substrate utilisation 515–17
theoretical problems and benefits
    of support 513–14
insulin
  amino acid stimulation 85
  cancer therapy 666
  carbohydrate homeostasis 83–4
  insulin resistance, liver disease 86
  and MR 68
  protein turnover modification
    46–7
  proteolysis effect 47
insulin-like growth factor (IGF-1),
    protein turnover effects
    47–8
intensive care 591–603
  body composition changes **594**
  carnitine deficiency 597
  EN vs PN 768–9
  future trends 598–9
  glutamine concentrations in muscle
    595
  history 593–4
  practical applications
    energy supply 596–7
    nitrogen supply 597–8
  practical guide for nutrition
    599–600
  protein synthesis rate **595**
interferon-gamma, fat metabolism
    effects 649
interleukins 95–104
  IL-1 97–104
    cancer cachexia 649
  IL-6 97–104
    elevation in cancer 649
    nitrogen metabolism 649
  inhibitors 97–8
  see also cytokines
intestinal barrier *see* gastrointestinal
    epithelium
intestinal metabolism 107–35
  amino acid metabolism 42
intestinal morphology 761–2
intestinal obstruction
  feeding tube leakage 336
  PEG complication 290
intestinal physiology 761
intestinal size *see* short bowel
intramural gas, imaging investigation
    339
iodine
  excess 141

RDA/effects 206–7
iron
  acute phase response **206**
  age and RDA 219
  deficiency 559
    paediatric 220–1
  and immune function 140
  RDA/effects 206–7
irradiation, taurine excretion 407
isotopes
  dilution techniques, body water
    volume assessment 172
  doubly-labelled water method,
    measurement of MR **64**
  extracellular water volume (ECW),
    assessment 171
  protein metabolism tracers 29–30
  radioactive and stable-isotope
    tracers, legal and ethical
    considerations 30
  turnover measurements, protein
    metabolism 31–7

jaundice, and steatorrhoea *see* liver
    disease
jejunal absorption, short bowel 705,
    705
jejunal biopsy, partial villous atrophy
    and crypt hyperplasia,
    weight loss in HIV
    infection **621**
jejunal feeding
  gastric stasis 155
  jejunal tubes
    advantages/disadvantages 357
    specifications **358**
jejunostomy 709–13
  button devices 293
  child 356–7
  cuffed-tube (CTJ) 293
  EN 292–3
  endoscopic 292, 293, 292
    see also percutaneous endoscopic
      jejunostomy
  jejunostomy tubes, HETF 371
  magnesium and potassium
    deficiency 710
  needle catheter (NCJ) 292–3
    feeding tube displacement 336–7
    patient selection 292
    standard-size jejunostomy
      conversion 292–3
  nutrient absorption, PN 712–13
  PEJ 291–2
  presentation 709
  subcutaneous (SCJ) 293
  surgical (SJ) 292
    patient selection 292

Witzel technique, complications 292
treatment 710–12
 antidiarrhoeal drugs 712
 antisecretory drugs 711–12
 magnesium supplements 712
 oral glucose-saline solution 711
 oral omeprazole **712**
 restrict oral fluids 710–11
 water and mineral losses 709–10
jugular veins, cannulation 385

ketogenesis
 3-hydroxybutyrate (beta-OHB) and acetoacetate (AcAc) **11–13**
  circulating concentration 10, **11**
  metabolism in obese subjects 10
  molar ratio **11**
  release in short-term starvation **12**, 71
 amino acids 84
 starvation 10–13
 storage costs 69
^{13}C-alpha-ketoisocaproate labelling, protein turnover measurement 44–5
Kleiber's law 109–10
Krebs' tricarboxylic acid cycle
 amino acid metabolism 41
 CoA 84
Kyte–Doolittle hydropathy plots 114–15

lactation, protein intake recommendations 42, 220
lactic acid, cancer 645
lactic acidosis, fructose administration rate 423
lactose intolerance 271, 337
lactulose, hepatic encephalopathy treatment 89, 112
lead, excess 141
lecithin–cholesterol acyltransferase (LCAT), hepatitis 86
leptin 230–2
 human/murine *ob* gene 229–32
 long-term regulation of appetite and body weight 229–32
 mutations in receptor 231
 relation between body fat and serum leptin **232**
 site of action 230–1
leucine tracer
 protein turnover measurement 32, 34–5
  fractional synthetic rate calculation 34

leukotrienes
 synthesis, EPA effects 421
 and thromboxane, inflammatory bowel disease **564**
line fracture, catheter-related sepsis 490
lipase, hormone-sensitive, REE stabilisation 650
lipid emulsions
 anabolic response 158
 ICU 597
 and lung 473
 MCT, proinflammatory cytokine reduction 158
 phospholipids, IV 437
 PN 452–3, 472–3
  hypercholesterolaemia 453
  hypertriglyceridaemia 453
  lipoprotein X (LPX) 453
 stability 437–8
  affecting factors 438–9
  assessment 439
  mechanisms 438
  Van der Waal's forces 437–8
lipid mediators, glutamine influence 412
lipid mobilising factor (LMF), catabolic factors, cancer cachexia 650
lipid nutrition substrates 418
 new preparations 418–22
 physiologic functions 418
lipids 69, 98–9, 140, 217, 472
 absorption 122–3
  emulsification 122
 assimilation 126–7
 cholesterol 99
 classification 98
 digestion and absorption disturbances, enteral feeding 337–8
 elderly requirements 685
 fish oil preparations 420–1
 healthy subjects 186
 hepatic metabolism 84, 86–7
 home PN 490
 and immune function 140
 influence of disease on non-esterified fatty acid (NEFA) **187**
lipogenesis and RQ 74
metabolism
 amino acid regulatory role 39
 cancer cachexia 646
 cytokine mediation 647–8
oxidation/turnover
 oxygen consumption and RQ **68**

sepsis, low and high REE, with i.v. glucose **74**
paediatric requirements 217
peroxidation, PN formulations 442
predigested elemental diets 319
requirements in disease 187
 in respiratory failure 545–6
sources, paediatric PN 472
structured 403, 422
 rapid plasma clearance 422
total kJ in storage 69
see also fatty acids; triglycerides
lipolysis stimulation, TNF-alpha 649
lipoprotein lipase 472
lipoproteins
 lipase inhibition, alcohol misuse 87
 lipoprotein X 87, 453
  cholestasis 87
lipostat theory, appetite control 230
liquid supplements, energy and protein content **271**
lithocholic acid 477
liver disease 499–510
 acute liver failure 320–1, 507
 ascites 506
 assessment of nutrition status 504–6
 carbohydrate metabolism 86
 cirrhosis
  fat-soluble vitamin deficiencies 86
  feeding tube insertion haemorrhage 337
  hyperinsulinaemia 86
  hypoglycaemia 86
  pancreas beta-cell response 86
  RQ **504**
  specialised enteral diet 311
 cysteine administration 407
 encephalopathy 506
  and coma 320
  complications 506
  enteral diets, branched chain amino acids 89, 320–1
  lactulose therapy 112
 energy expenditure, substrate utilization 503–4
 enteral diet 307, 311, 321
 fulminant hepatic failure (FHF) 320–1, 507
 future perspectives 508
 glucose homeostasis abnormalities 86
 hepatic failure, intracellular amino acids 30
 hepatitis, LCAT reduction 86
 hepatocellular carcinoma, protein turnover rate increase 646
 history 501

liver disease – *continued*
  HPN related 491
  inappropriate nutrients in PN 454
  jaundice and steatorrhoea 506–7
  lipid metabolism 86–7
  liver transplantation 507–8
  malnutrition 86, **503**, 506–7
  osteomalacia 87
  steatohepatitis, HPN related 491
  steatorrhoea, jaundice 506–7
  steatosis, excessive glucose
      administration in PN 451–2
  theoretical problems and benefits
      of support 502–3
  tyrosine 408
  tyrosine dipeptide TPN 417
  visceral proteins 505
  vitamin deficiencies 87
liver function
  amino acid metabolism 42, 88–9
  energy metabolism 83
  hepatic growth factors 90
  lipid metabolism 84, 86–7
  metabolic disturbances 86–9
  metabolism/metabolic rate 73,
      81–91
  and PN 477
  protein metabolism 88–9
  protein turnover effects 46
  regeneration, nutrition 89–90
  replication of hepatocytes 89
liver transplantation 507–8
  pre-transplant patient assessment 86
loperamide 709, 712
  diarrhoea therapy 338
lungs
  immune system, effects of
      malnutrition and refeeding
      542–3
  parenchyma 541–4
    altered microcirculation and
      interstitial water 543
    effects of malnutrition and
      refeeding 541–4
  see also respiratory disease/failure
lymphangiectasia, enteral diet 311
lymphatic system, lipid release 123
lymphocytes
  cysteine enhancement 407–8
  and macrophages, glutamine 139
  proliferation, glutamine effects 413
lysine, deprivation by arginine 406

macrocytic megaloblastic anaemia,
      vitamin B12 deficiency 156
alpha-2-macroglobulin 101–2
macronutrient requirements 177–91
  definition 179

see also named nutrients
macrophages
  cysteine transportation 407
  glutamine 139
  and smoking 100–1
magnesium
  age and RDA 219
  deficiency 140
    calcium absorption inhibition
      493
    jejunostomy 710
  osteoporosis 687
  supplements, jejunostomy 712
malabsorption
  cancer 651, 653
  causes 310
  classification 310, 311
malnutrition
  cost-effectiveness of treatment
      735–51
  cytokines 103
  delayed wound healing 350
  digestive tract secondary changes
      643
  disease-related
    cancer 642, 653–4
    causes **738**
    costs associated **740**
    liver disease 86, 502–3
    prevalence **736–7**
  elderly patients
    effects and consequences 688–9
    free-living and hospitalised 689
    management 691–3
  hospitalised patients 149–64
    clinical consequences 155–6
    immune system 155–6
    incidence 153–4
    metabolic problems 158
    pathogenesis 154–5
    prevalence 153–4
    recognition 151–3
    refeeding syndrome 158
    thermoregulation 156
  iatrogenic 651–3
  increased susceptibility to infection
      350
  malabsorption, cancer 651
  paediatric
    altered mood and depression
      350
    brain growth and
      neurodevelopment 349–50
    fetal/neonatal, and adult health
      220
    gastrointestinal function 350
    growth and delayed puberty 350
    long term health 350

peptide-based diets 116
protein–energy malnutrition
  albumin and 222
  IBD 555–8, **560**
  immune function 139
  increased intestinal protein losses
      557
  increased metabolism 556–7
  pathological factors **557**
  short bowel 706
  refeeding, and respiratory system
      540–4
  skeletal protein los 142–3
  specific nutrient deficiencies 350
  see also starvation
maltases, classification 118
maltodextrins, predigested elemental
      diets 318
maltotriose, carbohydrate end-
      product 117
manganese
  age and RDA 219
  in bile 474
  RDA/effects 204–5
mass isotope analysis, protein
      turnover 36
Mediterranean diet 419
medroxyprogesterone acetate, cancer
      therapy 665
megaloblastic anaemia
  alcohol misuse 87
  folate deficiency 156
  vitamin B12 deficiency 156
megestrol acetate, cancer therapy 665
melanin-concentrating hormone,
      appetite control 234
melanocyte-stimulating hormone,
      appetite control 235
melatonin, cancer therapy 667
mercury, excess 141
metabolic competition theory, cancer
      cachexia 642
metabolic inhibitors, cancer therapy
      667
metabolic manipulation, cancer
      therapy 669
metabolism/metabolic rate 61–79,
      179–83
  adipose tissue, brown/white **66**
  and BMI, predictive equations **66**
  clinical aspects 69–71
    chronic diseases 73
    fasting/starvation 69–71
    see also starvation
    in injury and sepsis 14–15, 71–3,
      517–18, **518**
  cytokines and amino acids 101–2
  energy expenditure, MEE 580–1

energy requirements, in respiratory failure 544–5
estimates **180**
exogenous nutrient utilization 74–5
and FFM 65
hormonal control 67–8
major metabolic processes 68–9
measurement 180–1
  bicarbonate–urea method 65, **65**
  direct and indirect calorimetry 181
  doubly-labelled water method **64**, 180
    isotope disappearance curves **64**
  paediatric energy requirements 216
  respiratory gas exchange 63–4
  standardizations of MR measurements and values 65–6
micronutrients 207–8
oxidation 68–9
  energy yields, oxygen consumption and RQ **68**
PN complications 445–59
REE, *see also* resting energy expenditure (REE)
surface area 65
and synthesis 69
TEE, *see also* total available energy (TEE)
tissues and organs 66–7, **66**
see also basal metabolic rate; injury and sepsis; starvation
metallothionein, and cytokines 97
methionine 477
methotrexate
  malabsorption 653
  mucositis 652
methyldopa, diarrhoea association 338
3-methylhistidine, protein turnover measurement 32–3, 43, 44–5
metoclopromide, gastric emptying 287
microbiologist, team role 246
micronutrients and minerals *see named minerals*; trace elements; vitamins
Mini-Nutritional Assessment (MNA), elderly patients 691
molybdenum
  age and RDA 219
  deficiency 450
  RDA/effects 204–5

monosaccharides
  carbohydrate hydrolysis 318
  liver utilisation 83
  transport 119–20
    GLUT2 and 5 119
    sodium-glucose linked transporter 1 (SGLT1) 119
    'solvent drag' 120
  unfermented, diarrhoea potentiation 124
monounsaturated fatty acids (MUFA), Mediterranean diet 419
motility *see* gastrointestinal function
motor neurone disease, enteral tube feeding 159
mucosal atrophy, TPN 762
mucosal injury, predictor, nosocomial pneumonia 766
mucosal permeability 123–4
mucositis, chemotherapy 652
multi-organ failure, bacterial translocation 610
myocardial infarction, fish oil emulsion 422
myocardial ischaemia, parenteral arginine 406
myopathy, selenium depletion 156

[15]N-glycine ammonia, protein turnover measurement 32
NADH:NAD ratio, alcohol misuse 86–7
nasoenteral tubes 281–302
  access routes 283–5
  administration techniques 293–6
  advantages/disadvantages 357
  blockage, dietary protein 112
  double-lumen (dual-function) 287–8
  feeding reservoirs and giving sets, hang time 294–5
  fine-bore (FBT) 284–6
    access, endotracheal tube 285
    complications 284–5, 287
    extubation, unplanned and non-elective 286
    infants 286
    PEG to PECJ conversion 291
    placement
      nasoduodenal or jejunal 286–7
      nasopharyngoscope 285
      techniques 287
      X-ray confirmation 285
    prokinetic drugs 287
    transnasal 285–6
  long-term
    ports 293
    tube composition 288

nasogastric, elderly patients 693
  oral supplements 272–3
  percutaneous gastrostomy 160
  pump-controlled 337
  reflux and tube position 339
  secretagogue bypass 311
  simultaneous gastric aspiration 159
  tube blockage prevention 293
  see also enteral tube feeding
nasogastric tubes
  advantages/disadvantages 357
  postoperative 273
  specifications **358**
nasojejunal tubes 357
  specifications **358**
nasopharyngoscope, flexible, FBT placement 285
NCJ *see* jejunostomy, needle catheter
necrosis, feeding tubes 336
necrotising enterocolitis, EN 339
needle catheters *see* catheters
neurocognitive disorders, vitamin deficiency relationship 685
neurodevelopmental disorders, indications for EN 351–2
neurologic deficit, and aspiration risks, EN 338
neuromotor deglutition disorders
  diet regurgitation and aspiration risks 286
  gastric atony 309
neuromuscular blocking agents, diet regurgitation and aspiration risks 286
neuropeptide Y, food intake, appetite control 233–4
neurosurgical patients
  diet regurgitation and aspiration risks 286
  gastric atony 309
neurotransmitters
  increasing food intake 233–4
  reducing food intake 235–6
  see also peptides
niacin, RDA/effects 202–3
nickel, excess 141
nicotinic acid, age and RDA 218
nitric oxide (NO), arginine substrate 406
nitrogen, *see also* protein metabolism
nitrogen assimilation
  comparative diets 117
  free amino acid transport 112–14
  intestinal 112–15
  peptide hydrolysis 116
  peptide transport 114–15
  protein, dietary and endogenous 112

nitrogen assimilation – *continued*
  urea utilisation 112
nitrogen balance *see* protein
        metabolism, nitrogen
        balance
nitrogen mustard, side effects 652
nitrogen requirements
  predigested elemental diets 318
  recommendations 308
  sources, paediatric PN 469–72
'nitrogen trap', neoplastic cells 642
non-Hodgkin's lymphoma, labelling
        index 663
non-steroidal anti-inflammatories,
        topical, PVT risk reduction
        392, 395
noradrenaline
  appetite control 234
  excretion 452
nuclear factor (NF) kappa-beta, HIV
        replication 96
nuclear transcription factors 96
nucleic acids, immune response
        modulation 322
nucleotides
  and immune function 139
  intestine utilisation 125–6
  PRPP salvage 125
  supplementation 126
nurse, team role 245
nutrition, postoperative *see*
        postoperative nutrition
nutritional assessment *see* assessment
        of nutrition
nutritional support team (NST) *see*
        support team roles

ob protein and *ob* receptor in mice,
        appetite control 230
obesity
  fat reduction 685
  human/murine *ob* gene 229–32
  ketone bodies, metabolism 10
  and prolonged starvation 4, **5**
    fuel availability/survival time **6**
    glucose and plasma FFA, ketone
        bodies **71**
    murine models 5, **229**
    TEE, fat, carbohydrate and
        protein **6**
octreotide 711
ODC *see* ornithine decarboxylase
oesophageal disease, indications for
        paediatric EN 351
oesophageal obstruction, PEG
        complication 290
oesophageal varices, feeding tube
        insertion haemorrhage 337

oesophagostomy, cervical, longer-
        term EN 288
oligosaccharidases, brush border 118
olive oil, lipid emulsions 419
omeprazole, jejunostomy 711, **712**
oral diet 255–65, 267–80
  liquid vs solid food, and energy
        density, satiety and intake
        270
  records of food intake 276–7
  undernourished patients,
        recommendations 263–4,
        277
  see also hospital food; oral
        supplements
oral supplements 270–6, 306, 307,
        313
  commercial drinks/liquid
        supplements, energy and
        protein content **271**
  cost-effectiveness studies **742**
  elderly/geriatric patients 274–5
  home made, recipe for quarg and
        cocoa quarg drink **271**
  hospitalised patients 159
  nasogastric tubes 272–3
  palatability studies 272
  post discharge from hospital 275
  post surgery 273–4
  preoperative feeding vs overnight
        fasting 274–5
  principles 272–6
  sip feeding, reduction in solid food
        consumption 276
  undernourished patients, studies
        276
organ function, malnutrition 155
ornithine decarboxylase (ODC),
        hepatic activation 90
oropharyngeal disease, enteral tube
        feeding 159
orthopaedic department, elderly
        patients, oral supplements
        274
osteomalacia
  chronic hepatic disease 87
  vitamin D-induced, HPN related
        492
osteoporosis 87, 492–3
  calcium intake 687
overfeeding *see* hyperalimentation
oxalate, absorption, short bowel 708
oxidants, and antioxidant status,
        modulation of cytokines
        100–1
oxygen consumption
  aerobic metabolism 68–9
  and RQ, energy yields **68**

paediatric(s), *see also* – nutrition
        assessment; – nutrition
        requirements; – parenteral
        nutrition; paediatric enteral
        nutrition
paediatric enteral nutrition 347–65
  choice of enteral feed 354–6
  complications of feeding 357
  elemental formula 356
  feeding routes 356–7, **357**
  home enteral tube feeding 357–61
    complications **360**
    ideal feeding tubes, pumps and
        devices **358**, 359
    psychological and social
        implications 359, 361
    training 357–9
  indications for EN 350–4
    cerebral palsy and neuro-
        developmental disorders
        351–2
    childhood malignancies 353
    congenital heart disease (CHD)
        353–4
    Crohn's disease 351
    cystic fibrosis (CF) 352–3
    inadequate oral intake 350–1
    inherited metabolic disease 351
    malignancies 353
    oesophageal disease/injury 351
    primary disease management
        351
    short bowel syndrome 351
    swallowing dysfunction 351
  infant formulae 354
    amino acid-based 356
  malnutrition 349–50
  modular feeds 356
  nutrition requirements 1–12, **349**
  oral feeding, maintaining skills 361
  polymeric feeds 354–5
    children 1–6 years 355
    children over 6 years 355
    infants 0–12 months 354
  protein hydrolysate formulae
        355–6
    children 0–2 years 355
    children over 2 years 355–6
  see also home enteral tube feeding
paediatric HIV infection 629–33
paediatric jejunostomy 356–7
paediatric nutrition assessment 221–2
  anthropometry 221–2
  cancer 642, 654
  clinical examination 221
  current perspectives 215–16
  dietary intake measurements 221
  laboratory 222

paediatric nutrition requirements
213–24
carbohydrate 217
energy 216, 349
fat 217
fatty acids, long chain
polyunsaturated 221
fetal and neonatal malnutrition,
effects on adult health 220
fluids and energy **216**
height velocity and height attained
curves for boys and girls
215
historical background 215
infants, energy requirements 349
iron deficiency 220–1
mineral and trace elements 219
protein 217–19
protein intake 42
starvation effects in infants and
young children 219–21
vitamins 218–19
vulnerability of infants 349
water **216**, 217–18
paediatric parenteral nutrition **349**,
461–84
calcium and phosphate sources 473
carbohydrate sources 469
catheter complications 475–6
mechanical catheter problems
476
replacing surgical central venous
catheters 476
sepsis 475–6
cholestasis associated with PN
477–8
energy requirements 469
fat sources 472
fat emulsion and lung 473
formulation of feeds **465**, 468
commercially available products
466–7
nutrients, electrolytes, minerals
and vitamins **465**, 474
Fresenius Kabi nutrition
programme **470**
history 463
indications 464–7, **464**
metabolic complications **468**
monitoring 468–9, **468**
composition of abnormal fluid
losses **469**
nitrogen sources 469–72
outcome 478
particulate contamination of PN
solutions 478
PN formulation 441
prescription worksheet **471**

psychosocial development 478
special considerations 463–4
techniques for administering PN
474–7
central venous access 474–5
delivery 476–7
peripheral venous access 474
vitamins and trace elements 474
pamidronate, osteoporosis, HPN-
related 493
pancreatectomy
postoperative malabsorption 653
starch assimilation 118
pancreatic cancer
REE 644
specialised enteral diet 311
pancreatitis 719–32
acute
intracellular amino acids 30
post-pyloric enteral feeding
benefit 769
algorithm for nutritional
hyperalimentation **728**
chronic, dietary LCT and MCT
127
EN and PN 727–9
future trends 729–30
graded balance of nutritional
management **727**
history 721–2
pancreatic secretory stimulants **726**
level of GI tract **725**
theoretical concepts and benefits
722–7
villous height, effect of duration of
TPN therapy **723–4**
parathormone secretion
HPN, overnight feeding pattern
492
HPN bone disorders 492–3
parenteral nutrition
bacterial translocation 765
bag design
Big Bag system 437, 441
multichambered bag (MCG) 441
multilayered bags 440, 441
cancer 658–66
commercially available products
466–7
controversial areas 441–2
cost-effectiveness 743
elderly patients 693
EN vs PN 759–73
morbidity and mortality 767–9
non-outcome studies 763–4
equipment and facilities 441
aseptic facility 441–2
formulations 435–44

application practicalities 442
chemical stability and
compatibility 439–40
drug administration 440–1
historical background 437
monitoring 441
particulate contamination 478
precipitation
calcium phosphate 439–40,
441
monitoring 440
trace elements 440
stability of lipids 437–9
glutamine 159
HIV infection and AIDS 628–9
hospitalised patients 160
IBD 560–1
immune dysfunction 143
intradialytic, MHD patients 532
monitoring guidelines (BAPEN)
340–1
nutrition teams 396
pancreatitis 727–9
pre- and post-operative 156–8
surgical patients 610
see also parenteral nutrition, central
venous route (CPN); –
nutrition, metabolic
complications; – nutrition,
peripheral (PPN); – –
substrates; paediatric – –
parenteral nutrition, central venous
route (CPN) 382–8
access 474–5, 477
catheters 382–5
complications 386–8
indications/contraindications 382
tunnelling 385
parenteral nutrition, metabolic
complications 445–59
acute metabolic deficiencies 447–9
hypocalcaemia 448–9
hypoglycaemia 447–8
hypophosphataemia 448
amino acids 453–4
hypercalcaemia 453–4
biochemical monitoring **455**
chronic deficiency syndromes
449–50, **449**
essential fatty acid deficiency
(EFAD) 449
trace minerals 449–50
vitamins 450
zinc 449
definition **448**
diagnostic criteria 447
excessive glucose administration
450–2

parenteral nutrition, metabolic
    complications – *continued*
  excessive glucose administration –
      continued
    fluid retention 452
    hepatic steatosis 451–2
    hypercapnia 451
    hyperglycaemia 450–1
    hyperosmolar dehydration 451
    increased sympathetic activity
      452
  inappropriate composition of
      nutrients 454–5
    hepatic dysfunction 454
    metabolic bone disease 454–5
    refeeding syndrome 455
  lipid emulsions 452–3
  nutrient deficiencies 447–50
  overfeeding of nutrients 450–4
parenteral nutrition, peripheral (PPN)
    388–95
  access 160, 474
  administration methods 393–4
  catheters, care 395–6
  contraindications 389
  current practice 389
  evolution 388–9
  feeding duration 390
  limitations 389–90
  nutrient solution 395
  PVT risks 390–3
  recommendations 394–5
  regimen 389–90
  venous access, rotation and cyclical
      PPN infusion 393–5
parenteral nutrition substrates 401–34
  carbohydrates 422–4
  historical development 403–5
  lipids 418–22
  proteins 405–18
Parkland formula, fluid requirements
    579
Patients on Intravenous and
    Nasogastric Nutritional
    Therapy (PINNT), pumps
    and stands 489
pectin supplements, predigested
    elemental diets 319
pentane production, free radicals
    100
pentoxifylline, cancer therapy 649,
    667
pepsins, secretion 111
peptides
  absorptive characteristics 115–17
    PepT1, feeding modes 117
  and neurotransmitters
    increasing food intake 233–4

reducing food intake 235–6
predigested elemental diets 318
transport
  nitrogen assimilation 114–15
  PepT1 structural requirements
    115
percutaneous endoscopic
    duodenostomy (PED) 292
  removal 291
percutaneous endoscopic gastrostomy
    (PEG) 160
  advantages/disadvantages 357, 371
  anatomy variations 291
  antibiotic prophylaxis 290
  complications 160, 290–1
  conversion to jejunostomies 281,
    292
  Crohn's disease 290
  direct stab technique 288
  elderly patients 692–3
    complications 693
  feeding tube displacement 336–7
  long-term EN 288–91
  prophylactic antibiotics 693
  pull or push-through technique
    288–9
  removal 291
  replacement 290–1
  Staphylococcus aureus colonisation
    336
percutaneous endoscopic jejunostomy
    (PEJ) 292
  removal 291
percutaneous gastrostomy,
    fluoroscopically guided
    (FPG) 291
peripheral vein thrombophlebitis
    (PVT) 390–3
  pathogenesis and aetiology 390
  predisposing factors and
    modification effects 391
  venous access rotation and cyclical
    PPN infusion 393–5
  venous trauma 393
peritoneal dialysis, continuous
    ambulatory, PN 532
pharmacist, team role 246
pharmaconutrition 610–12
  see also arginine; fatty acids;
    glutamine
pharyngeal flora 762
pharyngostomy, cervical, longer-term
    EN 288
phenylalanine–tyrosine tracer, protein
    turnover measurement 32
phenylketonuria, tyrosine 408
phlebitis, peripheral venous access
    474

phosphate
  age and RDA 219
  hypophosphataemia 341, 448, 530,
    544
  monitoring, EN 296
  precipitation in formulations, PN
    439–40, 441
  pyridoxal-5'-phosphate (PLP) 87
  sources, paediatric PN 473
phospholipids, intravenous lipid
    emulsions 437
5-phosphoribosyl-1-phosphate
    (PRPP), nucleotide salvage
    125
photodegradation of vitamins 440
PICCs (peripherally inserted central
    catheters) 384–5
pigeon, prolonged starvation,
    percentage loss of organs **5**
cis-platinum, side effects 652
PN *see* parenteral nutrition
pneumatosis intestinalis, EN 339
pneumonia
  aspiration, intermittent enteral
    feeding 295
  aspiration risks, EN 338
  nosocomial, gut mucosal injury
    predictor 766
pneumoperitoneum, PEG
    complication 290
pneumothorax, CPN complication
    386
polymeric enteral diets 305–6,
    313–14
  fibre source 317
  hypotonic 313
  low osmolality 314
  paediatric EN 354–5
polyribosome fraction, muscle protein
    synthesis 43
portal vein, neutral lipid
    transportation 123
postoperative nutrition 270–7
  cancer patients 275–6
  commercial drinks/liquid
    supplements **271**
  elderly/geriatric patients 274–5
  post discharge from hospital 275
  vs preoperative 609–10
  preoperative feeding vs overnight
    fasting 274–5
  respiratory disease 275
  sip feeding, reduction in solid food
    consumption 276
  studies 276, **742**
  surgical patients 156–8
potassium
  deficiency 341

jejunostomy 710
monitoring, EN 296
whole-body (WBK), TPN and EN 655–6
PPN *see* parenteral nutrition, peripheral
predigested chemically defined elemental diets 305–7, 311, 317–19
  fibre content 319
  lipid energy source 319
  nitrogen and carbohydrate source 318–19
    di/tripeptides 318
    maltodextrins 318
  sodium content 319
  trace elements and vitamins 319
pregnancy, protein intake recommendations 42
procarbazine, radiotherapy combination 653
prognostic nutritional index (PNI) 173–4
prokinetic drugs, FBT duodenal placement 287
propranolol, diarrhoea association 338
prostaglandins 473
  metabolism, PUFAs 545–6
protease inhibitors, acute phase proteins 18–20
proteases
  pancreatic, cascade 111
  protein hydrolysis 111
protein(s)
  acute phase proteins 18–20
  assimilation 126
    absorption 110–12
    quantitative aspects 115–17
  dietary and endogenous, nitrogen assimilation 112
  fatty-acid binding protein (iFABP) 123
  hepatic disease 88–9
  hydrolysis 111, 116
  partial enzymic hydrolysates 318
  structure 111
  total body protein (TBP) 170
  transport protein identification, Kyte–Doolittle hydropathy plots 114–15
  transporter systems 112–15
    dibasic amino acids 114
    hydropathy identification 114–15
protein assessment
  albumin and visceral proteins 169–70
  burns, predictions **583**

in respiratory failure 546
skeletal muscle 170–1
  critically ill patients in ICU **595**
visceral proteins 169–70
protein hydrolysates
  formulae, paediatric EN 355–6
  pulse-feeding 684
  short-chain 418
protein metabolism 25–59
  activity and energy cost, burn injury **16**
  and alpha-2-macroglobulin 101–2
  analysis 29–31
  bacteraemia and increased mortality 103
  cancer cachexia 646
    tumour interference 647
  cytokines 101–2, 647–8
    sepsis, low and high REE, with i.v. glucose **74**
  dynamic nature 27
  energy and protein balances, TEE post severe head injury **17**
  hepatic, cancer cachexia 647
  kinetic response, TPN, cancer 656
  lean body mass determination, deuterium dilution 29
  muscle synthesis and breakdown, cancer cachexia 646–7
  nitrogen balance
    critically ill patients 260–1, 597–8
    dietary energy and protein effects 44
    glutamine dipeptide TPN 411, 416
    loss, lean tissue proteolysis 49
    measurement 17
    renal disease 525–6
    starvation, lean/obese subjects **13**
    total body (TBN), TPN and EN 655–6
    trauma and sepsis 15–17, 517–18, **518**
    urinary, monitoring, EN 296
  nitrogen excretion
    BUN and UNA 526, 529–30
    starvation
      fed state and post starvation 13
      ratio of cumulative N loss to weight loss **7, 8**
      short term **4**
  radioactive and stable-isotope tracers 29–30
  recommended intakes 42–3
  TNF-alpha effects 649–50
  tumour interference 638

turnover/measurements 31–7, 69
  ageing effects 48–9
  amino acid free pool size 39
  amino acid intermediary metabolism 39–41
  arteriovenous (A–V) differences 32
  cancer 658
  catecholamines 48
  cellular biochemistry 43
  CO_2 32
  compartmental and stochastic analysis 31–2
  cytokines 48
  defined 27
  dynamic methods 32–5
  eukaryotic initiation factors (eIFs) 43
  fed/fasted state responses 45
  glucagon 47
  growth hormone 47–8
  growth-related synthesis 43
  IGF-1 47–8
  index, tracer amino acids 33–4
  indicator amino acids 32–3
  injured/burned subjects **16**, 72
  insulin modification 46–7
  ^{13}C-alpha-ketoisocaproate labelling 44–5
  mass isotope analysis 36
  muscle, disease and injury effects 49
  ^{15}N-glycine ammonia 32
  nutrient and hormonal modification 46–9
  short term starvation 4
  testosterone 48
  thyroid hormone 47
  tracer amino acid incorporation 34–5
  whole body 170
    nutrient supply responses 44–5
    physiological control 43–6
    skeletal muscle 45–6
protein mobilising factor (PMF), cancer cachexia 650–1
protein nutrition substrates 405–9
  alternatives 409–18
protein requirements
  amino acids **183**
  in disease 184–5
  elderly 684
  and energy intake 184
  healthy subjects 183–4
  hospital food 260–1
  in injury and sepsis 519
  oxygen consumption and RQ **68**, 181

protein requirements – *continued*
  paediatric requirements 217–19, 355
  total kJ in storage 69
protein synthesis 69
  coagulation system 85
  glutamine dipeptide TPN 411
  rate, intensive care **595**
  skeletal muscle 41–2, 43, 45
protein–energy malnutrition *see* malnutrition
proteolytic enzymes, protein catabolism 31
proton pump inhibitors 711–12
pseudomembranous colitis 338
psoriasis, fish oil preparations 420
psychosis, PEG contraindication 290
psychosocial development, paediatric PN 478
pulmonary aspiration *see* aspiration
pulmonary immune response, malnutrition and refeeding 542–3
pumps
  controlled feeding 337
  enteral tube feeding **358**, 359
  HPN 489
  portable EN pump **372**
  and stands 489
  volumetric 477
PVT *see* peripheral vein thrombophlebitis
pyridoxal–5'–phosphate (PLP), chronic hepatitis 87
pyridoxine *see* vitamin B$_6$
PYY, gastrointestinal effects 310–11

quality of life
  HETF 375–6
  HPN 494
  and performance status, cancer, TPN 660

radiation, taurine excretion 407
radiation enteritis, PN 155
radiotherapy
  and chemotherapy combination, cytotoxicity 653
  gastrointestinal tract tolerance 651–2
  head and neck 652
  nutrition complications 651
  TPN and EN 655, 660
ranitidine 711
  PN formulation, multilayered bag 440–1
rat
  prolonged starvation, percentage loss of organs **5**

weight loss, acute phase proteins **19**
recumbency *see* aspiration
REE *see* resting energy expenditure
refeeding syndrome 158
  effects on respiratory system 540–4
  PN 455
reference nutrient intake (RNI) 199
regurgitation, EN-related, incidence rates 337
renal disease 523–35
  administration method 531–2
  amino acid metabolism 42
  background 525
  clinical management of nutrition therapy 528–30
  enteral diets 307
  experimental studies 528
  minerals, trace elements and vitamin requirements 530–1
  nitrogen balance 525–6
  serine 405
  tyrosine 408
renal failure 321, 525
  intradialytic PN, MHD patients 532
  and MR 73
  nutrition management 526–8
  taurine concentrations 407
  tyrosine dipeptide TPN 416–17
renal MR **66**
respiratory disease/failure 537–52
  dehydration, elderly patients 689–90
  effects of malnutrition and refeeding 540–4
    altered microcirculation and interstitial lung water content 543
    cellular metabolism 543–4
    central ventilatory drive 540
    COPD 73, 319–20, 539, 541
    lung parenchyma 541–4
    pulmonary immune response 542–3
    respiratory muscle function 540–1
    structural changes 541–2
  enteral diets 319–20
  nutrition considerations 544–7
    administration route 547
    carbohydrates 545
    energy requirements 544–5
    hydration 547
    lipids 545–6
    micronutrients 546–7
    oral supplements 275
    pharmacology 547

postoperative nutrition 272–5, 609–10
  proteins 546
  status 539–40
  see also lungs
respiratory distress syndrome, fish oil emulsions 421
respiratory gas exchange, measurement of MR 63–4
respiratory muscles, effects of malnutrition and refeeding 540–1
respiratory quotient (RQ)
  cirrhosis, energy expenditure **504**
  lipogenesis and lipids 74
  major nutrients **68**
  oxygen consumption **68**
  refeeding 543
resting energy expenditure (REE)
  after elective surgery **15**
  after injury **14**, 72
  after short term starvation **3–4**
  basal hypermetabolism **14**, 72–3
  direct effects of disease 181–3, 544–5
    ARF 528
    post absorptive state after fasting **182**
    sepsis, low and high REE, i.v. glucose **74**
  estimates **180**
  Harris & Benedict equations 179, 260, 308
  indirect effects of disease 181–2
    fever and ambient temperature 181–2
    injury and sepsis 515
    loss of lean body mass 181
    respiratory failure 544
  low and high REE, with IV glucose **74**
  short term starvation **3–4**
resuscitation, Ringers lactate 579
retinol binding protein, as marker of nutrition 170
rheumatoid arthritis
  cytokines 97
  fish oil preparations 420
riboflavin *see* vitamin B$_2$
rickets, paradox, HPN 492
RNA, protein metabolism measurement 31
RNA intake, immune function 139
rough endoplasmic reticulum (RER), protein synthesis 85

saccharidases, brush-border disaccharidases, TPN 761

satiety, defined 227
scurvy, ascorbic acid deficiency 156
secretagogue release, enteral diets 311
selenium
    age and RDA 219
    deficiency 100, 140, 449–50, 546
        AIDS 625, 631
        HPN, cardiomyopathy
            association 490
        IBD 559
        myopathy and cardiomyopathy
            association 156
    supplements 474
    RDA/effects 204–5, 546
sepsis
    catheter-related 386–7
        catheter care 384
        diagnosis 387
    intracellular amino acids 30
    see also injury and sepsis
serine, protein nutrition substrate
        405
serotonin, food intake, appetite
        control 235
short bowel/syndrome 701–18
    anatomical and physiological
            considerations 703–5
        GI motility 704
        jejunal, ileal and colonic
            absorption 704–5
        small intestinal length 703–4
        sodium:glucose **704**
        types 705–6
        volume of GI secretions 704
    causes 706
    diarrhoea 708–9
    electrolyte and fluid losses 319
    enteral diets 311
    future treatments 714
        conjugated bile acid treatment
            714
        dietary or drug therapy to
            improve absorption 714
        mucosal growth factors 714
    gallstones 707
    glucose uptake 120–1
    history 703
    indications for EN, paediatric 351
    intestinal size
        adaptation, post-surgery 110
        metabolic body mass relationship
            109–10
    PN 155
    preserved colon 707–9
        carbohydrates 708
        fat 708
        nutrient absorption 707–8
        oxalate 708

    presentation 707
        water and mineral losses 708
    problems and treatments 706–7,
        706
    protein–energy malnutrition 706
    social problems 707
    steatorrhoea 319
    surgery 713–14
    transplantation 714
    vitamin B$_{12}$ deficiency 707
    see also jejunostomy
short-chain peptides
    synthetic 409, 416–17
    see also glutamine, glutamine
            dipeptides; tyrosine,
            tyrosine dipeptides
sip-feeds, elderly patients 692, 694
skeletal muscle
    amino acid metabolism 42
    ketone bodies 71
    loss
        ageing 683
        protein supplementation 684
    MR **66**
    protein assessment 170–1
    protein synthesis 41–3, 45
    protein turnover effects 45–6
small bowel
    amino acid metabolism 42
    anastomosis, oral feeding 273
    radiotherapy effects 653
    resection, dietary LCT and MCT
            127
small bowel transplantation 714
smoking
    acute phase proteins 101
    and antioxidants, in cytokines
            99–101
    catheter-related sepsis risks 489
    and macrophages 100–1
sodium
    hyper/hyponatraemia 341
    predigested elemental diets 319
sorbitol, risks 423
spirometry 63
splanchnic bed
    blood exchange, amino acids 32
    MR **66**
Staphylococcus aureus
    catheter-related sepsis 386
    PEG association 336
starch, oxygen consumption and RQ
        68
starvation, prolonged 4–13
    BMR, and fuel selection **10**
    body composition, fuel availability
            and survival time **6**
    clinical aspects 69–71

    energy expenditure, urinary N
            excretion **70**
        glucose and plasma FFA, obese
            subjects **71**
        increase in energy expenditure
            70
        metabolism/metabolic rate
            69–71
    intermediary metabolism 9–13
    ketone bodies (3-hydroxybutyrate
            (beta-OHB) and
            acetoacetate (AcAc)
        adults and children **11**
        blood glucose and non-esterified
            fatty acids **13**
        circulating concentration **12**
        molar ratio **11**
        obese subjects **71**
    N excretion **8**
        fed state and post starvation 13
        ratio of cumulative N loss to
            weight loss **7**
    obesity, effect on survival time,
            mice/humans **5**, **8**
    percentage loss of organs, various
            species 5
    protein deprivation 316
    protein oxidation, BMR, effect of
            BMI **9**
    total available energy derived from
            fat, carbohydrate and
            protein **6**
starvation, short-term 3–4
    clinical aspects 69–71
    effects in infants and young
            children 219–21
    energy metabolism 3–4
        changes in REE **3–4**
    gastrointestinal motility 309
    glutamine provision 127
    metabolic response 154
    nitrogen excretion decrease 44
    peptide absorption 115–16, 126
    protein metabolism 4
    protein synthesis depression 45
steatohepatitis, HPN related 491
steatorrhoea see liver disease
steroids
    anabolic
        cancer therapy 666
        protein turnover effects 48
stoma
    gastrostomy button **358**
    short bowel anastomosed to colon
            707
streptozotocin, side effects 652
subcutaneous tube (SCJ), jejunostomy
        293

substrate utilisation, injury and sepsis
515–17
sucrase, classification 118
sucrose, EN 120–2
support team roles 241–53, 396
   Calman modular training 251
   composition of Oldchurch team
247
   finance 251
   general hospital audit 248–50
   history of nutrition support 243
   multidisciplinary approach 244
   optimal nutrition 160
   primary/secondary care interface
250
   relationship to non-team clinicians
244–5
   safer IV feeding 243–4
   subsequent developments 250–1
   team members 245–7
surgical patients 605–16
   correction of nutrition depletion
608–9
      population at risk 609
   EN vs PN 610
   enteral feeding contraindication
296
   future trends 611–12
   gastric atony 309
   history 607
   malnourishment 154
      morbidity increase 156
   pharmaconutrition 610–12
      arginine 611
      glutamine 610–11
      n-3 fatty acids 611
   polymeric enteral diets 313–14
   practical applications 609–12
   pre- and postoperative nutrition
support
      EN vs PN 768
      PN 156–8
   preoperative vs postoperative
nutrition 272–5, 609–10
   surgical risk 608
   theoretical benefits of nutrition
support 607–9
   see also hospital patients;
postoperative nutrition;
specific surgical procedures
surgical procedures
   abdominal, enteral tube feeding 159
   gastrointestinal, enteral feeding
contraindication 296
   intestinal, oral regimen/
supplements **273**
   postabdominal, diet regurgitation
and aspiration risks 286

postoperative intracellular amino
acids 30
postoperative risk factors 608
preoperative vs postoperative
nutrition 272–5, 609–10
swallowing disorders 286, 309
   enteral tube feeding 159–60
   indications for paediatric EN 351

tachyphylaxis, TNF-alpha
administration 648
taurine 477
   conjugate hydrolysis 407
   intracellular 38
   protein nutrition substrate 406–7
taurine-enriched HPN 491
testosterone, protein turnover effects
48
thermoregulation, malnutrition
association 156
thiamin *see* vitamin B_1
thioguanine, malabsorption 653
thrombophlebitis, particulates 478
thrombosis
   catheter material 383
   central vein (CVT), catheter-
related sepsis 490
   CPN 387
   postoperative, fish oil emulsion 421
   see also peripheral vein
thrombophlebitis (PVT)
thromboxane, and leukotrienes **564**
thymic atrophy, protein energy
malnutrition 155–6
thyroid hormones
   MR 67
   protein turnover effects 47
   thyroxine, carbohydrate
homeostasis 83
thyroid-binding prealbumin,
monitoring, EN 296
thyrotropin-releasing hormone 236
tissue biopsy, body composition
determination 29
tissue wasting
   accelerated 155
   arm circumference measurement
151–2
total available energy (TEE)
   elderly patients 684
   estimates of metabolism/metabolic
rate **180**
   post severe head injury, energy and
protein balances **17**
   prolonged starvation, fat,
carbohydrate and protein **6**
   weight loss, HIV infection and
AIDS **623**

total parenteral nutrition
   historical landmarks 382
   see also parenteral nutrition
trace elements 193–212, **204–7**
   assessment and monitoring of status
199–207
   cellular metabolism **197**
   effects of disease 198
   elderly requirements 686–7
   EN, monitoring and replacement
340
   enteral and parenteral
differentiation 198–9, 208
   functions 197–8
   HPN 490
   metabolism and biochemistry
207–8
   oral dietary supplements 313
   PN formulation, extended shelf
lives 442
   PN mixture precipitation 440
   predigested elemental diets 319
   recommended intakes 199–207
      biological dose–response curves
199
      inadequate, progressive effect
195
      large intake effects 196–7
      suboptimal intake effects 195–6
   reference nutrient intake (RNI)
199
   requirements
      paediatric 219, 474
      renal disease 530–1
      respiratory failure 546–7
      short bowel 705
   ultra-trace elements 208
   see also named minerals
tracheal intubation, feeding tube
malposition 335
tracheostomy
   aspiration risks, EN 338
   PEG placement 290
transferrin
   monitoring, EN 296
   visceral protein marker 170
transgastric jejunal tube 358
transnasal nasoenteral tubes 285–6
transporter systems
   monosaccharide 119–20, 120
   proteins 112–15
triacylglycerol, storage costs 69
triceps skinfold thickness (TSF) 169,
173
triglyceride–fatty acid metabolism
   activity and energy cost, burn
injury **16**
   critical illness 74

during starvation 9–10
triglycerides 448
  emulsion (STG) 452
  hepatitis 86–7
  hydrolysis, colipase micellar
     binding 122
  hypertriglyceridaemia, lipid
     emulsions in PN 453
  long-chain (LCT) 122, 452, 456
  medium-chain (MCT) 122–3, 403,
     419–20, 452, 456
    LCT combination 420
    rate of administration 420
  synthesis 84
trophamine 472
trypsin, zymogen activation 111
tryptophan, encephalopathy
    association 89
tube feeding syndrome 340
tumour cells
  growth retardation, arginine 405–6
  proliferation, TPN 661–3
  stomal seeding, PEG complications
    290
tumour necrosis factor-alpha
  cancer cachexia 648–9
  capillary leak in injury and sepsis
    514
  fat metabolism 649
  glucose metabolism 649
  inhibitors 97–8, 648–9
  lipolysis stimulation 649
  nitrogen metabolism 649
  role 95
  and weight loss 101
  see also cytokines
tyrosine 408
  acetyltyrosine, renal clearance
    417–18
  tyrosine dipeptides 408, 416–17

ulceration, feeding tubes 336
ulcerative colitis 555–66
  fish oil preparations 420
  nutritional management 563–4
ultrasonography, FBT placement
    287
undernutrition, inpatients
  actual consumption 257–9
  immune dysfunction 142
  recommendations 263–4, 277
  see also malnutrition
uraemia
  hepatic encephalopathy 89
  histidine 405
  intracellular amino acids 30
  muscle fatigue, taurine depletion
    association 406–7

urea
  nitrogen assimilation 112
  synthesis
    amino acid metabolism 84
    hepatic disease 88
    inhibition, xylitol 423–4
urea nitrogen appearance (UNA)
    526, 529–30
ureagenesis, amino acid regulatory
    role 39
urinary catheterisation, laparoscopic
    gastrostomy 291–2
urinary infections, dehydration,
    elderly patients 689–90
ursodeoxycholic acid, intrahepatic
    cholestasis 491–2

Van der Waal's forces, lipid emulsion
    destabilisation 437–8
vanadium
  excess 141
  PTH secretion suppression 493
ventilated patients, diet regurgitation
    and aspiration risks 286
ventilatory drive
  effects of malnutrition and
    refeeding 540
  malnutrition in respiratory disease/
    failure 540
villous height, TPN in pancreatitis
    723–4
vinca alkaloids
  chemotherapy combination 653
  malabsorption 653
  mucositis 652
viruses, and cytokines 96
visceral proteins see albumin;
    transferrin
vitamin A
  age and RDA 218
  Crohn's 558
  hypervitaminosis A 686
  immune function 141
  and mother-to-child transmission
    of HIV **626**
  photodegradation 440
  RDA/effects 200–1
  renal failure 531
vitamin B$_1$
  deficiency
    alcohol misuse 109
    Wernicke's encephalopathy 156,
     686
  degradation, bisulphite 440
vitamin B$_1$ and B$_2$
  age and RDA 218
  deficiency 450
  ICU **196**

immune function 141
RDA/effects 200–1
vitamin B$_6$
  deficiency, and immune function
    141
  RDA/effects 202–3
  renal failure 531
vitamin B$_{12}$
  deficiency 707
    ageing 109
    macrocytic megaloblastic
     anaemia 156
  RDA/effects 202–3
vitamin C
  age and RDA 218
  degradation, PN formulation 440
  immune function 141
  RDA/effects 202–3
  scurvy 156
vitamin D
  age and RDA 218
  D-induced osteomalacia, HPN 492
  deficiency 558
    PBC 87
  RDA/effects 200–1
  renal failure 531
vitamin E
  age and RDA 218
  deficiency 100, 558
  immune function 141
  photodegradation 440
  RDA/effects 200–1
vitamin K
  deficiency
    bone metabolism 493
    prothrombin time 87–8, 89
  RDA/effects 200–1
  renal failure 531
vitamins 193–212, **200–3**
  assessment and monitoring of status
    199–207
  in cellular metabolism **197**
  deficiencies **195**
    causes and effects 686
    hepatic disease 87–8
    in IBD 558–9
    and immune function 141
    PN 450
    see also specified substances
  degradation, PN formulation 440
  effects of disease 198
  elderly requirements 685–6
  enteral and parenteral
    differentiation 198–9, 208
  fat-soluble, cirrhosis 86
  functions 197–8
  hepatic metabolism 85
  HPN 490

vitamins – *continued*
  inadequate intake, progressive effect **195**
  metabolism and biochemistry 207–8
  monitoring and replacement, EN 340
  neurocognitive disorder relationship 685
  oral dietary supplements 313
  paediatric requirements 218–19, 474
  PN formulation, extended shelf lives 442
  predigested elemental diets 319
  recommended intakes 199–207
    biological dose–response curves **199**
    inadequate, progressive effect **195**
    large intake effects 196–7
    renal disease 530–1
    suboptimal intake effects 195–6
  respiratory failure 546–7
  short bowel 705

water and fat-soluble, immune function 141
volunteers, help with hospital feeding 262
vomiting
  EN-related, incidence rates 337
  feeding tube malposition 337

ward staffing 262
warfarin, HPN 387
water
  doubly-labelled water method, measurement of MR **64**
  and electrolyte absorption 123–4
  extracellular water volume (ECW)
    albumin as marker 173
    assessment 171
  malabsorption and diarrhoea 124–5
  paediatric requirements 217–18
  requirements, elderly patients 689–90
weight gain/loss *see* appetite; body weight; obesity
Wernicke's encephalopathy
  alcoholic cirrhosis 87

thiamine deficiency 156
vitamin B$_1$ 686
WHO cholera solution 711

Xenopus laevis oocyte, transporter proteins 113–14
xylitol, liver metabolism 423–4

zinc
  acute phase response **206**
  age and RDA 219
  and casein 219
  and cytokines 97
  deficiency
    acrodermatitis 140
    HIV infection 625, 631
    IBD 559
    incidence rates 341
    PN 449
  and immune function 140
  RDA/effects 204–5
  RNI and RDA 199
  supplements 474
  TNF-alpha inhibitors 97–8, 648–9